BONE CANCER

PROGRESSION AND THERAPEUTIC APPROACHES

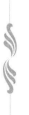

BONE CANCER

PROGRESSION AND THERAPEUTIC APPROACHES

Edited by

DOMINIQUE HEYMANN

ELSEVIER

AMSTERDAM • BOSTON • HEIDELBERG • LONDON • NEW YORK • OXFORD
PARIS • SAN DIEGO • SAN FRANCISCO • SINGAPORE • SYDNEY • TOKYO
Academic Press is an imprint of Elsevier

Academic Press is an imprint of Elsevier
32 Jamestown Road, London NW1 7BY, UK
30 Corporate Drive, Suite 400, Burlington, MA 01803, USA
525 B Street, Suite 1900, San Diego, CA 92101-4495, USA

First edition 2010

British Library Cataloguing in Publication Data
A catalogue record for this book is available from the British Library

Library of Congress Cataloguing in Publication Data
A catalogue record for this book is available from the Library of Congress

ISBN: 978-0-12-374895-9

For information on all Academic Press publications
visit our website at www.elsevierdirect.com

Printed and bound in United States of America
10 11 12 13   10 9 8 7 6 5 4 3 2 1

Working together to grow
libraries in developing countries

www.elsevier.com | www.bookaid.org | www.sabre.org

ELSEVIER   BOOK AID
            International   Sabre Foundation

Contents

Foreword

Our understanding of bone malignancies is following, with only a slight delay, that of the molecular bases of cell differentiation and function in the skeleton. As a result, it is increasing steadily and rapidly. What this timely book (edited by Dr. Heymann) does is to set the records straight and to define the questions and problems that bone biologists can now tackle through the use of modern molecular approaches and appropriate model organisms.

Most of the bone metastases are osteolytic, the main exception being prostate cancer bone metastases that form new bones. Thus, understanding the pathogenesis of bone metastases relies, to a very large extent, on understanding osteoclast differentiation. As very well illustrated in this volume, our knowledge of this aspect of bone biology has greatly progressed through the identification of RANKL as a master osteoclast differentiation factor, through the identification of its receptor, and of the complex signal transduction pathways it triggers in osteoclast progenitor cells. This body of work has also greatly advanced our understanding of bone metastases. This alone, however, would not have been enough. What is allowing us to get a better understanding of bone metastases is the more and more generalized ability to perform cell-specific and sometimes time-specific gene deletion in mice. These two types of advances, molecular and genetic, also supported by the progress of bioinformatics, are the pillar of the modern study of bone metastases. Going forward, it is likely that new aspects of molecular biology, such as the emerging biology of small RNAs, will join the group.

Molecules like RANKL, osteoprotegerin and PTHrP, tumor suppressor genes such as p53 and Rb are now central players in the study of osteoclast differentiation and proliferation. Furthermore, what is progressively emerging, beyond these genes and their functions are partial but nevertheless useful genetic pathways. In the face of this steady increase in knowledge one can ask: what is the use of such a book? As a matter of fact, and as a bone biologist not working directly on metastases, such a volume is extremely timely for several reasons. Firstly, it provides a very good picture of the state of the knowledge on this part of bone biology in 2009; secondly, and just as importantly, in doing so it also puts together a list of questions and problems that are now facing the field. It was always humbling and difficult to make a statement, as a book is, about a field that is still developing rapidly. In that respect, what Dr. Heymann and his co-workers have done is outstanding and certainly very useful. They deserve congratulations for this work which, I am sure, will generate a lot of interest in our community.

Professor Gérard Karsenty, MD PhD
Department of Genetics and Development
College of Physicians and Surgeons
Columbia University
New York, New York, USA

Preface

The past decade has witnessed an explosion in the field of bone biology. The topic of bone biology over this period has been marked by significant advances that have opened up entirely new areas for investigation. Indeed, the molecular mechanisms that control bone remodeling have been extensively investigated and some scientific fields have emerged. This is the case for osteoimmunology after identification of a set of molecules, allowing communication between bone cells (ostoclasts, osteoblasts) and immune cells (monocytes, lymphocytes, dendritic cells). Similarly, concepts based on the neuronal regulation of bone mass have emerged. Unfortunately, genetic or environmental deregulations lead to the development of bone cancer diseases such as primary bone tumors (osteosarcoma, Ewing's sarcoma, chondrosarcomas, giant cell tumors, etc.) that originate from bone cells or from mesenchymal stem cells. Bone is also a privileged site for metastases due to the migration and development of tumor cells derivating from non-bone cells such as breast cancer cells or prostate carcinomas cells. Some tumor cells such as myeloma cells initially proliferate in bone sites and then induce a deregulation of the bone apposition and resorption balance in favor of an osteolytic process.

This book gives an overview of the most up-to-date epidemiological data of these tumors and their biology including molecular aspects (protein and gene) allowing clear identification of new therapeutic targets and approaches. As well as the biological aspects of bone tissue, primitive bone tumors and bone metastases well described in this book, the clinical aspects are also addressed: histopathology, imaging of bone tumors, management of bone pain and conventional therapeutic care. Finally, better understanding of biological mechanisms associated with the development of many pre-clinical models allows the emergence of new therapeutic approaches of bone tumors. Therefore, this book, describing bone tumors, from their fundamental aspects to their clinical aspects, is specifically dedicated to medical students and scientists, to health professionals, researchers and teachers working in the osteo-articular domain and interested in the more recent data available. This review book consists of 38 chapters resulting from the work of 26 professional teams from 11 countries and who are specializing in the pathophysiology of bone. I would like to thank the authors for the work performed and to give their expertise to the students, to our colleagues and to all readers.

Professor Dominique Heymann, PhD
Nantes University Faculty of Medicine
INSERM
Nantes, France

List of Contributors

Kosei Ando, MD
Department of Orthopaedic Surgery, Shiga University of
Medical Science, Shiga, Japan

Coskun Arslandemir, MD
Department of Nuclear Medicine, University Hospital,
Kiel, Germany

Walter C. Bell, MD
University of Alabama at Birmingham, Birmingham, AL,
USA

Ariane Berdal, Professor, DDS–PhD
Centre de Recherche des Cordeliers, Oral Facial Biology
and Pathology, Paris, France

Dominik Berthold, MD
Centre Phiridisciplinaire d'Oncologie—Centre Hospitalier
Universitaire Vaudois, Lausanne, Switzerland

Bheem M. Bhat, PhD
Women's Health and Musculoskeletal Biology, Wyeth
Research, Collegeville, PA, USA

Ramesh A. Bhat, PhD
Women's Health and Musculoskeletal Biology, Wyeth
Research, Collegeville, PA, USA

Sudeepa Bhattacharyya, PhD
Center of Orthopaedic Research, Department of
Orthopaedic Surgery and Physiology and Biophysics,
UAMS College of Medicine, University of Arkansas for
Medical Sciences, Little Rock, AR, USA

Julia Billiard, PhD
Women's Health and Musculoskeletal Biology, Wyeth
Research, Collegeville, PA, USA

Frederic Blanchard, PhD
INSERM, Université de Nantes, Nantes Atlantique
Universités, Laboratoire de Physiopathologie de la
Résorption Osseuse et Thérapie des Tumeurs Osseuses
Primitives, EA3822, Nantes, France

Peter V.N. Bodine, PhD
Women's Health and Musculoskeletal Biology, Wyeth
Research, Collegeville, PA, USA

Tom Böhling, MD
Department of Pathology, Haartman Institute, University of
Helsinki, Finland

Aymann Bouattour, DDS
Centre de Recherche des Cordeliers, Oral Facial Biology
and Pathology, Odontology Department, Pitié-Salpêtrière
Hospital, Paris, France

Corinne Bouvier, MD, PhD
Service d'Anatomie et Cytologie Pathologiques, Hôpital La
Timone, Faculté de Médecine de Timone, Marseille, France

Bénédicte Brounais, PhD student
INSERM, Université de Nantes, Nantes Atlantique
Universités, Laboratoire de Physiopathologie de la
Résorption Osseuse et Thérapie des Tumeurs Osseuses
Primitives, Nantes, France

Giacomina Brunetti, PhD
Department of Human Anatomy and Histology, University
of Bari Medical School, Bari, Italy

Stephanie Byrum, PhD
Center of Orthopaedic Research, Department of
Orthopaedic Surgery and Physiology and Biophysics,
UAMS College of Medicine, University of Arkansas for
Medical Sciences, Little Rock, AR, USA

Daniel Chappard, MD, PhD
INSERM, U922-LHEA, Bone Remodeling and
Biomaterials, Faculté de Médecine, Angers, France

Edward Chow, MBBS, PhD, FRCPC
Department of Radiation Oncology, University of Toronto,
Rapid Response Radiotherapy Program, Odette Cancer
Centre, Sunnybrook Health Sciences Centre, Toronto,
Ontario, Canada

Philippe Clezardin, PhD
INSERM, Laennec School of Medicine, Lyon,
France

Gregory A. Clines, MD
Division of Endocrinology and Metabolism,
Department of Medicine, University of Virginia,
Charlottesville, VA, USA

Denis R. Clohisy, MD
Department of Orthopedic Surgery and Cancer Center,
School of Medicine, University of Minnesota, Minneapolis,
MN, USA

Silvia Colucci, MD
Department of Human Anatomy and Histology, University
of Bari Medical School, Bari, Italy

Emmanuelle David, PharmD
INSERM, Université de Nantes, Nantes Atlantique
Universités, Laboratoire de Physiopathologie de la
Résorption Osseuse et Thérapie des Tumeurs Osseuses
Primitives, Nantes, France

Gonzague de Pinieux, MD, PhD
Service d'Anatomie et Cytologie Pathologiques, Hôpital
Trousseau, Faculté de Médecine, Université François
Rabelais, Tours, France

Vianney Descroix, DDS, PharmD, PhD
Centre de Recherche des Cordeliers, Oral Facial Biology
and Pathology, Odontology Department, Pitié-Salpêtrière
Hospital, Paris, France

Sara DeDosso, MD
Oncology Institute of Southern Switzerland, Medical
Oncology, Bellinzona, Switzerland

William C. Dougall, PhD
Amgen Washington, Seattle, WA, USA

Lauren K. Dunn, MD
Division of Endocrinology and Metabolism,
Department of Medicine, University of Virginia,
Charlottesville, VA, USA

Alysa Fairchild, BSc, PGDip (Epi), MD, FRCPC
Department of Radiation Oncology, University of Alberta,
Cross Cancer Institute, Alberta, Canada

Stefano Ferrari, MD
Chemotherapy unit, Department of Musculoskeletal
Oncology, Istituti Orthpedici Rizzoli, Bologna,
Italy

Luis Filgueira, MD
University of Western Australia, Crawley, WA, Australia

Adrienne M. Flanagan, MB, PhD
University College London, Department of Histopathology,
Royal National Orthopaedic Hospital, Middlesex, United
Kingdom

Yannick Fortun, PhD
INSERM, Université de Nantes, Nantes Atlantique
Universités, Laboratoire de Physiopathologie de la
Résorption Osseuse et Thérapie des Tumeurs Osseuses
Primitives, Nantes, France, Université d'Angers, IUT,
France

Pierrick Fournier, PhD
Division of Endocrinology and Metabolism, Department of
Medicine, University of Virginia, Charlottesville, VA, USA

Sonia Ghoul-Mazgar, DDS-PhD
Laboratoire d'Histologie-Embryologie, Faculté de
Médecine Dentaire de Monastir, Tunisia

**Panagiotis D. Gikas, BSc(Hons), MBBS(Hons),
MRCS(Engl)**
Academic Clinical Fellow, Trauma and Orthopaedic
Surgery, Royal National Orthopaedic Hospital, Stanmore,
Middlesex, United Kingdom

Georg Gosheger, MD
Klinik and Poliklinikfür Allgemeine Orthopädie
Universitätsklinikum Münster, Münster, Germany

François Gouin, MD, PhD
INSERM, Physiopathologie de la Résorption Osseuse et
Thérapie des Tumeurs Osseuses Primitives, Faculté de
Médecine, Nantes, France

Maria Grano, PhD
Department of Human Anatomy and Histology, University
of Bari Medical School, Bari, Italy

Theresa A. Guise, MD
Division of Endocrinology and Metabolism, Department of
Medicine, University of Virginia, Charlottesville, VA, USA

Jendrik Hardes, MD
Klinik and Poliklinikür Allgemeine Orthopädie
Universitätsklinikum Münster, Münster Germany

Esther I. Hauben, MD, PhD
Department of Pathology, University of Leuve, Leuven,
Belgium

Eric J. Heffernan, MD
Vancouver General Hospital, Department of Radiology,
Vancouver, BC, Canada

Monica Herrera, MD
Department of Pharmacology, College of Medicine,
University of Arizona, Tucson, AZ, USA

Fernanda G. Herrera, MD
Oncology Institute of Southern Switzerland, Radiation
Oncology, Bellinzona, Switzerland

Dominique Heymann, PhD
INSERM, Physiopathologie de la Résorption Osseuse
et Thérapie des Tumeurs Osseuses Primitives Faculté de
Médecine, Nantes, France

David G. Hicks, MD
Department of Pathology and Laboratory Medicine,
University of Rochester, Rochester, NY, USA

Amanda Hird, BSc
Rapid Response Radiotherapy Program, Odette Cancer
Centre, Sunnybrook Health Sciences Centre, Toronto,
Ontario, Canada

Pancras C.W. Hogendoorn, MD, PhD
Department of Pathology, Leiden University Medical
Center Leiden, The Netherlands

Ingunn Holen, PhD
Academic Unit of Clinical Oncology, School of Medicine
and Biomedical Sciences, University of Sheffield,
Sheffield, United Kingdom

Juan Miguel Jimenez-Andrade, MD
Department of Pharmacology, College of Medicine,
University of Arizona, Tucson, AZ, USA

Robert G. Jones, MRCP(UK), FRCR
Vancouver General Hospital, Department of Radiology,
Vancouver, BC, Canada

Joseph Khoury, MD
Department of Pathology, Nevada Cancer Institute, Las
Vegas, NV, USA

Sakari Knuutila, MD
Department of Pathology, Haartman Institute, University of
Helsinki, Finland

Udo Kontny, MD
Division of Pediatric Hematology and Oncology, Center for
Pediatrics and Adolescent Medicine, University Medical
Center, Freiburg, Germany

François Lamoureux, PhD
INSERM, Physiopathologie de la Résorption Osseuse et
Thérapie des Tumeurs Osseuses Primitives, Faculté de
Médecine, Nantes, France

Ching C. Lau, MD, PhD
Texas Children's Cancer Center, Baylor College of
Medicine, Huston, TX, USA

Nathan Lawrentschuk, MD
University of Melbourne, Department of Surgery, Urology
Unit, Austin Hospital; Heidelberg, Melbourne, Australia

Michelle A. Lawson, PhD
Academic Unit of Bone Biology, School of Medicine and
Biomedical Sciences, University of Sheffield, Sheffield,
United Kingdom

Jiyun Lee, MD
Genetics Laboratory, Department of Pediatrics at the
University of Oklahoma Health Sciences Center, Oklahoma
City, OK, USA

Frederic Lezot, DDS-PhD
Centre de Recherche des Cordeliers, Oral Facial Biology
and Pathology, Paris, France

Shibo Li, MD
Genetics Laboratory, Department of Pediatrics at the
University of Oklahoma Health Sciences Center, Oklahoma
City, OK, USA

Robert D. Loberg, PhD
Department of Internal Medicine and Urology, University
of Michigan Comprehensive Cancer Center, The University
of Michigan, Ann Arbor, MI, USA

Tsz-Kwong Man, PhD
Texas Children's Cancer Center, Baylor College of
Medicine, Huston, TX, USA

Patrick W. Mantyh, PhD
Department of Pharmacology, College of Medicine,
University of Arizona, Tucson, AZ, USA

Mallory Martin, MD
Genetics Laboratory, Department of Pediatrics at the
University of Oklahoma Health Sciences Center, Oklahoma
City, OK, USA

Yoshitaka Matsusue, MD
Department of Orthopaedic Surgery, Shiga University of
Medical Science, Shiga, Japan

Mario Mercuri, MD
Fifth Division of Orthopaedic Surgery, Department of
Musculoskeletal Oncology, Istituti Orthpedici Rizzoli,
Bologna, Italy

Kanji Mori, MD, PhD
Department of Orthopaedic Surgery, Shiga University of
Medical Science, Shiga, Japan

Peter L. Munk, MD
Vancouver General Hospital and University of British
Columbia, Department of Radiology, Vancouver, BC,
Canada

Richard J. Murrills, PhD
Women's Health and Musculoskeletal Biology, Wyeth
Research, Collegeville, PA, USA

Marc Padrines, PhD
INSERM, Faculté de Médecine, Nantes, France

Emanuela Palmerini, MD
Chemotherapy Unit, Department of Musculoskeletal
Oncology, Istituti Orthpedici Rizzoli, Bologna, Italy

Paul C. Park, MD, PhD
Department of Pathology and Molecular Medicine,
Richardson Labs, Queen's University, Kingston, Ontario,
Canada

Alexander HG Paterson, MD
Department of Medicine, Tom Baker Cancer Centre,
University of Calgary, Alberta, Canada

Gaëlle Picarda, Engineer
INSERM, Physiopathologie de la Résorption Osseuse et
Thérapie des Tumeurs Osseuses Primitives, Faculté de
Médecine, Nantes, France

Kenneth J. Pienta, MD
Department of Internal Medicine and Urology, University
of Michigan Comprehensive Cancer Center, The University
of Michigan, Ann Arbor, MI, USA

Nieroshan Rajarubendra, MD
University of Melbourne, Department of Surgery, Urology
Unit, Austin Hospital; Heidelberg, Melbourne, Australia

Pulivarthi H. Rao, PhD
Texas Children's Cancer Center, Baylor College of
Medicine, Houston, TX, USA

Faisal Rashid, MD
Vancouver General Hospital, Department of Radiology,
Vancouver, BC, Canada

Françoise Rédini, PhD
INSERM, Physiopathologie de la Résorption Osseuse et
Thérapie des Tumeurs Osseuses Primitives, Faculté de
Médecine, Nantes, France

Carl D. Richards, PhD
Professor, Department of Pathology and Molecular
Medicine, McMaster University, Hamilton, Ontario, Canada

John A. Robinson, PhD
Women's Health and Musculoskeletal Biology, Wyeth
Research, Collegeville, PA, USA

Julie Rousseau, PhD student
INSERM, Physiopathologie de la Résorption Osseuse et
Thérapie des Tumeurs Osseuses Primitives, Faculté de
Médecine, Nantes, France

Blandine Ruhin, MD, PhD
Centre de Recherche des Cordeliers, Oral Facial Biology
and Pathology, Stomatology and Maxillofacial Surgery
Department, Pitié-Salpêtrière University Hospital, Pierre et
Marie Curie University, Paris, France

Velasco C. Ruiz, MD
INSERM, Université de Nantes, Nantes Atlantique
Universités, Laboratoire de Physiopathologie de la
Résorption Osseuse et Thérapie des Tumeurs Osseuses
Primitives, Nantes, France

Ma'Ann C. Sabino, DDS, PhD
Division of Oral and Maxillofacial Surgery, School
of Dentistry, University of Minnesota, University of
Minnesota, Minneapolis, MN, USA

Suvi Savola, MD
Department of Pathology, Haartman Institute, University of
Helsinki, Finland

Holger Schirrmeister, MD
Department Head, Department of Nuklearmedicine
Westküstenklinikum Heide, Heide, Germany

Markus J. Seibel, MD, PhD
PhD, FRACP, ANZAC Research Institute, The University
of Sydney, Concord Campus, Sydney, Australia

Shamini Selvarajah, PhD
Center for Medical Oncologic Pathology, Dana-Farber
Cancer Institute, Boston, MA, USA

Gene P. Siegal, MD, PhD
Robert W. Mowry Endowed Professor of Pathology and
Director, Division of Anatomic Pathology, Exec. Vice-
Chair of Pathology – UAB Health System, Sr. Scientist,
UAB Comprehensive Cancer Center and the Gene Therapy
Center, Department of Pathology, University of Alabama at
Birmingham, Birmingham, AL, USA

Eric R. Siegel, MS
Center of Orthopaedic Research, Department of
Biostatistics, UAMS College of Medicine, University of
Arkansas for Medical Sciences, Little Rock, AR, USA

David Smyth, MD
Professor, Department of Pathology and Molecular
Medicine, McMaster University, Hamilton, Ontario,
Canada

Jeremy A. Squire, PhD
Director of Translational Laboratory Research, NCIC-Clinical Trials Group, Research Chair in Molecular Pathology, Kingston General Hospital, Department of Pathology and Molecular Medicine, Queen's University, Kingston, ON, Canada

Eric L. Staals, MD
Fifth Division of Orthopaedic Surgery, Department of Musculoskeletal Oncology, Istituti Orthpedici Rizzoli, Bologna, Italy

Arne Steitbueger, MD
Klinik and Poliklinikfür Allgemeine Orthopädie Universitätsklinikum Münster, Münster, Germany

Larry J. Suva, PhD
Center of Orthopaedic Research, Department of Orthopaedic Surgery and Physiology and Biophysics, UAMS College of Medicine, University of Arkansas for Medical Sciences, Little Rock, AR, USA

Ping Tang, MD, PhD
Department of Pathology and Laboratory Medicine, University of Rochester, Rochester, NY, USA

Roberto Tirabosco, MD, FRCPath
Royal National Orthopaedic Hospital, Stanmore, Middlesex, United Kingdom

Valérie Trichet, PhD
INSERM, Physiopathologie de la Résorption Osseuse et Thérapie des Tumeurs Osseuses Primitives, Faculté de Médecine, Nantes, France

Marina Vardanyan, MD
Department of Pharmacology, College of Medicine, University of Arizona, Tucson, AZ, USA

Maria Zielenska, PhD
Genetics and Genome Biology, Department of Pediatric Laboratory, Medicine and Pathobiology, The Hospital for Sick Children, Toronto, Ontario, Canada, Kingston General Hospital, Department of Pathology and Molecular Medicine, Queen's University, Kingston, ON, Canada

Section I. Epidemiology and Economical Aspects of Bone Cancer

CHAPTER **1**

Epidemiology of Primary Bone Tumors and Economical Aspects of Bone Metastases

ESTHER I. HAUBEN[1] AND PANCRAS C.W. HOGENDOORN[2]

[1]*Department of Pathology, University of Leuven, Leuven, Belgium*
[2]*Department of Pathology, Leiden University Medical Center, Leiden, The Netherlands*

Contents

Primary bone tumors are rare and as such they form a difficult category of tumors for appropriate recognition and classification both for clinicians as well as pathologists. They account for less than 0.2% of the malignancies registered in the SEER database [1]. The occurrence of bone sarcomas ranges between 0.8 and 2 cases per person per year [1]. However, particularly children and adolescents are affected, which means that bone tumors have a major impact on the life of patients and their immediate surroundings. The incidence of benign bone tumors may be considerably higher, but a number of these are asymptomatic and often missed by patients and their doctors. Therefore, benign bone tumors are most likely underreported. But nevertheless they are, like other benign tumors, a rare event. Another confounding factor is the high discrepancy rate at histological review of bone tumors, which make most population-based series somewhat unreliable [2]. On the other hand, consultation series or expert center series are likely to over-report difficult/unusual cases.

Bone tumors can occur spontaneously. However, a substantial number of them do occur in the context of a hereditary disorder thus implicating a detailed family history in every new case. If a hereditary context is suspected, then a proper follow-up, often in close collaboration with clinical geneticists, is mandatory [3,4]. This hereditary aspect might explain the higher incidences in some regional populations.

A subgroup of primary bone malignancies occurs secondary to benign precursor lesions in the bone such as in a case of Ollier disease, fibrous dysplasia or Paget's disease of bone [5–9], so the incidence adds up to the occurrence of the primary condition in the population. For instance, there is a well-known regional incidence difference for Paget's disease of bone.

Both benign as well as malignant primary tumors of bone are greatly outnumbered by metastases to the bone from epithelial cancers or melanoma and hematological disorders like multiple myeloma/plasmacytoma.

I. INCIDENCES OF PRIMARY BONE TUMORS

The incidence of bone tumors—especially primary bone sarcomas compared to malignant tumors—in general is very low. Review of large series revealed that approximately 0.2% of all neoplasms are bone sarcomas [10–12]. In Europe about two new primary bone sarcomas arise per 100,000 persons a year. Interestingly, at childhood there is a steep shift in frequency of occurrence over the age span [13]. From the first year of life the incidence increases from 3.9 per 100,000 to a peak of 142.9 per 100,000 at the age of fifteen [13]. The archives of the Netherlands Committee of Bone Tumors hold details of over 14,000 cases of bone tumors and tumor-like lesions where the percentages of the sarcomas are given in decreasing order of frequency for malignant bone tumors: osteosarcoma (37%), chondrosarcoma (23.6%), Ewing sarcoma (12.2%), fibrosarcoma/malignant fibrous histiocytoma (10.9%), Non-Hodgkin's lymphoma of bone (3.3%), malignancy in giant cell tumor (2.3%), Paget's sarcoma 1%, and adamantinoma (0.8%) [10].

Fibrosarcoma and malignant fibrous histiocytoma are diagnoses which are infrequently encountered these days. This is reflected by a change of methods used to classify these tumors, which in practice commonly appear to be poorly differentiated osteosarcoma, or dedifferentiated chondrosarcoma. For benign tumors, enchondroma is the most frequent (27.7%) followed by giant cell tumors (21.5%), osteochondroma (14%), osteoid osteoma (10.5%), chondroblastoma (9%) and osteoblastoma (5.7%) [10]. However, an age-dependent frequency difference is present [13], as discussed below.

II. AGE

Bone tumors have an age-related presentation. There are two age-specific peaks in frequency in bone sarcomas. The first peak occurs in the second decade of life and consists of osteosarcoma and Ewing's sarcoma in cases of malignant tumors and osteochondroma in the benign group [13]. The second peak, slightly increasing from the fourth decade, peaks after the sixth decade and includes chondrosarcomas, MFH, chordoma and osteosarcoma, including Paget's and radiation-induced sarcomas. Chondrosarcomas are somewhat equally distributed over all decades, although rarely found in someone younger than 20, and slightly increasing thereafter. Malignant progression of osteochondroma, as in multiple osteochondroma, only presents itself a number of years after closure of the growth plate and can be recognized by a regrowth of the cartilaginous cap of a pre-existent osteochondroma [14].

The majority of benign bone tumors and tumor-like lesions in young patients are seen in the first and second decades of life. In about half, the median age occurs in the second decade (solitary bone cyst, aneurysmal bone cyst, non-ossifying fibroma, fibrous cortical defect, enchondroma, Langerhanscell histiocytosis, osteochondroma, chondroblastoma, osteoblastoma and osteoid osteoma). The median age incidence of the rest is not specifically age-related and may be seen in the first decade of life, extending even into the sixth or seventh decade (i.e. juxtacortical chondroma, parosteal osteosarcoma, desmoplastic fibroma). Giant cell tumors occur almost exclusively after closure of the epiphysial plate.

III. GENDER

The male–female ratio has little diagnostic contribution for most bone tumors, as in general there is no striking difference and both sexes are roughly equally affected. In osteosarcoma the male–female ratio is 1:1. In Ewing's sarcoma, Paget's sarcoma, chordoma and primary osseous non-Hodgkin lymphoma there is a higher prevalence in males (2:1). There is some male predominance seen in a number of benign lesions like osteochondroma, chondroblastoma, osteoid osteoma, solitary bone cyst, or osteoblastoma. Whether this correlates to a higher incidence of trauma in males which attracts attention to an underlying, previously asymptomatic tumor, is unknown.

IV. RACIAL DIFFERENCES IN INCIDENCES OF PRIMARY BONE TUMORS

While there are some differences reported in incidences between different national registries in the frequency of occurrence, most striking racial differences are reported with regard to Ewing's sarcoma [15] and giant cell tumor of the bone [16]. There is, as yet, an unexplained, extremely low, incidence of Ewing's sarcoma in those of African descent; while giant cell tumors of the bone tend to occur more frequently in the Asian population.

V. SITE DISTRIBUTION

Bone tumors have a preference for the long bones of the extremities. The metaphysis is the preferred site for malignant bone tumors; especially the metaphysis of the distal and proximal femur, the proximal tibia and proximal humerus, which are the affected sites in more than 80% of instances of osteosarcoma. Depending on the extent of the tumor, the epiphysis, and even diaphysis, might be affected as well.

The majority of central chondrosarcoma are restricted to the long bone marrow space, mostly in metaphysial and diaphysial locations. Malignant fibrous histiocytomas arise and extend mostly in the metaphysis, like osteosarcoma, prompting us to question whether this should be regarded as a poorly differentiated form of osteosarcoma. Ewing's sarcoma tends to arise more frequent in the diaphysis but may also extend in the metaphysis. Chordomas are sited exclusively in the sacrum, vertebra and skull, except for very rare casuistic presentations in the long bones. Sites other than the long bones for sarcomas are the flat bones like pelvis, scapula and ribs (chondrosarcoma and Ewing's sarcoma) and craniofacial bones (osteosarcoma). Adamantinoma is almost pre-eminently sited in the tibia and sometimes the fibula.

In benign tumors the epiphysial location is restricted for chondroblastoma, osteoblastoma and dysplasia epiphysialis hemimelica. Solitary and aneurysmal bone cysts occur metaphysically, usually close to the epiphysis. All osteochondroma originate in the metaphysis of long bones and increase the distance to the epiphysis during growth. Fibrous dysplasia can occur at all sites in all bones. Lesions

TABLE 1.1

Publication	Author	Type of cancer	# pt	SRE + %	RT %	Fr %	Surg %	Total cost	Cost RT %	Cost Fr %	Cost surg %
2003	Groot *et al.* [34]	Prostate	28	100	NA	14	11	6.973[1]	NA	NA	NA
2004	Delea *et al.* [35]	Lung	534	55	68	35	14	$11.979[2]	61	15	21
2006	Delea *et al.* [37]	Breast	617	52	56	34	14	$13.940[3]	50	22	20
2007	Felix *et al.* [13,41]	Breast	121	NA	75	13	1	5963[4]	25	NA	NA
2008	Lage *et al.* [42]	Prostate	342	50	89	23	12	$12.469[5]	47	25	18

pt: number of patients with bone metastasis; SRE +: number of patients with bone metastasis and 1 or more SREs; RT: number of patients with radiation therapy; FR: number of patients with fracture; Surg: number of patients with surgery; Cost: cost of treatment of SREs
[1]Over 24 months; [2]over 36 months; [3]over 60 months; [4]over 12 months; [5]first year of treatment.

in the phalangeal bones are statistically almost always enchondroma, with rare exceptions [17,18].

VI. INCIDENCES OF BONE TUMORS AS A SECONDARY EVENT

Both benign and malignant bone tumors can occur as a result of a pre-existing non-tumorous condition of bone or as a result of an external noxe like Morbus Paget [19,20], chronic inflammation [21], irradiation [22–24], bone infarction [25], prostheses [26].

VII. INCIDENCES OF BONE METASTASES

The incidence of malignant tumors metastasizing to the skeleton is dependent of the incidence of a given cancer and can vary demographically. After the lung and liver, the skeletal system is the most common site for a metastatic tumor [27] and metastatic carcinoma is the most frequent malignancy of bone [12]. Preferred sites are spine, pelvis, femur and rib in descending order [28].

The most common cancers metastasizing to the bone are breast, lung, prostate, kidney and thyroid cancer [29]. Skeletal metastases develop in 70–80% of patients with breast or prostate cancer and in 40% of patients with advanced lung cancer [30].

VIII. PATHOLOGY OF BONE METASTASES

Neoplastic involvement of the bone causes an increased bone turnover and uncoupling of bone formation and resorption. Clinically this results in pain, risk of fracture, hypercalcemia and sometimes spinal cord compression [28,30]. Treatment consists of pain-stilling medication, radiation therapy and, where necessary, surgery. The denominator skeletal related event (SRE) encompasses pain, radiotherapy, reduced mobility, symptoms of hypercalcemia, pathologic, fracture, spinal cord compression and bone

marrow infiltration. Approximately half of the patients with bony metastasis develop at least one SRE (Table 1.1). Consequences for the patients are severe and consist of impairment or loss of functionality, loss of quality of life, and decreased survival. SREs also have financial implications for the health care system, and thus the community, as well as for the patient. The financial impact of SREs is greater for cancers with prolonged survival. The median survival for a patient presenting with a bony metastasis is 2 to 3 years for those with breast cancer or prostate cancer and a median of 4 months for those with lung cancer [31].

IX. COST OF ILLNESS

Cost of illness (COI) is defined as the value of the resources that are expended or forgone as a result of a health problem. It includes health sector costs (direct costs), the value of decreased or lost productivity by the patient (indirect costs), and the cost of pain and suffering (intangible costs) [32,33]. Direct costs for the health sector are: hospitalization, medication, emergency transport, and medical care. Also the patients and family have costs directly related with the treatment of an illness as there are non-refunded payments for hospitalization, medical visits and drugs; transportation of patient and family for health visits; transportation of family for visiting the hospitalized patient; modifications made to a home as a result of the illness; costs for taking care of the patient at home, etc. [33].

Decreased or lost productivity can be the result of illness, premature death, side effects of illness or treatment, or time spent receiving treatment. This does not only affect the patient but also the family members who reduce or stop working so that they can take care of the patient. Premature death can mean an indirect cost for the loss of potential wages and benefits.

It is clear that it is difficult to estimate the impact the COI would have based on the above. Indeed, the easiest cost to calculate is the direct cost for the health care system. The direct costs for the patient may be hard to estimate, because data on the costs can often be insufficient or inexact. The most difficult to estimate are the intangible costs, and the cost of loss of productivity. Most studies on the economic burden of illness focus only on the direct medical costs for the health care sector, thus underestimating the total cost of illness.

Nevertheless, cost analysis gives an indication of the financial impact of disease and provides information to policy makers, researchers, and medical specialists. This information can be considered when making decisions based on more efficient use of resources. Additionally, on the basis of distinction between different cost components, it may be possible to estimate the financial aspect of various treatment strategies, which can influence the choice of treatment.

X. ECONOMICAL BURDEN OF BONE METASTASIS

Studies on the economical impact of bone metastasis are rare and only report on the costs for the health care sector. The first study on the subject was done in the Netherlands in 2003. Groot *et al.* [34] investigated the cost of treatment for an SRE in patients with prostate cancer metastatic to the bone. They followed 28 patients with an SRE because of prostate cancer metastatic to the bone for a period of 24 months. The overall cost of treatment per patient for this period was 13,051 of which 6973 (50%) was spent for the treatment of SREs. The overall cost was calculated on the whole of the medical care including manpower, material, overhead cost (housing, etc.). For the cost directly related to the treatment of SREs, the costs of radiation therapy, hospitalization and surgical intervention were taken in to account. Thus, this is the direct cost for the health care sector. Indirect costs are estimated to be limited in patients with prostate cancer; therefore, they did not look at the cost of patient care in a nursery, or direct or indirect costs for the patient. In their study on these 28 patients, bone metastases developed after the age of sixty with a mean age of 73 years. This is a non-active population from the viewpoint of employment.

In 2004 a second study was published, this time from the US on the cost of treating SREs in patients with lung cancer [35]. In a US health insurance claim database, 534 patients were identified with lung cancer and skeletal involvement. Costs were estimated on the basis of the claims made and did not include overhead costs. Of these 534 patients, 55% developed at least one SRE. In the SRE patient group, 68% received radiation therapy, 35% suffered a pathologic fracture and 14% had bone surgery. The mean age at first SRE was 66.4 years, which also indicates that indirect costs due to loss of productivity tend to be limited. The mean survival after the first SRE was 4.1 months.

The estimated life-time SRE-related cost after 36 months is $11,979 of which 61% goes to radiation therapy. These and other studies are summarized in Table 1.1. Data are difficult to compare due to the difference in costs included, the method of treatment (e.g. single fraction or multiple fraction radiation therapy), the period over which the costs are calculated, the method of calculation, and index changes over the years.

These studies give an idea of the cost of treatment of SREs but not of the impact of SREs on the total direct medical care of cancer patients. Delea *et al.* [36] repeated their study on lung cancer patients with bone metastases, then compared the costs of treatment for patients with SRE and with patients without SRE. The additional cost for SRE patients on the total cost for cancer treatment was $27,982 per patient. The same exercise was done for patients with breast cancer metastatic to the bone [37]. Total medical care costs over 60 months in patients with SREs were $48,173 greater than in non-SRE patients. For women younger than 65 years of age the additional cost for treatment of SREs was $62,286, and for women above 65 it was $36,452. These figures indicate the better survival rates that younger women experience. The lower additional cost for SRE treatment in lung patients is explained by the fact that patients with lung cancer metastatic to the bone have a median survival of 4.1 months, whereas women with breast cancer and metastatic bone disease experience a mean expected lifetime of 2 to 3 years.

The costs of treatment attributable to the treatment of SREs have been reduced due to the use of bisphosphonates and especially zoledronic acid [38,39], but they also come with a price tag. The studies above do not give an idea of the economic impact of metastastic bone disease (MBD). Patients with MBD are expected to cost more to the health care sector than patients without because of, for example, intensified follow-up, SRE preventive treatment with bisphosphonates. MBD still has a huge impact on health care costs. A good view of the economic impact of bone metastasis is given by Schulman *et al.* [40]. They estimated the share of bone metastasis on the whole of direct medical costs in the US for 2007. The cost burden for metastatic bone disease was thus estimated at $12.6 billion, which represents 17% of the estimated total direct medical costs.

Unfortunately, information on two components in the COI for MBD is missing in the literature, namely the indirect and intangible costs.

XI. CONCLUSIONS

Bone metastasis weighs heavily on the health care budget. The reports available thus far on the economical impact underestimate the total cost, since they only give an estimate of the direct costs, and not the indirect and intangible costs.

Available data are difficult to compare due to the difference in costs included—differences in treatment modalities, the period over which the costs are calculated, the method of calculation, and index changes over the years.

The financial impact is more substantial for patients with cancer at a younger age and for cancer types with prolonged survival rates even with bony metastasis.

References

1. H.D. Dorfman, B. Czerniak, R. Kotz, D. Vanel, Y.K. Park & K.K. Unni, WHO classification of tumors of bone: introduction, in: C.D.M. Fletcher, K.K. Unni & F. Mertens (Eds.) World Health Organization Classification of Tumors. Pathology and Genetics of Tumors of Soft Tissue and Bone, IARC Press, Lyon, 2002, pp. 226–232.

2. H. van den Berg, A. Slaar, H.M. Kroon, A.H. Taminiau & P. Hogendoorn, Results of diagnostic review in pediatric bone tumors and tumorlike lesions, J Pediatr Orthop 28 (5) (2008) 561–564.

3. E.I. Hauben, J. Arends, J.P. Vandenbroucke, C.J. van Asperen, E. Van Marck & P.C. Hogendoorn, Multiple primary malignancies in osteosarcoma patients. Incidence and predictive value of osteosarcoma subtype for cancer syndromes related with osteosarcoma, Eur J Hum Genet 11 (8) (2003) 611–618.

4. L. Hameetman, J.V.M.G. Bovée, A.H.M. Taminiau, H.M. Kroon & P.C.W. Hogendoorn, Multiple osteochondromas: clinicopathological and genetic spectrum and suggestions for clinical management, Hereditary Cancer in Clinical Practice 2 (4) (2004) 161–173.

5. F. Mertens & K.K. Unni, Enchondromatosis: Ollier disease and Maffucci syndrome, in: C.D.M. Fletcher, K.K. Unni & F. Mertens (Eds.) World Health Organization Classification of Tumors. Pathology and genetics of tumors of soft tissue and bone, IARC Press, Lyon, 2002, pp. 356–357.

6. H.S. Schwartz, N.B. Zimmerman, M.A. Simon, R.R. Wroble, E.A. Millar & M. Bonfiglio, The malignant potential of enchondromatosis, J Bone Joint Surg Am 69 (2) (1987) 269–274.

7. K.K. Unni & D.C. Dahlin, Premalignant tumors and conditions of bone, Am J Surg Pathol 3 (1) (1979) 47–60.

8. R. Amin & R. Ling, Malignant fibrous histiocytoma following radiation therapy of fibrous dysplasia, Br J Radiol 68 (1995) 1119–1122.

9. W.K. Taconis, Osteosarcoma in fibrous dysplasia, Skeletal Radiol 17 (1988) 163–170.

10. J.D. Mulder, H.E. Schütte, H.M. Kroon & W.K. Taconis, Radiologic Atlas of Bone Tumors, 2nd ed., Elsevier, Amsterdam, 1993.

11. A.G. Huvos, Bone Tumors. Diagnosis, Treatment, and Prognosis, 2nd ed., W.B. Saunders Company, Philadelphia, 1991.

12. Dahlin's Bone Tumors General Aspects and Data on 11,087 Cases. 5th ed. Philadelphia: Lippincott-Raven Publishers, 1996.

13. H. van den Berg, H.M. Kroon, A. Slaar & P. Hogendoorn, Incidence of biopsy-proven bone tumors in children: a report based on the Dutch pathology registration 'PALGA', J Pediatr Orthop 28 (1) (2008) 29–35.

14. J.V.M.G. Bovee, A.M. Cleton-Jansen, A.H.M. Taminiau & P.C.W. Hogendoorn, Emerging pathways in the development of chondrosarcoma of bone and implications for targeted treatment, Lancet Oncology 6 (8) (2005) 599–607.

15. S. Ushigome, R. Machinami & P.H. Sorensen, Ewing sarcoma/primitive neuroectodermal tumor (PNET), in: C.D.M. Fletcher, K.K. Unni & F. Mertens (Eds.) World Health Organization Classification of Tumors; Pathology & Genetics; Tumors of Soft Tissue and Bone, IARC Press, Lyon, 2002, pp. 298–300.

16. W. Guo, W. Xu, A.G. Huvos, J.H. Healey & C. Feng, Comparative frequency of bone sarcomas among different racial groups, Chin Med J (Engl) 112 (12) (1999) 1101–1104.

17. L.F. Oudenhoven, E. Dhondt, S. Kahn, A. Nieborg, H.M. Kroon & P.C. Hogendoorn, et al., Accuracy of radiography in grading and tissue-specific diagnosis—a study of 200 consecutive bone tumors of the hand, Skeletal Radiol 35 (2) (2006) 78–87.

18. K.J. Van Zwieten, P. Brys, F. Van Rietvelde, L. Oudenhoven, F. Vanhoenacker & F. Willemssens, et al., Imaging of the hand, techniques and pathology: a pictorial essay, JBR-BTR 90 (5) (2007) 395–455.

19. A. Hadjipavlou, P. Lander, H. Srolovitz & I.P. Enker, Malignant transformation in Paget disease of bone, Cancer 70 (1992) 2802–2808.

20. A.G. Huvos, A. Butler & S. Bretsky, Osteogenic sarcoma associated with Paget's disease of bone. A clinicopathologic study of 65 patients, Cancer 52 (1983) 1489–1495.

21. A. Giunti & M. Laus, Malignant tumors in chronic osteomyelitis. (A report of thirty nine cases, twenty six with long term follow up), Ital J Orthop Traumatol 4 (2) (1978) 171–182.

22. C. Rubino, A. Shamsaldin, M.G. Le, M. Labbe, J.M. Guinebretiere & J. Chavaudra, et al., Radiation dose and risk of soft tissue and bone sarcoma after breast cancer treatment, Breast Cancer Res Treat 89 (3) (2005) 277–288.

23. A.G. Huvos & H.Q. Woodard, Postradiation sarcomas of bone, Health Phys 55 (4) (1988) 631–636.

24. Y.M. Kirova, H. Rafi, M.C. Voisin, M. Rieux, M. Kuentz & S.L. Mouel, et al., Radiation-induced bone sarcoma following total body irradiation: role of additional radiation on localized areas, Bone Marrow Transplant 25 (9) (2000) 1011–1013.

25. G.F. Domson, A. Shahlaee, J.D. Reith, C.H. Bush & C.P. Gibbs, Infarct-associated bone sarcomas, Clin Orthop Relat Res 20 (2009).

26. W.J. Gillespie, C.M. Frampton, R.J. Henderson & P.M. Ryan, The incidence of cancer following total hip replacement, J Bone Joint Surg Br 70 (4) (1988) 539–542.

27. B.A. Berretoni & J.R. Carter, Mechanisms of cancer metastasis to bone, J Bone Joint Surg Am 68 (2) (1986) 308–312.

28. D.L. Xu, X.T. Zhang, G.H. Wang, F.B. Li & J.Y. Hu, Clinical features of pathologically confirmed metastatic bone tumors—a report of 390 cases, Ai Zheng 24 (11) (2005) 1404–1407.

29. S. Desai & N. Jambhekar, Clinicopathological evaluation of metastatic carcinomas of bone: a retrospective analysis of 114 cases over 10 years, Indian J Pathol Microbiol 38 (1) (1995) 49–54.

30. R.E. Coleman, Skeletal complications of malignancy, Cancer 80 (8 Suppl) (1997) 1588–1594.

31. L.S. Rosen, D. Gordon, S. Tchekmedyian, R. Yanagihara, V. Hirsh & M. Krzakowski, et al., Zoledronic acid versus placebo in the treatment of skeletal metastases in patients with lung cancer and other solid tumors: a phase III, double-blind, randomized trial—the Zoledronic Acid Lung Cancer and Other Solid Tumors Study Group, J Clin Oncol 21 (16) (2003) 3150–3157.

32. M.L. Brown, J. Lipscomb & C. Snyder, The burden of illness of cancer: economic cost and quality of life, Annu Rev Public Health 22 (2001) 91–113.

33. Cost Analysis: Cost of illness, CDC Econ Eval Tutorials (E), http://www.cdc.gov/owcd.EET/cost/fixed/3.html

34. M.T. Groot, C.G. Boeken Kruger, R.C. Pelger & C.A. Uyl-de Groot, Costs of prostate cancer, metastatic to the bone, in the Netherlands, Eur Urol 43 (3) (2003) 226–232.

35. T. Delea, C. Langer, J. McKiernan, M. Liss, J. Edelsberg & J. Brandman, et al., The cost of treatment of skeletal-related events in patients with bone metastases from lung cancer, Oncology 67 (5–6) (2004) 390–396.

36. T.E. Delea, J. McKiernan, J. Brandman, J. Edelsberg, J. Sung & M. Raut, et al., Impact of skeletal complications on total medical care costs among patients with bone metastases of lung cancer, J Thorac Oncol 1 (6) (2006) 571–576.

37. T. Delea, J. McKiernan, J. Brandman, J. Edelsberg, J. Sung & M. Raut, et al., Retrospective study of the effect of skeletal complications on total medical care costs in patients with bone metastases of breast cancer seen in typical clinical practice, J Support Oncol 4 (7) (2006) 341–347.

38. N. Kinnane, Burden of bone disease, Eur J Oncol Nurs 11 (Suppl 2) (2007) S28–S31.

39. P. Major, Optimal management of metastatic bone disease, Eur J Oncol Nurs 11 (Suppl 2) (2007) S32–S37.

40. K.L. Schulman & J. Kohles, Economic burden of metastatic bone disease in the US, Cancer 109 (11) (2007) 2334–2342.

41. J. Felix, V. Andreozzi, M. Soares, H. Gervasio, A. Moreira & L. Costa, et al., Direct hospital costs of skeletal-related events in Portuguese patients with breast cancer and bone metastases, J Clin Oncol 25 (18S) (2007) 17084.

42. M.J. Lage, B.L. Barber, D.J. Harrison & S. Jun, The cost of treating skeletal-related events in patients with prostate cancer, Am J Manag Care 14 (5) (2008) 317–322.

Section II. Bone Microenvironment and Bone Cancer

CHAPTER **2**

Tumor-Bone Cell Interactions in Bone Metastases

PIERRICK G.J. FOURNIER[1], LAUREN K. DUNN[1], GREGORY A. CLINES[1] AND THERESA A. GUISE[1]

[1]*Division of Endocrinology and Metabolism, Department of Medicine, University of Virginia, Charlottesville, Virginia, USA.*

Contents

Grant Support

The authors acknowledge financial support from the US Department of Defense BCRP and PCRP (grants PC061185 to PGJF, BC073157 to LAK, PC073756 to GAC and PC040341 to TAG); the National Institutes of Health (grants CA118428 to GAC, CA69158, DK067333, and DK065837 to TAG); the Bone and Cancer Foundation (PGJF); the Prostate Cancer Foundation (TAG); the Mellon Institute (TAG); the Research and Development Committee of the University of Virginia (PGFJ); and the Gerald D. Aurbach Endowment of the University of Virginia (TAG).

I. INTRODUCTION

The development of bone metastasis is an organized multi-step process in which some organs are preferential targets. In patients with advanced cancer, bone is the third most common site for metastases after lung and liver [1]. Some cancers are particularly osteophilic, such as cancers of the breast and prostate where bone metastases occur in 60 to 70% of patients [1]. Bone metastases occurrence can be explained by the expression of different malignant factors such as the chemokine receptors CXCR4 [2–4] or CX3CR1 [5], or the integrin $\alpha_V\beta_3$ [6,7] promoting cancer cell homing to bone. Another critical parameter of tumor cell development in bone is their ability to survive and grow in the bone microenvironment. This exemplifies the 'seed and soil' theory from

Sir Stephen Paget: 'When a plant goes to seed, its seeds are carried in all directions; but they can only grow if they fall on congenial soil' [8]. Cancer cells (the seeds) arriving in the bone marrow cavity will not grow if they are not properly responsive or adapted to the bone environment (the soil).

Bone is a unique and rich environment whose integrity relies on the balance between osteoclastic bone resorption and osteoblastic bone formation to renew and adapt. The arrival of tumor cells and their interactions with bone cells disrupts normal bone remodeling causing abnormal new bone formation or bone destruction that characterizes osteoblastic and osteolytic metastases, respectively. Osteoblastic metastases are common with advanced prostate cancer while breast cancer bone metastases are typically osteolytic. However, many bone metastases are mixed and contain both osteoblastic and osteolytic characteristics. These skeletal complications have significant clinical consequences (hypercalcemia, intractable pain, fractures, nerve compression syndromes) that reduce the quality of life of these patients [9]. More importantly, unbalanced bone remodeling provides metastatic tumor cells the means to grow and survive in bone.

II. MECHANISMS OF OSTEOLYTIC METASTASES FROM SOLID TUMORS

A. The 'Vicious Cycle'

Paracrine interactions between cancer cells and the bone microenvironment are the basis for the 'seed and soil' hypothesis of Stephen Paget. Parathyroid hormone-related protein (PTHrP) and transforming growth factor-β (TGF-β) are secreted regulatory factors that promote breast cancer osteolysis. PTHrP secreted by breast cancer cells in the bone microenvironment drives receptor activator of NF-κB ligand (RANKL) expression and inhibits osteoprotegerin (OPG) secretion from osteoblasts and stromal cells, thereby activating osteoclastogenesis via the receptor activator of

NF-κB (RANK) located on osteoclast precursors [10]. In normal bone remodeling, a balance between RANKL and OPG is carefully regulated to prevent excessive bone loss [11]. The shift in the RANKL/OPG balance results in increased bone resorption and the release of factors, such as TGF-β, embedded within the bone matrix. The release of TGF-β further stimulates breast cancer cells [12]. Thus the vicious cycle begins: tumor cell production of PTHrP stimulates osteoclastic bone resorption and release of more TGF-β, which in turn stimulates more tumor-produced PTHrP (Figure 2.1). The reciprocal interactions between PTHrP and TGF-β have served as a model for discovering other signaling pathways that regulate cancer metastasis to bone. Furthermore, blockade of PTHrP and/or TGF-β to reduce bone metastasis represents an ideal strategy in the treatment of bone metastasis and has been a focus of research in preclinical models.

B. Transforming Growth Factor-β

1. THE BASICS OF TGF-β

The bone mineral matrix consists of hydroxyapatite crystals and matrix proteins. Ninety percent of the matrix protein component is type I collagen [13]. Among the other 10% of proteins embedded in bone are growth factors such as insulin-like growth factors (IGFs), TGF-βs, fibroblast growth factors (FGFs), platelet derived growth factor (PDGF) and bone morphogenetic proteins (BMPs) [14]. Bone is a major storehouse of TGF-β1 (200 μg/kg) [15] with a concentration only second to platelets [16]. Even though it is not the most abundant of the bone growth factors, it is one of the most studied and is of chief importance in osteolytic metastases. TGF-β is a multifunctional growth factor involved in cell growth, survival, differentiation and migration [17,18]. Three highly homologous isoforms of

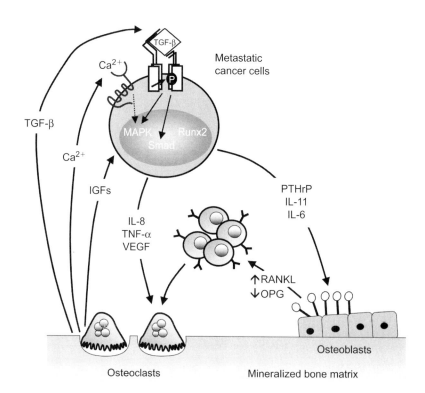

FIGURE 2.1 Mechanisms of cancer cell-induced bone resorption in the vicious cycle of osteolytic metastasis. After invading into the bone microenvironment, cancer cells secrete factors that support osteoclastogenesis. Factors such as PTHrP, IL-11 and IL-6 increase osteoblast RANKL and decrease OPG, inducing osteoclast differentiation and activity. Other factors, including IL-8, TNF-α or VEGF, can also induce osteoclastogenesis and bone resorption independently of the RANKL/RANK axis. The increased bone resorption is associated with an increased release of Ca^{2+} and growth factors, such as TGF-β and IGFs, contained in the mineralized bone matrix. TGF-β triggers a further increase of the secretion of osteolytic factors signaling through the TGF-β receptor-Smad pathway and the transcription factor Runx2. Additionally, IGFs can increase tumor growth, and Ca^{2+} through the Ca^{2+} sensing-receptor activates the MAPK pathway and cancer cell growth. The TGF-β receptor can also activate MAPK. IGF, insulin-like growth factor; IL, interleukin; MAPK, mitogen activated protein kinase; PTHrP, parathyroid hormone-related protein; RANK, receptor activator of NF-κB; RANKL, RANK ligand; Runx2, runt-related transcription factor 2; Smad, mothers against decapentalegic homologue protein; TGF-β, transforming growth factor-β; TNF-α, tumor necrosis factor α; VEGF, vascular endothelial growth factor.

TGF-β exist (TGF-β1, TGF-β2 and TGF-β3), of which TGF-β1 is the prototype. TGF-β is a critical factor in bone remodeling (for review, see Ref. 16). In bone, TGF-β1 is deposited and stored in the bone mineral matrix by osteoblasts. During osteoclastic bone resorption, TGF-β is released and acts on local cells within the bone microenvironment. TGF-β inhibits osteoclast maturation and survival [16]. Conversely, active TGF-β promotes the early stage of bone formation by increasing the recruitment and proliferation of osteoblast progenitors, while it blocks later stage of osteoblast differentiation regulated by BMPs [16].

In cancer, the role of TGF-β is complex and its effects are often referred to as a 'double-edged sword'. In early stages of cancer, TGF-β activates a cytostatic program and cell death, and acts as a tumor suppressor. In the later stages of disease, tumor cells elude TGF-β mediated cytostasis and TGF-β becomes a major mediator of metastasis. TGF-β activates the epithelial-mesenchymal transition (EMT) [19] and tumor cell invasion [20], increases angiogenesis [21] and induces immunosuppression [22].

Active TGF-β1 is a homodimer of 112 amino acids that binds to the TGF-β type II receptor (TβRII) that then promotes the association with the TGF-β type I receptor (TβRI, also known as ALK5) [23,24]. The constitutively active kinase domain of the TβRII transphosphorylates multiple serine and threonine residues of the TβRI cytoplasmic domain. Its subsequent activation exposes a binding site for the receptor-associated Smads proteins (RSmad), Smad2 and Smad3, which are then phosphorylated by the TβRI serine kinase domain to propagate the signal. The heterodimer formed by Smad2 and Smad3 interacts with nucleoporin and then translocates to the nucleus [25]. The recruitment of the Co-Smad, Smad4 (also known as DPC4), creates a core Smad complex that can bind differing DNA sequences, either the Smad-binding elements (defined as 5'-GTCT-3', or the complementary sequence 5'-CAGA-3') [26] or the GC-rich elements (as 5'-GCCGnCGC-3') [27,28]. The association of the RSmad-Smad4 complex with DNA-binding partner, such as FoxH1 [29], p300/CBP [30,31], or Runx2 [32] increases the specificity and affinity for DNA. The RSmad-Smad4 core can also interact with negative regulators such as TGIF, Ski or SnoN, repressing the transcription of TGF-β target genes [33,34]. The multiprotein Smad transcriptional complex may function either as an inducer or inhibitor of gene transcription [35]. The TGF-β signaling pathway is blocked by the inhibitory Smad, Smad7. Smad7 can bind the TGF-β receptor, competing with the RSmads, preventing their phosphorylation [36,37]. Smad7 recruits HECT domain E3 ubiquitin ligases such as Smurf1 [38,39], Smurf2 [40], Nedd4-2 [41] and Tiu11 (also named WWP1) [42] to the TβRI inducing its ubiquitylation and its subsequent degradation by the proteasome. A similar mechanism has been demonstrated in which Smad7 mediates the poly-ubiquitylation and degradation of Smad4 [43]. Smurf2 and Nedd4-2 can also directly

interact with Smad2 to induce their degradation [41,44,45]. TGF-β and its receptor activate ERK, JNK and p38 MAPK, either directly to control gene transcription or to regulate Smad activation [46].

2. INTEGRITY OF THE TGF-β SIGNALING PATHWAY IN BONE METASTASES

Mutations that inactivate mediators of the TGF-β signaling pathway (i.e. Smad2, Smad4, TβRII) have been identified in various types of cancer [23]. Approximately 30% of colorectal cancers contain mutations of *TGFBR2* resulting in inactivation of TβRII [47]. The mutation rate of *TGFBR2* is close to 90% in colorectal cancer due to DNA microsatellite instability [48]. In pancreatic cancer, only 4% of tumors contain *TGFBR2* mutations [49], while the *SMAD4* gene is inactivated either by loss of heterozygosity (LOH) or intragenic mutations in about 50% of tumors [50].

In breast cancer, *TGFBR2* mutations are a rare event. In samples from 72 patients with breast tumor, mutations of the *TGFBR2* were not more prevalent compared to normal cells [51]. The transgenic overexpression of a dominant negative form of the TβRII under the control of the mouse mammary tumor virus (MMTV) accelerates the outcome of mammary tumors and decreases the frequency of lung metastases [20]. Conversely, increased expression of TβRII in cancer cells was associated with an increased aggressiveness of the tumors in patients [51]. Two other independent studies demonstrated that overexpression of TGF-β1 or of a constitutively active form of TβRI in mouse epithelium in MMTV-Neu transgenic mice, while delaying mammary tumor occurrence, increased the frequency of lung metastases [20,52]. These results illustrate the dual role of the TGF-β signaling pathway as tumor suppressor in the early stages and as an activator of malignant progression in later stages of cancer progression. None of these studies analyzed the effect of TGF-β signaling pathway modulation on the occurrence of bone metastases. However, immunostaining demonstrated that Smad2 is phosphorylated and localized to the nucleus of cancer cells in 12 of 16 bone metastasis samples from breast cancer patients, exhibiting the expression of a functional TGF-β receptor and active Smad signaling at sites of bone metastases [27].

The TGF-β signaling pathway is critical for the establishment and development of skeletal tumor burden. Animal models of bone metastasis have significantly increased understanding of the importance of TGF-β. The MDA-MB-231 human breast cancer cell line forms osteolytic metastases in immunodeficient mice when inoculated into the left cardiac ventricle [53]. Kang *et al.* transduced MDA-MB-231 cells with a retroviral vector expressing the HSV-1 thymidine kinase under the control of a TGF-β sensitive promoter [27]. Metastases caused by these cells showed thymidine kinase activity specifically in bone by microPET (positron emission tomography), not in adrenal glands, demonstrating TGF-β signaling activity in cancer cells at bone sites. When the TGF-β signaling pathway was neutralized by Smad4 knockdown using shRNA expressing retrovirus in MDA-MB-231 cells, the formation of bone metastases in athymic nude mice was delayed and the skeletal tumor burden was decreased when compared to control transduced cells [27,54]. Similarly the inhibition of Smad signaling by the overexpression of Smad7 in 1205Lu melanoma cells inhibited the occurrence of bone metastases and increased the survival of immunodeficient mice [55]. Mice containing skeletal lesions had significantly less expression of bone metastases factors IL-11, PTHrP and CTGF when compared to the parental cells [55].

Manipulation of Smad4 and Smad7 expression not only targeted the TGF-β/Smad pathway but also the BMP/Smad pathway mediated by the BMP receptors [335] involved in cancers of the breast [56,57] and prostate [58,59]. TGF-β signaling pathway is specifically targeted by expressing an inactive form of the TβRII (TβRIIΔcyt) containing a deletion of the cytoplasmic TβRII, including the kinase domain [60]. MDA-MB-231 cells expressing the kinase deleted receptor did not respond to TGF-β treatment showing that TβRIIΔcyt constitutes a dominant-negative form [61]. Mice inoculated with TGF-β unresponsive MDA-MB-231 (MDA/TβRIIΔcyt) cells showed increased survival, and decreased osteolytic lesion number and area when compared to cells transfected with an empty vector [12]. The histological analysis confirmed that the skeletal tumor burden was significantly reduced, as well as the number of osteoclasts at the tumor/bone interface [12]. This effect is not specific to breast cancer and similar results were obtained by expressing TβRIIΔcyt in a cell line established from a renal cell carcinoma [62]. Expression of TβRI(T204D), a mutated form of the TβRI with a constitutively activated kinase domain [63], restored TGF-β signaling and reversed the effect of TβRIIΔcyt in MDA/TβRIIΔcyt cells [12]. Mice had increased osteoclast recruitment, bone lesions and skeletal tumor burden, and decreased survival compared to mice inoculated with MDA/TβRIIΔcyt cells [12]. When MDA-MB-231 or renal carcinoma cells expressing or not expressing TβRIIΔcyt were inoculated intramuscularly or subcutaneously, there was no significant difference in the tumor growth [12,62].

Using a CAGA-luciferase construct, whose activity is increased in response to TGF-β, Buijs *et al.* demonstrated that treatment with BMP-7 decreased TGF-β signaling in breast and prostate cancer cells *in vitro* [64,65]. *In vivo*, the engineered overexpression of BMP-7 in breast and prostate cancer cells decreased the development of the skeletal tumor burden after intracardiac inoculation of the mice. Similarly, a treatment with BMP-7 decreased tumor burden in bone, but had no effect on orthotopic tumors, and suggests that BMP-7 may be useful as an inhibitor of osteolytic bone metastases, possibly through inhibiting the action of TGF-β in bone [64,65].

Different small-molecule inhibitors of the TβRI kinase activity have been synthesized and some have been successfully tested in mouse models where bone metastases were induced with human cancer cells [66–68]. A pteridine-derivative, SD-208, has been tested on MDA-MB-231 bone metastases *in vivo*. While SD-208 did not affect tumor cell proliferation *in vitro*, it inhibited RSmad phosphorylation. *In vivo* SD-208 reduced the development and progression of osteolytic metastases, and prolonged mouse survival [68]. Similar results were obtained using PC-3 prostate cancer cells that also induced osteolytic metastases (Fournier *et al.*, unpublished results).

These studies collectively demonstrate that bone-derived TGF-β is a critical factor for the establishment and the development of skeletal tumor burden, and support a role for the TGF-β signaling pathway in the treatment of bone metastases. Different strategies are being carried out, not only on small-molecule inhibitors, but also on antibodies directed against TGF-β or stabilized antisense RNA against TGF-β2—the latter already being tested in clinical trials although not to treat bone metastases.

However, the importance of TGF-β in bone metastases is puzzling, since TGF-β does not direct proliferative effect on the cells in these mouse models [12,62]. It appears to promote bone metastasis by stimulating the secretion of cancer cell prometastatic proteins that act on bone cells.

3. TGF-β and the Parathyroid Hormone-Related Protein (PTHrP)

PTHrP is a key factor in osteolytic bone metastasis. Its direct effects on osteoclasts remain elusive; however, by decreasing the production of RANKL and increasing the secretion of OPG from the osteoblasts and stromal cells [16]. RANKL and OPG are two crucial factors of osteoclastogenesis. RANKL activates its receptor RANK to induce preosteoclasts fusion as well as the synthesis of proteins involved in osteoclastic resorption, such as the integrin $\alpha_v\beta_3$ or the cathepsin K [69]. Mice knocked out for RANK [70] or RANKL [71] are osteopetrotic due to lack of osteoclasts. The OPG is a soluble decoy receptor of RANK that prevents RANK-RANKL interaction [72], and OPG deficient mice show an increase of the number of osteoclasts as well as severe osteoporosis [73].

PTHrP was first described as a factor responsible for humoral hypercalcemia of malignancy [74]. A product of a complex gene, PTHrP is secreted as three different isoforms (1-139), (1-141) and (1-173) of which the N-terminal (1-34) region has high homology with parathyroid hormone (PTH) [75]. PTH and PTHrP both bind to the PTH type 1 receptor (PTH1R) [76], activating protein kinase A (PKA) and protein kinase C (PKC) pathways in kidney and bone where they decrease renal calcium resorption and increase bone resorption, respectively [75]. PTHrP was detected in 83–92% of breast cancer bone metastases by immunohistochemistry but only 17–38% of non-osseous metastases

[77,78]. In prostate patients, only 50% of bone metastases were positive for PTHrP by immunostaining [79,80]. *In vitro*, breast and prostate cancer cells that form osteolytic metastases (i.e., MDA-MB-231, MDA-MB-435s, PC-3) secreted PTHrP [81,82]. These results suggest that PTHrP could play an important role in bone metastases formation or development.

In a mouse model, Guise *et al.* showed that a treatment with a monoclonal antibody directed against PTHrP(1-34) drastically decreased the amount of bone destruction (60% inhibition) induced by MDA-MB-231 cells, when compared to treatment with a control antibody. This inhibition was associated with a decreased skeletal tumor burden (85% inhibition) as well as a decrease of osteoclast number [81]. Treatment with guanosine nucleotide compounds that specifically inhibit the transcription of the *PTHLH* gene and production of PTHrP in MDA-MB-231 cells reduced osteolytic metastasis in nude mice [83]. The role of PTHrP is not specific to breast cancer. When HARA or SBC-5 human lung cancer cells that strongly express PTHrP were studied in an animal model of bone metastases, PTHrP-neutralizing antibodies were also an effective therapy [84,85]. Conversely, engineered overexpression of PTHrP in breast (MDA-M-231, MCF-7) or prostate (Mat Ly Lu) cancer cells increased metastases to bone and osteoclast-mediated bone destruction at the tumor/bone interface [10,86,87]. The overexpression of PTHrP did not affect the formation of metastases to non-bone sites [86], and a PTHrP neutralizing antibody had no effect on visceral metastases caused by SBC-5 cells [85], suggesting that PTHrP only affects metastases to bone.

Expression of PTHrP at sites of primary tumor is not a predictor for the formation of bone metastases. Transgenic mice with mammary gland PTHrP overexpression did not have enhanced bone metastases or other tissue metastases when treated with the carcinogenic compound 9,10-dimethyl-1,2-benz-anthracene or DMBA [88]. PTHrP was well expressed and functional in these mice as they developed hypercalcemia due to high systemic PTHrP levels [88]. However, PTHrP was not identified in a pre-clinical model of bone metastasis as a protein involved in the bone metastatic 'multigenic program' [4]. These results are consistent with data of more than 350 patient primary tumor samples demonstrating that PTHrP expression predicted improved survival and decreased development of metastases including metastases to bone [89]. The role of PTHrP as prognostic factor has yet to be elucidated, but preliminary results suggest action as an autocrine factor to prevent DNA mutations and decrease cell apoptosis [90,91]. These results emphasize the importance of PTHrP specifically in the local destruction in bone metastases, as well as its preferential expression in the bone microenvironment [77,78].

Among all of the growth factors trapped in the bone mineral matrix and released during osteoclastic bone resorption, IGFs, FGFs or PDGF did not affect PTHrP secretion in MDA-MB-231 cells *in vitro*; only TGF-β increased PTHrP expression [12]. This regulation was totally reversed by expressing TβRIIΔcyt [12,61]; and partially reversed using: (1) dominant negative forms of Smad proteins (Smad2, Smad3 and Smad4); (2) inhibitors of p38 MAP kinase; and (3) inhibitors of MEK1/2 kinase [61]. PTHrP expression is, therefore, regulated by TGF-β through Smad-dependent and independent pathways. This regulation of PTHrP by bone-derived TGF-β was proven to be essential for malignant osteolysis. Inhibition of osteolysis induced by MDA/TβRIIΔcyt was reversed by the engineered overexpression of PTHrP [12]. Conversely, in MDA/TβRIIΔcyt overexpressing TβRI(T204D), a PTHrP-neutralizing antibody reduced skeletal tumor burden, osteolysis and the number of osteoclasts [61].

When MDA-MB-231 cells form bone metastases in mice, PTHrP concentrations were increased in metastatic bone marrow extract compared to normal bone marrow, while there was no detectable variation of PTHrP levels in blood [81]. The effects of PTHrP on osteolysis are likely to be locally mediated. Among cells in bone, osteoclasts express a functional PTH1R [92,93], but it is unlikely that tumor-secreted PTHrP acts directly on osteoclasts. Primary osteoblasts cultivated with mouse bone marrow in the presence of vitamin D_3 and PGE_2 induce the formation of osteoclasts [10]. In similar conditions, MDA-MB-231 cells or MCF7 cells transfected to express PTHrP (MCF-7 PTHrP), which induces osteolytic metastases in mice, failed to induce the formation of osteoclasts on their own. The addition of osteoblasts, in the absence of vitamin D_3 or PGE_2, restored osteoclastogenesis mediated by MCF-7-secreted PTHrP [10]. Co-culture of primary osteoblasts with MCF-7 PTHrP showed an increased expression of the RANKL mRNA and a decreased expression of OPG mRNA when compared to culture with regular MCF-7 cells [10]. Increase of the RANKL/OPG ratio is mediated by the PTH1R through the PKA and PKC pathways [94,95]. PTHrP can also induce an increased production of IL-6 and leukemia inhibitory factor (LIF) in osteoblasts, and subsequently increased bone resorption through RANKL and OPG [96–98].

Overall, these studies describe a comprehensive mechanism that places TGF-β and PTHrP at the heart of bone metastases formation and development. Cancer cells directed to bone by osteotropic factors will secrete PTHrP and modulate the RANKL/OPG ratio from osteoblasts and stromal cells. This environment promotes osteoclast maturation, activity and bone resorption. This results in hypercalcemia from release of Ca^{2+} from bone as well as the release of growth factors, such as activated TGF-β. TGF-β responsive cancer cells will produce, in turn, increased amount of PTHrP that could protect cancer cells in an autocrine loop or further induce bone resorption. Tumor cell activation and osteoclastic bone resorption are then sustaining each others in what has since been described as the vicious cycle of bone metastases. TGF-β-induced PTHrP is, however, not the only tumor factor that can modulate bone cells and other vicious cycles have been proposed.

4. TGF-β, COX-2 AND IL-8

Among the proteins secreted by malignant cells, IL-8 (CXCL8) expressed by breast, prostate and lung cancers regulate numerous steps of the metastatic cascade such as invasion, angiogenesis and tumorigenesis [99,100]. IL-8 was also associated with bone metastases development [101,102]. The MDA-MET cells were selected *in vivo* for their capacity to induce more osteolytic metastases when compared to their parental MDA-MB-231 breast cancer cells. However, this bone metastases phenotype is not correlated with PTHrP expression or an increased proliferation [103,104]. Based on the analysis of its transcriptome, the authors reported an increase of IL-8 expression in MDA-MET, and observed a correlation between IL-8 production and the propensity of different cancer cells to induce bone metastases [101,102]. Independently, Singh e*t al.* isolated a similar bone-seeking subclone of MDA-MB-231 cells that also present an increased secretion of IL-8 [105]. Since MDA-MET cells do not express IL-8 receptors, CXCR1 and CXCR2, this cytokine may not have autocrine but paracrine effects [101]. *In vitro*, rhIL-8 induced the expression of RANKL by an osteoblastic cell line that could indirectly increase osteoclastogenesis [104]. However, if rhIL-8 increased the formation of osteoclasts from human peripheral blood mononuclear cells (PBMC), neutralization of RANKL by a RANK-Fc chimera did not reverse the induction of osteoclastogenesis mediated by IL-8 [104]. Similarly conditioned media of MDA-MET increased the formation of osteoclasts from human peripheral blood mononuclear cells when compared to the parental MDA-MB-231 [103]. This induction was not affected by RANK-Fc or by antibodies against TGF-β, IL-1 or IL-6, but was decreased by IL-8 neutralizing antibodies [103,104]. Moreover immunofluorescence staining demonstrated that mature osteoclasts (multinucleated cells expressing $\alpha_V\beta_3$) express the IL-8 receptor CXCR1 but not CXCR2 [104]. These experiments suggest that tumor-secreted IL-8 directly activates the osteoclasts independently of the RANK/RANKL system. IL-8 can induce NF-κB activation in different cell lines including RAW264.7—a mouse pre-osteoclast cell line [106]. However, T cells may mediate IL-8-dependent independent of RANKL [107] and further studies are needed to understand the precise mechanisms.

Bendre *et al.* suggested that increased IL-8 expression was inherent to the cells, naturally expressing higher amounts of IL-8 in basal conditions, *in vitro* [101]. Other studies can be associated with this work to suggest an *in situ* regulation of IL-8 at sites of bone metastases. Singh *et al.* observed that the overexpression of a functional cyclo-oxygenase-2 (COX-2) induced an increase of IL-8 production in the breast cancer cells MDA-MB-231 and MCF10A.

Moreover, MDA-MB-231 bone-seeking subclones have increased COX-2 activity, measured by PGE_2 production, and correlated with IL-8 secretion [105,108]. COX-2 was identified as an inducer of breast cancers and its activity is correlated with the metastatic potential [109,110]. In patient biopsies, 87% of the bone metastases were positives for COX-2 by immunostaining [111]. More interestingly, immunostaining revealed stronger COX-2 expression in MDA-MB-231 bone metastases when compared to orthotopic mammary fat pad tumors [111]. This increased expression in bone metastases is likely due to bone-derived growth factors, since COX-2 was decreased *in vivo* when mice were treated with an inhibitor of osteoclastic bone resorption, the bisphosphonate risedronate. *Ex vivo* and *in vitro*, the authors demonstrated that TGF-β induced COX-2 expression in MDA-MB-231, but also in bone marrow stromal cells and osteoblasts [111]. In addition, the increased osteoclastogenesis induced by conditioned media of MDA-MB-231 cells treated with TGF-β was partially reversed when using a COX-2 inhibitor, NS-398. The effect of COX-2 is PTHrP-independent since *in vitro* the NS-398 did not change TGF-β-mediated PTHrP expression in MDA-MB-231 [111]. Bone-derived TGF-β could also increase osteolytic metastases by increasing COX-2 expression in bone. Consequently, the overexpression of COX-2 in the MDA-MB-435s breast cancer cells significantly increased the skeletal tumor burden after intracardiac inoculation of the cells in nude mice [108]. Different COX-2 inhibitors, NS-398, nimesulfide and MF-tricyclic, decreased bone metastases from MDA-MB-231 [111] and MDA-MB-435s [108].

Although the relationships between TGF-β, COX-2 and IL-8 remain to be further demonstrated *in vivo* at sites of bone metastases, these results suggest the existence of a new bone metastases vicious cycle where bone-derived TGF-β stimulates malignant IL-8 secretion through COX-2 to increase osteoclast maturation and resorption. The mechanisms through which TGF-β and COX-2 regulates IL-8 expression have not been totally addressed, and involvement of the NF-κB or β-catenin pathways have been suggested [105,112–114]. Interestingly, COX-2-mediated induction of IL-8 was prevented by the estrogen receptor. Estrogen receptor-positive breast cancer cells, MCF-7, when transfected to overexpress COX-2 did not show an increase of IL-8 expression [105].

IL-8 expression is also regulated by other factors such as hypoxia and acidosis [115] that may alter the bone microenvironment [116]. Another characterized factor is platelet aggregation. Platelet aggregation induced by cancer cells is a critical event during the metastases cascade [117,118]. Activated platelets release lysophosphatidic acid (LPA), recognized by the LPA receptor 1, increases cancer cell proliferation *in vitro* and *in vivo*, either in bone or subcutaneously in breast cancer models [119]. Therefore, this effect is not specific to bone metastases. However, LPA-treated breast cancer cells secrete increased amounts of cytokines that may increase osteoclastogenesis and bone resorption, including IL-8 [119,120].

Finally, the role of IL-8 in bone metastases may not just be a matter of quantity. Mass spectrometry revealed that the bone-seeking MDA-MET secrete a full-length isoform of IL-8 (1-77) when compared to the parental MDA-MB-231 that secrete a truncated form (6-77) [103,107]. Secretion of different isoforms of IL-8 by MDA-MB-231 clones has not been elucidated and is unlikely to involve protease maturation since protease inhibitors did not affect IL-8 secreted by these cells [103]. The potency of the IL-8 isoforms on osteoclastogenesis still has to be studied.

5. EFFECTS OF IL-11 INDUCED BY TGF-β

IL-11 is a multifunctional cytokine that was isolated from a bone marrow-derived stromal cell line and identified as part of the genes predicting bone metastases in breast cancer [4]. The IL-11 promoter region contains two activator protein-1 (AP-1) sites adjacent to a GC-rich region where Smad proteins can bind [27]. Thus IL-11 expression is increased by TGF-β as it was demonstrated in osteoblasts [121] and in cancer cells [4,27,122]. IL-11 production is also induced by COX-2 and its product PGE_2 in breast cancer cells *in vitro*, through a mechanism which unlike IL-8 is not subject to the estrogen receptor [123]. Due to bone-derived TGF-β and the induction of COX-2, malignant IL-11 expression is likely to be increased at sites of bone metastases. Moreover, cancer cells can also increase the expression of IL-11 from the osteoblasts through the secretion of TGF-β1 [121] or PTHrP [124].

IL-11 acts on cells through its specific receptor that combines the common β-subunit glycoprotein 130 (gp130) and the specificity-determining α-subunit (IL-11Rα), which are both expressed by osteoblasts and mature osteoclasts [125]. The receptors for IL-11 and IL-6 share gp130, and have many common biological properties [126]. Since IL-6 is known to induce bone resorption through modulation of the RANKL/OPG ratio [98], the effects of IL-11 on osteoclasts have then been studied. In mouse calvarial models with or without addition of bone marrow cells, IL-11 increased osteoclast formation as well as the resorption area on dentine or ivory slices [126,127]. IL-11 effects on osteoclasts were reversed by antibodies neutralizing IL-11, gp130 or IL-11Rα [124,126,128]. However, IL-11 failed to increase the resorption activity of isolated osteoclasts [127]. Similarly, conditioned media from TGF-β-treated breast cancer cells known to induce osteolysis in mice failed to induce the formation of osteoclasts from spleen cells on their own suggesting the mediation of another cellular partner [124]. Addition of primary osteoblasts was indeed required to allow osteoclast formation [124].

The downstream effects of IL-11 to induce osteoclastogenesis have not been totally explained and the results from different studies are contradictory. In mouse primary osteoblasts, IL-11-treatment increased the expression of the osteoclast differentiation factor RANKL [129]. Tsuda *et al.* also demonstrated that IL-11-induced osteoclastogenesis was inhibited by OPG [130]. OPG expression was, however, induced, to a lower extent, by IL-11 in calvaria osteoblasts, and, overall, the RANKL/OPG ratio is increased by IL-11 [131]. Despite these evidences of a RANK/RANKL/OPG mediated mechanism, Kudo *et al.* observed that neither the formation of osteoclasts from PBMCs nor the osteoclastic resorption induced by IL-11 were inhibited by OPG or RANK:Fc [128]. Another mechanism involves prostaglandin production. IL-11 increased PGE_2 production in calvarial cultures [124,132]. IL-11-induced PGE_2 secretion and osteoclastogenesis were both inhibited by the cyclooxygenase inhibitors, indomethacin and NS-398 [124,126,132]. Secretion of PGE_2 by the osteoblasts treated with MDA-MB-231 conditioned media or IL-11 decreased GM-CSF secretion in the spleen cells used for osteoclast formation assay [124]. Neutralization and decrease of GM-CSF in this assay significantly increased the formation of osteoclasts while addition of GM-CSF decreased osteoclastogenesis [124]. The role of GM-CSF in osteoclast formation and activity is also, unfortunately, unclear. While GM-CSF production as been demonstrated to inhibit osteoclast formation [133,134], it has also been reported to support osteoclastogenesis [135,136]. Recently it was shown that GM-CSF produced by breast cancer cells is a critical factor for osteolytic metastases since its knockdown using short hairpin RNA significantly reduced osteolysis and tumor burden in a mouse model [137].

The role of IL-11 in bone metastases requires more study. Different models to simulate *in vitro* or *ex vivo* osteoclast function and bone metastases environment may explain the different results encountered. It is also possible that IL-11 does not act independently but requires other factors to have a significant role. Osteopontin (OPN) is a glycosylated protein of the bone matrix, produced by osteoblasts and involved in the mineralization [138]. OPN also contains an Arg-Gly-Asp (RGD) motif recognized by the $\alpha_V\beta_3$ integrin expressed by osteoclasts. Binding of osteoclasts to OPN allows them to adhere to and resorb bone [139,140]. OPN is also expressed by cancer cells and play a role in metastases formation [141–144]. The constitutive overexpression of IL-11 or OPN only did not increase bone metastases induced by MDA-MB-231 as it would have been expected [4]. However, the combination of IL-11 and osteopontin (OPN) drastically accelerated the development of bone metastases in mice [27]. Bone metastases were further increased by overexpressing a third protein such as CXCR4 involved in the homing of cancer cells to bone, or the connective tissue growth factor (CTGF) [27]. CTGF is a member of the CCN family, whose expression is increased by TGF-β or PTHrP [145,146]. CTGF is a well-known pro-angiogenic protein also involved in skeletal development [147]. CTGF knockdown inhibit osteoclastogenesis *in vitro* and a CTGF-neutralizing antibody decreased bone metastases in mice [146]. We would hypothezise that the effect of CTGF on osteoclasts is mediated by its interaction with the $\alpha_V\beta_3$ integrin [148].

6. TGF-β, Runx2 and the Osteomimetism

TGF-β can enhance tumor cell invasiveness [149,150] by regulating the expression of different matrix metalloproteinases (MMP) including MMP-13. MMP-13, also known as collagenase-3, is a member of a family of homologous collagenases that includes MMP-1 and -8. It is a secreted proteinase that recognizes a broad spectrum of substrates including collagens, fibronectin, osteonectin, and tenascin-C [151]. MMP-13 is highly expressed by osteoblasts and is essential for long bone development [152,154]. It is also expressed in breast carcinoma where it was originally identified [155]. Its expression is increased by TGF-β in the breast cancer cells MDA-MB-231 [156], but also in head and squamous carcinoma cells [157] and osteoblasts [154]. TGF-β induction of MMP-13 was inhibited by ERK1/2 and p38 MAPK blockade, and with a dominant negative form of Smad3 involving both Smad and MAPK pathways [156]. The transcription inhibitor cycloheximide also inhibited TGF-β-induced MMP-13 indicating the need of *de novo* protein synthesis [156]. TGF-β induces first the synthesis of JunB and Runx2 that are then recruited by Smad3. This protein complex allows *MMP-13* transcription by binding to the osteoblast-specific element 2 (OSE2, also named runt domain) through Runx2, as shown by chromatin immunoprecipitation [158].

Runx2, also named Cbfa1 and Osf2, is a runt homology domain transcription factor induced by BMP-2, -4 or -7 that is critical in the first steps of osteoblast maturation [159]. Transgenic mice containing a targeted-deletion of *Runx2* lack ossification and mature osteoblasts [160]. Runx2 is also expressed in the mammary gland where it regulates the production of the milk protein, β-casein [161], but more importantly it is expressed and active in breast and prostate cancer cells and in melanoma cells that metastasize to bone [162–165]. In MDA-MB-231 breast cancer cells, the expression of an inactivated Runx2 inhibited the tumor-induced formation of osteoclasts *in vitro* [166]. Accordingly, *in vivo*, the inhibition of Runx2 activity in MDA-MB-231 cells decreased the development of bone metastases after intratibial injection in mice [166,167]. Modulation of Runx2 most likely affected the production of tumor-secreted factors mediating malignant osteoclast activity; however, these factors have not been identified yet. Meanwhile, it is clear that the overexpression of Runx2 in MDA-MB-231 induced in bone marrow stromal cells an increased expression of pro-osteoclastic genes such as M-CSF, IL-6, RANKL, or TNF [166,167]. Conversely, the expression of an inactivated Runx2 in cancer cells reduced the production of the same factors from bone cells [166,167].

Comparison of the transcriptome of MDA-MB-231 overexpressing a wild-type Runx2 or a mutated form also showed an increase in the expression of vascular endothelial growth factor, VEGF [167]. VEGF is not only an inducer of angiogenesis, it also promotes bone formation and fracture healing [168], and increases osteoclast recruitment, survival and activity [169–171]. VEGF expression is also regulated by TGF-β [172–174]. Therefore, the VEGF axis could be used as a target in bone metastases treatment. Mohamedali *et al.* used a fusion protein named VEGF$_{121}$/rGel between the VEGF$_{121}$ and the highly cytotoxic plant toxin gelonin (rGel) to target cells expressing the receptor binding VEGF$_{121}$: FLK-1 (VEGFR-2) [175–177]. FLK-1 as well as FLT-1 (VEGFR-1) is expressed on the endothelium of tumor vasculature and by the osteoclasts, and the VEGF$_{121}$/rGel is not then directly toxic for cancer cells [169,175,178]. VEGF$_{121}$/rGel was able to drastically delay and decrease the osteolysis induced by PC-3 prostate cancer cells injected in the femur of athymic mice, and the tumor burden in treated mice was considerably reduced [175].

The role of Runx2 expression induced by bone-derived TGF-β is also particularly interesting when considering the osteomimetism theory in bone metastases development [179]. The prostate cancer cell line LnCaP was used in mice to generate derived cells that reproduce prostate cancer progression such as the acquisition of the androgen-independent and metastatic phenotypes [180]. The propensity to form bone metastases was associated here with the expression of genes such as OPN, bone sialoprotein (BSP) and osteocalcin (OCN) [179]. This evolution retraces the maturation of osteoblasts and suggested that cancer cells when acquiring the capacity to 'home' to bone, become 'bone-like', hence the osteomimetic designation. Interestingly, the expression of OPN, BSP and OCN is known to be increased by or associated with Runx2 in osteoblasts and cancer cells [162,165,181–184].

The role of OCN produced by tumor cells in bone metastases development has not been properly addressed so far. But OCN secreted by mature osteoblasts may stop the mineralization process and induce osteoclast recruitment [185,186]. It was then hypothesized that tumor-secreted OCN would help to recruit osteoclasts in bone metastases [179]. BSP is a glycosylated protein, like OPN, that was thought to be bone-specific. However, BSP is also produced by cancer cells and its expression in breast, prostate or lung primary tumors of patients was associated with an increased risk of bone metastases development [187–190]. Interestingly, in subcutaneous tumors formed by MDA-MB-231 in mice, a stronger staining for BSP was noticed next to mineral structure or deposits [191]. In bone, BSP synthesized by the osteoblasts initiates the nucleation step of hydroxyapatite during matrix mineralization [138]. BSP is also preferentially expressed in cancer cells close to bone, at sites of breast or prostate cancer bone metastases, when compared to visceral metastases [192]. Based on the data we provided so far, this regulation of BSP in bone could be induced by TGF-β *via* Runx2. TGF-β could also directly induce BSP expression through a TGF-β activation element determined to be 5'-TTGGC-3' in the gene promoter [193]. Accordingly, an antibody directed against TGF-β was also shown to decrease BSP production in the 4T1 murine breast cancer cell line [194]. Wild-type BSP increased the invasiveness of bone marrow or cancer cells [195–198] while a form where the RGD peptide was mutated (BSP-KAE) did not [197]. This RGD-dependent mechanism points out to integrins and particularly to the $\alpha_v\beta_3$ integrin that can bind the BSP [199,200]. BSP also binds MMP-2 [201] and a MMP-2 neutralizing antibody decreased BSP-mediated invasion [197]. The $\alpha_v\beta_3$ integrin also mediates the activation of pro-MMP-2 [202], and Karadag *et al.* showed that BSP recruits both $\alpha_v\beta_3$ and MMP-2, creating a ternary complex to activate MMP-2 and promote tumor invasion [197]. Hence the overexpression of BSP in MDA-MB-231 cells increased osteotropism and the formation of bone metastases [203,204] while the knockdown of BSP with antisense strategy [203] or its neutralization with antibodies [205] decreased bone metastases. The effects of BSP may, however, not be totally bone metastases specific since in some studies BSP increased the growth of subcutaneous tumors and of soft tissue metastases [198], and BSP knockdown decreased metastases to the lung in the 4T1 model [194].

The secretion of OPN, OC or BSP by cancer cells in bone is parallel to osteoblast function. However, cancer cells express other factors relating them to osteoclasts and osteoclastic resorption. The modulation of Runx2 activity using knockdown or overexpression demonstrated that Runx2 regulates the expression of the gelatinase MMP-9 in breast and prostate cancer cells [164]. MMP-9 is involved in numerous steps of the metastatic cascade such as promoting cell invasion and angiogenesis by increasing VEGF bioavailability [206,207] but also in bone remodeling. In transgenic mice osteoclasts deficient in MMP-9 were still able to degrade bone but the migration of osteoclasts to the sites of resorption was delayed [170]. This suggests that osteoclasts, under the action of tumor-secreted MMP-9, are recruited close to cancer cells to resorb bone. Moreover MMP-9 increases collagen-degradation by MMP-13 [170]; and both of these MMPs are increased by Runx2 in cancer cells [158,164]. Considering that cancer cells also produce Cathepsin K, a key proteinase for bone matrix solubilization [208,209], these results raise the question whether cancer cells can resorb bone. Different studies reported the direct degradation of bone matrix by cancer cells, through MMPs, *in vitro* [209–212]. However, this phenomenon has not been observed *in vivo*. In bone metastasis biopsies of patients with breast cancer, histomorphometric analysis showed that malignant osteolysis is a local phenomenon, associated with the presence of osteoclasts [213]. Moreover, bone destruction induced by the intra-tibial injection of B16-F10 melanoma cells was totally prevented in *itgb3*$^{-/-}$ mice where the

osteoclasts are inactive due to the absence of $\alpha_v\beta_3$ integrin [118]. Similarly, in *src*$^{-/-}$ mice, in the absence of active osteoclasts, bone metastases induced by B16-F10 cells via intra-cardiac inoculation failed to induce significant bone loss [118]. Tumor cells in bone require then osteoclasts for bone destruction.

Finally, it was demonstrated in osteoblasts that Runx2 could induce the production of TβRI [214] and of RANKL [215]. It would then be interesting to study if such regulations happen in bone metastases cancer cells since they would increase TGF-β sensitivity or the induction of osteoclastogenesis.

C. The Insulin-Like Growth Factors

IGF-I and -II are the most abundant growth factors in bone. They bind the IGF-I receptor (IGF-IR), a tyrosine kinase domain receptor with a high homology to the insulin receptor. The IGF signaling is of crucial importance in development, and mice containing a targeted deletion of IGF-I, IGF-II or IGF-IR have a 45–60% decrease of the body weight [216]. Overproduction of IGF-I increases bone formation [217] while *igf1*$^{-/-}$ mice present shorter bones [218]. Targeted knockout of the IGF-IR in osteoblasts decreased osteoblastogenesis and induced bone defects [219]. Although IGF-I and IGF-IR are important in bone development, IGF-II does not seem to be involved [216]. The IGF-IR axis is also critical in cancer and metastases by promoting transformation and angiogenesis, inducing cell proliferation and invasion, or protecting from apoptosis [220,221]. However, the role of IGF in osteolytic metastases development has not been extensively studied, probably due to the lack of models.

In paired prostate cancer and bone metastases biopsies from patients, IGF-IR and its main protein partner, the insulin receptor substrate-1 (IRS-1), were more frequently upregulated than downregulated [222]. Moreover bone-seeking subclones from MDA-MB-231 had an increased expression of the IGF-IR when compared to the parental cell line and an increased phosphorylation of IRS-2 [223]. These cells were then more sensitive to IGF-I in migration and anchorage-independent growth assays [223,224]. Unpublished data demonstrate that conditioned media from mouse calvaria with active bone resorption had increased proliferation of MDA-MB-231 cells that was reversed with an IGF-IR neutralizing antibody [225]. Moreover the expression of an IGF-IR dominant negative receptor in MDA-MB-231 decreased bone metastases while the overexpression of the wild-type receptor increased bone metastases [226]. Using neuroblastoma cell lines, van Goelen *et al.* showed that increased expression of the IGF-IR was associated with an increased tumor rate and osteolysis when these cells were directly injected in the tibia [227]. All these data suggest that a functional IGF-signaling pathway promotes osteolytic bone metastases.

D. RANK, RANKL and OPG

Tumor cells at sites of bone metastases induce an increase in RANKL production by bone cells and bone resorption. Studies show that RANKL may have paracrine effects on cancer cells. Its receptor, RANK, is expressed not only on the membrane of prostate and breast cancer cell lines but also in primary tumors and metastases of patients with breast or prostate cancer [10,228–231]. This receptor is functional since a RANKL treatment induced the phosphorylation of IκB, activating the NF-κB pathway, as well as the phosphorylation of p38 MAPK and ERK1/2 [230,231]. RANKL-induced phosphorylation was blocked by the RANK decoy receptor, OPG, *in vitro* [231]. RANKL also increased the migration of prostate (DU145) and breast cancer cell lines (MDA-MB-231, MCF-7, Hs578T), and primary mammary epithelial cells which was also inhibited by OPG [229,230]. However, RANK activation did not increase DU145 cell proliferation [230]. Moreover, RANK/RANKL interaction increased the expression of genes inducing osteoclastogenesis or osteoclastic resorption, such as COX-2, IL-1, IL-6, IL-8 and MMP-9 [231].

Although the RANKL/OPG ratio is increased by cancer cells in bone, cancer cells can increase OPG expression from stromal cells in some situations [131]. OPG is also a decoy receptor for the TNF-related apoptosis-inducing ligand (TRAIL, also named Apo2L), preventing TRAIL binding to the receptors DR4 and DR5, and the subsequent apoptosis. The role of TRAIL and OPG in bone is not understood but it seems that OPG can inhibit osteoblast apoptosis [232]. Recombinant OPG or OPG from bone marrow stromal cells can also prevent TRAIL-induced apoptosis in prostate and breast cancer cells [233–235]. This protection was inhibited by either OPG-neutralizing antibodies or soluble RANKL [234]. Since RANKL is increased by tumor-secreted factors in bone metastases, the question remains whether local concentrations of OPG are high enough to protect cells from apoptosis. Interestingly, breast and prostate cancer cells *in vitro* or in tumors can also produce OPG which could have an autocrine effect [228,233–238]. OPG blood levels were also increased in patients with advanced prostate cancer and its expression was increased in bone metastases from prostate cancer when compared to lymph node metastases [228,239]. When MCF-7 cells overexpressing PTHrP (MCF-7 + PTHrP) were transfected to produce OPG and injected in the tibia of immunodeficient mice, osteolysis and skeletal tumor burden were significantly increased when compared to MCF-7 + PTHrP cells [240]. The full-length OPG protein secreted by MCF-7 + PTHrP + OPG cells was, however, inhibiting osteoclastogenesis *in vitro* as expected, and treatment of MCF-7 + PTHrP + OPG metastases with a fusion protein OPG-Fc reduced the osteolysis [240]. Malignant OPG did not protect MCF-7 cells from TRAIL-induced apoptosis and at sites of bone metastases the number of apoptotic cells (TUNEL staining) remained unchanged, enhancement of bone metastases development by malignant OPG was not due to an anti-apoptotic effect. The proliferative index measured by Ki67 immunostaining was, however, increased when OPG was expressed. OPG, whether it is produced by tumor cells or by stromal cells, or used as a therapeutic agent, has drastically different effects. Moreover, exogenous OPG as an anti-apoptotic agent has not been recommend for use in the treatment of bone metastases since it has not proven effective in mouse models [229,241,242].

RANKL is also secreted directly by cancer cells in bone. A study comparing prostatic tissues from normal patients or patients with metastatic prostate cancer showed that RANKL expression is correlated with the development of bone metastases [236]. Expression of RANKL on the membrane was shown in prostate cancer cells PC-3, DU145, LnCaP and C4-2B [228,242], and a soluble form of RANKL was further characterized in LnCaP and C4-2B [242]. These cells could then directly induce the formation of osteoclasts from RAW 264.7 mouse macrophages, in the absence of osteoblasts, with or without cell contact [242]. *In vitro*, breast cancer cells MDA-MB-231, T47D or MCF-7 do not support osteoclastogenesis on their own [10,124], which is consistent with lack of RANKL expression [10]. However, *in vitro* models utilizing co-cultures of osteoblasts and MDA-MB-231 breast cancer cells synthesize detectable amounts of RANKL [237]. Consistent with this finding, 60% of invasive tumors from breast cancer patients were positive for RANKL [238] suggesting that the tumor local environment induces RANKL expression. TGF-β increased the expression of RANKL in C4-2B prostate cancer cells *in vitro* and the RANKL promoter was active *in vivo* at bone metastatic sites [243]. In osteoblasts, Runx2 activated RANKL transcription [244]. It would then be interesting to confirm whether bone-derived TGF-β can induce RANKL expression via Runx2 in breast and prostate cancer bone metastases.

E. Extracellular Calcium and the Calcium Sensing Receptor

Osteoclastic bone resorption not only releases growth factors but also the mineral components of the bone matrix such as phosphate and calcium (Ca^{2+}) resulting in hypercalcemia. Extracellular calcium (Ca_o^{2+}) can also regulate cellular activity through the calcium-sensing receptor (CaSR), a G protein-coupled cell-surface receptor (GPCR) [245]. CaSR responding to Ca_o^{2+} exerts negative control of PTH production from parathyroid cells to regulate serum calcium [246]; it can also regulate the production of PTHrP.

During lactation, higher quantities of Ca^{2+} are needed to produce breast milk [247]. A low-calcium diet in lactating mice, mimicking hypocalcemia caused by transfer of Ca^{2+} to the milk, increased the circulating levels of PTHrP

[248]. In women, it was also observed that PTHrP levels were elevated during breast-feeding which was associated with a temporary 5 to 10% bone loss [247,249]. The specific knockout of PTHrP in mammary epithelial cells during late pregnancy and lactation significantly decreased PTHrP levels and prevented the lactation associated bone loss [250]. Secretion of PTHrP by mammary epithelial cells was specifically regulated by the CaSR whose expression is maximal during lactation [248]. These results demonstrate that mammary gland cells, responding to lower Ca_o^{2+} and signaling through the CaSR, increase PTHrP production to activate bone resorption and the release of bone matrix calcium. Conversely, higher concentrations of Ca_o^{2+} or CaSR agonists repress PTHrP production from primary mammary epithelial cells [248].

Considering CaSR is expressed by prostate and breast cancer cells [251,252], and that Ca_o^{2+} can reach concentrations as high as 8 to 40 mM adjacent to resorbing osteoclasts or in the resorption pit [253], it was conceivable that Ca_o^{2+} represses PTHrP synthesis from cancer cells in bone based on the lactation model. On the contrary, prostate and breast cancer cells *in vitro* exposed to increasing concentrations of Ca_o^{2+} and CaSR agonists induced a dose-dependent increase of PTHrP secretion [251,252]. In PC-3 cells the expression of a dominant-negative form of the CaSR partially decreased Ca_o^{2+}-stimulated PTHrP [251]. Human embryonic kidney cells, HEK293, do not express the CaSR and Ca_o^{2+} does not induce PTHrP expression. But, Ca_o^{2+}-induced PTHrP production developed after transfection with CaSR [254]. Although Sanders *et al.* did not detect any effect of Ca_o^{2+} on cell proliferation during short experiments (up to 24 hour treatment) [251,252], after 6 days of culture the proliferation of PC-3 and C4-2B cells was increased by 2.5 mM of Ca_o^{2+} when compared to 0.5 mM [255]. The proliferation of LnCaP cells was not changed by Ca_o^{2+}, but these cells appear to have a much lower expression of the CaSR when compared to PC-3 and C4-2B [255]. This Ca_o^{2+}-induced proliferation of PC-3 cells was reversed when using shRNA to decrease CaSR expression. Furthermore, the stable expression of a CaSR shRNA in PC-3 reduced the development of bone metastases compared to control cells in mice [255]. Clinical studies revealed that higher expression of CaSR is associated with bone metastases in breast cancer [256]. Apart from its role in calcium homeostasis, the CaSR appeared then to be involved in the development of bone metastases probably by promoting osteolysis. Interestingly, cotreatment of breast and prostate cells with Ca^{2+} and TGF-β induced a higher increase of PTHrP secretion than either treatment alone [251,252].

To further understand the mechanisms through which Ca^{2+} and the CaSR induce PTHrP, it was shown that inhibitors of MEK, p38 MAPK and JNK prevented Ca^{2+}-mediated PTHrP in HEK293 cells and H-500 Leydig cancer cells known to produce PTHrP and induce humoral

hypercalcemia [254,257]. Moreover activation of the CaSR by Ca^{2+} induced the phosphorylation of ERK1/2, p38 MAPK and of SEK1 (upstream of JNK) confirming the role of MAPK signaling in CaSR-induced PTHrP [254,257]. MAPK cascades are known to be activated by GPCRs through transactivation of tyrosine kinase receptors (TKR), such as the IGF-IR, the VEGF receptor, the platelet derived growth factor (PDGF) receptor and the epidermal growth factor (EGF) receptor [258]. In PC-3 prostate cancer cells, a PDGF receptor kinase inhibitor did not alter Ca^{2+}-induced PTHrP, while neither an EGF receptor kinase inhibitor, an EGF receptor neutralizing antibody nor an antibody against heparin-binding EGF (HB-EGF) prevented PTHrP secretion [259]. Consequently, a similar treatment neutralizing the EGF pathway inhibited Ca_o^{2+}-induced phosphorylation of ERK1/2, and Ca^{2+}-induced EGF receptor phosphorylation [259]. Different mechanisms for TKR transactivation by GPCRs have been suggested and the CaSR appears to activate the EGF receptor via triple-membrane-passing-signaling [258]. This particular type of transactivation involves a sequence of three transmembrane signaling events: CaSR activation, membrane metalloproteinase activation leading to the shedding of the membrane bound proHB-EGF, and finally activation of the EGF receptor. In PC-3 cells, a pan MMP inhibitor prevented indeed ERK1/2 phosphorylation and PTHrP secretion induced by Ca_o^{2+} [259]. The possible involvement of the EGF receptor in bone metastases through CaSR response and PTHrP production is interesting since it had already been shown that EGF could induce PTHrP in prostatic epithelial cells [260]. Moreover, Zhu *et al.* demonstrated that EGF-like ligands secreted by MDA-MB-231 cells activate the EGFR on osteoblasts [261]. These responded by secreting less OPG and more monocyte chemoattractant protein 1 (MCP1), resulting in increased osteoclastogenesis and osteoclast activity. A direct activation of the osteoclasts and their precursors by EGF-like ligands appeared unlikely since they did not express the EGFR [261]. Inversely, inhibitors of the EGF receptor such as gefitinib or PKI166 were shown to reduce osteoclastogenesis induced by bone marrow stromal cells [262] and malignant osteolysis as well as the growth of cancer cells and in bone [263,264].

III. SKELETAL COMPLICATIONS OF MULTIPLE MYELOMA

Multiple myeloma (MM) is a malignancy of plasma cells that leads to anemia, kidney failure, hypercalcemia and osteolytic bone destruction. MM is considered to be different from bone metastases since it is not originating from solid tumors. Although MM shares similar mechanisms with bone metastases to induce osteolysis (i.e., imbalance in the RANKL/OPG system), the models are different. While bone metastases are usually mixed, inducing both

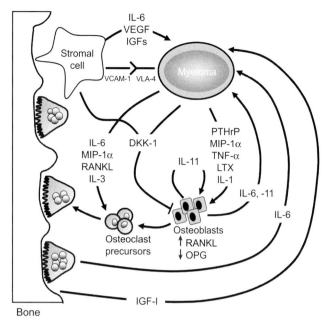

Bone

FIGURE 2.2 Bone resorption in multiple myeloma. Similarly to bone metastatic cells, myeloma cells produce multiple factors that can directly or indirectly induce bone resorption. Production of osteoclastic factors is enhanced by the interaction with bone marrow stromal cells through VCAM-1 and VLA-4. In addition, stromal cells and the bone microenvironment provide IL-6, IGFs and VEGFs supporting myeloma proliferation and survival. Myeloma cells also secrete DKK1 resulting in suppression of osteoblast activity. DKK-1, dickkopf homolog 1; IGF, insulin-like growth factor; IL, interleukin; VCAM-1, vascular adhesion molecule-1; VEGF, vascular endothelial growth factor; VLA-4, very late antigen-4.

bone destruction and bone formation, MM enhances bone destruction and decreases bone formation as shown by the decrease of osteocalcin and bone-specific alkaline phosphatase levels, bone formation markers, in patients with MM [265]. Similarly to bone metastases, MM cells flourish in bone because of the proper microenvironment that provides many growth factors including IL-6, IGF-I, VEGF, B-cell activating factor and TNFα [266,267] (Figure 2.2).

A. Bone Microenvironment Supports Multiple Myeloma Growth

Among the first factors identified was the B-cell stimulatory factor-2 (BSF-2), later renamed IL-6, shown to increase MM cell proliferation in an autocrine loop [268]. Later it appeared that only a fraction of MM cells secrete IL-6 [269] but that they can stimulate IL-6 secretion from osteoblasts [270], osteoclasts [271] and bone marrow stromal cells (BMSC) [272]. The direct interaction of MM cells with BMSCs activates NF-κB and increases IL-6 secretion [272,273]. NF-κB inhibitors can also inhibit IL-6 secretion from osteoblasts cultivated with the RPMI-8226 MM cells [274]. Cellular interactions between MM and bone cells appear important for IL-6 induction via CD44 or CD56

[275], but also via a disintegrin and metalloproteinase, ADAM-9 [274]. ADAM-9 shed or bound to MM cell membrane can interact with the integrin $\alpha_V\beta_5$ from osteoblasts, inducing p38 MAPK activation and IL-6 secretion, independently of NF-κB.

This induction of IL-6 secretion in the tumor microenvironment results in increased levels of IL-6 in the blood of MM patients and is correlated with the disease severity as well as the prognostic, underlining the role of the cytokine [276,277]. Indeed, the growth of MM cell extracted from most of the patients depends on IL-6 [278,279]. Inversely, antibodies against IL-6 can inhibit the proliferation of MM cells *ex vivo* [268,280] and transiently in patients [280,281]. IL-6 exerts its effects through the specific receptor IL-6R or gp80 that interacts with and phosphorylates the common receptor gp130. Interestingly, IL-6R can be shed from the cell membrane by a non-matrix metalloproteinase inhibited by TIMP-3 and a hydroxamate-based metalloproteinase inhibitor [282] resulting in higher levels of circulating soluble IL-6R in MM patients [283]. This soluble receptor retains its ability to bind IL-6 and gp130, and acts as an agonist, increasing MM cell sensitivity to IL-6 [283]. IL-6 through its receptor triggers three different signaling pathways: the Ras/Raf/MEK/ERK and PI3K/Akt cascades induce cell proliferation, while JAK2/STAT3 signaling increases MM cells survival [267,284–286]. IL-6 is therefore a potent survival and anti-apoptotic agent for MM cells.

MM is also associated with increased microvessel density in bone marrow correlated with a bad prognosis [287,288]. Among the different angiogenic agents, VEGF raised interest and although the blood levels seemed to remain low for patients with active MM [288], different studies showed increased levels of VEGF in the bone marrow from MM patients [289,290]. VEGF in these bones may have different sources: MM cells were shown to express VEGF on their own, but BMSCs are likely to be a major provider, and VEGF secretion is increased by MM and BMSC contact [291]. This secretion is further increased when BMSCs are treated with IL-6 that would act as an autocrine factor [291,292]. MM cells from patients or from established cell lines express the VEGF receptor (VEGFR) 1 or Flt1 and some were shown to also express the VEGFR2 or Kdr [293–296]. Treatment of MM cells with VEGF triggers VEGFR1 tyrosine-phosphorylation, inducing cell growth, adhesion to fibronectin and migration [295,296]. VEGF-mediated myeloma cell growth and migration were inhibited by PTK787/ZK222584, a tyrosine kinase inhibitor most specific for VEGFR1 and 2 [295]. The VEGFR1 activates the Ras/Raf/MEK/ERK pathway but not p38, JNK or STAT3, and a MEK-1 inhibitor prevented the VEGF-induced proliferation of myeloma cells [296]. Cell migration triggered by VEGF was not reversed by MEK-1 inhibition but was abolished by a PKC inhibitor [296]. Further studies demonstrated that the VEGF induced a PI3K-dependent activation of the PKCα isoform specifically [297]. PKCα activation is associated with a transfer from the cytosol to the cell membrane [298] where they interact with the integrin subunit β_1, which can heterodimerize to form the integrins $\alpha_4\beta_1$ (also named VLA-4) and $\alpha_5\beta_1$ (VLA-5), stimulating cell adhesion on fibronectin and migration [297]. A PKC inhibitor, named enzastaurin, reverted these VEGF-mediated effects and inhibited the subcutaneous growth of myeloma cells, MM.S1, in mice [299].

The IGF-IR is expressed by a wide variety of MM cell lines tested and detected in fresh samples from MM patients [300]. Inhibition of IGF-IR can also abrogate IL-6-induced proliferation in some MM cell lines suggesting a pivotal role for IGF-I [300]. The cell responses to IGF-I and IL-6 are not inhibited by antibodies neutralizing gp130 and IGF-IR or IGF-I, respectively, suggesting that they are mediated through independent pathways, and that combination of IGF-I and IL-6 can induce an additive increase of MM cell survival [301]. However, in the NOP2 cell line, IL-6R and IGF-IR exist in close proximity on the cell membrane and IL-6 induced the phosphorylation of the IGF-IR [302], while the inhibition of the IGF-I axis inhibited the IL-6-mediated survival of INA-6 MM cells [300]. The relationship between IL-6 and IGF-I in MM cells remains poorly understood.

In vitro, IGF-I induces the migration and the adhesion of MM cells through PI3K [303,304], as well as cell growth and survival [300,301,305]. In a mouse model, the selective IGF-IR kinase inhibitor, NVP-ADW742, inhibited the growth of MM-1S orthotopic tumors and increased mouse survival [300]. Although IGF-I blood levels are not increased in MM patients compared to healthy individuals [306], IGF-I is abundant in bone matrix and the local concentrations in bones where the resorption is increased could be sufficient to trigger the IGF-I axis. In a mouse model where RPMI8226 MM cells are inoculated in a fragment of human adult bone implanted in NOD/SCID mice, Araki *et al.* showed that KM1468, an anti-IGF-I/II antibody, inhibited MM growth [307]. Since KM1468 is human specific and does not recognize the mouse IGF-I, it is likely that it is not mouse circulating IGF-I but human bone-derived IGF-I that contributed to MM development.

The potential role of bone-derived IGF-I in MM development raises the question whether bone-derived TGF-β could also be involved since it has such a pivotal role in bone metastases from solid tumors. TGF-β is known for its immunosuppressive properties and inhibition of immunoglobulin secretion and proliferation in normal splenic B cells [308]. On the contrary MM cells secrete TGF-β and BMSCs from MM patients secrete more TGF-β than BMSCs from normal patients. However, cell proliferation of MM cells was unaffected by TGF-β [309]. These results suggest that MM cells became TGF-β insensitive compared to normal B cells during the malignant process. This insensitivity can be explained by the low expression of the TβRII in some MM cells [309] but also by a ligand-dependent mechanism demonstrated in plasmacytoma (PCT) cells. While MM affects different locations in the body, PCT is a solitary lesion which can be considered as an early stage of MM. Similarly to MM cells, TGF-β does not inhibit PCT cell proliferation or induce their apoptosis compared to B cells, despite the expression of TβRI and TβRII as detected by RT-PCR and on western blot of whole cell lysate [310]. The TβRII was sequenced from mRNA of PCTs and did not show consistent mutations and the kinase domain was still active [311]; however, exogenous TGF-β could not bind to the TβRII [310]. This phenomenon is due to the secretion of active TGF-β by PCT cells that binds the TβRII in the cytosol and precludes its translocation to the plasma membrane. Reduction of TGF-β expression by antisense strategy allowed the detection of TβRII on the membrane [311]. This ligand-receptor complex although present in the PCT cells did not induce Smad2 phosphorylation and the TGF-β pathway remained inactivated [311]. However TGF-β appears to be an important factor in the pathogenesis of MM since it: (1) contributes to the functional impairment of the immune system [312]; and (2) induces IL-6 and VEGF secretion from BMSCs [309,313].

B. Mechanisms of Multiple Myeloma-Induced Bone Resorption

The importance of osteoclasts and bone resorption in MM was demonstrated in the 5T2MM mouse model [314] and in the SCID-hu-MM model, where fragments of human long bones inoculated with MM cells are grafted in SCID mice [315], using bisphosphonates which inhibit osteoclast activity. Zoledronic acid and pamidronate successfully decreased bone resorption induced by MM cells as well as the tumor burden and increased mouse survival. However, bisphosphonate effects on myeloma cells in bones could be attributed to direct anti-tumor properties that have been shown *in vitro* on MM cells [316–318].

Among the different factors expressed by MM cells, RANKL appears to be an important inducer of osteoclastogenesis. The engineered overexpression of the RANKL inhibitor OPG, the RANK decoy receptor, in ARH-77 myeloma cells with lentiviral particle resulted in decreased bone destruction when the cells were inoculated in mice [319]. Similarly treatments with a recombinant OPG (Fc-OPG) inhibited osteoclast formation and malignant osteolysis, and resulted in increased bone mineral density in the 5T2MM and 5T33MM mouse models [320–321]. In the 5T2MM model, recombinant OPG also decreased the tumor burden and increased mouse survival [321]. The use of OPG in patients may, however, not be advised since it can inhibit MM cell apoptosis induced by TRAIL [322] similarly to what was observed in prostate and breast cancer cells as we have described previously. To overcome this side effect of OPG, RANK-Fc, a RANKL antagonist, was developed, consisting of the extracellular domain of RANK fused to the constant region of human IgG1 [323]. RANK-Fc has a higher affinity for RANKL than OPG, does not interfere with TRAIL and prevents osteoclasto-genesis [323]. RANK-Fc was tested in two different mouse myeloma models, SCID/ARH-77 and SCID-hu-MM, and inhibited bone MM-induced bone destruction as well as the tumor burden [315,323,324].

Another myeloma-produced factor important in bone destruction is macrophage inflammatory protein-1α (MIP-1α), a member of the RANTES family of chemokines. MIP-1α is a potent osteoclast stimulatory factor with an increased marrow plasma concentration in 70% of myeloma patients [325]. MIP-1α enhances osteoclast formation induced by IL-6, PTHrP and RANK [326]. MIP-1α neu-tralizing antibodies blocked osteoclast formation in bone marrow cultures treated with human myeloma bone marrow plasma [327] and reduced osteolysis in an *in vivo* mouse myeloma model [328].

MM cells induce bone destruction via cell-cell interac-tions with BMSCs through cell adhesion molecules. The integrin $\alpha_4\beta_1$, also named very late antigen-4 (VLA-4), is expressed at the surface of myeloma cells [329,330] and interacts with the vascular adhesion molecule-1 (VCAM-1) constitutively expressed on BMSCs [331,332]. This inter-action presumably promotes the recruitment of myeloma cells to bone and enhances osteoclastogenesis and osteo-clastic resorption *in vitro* independently of IL-1, IL-6, TNF-α and PTHrP [333]. The VLA-4/VCAM-1 system upregulates the production of RANKL and decreases the expression of OPG by BMSCs and pre-osteoblasts [334]. Disruption of this cell-cell interaction with an antibody against the subunit α_4 of VLA-4 prevented RANKL induc-tion [333]. *In vivo*, a treatment with an antibody neutral-izing the subunit α_4 decreased the development of 5TGM1 myeloma cells in bones, as well as bone destruction in mice [335,336].

C. Multiple Myeloma Suppresses Osteoblastic Bone Formation

Breast cancer osteolytic bone metastasis is character-ized by high bone turnover—increased osteoclast and osteoblast activity. However, a puzzling feature of MM is uncoupled bone turnover—high osteoclastic bone resorp-tion and suppressed osteoblast bone formation. Dickkopf homolog 1 (DKK-1) is increased in the bone microen-vironment of MM patients and was proposed to be an underlying mechanism of osteoblast suppression [337]. DKK-1 is a secreted inhibitor of the Wnt signaling path-way that binds to the LDL-receptor-related proteins 5 and 6 (LRP5 and 6), preventing interaction of these co-receptors with the frizzled (Frz) receptor family [338]. The importance of the Wnt signaling pathway in human osteoblast biology was found with the discovery that acti-vating mutations of LRP5 cause high bone mass [339,340] and loss-of-function mutations result in osteoporosis-pseudoglioma syndrome [341]. DKK-1 mRNA concen-trations were increased in plasma cells of patients with more advanced disease; and DKK-1 protein levels were higher in the bone marrow plasma and peripheral blood of patients with myeloma bone disease compared to controls [337]. However, whether enhanced DKK-1 production originates from myeloma cells themselves or host stro-mal cells or osteoblasts as a consequence of the myeloma cells is unclear. Irrespective of the source of DKK-1, this factor may prove as a MM therapeutic target. In a mouse model of myeloma bone disease, an anti-DKK-1 antibody increased osteoblast activation and osteoclast inactivation, and decreased bone loss and tumor burden [342]. Another secreted Wnt antagonist, secreted frizzled-related protein-2 (sFRP2), was found expressed in myeloma cells and may cooperate with DKK-1 to promote maximal osteo-blast suppression [343].

Increased concentrations of interleukin-3 (IL-3) in the bone marrow plasma of myeloma patients stimulate osteo-clast formation, but may also inhibit osteoblast differentia-tion. In a report, IL-3 decreased osteoblast differentiation of murine stromal cell cultures and human bone marrow aspi-rates, and blocked BMP-2-mediated osteoblast differentia-tion. Additionally, an IL-3 neutralizing antibody enhanced osteoblast differentiation from bone marrow plasma derived from myeloma patients [344].

IV. OSTEOBLASTIC BONE METASTASES

Advanced prostate and some breast cancers commonly form osteoblastic bone metastases. Tumor-secreted factors act on bone cells to increase osteoblast activity, decrease osteoclast activity, or both, shifting the balance of bone for-mation and resorption in favor of net new bone formation (Figure 2.3). However, osteoblastic bone lesions are often heterogeneous and may include regions of osteoclastic bone resorption intermixed with osteoblast-stimulated new bone [345]. Interactions between tumor cells and bone cells pro-mote osteoblastic bone metastases. Tumor cells secrete fac-tors, such as ET-1, which induces new bone formation, and proteases, such as PSA, which may activate growth factors in bone. Bone-secreted factors, such as TGF-β and Notch, have reciprocal actions on tumor cells to induce prolifera-tion in osteoblastic metastases.

A. Factors Secreted by Tumor Cells

1. ENDOTHELIN-1 AND DKK-1

Endothelin-1 (ET-1) is a 21-amino acid peptide, a potent vasoconstrictor, and an important mediator of osteoblas-tic bone metastases. The peptide binds to and activates

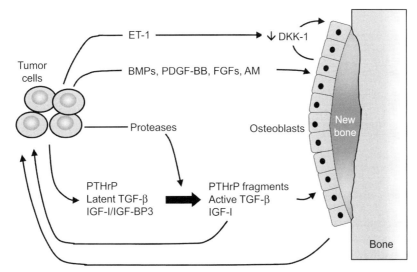

FIGURE 2.3 Model of interactions at sites of osteoblastic metastasis. Multiple factors, such as ET-1, BMPs or PDGF, are secreted by cancer cells in the bone microenvironment to induce osteoblast proliferation and new bone formation. ET-1 produced by cancer cells stimulates osteoblasts by repressing the expression of DKK-1, an inhibitor of the Wnt/β-Catenin pathway. In turn, proteins produced by the osteoblasts support cancer cell development in bone. Other factors secreted by cancer cells, including PTHrP, IGF and TGF-β, require processing by proteases such as PSA to acquire their osteoblastic/active state. Mature IGF-I does not only promote bone formation but can also promote cancer cell growth. BMP, bone morphogenetic protein; DKK-1, dickkopf homolog-1; ET-1, endothelin-1; IGF, insulin-like growth factor; PDGF, platelet-derived growth factor; PTHrP, parathyroid hormone-related protein; TGF-β, transforming growth factor-β.

two G-coupled protein receptors, the endothelin A receptor (ETAR) and endothelin B receptor (ETBR). The effects of ET-1 in bone are primarily mediated through the ETAR [346], which is expressed on osteoblasts. Treatment with a selective inhibitor of the ETAR prevented ET-1 stimulated IL-6 expression by osteoblasts, while a selective inhibitor of the ETBR had no effect [347]. ET-1 stimulates proliferation and differentiation of osteoprogenitor cells towards the osteoblast lineage. Treatment of rat calvarial organ cultures with ET-1 led to a 140-fold increase in bone nodule formation compared to untreated cultures [348]. This also resulted in increased alkaline phosphatase activity and increased mRNA expression of the osteoblast marker osteocalcin [348,349].

ET-1 is an important mediator of osteoblastic bone metastases. Men with prostate cancer bone metastases were found to have higher levels of circulating ET-1 in plasma [349]. In addition, ET-1 mRNA and protein are expressed in human prostate cancer tumor lines and stimulate tumor cell proliferation *in vitro* [349]. A human tumor cell line, derived from amnion and transfected to overexpress ET-1 cDNA, inoculated into the lower leg of mice, resulted in increased new bone growth, while treatment with a selective antagonist of the ETAR blocked new bone formation. Similarly, in models for breast cancer, tumor cell lines that form osteoblastic bone metastases, ZR-75-1, MCF-7, and T47D, secreted high levels of ET-1. Treatment with an ETAR antagonist decreased bone metastases in animals bearing tumors from these cell lines [82].

ET-1 mediates interactions between tumor and bone cells. Bone microenvironment factors, such as IL-1β, TNF-α, and TGF-β, promote the secretion of ET-1 from tumor cells [350]. ET-1 secreted from tumor cells acts on osteoblasts to stimulate the production of numerous factors, including IL-6, IL-11, CCN proteins: CYR61 and CTGF, receptor activator of nuclear factor B ligand (RANKL), all of which have been implicated in bone metastasis [351]. ET-1 may also promote bone metastases by suppressing osteoblast expression of dickkopf homolog-1, DKK-1, an inhibitor of Wnt signaling. Wnt signaling results in activation and translocation of β-catenin to the nucleus to mediate the transcription of genes, such as osteocalcin. Expression of these genes to promote differentiation and activation of osteoblasts is inhibited by DKK-1. Treatment of calvarial organ cultures with ET-1 decreased DKK-1 mRNA expression and secretion of DKK-1 protein into conditioned medium. Conversely, treatment with recombinant DKK-1 blocked ET-1-mediated osteoblast proliferation and new bone formation, while a neutralizing antibody to DKK-1 had the opposite effects [351].

Cancer cell analysis of DKK-1 expression has revealed an inverse correlation between the appearance of osteoblastic lesions detected by radiography and the expression of DKK-1 that may at least partially determine whether tumor cells in bone produce osteoblastic lesions. The breast cancer cell lines ZR-75-1 and T47D have low DKK-1 expression and produce osteoblastic lesions [352,353]. Conversely, the breast cancer cell line MDA-MB-231 and the prostate cancer cell line PC-3 have high DKK-1 expression and produce osteolytic lesions in mouse models of bone metastasis [352–354]. PC-3 prostate cancer cells, which secrete DKK-1, stably transfected with *DKK-1* shRNA were converted from an osteolytic to an osteoblastic phenotype in an animal model of bone metastasis [355]. Conversely, DKK-1 overexpression in the mixed osteoblastic/osteolytic prostate cancer cell line C4-2B produced osteolytic lesions in an animal model [355]. These studies show a clear *inverse* relationship between DKK-1 and osteoblast activity. DKK-1 is a central regulator of osteoblast activity and osteoblastic bone metastasis and is likely dually dependent on the downregulation of microenvironment DKK-1 secretion from: (1) osteoblasts via tumor-produced ET-1; and (2) prostate cancer cells themselves. These mechanisms are complementary, each representing an important pathway of DKK-1 regulation in prostate cancer bone metastasis.

ET-1, in addition to stimulating osteoblast differentiation and proliferation, also has direct and indirect effects on osteoclasts. ET-1 prevented osteoclast-mediated bone resorption and prevented cell motility, which was reversed upon removal of the peptide [356]. In addition, co-culture of bone slices with androgen-independent prostate cancer cells blocked osteoclast-mediated bone resorption without effects on osteoclast proliferation or apoptosis. This effect was prevented by treatment with an ET-1 neutralizing antibody [357]. This may be an indirect effect due to ET-1 action to prevent osteoblast production of the osteoclast stimulator IL-6 [347,351]. However, the effects of ET-1 may be more complex, as some models have demonstrated that ET-1 actually stimulates osteoclastic bone resorption in calvarial organ culture models [358].

Inhibitors of ET-1 signaling have been tested for the treatment of bone metastases. In a phase II clinical study, atrasentan, an ETAR antagonist, was demonstrated to slow progression and decrease PSA production compared to control in men with hormone refractory prostate cancer [359]. In phase III trials, atrasentan decreased bone metastasis but had no effect on overall disease progression in men with advanced disease [360]. Results of a phase II trial of the ETAR antagonist ZD4054 in men with advanced prostate cancer demonstrate that ETAR blockade may have mortality benefit as well [361]. Thus, the effects of ET-1 may be bone specific and inhibitors may be useful in the prevention of bone metastases [362].

2. PROTEASE ACTIVATION OF GROWTH FACTORS

Prostate Specific Antigen Proteases released by tumor cells may activate growth factors within the bone microenvironment to promote osteoblastic bone metastases. Prostate specific antigen, PSA, is a serine protease whose expression is regulated by androgens and is increased in advanced prostate cancer [345]. PSA proteolytically cleaves and activates bone-derived growth factors, such as

TGF-β, or PTHrP that contribute to bone metastasis. Inactive TGF-β is secreted from tumor and bone cells and can be activated by tumor-secreted PSA [363,364]. TGF-β1 modulates cell proliferation, differentiation, angiogenesis and immune response and is more highly expressed in advanced prostate tumors [365]. Early in tumorigenesis, TGF-β acts as a tumor suppressor. Later in cancer progression, tumor cells are no longer growth inhibited by TGF-β and can instead be stimulated to metastasize [345].

PSA has also been demonstrated to activate insulin-like growth factors (IGFs). Two forms of IGF, IGF-I and IGF-II, are secreted by osteoblasts and stored in high levels in bone. IGF-I is also secreted at high levels by prostate cancer cells and can promote tumor cell proliferation through the IGF-I receptor [366]. IGF-I and -II are secreted as prepropeptides, which are bound to IGF binding proteins (IGFBPs). In the case of IGF-I, IGFBP-3 modulates the amount of free peptide that is available for interacting with the IGF-IR. PSA secreted by tumor cells proteolytically cleaves IGFBP-3 thus releasing IGF-I. Increased IGF-I signaling promoted osteoblast proliferation in cells co-cultured with MDA-PCa-2b human prostate carcinoma cells [367]. In addition to stimulating cell proliferation, IGFs also protect against apoptosis. Thus, IGF-I may have autocrine effects on tumor cells, promoting cell survival and growth [366]. Treatment of mice with MDA PCa 2b prostate cancer bone metastases with an antibody to IGF-I and -II decreased tumor growth in bone and prevented development of new tumors [368].

A third factor cleaved by PSA [369] and activated in the bone microenvironment is PTHrP. Cleavage within the PTH-like domain blocked PTHrP-stimulated cAMP production in osteoblasts [370]. PTHrP fragments stimulate osteoclasts to resorb bone and may contribute to osteolytic bone metastases observed with breast cancers. Inactivation of PTHrP by PSA in prostate cancer may contribute to osteoblastic bone metastases through inhibition of PTHrP-stimulated osteoclastic bone resorption. In addition, an N-terminal PTHrP cleavage product lacking the PTH/PTHrP-receptor domain has been demonstrated to bind and activate the cardiac ETAR [371]. PTHrP binding to the ETAR on osteoblasts may stimulate osteoblast proliferation and differentiation, potentially contributing to osteoblastic bone metastases.

Urokinase type plasminogen activator Proteases other than PSA may also contribute to prostate cancer bone metastases, such as urokinase type plasminogen activator, uPA. uPA is expressed on the surface of normal and tumor cells and activates matrix metalloproteinases in the extracellular milieu. Conditioned media from osteoblasts cultures induced chemotaxis and invasion by prostate carcinoma cells by matrigel invasion assay and stimulated the release of uPA and MMP-9. Inhibition of uPA by treatment with urokinase inhibitors and a uPA neutralizing antibody decreased tumor cell invasion [372,373]. The role of uPA in osteoblastic bone metastases was demonstrated in animal models. Mice inoculated via intracardiac injection with prostate cancer cells transfected to overexpress uPA developed increased osteoblastic bone metastases compared to control [374]. This effect was mediated by the amino terminal fragment of uPA, which increased expression of c-fos, c-jun, and c-myc in human-osteoblast derived osteosarcoma cells (SaOS2) [375].

3. PLATELET-DERIVED GROWTH FACTOR

Other tumor-derived growth factor may also contribute to osteoblastic bone metastases. An isoform of platelet-derived growth factor, PDGF-BB, was demonstrated to promote osteoblastic bone metastases in breast cancer models. Mice inoculated with MCF-7 human breast cancer cells overexpressing the *Neu* oncogene developed osteoblastic bone metastases and had high levels of PDGF-BB in serum [376]. Treatment of calvarial organ cultures with conditioned medium from MCF-7 cells led to increased bone formation, which was blocked by an inhibitor of PDGF-BB. Knockdown of hPDGF-BB in MCF-7/Neu cells decreased bone metastases and plasma hPDGF-BB levels while stable expression of PDGF-bb in MDA-MB-231, which characteristically form osteolytic bone metastases, changed the phenotype of these cells to induce osteoblastic lesions at the sites of osteolysis [376].

4. BONE MORPHOGENETIC PROTEINS

Bone morphogenetic proteins (BMPs) are members of the TGF-β superfamily and, like TGF-β, may also contribute to bone metastases. BMPs bind to a combination of type I receptors (type IA and IB BMP receptors and type IA activin receptor) and type II receptors (type II BMP receptor, and type II and IIB activin receptors) to receptors of the TGF-β superfamily and activate the Smad signaling cascade. This results in transcription of BMP target genes, such as OPG and Cbfa-1, which are important osteoblastic factors [377,378]. In the setting of prostate cancer, two bone metastatic prostate cancer cell lines, LAPC-4 and -9, were demonstrated to express BMP receptor mRNA and protein. Treatment with BMP-2 and -7, but not BMP-4, increased LAPC-4 cell migration and invasion *in vitro* [58]. LAPC-9 cells formed osteoblastic bone metastases when implanted into the tibias of immunodeficient mice. Osteoblastic lesion formation was prevented by expression of the BMP-inhibitor noggin in prostate cancer cells [58]. BMP-6 may also be important for osteoblastic bone metastases. Prostate cancer cell lines and tumor specimens were demonstrated to have increased BMP-6 expression, which correlated with increased tumor aggressiveness [379]. Conditioned media from prostate cancer cells increased Smad phosphorylation and mineralization in preosteoblast MC3T3 cells, which was decreased by treatment with the BMP inhibitor noggin and by an anti-BMP-6 antibody [379]. Mice implanted with

human fetal bones and injected with LuCaP 23.1 prostate cancer cells developed bone metastases. Treatment with an anti-BMP-6 antibody decreases osteoblastic activity, but not osteolytic activity induced by the tumor cells [379]. BMP-6 also increased invasiveness of tumor cells into bone, thus promoting osteoblastic bone metastases through effects on both bone and tumor cells. Conversely, studies indicate that BMPs may have an opposite effect on osteolytic bone metastases from breast and prostate cancer in mice, decreasing tumor growth by acting as antagonists of the TGF-β signaling pathway [64,65]. The role of BMPs in bone metastases remains poorly understood and merits further study.

C. Bone Factors Stimulate Tumor Cell Proliferation

Factors from the bone microenvironment induce tumor cell proliferation in osteoblastic metastases. One such factor is TGF-β. TGF-β is secreted by osteoblasts and is found abundantly in the mineralized bone matrix. As discussed previously, TGF-β is activated by PSA from tumor cells and induces the secretion of IGF-I and IGFBP-3 by osteoblasts [380]. Degradation of IGFBP-3 by PSA [367], MMP-3 [381], MMP-7 [382], or MMP-9 [383], may contribute to increased IGF-I in the bone microenvironment which may in turn, have paracrine effects on cancer cell growth [368]. Interestingly, conditioned media from osteoblasts induces MMP-9 secretion, as well as uPA secretion from cancer cells [372], which increased migration and invasiveness of prostate cancer cells [372,373]. IGFBP-3 functions to induce apoptosis of cancer cells [384,385], thus, degradation of IGFBP-3 by these proteases may promote tumor cell survival.

Two other bone-derived factors that may promote osteoblastic metastases are Jagged1 and Delta1. These membrane-bound proteins bind to their receptor, Notch1, to induce osteoblast-mediated new bone formation [386,387]. A functional Notch1 receptor is expressed by cancer cell lines, including MDA-PCA-24 and C4-2B [388]. Interactions between osteoblasts and tumor cells stimulate tumor cell growth and osteomimetism, including expression of the transcription factor Runx2 that has important functions in osteoblasts. Delta1 may also have autocrine effects on C4-2B cells, which themselves express this factor [388]. Osteoblast expression of Jagged1 is increased by activation of the PTH/PTHrP receptor on these cells [389]. PTHrP secreted by tumors cells and promotes osteolytic bone metastases. Tumor-secreted PTHrP may have secondary effects in bone to increase Jagged1 expression, thus resulting in further activation of Notch1.

Osteoblastic bone metastases result from complex interactions between osteoblasts and tumor cells within the bone microenvironment. Tumor-secreted factors, such as ET-1 and BMPs, promote osteoblast proliferation and stimulate new bone formation. Proteases, including PSA and uPA, activate bone matrix growth factors, such as TGF-β, which are important for tumor cell growth and survival. Understanding their role in regulating osteoblast activating and tumor cell growth may provide novel targets for the treatment of osteoblastic bone metastases.

References

1. T. Yoneda, A. Sasaki & G.R. Mundy, Osteolytic bone metastasis in breast cancer, Breast Cancer Res Treat 32 (1994) 73–84.
2. A. Muller, B. Homey & H. Soto, et al., Involvement of chemokine receptors in breast cancer metastasis, Nature 410 (2001) 50–56.
3. Y.X. Sun, A. Schneider & Y. Jung, et al., Skeletal localization and neutralization of the SDF-1(CXCL12)/CXCR4 axis blocks prostate cancer metastasis and growth in osseous sites *in vivo*, J Bone Miner Res 20 (2005) 318–329.
4. Y. Kang, P.M. Siegel & W. Shu, et al., A multigenic program mediating breast cancer metastasis to bone, Cancer Cell 3 (2003) 537–549.
5. S.A. Shulby, N.G. Dolloff & M.E. Stearns, et al., CX3CR1-fractalkine expression regulates cellular mechanisms involved in adhesion, migration and survival of human prostate cancer cells, Cancer Res 64 (2004) 4693–4698.
6. J.F. Harms, D.R. Welch & R.S. Samant, et al., A small molecule antagonist of the alpha(v)beta3 integrin suppresses MDA-MB-435 skeletal metastasis, Clin Exp Metastasis 21 (2004) 119–128.
7. I. Pécheur, O. Peyruchaud & C.M. Serre, et al., Integrin $\alpha_v\beta_3$ expression confers on tumor cells a greater propensity to metastasize to bone, Faseb J 16 (2002) 1266–1268.
8. S. Paget, The distribution of secondary growths in cancer of the breast, The Lancet 133 (1889) 571–573.
9. R.E. Coleman, Metastatic bone disease: clinical features, pathophysiology and treatment strategies, Cancer Treat Rev 27 (2001) 165.
10. R.J. Thomas, T.A. Guise & J.J. Yin, et al., Breast cancer cells interact with osteoblasts to support osteoclast formation, Endocrinology 140 (1999) 4451–4458.
11. B.F. Boyce, L. Xing & W. Shakespeare, et al., Regulation of bone remodeling and emerging breakthrough drugs for osteoporosis and osteolytic bone metastases, Kidney International Supplement 85 (2003) S2–S5.
12. J.J. Yin, K. Selander & J.M. Chirgwin, et al., TGF-beta signaling blockade inhibits PTHrP secretion by breast cancer cells and bone metastases development, J Clin Invest 103 (1999) 197–206.
13. S. Viguet-Carrin, P. Garnero & P.D. Delmas, The role of collagen in bone strength, Osteoporos Int 17 (2006) 319–336.
14. S. Mohan & D.J. Baylink, Bone growth factors, Clin Orthop Relat Res (1991) 30–48.
15. S.M. Seyedin, T.C. Thomas & A.Y. Thompson, et al., Purification and characterization of two cartilage-inducing factors from bovine demineralized bone, Proc Natl Acad Sci USA 82 (1985) 2267–2271.
16. K. Janssens, P. ten Dijke & S. Janssens, et al., Transforming growth factor-beta1 to the bone, Endocr Rev 26 (2005) 743–774.
17. J. Massague & R.R. Gomis, The logic of TGFβ signaling, FEBS Letters 580 (2006) 2811–2820.
18. P.M. Siegel & J. Massague, Cytostatic and apoptotic action of TGF-β in homeostasis and cancer, Nat Rev Cancer 3 (2003) 807–820.
19. Y. Kang & J. Massague, Epithelial-mesenchymal transitions: twist in development and metastasis, Cell 118 (2004) 277–279.
20. P.M. Siegel, W. Shu & R.D. Cardiff, et al., Transforming growth factor beta signaling impairs Neu-induced mammary tumorigenesis while promoting pulmonary metastasis, Proc Natl Acad Sci USA 100 (2003) 8430–8435.
21. P. Bertolino, M. Deckers & F. Lebrin, et al., Transforming growth factor-β signal transduction in angiogenesis and vascular disorders, Chest 128 (2005) 585S–590S.
22. L. Gorelik & R.A. Flavell, Transforming growth factor-beta in T-cell biology, Nat Rev Immunol 2 (2002) 46–53.
23. B. Bierie & H.L. Moses, Tumour microenvironment: TGFβ: the molecular Jekyll and Hyde of cancer, Nat Rev Cancer 6 (2006) 506.
24. Y. Shi & J. Massague, Mechanisms of TGF-beta signaling from cell membrane to the nucleus, Cell 113 (2003) 685–700.
25. L. Xu, Y. Kang, S. Col & J. Massague, Smad2 nucleocytoplasmic shuttling by nucleoporins CAN/Nup214 and Nup153 feeds TGFbeta signaling complexes in the cytoplasm and nucleus, Mol Cell 10 (2002) 271–282.
26. Y. Shi, Y.F. Wang & L. Jayaraman, et al., Crystal structure of a Smad MH1 domain bound to DNA: insights on DNA binding in TGF-beta signaling, Cell 94 (1998) 585–594.
27. Y. Kang, W. He & S. Tulley, et al., Breast cancer bone metastasis mediated by the Smad tumor suppressor pathway, Proc Natl Acad Sci USA 102 (2005) 13909–13914.
28. J. Kim, K. Johnson & H.J. Chen, et al., Drosophila Mad binds to DNA and directly mediates activation of vestigial by Decapentaplegic, Nature 388 (1997) 304–308.
29. X. Chen, M.J. Rubock & M. Whitman, A transcriptional partner for MAD proteins in TGF-beta signalling, Nature 383 (1996) 691–696.
30. R. Janknecht, N.J. Wells & T. Hunter, TGF-beta-stimulated cooperation of Smad proteins with the coactivators CBP/p300, Genes Dev 12 (1998) 2114–2119.
31. X. Shen, P.P. Hu & N.T. Liberati, et al., TGF-beta-induced phosphorylation of Smad3 regulates its interaction with coactivator p300/CREB-binding protein, Mol Biol Cell 9 (1998) 3309–3319.
32. J.-I. Hanai, L.F. Chen & T. Kanno, et al., Interaction and functional cooperation of PEBP2/CBF with Smads. Synergistic induction of the immunoglobulin germline Calpha promoter, J Biol Chem 274 (1999) 31577–31582.
33. K. Luo, Ski and SnoN: negative regulators of TGF-beta signaling, Curr Opin Genet Dev 14 (2004) 65–70.
34. D. Wotton, R.S. Lo, S. Lee & J. Massague, A Smad transcriptional corepressor, Cell 97 (1999) 29–39.
35. J. Massague, J. Seoane & D. Wotton, Smad transcription factors, Genes Dev 19 (2005) 2783–2810.
36. H. Hayashi, S. Abdollah & Y. Qiu, et al., The MAD-related protein Smad7 associates with the TGFbeta receptor and functions as an antagonist of TGFbeta signaling, Cell 89 (1997) 1165–1173.

37. A. Nakao, M. Afrakhte & A. Moren, et al., Identification of Smad7, a TGFbeta-inducible antagonist of TGF-beta signalling, Nature 389 (1997) 631–635.

38. T. Ebisawa, M. Fukuchi & G. Murakami, et al., Smurf1 interacts with transforming growth factor-beta type I receptor through Smad7 and induces receptor degradation, J Biol Chem 276 (2001) 12477–12480.

39. C. Suzuki, G. Murakami & M. Fukuchi, et al., Smurf1 regulates the inhibitory activity of Smad7 by targeting Smad7 to the plasma membrane, J Biol Chem 277 (2002) 39919–39925.

40. P. Kavsak, R.K. Rasmussen & C.G. Causing, et al., Smad7 binds to Smurf2 to form an E3 ubiquitin ligase that targets the TGF beta receptor for degradation, Mol Cell 6 (2000) 1365–1375.

41. G. Kuratomi, A. Komuro & K. Goto, et al., NEDD4-2 (neural precursor cell expressed, developmentally downregulated 4-2) negatively regulates TGF-beta (transforming growth factor-beta) signalling by inducing ubiquitin-mediated degradation of Smad2 and TGF-beta type I receptor, Biochem J 386 (2005) 461–470.

42. S.R. Seo, F. Lallemand & N. Ferrand, et al., The novel E3 ubiquitin ligase Tiul1 associates with TGIF to target Smad2 for degradation, Embo J 23 (2004) 3780–3792.

43. A. Moren, T. Imamura & K. Miyazono, et al., Degradation of the tumor suppressor Smad4 by WW and HECT domain ubiquitin ligases, J Biol Chem 280 (2005) 22115–22123.

44. X. Lin, M. Liang & X.H. Feng, Smurf2 is a ubiquitin E3 ligase mediating proteasome-dependent degradation of Smad2 in transforming growth factor-beta signaling, J Biol Chem 275 (2000) 36818–36822.

45. Y. Zhang, C. Chang & D.J. Gehling, et al., Regulation of Smad degradation and activity by Smurf2, an E3 ubiquitin ligase, Proc Natl Acad Sci USA 98 (2001) 974–979.

46. R. Derynck & Y.E. Zhang, Smad-dependent and Smad-independent pathways in TGF-beta family signalling, Nature 425 (2003) 577–584.

47. N.M. Munoz, M. Upton & A. Rojas, et al., Transforming growth factor β receptor type II inactivation induces the malignant transformation of intestinal neoplasms initiated by Apc mutation, Cancer Res 66 (2006) 9837–9844.

48. R. Parsons, L.L. Myeroff & B. Liu, et al., Microsatellite instability and mutations of the transforming growth factor β Type II receptor gene in colorectal cancer, Cancer Res 55 (1995) 5548–5550.

49. M. Goggins, M. Shekher & K. Turnacioglu, et al., Genetic alterations of the transforming growth factor beta receptor genes in pancreatic and biliary adenocarcinomas, Cancer Res 58 (1998) 5329–5332.

50. S.A. Hahn, M. Schutte & A.T.M.S. Hoque, et al., DPC4, a candidate tumor suppressor gene at human chromosome 18q21.1, Science 271 (1996) 350–353.

51. J. Barlow, D. Yandell & D. Weaver, et al., Higher stromal expression of transforming growth factor-beta type II receptors is associated with poorer prognosis breast tumors, Breast Cancer Res Treat 79 (2003) 149–159.

52. R.S. Muraoka, Y. Koh & L.R. Roebuck, et al., Increased malignancy of Neu-induced mammary tumors overexpressing active transforming growth factor beta1, Mol Cell Biol 23 (2003) 8691–8703.

53. A. Sasaki, B.F. Boyce & B. Story, et al., Bisphosphonate risedronate reduces metastatic human breast cancer burden in bone in nude mice, Cancer Res 55 (1995) 3551–3557.

54. M. Deckers, M. van Dinther & J. Buijs, et al., The tumor suppressor Smad4 is required for transforming growth factor β-induced epithelial to mesenchymal transition and bone metastasis of breast cancer cells, Cancer Res 66 (2006) 2202–2209.

55. D. Javelaud, K.S. Mohammad & C.R. McKenna, et al., Stable overexpression of Smad7 in human melanoma cells impairs bone metastasis, Cancer Res 67 (2007) 2317–2324.

56. M.W. Helms, J. Packeisen & C. August, et al., First evidence supporting a potential role for the BMP/SMAD pathway in the progression of oestrogen receptor-positive breast cancer, J Pathol 206 (2005) 366–376.

57. F. Pouliot, A. Blais & C. Labrie, Overexpression of a dominant negative type II bone morphogenetic protein receptor inhibits the growth of human breast cancer cells, Cancer Res 63 (2003) 277–281.

58. B.T. Feeley, S.C. Gamradt & W.K. Hsu, et al., Influence of BMPs on the formation of osteoblastic lesions in metastatic prostate cancer, J Bone Miner Res 20 (2005) 2189–2199.

59. L. Ye, J.M. Lewis-Russell & G. Davies, et al., Hepatocyte growth factor upregulates the expression of the bone morphogenetic protein (BMP) receptors, BMPR-IB and BMPR-II, in human prostate cancer cells, Int J Oncol 30 (2007) 521–529.

60. R. Wieser, L. Attisano & J.L. Wrana, et al., Signaling activity of transforming growth factor beta type II receptors lacking specific domains in the cytoplasmic region, Mol Cell Biol 13 (1993) 7239–7247.

61. S.M. Kakonen, K.S. Selander & J.M. Chirgwin, et al., Transforming growth factor-beta stimulates parathyroid hormone-related protein and osteolytic metastases via Smad and mitogen-activated protein kinase signaling pathways, J Biol Chem 277 (2002) 24571–24578.

62. S.L. Kominsky, M. Doucet & K. Brady, et al., TGF-β promotes the establishment of renal cell carcinoma bone metastasis, J Bone Miner Res 22 (2007) 37–44.

63. R. Wieser, J.L. Wrana & J. Massague, GS domain mutations that constitutively activate T beta R-I, the downstream signaling component in the TGF-beta receptor complex, Embo J 14 (1995) 2199–2208.

64. J.T. Buijs, N.V. Henriquez & P.G. van Overveld, et al., Bone morphogenetic protein 7 in the development and treatment of bone metastases from breast cancer, Cancer Res 67 (2007) 8742–8751.

65. J.T. Buijs, C.A. Rentsch & G. van der Horst, et al., BMP7, a putative regulator of epithelial homeostasis in the human prostate, is a potent inhibitor of prostate cancer bone metastasis *in vivo*, Am J Pathol 171 (2007) 1047–1057.

66. A. Bandyopadhyay, J.K. Agyin & L. Wang, et al., Inhibition of pulmonary and skeletal metastasis by a transforming growth factor-beta type I receptor kinase inhibitor, Cancer Res 66 (2006) 6714–6721.

67. S. Ehata, A. Hanyu & M. Fujime, et al., Ki26894, a novel transforming growth factor-β; type I receptor kinase inhibitor, inhibits *in vitro* invasion and *in vivo* bone metastasis of a human breast cancer cell line, Cancer Science 98 (2007) 127–133.

68. E.G. Stebbins, K.S. Mohammad & M. Niewolna, et al., SD-208, a small molecule inhibitor of transforming growth

factor-βreceptor I kinase reduces breast cancer metastases to bone and improves survival in a mouse model, J Bone Miner Res 20 (2005) S55.

69. W.J. Boyle, W.S. Simonet & D.L. Lacey, Osteoclast differentiation and activation, Nature 423 (2003) 337–342.

70. J. Li, I. Sarosi & X.-Q. Yan, et al., RANK is the intrinsic hematopoietic cell surface receptor that controls osteoclastogenesis and regulation of bone mass and calcium metabolism, Proc Natl Acad Sci USA 97 (2000) 1566–1571.

71. Y.-Y. Kong, H. Yoshida & I. Sarosi, et al., OPGL is a key regulator of osteoclastogenesis, lymphocyte development and lymph-node organogenesis, Nature 397 (1999) 315–323.

72. T. Akatsu, T. Murakami & K. Ono, et al., Osteoclastogenesis inhibitory factor exhibits hypocalcemic effects in normal mice and in hypercalcemic nude mice carrying tumors associated with humoral hypercalcemia of malignancy, Bone 23 (1998) 495–498.

73. N. Bucay, I. Sarosi & C.R. Dunstan, et al., Osteoprotegerin-deficient mice develop early onset osteoporosis and arterial calcification, Genes Dev 12 (1998) 1260–1268.

74. J.J. Wysolmerski & A.E. Broadus, Hypercalcemia of malignancy: the central role of parathyroid hormone-related protein, Annu Rev Med 45 (1994) 189–200.

75. A.C. Karaplis & D. Goltzman, PTH and PTHrP effects on the skeleton, Rev Endocr Metab Disord 1 (2000) 331–341.

76. H. Juppner, A.B. Abou-Samra & M. Freeman, et al., A G protein-linked receptor for parathyroid hormone and parathyroid hormone-related peptide, Science 254 (1991) 1024–1026.

77. N. Kohno, S. Kitazawa & M. Fukase, et al., The expression of parathyroid hormone-related protein in human breast cancer with skeletal metastases, Surg Today 24 (1994) 215–220.

78. G. Powell, J. Southby & J. Danks, et al., Localization of parathyroid hormone-related protein in breast cancer metastases: increased incidence in bone compared with other sites, Cancer Res 51 (1991) 3059–3061.

79. A.A. Bryden, S. Islam & A.J. Freemont, et al., Parathyroid hormone-related peptide: expression in prostate cancer bone metastases, Prostate Cancer Prostatic Dis 5 (2002) 59–62.

80. J. Iddon, N.J. Bundred & J. Hoyland, et al., Expression of parathyroid hormone-related protein and its receptor in bone metastases from prostate cancer, J Pathol 191 (2000) 170–174.

81. T.A. Guise, J.J. Yin & S.D. Taylor, et al., Evidence for a causal role of parathyroid hormone-related protein in the pathogenesis of human breast cancer-mediated osteolysis, J Clin Invest 98 (1996) 1544–1549.

82. J.J. Yin, K.S. Mohammad & S.M. Kakonen, et al., A causal role for endothelin-1 in the pathogenesis of osteoblastic bone metastases, Proc Natl Acad Sci USA 100 (2003) 10954–10959.

83. W.E. Gallwitz, T.A. Guise & G.R. Mundy, Guanosine nucleotides inhibit different syndromes of PTHrP excess caused by human cancers *in vivo*, J Clin Invest 110 (2002) 1559–1572.

84. H. Iguchi, S. Tanaka & Y. Ozawa, et al., An experimental model of bone metastasis by human lung cancer cells: the role of parathyroid hormone-related protein in bone metastasis, Cancer Res 56 (1996) 4040–4043.

85. T. Miki, S. Yano & M. Hanibuchi, et al., Parathyroid hormone-related protein (PTHrP) is responsible for production of bone metastasis, but not visceral metastasis, by human small cell lung cancer SBC-5 cells in natural killer cell-depleted SCID mice, Int J Cancer 108 (2004) 511–515.

86. T.A. Guise, J.J. Yin & R.J. Thomas, et al., Parathyroid hormone-related protein (PTHrP)-(1-139) isoform is efficiently secreted *in vitro* and enhances breast cancer metastasis to bone *in vivo*, Bone 30 (2002) 670–676.

87. S.A. Rabbani, J. Gladu & P. Harakidas, et al., Over-production of parathyroid hormone-related peptide results in increased osteolytic skeletal metastasis by prostate cancer cells *in vivo*, Int J Cancer 80 (1999) 257–264.

88. J.J. Wysolmerski, P.R. Dann & E. Zelazny, et al., Overexpression of parathyroid hormone-related protein causes hypercalcemia but not bone metastases in a murine model of mammary tumorigenesis, J Bone Miner Res 17 (2002) 1164–1170.

89. M.A. Henderson, J.A. Danks & J.M. Moseley, et al., Parathyroid hormone-related protein production by breast cancers, improved survival and reduced bone metastases, J Natl Cancer Inst 93 (2001) 234–237.

90. A. Dittmer, M. Vetter & D. Schunke, et al., Parathyroid hormone-related protein regulates tumor-relevant genes in breast cancer cells, J Biol Chem 281 (2006) 14563–14572.

91. N. Ilievska, S. Bouralexis & R.J. Thomas-Mudge, et al., PTHrP as a mediator of DNA repair in cancer, J Bone Miner Res 19 (2004) S194.

92. C. Faucheux, M.A. Horton & J.S. Price, Nuclear localization of type I parathyroid hormone/parathyroid hormone-related protein receptors in deer antler osteoclasts: evidence for parathyroid hormone-related protein and receptor activator of NF-kappaB-dependent effects on osteoclast formation in regenerating mammalian bone, J Bone Miner Res 17 (2002) 455–464.

93. C.V. Gay, B. Zheng & V.R. Gilman, Co-detection of PTH/PTHrP receptor and tartrate resistant acid phosphatase in osteoclasts, J Cell Biochem 89 (2003) 902–908.

94. H. Fukushima, E. Jimi & H. Kajiya, et al., Parathyroid-hormone-related protein induces expression of receptor activator of NF-κB ligand in human periodontal ligament cells via a cAMP/protein kinase A-independent pathway, J Dent Res 84 (2005) 329–334.

95. H. Kondo, J. Guo & F.R. Bringhurst, Cyclic adenosine monophosphate/protein kinase A mediates parathyroid hormone/parathyroid hormone-related protein receptor regulation of osteoclastogenesis and expression of RANKL and osteoprotegerin mRNAs by marrow stromal cells, J Bone Miner Res 17 (2002) 1667–1679.

96. C. Guillen, P. Martinez & A.R. de Gortazar, et al., Both N- and C-terminal domains of parathyroid hormone-related protein increase Interleukin-6 by Nuclear Factor-kappa B activation in osteoblastic cells, J Biol Chem 277 (2002) 28109–28117.

97. P. Palmqvist, E. Persson & H.H. Conaway, et al., IL-6, leukemia inhibitory factor and oncostatin M stimulate bone resorption and regulate the expression of receptor activator of NF-kappa B ligand, osteoprotegerin and receptor activator of NF-kappa B in mouse calvariae, J Immunol 169 (2002) 3353–3362.

98. J.H. Pollock, M.J. Blaha & S.A. Lavish, et al., *In vivo* demonstration that parathyroid hormone and parathyroid hormone-related protein stimulate expression by osteoblasts of interleukin-6 and leukemia inhibitory factor, J Bone Miner Res 11 (1996) 754–759.

99. J.A. Belperio, M.P. Keane & D.A. Arenberg, et al., CXC chemokines in angiogenesis, J Leukoc Biol 68 (2000) 1–8.

100. A. Nicolini, A. Carpi & G. Rossi, Cytokines in breast cancer, Cytokine Growth Factor Rev 17 (2006) 325–337.

101. M.S. Bendre, D. Gaddy-Kurten & T. Mon-Foote, et al., Expression of interleukin 8 and not parathyroid hormone-related protein by human breast cancer cells correlates with bone metastasis *in vivo*, Cancer Res 62 (2002) 5571–5579.

102. J.E. De Larco, B.R.K. Wuertz & K.A. Rosner, et al., A potential role for interleukin-8 in the metastatic phenotype of breast carcinoma cells, Am J Pathol 158 (2001) 639–646.

103. M.S. Bendre, A.G. Margulies & B. Walser, et al., Tumor-derived interleukin-8 stimulates osteolysis independent of the receptor activator of nuclear factor-kappaB ligand pathway, Cancer Res 65 (2005) 11001–11009.

104. M.S. Bendre, D.C. Montague & T. Peery, et al., Interleukin-8 stimulation of osteoclastogenesis and bone resorption is a mechanism for the increased osteolysis of metastatic bone disease, Bone 33 (2003) 28–37.

105. B. Singh, J.A. Berry & L.E. Vincent, et al., Involvement of IL-8 in COX-2-mediated bone metastases from breast cancer, J Surg Res 134 (2006) 44–51.

106. S.K. Manna & G.T. Ramesh, Interleukin-8 induces nuclear transcription factor-κB through a TRAF6-dependent pathway, J Biol Chem 280 (2005) 7010–7021.

107. L.J. Suva, T. Kelly & R.D. Sanderson, The role of IL-8 in the complex phenotype of osteolytic breast cancer, Cancer Treat Rev 32 (2006) S27.

108. B. Singh, J.A. Berry & A. Shoher, et al., COX-2 involvement in breast cancer metastasis to bone, Oncogene 26 (2007) 3789–3796.

109. N. Kundu, Q. Yang & R. Dorsey, et al., Increased cyclooxygenase-2 (cox-2) expression and activity in a murine model of metastatic breast cancer, Int J Cancer 93 (2001) 681–686.

110. C.H. Liu, S.H. Chang & K. Narko, et al., Overexpression of cyclooxygenase-2 is sufficient to induce tumorigenesis in transgenic mice, J Biol Chem 276 (2001) 18563–18569.

111. T. Hiraga, A. Myoui & M.E. Choi, et al., Stimulation of cyclooxygenase-2 expression by bone-derived transforming growth factor-beta enhances bone metastases in breast cancer, Cancer Res 66 (2006) 2067–2073.

112. M.D. Castellone, H. Teramoto & J.S. Gutkind, Cyclooxygenase-2 and colorectal cancer chemoprevention: the beta-catenin connection, Cancer Res 66 (2006) 11085–11088.

113. Y.C. Fong, M.C. Maa & F.J. Tsai, et al., Osteoblast-derived TGF-beta1 stimulates IL-8 release through AP-1 and NF-kappaB in human cancer cells, J Bone Miner Res 23 (2008) 961–970.

114. L. Levy, C. Neuveut & C.-A. Renard, et al., Transcriptional activation of interleukin-8 by beta-catenin-Tcf4, J Biol Chem 277 (2002) 42386–42393.

115. K. Xie, Interleukin-8 and human cancer biology, Cytokine Growth Factor Rev 12 (2001) 375–391.

116. L.A. Kingsley, P.G. Fournier & J.M. Chirgwin, et al., Molecular biology of bone metastasis, Mol Cancer Ther 6 (2007) 2609–2617.

117. A. Amirkhosravi, S.A. Mousa & M. Amaya, et al., Inhibition of tumor cell-induced platelet aggregation and lung metastasis by the oral GpIIb/IIIa antagonist XV454, Thromb Haemost 90 (2003) 549–554.

118. S.J. Bakewell, P. Nestor & S. Prasad, et al., Platelet and osteoclast beta3 integrins are critical for bone metastasis, Proc Natl Acad Sci USA 100 (2003) 14205–14210.

119. A. Boucharaba, C.M. Serre & S. Gres, et al., Platelet-derived lysophosphatidic acid supports the progression of osteolytic bone metastases in breast cancer, J Clin Invest 114 (2004) 1714–1725.

120. A. Boucharaba, C.M. Serre & J. Guglielmi, et al., The type 1 lysophosphatidic acid receptor is a target for therapy in bone metastases, Proc Natl Acad Sci USA 103 (2006) 9643–9648.

121. Y. Morinaga, N. Fujita & K. Ohishi, et al., Stimulation of interleukin-11 production from osteoblast-like cells by transforming growth factor-beta and tumor cell factors, Int J Cancer 71 (1997) 422–428.

122. M. Lacroix, B. Siwek & P.J. Marie, et al., Production and regulation of interleukin-11 by breast cancer cells, Cancer Lett 127 (1998) 29–35.

123. B. Singh, J.A. Berry & A. Shoher, et al., COX-2 induces IL-11 production in human breast cancer cells, J Surg Res 131 (2006) 267–275.

124. H. Morgan, A. Tumber & P.A. Hill, Breast cancer cells induce osteoclast formation by stimulating host IL-11 production and downregulating granulocyte/macrophage colony-stimulating factor, Int J Cancer 109 (2004) 653–660.

125. E. Romas, N. Udagawa & H. Zhou, et al., The role of gp130-mediated signals in osteoclast development: regulation of interleukin 11 production by osteoblasts and distribution of its receptor in bone marrow cultures, J Exp Med 183 (1996) 2581–2591.

126. G. Girasole, G. Passeri & R.L. Jilka, et al., Interleukin-11: a new cytokine critical for osteoclast development, J Clin Invest 93 (1994) 1516–1524.

127. P.A. Hill, A. Tumber & S. Papaioannou, et al., The cellular actions of interleukin-11 on bone resorption *in vitro*, Endocrinology 139 (1998) 1564–1572.

128. O. Kudo, A. Sabokbar & A. Pocock, et al., Interleukin-6 and interleukin-11 support human osteoclast formation by a RANKL-independent mechanism, Bone 32 (2003) 1–7.

129. H. Yasuda, N. Shima & N. Nakagawa, et al., Osteoclast differentiation factor is a ligand for osteoprotegerin/osteoclastogenesis-inhibitory factor and is identical to TRANCE/RANKL, Proc Natl Acad Sci USA 95 (1998) 3597–3602.

130. E. Tsuda, M. Goto & S.-I. Mochizuki, et al., Isolation of a novel cytokine from human fibroblasts that specifically inhibits osteoclastogenesis, Biochem Biophys Res Commun 234 (1997) 137–142.

131. N.J. Horwood, J. Elliott & T.J. Martin, et al., Osteotropic agents regulate the expression of osteoclast differentiation factor and osteoprotegerin in osteoblastic stromal cells, Endocrinology 139 (1998) 4743–4746.

132. Y. Morinaga, N. Fujita & K. Ohishi, et al., Suppression of interleukin-11-mediated bone resorption by cyclooxygenases inhibitors, J Cell Physiol 175 (1998) 247–254.

133. G. Gorny, A. Shaw & M.J. Oursler, IL-6, LIF and TNF-alpha regulation of GM-CSF inhibition of osteoclastogenesis *in vitro*, Exp Cell Res 294 (2004) 149–158.

134. N. Udagawa, N.J. Horwood & J. Elliott, et al., Interleukin-18 (interferon-gamma-inducing factor) is produced by osteoblasts and acts via granulocyte/macrophage

colony-stimulating factor and not via interferon-gamma to inhibit osteoclast formation, J Exp Med 185 (1997) 1005–1012.

135. Y. Fujikawa, A. Sabokbar & S.D. Neale, et al., The effect of macrophage-colony stimulating factor and other humoral factors (interleukin-1, -3, -6 and -11, tumor necrosis factor-alpha and granulocyte macrophage-colony stimulating factor) on human osteoclast formation from circulating cells, Bone 28 (2001) 261–267.

136. J.M. Hodge, M.A. Kirkland & C.J. Aitken, et al., Osteoclastic potential of human CFU-GM: biphasic effect of GM-CSF, J Bone Miner Res 19 (2004) 190–199.

137. B.K. Park, H. Zhang & Q. Zeng, et al., NF-kappaB in breast cancer cells promotes osteolytic bone metastasis by inducing osteoclastogenesis via GM-CSF, Nat Med 13 (2007) 62–69.

138. P. Gehron Robey & A.L. Boskey, Extracellular matrix and biomineralization of bone, in: M.I. Favus (Ed.), Primer on the metabolic bone diseases and disorders of mineral metabolism, 5th ed., American Society for Bone and Mineral Research, Washington, DC, 2003, pp. 38–46.

139. A. Miyauchi, J. Alvarez & E.M. Greenfield, et al., Recognition of osteopontin and related peptides by an alpha v beta 3 integrin stimulates immediate cell signals in osteoclasts, J Biol Chem 266 (1991) 20369–20374.

140. F.P. Ross, J. Chappel & J.I. Alvarez, et al., Interactions between the bone matrix proteins osteopontin and bone sialoprotein and the osteoclast integrin alpha v beta 3 potentiate bone resorption, J Biol Chem 268 (1993) 9901–9907.

141. H. Adwan, T.J. Bauerle & M.R. Berger, Downregulation of osteopontin and bone sialoprotein II is related to reduced colony formation and metastasis formation of MDA-MB-231 human breast cancer cells, Cancer Gene Ther 11 (2004) 109–120.

142. N. Dornhofer, S. Spong & K. Bennewith, et al., Connective tissue growth factor-specific monoclonal antibody therapy inhibits pancreatic tumor growth and metastasis, Cancer Res 66 (2006) 5816–5827.

143. K.A. Furger, R.K. Menon & A.B. Tuck, et al., The functional and clinical roles of osteopontin in cancer and metastasis, Curr Mol Med 1 (2001) 621–632.

144. G.N. Thalmann, R.A. Sikes & R.E. Devoll, et al., Osteopontin: possible role in prostate cancer progression, Clin Cancer Res 5 (1999) 2271–2277.

145. A. Leask, A. Holmes & C.M. Black, et al., Connective tissue growth factor gene regulation. Requirements for its induction by transforming growth factor-beta 2 in fibroblasts, J Biol Chem 278 (2003) 13008–13015.

146. T. Shimo, S. Kubota & N. Yoshioka, et al., Pathogenic role of connective tissue growth factor (CTGF/CCN2) in osteolytic metastasis of breast cancer, J Bone Miner Res 21 (2006) 1045–1059.

147. S. Ivkovic, B.S. Yoon & S.N. Popoff, et al., Connective tissue growth factor coordinates chondrogenesis and angiogenesis during skeletal development, Development 130 (2003) 2779–2791.

148. R. Gao & D.R. Brigstock, Connective tissue growth factor (CCN2) induces adhesion of rat activated hepatic stellate cells by binding of its C-terminal domain to integrin alpha(v)beta(3) and heparan sulfate proteoglycan, J Biol Chem 279 (2004) 8848–8855.

149. D. Javelaud, V. Delmas & M. Moller, et al., Stable over-expression of Smad7 in human melanoma cells inhibits their tumorigenicity *in vitro* and *in vivo*, Oncogene 24 (2005) 7624–7629.

150. Y. Kang, Pro-metastasis function of TGFbeta mediated by the Smad pathway, J Cell Biochem 98 (2006) 1380–1390.

151. R. Ala-aho & V.M. Kahari, Collagenases in cancer, Biochimie 87 (2005) 273–286.

152. N. Fratzl-Zelman, H. Glantschnig & M. Rumpler, et al., The expression of matrix metalloproteinase-13 and osteocalcin and is modulated by 1,25-dihydroxyvitamin D3 and thyroid hormones, Cell Biol Int 27 (2003) 459–468.

153. M. Inada, Y. Wang & M.H. Byrne, et al., Critical roles for collagenase-3 (Mmp13) in development of growth plate cartilage and in endochondral ossification, Proc Natl Acad Sci USA 101 (2004) 17192–17197.

154. N. Selvamurugan, S. Kwok & T. Alliston, et al., Transforming growth factor-beta 1 regulation of collagenase-3 expression in osteoblastic cells by cross-talk between the Smad and MAPK signaling pathways and their components, Smad2 and Runx2, J Biol Chem 279 (2004) 19327–19334.

155. J.M. Freije, I. Diez-Itza & M. Balbin, et al., Molecular cloning and expression of collagenase-3, a novel human matrix metalloproteinase produced by breast carcinomas, J Biol Chem 269 (1994) 16766–16773.

156. N. Selvamurugan, Z. Fung & N.C. Partridge, Transcriptional activation of collagenase-3 by transforming growth factor-beta1 is via MAPK and Smad pathways in human breast cancer cells, FEBS Lett 532 (2002) 31–35.

157. S.K. Leivonen, R. Ala-aho & K. Koli, et al., Activation of Smad signaling enhances collagenase-3 (MMP-13) expression and invasion of head and neck squamous carcinoma cells, Oncogene 25 (2006) 2588–2600.

158. N. Selvamurugan, S. Kwok & N.C. Partridge, Smad3 interacts with JunB and Cbfa1/Runx2 for transforming growth factor-beta1-stimulated collagenase-3 expression in human breast cancer cells, J Biol Chem 279 (2004) 27764–27773.

159. P. Ducy, R. Zhang & V. Geoffroy, et al., Osf2/Cbfa1: a transcriptional activator of osteoblast differentiation, Cell 89 (1997) 747–754.

160. T. Komori, H. Yagi & S. Nomura, et al., Targeted disruption of cbfa1 results in a complete lack of bone formation owing to maturational arrest of osteoblasts, Cell 89 (1997) 755–764.

161. P. Shore, A role for Runx2 in normal mammary gland and breast cancer bone metastasis, J Cell Biochem 96 (2005) 484–489.

162. G.L. Barnes, A. Javed & S.M. Waller, et al., Osteoblast-related transcription factors Runx2 (Cbfa1/AML3) and MSX2 mediate the expression of bone sialoprotein in human metastatic breast cancer cells, Cancer Res 63 (2003) 2631–2637.

163. K.D. Brubaker, R.L. Vessella & L.G. Brown, et al., Prostate cancer expression of runt-domain transcription factor Runx2, a key regulator of osteoblast differentiation and function, Prostate 56 (2003) 13–22.

164. J. Pratap, A. Javed & L.R. Languino, et al., The Runx2 osteogenic transcription factor regulates matrix metalloproteinase 9 in bone metastatic cancer cells and controls cell invasion, Mol Cell Biol 25 (2005) 8581–8591.

165. M. Riminucci, A. Corsi & K. Peris, et al., Coexpression of bone sialoprotein (BSP) and the pivotal transcriptional

regulator of osteogenesis, Cbfa1/Runx2, in malignant melanoma, Calcif Tissue Int 73 (2003) 281–289.

166. G.L. Barnes, K.E. Hebert & M. Kamal, et al., Fidelity of Runx2 activity in breast cancer cells is required for the generation of metastases-associated osteolytic disease, Cancer Res 64 (2004) 4506–4513.

167. A. Javed, G.L. Barnes & J. Pratap, et al., Impaired intranuclear trafficking of Runx2 (AML3/CBFA1) transcription factors in breast cancer cells inhibits osteolysis *in vivo*, Proc Natl Acad Sci USA 102 (2005) 1454–1459.

168. J. Street, M. Bao & L. deGuzman, et al., Vascular endothelial growth factor stimulates bone repair by promoting angiogenesis and bone turnover, Proc Natl Acad Sci USA 99 (2002) 9656–9661.

169. S.E. Aldridge, T.W. Lennard & J.R. Williams, et al., Vascular endothelial growth factor acts as an osteolytic factor in breast cancer metastases to bone, Br J Cancer 92 (2005) 1531–1537.

170. M.T. Engsig, Q.J. Chen & T.H. Vu, et al., Matrix metalloproteinase 9 and vascular endothelial growth factor are essential for osteoclast recruitment into developing long bones, J Cell Biol 151 (2000) 879–889.

171. M. Nakagawa, T. Kaneda & T. Arakawa, et al., Vascular endothelial growth factor (VEGF) directly enhances osteoclastic bone resorption and survival of mature osteoclasts, FEBS Letters 473 (2000) 161–164.

172. G. Breier, S. Blum & J. Peli, et al., Transforming growth factor-beta and Ras regulate the VEGF/VEGF-receptor system during tumor angiogenesis, Int J Cancer 97 (2002) 142–148.

173. J.H. Harmey, E. Dimitriadis & E. Kay, et al., Regulation of macrophage production of vascular endothelial growth factor (VEGF) by hypoxia and transforming growth factor beta-1, Ann Surg Oncol 5 (1998) 271–278.

174. H. Teraoka, T. Sawada & T. Nishihara, et al., Enhanced VEGF production and decreased immunogenicity induced by TGF-beta 1 promote liver metastasis of pancreatic cancer, Br J Cancer 85 (2001) 612–617.

175. K.A. Mohamedali, A.T. Poblenz & C.R. Sikes, et al., Inhibition of prostate tumor growth and bone remodeling by the vascular targeting agent VEGF121/rGel, Cancer Res 66 (2006) 10919–10928.

176. S. Ran, K.A. Mohamedali & T.A. Luster, et al., The vascular-ablative agent VEGF(121)/rGel inhibits pulmonary metastases of MDA-MB-231 breast tumors, Neoplasia 7 (2005) 486–496.

177. L.M. Veenendaal, H. Jin & S. Ran, et al., *In vitro* and *in vivo* studies of a VEGF121/rGelonin chimeric fusion toxin targeting the neovasculature of solid tumors, Proc Natl Acad Sci USA 99 (2002) 7866–7871.

178. G. McMahon, VEGF receptor signaling in tumor angiogenesis, Oncologist 5 (suppl 1) (2000) 3–10.

179. K.S. Koeneman, F. Yeung & L.W. Chung, Osteomimetic properties of prostate cancer cells: a hypothesis supporting the predilection of prostate cancer metastasis and growth in the bone environment, Prostate 39 (1999) 246–261.

180. G.N. Thalmann, P.E. Anezinis & S.M. Chang, et al., Androgen-independent cancer progression and bone metastasis in the LNCaP model of human prostate cancer, Cancer Res 54 (1994) 2577–2581.

181. C.K. Inman & P. Shore, The osteoblast transcription factor Runx2 is expressed in mammary epithelial cells and mediates osteopontin expression, J Biol Chem 278 (2003) 48684–48689.

182. H. Roca, M. Phimphilai & R. Gopalakrishnan, et al., Cooperative interactions between RUNX2 and homeodomain protein-binding sites are critical for the osteoblast-specific expression of the bone sialoprotein gene, J Biol Chem 280 (2005) 30845–30855.

183. M. Sato, E. Morii & T. Komori, et al., Transcriptional regulation of osteopontin gene *in vivo* by PEBP2alphaA/CBFA1 and ETS1 in the skeletal tissues, Oncogene 17 (1998) 1517–1525.

184. F. Yeung, W.K. Law & C.H. Yeh, et al., Regulation of human osteocalcin promoter in hormone-independent human prostate cancer cells, J Biol Chem 277 (2002) 2468–2476.

185. J. Glowacki & J.B. Lian, Impaired recruitment and differentiation of osteoclast progenitors by osteocalcin-deplete bone implants, Cell Differ 21 (1987) 247–254.

186. H.I. Roach, Why does bone matrix contain non-collagenous proteins? The possible roles of osteocalcin, osteonectin, osteopontin and bone sialoprotein in bone mineralisation and resorption, Cell Biol Int 18 (1994) 617–628.

187. A. Bellahcene, M. Kroll & F. Liebens, et al., Bone sialoprotein expression in primary human breast cancer is associated with bone metastases development, J Bone Miner Res 11 (1996) 665–670.

188. A. Bellahcene, N. Maloujahmoum & L.W. Fisher, et al., Expression of bone sialoprotein in human lung cancer, Calcif Tissue Int 61 (1997) 183–188.

189. I.J. Diel, E.F. Solomayer & M.J. Seibel, et al., Serum bone sialoprotein in patients with primary breast cancer is a prognostic marker for subsequent bone metastasis, Clin Cancer Res 5 (1999) 3914–3919.

190. D. Waltregny, A. Bellahcene & I. Van Riet, et al., Prognostic value of bone sialoprotein expression in clinically localized human prostate cancer, J Natl Cancer Inst 90 (1998) 1000–1008.

191. T. Ibrahim, I. Leong & O. Sanchez-Sweatman, et al., Expression of bone sialoprotein and osteopontin in breast cancer bone metastases, Clin Exp Metastasis 18 (2000) 253–260.

192. D. Waltregny, A. Bellahcene & X. de Leval, et al., Increased expression of bone sialoprotein in bone metastases compared with visceral metastases in human breast and prostate cancers, J Bone Miner Res 15 (2000) 834–843.

193. Y. Ogata, N. Niisato & S. Furuyama, et al., Transforming growth factor-beta 1 regulation of bone sialoprotein gene transcription: identification of a TGF-beta activation element in the rat BSP gene promoter, J Cell Biochem 65 (1997) 501–512.

194. J.S. Nam, A.M. Suchar & M.J. Kang, et al., Bone sialoprotein mediates the tumor cell-targeted prometastatic activity of transforming growth factor beta in a mouse model of breast cancer, Cancer Res 66 (2006) 6327–6335.

195. J. Chen, J.A. Rodriguez & B. Barnett, et al., Bone sialoprotein promotes tumor cell migration in both *in vitro* and *in vivo* models, Connect Tissue Res 44 (suppl 1) (2003) 279–284.

196. A. Karadag & L.W. Fisher, Bone sialoprotein enhances migration of bone marrow stromal cells through matrices

by bridging MMP-2 to αvβ3-integrin, J Bone Miner Res 21 (2006) 1627–1636.

197. A. Karadag, K.U.E. Ogbureke & N.S. Fedarko, et al., Bone sialoprotein, matrix metalloproteinase 2 and $\alpha_v\beta_3$ integrin in osteotropic cancer cell invasion, J Natl Cancer Inst 96 (2004) 956–965.

198. J.A. Sharp, M. Waltham & E.D. Williams, et al., Transfection of MDA-MB-231 human breast carcinoma cells with bone sialoprotein (BSP) stimulates migration and invasion *in vitro* and growth of primary and secondary tumors in nude mice, Clin Exp Metastasis 21 (2004) 19–29.

199. T.V. Byzova, W. Kim & R.J. Midura, et al., Activation of integrin alpha(V)beta(3) regulates cell adhesion and migration to bone sialoprotein, Exp Cell Res 254 (2000) 299–308.

200. A. Oldberg, A. Franzen & D. Heinegard, et al., Identification of a bone sialoprotein receptor in osteosarcoma cells, J Biol Chem 263 (1988) 19433–19436.

201. A. Teti, A.R. Farina & I. Villanova, et al., Activation of MMP-2 by human GCT23 giant cell tumour cells induced by osteopontin, bone sialoprotein and GRGDSP peptides is RGD and cell shape change dependent, Int J Cancer 77 (1998) 82–93.

202. E.I. Deryugina, B. Ratnikov & E. Monosov, et al., MT1-MMP initiates activation of pro-MMP-2 and integrin alphav-beta3 promotes maturation of MMP-2 in breast carcinoma cells, Exp Cell Res 263 (2001) 209–223.

203. J.H. Zhang, J. Tang & J. Wang, et al., Over-expression of bone sialoprotein enhances bone metastasis of human breast cancer cells in a mouse model, Int J Oncol 23 (2003) 1043–1048.

204. J.H. Zhang, J. Wang & J. Tang, et al., Bone sialoprotein promotes bone metastasis of a non-bone-seeking clone of human breast cancer cells, Anticancer Res 24 (2004) 1361–1368.

205. T. Bauerle, J. Peterschmitt & H. Hilbig, et al., Treatment of bone metastasis induced by MDA-MB-231 breast cancer cells with an antibody against bone sialoprotein, Int J Oncol 28 (2006) 573–583.

206. G. Bergers, R. Brekken & G. McMahon, et al., Matrix metalloproteinase-9 triggers the angiogenic switch during carcinogenesis, Nat Cell Biol 2 (2000) 737–744.

207. E.I. Deryugina & J.P. Quigley, Matrix metalloproteinases and tumor metastasis, Cancer Metastasis Rev 25 (2006) 9–34.

208. K.D. Brubakcr, R.L. Vcssclla & L.D. True, et al., Cathepsin K mRNA and protein expression in prostate cancer progression, J Bone Miner Res 18 (2003) 222–230.

209. A.J. Littlewood-Evans, G. Bilbe & W.B. Bowler, et al., The osteoclast-associated protease cathepsin K is expressed in human breast carcinoma, Cancer Res 57 (1997) 5386–5390.

210. G. Eilon & G.R. Mundy, Direct resorption of bone by human breast cancer cells *in vitro*, Nature 276 (1978) 726–728.

211. O.H. Sanchez-Sweatman, J. Lee & F.W. Orr, et al., Direct osteolysis induced by metastatic murine melanoma cells: role of matrix metalloproteinases, Eur J Cancer 33 (1997) 918–925.

212. O.H. Sanchez-Sweatman, F.W. Orr & G. Singh, Human metastatic prostate PC3 cell lines degrade bone using matrix metalloproteinases, Invasion Metastasis 18 (1998) 297–305.

213. T. Taube, I. Elomaa & C. Blomqvist, et al., Histomorphometric evidence for osteoclast-mediated bone resorption in metastatic breast cancer, Bone 15 (1994) 161–166.

214. C. Ji, S. Casinghino & D.J. Chang, et al., CBFa(AML/PEBP2)-related elements in the TGF-beta type I receptor promoter and expression with osteoblast differentiation, J Cell Biochem 69 (1998) 353–363.

215. V. Geoffroy, M. Kneissel & B. Fournier, et al., High bone resorption in adult aging transgenic mice overexpressing cbfa1/runx2 in cells of the osteoblastic lineage, Mol Cell Biol 22 (2002) 6222–6233.

216. J. Dupont & M. Holzenberger, Biology of insulin-like growth factors in development, Birth Defects Res C Embryo Today 69 (2003) 257–271.

217. G. Zhao, M.C. Monier-Faugere & M.C. Langub, et al., Targeted overexpression of insulin-like growth factor I to osteoblasts of transgenic mice: increased trabecular bone volume without increased osteoblast proliferation, Endocrinology 141 (2000) 2674–2682.

218. L. Powell-Braxton, P. Hollingshead & C. Warburton, et al., IGF-I is required for normal embryonic growth in mice, Genes Dev 7 (1993) 2609–2617.

219. M. Zhang, S. Xuan & M.L. Bouxsein, et al., Osteoblast-specific knockout of the insulin-like growth factor (IGF) receptor gene reveals an essential role of IGF signaling in bone matrix mineralization, J Biol Chem 277 (2002) 44005–44012.

220. C. Bahr & B. Groner, The IGF-1 receptor and its contributions to metastatic tumor growth-novel approaches to the inhibition of IGF-1R function, Growth Factors 23 (2005) 1–14.

221. R. Baserga, F. Peruzzi & K. Reiss, The IGF-1 receptor in cancer biology, Int J Cancer 107 (2003) 873–877.

222. G.O. Hellawell, G.D. Turner & D.R. Davies, et al., Expression of the type 1 insulin-like growth factor receptor is upregulated in primary prostate cancer and commonly persists in metastatic disease, Cancer Res 62 (2002) 2942–2950.

223. J.G. Jackson, X. Zhang & T. Yoneda, et al., Regulation of breast cancer cell motility by insulin receptor substrate-2 (IRS-2) in metastatic variants of human breast cancer cell lines, Oncogene 20 (2001) 7318–7325.

224. T. Yoneda, P.J. Williams & T. Hiraga, et al., A bone-seeking clone exhibits different biological properties from the MDA-MB-231 parental human breast cancer cells and a brain-seeking clone *in vivo* and *in vitro*, J Bone Miner Res 16 (2001) 1486–1495.

225. T. Yoneda, P.J. Williams & C.R. Dunstan, et al., Growth of metastatic cancer cells in bone is enhanced by bone-derived insulin-like growth factors (IGFs), J Bone Miner Res 10 (1995) S269.

226. T. Hiraga, A. Myoui & P. Williams, et al., Suppression of IGF signaling propagation and NF-κB activation reduces bone metastases in breast cancer, J Bone Miner Res 16 (2001) S200.

227. C.M. van Golen, T.S. Schwab & B. Kim, et al., Insulin-like growth factor-I receptor expression regulates neuroblastoma metastasis to bone, Cancer Res 66 (2006) 6570–6578.

228. G. Chen, K. Sircar & A. Aprikian, et al., Expression of RANKL/RANK/OPG in primary and metastatic human prostate cancer as markers of disease stage and functional regulation, Cancer 107 (2006) 289–298.

229. D.H. Jones, T. Nakashima & O.H. Sanchez, et al., Regulation of cancer cell migration and bone metastasis by RANKL, Nature 440 (2006) 692–696.

230. K. Mori, B. Le Goff & C. Charrier, et al., DU145 human prostate cancer cells express functional receptor activator of NF[kappa]B: New insights in the prostate cancer bone metastasis process, Bone 40 (2007) 981–990.

231. M. Tometsko, A. Armstrong & R. Miller, et al., RANK ligand directly induces osteoclastogenic, angiogenic, chemoattractive and invasive factors on RANK-expressing human cancer cells MDA-MB-231 and PC3, J Bone Miner Res 19 (2004) S25.

232. G.J. Atkins, S. Bouralexis & A. Evdokiou, et al., Human osteoblasts are resistant to Apo2L/TRAIL-mediated apoptosis, Bone 31 (2002) 448–456.

233. I. Holen, S.S. Cross & H.L. Neville-Webbe, et al., Osteoprotegerin (OPG) expression by breast cancer cells *in vitro* and breast tumours *in vivo*—a role in tumour cell survival?, Breast Cancer Res Treat 92 (2005) 207–215.

234. I. Holen, P.I. Croucher & F.C. Hamdy, et al., Osteoprotegerin (OPG) is a survival factor for human prostate cancer cells, Cancer Res 62 (2002) 1619–1623.

235. H.L. Neville-Webbe, N.A. Cross & C.L. Eaton, et al., Osteoprotegerin (OPG) produced by bone marrow stromal cells protects breast cancer cells from TRAIL-induced apoptosis, Breast Cancer Res Treat 86 (2004) 269–279.

236. J.M. Brown, E. Corey & Z.D. Lee, et al., Osteoprotegerin and rank ligand expression in prostate cancer, Urology 57 (2001) 611–616.

237. H.R. Park, S.K. Min & H.D. Cho, et al., Expression of osteoprotegerin and RANK ligand in breast cancer bone metastasis, J Korean Med Sci 18 (2003) 541–546.

238. C. van Poznak, S.S. Cross & M. Saggese, et al., Expression of osteoprotegerin (OPG), TNF related apoptosis inducing ligand (TRAIL) and receptor activator of nuclear factor kappaB ligand (RANKL) in human breast tumours, J Clin Pathol 59 (2006) 56–63.

239. J.M. Brown, R.L. Vessella & P.J. Kostenuik, et al., Serum osteoprotegerin levels are increased in patients with advanced prostate cancer, Clin Cancer Res 7 (2001) 2977–2983.

240. J.L. Fisher, R.J. Thomas-Mudge & J. Elliott, et al., Osteoprotegerin overexpression by breast cancer cells enhances orthotopic and osseous tumor growth and contrasts with that delivered therapeutically, Cancer Res 66 (2006) 3620–3628.

241. J.E. Quinn, L.G. Brown & J. Zhang, et al., Comparison of Fc-osteoprotegerin and zoledronic acid activities suggests that zoledronic acid inhibits prostate cancer in bone by indirect mechanisms, Prostate Cancer Prostatic Dis 8 (2005) 253–259.

242. J. Zhang, J. Dai & Y. Qi, et al., Osteoprotegerin inhibits prostate cancer-induced osteoclastogenesis and prevents prostate tumor growth in the bone, J Clin Invest 107 (2001) 1235–1244.

243. J. Zhang, Y. Lu & J. Dai, et al., *In vivo* real-time imaging of TGF-beta-induced transcriptional activation of the RANK ligand gene promoter in intraosseous prostate cancer, Prostate 59 (2004) 360–369.

244. H. Enomoto, S. Shiojiri & K. Hoshi, et al., Induction of osteoclast differentiation by Runx2 through receptor activator

245. of nuclear factor-kappa B ligand (RANKL) and osteoprotegerin regulation and partial rescue of osteoclastogenesis in Runx2 −/− mice by RANKL transgene, J Biol Chem 278 (2003) 23971–23977.

245. E.M. Brown, G. Gamba & D. Riccardi, et al., Cloning and characterization of an extracellular Ca(2+)-sensing receptor from bovine parathyroid, Nature 366 (1993) 575–580.

246. E.M. Brown & H. Juppner, Parathyroid hormone: synthesis, secretion and action, in: M.J. Favus (Ed.), Primer on the Metabolic Bone Diseases and Disorders of Mineral Metabolism, 6th ed., American Society for Bone and Mineral Research, Washington, DC, 2006, pp. 90–99.

247. C.S. Kovacs, Calcium and bone metabolism during pregnancy and lactation, J Mammary Gland Biol Neoplasia 10 (2005) 105–118.

248. J. VanHouten, P. Dann, G. McGeoch & E.M. Brown, et al., The calcium-sensing receptor regulates mammary gland parathyroid hormone-related protein production and calcium transport, J Clin Invest 113 (2004) 598–608.

249. M.F. Sowers, B.W. Hollis & B. Shapiro, et al., Elevated parathyroid hormone-related peptide associated with lactation and bone density loss, JAMA 276 (1996) 549–554.

250. J.N. VanHouten, P. Dann & A.F. Stewart, et al., Mammary-specific deletion of parathyroid hormone-related protein preserves bone mass during lactation, J Clin Invest 112 (2003) 1429–1436.

251. J.L. Sanders, N. Chattopadhyay & O. Kifor, et al., Ca(2+)-sensing receptor expression and PTHrP secretion in PC-3 human prostate cancer cells, Am J Physiol Endocrinol Metab 281 (2001) E1267–E1274.

252. J.L. Sanders, N. Chattopadhyay & O. Kifor, et al., Extracellular calcium-sensing receptor expression and its potential role in regulating parathyroid hormone-related peptide secretion in human breast cancer cell lines, Endocrinology 141 (2000) 4357–4364.

253. I.A. Silver, R.J. Murrills & D.J. Etherington, Microelectrode studies on the acid microenvironment beneath adherent macrophages and osteoclasts, Exp Cell Res 175 (1988) 266–276.

254. R.J. MacLeod, N. Chattopadhyay & E.M. Brown, PTHrP stimulated by the calcium-sensing receptor requires MAP kinase activation, Am J Physiol Endocrinol Metab 284 (2003) E435–E442.

255. J. Liao, A. Schneider & N.S. Datta, et al., Extracellular calcium as a candidate mediator of prostate cancer skeletal metastasis, Cancer Res 66 (2006) 9065–9073.

256. R. Mihai, J. Stevens & C. McKinney, et al., Expression of the calcium receptor in human breast cancer—a potential new marker predicting the risk of bone metastases, Eur J Surg Oncol 32 (2006) 511–515.

257. J. Tfelt-Hansen, R.J. MacLeod & N. Chattopadhyay, et al., Calcium-sensing receptor stimulates PTHrP release by pathways dependent on PKC, p38 MAPK, JNK and ERK1/2 in H-500 cells, Am J Physiol Endocrinol Metab 285 (2003) E329–E337.

258. R. Wetzker & F.D. Bohmer, Transactivation joins multiple tracks to the ERK/MAPK cascade, Nat Rev Mol Cell Biol 4 (2003) 651–657.

259. S. Yano, R.J. Macleod & N. Chattopadhyay, et al., Calcium-sensing receptor activation stimulates parathyroid hormone-related protein secretion in prostate cancer cells: role of

epidermal growth factor receptor transactivation, Bone 35 (2004) 664–672.

260. S.D. Cramer, D.M. Peehl & M.G. Edgar, et al., Parathyroid hormone-related protein (PTHrP) is an epidermal growth factor-regulated secretory product of human prostatic epithelial cells, Prostate 29 (1996) 20–29.

261. J. Zhu, X. Jia & G. Xiao, et al., EGF-like ligands stimulate osteoclastogenesis by regulating expression of osteoclast regulatory factors by osteoblasts: Implications for osteolytic bone metastases, J Biol Chem 282 (2007) 26656–26664.

262. N. Normanno, A. De Luca & D. Aldinucci, et al., Gefitinib inhibits the ability of human bone marrow stromal cells to induce osteoclast differentiation: implications for the pathogenesis and treatment of bone metastasis, Endocr Relat Cancer 12 (2005) 471–482.

263. S.J. Kim, H. Uehara & T. Karashima, et al., Blockade of epidermal growth factor receptor signaling in tumor cells and tumor-associated endothelial cells for therapy of androgen-independent human prostate cancer growing in the bone of nude mice, Clin Cancer Res 9 (2003) 1200–1210.

264. K.L. Weber, M. Doucet & J.E. Price, et al., Blockade of epidermal growth factor receptor signaling leads to inhibition of renal cell carcinoma growth in the bone of nude mice, Cancer Res 63 (2003) 2940–2947.

265. U. Heider, C. Fleissner & I. Zavrski, et al., Bone markers in multiple myeloma, Eur J Cancer 42 (2006) 1544–1553.

266. T. Hideshima, C. Mitsiades & G. Tonon, et al., Understanding multiple myeloma pathogenesis in the bone marrow to identify new therapeutic targets, Nat Rev Cancer 7 (2007) 585–598.

267. H. Yasui, T. Hideshima & P.G. Richardson, et al., Novel therapeutic strategies targeting growth factor signalling cascades in multiple myeloma, Br J Haematol 132 (2006) 385–397.

268. M. Kawano, T. Hirano & T. Matsuda, et al., Autocrine generation and requirement of BSF-2/IL-6 for human multiple myelomas, Nature 332 (1988) 83–85.

269. H. Hata, H. Xiao & M.T. Petrucci, et al., Interleukin-6 gene expression in multiple myeloma: a characteristic of immature tumor cells, Blood 81 (1993) 3357–3364.

270. A. Karadag, B.O. Oyajobi & J.F. Apperley, et al., Human myeloma cells promote the production of interleukin 6 by primary human osteoblasts, Br J Haematol 108 (2000) 383–390.

271. M. Abe, K. Hiura & J. Wilde, et al., Osteoclasts enhance myeloma cell growth and survival via cell-cell contact: a vicious cycle between bone destruction and myeloma expansion, Blood 104 (2004) 2484–2491.

272. D. Chauhan, H. Uchiyama & Y. Akbarali, et al., Multiple myeloma cell adhesion-induced interleukin-6 expression in bone marrow stromal cells involves activation of NF-kappa B, Blood 87 (1996) 1104–1112.

273. T. Hideshima, D. Chauhan & P. Richardson, et al., NF-kappa B as a therapeutic target in multiple myeloma, J Biol Chem 277 (2002) 16639–16647.

274. A. Karadag, M. Zhou & P.I. Croucher, ADAM-9 (MDC-9/ meltrin-gamma), a member of the disintegrin and metalloproteinase family, regulates myeloma-cell-induced interleukin-6 production in osteoblasts by direct interaction with the alpha(v)beta5 integrin, Blood 107 (2006) 3271–3278.

275. S. Barille, M. Collette & R. Bataille, et al., Myeloma cells upregulate interleukin-6 secretion in osteoblastic cells

276. R. Bataille, M. Jourdan & X.G. Zhang, et al., Serum levels of interleukin 6, a potent myeloma cell growth factor, as a reflection of disease severity in plasma cell dyscrasias, J Clin Invest 84 (1989) 2008–2011.

277. H. Ludwig, D.M. Nachbaur & E. Fritz, et al., Interleukin-6 is a prognostic factor in multiple myeloma, Blood 77 (1991) 2794–2795.

278. K.C. Anderson, R.M. Jones & C. Morimoto, et al., Response patterns of purified myeloma cells to hematopoietic growth factors, Blood 73 (1989) 1915–1924.

279. X.G. Zhang, J.P. Gaillard & N. Robillard, et al., Reproducible obtaining of human myeloma cell lines as a model for tumor stem cell study in human multiple myeloma, Blood 83 (1994) 3654–3663.

280. R. Bataille, B. Barlogie & Z.Y. Lu, et al., Biologic effects of anti-interleukin-6 murine monoclonal antibody in advanced multiple myeloma, Blood 86 (1995) 685–691.

281. M. Trikha, R. Corringham & B. Klein, et al., Targeted anti-interleukin-6 monoclonal antibody therapy for cancer: a review of the rationale and clinical evidence, Clin Cancer Res 9 (2003) 4653–4665.

282. P.G. Hargreaves, F. Wang & J. Antcliff, et al., Human myeloma cells shed the interleukin-6 receptor: inhibition by tissue inhibitor of metalloproteinase-3 and a hydroxamate-based metalloproteinase inhibitor, Br J Haematol 101 (1998) 694–702.

283. J.P. Gaillard, R. Bataille & H. Brailly, et al., Increased and highly stable levels of functional soluble interleukin-6 receptor in sera of patients with monoclonal gammopathy, Eur J Immunol 23 (1993) 820–824.

284. R. Catlett-Falcone, T.H. Landowski & M.M. Oshiro, et al., Constitutive activation of Stat3 signaling confers resistance to apoptosis in human U266 myeloma cells, Immunity 10 (1999) 105–115.

285. D. Loffler, K. Brocke-Heidrich & G. Pfeifer, et al., Interleukin-6-dependent survival of multiple myeloma cells involves the Stat3-mediated induction of microRNA-21 through a highly conserved enhancer, Blood 110 (2007) 1330–1333.

286. A. Ogata, D. Chauhan & G. Teoh, et al., IL-6 triggers cell growth via the Ras-dependent mitogen-activated protein kinase cascade, J Immunol 159 (1997) 2212–2221.

287. D. Ribatti, A. Vacca & B. Nico, et al., Bone marrow angiogenesis and mast cell density increase simultaneously with progression of human multiple myeloma, Br J Cancer 79 (1999) 451–455.

288. A. Vacca, D. Ribatti & M. Presta, et al., Bone marrow neovascularization, plasma cell angiogenic potential and matrix metalloproteinase-2 secretion parallel progression of human multiple myeloma, Blood 93 (1999) 3064–3073.

289. F. Di Raimondo, M.P. Azzaro & G. Palumbo, et al., Angiogenic factors in multiple myeloma: higher levels in bone marrow than in peripheral blood, Haematologica 85 (2000) 800–805.

290. T. Wrobel, G. Mazur & P. Surowiak, et al., Increased expression of vascular endothelial growth factor in bone marrow of multiple myeloma patients, Eur J Intern Med 14 (2003) 98–100.

through cell-to-cell contact but downregulate osteocalcin, Blood 86 (1995) 3151–3159.

291. D. Gupta, S.P. Treon & Y. Shima, et al., Adherence of multiple myeloma cells to bone marrow stromal cells upregulates vascular endothelial growth factor secretion: therapeutic applications, Leukemia 15 (2001) 1950–1961.

292. B. Dankbar, T. Padro & R. Leo, et al., Vascular endothelial growth factor and interleukin-6 in paracrine tumor-stromal cell interactions in multiple myeloma, Blood 95 (2000) 2630–2636.

293. W.T. Bellamy, L. Richter & Y. Frutiger, et al., Expression of vascular endothelial growth factor and its receptors in hematopoietic malignancies, Cancer Res 59 (1999) 728–733.

294. S. Kumar, T.E. Witzig & M. Timm, et al., Expression of VEGF and its receptors by myeloma cells, Leukemia 17 (2003) 2025–2031.

295. B. Lin, K. Podar & D. Gupta, et al., The vascular endothelial growth factor receptor tyrosine kinase inhibitor PTK787/ZK222584 inhibits growth and migration of multiple myeloma cells in the bone marrow microenvironment, Cancer Res 62 (2002) 5019–5026.

296. K. Podar, Y.T. Tai & F.E. Davies, et al., Vascular endothelial growth factor triggers signaling cascades mediating multiple myeloma cell growth and migration, Blood 98 (2001) 428–435.

297. K. Podar, Y.T. Tai & B.K. Lin, et al., Vascular endothelial growth factor-induced migration of multiple myeloma cells is associated with beta 1 integrin- and phosphatidylinositol 3-kinase-dependent PKC alpha activation, J Biol Chem 277 (2002) 7875–7881.

298. A.C. Newton & J.E. Johnson, Protein kinase C: a paradigm for regulation of protein function by two membrane-targeting modules, Biochim Biophys Acta 1376 (1998) 155–172.

299. K. Podar, M.S. Raab & J. Zhang, et al., Targeting PKC in multiple myeloma: *in vitro* and *in vivo* effects of the novel, orally available small-molecule inhibitor enzastaurin (LY317615, HCl), Blood 109 (2007) 1669–1677.

300. C.S. Mitsiades, N.S. Mitsiades & C.J. McMullan, et al., Inhibition of the insulin-like growth factor receptor-1 tyrosine kinase activity as a therapeutic strategy for multiple myeloma, other hematologic malignancies and solid tumors, Cancer Cell 5 (2004) 221–230.

301. M. Ferlin, N. Noraz & C. Hertogh, et al., Insulin-like growth factor induces the survival and proliferation of myeloma cells through an interleukin-6-independent transduction pathway, Br J Haematol 111 (2000) 626–634.

302. S. Abroun, H. Ishikawa & N. Tsuyama, et al., Receptor synergy of interleukin-6 (IL-6) and insulin-like growth factor-I in myeloma cells that highly express IL-6 receptor alpha, Blood 103 (2004) 2291–2298.

303. Y.W. Qiang, L. Yao & G. Tosato, et al., Insulin-like growth factor I induces migration and invasion of human multiple myeloma cells, Blood 103 (2004) 301–308.

304. Y.T. Tai, K. Podar & L. Catley, et al., Insulin-like growth factor-1 induces adhesion and migration in human multiple myeloma cells via activation of beta1-integrin and phosphatidylinositol 3′-kinase/AKT signaling, Cancer Res 63 (2003) 5850–5858.

305. P. Georgii-Hemming, H.J. Wiklund & O. Ljunggren, et al., Insulin-like growth factor I is a growth and survival factor in human multiple myeloma cell lines, Blood 88 (1996) 2250–2258.

306. T. Standal, M. Borset & S. Lenhoff, et al., Serum insulin-like growth factor is not elevated in patients with multiple myeloma but is still a prognostic factor, Blood 100 (2002) 3925–3929.

307. K. Araki, T. Sangai & S. Miyamoto, et al., Inhibition of bone-derived insulin-like growth factors by a ligand-specific antibody suppresses the growth of human multiple myeloma in the human adult bone explanted in NOD/SCID mouse, Int J Cancer 118 (2006) 2602–2608.

308. J.H. Kehrl, A.B. Roberts & L.M. Wakefield, et al., Transforming growth factor beta is an important immunomodulatory protein for human B lymphocytes, J Immunol 137 (1986) 3855–3860.

309. M. Urashima, A. Ogata & D. Chauhan, et al., Transforming growth factor-beta1: differential effects on multiple myeloma versus normal B cells, Blood 87 (1996) 1928–1938.

310. S.R. Amoroso, N. Huang & A.B. Roberts, et al., Consistent loss of functional transforming growth factor beta receptor expression in murine plasmacytomas, Proc Natl Acad Sci USA 95 (1998) 189–194.

311. T. Fernandez, S. Amoroso & S. Sharpe, et al., Disruption of transforming growth factor beta signaling by a novel ligand-dependent mechanism, J Exp Med 195 (2002) 1247–1255.

312. D.J. Berg & R.G. Lynch, Immune dysfunction in mice with plasmacytomas. *I.* Evidence that transforming growth factor-beta contributes to the altered expression of activation receptors on host B lymphocytes, J Immunol 146 (1991) 2865–2872.

313. T. Hayashi, T. Hideshima & A.N. Nguyen, et al., Transforming growth factor beta receptor I kinase inhibitor downregulates cytokine secretion and multiple myeloma cell growth in the bone marrow microenvironment, Clin Cancer Res 10 (2004) 7540–7546.

314. P.I. Croucher, R. De Hendrik & M.J. Perry, et al., Zoledronic acid treatment of 5T2MM-bearing mice inhibits the development of myeloma bone disease: evidence for decreased osteolysis, tumor burden and angiogenesis and increased survival, J Bone Miner Res 18 (2003) 482–492.

315. S. Yaccoby, R.N. Pearse & C.L. Johnson, et al., Myeloma interacts with the bone marrow microenvironment to induce osteoclastogenesis and is dependent on osteoclast activity, Br J Haematol 116 (2002) 278–290.

316. A. Aparicio, A. Gardner & Y. Tu, et al., *In vitro* cytoreductive effects on multiple myeloma cells induced by bisphosphonates, Leukemia 12 (1998) 220–229.

317. C.M. Shipman, P.I. Croucher & R.G. Russell, et al., The bisphosphonate incadronate (YM175) causes apoptosis of human myeloma cells *in vitro* by inhibiting the mevalonate pathway, Cancer Res 58 (1998) 5294–5297.

318. R. Takahashi, C. Shimazaki & T. Inaba, et al., A newly developed bisphosphonate, YM529, is a potent apoptosis inducer of human myeloma cells, Leuk Res 25 (2001) 77–83.

319. P.M. Doran, R.T. Turner & D. Chen, et al., Native osteoprotegerin gene transfer inhibits the development of murine osteolytic bone disease induced by tumor xenografts, Exp Hematol 32 (2004) 351–359.

320. P.I. Croucher, C.M. Shipman & J. Lippitt, et al., Osteoprotegerin inhibits the development of osteolytic bone disease in multiple myeloma, Blood 98 (2001) 3534–3540.

321. K. Vanderkerken, E. De Leenheer & C. Shipman, et al., Recombinant osteoprotegerin decreases tumor burden and increases survival in a murine model of multiple myeloma, Cancer Res 63 (2003) 287–289.

322. C.M. Shipman & P.I. Croucher, Osteoprotegerin is a soluble decoy receptor for tumor necrosis factor-related apoptosis-inducing ligand/Apo2 ligand and can function as a paracrine survival factor for human myeloma cells, Cancer Res 63 (2003) 912–916.

323. E.M. Sordillo & R.N. Pearse, RANK-Fc: a therapeutic antagonist for RANK-L in myeloma, Cancer 97 (2003) 802–812.

324. R.N. Pearse, E.M. Sordillo & S. Yaccoby, et al., Multiple myeloma disrupts the TRANCE/osteoprotegerin cytokine axis to trigger bone destruction and promote tumor progression, Proceedings of the National Academy of Sciences 98 (2001) 11581–11586.

325. G.D. Roodman, Mechanisms of bone destruction in myeloma. In Skeletal Complications of Malignancy IV, Bethesda, MD, 2005.

326. J.H. Han, S.J. Choi & N. Kurihara, et al., Macrophage inflammatory protein-1alpha is an osteoclastogenic factor in myeloma that is independent of receptor activator of nuclear factor kappaB ligand, Blood 97 (2001) 3349–3353.

327. S.J. Choi, J.C. Cruz & F. Craig, et al., Macrophage inflammatory protein 1-alpha is a potential osteoclast stimulatory factor in multiple myeloma, Blood 96 (2000) 671–675.

328. B.O. Oyajobi & G.R. Mundy, Receptor activator of NF-kappaB ligand, macrophage inflammatory protein-1alpha and the proteasome, Cancer 97 (2003) 813–817.

329. I. Kim, H. Uchiyama & D. Chauhan, et al., Cell surface expression and functional significance of adhesion molecules on human myeloma-derived cell lines, Br J Haematol 87 (1994) 483–493.

330. K. Miyake, K. Medina & K. Ishihara, et al., A VCAM-like adhesion molecule on murine bone marrow stromal cells mediates binding of lymphocyte precursors in culture, J Cell Biol 114 (1991) 557–565.

331. K. Jacobsen, J. Kravitz & P.W. Kincade, et al., Adhesion receptors on bone marrow stromal cells: *in vivo* expression of vascular cell adhesion molecule-1 by reticular cells and sinusoidal endothelium in normal and gamma-irradiated mice, Blood 87 (1996) 73–82.

332. H. Uchiyama, B.A. Barut & D. Chauhan, et al., Characterization of adhesion molecules on human myeloma cell lines, Blood 80 (1992) 2306–2314.

333. T. Michigami, N. Shimizu & P.J. Williams, et al., Cell-cell contact between marrow stromal cells and myeloma cells via VCAM-1 and alpha(4)beta(1)-integrin enhances production of osteoclast-stimulating activity, Blood 96 (2000) 1953–1960.

334. N. Giuliani, R. Bataille & C. Mancini, et al., Myeloma cells induce imbalance in the osteoprotegerin/osteoprotegerin ligand system in the human bone marrow environment, Blood 98 (2001) 3527–3533.

335. Y. Mori, N. Shimizu & M. Dallas, et al., Anti-alpha4 integrin antibody suppresses the development of multiple myeloma and associated osteoclastic osteolysis, Blood 104 (2004) 2149–2154.

336. D.L. Olson, L.C. Burkly & D.R. Leone, et al., Anti-alpha4 integrin monoclonal antibody inhibits multiple myeloma growth in a murine model, Mol Cancer Ther 4 (2005) 91–99.

337. E. Tian, F. Zhan & R. Walker, et al., The role of the Wnt-signaling antagonist DKK1 in the development of osteolytic lesions in multiple myeloma, New England Journal of Medicine 349 (2003) 2483–2494.

338. B. Mao, W. Wu & Y. Li, et al., LDL-receptor-related protein 6 is a receptor for Dickkopf proteins, Nature 411 (2001) 321–325.

339. L.M. Boyden, J. Mao & J. Belsky, et al., High bone density due to a mutation in LDL-receptor-related protein 5, New England Journal of Medicine 346 (2002) 1513–1521.

340. R.D. Little, J.P. Carulli & R.G. Del Mastro, et al., A mutation in the LDL receptor-related protein 5 gene results in the autosomal dominant high-bone-mass trait, American Journal of Human Genetics 70 (2002) 11–19.

341. Y. Gong, R.B. Slee & N. G. Fukai, et al., The Osteoporosis-Pseudoglioma Syndrome Collaborative, LDL receptor-related protein 5 (LRP5) affects bone accrual and eye development, Cell 107 (2001) 513–523.

342. S. Yaccoby, F. Zhan & B. Barlogie, et al., Blocking Dkk1 activity in primary myeloma-bearing SCID-rab mice is associated with increased osteoblast activity and bone formation and inhibition of tumor growth, Journal of Bone & Mineral Research 20 (2005) S33.

343. T. Oshima, M. Abe & J. Asano, et al., Myeloma cells suppress bone formation by secreting a soluble Wnt inhibitor, sFRP-2, Blood 106 (2005) 3160–3165.

344. L.A. Ehrlich, H.Y. Chung & I. Ghobrial, et al., IL-3 is a potential inhibitor of osteoblast differentiation in multiple myeloma, Blood 106 (2005) 1407–1414.

345. J.M. Chirgwin & T.A. Guise, Does prostate-specific antigen contribute to bone metastases?, Clin Cancer Res 12 (2006) 1395–1397.

346. A. Suzuki, J. Shinoda & Y. Watanabe-Tomita, et al., ETA receptor mediates the signaling of endothelin-1 in osteoblast-like cells, Bone 21 (1997) 143–146.

347. S.L. Perkins, E. Sarraj & S.J. Kling, et al., Endothelin stimulates osteoblastic production of IL-6 but not macrophage colony-stimulating factor, Am J Physiol Endocrinol Metab 272 (1997) E461–E468.

348. H.P. von Schroeder, C.J. Veillette & J. Payandeh, et al., Endothelin-1 promotes osteoprogenitor proliferation and differentiation in fetal rat calvarial cell cultures, Bone 33 (2003) 673–684.

349. J.B. Nelson, S.P. Hedican & D.J. George, et al., Identification of endothelin-1 in the pathophysiology of metastatic adenocarcinoma of the prostate, Nat Med 1 (1995) 944–949.

350. G. Le Brun, P. Aubin & H. Soliman, et al., Upregulation of endothelin-1 and its precursor by Il-1β, TNF-α and TGF-β in the PC3 human prostate cancer cell line, Cytokine 11 (1999) 157–162.

351. G.A. Clines, K.S. Mohammad & Y. Bao, et al., Dickkopf homolog 1 mediates endothelin-1-stimulated new bone formation, Mol Endocrinol 21 (2007) 486–498.

352. R. Schwaninger, C.A. Rentsch & A. Wetterwald, et al., Lack of noggin expression by cancer cells is a determinant of the osteoblast response in bone metastases, American Journal of Pathology 170 (2007) 160–175.

353. N. Voorzanger-Rousselot, D. Goehrig & F. Journe, et al., Increased Dickkopf-1 expression in breast cancer bone metastases, Br J Cancer 97 (2007) 964–970.

354. M.A. Forget, S. Turcotte & D. Beauseigle, et al., The Wnt pathway regulator DKK1 is preferentially expressed in hormone-resistant breast tumours and in some common cancer types, Br J Cancer 96 (2007) 646–653.

355. C.L. Hall, A. Bafico & J. Dai, et al., Prostate cancer cells promote osteoblastic bone metastases through Wnts, Cancer Research 65 (2005) 7554–7560.

356. A.S. Alam, A. Gallagher & V. Shankar, et al., Endothelin inhibits osteoclastic bone resorption by a direct effect on cell motility: implications for the vascular control of bone resorption, Endocrinology 130 (1992) 3617–3624.

357. J.W. Chiao, B.S. Moonga & Y.M. Yang, et al., Endothelin-1 from prostate cancer cells is enhanced by bone contact which blocks osteoclastic bone resorption, Br J Cancer 83 (2000) 360–365.

358. A. Tatrai, S. Foster & P. Lakatos, et al., Endothelin-1 actions on resorption, collagen and noncollagen protein synthesis and phosphatidylinositol turnover in bone organ cultures, Endocrinology 131 (1992) 603–607.

359. M.A. Carducci, Prostate cancer update: advanced disease, Rev Urol 5 (Suppl 6) (2003) S47–S53.

360. J.B. Nelson, Endothelin receptor antagonists, World Journal of Urology 23 (2005) 19–27.

361. N.D. James, M. Borre, B. Zonnenberg, et al., ZD4054, a potent, specific endothelin A receptor antagonist, improves overall survival in pain-free or mildly symptomatic patients with hormone-resistant prostate cancer (HRPC) and bone metastases. In *ECCO 14 – the European Cancer Conference*. Barcelona, Spain, 2007.

362. A. Jimeno & M. Carducci, Atrasentan: a novel and rationally designed therapeutic alternative in the management of cancer, Expert Rev Anticancer Ther 5 (2005) 419–427.

363. S.L. Dallas, J.L. Rosser & G.R. Mundy, et al., Proteolysis of latent Transforming Growth Factor-beta (TGF-β)-binding protein-1 by osteoclasts. A cellular mechanism for release of TGF-β from bone matrix, J Biol Chem 277 (2002) 21352–21360.

364. C.S. Killian, D.A. Corral & E. Kawinski, et al., Mitogenic response of osteoblast cells to prostate-specific antigen suggests an activation of latent TGF-beta and a proteolytic modulation of cell adhesion receptors, Biochemical and Biophysical Research Communications 192 (1993) 940–947.

365. M. Steiner, Z. Zhou & D. Tonb, et al., Expression of transforming growth factor-beta 1 in prostate cancer, Endocrinology 135 (1994) 2240–2247.

366. R. Baserga, A. Hongo & M. Rubini, et al., The IGF-I receptor in cell growth, transformation and apoptosis, Biochim Biophys Acta 1332 (1997) F105–F126.

367. K. Fizazi, J. Yang & S. Peleg, et al., Prostate cancer cells-osteoblast interaction shifts expression of growth/survival-related genes in prostate cancer and reduces expression of osteoprotegerin in osteoblasts, Clin Cancer Res 9 (2003) 2587–2597.

368. M. Goya, S.I. Miyamoto & K. Nagai, et al., Growth inhibition of human prostate cancer cells in human adult bone implanted into nonobese diabetic/severe combined immunodeficient mice by a ligand-specific antibody to human insulin-like growth factors, Cancer Res 64 (2004) 6252–6258.

369. M. Iwamura, J. Hellman & A.T. Cockett, et al., Alteration of the hormonal bioactivity of parathyroid hormone-related protein (PTHrP) as a result of limited proteolysis by prostate-specific antigen, Urology 48 (1996) 317–325.

370. S.D. Cramer, Z. Chen & D.M. Peehl, Prostate specific antigen cleaves parathyroid hormone-related protein in the PTH-like domain: inactivation of PTHrP-stimulated cAMP accumulation in mouse osteoblasts, J Urol 156 (1996) 526–531.

371. K.D. Schluter, C. Katzer & H.M. Piper, A N-terminal PTHrP peptide fragment void of a PTH/PTHrP-receptor binding domain activates cardiac ET(A) receptors, Br J Pharmacol 132 (2001) 427–432.

372. C. Festuccia, D. Giunciuglio & F. Guerra, et al., Osteoblasts modulate secretion of urokinase-type plasminogen activator (uPA) and matrix metalloproteinase-9 (MMP-9) in human prostate cancer cells promoting migration and matrigel invasion, Oncol Res 11 (1999) 17–31.

373. C. Festuccia, A. Teti & P. Bianco, et al., Human prostatic tumor cells in culture produce growth and differentiation factors active on osteoblasts: a new biological and clinical parameter for prostatic carcinoma, Oncol Res 9 (1997) 419–431.

374. A. Achbarou, S. Kaiser & G. Tremblay, et al., Urokinase overproduction results in increased skeletal metastasis by prostate cancer cells *in vivo*, Cancer Res 54 (1994) 2372–2377.

375. S.A. Rabbani, J. Gladu & A.P. Mazar, et al., Induction in human osteoblastic cells (SaOS2) of the early response genes fos, jun and myc by the amino terminal fragment (ATF) of urokinase, J Cell Physiol 172 (1997) 137–145.

376. B. Yi, P.J. Williams & M. Niewolna, et al., Tumor-derived platelet-derived growth factor-BB plays a critical role in osteosclerotic bone metastasis in an animal model of human breast cancer, Cancer Res 62 (2002) 917–923.

377. F. Gori, T. Thomas & K.C. Hicok, et al., Differentiation of human marrow stromal precursor cells: bone morphogenetic protein-2 increases OSF2/CBFA1, enhances osteoblast commitment and inhibits late adipocyte maturation, J Bone Miner Res 14 (1999) 1522–1535.

378. K. Tsuji, Y. Ito & M. Noda, Expression of the PEBP2alphaA/AML3/CBFA1 gene is regulated by BMP4/7 heterodimer and its overexpression suppresses type I collagen and osteocalcin gene expression in osteoblastic and nonosteoblastic mesenchymal cells, Bone 22 (1998) 87–92.

379. J. Dai, J. Keller & J. Zhang, et al., Bone morphogenetic protein-6 promotes osteoblastic prostate cancer bone metastases through a dual mechanism, Cancer Res 65 (2005) 8274–8285.

380. M. Kveiborg, A. Flyvbjerg & E. Eriksen, et al., Transforming growth factor-beta1 stimulates the production of insulin-like growth factor-I and insulin-like growth factor-binding protein-3 in human bone marrow stromal osteoblast progenitors, J Endocrinol 169 (2001) 549–561.

381. J.L. Fowlkes, D.M. Serra & R.C. Bunn, et al., Regulation of insulin-like growth factor (IGF)-I action by matrix metalloproteinase-3 involves selective disruption of IGF-I/IGF-binding protein-3 complexes, Endocrinology 145 (2004) 620–626.

382. S. Mochizuki, M. Shimoda & T. Shiomi, et al., ADAM28 is activated by MMP-7 (matrilysin-1) and cleaves insulin-like growth factor binding protein-3, Biochem Biophys Res Commun 315 (2004) 79–84.

383. S. Manes, M. Llorente & R.A. Lacalle, et al., The matrix metalloproteinase-9 regulates the insulin-like growth factor-triggered autocrine response in DU-145 carcinoma cells, J Biol Chem 274 (1999) 6935–6945.

384. J. Hong, G. Zhang & F. Dong, et al., Insulin-like growth factor (IGF)-binding protein-3 mutants that do not bind IGF-I or IGF-II stimulate apoptosis in human prostate cancer cells, J Biol Chem 277 (2002) 10489–10497.

385. H.S. Kim, A.R. Ingermann & J. Tsubaki, et al., Insulin-like growth factor-binding protein 3 induces caspase-dependent apoptosis through a death receptor-mediated pathway in MCF-7 human breast cancer cells, Cancer Res 64 (2004) 2229–2237.

386. M. Nobta, T. Tsukazaki & Y. Shibata, et al., Critical regulation of bone morphogenetic protein-induced osteoblastic differentiation by delta1/jagged1-activated notch1 signaling, J Biol Chem 280 (2005) 15842–15848.

387. K. Tezuka, M. Yasuda & N. Watanabe, et al., Stimulation of osteoblastic cell differentiation by Notch, J Bone Miner Res 17 (2002) 231–239.

388. M. Zayzafoon, S.A. Abdulkadir & J.M. McDonald, Notch signaling and ERK activation are important for the osteomimetic properties of prostate cancer bone metastatic cell lines, J Biol Chem 279 (2004) 3662–3670.

389. L.M. Calvi, G.B. Adams & K.W. Weibrecht, et al., Osteoblastic cells regulate the haematopoietic stem cell niche, Nature 425 (2003) 841–846.

CHAPTER 3

Early Bone Metastasis-Associated Molecular and Cellular Events

PHILIPPE CLÉZARDIN[1,2]

[1]*INSERM, UMR 664, Lyon, France*
[2]*Université Claude Bernard Lyon-1, Villeurbanne, France*

Contents

I. INTRODUCTION

Bone metastases are common complications of several solid tumors, including carcinomas of the breast, prostate and lung [1]. They can be fatal or may rapidly impede the quality of life, causing intractable bone pain, nerve compression syndromes, hypercalcemia and pathological fractures. Bone metastases from breast and lung carcinomas are generally osteolytic, whereas those from prostate carcinoma are most often osteoblastic [1]. In osteolytic metastases, bone-residing metastatic cells do not directly destroy bone. Instead, they secrete different molecules, such as parathyroid hormone-related protein, interleukins (IL-6, IL-8, and IL-11), cytokines (MG-CSF, M-CSF) and prostaglandins that stimulate the activity of bone-resorbing cells (osteoclasts) [1,2]. Breast cancer cells also coopt on to lysophosphatidic acid released from activated platelets as a tumor mitogen and inducer of tumor-derived IL-6 and IL-8 [3]. In addition, they secrete factors (dickkopf-1, Noggin) that inhibit the activity of bone-forming cells (osteoblasts) [4]. This leads to an imbalance between bone resorption and bone formation, resulting in enhanced skeletal destruction and, as a consequence of osteolysis, frequent occurrence of pathological fractures [1]. Conversely, prostate cancer cells secrete factors that activate osteoblasts (endothelin-1,

BMPs, VEGF, Wnts, IGFs) and inhibit osteoclasts (endothelin-1), yielding osteoblastic lesions [1]. However, osteoblastic lesions are also accompanied by pathologic fractures because of the poor quality of bone produced by osteoblasts [1,5]. In addition, secondary resorption of bone may occur in response to abnormal bone formation in osteoblastic lesions, while there is some attempt of bone repair in osteolytic lesions. Indeed, osteolytic and osteoblastic lesions are two extremes of a continuum, and patients can have mixed lesions containing both osteolytic and osteoblastic elements [1].

Given that osteoclasts play a pivotal role in bone metastasis formation, bisphosphonates (as inhibitors of osteoclast-mediated bone resorption) are used extensively to treat patients with bone metastases [6]. Yet, these treatments are only palliative and do not provide a life-prolonging benefit to patients with advanced disease [6]. A better understanding of the molecular mechanisms that precede the overt development of skeletal lesions is therefore required to identify new targets for cancer therapeutics. Gene expression profiling using DNA microarrays has provided insights into the genetic basis of metastasis, showing that organ-specific gene signatures for metastasis formation exist [7–11]. Among genes included in the bone metastasis signature, the focus here is on those that draw metastatic cells to colonize bone. Evidence that cancer cells acquire bone-like properties to adapt and thrive in the bone microenvironment is also presented. Finally, we discuss the possible contribution of stem cell niches in the early development of bone metastases.

II. BONE TROPISM OF CANCER CELLS

A. Chemokines

The tropism of cancer cells to distant organs depends on attraction signals that are conveyed by chemotactic factors called chemokines. Chemokines are a family of low molecular weight (8–10 kDa) pro-inflammatory cytokines which bind to G-protein coupled seven-span transmembrane receptors [12]. The human chemokine system includes more than 50 chemokines which are structurally divided into four groups (C, CC, CXC and CX3C) based upon the arrangement of conserved cysteine residues (C) of the mature proteins. CC, CXC and CX3C chemokines all have four conserved cysteine residues, whereas C chemokines have only two. The first two cysteine residues in CC chemokines are adjacent, whereas one and three amino acids separate the first two cysteine residues in CXC and CX3C chemokines, respectively [12].

The chemokine receptor CXCR4 is included in both the lung and bone metastasis signatures for breast cancer [9,11]. CXCR4 controls the metastatic destination of breast cancer cells in certain organs (lung, liver, and bone marrow) where its ligand, the chemokine CXCL-12, is produced in high quantity [13,14]. For instance, the overexpression of CXCR4 in MDA-MB-231 breast cancer cells promotes bone metastasis formation in nude mice [11]. Just as in breast cancer, high-level expression of CXCR4 has been reported in prostate cancer, and CXCR4 signaling in response to CXCL-12 induces the migration of prostate cancer cells to bone [15]. Consistent with this, the blockade of CXCR4 using antibodies, synthetic peptidic antagonist or small interfering RNA gene silencing reduces the formation of experimental lung and bone metastases caused by CXCR4-expressing breast or prostate cancer cells [16–18], thus validating this chemokine receptor as a metastasis gene. However, other chemokines could be involved in mediating the attraction of cancer cells to bone *in vivo*. For instance, the human lung cancer cell line SBC-5 that efficiently metastasizes to bone *in vivo* expresses the chemokine receptor CCR4. Interestingly, its ligand, the chemokine CCL22, is produced by osteoclasts and stimulates SBC-5 cell migration *in vitro*, suggesting a possible contribution of CCL22 in the bone tropism of lung cancer cells [19]. Similarly, a soluble form of the plasma membrane-bound chemokine CX3CL-1 (fractalkine), which is expressed by osteoblasts and bone marrow-derived endothelial cells, stimulates *in vitro* the migration of prostate cancer cells (PC3-ML, LNCaP, MDA-Pca 2b) that express its receptor CX3CR1 [20]. Thus, stromal cells, osteoclasts and osteoblasts most probably produce different chemokines that enable several types of carcinoma cells to home to bone. However, inhibition of the interaction of chemokines with their cognate receptors only partially blocks metastasis formation *in vivo*, suggesting that additional factors are involved in the bone tropism of cancer cells.

B. RANKL

The cytokine receptor activator of nuclear factor-κB ligand (RANKL), RANK and osteoprotegerin (OPG) have been described as key regulators of osteoclast-mediated bone resorption [21]. RANKL is a transmembrane protein expressed on the surface of osteoblasts [21] that can be shed from the plasma membrane by osteoclast-derived MMP-7 [22]. Both the membrane-bound and soluble form of RANKL attach to RANK, a receptor on the cell surface of osteoclast precursors, to stimulate the formation, activation, migration and survival of osteoclasts [21,23]. Conversely, OPG is a soluble RANKL inhibitor produced by osteoblasts that inhibits RANKL/RANK interaction [21]. Hence, the balance between RANKL and OPG regulates the process of bone resorption.

RANK is not only expressed by osteoclasts, but also by some primary tumors and cancer cell lines (breast, prostate, myeloma, melanoma) [24,25]. In addition, primary tumors are often infiltrated with T cells and macrophages, which are a major source of RANKL [26], and high levels of soluble RANKL have been detected in the serum of patients with osteolytic bone metastases [25]. Taken together, these observations suggest that RANKL levels in the tumor microenvironment and blood circulation could play a critical role in tumor cell dissemination. For instance, prostate tumor infiltration by RANKL-expressing inflammatory cells leads to the repression of maspin, a metastasis suppressor gene, in RANK-expressing prostate carcinoma cells, thereby promoting metastasis formation in animals [26]. Soluble RANKL also triggers the migration of RANK-expressing breast and prostate cancer cells *in vitro*, and OPG blocks the bone tropism of melanoma cells *in vivo* [24]. Thus, RANKL may act as another bone-derived factor that draws cancer cells to metastasize to bone.

III. INTERACTION OF CANCER CELLS WITH THE BONE MARROW ENDOTHELIUM

It is generally accepted that circulating cancer cells have to attach to the endothelium of blood vessels in order to penetrate into surrounding tissues, but there is controversy as to how cancer cells escape from the lumina of these vessels. There is experimental evidence that endothelium-attached cancer cells proliferate within the lumen of the vessel, creating an intravascular tumor that subsequently destroys the vascular walls and grows in the surrounding tissue parenchyma [27]. At the same time, other observations suggest that endothelium-attached cancer cells quickly extravasate in the tissue parenchyma following a process that resembles the transmigration of leukocytes upon inflammatory response [28]. Endothelium transmigration of cancer cells has been frequently observed in sinusoids of the liver using intravital fluorescence microscopy [29,30]. This may be related to the fenestrated nature of liver sinusoidal vessels which facilitates the passage of cancer cells into the parenchyma. Cancer cell extravasation could therefore also occur in sinusoidal vessels of the bone marrow. Indeed, substantial *in vitro* data provide evidence that tumor cells depend on selectins, vascular cell adhesion molecules and integrins to attach to the bone marrow endothelium and extravasate [28]. Importantly, using dynamic *in vivo* confocal imaging, Sipkins *et al.* [31] have shown that cancer cells (leukemia, myeloma, prostate carcinoma) specifically attach to spatially restricted bone marrow endothelial microdomains, allowing the extravasation of these cancer cells in the parenchyma. These vascular microdomains express a unique combination of molecules (E-selectin, CXCL-12) enabling the attachment, then the transendothelial migration of CXCR4-expressing cancer cells [31]. Moreover, hematopoietic stem cells also localize to these microdomains [31], suggesting that there exists vascular gateways with specific 'molecular ZIP codes', enabling the entry of normal and malignant cells into the marrow space.

IV. INVASION OF CANCER CELLS INTO THE BONE

Once cancer cells have arrived within the bone marrow, they have to invade the marrow stroma and travel to the endosteal bone surface. This invasive process requires the coordinated action of integrins with proteases. Integrins serve to attach the cells to the extracellular matrix proteins, whereas proteases degrade the extracellular matrix in the immediate vicinity of these cells, thereby promoting cell motility.

A. Integrins

Integrins constitute a family of cell surface receptors that are heterodimers composed of non-covalently associated α and β subunits [32]. The integrin family is composed of 18 α and 8 β subunits that form heterodimers in various combinations to produce some 24 different integrins [32]. There is a growing body of evidence from preclinical research showing that integrins mediate metastasis to bone [33–37]. For instance, a direct role of α2β1 integrin in prostate cancer bone metastasis has been reported [33]. Prostate cancer cells expressing α2β1 attach and migrate toward type I collagen *in vitro*, and selectively grow within the bone *in vivo* [33]. In a similar vein, Chinese hamster ovarian (CHO) cancer cells transfected to *de novo* express α4β1 integrin specifically metastasize to bone by interacting with vascular cell adhesion molecule (VCAM)-1 which is expressed on bone marrow stromal cells [34]. There is also evidence that αvβ3 integrin expression by breast cancer cells is associated with the ability of these cells to metastasize to bone [35–37]. For instance, the *de novo* expression of αvβ3 in 66cl4 breast cancer and CHO ovarian cancer cells that metastasize to lungs, but not to bone, is sufficient to promote their dissemination to bone [35,36]. Following *in vivo* selection of MDA-MB-231 breast cancer cells, we

have isolated a bone metastatic cell subpopulation (called B02) which constitutively and specifically overexpresses αvβ3 integrin [35], and the overexpression of αvβ3 integrin in the parental MDA-MB-231 cells reproduces the bone metastatic phenotype of B02 cells *in vivo* [37]. In addition, the treatment of animals with a non-peptide αvβ3 integrin antagonist causes a profound and specific inhibition of bone colonization by αvβ3-expressing cancer cells *in vivo* [37]. Indeed, αvβ3 integrin increases the adhesiveness and invasiveness of metastatic breast cancer cells toward bone extracellular matrix proteins [35–37]. For instance, αvβ3 cooperates with bone sialoprotein, osteonectin, and matrix metalloproteinase (MMP)-2 in promoting breast and prostate cancer cell invasion *in vitro* [38–40]. Moreover, αvβ3 and β1 integrins also associate with the urokinase plasminogen activator receptor (uPAR), providing an additional mechanism to recruit proteolytic activity (urokinase, plasmin) to the leading edge of invading cancer cells [32,41]. Taken together, these findings [35–41] strongly suggest that αvβ3, in promoting cell adhesion and invasion, is playing a causal role in the colonization of bone by cancer cells.

B. Proteases

Other proteases (MT1-MMP, MMP-1, cathepsin K) produced by cancer cells could promote invasion of the bone matrix *in vivo*. For instance, membrane type 1-matrix metalloproteinase (MT1-MMP) is a membrane-anchored protease that is expressed *in situ* by prostate cancer cells in human bone metastatic specimens; its ectopic expression in MT1-MMP-deficient LNCaP prostate cancer cells promotes skeletal tumor growth and osteolysis *in vivo* [42]. MMP-1, which specifically degrades the collagen, is overexpressed by breast cancer cells that preferentially metastasize to bone, and is one of the genes included in the bone metastasis signature [11]. Cathepsin K is a cysteine proteinase secreted by osteoclasts that degrades the collagenous matrix of bone. Cathepsin K is also expressed in primary breast and prostate tumors, and overproduced in bone-residing breast and prostate cancer cells [43–45]. The function of cathepsin K in cancer cells is unknown. However, we have observed that a cathepsin K inhibitor blocks B02 breast cancer cell invasion *in vitro*, suggesting cathepsin K could contribute to the invasiveness of B02 cells within bone *in vivo* [45].

V. OSTEOMIMETISM

Once metastatic cells have invaded the bone marrow, they may start to grow and form small clumps of cancer cells called micrometastases. Then, these micrometastases need to adapt to the bone microenvironment in order to survive and acquire the ability to grow into a clinically detectable bone metastasis. In order to adapt to the microenvironment, metastatic cancer cells must acquire bone-like or osteomimetic properties [46]. Using clinical bone metastasis specimens and human breast and prostate cancer cell lines, different studies have reported the expression of several bone-specific proteins (osteocalcin, bone sialoprotein, osteonectin, cathepsin K, notch) in cancer cells that metastasize to the skeleton [45–51]. The expression of these bone-related proteins in cancer cells is regulated by transcription factors (Runx2, MSX2) that have an indispensable role in osteogenesis [47,48,52]. The inactivation of Runx2 in osteotropic breast cancer cells blocks the invasive and osteolytic properties of these cells *in vivo* [52], suggesting that Runx2 plays also a pivotal role in breast cancer bone metastasis. In order to further reveal the osteomimetic properties of bone metastatic cancer cells, we have compared the gene profile of the MDA-MB-231 human breast cancer cell line with that of a variant (B02) selected for its unique ability to metastasize to bone *in vivo* [35]. We found that B02 cells overexpress a set of osteoblastic genes, including cadherin 11 (*CDH11*), cyclooxygenase (*COX-2*), connective tissue growth factor (*CTGF*), connexin 43 (*Cx43*), follistatin (*FST*) and osteonectin (*SPARC*), and that these bone-related proteins are also selectively overexpressed in human breast cancer bone metastases relative to the primary tumor and visceral (liver) metastases [53]. Interestingly, cadherin 11 expression in MDA-MB-231 breast cancer cells promotes bone metastasis formation [54], and osteonectin enhances the invasiveness of breast and prostate cancer cells [39,55]. In addition, CTGF is one of the genes included in the bone metastasis signature and it promotes experimental bone metastasis formation [11]. Taken together, these findings [11,39,45–55] demonstrate that bone-related proteins and skeletal transcription factors that are aberrantly expressed at high levels in metastatic cancer cells play a crucial role in the development of bone metastases.

VI. IMPACT OF BONE MARROW STEM CELL NICHES

A stem cell niche is a specific site in adult tissues where stem cells reside and undergo self-renewal and produce their progeny. In the bone marrow, hematopoietic stem cells reside either next to the bone endosteal surface (osteoblastic niche) or adjacent to sinusoidal vessels (vascular niche) [56]. The osteoblastic niche is maintaining the hematopoietic stem cells in a quiescent state, whereas the vascular niche is regulating the mobilization, proliferation and differentiation of these stem cells [56].

It is generally agreed that cancer cells residing in the bone marrow may remain dormant for many years until some, as yet unknown, signals promote their growth and metastasis formation. Moreover, because of their quiescence, cancer cells may become resistant to chemotherapies, probably explaining the persistence in the bone marrow of a 'minimal residual disease' following treatment.

Indeed, there is an emerging concept that the bone marrow may provide specific anti-apoptotic niches in which cancer cells remain dormant. For instance, bone marrow-derived hematopoietic progenitors which express vascular endothelial growth factor receptor (VEGFR)-1 and α4β1 integrin form cellular clusters that produce CXCL-12, creating a pre-metastatic niche for the arrival of CXCR4-expressing cancer cells [57]. This concept is also supported by the observation that N-cadherin and osteopontin, which are involved in promoting metastasis formation [32,58], are expressed by spindle-shaped N-cadherin$^+$CD45$^-$ osteoblastic (SNO) cells and contribute to the retention of hematopoietic stem cells in the osteoblastic niche [56]. N-cadherin and osteopontin could also mediate the anchoring of cancer cells in osteoblastic niches in a manner that mimics the mechanisms used by SNO cells to retain hematopoietic stem cells in these niches. Moreover, breast and prostate tumor stem cells have been identified [59,60], which could also explain resistance to chemotherapies.

VII. CONCLUSION AND PERSPECTIVES

In this review we have focused on the mechanisms that draw metastatic cells to colonize bone. We have also discussed the possible contribution of osteoblastic and vascular stem cell niches in the early development of bone metastases. Several factors expressed by metastatic cells and other cells from the bone marrow microenvironment (CXCR4/CXCL-12, RANK/RANKL, E-selectin, integrins, proteases, Runx2) have been identified as being capable of mediating the early development of bone metastases. Undoubtedly, these factors provide attractive new targets for cancer therapeutics. However, cancer (stem) cells and bone marrow stem cells use overlapping molecular features to interact with the vascular endothelium, and invade and thrive in the bone marrow, suggesting that therapies targeting some of these factors expressed by cancer cells could also have detrimental effects on bone marrow cells.

References

1. V.A. Siclari, T.A. Guise & J.M. Chirgwin, Cancer Metastasis Rev 25 (2006) 621–633.
2. B.K. Park, H. Zhang & Q. Zeng, et al., Nat Med 13 (2007) 62–69.
3. A. Boucharaba, C.M. Serre & J. Guglielmi, et al., Proc Natl Acad Sci USA 103 (2006) 9643–9648.
4. R. Schwaninger, C.A. Rentsch & A. Wetterwald, et al., Am J Pathol 170 (2007) 160–175.
5. R.D. Loberg, C.J. Logothetis, E.T. Keller & K.J. Pienta, J Clin Oncol 23 (2005) 8232–8241.
6. B.E. Hilner, J.N. Ingle & J.R. Berenson, et al., J Clin Oncol 18 (2000) 1378–1391.
7. M.J. van de Vijver, Y.D. He & L.J. van't Veer, et al., N Engl J Med 347 (2002) 1999–2009.

8. G.V. Glinsky, A.B. Glinskii & A.J. Stephenson, et al., J Clin Invest 113 (2004) 913–923.
9. A.J. Minn, Y. Kang & I. Serganova, et al., J Clin Invest 115 (2005) 44–55.
10. M. Smid, Y. Wang & J.G.M. Klijn, et al., J Clin Oncol 24 (2006) 2261–2267.
11. Y. Kang, P.M. Siegel & W. Shu, et al., Cancer Cell 3 (2003) 537–549.
12. F. Balkwill, Nature Rev Cancer 4 (2004) 540–550.
13. P. Staller, J. Sulitkova & J. Lisztwan, et al., Nature 425 (2003) 307–311.
14. A. Müller, B. Homey & H. Soto, et al., Nature 410 (2001) 50–56.
15. J. Wang, R. Loberg & R.S. Taichman, Cancer Metastasis Rev 25 (2006) 573–587.
16. Z. Liang, T. Wu & H. Lou, et al., Cancer Res 64 (2004) 4302–4308.
17. Y.X. Sun, A. Schneider & Y. Jung, et al., J Bone Miner Res 20 (2005) 318–329.
18. Z. Liang, Y. Yoon & J. Votaw, et al., Cancer Res 65 (2005) 967–971.
19. E.S. Nakamura, K. Koizumi & M. Kobayashi, et al., Clin Exp Metastasis 23 (2006) 9–18.
20. S.A. Shulby, N.G. Dolloff & M.E. Stearns, et al., Cancer Res 64 (2004) 4693–4698.
21. W.J. Boyle, W.S. Simonet & D.L. Lacey, Nature 423 (2003) 337–342.
22. K. Henriksen, M. Karsdal & J.M. Delaissé, et al., J Biol Chem 278 (2003) 48745–48753.
23. C.C. Lynch, A. Hikosaka & H.B. Acuff, et al., Cancer Cell 7 (2005) 485–496.
24. D.H. Jones, T. Nakashima & O.H. Sanchez, et al., Nature 440 (2006) 692–696.
25. W.C. Dougall & M. Chaisson, Cancer Metastasis Rev 25 (2006) 541–549.
26. J.L. Luo, W. Tan & J.M. Ricono, et al., Nature 446 (2007) 690–694.
27. A.B. Al-Medhi, K. Tozawa & A.B. Fisher, et al., Nat Med 6 (2000) 100–102.
28. V.V. Glinsky, Cancer Metastasis Rev 25 (2006) 531–540.
29. S. Ito, H. Nakanishi & Y. Ikehara, et al., Int J Cancer 93 (2001) 212–217.
30. K. Schlüter, P. Gassmann & A. Enns, et al., Am J Pathol 169 (2006) 1064–1073.
31. D.A. Sipkins, X. Wei & J.W. Wu, et al., Nature 435 (2005) 969–973.
32. W. Guo & F.G. Giancotti, Nature Rev Mol Cell Biol 5 (2004) 816–826.
33. C.L. Hall, J. Dai & K.L. van Golen, et al., Cancer Res 66 (2006) 86488654.
34. N. Matsuura, W. Puzon-McLaughlin & A. Irie, et al., Am J Pathol 148 (1996) 55–61.
35. I. Pécheur, O. Peyruchaud & C.M. Serre, et al., FASEB J 16 (2002) 1266–1268.
36. E.K. Sloan, N. Pouliot & K.L. Stanley, et al., Breast Cancer Res 8 (2006) R20.
37. Y. Zhao, R. Bachelier & I. Treilleux, et al., Cancer Res 67 (2007) 5821–5830.
38. A. Karadag, K.U.E. Ogbureke & N.S. Fedarko, et al., J Natl Cancer Inst 96 (2004) 956–965.
39. S. De, J. Chen & N.V. Narizhneva, et al., J Biol Chem 278 (2003) 39044–39050.
40. K. Jacob, M. Webber & D. Benayahu, et al., Cancer Res 59 (1999) 4453–4457.
41. G. van der Pluijm, B. Sijmons & H. Vloedgraven, et al., Am J Pathol 159 (2001) 971–982.
42. R.D. Bonfil, Z. Dong & J.C.T. Filho, et al., Am J Pathol 170 (2007) 2100–2111.
43. A.J. Littlewood-Evans, G. Bilbe & W.B. Bowler, et al., Cancer Res 57 (1997) 5386–5390.
44. K.D. Brubaker, R.L. Vessella & L.D. True, et al., J Bone Min Res 18 (2003) 222–230.
45. C. Le Gall, A. Bellahcène, E. Bonnelye, et al., Cancer Res (2007) 9894–9902.
46. K.S. Koeneman, F. Yeung & L.W. Chung, Prostate 39 (1999) 246–261.
47. J. Yang, K. Fizazi & S. Peleg, et al., Cancer Res 61 (2001) 5652–5659.
48. G.L. Barnes, A. Javed & S.M. Waller, et al., Cancer Res 63 (2003) 2631–2637.
49. M. Zayzafoon, S.A. Abdulkadir & J.M. McDonald, J Biol Chem 279 (2004) 3662.
50. W.C. Huang, Z. Xie & H. Konaka, et al., Cancer Res 65 (2005) 2303–2313.
51. D.A. Campo McKnight, D.M. Sosnoski & J.E. Koblinski, et al., J Cell Biochem 97 (2006) 288–302.
52. A. Javed, G.L. Barnes & J. Pratap, et al., Proc Natl Acad Sci USA 102 (2005) 1454–1459.
53. A. Bellahcène, R. Bachelier & C. Detry, et al., Breast Cancer Res Treat 101 (2007) 135–148.
54. T. Yoneda & T. Hiraga, Biochem Biophys Res Com 328 (2005) 679–687.
55. N. Chen, X.C. Ye & K. Chu, et al., Cancer Res 67 (2007) 6544–6548.
56. T. Yin & L. Li, J Clin Invest 116 (2006) 1195–1201.
57. R.N. Kaplan, R.D. Riba & S. Zacharoulis, et al., Nature 438 (2005) 820–827.
58. R.B. Hazan, G.R. Philipps & R.F. Qiao, et al., J Cell Biol 148 (2000) 779–790.
59. M. Al-Hajj, M.S. Wicha & A. Benito-Hernandez, et al., Proc Natl Acad Sci USA 100 (2003) 3983–3988.
60. A.T. Collins, P.A. Berry & C. Hyde, et al., Cancer Res 65 (2005) 10946–10951.

CHAPTER **4**

Regulation of Osteoblast Differentiation and Bone Cancers by Wnt and PTH Signaling Pathways

JULIA BILLIARD[1], JOHN A. ROBINSON[1], RAMESH A. BHAT[1], BHEEM M. BHAT[1], RICHARD J. MURRILLS[1] AND PETER V.N. BODINE[1]

[1] Women's Health and Musculoskeletal Biology, Wyeth Research, Collegeville, PA, USA.

Contents

I. INTRODUCTION

Bone formation is a dynamic process involving several different cell types including osteoprogenitors, osteoblasts and osteocytes. Osteoblasts arise from mesenchymal stem cells, and the differentiation of these progenitors to osteoblasts is controlled by many growth factors and hormones including Wnts and parathyroid hormone (PTH). The Wnt signaling pathway modulates many cell-fate decisions throughout development by controlling gene expression, cell behavior, adhesion and polarity. Aberrant regulation of the Wnt pathway results in inappropriate expression of target genes that leads to a variety of abnormalities and degenerative diseases and is implicated in several human cancers including osteosarcoma. Studies have indicated that the secreted Wnt antagonist dickkopf-1 inhibits osteoblastic activity, promotes osteoclastic function and plays a role in the pathophysiology of multiple myeloma. Another Wnt antagonist, secreted frizzled-related protein-2, also appears to be involved in this disease. Osteosarcoma is a rare, sporadic malignancy that is found in only 4–5 people per million.

These tumors are malignant mesenchymal cancers that produce osteoid and bone, occasionally in a trabecular pattern. Unlike most cancers, osteosarcoma is predominantly a disease of young people that peaks in the second and third decades of life and appears to be associated with the adolescent growth spurt. This cancer is also more common in patients with Paget's disease, and some studies suggest an additional peak after the age of 50. Pre-clinical safety studies with PTH revealed a link between long-term treatment with the peptide and the development of bone neoplasias. The mechanisms for the induction of osteosarcoma by PTH are not well understood but may involve stimulation of osteoblastic cell proliferation and/or prevention of cellular apoptosis. Since the Wnt signaling pathway also regulates many aspects of normal osteoblast physiology, a better understanding of the role that these growth factors play in bone cancer is also warranted.

II. CONTROL OF OSTEOBLAST DIFFERENTIATION BY PARATHYROID HORMONE AND WNT

Bone formation is a highly dynamic process involving many cell types including osteoprogenitor cells, osteoblasts (OBs), and osteocytes. OBs play a primary role in extracellular matrix (ECM) deposition and mineralization [1], while osteocytes, which express some ECM proteins, are believed to act as mechanosensors signaling to the OBs and other bone cells to regulate their activity [2,3]. OBs arise from mesenchymal stem cells (MSCs) of the colony-forming unit-fibroblast lineage. The MSCs have classically been viewed as derived from the bone marrow [4], although one study suggests that they are also circulating in whole blood [5]. Bone marrow-derived MSCs are the most

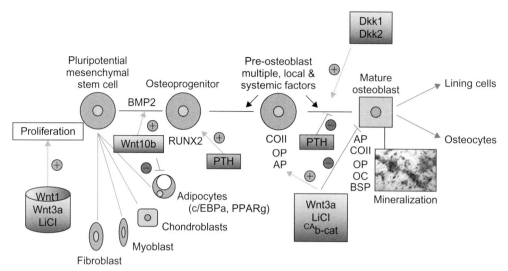

FIGURE 4.1   A model for osteoblast differentiation. Please refer to the text for a discussion of this model.

widely studied and express the surface antigen Stro-1 [1,6]. Although these cells can differentiate to OBs, they can also give rise to other cell lineages, including chondrocytes and adipocytes (Figure 4.1). The early osteoprogenitors are highly proliferative and express the bone-specific transcription factor Runx2, which is required for subsequent differentiation to OBs [1,7]. These cells continue to differentiate to pre-osteoblasts, which are characterized by expression of collagen 1α1 (Col1α1) and alkaline phosphatase (AP) [1]. Pre-osteoblasts eventually cease to proliferate and become mature OBs that synthesize the bone matrix and are characterized by expression of osteocalcin and bone sialoprotein [1,8]. Finally, mature OBs have one of three fates [1,4]: they can differentiate into osteocytes upon entrapment within the ECM; they can differentiate into lining cells; or they can undergo apoptosis. The differentiation of OBs is highly regulated and controlled not only by bone morphogenetic protein 2 (BMP2) [9], but also by other hormones and growth factors including parathyroid hormone (PTH) and Wnt.

The effects of PTH on OB differentiation have been studied extensively both *in vivo* and *in vitro*, but still remain controversial. Treatment with PTH *in vivo* has diverse effects on the bone tissue depending on the mode of administration: continuous infusion causes bone loss, whereas intermittent exposure increases bone formation (reviewed in [10–12]). It is tempting to speculate that these effects of PTH are mediated at least in part by its effects on OB differentiation, but experimental evidence does not necessarily support this hypothesis. Continuous PTH treatment increased [13] or decreased [14] OB number in the rat bone depending on the dosing and the site examined. But in all cases, persistent exposure to PTH greatly increased markers of osteoclastogenesis [15,16] that most likely accounts for the observed catabolic effects of prolonged PTH treatment. The anabolic effects of PTH are mediated in part through

a large increase in the OB number [14,17–19], but whether this increase reflects stimulated OB differentiation remains controversial. Intermittent treatment of rats with PTH increased the percentage of cells in bone marrow that gave rise to AP-positive colonies in culture [20], suggesting that this regimen, directly or indirectly, promotes the early step of differentiation from MSC to osteoprogenitors. However, using electron microscopy, Leaffer *et al.* [18] demonstrated that the number of mature OBs with large cytoplasmic volume increases at the expense of flat lining cells without the increase in total cell number, suggesting that PTH-produced OBs arise from activation of lining cells rather than the differentiation of osteoprogenitors. Alternatively, Jilka *et al.* proposed that the increase in OB number can be accounted for by PTH-induced decrease in OB apoptosis [21].

Studies of direct PTH effects on OB differentiation *in vitro* are complicated, and their outcomes depend primarily on the cell type, the stage of differentiation, and the duration of treatment. Treatment duration seems to be one of the major determinants of PTH effects *in vitro*. A majority of evidence suggests that prolonged exposure to PTH inhibits OB differentiation, whereas shorter exposure stimulates it. Continuous treatment with PTH suppressed matrix mineralization of murine MC3T3-E1 osteoblast-like cells after 30 days [22] and strongly reduced the number of mineralized nodules in primary OB cultures from both rat [23] and mouse [24] calvariae after 17–22 days. In MC3T3-E1 cells, PTH promoted expression of osteocalcin mRNA after 1–6 hr exposure [25], but suppressed AP activity and osteocalcin expression after 72–96 hr of incubation [26]. Similarly, PTH induced bone sialoprotein expression in ROS 17/2.8 rat osteosarcoma cells after 3–12 hr [27], but reduced AP activity in these cells after 3 days of treatment [28].

Several lines of evidence suggest that continuous exposure to PTH in culture inhibits, while intermittent exposure promotes OB differentiation, mimicking anabolic versus catabolic effects of PTH *in vivo*. Continuous PTH treatment of neonatal mouse calvarial cells blocked OB differentiation monitored by green fluorescent protein marker gene driven by differentiation stage-specific *Col1α1* promoter fragments [29]. In contrast, transient PTH exposure resulted in enhanced differentiation and mineralized nodule formation in this system [29]. In a mouse bone marrow culture, intermittent PTH treatment (two cycles of 6 hr on/42 hr off) increased mRNA for OB differentiation markers (Runx2, AP, and type I procollagen), whereas continuous treatment for 96 hr resulted in production of large numbers of TRAP-positive multinucleated osteoclasts [30].

Using mouse osteoblast-like cells isolated from calvarial bones, Isogai *et al.* demonstrated that PTH exerts disparate effects depending on the stage of OB differentiation [31]. Mouse calvarial cells acquire osteoblastic phenotype as they progress through culture, demonstrating increased AP activity and osteocalcin production only after they reach confluence [32]. When PTH was added to these cells for 7 days in the pre-confluent state, it stimulated AP activity [31]. In contrast, PTH addition to confluent cultures for the same length of time inhibited both AP activity and osteocalcin production [31]. These data suggest that PTH promotes differentiation in immature OBs but inhibits it in more mature cells. In support of this hypothesis, PTH increased the proportion of AP-positive colonies [31] and promoted osteocalcin expression [25] in bone marrow cells isolated from mouse tibiae. Furthermore, when mouse calvarial OBs [24] and MC3T3-E1 cells [22] were exposed to PTH for a period of time and then switched to medium without PTH, mineralized nodules appeared very quickly upon PTH withdrawal, and for MC3T3-E1 cells, were 5-fold more pronounced than in the control cultures. These results again suggest that PTH likely promotes early stages of OB differentiation, but inhibits a late stage of this process, perhaps a transition from pre-osteoblasts to mature OBs. This hypothesis, summarized in Figure 4.1, may help explain the disparate effects of PTH depending on treatment duration and whether or not the treatment was removed during differentiation.

It has been shown that PTH can regulate Wnt pathway components and activate β-catenin signaling [33]. Additionally, over the last several years, it has become evident that Wnt/β-catenin signaling may play an important role not only in regulating osteoblastogenesis, but is also involved in controlling MSC cell fate, as well as proliferation and regeneration of these cells (Figure 4.1). Significant effort in this area was initiated when low-density lipoprotein related protein 5 (LRP5) was identified as playing an important role in regulating bone mass [34–37]. Furthermore, recent expression profiling studies of OBs and mesenchymal progenitors (MC3T3-E1, primary mouse calvarial OBs, murine C2C12, human bone marrow derived MSCs) have demonstrated that many components of Wnt signaling including LRP5, LRP6, various Wnts, frizzled receptors,

kremens, and antagonists of the pathway like secreted frizzled related proteins (sFRPs), dickkopfs (Dkks) and Wnt inhibitory factor (Wif) are expressed by these cells [38–40].

Suggestive of the importance of activation of the Wnt/β-catenin pathway in stem cell growth, treatment of mouse and human embryonic stem cells with an inhibitor of glycogen synthase kinase-3 (GSK-3) has been shown to maintain both self-renewal and pluripotency of those cells [41]. Similarly, in murine C3H10T1/2 embryonic stem cells and human bone marrow derived MSCs, Wnt3a or low concentrations of lithium chloride (a non-specific inhibitor of GSK-3) also promoted cell proliferation [42–44]. In addition to these effects on growth and proliferation, activation of Wnt/β-catenin signaling has also been shown to influence differentiation of the MSCs to OBs; however, the actions of Wnt signaling on differentiation are complex as both stimulatory and inhibitory activities like PTH have been reported. With this said, there is increasing support for the concept that activation of Wnt/β-catenin signaling induces early stages of osteoblast differentiation but may inhibit late stage differentiation.

In support of this hypothesis, we have shown that transcription of Runx2 (an early marker of osteoblast differentiation) is upregulated by Wnt1 in MC3T3-E1 osteoprogenitors and embryonic MSCs [45]. In another study, induction of β-catenin signaling using a constitutively active β-catenin expression retrovirus or lithium chloride was shown to induce AP expression similar to BMP2 treatment in C3H10T1/2 cells [46]. However, there was no increase in osteocalcin expression, a marker of late stage of OB differentiation. Similarly, Wnt1, Wnt2 and Wnt3a, which are activators of canonical Wnt/β-catenin signaling, induced AP expression in short-term cultures of C3H10T1/2, ST2 and C2C12 cells but had no effect on other markers of osteoblast differentiation such as Runx2, type I collagen and osteocalcin [44]. In contrast, prolonged exposure to Wnt3a or lithium chloride has been shown to inhibit dexamethosone-induced AP expression and mineralization in human MSCs [42] as well as in murine K5483 pre-osteoblastic cells [47]. Interestingly, expression of Dkk1 and Dkk2, both of which can antagonize Wnt/β-catenin signaling, is increased during osteoblast differentiation [47,48] and silencing of either Dkk1 or Dkk2 expression in long-term cultures of KS483 cells inhibited mineralization and suppressed AP expression [47]. Furthermore, Dkk2 overexpression in calvarial cultures from Dkk2 null mice increased osteocalcin and osteopontin expression that was suppressed in the cells prior to overexpression [48]. In addition, overexpression of Dkk1 or Dkk2 in mouse bone marrow-derived MSCs induced mineralization of these cultures. Collectively, these data suggest that downregulation of Wnt/β-catenin signaling may be required to induce late stage OB differentiation necessary for subsequent mineralization.

Although the extent to which Wnt/β-catenin signaling influences osteoblast differentiation is far from clear, it is evident that this pathway plays an important role in cell fate determination. Specifically, Wnt1 and Wnt10b, which are canonical Wnt pathway activators, have been shown to inhibit adipocyte differentiation of 3T3-L1 pre-adipocytes [49]. This effect was in part due to suppressed expression of the adipocyte markers C/EBPα and PPARγ. In support of this observation, Wnt1 and Wnt10b were shown to increase AP expression and mineralization (in presence of osteogenic media) in ST2 cells, and in presence of adipogenic media, they inhibited adipogenesis as demonstrated by the absence of Oil red O staining and suppressed expression of C/EBPα and PPARγ [50]. Similar effects were seen following Wnt3a overexpression in C3H10T1/2 cells cultured in adipogenic medium as lipidic vacuole formation and expression of PPARγ and aP2 (another marker of adipocyte differentiation) were inhibited [44].

It is well accepted that the process of OB differentiation is controlled by the coordinated efforts of many signaling pathways, and the more we learn about the potential cross-talk between PTH, Wnt, BMP2 and other factors, the greater the likelihood that therapies for bone related disorders will be identified.

III. WNT SIGNALING AND CANCER

The highly regulated Wnt signaling pathway determines many important cell-fate decisions throughout development by controlling gene expression, cell behavior, cell adhesion and cell polarity. Misregulation of the Wnt pathway results in inappropriate expression of the Wnt target genes that leads to a variety of abnormalities and degenerative diseases and is implicated in several human cancers [51]. The role of Wnt in cancer was first suggested with the discovery of Wnt1 as an integration site for mouse mammary tumor virus in mouse mammary carcinoma [52]. Animals ectopically expressing Wnt1 develop mammary and salivary adenocarcinomas. Wnt2 has also been implicated in mouse mammary tumorigenesis through gene amplification [53] and is upregulated in gastric cancers, colorectal cancers, melanoma and in non-small cell lung cancer [54–56]. Overexpression of Wnt2, Wnt5A and Wnt7B is also seen in a subset of human breast carcinomas [57,58]. However, to date, documentation of mutations in Wnt itself in human cancers is rare, but instead mutations in the Wnt signaling pathway components are frequently seen in tumors [59,60]. It is perhaps not surprising, since the Wnt signaling pathway is tightly regulated and overexpression of the Wnt ligand may not necessarily lead to constitutive activation of the pathway; however, dysfunction of the downstream components leads to activation of the pathway in the absence of Wnt. The three most frequently mutated Wnt regulatory proteins are adenomatous polyposis coli (APC), β-catenin, and Axin. The majority of these mutations result in accumulation of the unphosphorylated β-catenin, thereby

constitutively activating gene transcription and potentially promoting carcinogenesis [60,61].

The APC protein acts as a tumor suppressor and was originally discovered as the genetic cause for familial adenomatous polyposis (FAP). FAP patients develop large numbers of colorectal polyps in early adulthood, and without intervention, many of the polyps can further develop into carcinomas and metastatic colorectal cancers [60,62,63]. The APC gene encodes a 2843 amino acid multifunctional protein that plays an integral role in the Wnt signaling pathway and in intracellular adhesion. The N-terminus of APC contains an oligomerization domain followed by the seven repeats of the armadillo motif. The armadillo motif binds to Asef, which is a GDP/GTP exchange protein for the small G protein Rac [64]. The armadillo motif also binds KIF3, which is known to bind to kinesin and regulate vesicle transport on microtubules [65]. Thus, APC may play a role in stabilization and motility of the actin cytoskeleton network [66]. The armadillo region is also known to bind to the regulatory B56 subunit of protein phosphatase 2A, an enzyme that may be involved in the dephosphorylation of specific components of the APC signaling complex [67]. Although the armadillo region is essential for cellular survival and is invariably retained in mutant APC proteins, it is unlikely that it plays an integral role in the tumor suppressor function of APC. The middle portion of APC contains the domains important for interaction with the proteins in the Wnt signaling pathway and is sufficient on its own to function in the pathway. This portion contains seven related, but distinct, 20 amino acid repeat motifs, each of which carries the signature TPxxxFSxxxSL amino acid motif. β-catenin binds to these sites subsequent to phosphorylation of the serine/threonine residues by GSK3β leading to formation of a complex marked for degradation by ubiquitin-mediated proteolysis [62,63]. Downregulation of β-catenin is dependent on the presence of at least three of the seven 20 amino acid repeats in APC, and the majority of APC mutants found in tumors lack all, or most, of these repeats. The central domain also binds Axin via several binding regions containing a characteristic SAMP amino acid sequence that, when altered, results in abolition of Axin binding. Following the 20 amino acid repeats, there are several regions that are involved in binding to the microtubules: the basic amino acid cluster that binds tubulin and promotes tubulin assembly *in vitro*; an S/TXV motif that interacts with the PDZ domain-containing human Dlg homolog; and a binding site for the End-Binding protein, EB1, which is known to be closely associated with the centromere, the mitotic spindle and the distal tip of microtubules at all stages of the cell cycle [62,63].

The majority of FAP patients contain germ line mutations in APC, most of which are nonsense or frameshift mutations that result in a truncated protein with abnormal functions. These patients generally carry additional somatic mutations or loss of heterozygocity at this locus in addition to the original germ line mutation. Somatic mutations in the APC gene are also found in many colorectal adenomas and carcinomas. APC mutations occur early during colorectal tumorigenesis and often result in truncated APC proteins that lack all of the Axin binding sites and all but one or two of the β-catenin binding sites. It is likely that the function of APC in Wnt signaling is responsible for its role in colorectal carcinoma. However, mutant APC may also disrupt the intracellular adhesion and the stability of the cytoskeleton, both of which play a part in cancer progression. Mutations in APC are also detected in other cancers, most notably breast cancer [59,68,69].

The transcription factor β-catenin contains three main domains. The first is the N-terminal portion of approximately 130 amino acids including the $D^{32}SGxxSxxxTxxxS^{45}$ motif that contains putative phosphorylation sites for Casein KinaseIα (CKIα) and GSK3β. The second domain is the central region of 550 amino acids containing 12 segments of 42 amino acids known as armadillo repeats [70]. These repeats form an elongated superstructure with a basically charged groove running along its side. This groove functions as a binding region for Axin, APC, Cadherin, and T-cell Factor [71]. Finally, the C-terminal 110 amino acids harbor a potent transactivation domain that binds essential transcription co-activators such as CBP and Brg-1 [72].

The critical role of β-catenin in tumorigenesis has been demonstrated in humans as well as in animal models. Mutations in the β-catenin gene have been frequently identified in many tumors induced by carcinogens or activated oncogenes, and transgenic animals expressing dominant, stable forms of β-catenin develop tumors [73]. Disregulation of β-catenin signaling is also involved in the development of a broad range of human malignancies. The β-catenin mutants lacking the CKIα and GSK3β phosphorylation sites are more stable than the wild-type protein and can constitutively activate Wnt signaling [74]. Consequently, point mutations in or near the four serine/threonine phosphorylation sites are found in a variety of human cancers, including colon cancers, desmoids tumors, gastric cancers, hepatocarcinoma, medulloblastoma, melanoma, ovarian cancer, uterine endometrial carcinoma, thyroid carcinoma, renal cancer, osteosarcoma, pancreatic cancer and prostate cancer [59,60,68]. Other mutations affecting the N-terminal region of β-catenin make it refractory to regulation by APC. Overexpression of c-myc and cyclin D1 genes that are downstream targets of β-catenin has also been extensively documented in human tumors [75]. Mutations in either APC or β-catenin account for over 90% of colorectal cancers [59]. Furthermore, a significant percentage of non-colon cancers also show apparent accumulation of the β-catenin protein. However, the cause of this β-catenin accumulation is unknown, as these tumors show no mutations in APC and very low incidence of mutations in β-catenin [59,68].

The tumor suppressor Axin is an intracellular protein that binds to the APC/GSK3β/CKIα complex and is pivotal in regulating β-catenin degradation. Axin is an 863 amino acid protein that binds APC via an N-terminal RGS (regulator of the G protein signaling) domain. The central region of Axin contains GSK3β, CKIα and β-catenin binding sites, while the C-terminal region contains a disheveled binding domain. Axin appears to act as a scaffold protein in the formation of a multiprotein complex with APC and β-catenin, which facilitates phosphorylation of both APC and β-catenin by GSK3β and the subsequent degradation of β-catenin. Axin thus acts as a negative regulator of the Wnt signaling pathway by reducing the amount of β-catenin available for transcription activation [74,76]. Mutations of Axin genes and/or its loss of expression have been linked to numerous neoplasms such as colorectal cancer, esophageal squamous cell carcinoma, and medulloblastoma. Mutations in Axin have also been reported in hepatocellular carcinoma with intact genes for β-catenin and APC. All of these mutations generate a truncated form of Axin in which the β-catenin binding site is eliminated [59,68].

Wnt-mediated signals are modulated extracellularly by secreted atagonists. These antagonists, such as sFRP family members, Wif1 and Cerberus, bind to Wnts or frizzled receptors to form inactive complexes, while Dkk1 family members inhibit Wnt signaling by binding to the LRP5 or 6 component of the receptor complex [77,78]. Downregulation of these inhibitor levels has been demonstrated in cervical carcinomas [77–79], breast cancer [80], gastric cancers [81], colorectal cancers, and lung cancers [82]. In most cases, hypermethylation of CpG islands in the promoter region of these antagonists results in transcriptional silencing and is likely to be one of the mechanisms for aberrant activation of the Wnt signaling pathway in cancer [83].

IV. WNT SIGNALING AND OSTEOSARCOMA

Canonical Wnt signaling has been shown to play a role in osteosarcoma. Haydon *et al.* examined β-catenin protein levels in 47 human osteosarcoma samples [84]. These authors found that cytoplasmic and/or nuclear β-catenin levels were elevated in 70% of these tumor samples, and that this correlated with younger age at presentation. However, this accumulation did not result from activating mutations in exon 3 of the gene, indicating that other mechanisms lead to the increase in cellular β-catenin. Consistent with these findings, Hoang *et al.* reported that 50% of human osteosarcoma samples examined (22 of 44) expressed the Wnt co-receptor LRP5 [85]. Moreover, these authors observed that expression of this gene correlated with tumor metastasis. This research group also studied the effects of the Wnt antagonist, Dkk3, on invasive activity and motility of the human osteosarcoma cell line Saos-2 [86]. Overexpression of Dkk3 by Saos-2 cells reduced cytoplasmic β-catenin levels and prevented nuclear translocation of the protein, indicating that canonical Wnt signaling was suppressed. Overexpression of Dkk3 and a dominant negative LRP5 also suppressed the *in vitro* invasive index and motility of the cells, suggesting a potential role for canonical Wnt signaling in tumor metastasis. However, overexpression of Dkk3 also improved the ability of Saos-2 cells to survive treatment with cisplatin and doxorubicin, implying that downregulation of canonical Wnt signaling may increase drug resistance.

V. DKK1 AND CANCER METASTASES TO BONE

Dkk1 is the first identified and the most studied member of the Dkk family of secreted proteins, which contains a total of four members, Dkk1-4. Dkk1 binds to LRP5/6 and a transmembrane receptor Kremen, and this ternary complex becomes internalized removing LRP5/6 from the cell surface and inhibiting canonical Wnt-LRP5-Frizzled signaling [87]. Among Dkks, Dkk1, 2, and 4 inhibit canonical Wnt signaling, while Dkk2 can also act as an activator of the signal depending on the cellular context [88,89]. Since its discovery as an embryonic head inducer in Xenopus [90], Dkk1 has been identified in humans and various vertebrates and invertebrates [91]. Human Dkk1 is a 256 amino acid protein that migrates at ~45 kDa due to glycosylation [92]. Dkk1 contains two cysteine-rich domains, and the C-terminal cysteine-rich domain folds in a distinct pattern known as colipase fold [93]. Deletion analysis of Dkk1 revealed that this colipase domain is essential and sufficient for the Wnt-inhibitory activity in cell culture systems, although its potential significance *in vivo* is yet to be determined [89,94]. Furthermore, the C-terminal 21 amino acids within the colipase domain as well as proper glycosylation are necessary for full activity [95]. Deletion and mutation analysis of LRP5/6 indicates that among four distinct β-propeller/EGF-like domains in the extracellular region, Dkk1 binds to the 3rd and 4th propellers [96], and the 1st propeller can confer resistance to Dkk1 [97–99]. Conversely, the entire extracellular domain of Kremen is necessary for Dkk1-mediated endocytosis of the receptor complex and inhibition of Wnt-LRP5-TCF signal [87,95,100]. Dkk1 can also inhibit LRP5-β-catenin signal that is mediated by other, Wnt-unrelated, ligands, such as Norrin [101,102].

Dkk1 is expressed in various organs including brain, skin, gastrointestinal track, kidney, pancreas, lungs, and bone [103]. The role of Dkk1 in regulating bone maintenance was first suggested when the LRP5 G171V mutation that causes high bone mass in humans and in animal models showed resistance to Dkk1-mediated inhibition *in vitro* [34,35,37,97,104]. This role was confirmed when

mice heterozygous for the Dkk1 deletion were found to have increased bone density [105]. Homozygous deletion of Dkk1 is embryonic lethal [106]. Furthermore, ovariectomy-induced bone loss is accompanied by increased levels of Dkk1, and treatment of ovariectomized rats with Dkk1 antisense oligonucleotide *in vivo* increases bone mineral density [107].

More recent studies indicate that in addition to inhibiting the Wnt-mediated osteoblastic activity, Dkk1 also could promote osteoclastic function [107–109]. Osteoclasts (OCs) are derived from bone marrow macrophages through a differentiation process controlled by receptor activator of nuclear factor-κB ligand (RANKL) and osteoprotegerin (OPG) [110]. RANKL is expressed by OBs, binds to RANK on OCs and is the primary mediator of OC differentiation, activation, and survival. OPG inhibits RANKL activity by binding to it and acting as a decoy receptor. Activation of β-catenin in OBs induces OPG expression and thus prevents OC formation [111]. In keeping with its role as a Wnt-β-catenin antagonist, Dkk1 increases the number and activity of OCs *in vitro* [107]. Furthermore, monoclonal antibodies against Dkk1 block or reduce osteoclastogenesis in animal models [112]. Given that Dkk1 regulates bone homeostasis, it is perhaps not surprising that it plays a role in a variety of cancers that metastasize to bone.

The first cancer shown to have abnormal levels of Dkk1 expression was multiple myeloma (MM) [113]. MM is a highly debilitating and fatal neoplastic disease of B cell origin. This disease is characterized by severe bone pain and pathologic fractures in >80% of patients due to increased osteolysis and suppressed bone formation that lead to bone-lysing (osteolytic) lesions [108,114]. Myeloma cells from MM patients with focal osteolytic lesions show markedly higher expression of Dkk1 and RANKL as compared to the cells from patients without detectable bone lesions [113], and serum levels of Dkk1 and RANKL are also increased in MM patients with osteolytic lesions [115,116]. Since elevated levels of Dkk1 suppress Wnt signaling and decrease OB activity, whereas elevated RANKL enhances OC activity, together they could promote formation of osteolytic lesions and favor the growth of tumor cells. In fact, reducing the serum levels of Dkk1 and RANKL with Bortezomib (a clinically approved proteosome inhibitor for MM) leads to increased bone formation and decreased bone resorption [116]. Furthermore, in animal models of MM, treatment with Dkk1 antibodies increases OB numbers and bone mineral density, decreases OC numbers and stops lesion progression [112]. However, unlike MM, Dkk1 is not overexpressed in patients with chronic lymphocytic leukemia who have osteolytic syndrome very similar to that observed in MM [117].

In addition to MM, a number of solid tumors frequently metastasize to bone, including breast and prostate. These cancers can generate two types of bone metastases. They can cause formation of bone-lysing (osteolytic) lesions similar to MM or give rise to bone-forming (osteoblastic) lesions with enhanced OB activity [118]. Clinically, tumor growth in bone can cause fractures, pain associated with nerve compression, and paralysis. The seriousness of this phenomenon has been documented in prostate cancer, where greater than 80% of men who die of the disease have skeletal metastases [119]. It has recently been suggested that the level of Dkk1 expression by the tumor cells determines the phenotype of bone lesions [120]. Dkk1 is abundantly expressed in human PC-3 prostate cancer cells, which are very osteolytic, but not in a variety of other prostate cancer cell lines, which produce mixed lytic/blastic lesions [120]. Stable overexpression of Dkk1 in the prostate cancer cell lines that normally do not express this protein, significantly increases osteolysis following injection of the cells into the marrow space of immunodeficient mice [120]. Conversely, shRNA-mediated inhibition of Dkk1 in PC-3 cells confers osteoinductive properties upon this cell line. Based on these results, Hall and co-workers propose that high levels of Dkk1 block Wnt-induced OB differentiation, and also supress Wnt-mediated inhibition of osteoclastogenesis resulting in increased osteolysis. Low expression of Dkk1 results in increased OB differentiation and switches the lesion phenotype to bone-forming.

In addition to production of Dkk1 by cancer cells, this Wnt inhibitor is also expressed in OBs, wherein its expression is regulated by endothelin-1 (ET-1) [121]. ET-1 is a 21 amino acid peptide produced by tumor cells, which is considered to be one of the primary regulators of osteoblastic bone metastases of prostate and breast cancers [122]. ET-1 acts through a pair of G-protein-coupled receptors expressed in OBs, ETAR and ETBR [123,124]. Oral administration of an ETAR inhibitory compound (ABT-627) prevents development of osteoblastic bone lesions by ET-1-producing human breast cancer cell lines when infused into nude mice [122]. Similar effects of the compound was reported in men with advanced prostate cancer with bone metastasis [125]. ET-1 has been shown to decrease Dkk1 expression in OBs [121]. Furthermore, addition of recombinant Dkk1 blocked ET-1-mediated OB proliferation and new bone formation in calvarial organ cultures, whereas a Dkk1-neutralizing antibody increased OB numbers and new bone formation [121]. Thus reduction of Dkk1 expression in OBs appears to mediate ET-1-stimulated new bone formation.

In summary, current evidence suggests that Dkk1, produced by both cancer cells and the bone microenvironment, promotes formation of osteolytic lesions but inhibits bone-forming metastases.

VI. SFRP-2 AND MULTIPLE MYELOMA

Another secreted Wnt antagonist, sFRP-2, also appears to play a role in MM. Oshima *et al.* examined conditioned media from the human MM cell lines, RPMI8226 and U266 for secreted factors that suppress *in vitro* bone

formation [126]. Treatment of mouse MC3T3-E1 osteoblasts with BMP-2 increased AP activity and mineralized nodule formation, but this was reduced by co-treatment with RPMI8226 and U266 cell conditioned media. Of the secreted Wnt antagonists examined (sFRP-1, -2, -3 and Dkk1), sFRP-2 mRNA and protein levels were elevated in the MM cell lines, and conditioned media also contained this inhibitor. The authors went on to show that primary human MM cells also expressed sFRP-2 protein, and that immunodepletion of sFRP-2 from RPMI8226 and U266 cell conditioned media restored the ability of BMP-2 to promote *in vitro* bone formation by the MC3T3-E1 cells. Moreover, removal of sFRP-2 from the conditioned medium of RPMI8226 cells correlated with an elevation of canonical Wnt signaling in the primary murine osteoblasts.

VII. PTH AND OSTEOSARCOMA

A. Osteosarcoma

Osteosarcoma (osteogenic sarcoma) is a rare malignancy, being found only in 4–5 people per million [127]. Unlike most cancers, osteosarcoma is predominantly a disease of young people that peaks in the second and third decades of life and appears to be associated with the adolescent growth spurt [128]. It is more common in patients with Paget's disease [129], and some studies suggest an additional peak after the age of 50 [128,130] which is absent in regions where Paget's is infrequently reported [129].

Osteosarcomas are malignant mesenchymal cancers that produce osteoid and bone, sometimes in a trabecular pattern [128,131]. These tumors are typically present as bony masses arising in the metaphysis of rapidly growing long bones, with about 50% being found in the proximal tibia or distal femur [131]. The predominant cell type in osteosarcoma is osteoblastic (50–80%) with fibroblastic-fibrohistiocytic or chondroblastic components [128]. Some osteosarcomas can be osteolytic or mixed, and they can destroy cortical bone [131].

B. Pathogenesis of Osteosarcoma

Current theories suggest that cancer results from accumulation of genetic damage in genes controlling the cell cycle, particularly tumor suppressor genes. This can occur because of a high rate of genetic instability, a reduction in the cell's ability to repair genetic errors, or through an enhanced rate of cell division that limits the amount of time available for repair prior to the next division. Risk factors for osteosarcoma include radiation, which induces genetic damage [132]; the adolescent growth spurt, which increases the rate of cell division; and Paget's disease [129], which increases the local rate of bone turnover.

Some genetic conditions are associated with a predisposition to osteosarcoma. Hereditary retinoblastoma, for example, increases the incidence of osteosarcoma to 500 times that of the general population [133,134], and other syndromes such as Li-Fraumeni syndrome, Rothmund-Thomson syndrome, Werner syndrome and Blooms syndrome cause similar predispositions. The mutations responsible for these hereditary syndromes are known and play roles in the cell cycle and function as recessive tumor suppressors [128,135].

However, a majority of osteosarcoma cases are not due to inherited syndromes and are sporadic. It is noteworthy that the genes mutated in the hereditary syndromes (i.e. RB1, p53, RTS, WRN, BLM) are also altered in many sporadic cases of osteosarcoma. For example, RB1, the gene altered in hereditary retinoblastoma, is also altered in 50–90% of sporadic osteosarcomas [39,128,136], and p53 (Li-Fraumeni syndrome) is mutated in 15–30% of osteosarcomas [39]. For a more complete survey of genetic alterations in osteosarcoma the reader is referred to the recent excellent review by Kansara & Thomas [128].

C. Osteosarcoma Observed in Animal Studies with PTH

Three separate animal toxicity trials, two with subcutaneous PTH(1-34) (teriparatide, Forteo) [137,138] and one with full-length PTH(1-84) [139], revealed a strong, dose-related link between long-term treatment with PTH and the development of bone neoplasms in Fischer 344 rats. Osteosarcomas were by far the most common bone neoplasm observed in each study, while osteoma, osteoblastoma, fibrosarcoma and focal OB hyperplasia, although observed, were rare [137,139]. The tibia was the most common site for osteosarcoma, although tumors were found all over the skeleton except the feet and paws [137,139]. No tumor induction was noted in non-osseous tissues, even those known to have PTH receptors (e.g., kidney) suggesting a possibility of the bone targeting of PTH, presumably through PTH receptors on bone cells.

Prolonged treatment of at least 11 months was required for tumor induction. In female rats, the lag period before tumor production upon PTH(1-34) treatment was 530 days (at the 75 µg/kg dose), 560 days (at 30 µg/kg), or 600 days (at 5 µg/kg) [138]. In males, the lag period was shorter, being only 347 days at the highest dose (75 µg/kg) and 507 days at the intermediate dose (30 µg/kg), while an insufficient number of tumors was observed at the lowest dose (5 µg/kg) [138]. A 6-month treatment commencing at a young age (2 months) followed by no treatment for up to 18 months was insufficient to induce significant tumorigenesis [138]. For PTH(1-84), a delayed start to dosing, which avoided dosing animals until they were approximately 34 weeks old, appeared to protect males but not females from tumorigenesis [139]. Hence, it was not possible to show a convincing effect of young age as a co-factor for the induction of osteosarcoma by PTH, perhaps because, unlike

the human, most of the rat's growth plates do not close until very late in its life, if at all.

D. Mechanism of Induction of Osteosarcoma by PTH

PTH is not mutagenic or genotoxic [140], so we must seek alternative explanations for the induction of osteosarcoma. Possible mechanisms for oncogenesis could involve a stimulation of proliferation or a prevention of apoptosis by PTH. However, the literature on whether or not PTH induces OB proliferation or delays apoptosis is complex.

In some *in vitro* studies, PTH has been reported to directly stimulate proliferation of OBs or OB-like cells, but the effect appears to be concentration-, cell density- and cell-type-dependent. For example, while PTH-stimulated proliferation has been reported in TE-85 cells [141,142] and in chick bone cells [143], proliferation was only detected in UMR 106-01 rat osteosarcoma cells at low concentrations of PTH [144], and only in high density cell cultures in OBs derived from human trabecular bone [145]. In one study using chick cells, PTH had no effect alone but potentiated the mitogenic effect of IGF-1 [146]. There is evidence that activation of the PLC/PKC/ERK pathways is favorable to proliferation of PTH receptor-bearing bone and kidney cells [143,144,147], and consistent with this, no cAMP response was noted in TE-85 cells that nonetheless proliferated in response to PTH [142]. Activation of the cAMP pathway has been reported to result in either inhibition or stimulation of proliferation depending upon the expression level of B-Raf in the cells, which directs cAMP signaling toward the mitogenic ERK pathway [148].

Although it may appear that there is a substantial body of *in vitro* evidence supporting a direct proliferative effect of PTH on bone cells, it should be noted that several *in vitro* studies using UMR 106 rat osteosarcoma cells have shown that PTH inhibited proliferation [141,149–152], and inhibition of proliferation was also noted in mouse MC3T3 cells [153], human Saos-2 osteosarcoma cells [154], rat calvarial cells [155] and in proliferating OB progenitors recovered from the primary spongiosa of young rats (3–5 weeks old) [156].

In vivo studies have shown that an osteogenic regimen of PTH increases bone marrow osteoprogenitor cell numbers [20,157], and a continuous PTH infusion induces peri-trabecular fibrosis that has been interpreted as indicating mesenchymal cell proliferation [158]. In contrast, *in vivo* studies failed to detect a stimulatory effect of PTH on OB proliferation, and the bone anabolic effect of PTH has been attributed to an increase in differentiation of OBs, activation of lining cells, and/or an increase in longevity of the OB (discussed in the first section of this chapter).

A plausible explanation for the induction of osteosarcoma has been proposed by Whitfield [159], based upon PTH inducing proliferation of primitive OB precursors, via mitogenic growth factors emanating from PTH-responsive osteoblasts; for example, IGF-1, FGF-2 and TGF-β [157,159]. Such indirect proliferative effects might result in the perpetuation and proliferation of progenitor cells containing oncogenic mutations and thus be responsible for the induction of osteosarcoma [159].

An alternative hypothesis is that PTH prevents the apoptosis of OBs. The effects of PTH on apoptosis are also complex. *In vitro*, PTH has been reported to have either inhibitory or stimulatory effects on apoptosis [21,160–162]. *In vivo*, using PTH(1-34), a decrease in apoptosis has been reported in mice [21], but the opposite appears to be true in rats [163] and humans [164], where PTH(1-34) increased the number of apoptotic osteocytes or bone cells. At one point it was hypothesized that the full-length PTH(1-84) might differ in its effects on apoptosis from PTH(1-34), because PTH-(1-84) induced apoptosis in osteocytes that did not express the PTH1 receptor, but instead expressed a receptor for the C-terminal region of PTH [165]. As PTH(1-34) lacks this C-terminal region, the hypothesis predicted that PTH(1-34) would not exert this apoptotic effect and the lack of apoptosis would result in, or fail to block, the development of osteosarcoma. However, subsequent animal studies showed that PTH(1-84) did induce osteosarcoma and other bone cancers, just as PTH(1-34) did, and this effect differed only in that the PTH(1-84) study found a single dose (10 μg/kg) that induced bone formation without inducing osteosarcoma [139]. Hence, there does not seem to be strong evidence at this point for delayed apoptosis playing a role in the development of osteosarcoma in PTH-treated rats.

E. The Risk of Osteosarcoma for Patients Treated with PTH

Following the appearance of osteosarcomas in animals, and the simultaneous termination of the ongoing clinical trial, the FDA ruled that patient populations with a predisposition to osteosarcoma (i.e., those with a history of radiation exposure, young adults with open epiphyses, and Paget's disease patients) were contraindicated for PTH osteoporosis treatment. The early termination of the clinical trial after 18 months also means that the safety of PTH is only established for 18 months; hence, patients cannot be treated for longer than this time period.

Several authorities appear confident that there is little risk of osteosarcoma to patients, based on a variety of arguments:

1. In safety studies, rats were dosed for almost all their lives, whereas patients would only be dosed for 18 months [138,140]. There is a correlation between an animal's maximal lifespan and its rate of DNA repair, such that short-lived species (e.g., rat) have less efficient DNA repair mechanisms than longer-lived ones (e.g., human) [166]. Consequently, during 18 months, a rat might be expected to retain more potential cancer-causing mutations

than a human patient. A review of available data suggested that humans have 5.3 times the rate of DNA repair of a rat [167], lending support to the assumption that 18 months in a rat's life is more cancer-prone than 18 months in a human's life. However, the precise margin of safety for this assumption, which should also include an allowance for differing rates at which mutations may occur, is not known.

2. The dose used in the rat studies is 150–200 times higher than that used for humans [159]. However, when we take into account a longer PTH half-life in humans and other differences in pharmacokinetic parameters between the species [168], the exposure multiple is only 3-fold greater in the rats for the 5 μg/kg dose, which was oncogenic [169].

3. The incidence of osteosarcoma in older people being treated for osteoporosis is low [140]. However, we have seen that even though this is true, the addition of an extra risk factor (e.g., the high turnover of Paget's disease) may trigger osteosarcoma in older patients. In fact, one study suggests that the incidence of osteosarcoma in older Paget's patients, as deduced from autopsy studies, may actually be as high as 30% [129].

4. Patients with hyperparathyroidism who have been exposed to chronically elevated levels of PTH do not have a higher incidence of osteosarcoma [140]; Conversely, patients with osteosarcoma do not have high circulating levels of PTH. Retrospective analyses have indicated that each of these statements is true [127,170]. However, while these studies are reassuring, the differing plasma profiles of PTH in hyperparathyroidism (persistent elevation of PTH levels) and during PTH therapy (transient elevation of PTH levels following injection) suggest that these data should be interpreted cautiously [165].

Hence, although monitoring of patients treated with PTH(1-34) has to date shown no evidence of osteosarcoma induction [169], there remain several theoretical reasons why vigilance should be maintained, and the current data should most wisely be interpreted as an encouraging progress report, and not necessarily as conclusive proof of the long-term safety of PTH treatment [169].

VIII. CONCLUSIONS AND PERSPECTIVES

It has been known for many years that intermittent administration of PTH stimulates bone formation *in vivo*. Moreover, *in vitro* studies have shown that PTH regulates many aspects of osteoblast physiology including proliferation, differentiation and apoptosis. Canonical Wnt signaling has also been discovered to play a vital role in the control of bone formation through modulation of the osteoblast. Thus, it is perhaps not entirely surprising that potential points of intersection have been found in bone cells between these two important pathways. However, additional research is needed to more firmly establish this crosstalk as a mechanism for bone anabolism.

Likewise, although PTH appears to control osteoblast proliferation, differentiation and apoptosis, it is not clear which of these events is key to the development of osteosarcoma. Similarly, while canonical Wnt signaling is known to contribute to the development of non-skeletal tumors like colorectal cancer, links between this pathway and bone neoplasias are less well established. Consequently, further studies are also required to more fully refine not only the molecular actions by which PTH and Wnts control bone formation, but also the relationships between these events and tumor development.

References

1. J.B. Lian, G.S. Stein, E. Canalis, et al., Primer on the Metabolic Bone Diseases and Disorders of Mineral Metabolism, in: M.J. Favus, (Ed.), Lippincott Williams & Wilkins, Philadelphia (1999), pp. 14–29.

2. C.T. Rubin & L.E. Lanyon, J Orthop Res 5 (1987) 300–310.

3. A.F. Taylor, M.M. Saunders & D.L. Shingle, et al., Am J Physiol Cell Physiol 292 (2007) C545–C552.

4. J.E. Aubin, Journal of Cellular Biochemistry Supplements 30/31 (1998) 73–82.

5. S. Khosla & G.Z. Eghbali-Fatourechi, Ann NY Acad Sci 1068 (2006) 489–497.

6. P. Bianco, M. Riminucci & S. Kuznetsov, et al., Critical Reviews in Eukaryotic Gene Expression 9 (1999) 159–173.

7. A. Yamaguchi, T. Komori & T. Suda, Endocrine Reviews 21 (2000) 393–411.

8. P. Gehron Robey, P. Bianco & J.D. Termine, Disorders of Bone and Mineral Metabolism, in: F.L. Coe & M.J. Favus, (eds), Raven Press, New York (1992), pp. 241–264.

9. J.M. Wozney, Spine 27 (2002) S2–S8.

10. L. Qin, L.J. Raggatt & N.C. Partridge, Trends Endocrinol Metab 15 (2004) 60–65.

11. C.J. Rosen & J.P. Bilezikian, J Clin Endocrinol Metab 86 (2001) 957–964.

12. R. Murrills, Clinical Reviews in Bone and Mineral Metabolism 4 (2007) 233–257.

13. P.H. Watson, L.J. Fraher & M. Kisiel, et al., Bone 24 (1999) 89–94.

14. H. Dobnig & R.T. Turner, Endocrinology 138 (1997) 4607–4612.

15. A.B. Hodsman, L.J. Fraher & T. Ostbye, et al., J Clin Invest 91 (1993) 1138–1148.

16. Y.L. Ma, R.L. Cain & D.L. Halladay, et al., Endocrinology 142 (2001) 4047–4054.

17. H. Dobnig & R.T. Turner, Endocrinology 136 (1995) 3632–3638.

18. D. Leaffer, M. Sweeney & L.A. Kellerman, et al., Endocrinology 136 (1995) 3624–3631.

19. I.U. Schmidt, H. Dobnig & R.T. Turner, Endocrinology 136 (1995) 5127–5134.

20. S. Nishida, A. Yamaguchi & T. Tanizawa, et al., Bone 15 (1994) 717–723.

21. R.L. Jilka, R.S. Weinstein & T. Bellido, et al., J Clin Invest 104 (1999) 439–446.

22. P.C. Schiller, G. D'Ippolito & B.A. Roos, et al., J Bone Miner Res 14 (1999) 1504–1512.

23. A.J. Koh, B. Demiralp & K.G. Neiva, et al., Endocrinology 146 (2005) 4584–4596.

24. C.G. Bellows, H. Ishida & J.E. Aubin, et al., Endocrinology 127 (1990) 3111–3116.

25. D. Jiang, R.T. Franceschi & H. Boules, et al., J Biol Chem 279 (2004) 5329–5337.

26. J.A. Robinson, V. Susulic & Y.B. Liu, et al., J Cell Biochem 98 (2006) 1203–1220.

27. Y. Ogata, S. Nakao & R.H. Kim, et al., Matrix Biol 19 (2000) 395–407.

28. S.B. Rodan, M. Noda & G. Wesolowski, et al., J Clin Invest 81 (1988) 924–927.

29. Y.H. Wang, Y. Liu & K. Buhl, et al., J Bone Miner Res 20 (2005) 5–14.

30. R.M. Locklin, S. Khosla & R.T. Turner, et al., J Cell Biochem 89 (2003) 180–190.

31. Y. Isogai, T. Akatsu & T. Ishizuya, et al., J Bone Miner Res 11 (1996) 1384–1393.

32. T.A. Owen, M. Aronow & V. Shalhoub, et al., J Cell Physiol 143 (1990) 420–430.

33. N.H. Kulkarni, D.L. Halladay & R.R. Miles, et al., J Cell Biochem 95 (2005) 1178–1190.

34. P. Babij, W. Zhao & C. Small, et al., J Bone Miner Res 18 (2003) 960–974.

35. L.M. Boyden, J. Mao & J. Belsky, et al., N Engl J Med 346 (2002) 1513–1521.

36. M. Kato, M.S. Patel & R. Levasseur, et al., J Cell Biol 157 (2002) 303–314.

37. R.D. Little, J.P. Carulli & R.G. Del Mastro, et al., Am J Hum Genet 70 (2002) 11–19.

38. S.L. Etheridge, G.J. Spencer & D.J. Heath, et al., Stem Cells 22 (2004) 849–860.

39. I. Kalajzic, A. Staal & W.P. Yang, et al., J Biol Chem 280 (2005) 24618–24626.

40. B.L. Vaes, K.J. Dechering & E.P. van Someren, et al., Bone 36 (2005) 803–811.

41. N. Sato, L. Meijer & L. Skaltsounis, et al., Nat Med 10 (2004) 55–63.

42. J. de Boer, R. Siddappa & C. Gaspar, et al., Bone 34 (2004) 818–826.

43. J. De Boer, H.J. Wang & C. Van Blitterswijk, Tissue Eng 10 (2004) 393–401.

44. G. Rawadi, B. Vayssiere & F. Dunn, et al., J Bone Miner Res 18 (2003) 1842–1853.

45. T. Gaur, C.J. Lengner & H. Hovhannisyan, et al., J Biol Chem 280 (2005) 33132–33140.

46. G. Bain, T. Muller & X. Wang, et al., Biochem Biophys Res Commun 301 (2003) 84–91.

47. G. van der Horst, S.M. van der Werf & H. Farih-Sips, et al., J Bone Miner Res 20 (2005) 1867–1877.

48. X. Li, P. Liu & W. Liu, et al., Nat Genet 37 (2005) 945–952.

49. S.E. Ross, N. Hemati & K.A. Longo, et al., Science 289 (2000) 950–953.

50. C.N. Bennett, K.A. Longo & W.S. Wright, et al., Proc Natl Acad Sci USA 102 (2005) 3324–3329.

51. P. Polakis, Curr Opin Genet Dev 17 (2007) 45–51.
52. R. Nusse & H.E. Varmus, Cell 31 (1982) 99–109.
53. M.C. Yoshida, M. Wada & H. Satoh, et al., Proc Natl Acad Sci USA 85 (1988) 4861–4864.
54. M. Katoh, Int J Mol Med 12 (2003) 811–816.
55. R.F. Holcombe, J.L. Marsh & M.L. Waterman, et al., Mol Pathol 55 (2002) 220–226.
56. K. Pham, T. Milovanovic & R.J. Barr, et al., Mol Pathol 56 (2003) 280–285.
57. E.L. Huguet, J.A. McMahon & A.P. McMahon, et al., Cancer Res 54 (1994) 2615–2621.
58. R.V. Iozzo, I. Eichstetter & K.G. Danielson, Cancer Res 55 (1995) 3495–3499.
59. R.H. Giles, J.H. van Es & H. Clevers, Biochim Biophys Acta 1653 (2003) 1–24.
60. H. Clevers, Cell 127 (2006) 469–480.
61. R.T. Moon, A.D. Kohn & G.V. De Ferrari, et al., Nat Rev Genet 5 (2004) 691–701.
62. N.S. Fearnhead, M.P. Britton & W.F. Bodmer, Hum Mol Genet 10 (2001) 721–733.
63. I.S. Nathke, Annu Rev Cell Dev Biol 20 (2004) 337–366.
64. Y. Kawasaki, T. Senda & T. Ishidate, et al., Science 289 (2000) 1194–1197.
65. T. Jimbo, Y. Kawasaki & R. Koyama, et al., Nat Cell Biol 4 (2002) 323–327.
66. Y. Kawasaki, R. Sato & T. Akiyama, Nat Cell Biol 5 (2003) 211–215.
67. J.M. Seeling, J.R. Miller & R. Gil, et al., Science 283 (1999) 2089–2091.
68. P. Polakis, Genes Dev 14 (2000) 1837–1851.
69. S. Segditsas & I. Tomlinson, Oncogene 25 (2006) 7531–7537.
70. T. Akiyama, Cytokine Growth Factor Rev 11 (2000) 273–282.
71. L. Shapiro, Nat Struct Biol 8 (2001) 484–497.
72. N. Barker, A. Hurlstone & H. Musisi, et al., Embo J 20 (2001) 4935–4943.
73. N. Harada, Y. Tamai & T. Ishikawa, et al., Embo J 18 (1999) 5931–5942.
74. A. Kikuchi, Cancer Sci 94 (2003) 225–229.
75. H.H. Luu, R. Zhang & R.C. Haydon, et al., Curr Cancer Drug Targets 4 (2004) 653–671.
76. S. Ikeda, S. Kishida & H. Yamamoto, et al., Embo J 17 (1998) 1371–1384.
77. Y. Kawano & R. Kypta, J Cell Sci 116 (2003) 2627–2634.
78. J.S. Rubin, M. Barshishat-Kupper & F. Feroze-Merzoug, et al., Front Biosci 11 (2006) 2093–2105.
79. J. Ko, K.S. Ryu & Y.H. Lee, et al., Exp Cell Res 280 (2002) 280–287.
80. F. Ugolini, E. Charafe-Jauffret & V.J. Bardou, et al., Oncogene 20 (2001) 5810–5817.
81. K.F. To, M.W. Chan & W.K. Leung, et al., Life Sci 70 (2001) 483–489.
82. J. Mazieres, B. He, L. You & Z. Xu, et al., Cancer Lett 222 (2005) 1–10.
83. O. Aguilera, A. Munoz & M. Esteller, et al., Endocr Metab Immune Disord Drug Targets 7 (2007) 13–21.
84. R.C. Haydon, A. Deyrup & A. Ishikawa, et al., International Journal of Cancer 102 (2002) 338–342.
85. B.H. Hoang, T. Kubo & J.H. Healey, et al., International Journal of Cancer 109 (2004) 106–111.
86. B.H. Hoang, T. Kubo & J.H. Healey, et al., Cancer Research 64 (2004) 2734–2739.
87. B. Mao, W. Wu & G. Davidson, et al., Nature 417 (2002) 664–667.
88. P. Fedi, A. Bafico & A. Nieto Soria, et al., J Biol Chem 274 (1999) 19465–19472.
89. B.K. Brott & S.Y. Sokol, Mol Cell Biol 22 (2002) 6100–6110.
90. A. Glinka, W. Wu & H. Delius, et al., Nature 391 (1998) 357–362.
91. C. Guder, S. Pinho, T.G. Nacak, H.A. Schmidt, B. Hobmayer, C. Niehrs & T.W. Holstein, Development 133 (2006) 901–911.
92. V.E. Krupnik, J.D. Sharp & C. Jiang, et al., Gene 238 (1999) 301–313.
93. L. Aravind & E.V. Koonin, Curr Biol 8 (1998) R477–R478.
94. B. Mao & C. Niehrs, Gene 302 (2003) 179–183.
95. B.M. Bhat, H. Lam & V. Coleburn, et al., J Bone Miner Res 20 (2005) S364.
96. B. Mao, W. Wu & Y. Li, et al., Nature 411 (2001) 321–325.
97. B.M. Bhat, K.M. Allen & J. Graham, et al., J Bone Miner Res 18 (2003) S46.
98. M. Ai, S.L. Holmen & W. Van Hul, et al., Mol Cell Biol 25 (2005) 4946–4955.
99. B.M. Bhat, K.M. Allen & W. Liu, et al., Gene 391 (2007) 103–112.
100. G. Davidson, B. Mao & I. del Barco Barrantes, et al., Development 129 (2002) 5587–5596.
101. Q. Xu, Y. Wang & A. Dabdoub, et al., Cell 116 (2004) 883–895.
102. B.M. Bhat, H. Lam & V. Coleburn, et al., Mol Biol Cell 17 (suppl) (2006) 68.
103. K. Fjeld, P. Kettunen & T. Furmanek, et al., Dev Dyn 233 (2005) 161–166.
104. Y. Zhang, Y. Wang & X. Li, et al., Mol Cell Biol 24 (2004) 4677–4684.
105. F. Morvan, K. Boulukos & P. Clement-Lacroix, et al., J Bone Miner Res 21 (2006) 934–945.
106. M. Mukhopadhyay, S. Shtrom & C. Rodriguez-Esteban, et al., Dev Cell 1 (2001) 423–434.
107. F.S. Wang, J.Y. Ko & C.L. Lin, et al., Bone 40 (2007) 485–492.
108. G.D. Roodman, Clin Cancer Res 12 (2006) 6270s–6273s.
109. D. Diarra, M. Stolina & K. Polzer, et al., Nat Med 13 (2007) 156–163.
110. T. Suda, N. Takahashi, N. Udagawa & E. Jimi, et al., Endocr Rev 20 (1999) 345–357.
111. D.A. Glass II, P. Bialek & J.D. Ahn, et al., Dev Cell 8 (2005) 751–764.
112. S. Yaccoby, W. Ling & F. Zhan, et al., Blood 109 (2007) 2106–2111.
113. E. Tian, F. Zhan & R. Walker, et al., N Engl J Med 349 (2003) 2483–2494.
114. M.G. Alexandrakis, F.H. Passam & N. Malliaraki, et al., Clin Chim Acta 325 (2002) 51–57.
115. M.C. Politou, D.J. Heath & A. Rahemtulla, et al., Int J Cancer 119 (2006) 1728–1731.
116. E. Terpos, D.J. Heath & A. Rahemtulla, et al., Br J Haematol 135 (2006) 688–692.

117. V. Lazarevic, A. Wahlin & M. Hultdin, et al., Leuk Lymphoma 47 (2006) 1987–1988.
118. C.L. Hall, A. Bafico & J. Dai, et al., Cancer Res 65 (2005) 7554–7560.
119. L. Bubendorf, A. Schopfer & U. Wagner, et al., Hum Pathol 31 (2000) 578–583.
120. C.L. Hall, S. Kang & O.A. MacDougald, et al., J Cell Biochem 97 (2006) 661–672.
121. G.A. Clines, K.S. Mohammad & Y. Bao, et al., Mol Endocrinol 21 (2007) 486–498.
122. K.S. Mohammad & T.A. Guise, Clin Orthop Relat Res 415 (Suppl) (2003) S67–S74.
123. H. Arai, S. Hori & I. Aramori, et al., Nature 348 (1990) 730–732.
124. T. Sakurai, M. Yanagisawa & Y. Takuwa, et al., Nature 348 (1990) 732–735.
125. M.A. Carducci & A. Jimeno, Clin Cancer Res 12 (2006) 6296s–6300s.
126. T. Oshima, M. Abe & J. Asano, et al., Blood 106 (2005) 3160–3165.
127. C. Jimenez, Y. Yang & H.W. Kim, et al., J Bone Miner Res 20 (2005) 1562–1568.
128. M. Kansara & D.M. Thomas, DNA Cell Biol 26 (2007) 1–18.
129. M.F. Hansen, M. Seton & A. Merchant, J Bone Miner Res 21 (Suppl 2) (2006) P58–P63.
130. H.D. Dorfman & B. Czerniak, Cancer 75 (1995) 203–210.
131. M. Whyte, Primer on the metabolic bone diseases and disorders of mineral metabolism, in: M.J. Favus, (ed.), American Society for Bone and Mineral Research, Washington, DC (2006), pp. 368–375.
132. B. Fuchs & D.J. Pritchard, Clin Orthop Relat Res 397 (2002) 40–52.
133. M.F. Hansen, A. Koufos & B.L. Gallie, et al., Proc Natl Acad Sci USA 82 (1985) 6216–6220.
134. F.L. Wong, J.D. Boice Jr. & D.H. Abramson, et al., JAMA 278 (1997) 1262–1267.
135. L.L. Wang, Cancer J 11 (2005) 294–305.
136. A. Deshpande & P.W. Hinds, Curr Mol Med 6 (2006) 809–817.
137. J.L. Vahle, M. Sato & G.G. Long, et al., Toxicol Pathol 30 (2002) 312–321.
138. J.L. Vahle, G.G. Long & G. Sandusky, et al., Toxicol Pathol 32 (2004) 426–438.
139. J. Jolette, C.E. Wilker & S.Y. Smith, et al., Toxicol Pathol 34 (2006) 929–940.
140. R.M. Neer, C.D. Arnaud & J.R. Zanchetta, et al., N Engl J Med 344 (2001) 1434–1441.
141. T. Onishi & K. Hruska, Endocrinology 138 (1997) 1995–2004.
142. R.D. Finkelman, S. Mohan & T.A. Linkhart, et al., Bone Miner 16 (1992) 89–100.
143. C. Duvos, A. Scutt & H. Mayer, Bone 17 (1995) 403–406.
144. J.T. Swarthout, T.A. Doggett & J.L. Lemker, et al., J Biol Chem 276 (2001) 7586–7592.
145. B.R. MacDonald, J.A. Gallagher & R.G. Russell, Endocrinology 118 (1986) 2445–2449.
146. E.M. Spencer, E.C. Si & C.C. Liu, et al., Acta Endocrinol (Copenh) 121 (1989) 435–442.
147. D. Somjen, I. Binderman & K.D. Schluter, et al., Biochem J 272 (1990) 781–785.
148. T. Fujita, T. Meguro & R. Fukuyama, et al., J Biol Chem 277 (2002) 22191–22200.
149. K.K. Pun, J Biochem (Tokyo) 106 (1989) 1090–1093.
150. A.J. Felsenfeld, A. Iida-Klein & T.J. Hahn, J Bone Miner Res 7 (1992) 1319–1325.
151. M. Nasu, T. Sugimoto & H. Kaji, et al., Endocr J 45 (1998) 229–234.
152. N.C. Partridge, A.L. Opie & R.T. Opie, et al., Calcif Tissue Int 37 (1985) 519–525.
153. V.K. Tam, T.L. Clemens & J. Green, Endocrinology 139 (1998) 3072–3080.
154. M. Nasu, T. Sugimoto & H. Kaji, et al., J Endocrinol 167 (2000) 305–313.
155. L. Qin, J. Tamasi & L. Raggatt, et al., J Biol Chem 280 (2005) 3974–3981.
156. J.E. Onyia, B. Miller & J. Hulman, et al., Bone 20 (1997) 93–100.
157. P.J. Kostenuik, J. Harris & B.P. Halloran, et al., J Bone Miner Res 14 (1999) 21–31.
158. R. Kitazawa, Y. Imai & M. Fukase, et al., Bone Miner 12 (1991) 157–166.
159. J.F. Whitfield, Medscape Womens Health 6 (2001) 7.
160. H.L. Chen, B. Demiralp & A. Schneider, et al., J Biol Chem 277 (2002) 19374–19381.
161. H. Sowa, H. Kaji & M.F. Iu, et al., J Biol Chem 278 (2003) 52240–52252.
162. P.R. Turner, S. Mefford & S. Christakos, et al., Mol Endocrinol 14 (2000) 241–254.
163. D. Stanislaus, X. Yang & J.D. Liang, et al., Bone 27 (2000) 209–218.
164. R. Lindsay, H. Zhou & F. Cosman, et al., J Bone Miner Res 22 (2007) 495–502.
165. J. Fox, Curr Opin Pharmacol 2 (2002) 338–344.
166. R.W. Hart & R.B. Setlow, Basic Life Sci 5B (1975) 801–804.
167. G.A. Cortopassi & E. Wang, Mech Ageing Dev 91 (1996) 211–218.
168. C.A. Frolik, E.C. Black & R.L. Cain, et al., Bone 33 (2003) 372–379.
169. A.H. Tashjian Jr. & R.F. Gagel, J Bone Miner Res 21 (2006) 354–365.
170. U. Cinamon & R.E. Turcotte, Bone 39 (2006) 420–423.

CHAPTER **5**

Osteoclast Differentiation and Function

LUIS FILGUEIRA[1]

[1] School of Anatomy and Human Biology, University of Western Australia, Australia

Contents

I. OSTEOCLASTS IN HEALTH AND DISEASE

Osteoclasts are the only bone resorptive cells (Figure 5.1). They are essential for healthy bone development, bone growth and bone remodeling. Consequently, most conditions affecting osteoclasts interfere with bone metabolism. However, under physiological conditions, osteoclast recruitment, differentiation and function are under the tight control of osteoblasts (bone forming cells). Therefore, conditions affecting osteoblasts may well result in dysfunction of osteoclasts.

II. OSTEOCLAST RECRUITMENT

Osteoclasts are recruited to the site of bone resorption as they are resident in the bone resorption area only as long as they are needed for their function. Cells are recruited from the blood microcirculation or directly from the red bone marrow at a precursor stage. The mechanism and regulation of recruitment is, at present, not well understood. However, osteoclast precursor cells derive from the myeloid lineage and the cells form part of the large macrophage family that includes Kupffer cells of liver and other tissue macrophages, as well as myeloid dendritic cells [1–5]. Human blood osteoclast precursors express DC45 (leucocyte marker), CD33 (myeloid marker), CD14 (monocyte marker), RANK (receptor activator of NFκB) and M-CSF (macrophage colony stimulating factor, CSF1) receptor [1] and OSCAR (osteoclast associate receptor) [6]. Depending on the specific tissue-related micro-environment and corresponding factors, the precursor cells differentiate into a variety of macrophage-related cells including myeloid dendritic cells and osteoclasts [7,8]. Chemokines that are produced by bone lining cells, or osteoblasts of the endosteum or periosteum, attract precursor cells expressing corresponding chemokine receptors to the bone resorption site. The chemokine CCL9/MIP-1γ and its receptor CCR1 are the most important osteoclast recruitment factors [9–11]. The mechanisms and signals leading to chemokine secretion and subsequent osteoclast recruitment are still not known. It is postulated

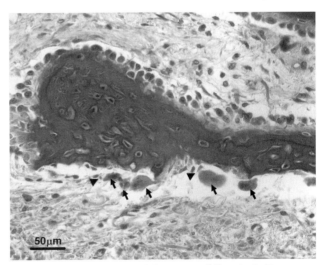

FIGURE 5.1 Histology of bone remodeling including osteoclasts (azan stain). This histological sample shows primary foetal spongiosa. On the upper site, osteoblasts deposit new bone matrix onto the surface of the bone. On the lower site, osteoclasts (arrows) seen as large, multinucleated cells are resorbing bone matrix. Note that some osteoblastic cells are in close contact with the osteoclasts (arrow heads).

Bone Cancer
ISBN: 978-0-12-374895-9

that osteocytes may be the initiators of a signal cascade that includes the sensing of biomechanical changes in the bone matrix by osteocytes or cell death of osteocytes. This is followed by interaction and communication of this sensing between the osteocytes and the bone lining cells which results in chemokine secretion and the subsequent attraction of the osteoclast precursor cells [12]. Most interestingly, in cases of functional osteoclast deficiency, increased recruitment of precursor cells and elevated osteoclast numbers have been documented, probably as a compensatory mechanism [13,14]. Once recruited to the site of action, the osteoclast precursor cells will further differentiate, mature and become fully functional. This process of osteoclast differentiation and maturation is called 'osteoclastogenesis'.

A. Osteoclastogenesis

Osteoclast differentiation and function is under the control of neighboring immature osteoblasts or bone lining cells of the endosteum or periosteum [15]. Thereby tight cell-to-cell contact and interaction between the osteoblasts and the newly recruited osteoclast precursor cells are needed. Membrane bound RANK-L (RANK-ligand, also known as osteoprotegerin-ligand or TRANCE) and M-CSF, expressed by the osteoblastic cells, are essential factors for further differentiation, maturation, function and survival of osteoclasts [16,17]. Consequently, osteoblast pathologies, including genetic related changes in M-CSF and RANK-L expression, certainly influence osteoclast differentiation. Under physiological conditions, Wnt signaling has also been shown to influence osteoblasts in their osteoclastogenic function [18,19]. Furthermore, corticosteroids, estrogens, testosterone and other factors play a regulatory role in osteoclastogenesis, mainly in an indirect manner through influencing the osteoblasts [14,20–22]. Finally, a variety of neoplasms able to form osteoclastic bone metastases are able to mimic or influence the osteoblastic function of osteoclast differentiation and activation [23,24]. Genetically modified mouse models have been very helpful in elucidating osteoclastogenesis. Thereby, deficiency of M-CSF, RANK-L or RANK indicate that these factors are essential for osteoclastogenesis [25–29]. In addition, co-stimulatory receptors signaling through ITAM motifs also contribute to osteoclastogenesis [30].

Differentiation of osteoclasts works in parallel with an expression of the vitronectin receptor $\alpha v\beta 3$, and calcitonin receptor [31,32]. The vitronectin receptor $\alpha v\beta 3$ mediates the attachment of the cells to the bone matrix surface and delivers an additional signal of differentiation and survival [33,34]. The calcitonin receptor regulates the resorptive function of the cells depending on blood calcium concentration and the secretion of calcitonin by the C-cells (parafollicular cells) of the thyroid gland [35].

Produced by osteoblasts, M-CSF acts through binding to its c-Fms surface membrane receptor, expressed by the osteoclasts. Functional loss of c-Fms leads to deficient

osteoclastogenesis resulting in osteopetrosis, as shown by the op/op and the cfslr-deficient mouse models [16]. However, Flt3-ligand acting through Flt3, belonging to the same receptor family of the class III receptor tyrosine kinases, may compensate for M-CSF and c-Fms deficiency, as well as IL-3 and GM-CSF, binding to their receptors, which belong to the hematopoietin receptor superfamily [36–42]. However, GM-CSF, as well as IL-3 and FLt3-ligand may well redirect osteoclast precursor cell towards dendritic cell differentiation depending on the differentiation stage, but the detailed mechanisms and the stage where the two cell types separate are still not known [43–45].

Interaction between membrane bound RANK-L and RANK is tightly regulated by the osteoblastic expression of osteoprotegerin (OPG), a soluble decoy receptor that is a member of the TNF receptor family [46]. OPG binds RANK-L and prevents RANK-L from binding to RANK. Consequently, the ratio between RANK-L and OPG is determining whether there is enough free RANK-L available, binding to RANK and finally acting on the osteoclasts. As OPG and soluble RANK-L are also expressed by other cells, including immune cells and neoplastic cells, the OPG to RANK-L ratio may be influenced by extraosseous factors [47,48]. Induction of RANK signaling, upon binding of its ligand, results in activation of AKT/PKP through src and TRAF-6 (TNF receptor-associated factor 6) [49–53]. However, RANK signaling may be even more complicated and there seems to be additional signaling pathways involved [54]. Furthermore, the RANK signaling pathway integrates multiple other cytokines and factors through their receptors. Most of those factors are immune related and manifest the close relationship between osteoclasts and the immune system and inflammatory processes. However, a multitude of other factors and receptor activation are able to influence and modify RANK signaling, including TNFα, IL-17, IL-25, IFNγ, TLR-2 ligands, TLR-4 ligands [55–59]. In addition to interfering with the RANK signaling pathways in osteoclasts, immune cells express and use OPG/RANK/RANK-L as signaling molecules in many ways and therefore may interfere with osteoclastogenesis or osteoclast function [60–63].

Since M-CSF and RANK-L are available as recombinant proteins, osteoclasts can also be generated *in vitro* from blood or bone marrow derived precursor cells in the presence of these cytokines in a variety of species, including avian, mouse, and human cells [7,31,64,65] (Figure 5.2). Consequently, *in vitro* investigation of osteoclastogenesis and osteoclast function has become possible (Figures 5.3 and 5.4).

Finally, there is one morphological peculiar process of osteoclastogenesis: fusion of mononucleated cells to giant multinucleated syncytia. The reason why the cells fuse and the mechanism is unknown. For fusion, expression of macrophage fusion receptor (MFR) and CD47 are required [66]. However, for the bone resorptive function, cell fusion seems

Dermal-like dendritic cell

GM-CSF
IL-4

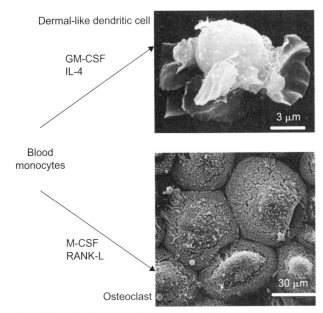

Blood
monocytes

M-CSF
RANK-L

Osteoclast

FIGURE 5.2 *In vitro* differentiation of human monocyte to osteoclasts and dendritic cells *in vitro* under the influence of different cytokines.

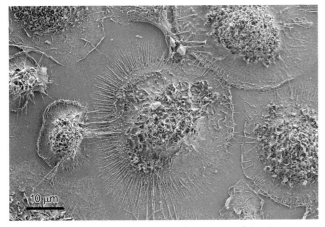

FIGURE 5.3 Scanning electron microscopy of *in vitro* generated human osteoclasts.

not to be required, as active mononucleated osteoclasts are detected in histological specimens of bone. On the other hand, giant cells may well be more active and efficient in their bone resorptive function.

III. OSTEOCLAST FUNCTION

Bone resorption is the main function of osteoclasts. In addition, and related to bone resorption, osteoclasts influence calcium homeostasis. Calcium metabolism and physiological calcium blood serum concentrations are essential to life. Consequently, osteoclast function and bone resorption are included in the sophisticated regulatory mechanisms of calcium homeostasis [67,68]. However, calcium homeostasis will not be covered here.

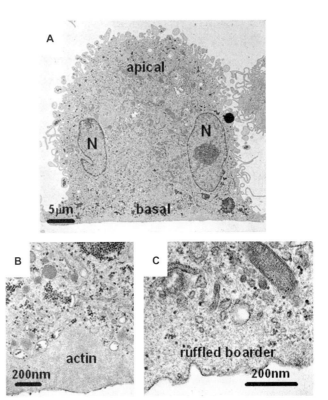

FIGURE 5.4 Transmission electron microscopy of *in vitro* generated human osteoclasts. (a) Lower magnification showing a cross-section through a human osteoclast and two of its nuclei (N); (b) Higher magnification of the basal area of a human osteoclast focusing on the actin ring; (c) Higher magnification of the basal area of a human osteoclast focusing on the ruffled border.

To understand osteoclast function one has first to understand how the cells are morphologically organized. They are polarized cells. They enter in contact with the bone matrix through their basal membrane. They stabilize their peripheral basal membrane, called the sealing zone, through binding to matrix vitronectin by the $\alpha v \beta 3$ receptor and forming a strong sub-membranous actin-containing cytoskeleton ring [69–71]. Through tight attachment to the matrix, the cells enclose in the center of the basal membrane a resorption lacuna or resorption pit. The basal membrane covering the resorption lacuna is called the ruffled border because of its irregular surface as seen with transmission electron microscopy. The ruffled border is a very dynamic cellular compartment as secretion and phagocytosis processes are going on at the same time. Between the ruffled border and the bone matrix, within the lacuna, the osteoclasts generate a specific resorptive environment. A variety of enzymes are continually synthesized, transported towards and secreted into the lacuna. In addition, protons are released for the acidification of the lacunar area through vacuolar-type H+-ATPase [71]. Low pH is essential for dissolving the calcium apatite crystals and thus decalcification of the bone matrix [72,73]. In addition, the low pH optimizes the working conditions for multiple enzymes involved in bone matrix degradation [74].

Cathepsin K (catK) is one of the enzymes secreted into the resorption pit. CatK is essential for degradation of the bone matrix. However, it is expressed not only in osteoclasts, but also in osteoblasts [13,75]. Mutations in the corresponding gene and subsequent catK deficiency in mouse models and in humans result not only in impairment of bone resorption and consequently osteopetrotic syndromes, but also in osteoblast function disruption, which is not yet well understood [76]. In parallel with secretion of the resorptive enzymes into the pit, the osteoclasts resorb the disrupted bone matrix components [77,78]. Osteoclasts have highly organized and separated vesicular compartments, separating vesicles directed towards the lacuna from vesicles deriving from the lacuna and phagolysosomal vesicles derived from the apical surface membrane [79]. The resorption products are further processed by the cells in an intracellular acid vesicular compartment [75,77,78]. There, collagen fragments will be further cut into smaller parts with the help of the tartrate resistant acid phosphatase (Figure 5.5).

Finally, the resorption products and probably also resorption enzymes, including catK, will be transported through the cell by transcytosis and secreted through the secretory domain of the apical membrane into the paracellular space. Apically secreted products of bone resorption end up in the systemic blood circulation and may eventually be excreted through the urinary system, including pyridinoline, deoxypyridinoline and type I collagen cross-linked N-telopeptide [80,81]. These products can be measured and are significantly increased in the urine in the course of increased bone resorption [82,83]. Of note is also the fact that osteoclasts come across bone embedded osteocytes during bone resorption which are taken up as well [84].

The resorptive function of mature osteoclasts is specifically regulated. As already mentioned, regulatory processes of the calcium homeostasis act through the calcitonin receptor. Again, bone resorptive function and activity of mature osteoclasts are regulated by cell-to-cell contacts between the osteoclasts and the surrounding osteoblasts. More recently, a variety of factors have been identified that influence osteoclast activity, including the OPG/RANK-L/RANK mechanism and leptin [19,85,86]. However, it is not known what makes osteoclast stop and die after the resorptive phase of bone remodeling is over, and the osteoblastic bone forming phase is initiated. Finally, cellular communication between osteoblasts and osteoclasts are essential during the process of osteoclast recruitment, osteoclastogenesis and bone resorption. As mentioned above, various molecules and signaling pathways have been discovered that are important in the cross-talk between osteoblasts and osteoclasts. However, little is known about feedback communication from osteoclasts to osteoblasts.

IV. CONTROLLING OSTEOCLAST FUNCTION IN THE CONTEXT OF OSTEOPOROSIS

Osteoporosis is the most frequent and serious bone-related condition [87]. Although there may be diverse causes responsible for osteoporosis, often a misbalance between bone formation and bone resorption over a long period of time seems to result in the pathologic and irreversible decline of bone mass. Consequently, controlling and down-regulating the osteoclast function may be a good approach in slowing down or even reversing the osteoporotic process. Therefore, a variety of chemical compounds have been evaluated, some with promising success, including biphosphonates, for the treatment of postmenopausal and corticosteroid-induced osteoporosis [88–90]. Another possibility of influencing the resorptive function of osteoclasts is interfering with RANK/RANK-L mechanisms. In that respect, RANK-L binding and inactivating antibodies are being evaluated [91,92].

However, one has to be aware that therapeutical interfering with bone resorption also means interfering with bone remodeling. In that respect, suppression of bone resorption may not necessarily result in improving formation of new bone and bone quality, but may induce osteopetrosis-like conditions, especially in osteoporotic cases where osteoblasts may be affected and the primary reason for the disease. Therefore, more research is needed to better understand the role of osteoclasts in osteoporosis.

V. OSTEOCLAST IN BONE MALIGNANCIES

A variety of malignant tumors affect bone or metastasize into bone, including osteosarcomas, plasmocytomas, melanoma, breast and prostate cancer. In some cases, these malignant bone diseases induce bone resorption resulting in lytic lesions. Usually, the cancer cells themselves express factors that induce osteoclast recruitment, osteoclastogenesis

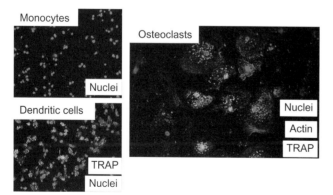

FIGURE 5.5 Expression of tartrate resistant acid phosphatase (TRAP) in human monocytes, dendritic cells and osteoclasts documented with confocal fluorescence microscopy.

and upregulation of osteoclast function. Uncontrolled activation of bone resorption not only provides space for the growing tumor, but it often weakens the bone to a degree that its function is no longer provided, culminating in spontaneous bone fractures [93–98].

More recently, biphosphonates have emerged as a very promising therapeutical option for the treatment of various lytic malignancies. On the one hand, biphosphonates may act on osteoclasts; on the other, there is evidence that they also act on the tumor cells themselves [99–103].

VI. OSTEOCLASTS IN INFLAMMATORY DISEASES

Chronic inflammatory diseases, including rheumatoid arthritis, inflammatory bowel disease, asthma and skin diseases, as well as chronic infectious diseases, are associated with systemic or local decreased bone mass, as well as with destruction of articular cartilage [67,104–110]. Long-term and systemic corticosteroid treatment of these inflammatory diseases may also play a role in chronic inflammation related osteoporosis. However, more recently, factors acting on osteoclastogenesis and increasing osteoclast functions have been identified. One reason for increased bone resorption is a misbalance between OPG and RANK-L, due to interference of immune cells that are able to produce RANK-L [111]. Consequently, besides treating the infection and/or inflammation related symptoms, prevention of osteoporosis or osteolysis has to be considered by influencing the osteoclast function.

VII. SUMMARY AND CONCLUSION

Osteoclasts are the only bone resorbing cells. They are essential in healthy bone development and bone remodeling. Dysfunction of osteoclasts results in deficiency of bone turnover and in osteopetrotic-like diseases.

Osteoclasts are unique in their function, but closely related to the macrophage family, cells of the immune system. Therefore, immune related diseases and certain chronic inflammatory processes may influence the osteoclastogenesis and osteoclast functions, often resulting in a loss of bone mass and osteoporosis, or bone lysis.

Osteoclast recruitment, development and function are under tight control of osteoblast-like cells. Cell-to-cell communication between the two cell types plays a crucial role. Altered cellular communication or signaling often results in a misbalance of bone remodeling, where bone resorption prevails, leading to an increased and uncoupled osteoclast function and, finally, in the loss of bone mass and osteoporosis. Understanding the osteoclast function thus includes an understanding of the interaction between osteoblasts and osteoclasts, and therefore an understanding of osteoblasts themselves. Better knowledge of the cell-to-cell interaction between osteoblasts and osteoclasts will also certainly improve the understanding of neoplastic and metastatic bone lysis.

References

1. V. Shalhoub, G. Elliott & L. Chiu, et al., Characterization of osteoclast precursors in human blood, Brit J Haematol 111 (2000) 501–512.
2. S. Takeshita, K. Kaji & A. Kudo, Identification and characterization of the new osteoclast progenitor with macrophage phenotypes being able to differentiate into mature osteoclasts, J Bone Min Res 15 (2000) 1477–1488.
3. T. Toyosaki-Maeda, H. Takano & T. Tomita, et al., Differentiation of monocytes into multinucleated giant bone-resorbing cells: two-step differentiation induced by nurse-like cells and cytokines, Arthrit Res 3 (2001) 306–310.
4. J. Banchereau & R.M. Steinman, Dendritic cells and the control of immunity, Nature 392 (1998) 245–252.
5. M. Naito, G. Hasegawa & Y. Ebe, et al., Differentiation and function of Kupffer cells, Med Electr Mic 37 (2004) 16–28.
6. N. Kim, M. Takami & J. Rho, et al., A novel member of the leukocyte receptor complex regulates osteoclast differentiation, J Exp Med 195 (2002) 201–209.
7. L. Filgueira, Fluorescence-based staining for tartrate-resistant acidic phosphatase (TRAP) in osteoclasts combined with other fluorescent dyes and protocols, J Histochem Cytochem 52 (2004) 411–414.
8. J.L. Kramer, I. Baltathakis & O.S.F. Alcantara, et al., Differentiation of functional dendritic cells and macrophages from human peripheral blood monocyte precursors is dependent on expression of p21 (WAF1/CIP1) and requires iron, Brit J Haematol 117 (2002) 727–734.
9. J.M. Lean, C. Murphy & K. Fuller, et al., CCL9/MIP-1gamma and its receptor CCR1 are the major chemokine ligand/receptor species expressed by osteoclasts, J Cell Biochem 87 (2002) 386–393.
10. N. Ishida, K. Hayashi & A. Hattori, et al., CCR1 acts downstream of NFAT2 in osteoclastogenesis and enhances cell migration, J Bone Min Res 21 (2006) 48–57.
11. M. Yang, G. Mailhot & C.A. MacKay, et al., Chemokine and chemokine receptor expression during colony stimulating factor-1-induced osteoclast differentiation in the toothless osteopetrotic rat: a key role for CCL9 (MIP-1gamma) in osteoclastogenesis *in vivo* and *in vitro*, Blood 107 (2006) 2262–2270.
12. G. Gu, M. Mulari & Z. Peng, et al., Death of osteocytes turns off the inhibition of osteoclasts and triggers local bone resorption, Biochem Biophys Res Com 335 (2005) 1095–1101.
13. C.Y. Li, K.J. Jepsen & R.J. Majeska, et al., Mice lacking cathepsin K maintain bone remodeling but develop bone fragility despite high bone mass, J Bone Min Res 21 (2006) 865–875.
14. K.M. Robertson, M. Norgard & S.H. Windahl, et al., Cholesterol-sensing receptors, liver X receptor alpha and beta, have novel and distinct roles in osteoclast differentiation and activation, J Bone Min Res 21 (2006) 1276–1287.

15. S.L. Teitelbaum & F.P. Ross, Genetic regulation of osteoclast development and function, Nature Rev Gen 4 (2003) 638–649.

16. F.P. Ross, M-CSF, c-Fms, and signaling in osteoclasts and their precursors, Ann NY Acad Sci 1068 (2006) 110–116.

17. Y. Yamamoto, N. Udagawa & S. Matsuura, et al., Osteoblasts provide a suitable microenvironment for the action of receptor activator of nuclear factor-kappaB ligand, Endocrinology 147 (2006) 3366–3374.

18. G.J. Spencer, J.C. Utting & S.L. Etheridge, et al., Wnt signaling in osteoblasts regulates expression of the receptor activator of NFkappaB ligand and inhibits osteoclastogenesis in vitro, J Cell Sci 119 (2006) 1283–1296.

19. K. Henriksen, J. Gram & P. Hoegh-Andersen, et al., Osteoclasts from patients with autosomal dominant osteopetrosis type I caused by a T253I mutation in low-density lipoprotein receptor-related protein 5 are normal in vitro, but have decreased resorption capacity in vivo, Am J Pathol 167 (2005) 1341–1348.

20. C. Swanson, M. Lorentzon & H.H. Conaway, et al., Glucocorticoid regulation of osteoclast differentiation and expression of receptor activator of nuclear factor-kappaB (NF-kappaB) ligand, osteoprotegerin, and receptor activator of NF-kappaB in mouse calvarial bones, Endocrinology 147 (2006) 3613–3622.

21. H. Michael, P.L. Harkonen & H.K. Vaananen, et al., Estrogen and testosterone use different cellular pathways to inhibit osteoclastogenesis and bone resorption, J Bone Min Res 20 (2005) 2224–2232.

22. M.L. Yen, H.F. Tsai & Y.Y. Wu, et al., TNF-related apoptosis-inducing ligand (TRAIL) induces osteoclast differentiation from monocyte/macrophage lineage precursor cells, Mol Immunol 45 (2008) 2205–2213.

23. I. Roato, M. Grano & G. Brunetti, et al., Mechanisms of spontaneous osteoclastogenesis in cancer with bone involvement, FASEB J 19 (2005) 228–230.

24. Y. Sohara, H. Shimada & C. Minkin, et al., Bone marrow mesenchymal stem cells provide an alternate pathway of osteoclast activation and bone destruction by cancer cells, Cancer Res 65 (2005) 1129–1135.

25. N. Kim, P.R. Odgren & D.K. Kim, et al., Diverse roles of the tumor necrosis factor family member TRANCE in skeletal physiology revealed by TRANCE deficiency and partial rescue by a lymphocyte-expressed TRANCE transgene, PNAS 97 (2000) 10905–10910.

26. R.P. Kapur, Z. Yao & M.H.K. Iida, et al., Malignant autosomal recessive osteopetrosis caused by spontaneous mutation of murine Rank, J Bone Min Res 19 (2004) 1689–1697.

27. J.M. Lean & K. Fuller, FLT3 ligand can substitute for macrophage colony-stimulating factor in support of osteoclast differentiation and function, Blood 98 (2001) 2702–2713.

28. G.J. Lieschke, E. Stanley & D. Grail, et al., Mice lacking both macrophage- and granulocyte-macrophage colony-stimulating factor have macrophages and coexistent osteopetrosis and severe lung disease, Blood 84 (1994) 27–35.

29. R. Felix, M.G. Cecchini & H. Fleisch, Macrophage colony stimulating factor restores in vivo bone resorption in the op/op osteopetrotic mouse, Endocrinology 127 (1990) 2592–2594.

30. T. Koga, M. Inui & K. Inoue, et al., Costimulatory signals mediated by the ITAM motif cooperate with RANKL for bone homeostasis, Nature 428 (2004) 758–763.

31. C.S. Lader, J. Scopes & M.A. Horton, et al., Generation of human osteoclasts in stromal cell-free and stromal cell-rich cultures: differences in osteoclast CD11c/CD18 integrin expression, Brit J Haematol 112 (2001) 430–437.

32. M.A. Horton, H.M. Massey & N. Rosenberg, et al., Upregulation of osteoclast alpha2beta1 integrin compensates for lack of alphavbeta3 vitronectin receptor in Iraqi-Jewish-type Glanzmann thrombasthenia, Brit J Haematol 122 (2003) 950–957.

33. L.T. Duong, P. Lakkakorpi & I. Nakamura, et al., Integrins and signaling in osteoclast function, Matrix Biol 19 (2000) 97–105.

34. S.L. Teitelbaum, Osteoclasts and integrins, Ann NY Acad Sci 1068 (2006) 95–99.

35. P.H. Carter & E. Schipani, The roles of parathyroid hormone and calcitonin in bone remodeling: prospects for novel therapeutics, Endo Met Immun Dis Drug Targ 6 (2006) 59–76.

36. F.M. Abu-Duhier, A.C. Goodeve & R.S. Care, et al., Mutational analysis of class III receptor tyrosine kinases (C-KIT, C-FMS, FLT3) in idiopathic myelofibrosis, Brit J Haematol 120 (2003) 464–470.

37. J.M. Lean, K. Fuller & T.J. Chambers, FLT3 ligand can substitute for macrophage colony-stimulating factor in support of osteoclast differentiation and function, Blood 98 (2001) 2707–2713.

38. J.M. Hodge, M.A. Kirkland & G.C. Nicholson, GM-CSF cannot substitute for M-CSF in human osteoclastogenesis, Biochem Biophys Res Com 321 (2004) 7–12.

39. J.M. Hodge, M.A. Kirkland & C.J. Aitken, et al., Osteoclastic potential of human CFU-GM: biphasic effect of GM-CSF, J Bone Min Res 19 (2004) 190–199.

40. S.D. Yogesha, S.M. Khapli & M.R. Wani, Interleukin-3 and granulocyte-macrophage colony-stimulating factor inhibits tumor necrosis factor (TNF)-alpha-induced osteoclast differentiation by down-regulation of expression of TNF receptors 1 and 2, J Biol Chem 280 (2005) 11759–11769.

41. J.W. Lee, H.Y. Chung & L.A. Ehrlich, et al., IL-3 expression by myeloma cells increases both osteoclast formation and growth of myeloma cells, Blood 103 (2004) 2308–2315.

42. M. Martinez-Moczygemba & D.P. Huston, Biology of common beta receptor-signaling cytokines: IL-3, IL-5, and GM-CSF, J Allergy Clin Immunol 112 (2003) 653–666.

43. G.S. Angelov, M. Tomkowiak & A. Marcais, et al., Flt3 ligand-generated murine plasmacytoid and conventional dendritic cells differ in their capacity to prime naive CD8T cells and to generate memory cells in vivo, J Immunol 175 (2005) 189–195.

44. K. Breckpot, J. Corthals & A. Bonehill, et al., Dendritic cells differentiated in the presence of IFN-beta and IL-3 are potent inducers of an antigen-specific CD8+ T cell response, J Leukoc Biol 78 (2005) 898–908.

45. A. Berhanu, J. Huang & S.M. Alber, et al., Combinational FLt3 ligand and granulocyte macrophage colony-stimulating factor treatment promotes enhanced tumor infiltration by dendritic cells and antitumor CD8 T-cell cross-priming but is ineffective as a therapy, Cancer Res 66 (2006) 4895–4903.

46. S. Kanzaki, M. Ito & Y. Takada, et al., Resorption of auditory ossicles and hearing loss in mice lacking osteoprotegerin, Bone 32 (2006) 414–419.

47. L.A. Schneeweis, D. Willard & M.E. Milla, Functional dissection of osteoprotegerin and its interaction with receptor activator of NF-kappaB ligand, J Biol Chem 280 (2005) 41155–41164.

48. P. Palmqvist, P. Lundberg & E. Persson, et al., Inhibition of hormone and cytokine-stimulated osteoclastogenesis and bone resorption by interleukin-4 and interleukin-13 is associated with increased osteoprotegerin and decreased RANKL and RANK in a STAT6-dependent pathway, J Biol Chem 281 (2006) 2414–2429.

49. B.G. Darnay, V. Haridas & J. Ni, et al., Characterization of the intracellular domain of receptor activator of NF-kappaB (RANK): interaction with tumor necrosis factor receptor-associated factors and activation of NF-kappaB and c-JUN N-terminal kinase, J Biol Chem 273 (1998) 20551–20555.

50. B.R. Wong, D. Besser & N. Kim, et al., TRANCE, a TNF family member, activates Akt/PKB through a signaling complex involving TRAF6 and c-Src, Molec Cell 4 (1999) 1041–1049.

51. N. Kobayashi, Y. Kadono & A. Naito, et al., Segregation of TRAF6-mediated signaling pathways clarifies its role in osteoclastogenesis, EMBO J 20 (2001) 1271–1280.

52. Y.H. Zhang, A. Heulsmann & M.M. Tondravi, et al., Tumor necrosis factor-alpha (TNF) stimulates RANKL-induced osteoclastogenesis via coupling of TNF type 1 receptor and RANK signaling pathways, J Biol Chem 276 (2001) 563–568.

53. T. Wada, T. Nakashima & N. Hiroshi, et al., RANKL-RANK signaling in osteoclastogenesis and bone disease, Trends Mol Med 12 (2006) 17–25.

54. D. Xu, S. Wang & W. Liu, et al., A novel receptor activator of NF-kappaB (RANK) cytoplasmic motif plays an essential role in osteoclastogenesis by committing macrophages to the osteoclast lineage, J Biol Chem 281 (2006) 4678–4690.

55. Y. Maezawa, H. Nakajima & K. Suzuki, et al., Involvement of TNF receptor-associated factor 6 in IL-25 receptor signaling, J Immunol 176 (2006) 1013–1018.

56. A. Mansell, E. Brint & J.A. Gould, et al., Mal interacts with tumor necrosis factor receptor-associated factor (TRAF)-6 to mediate NF-kappaB activation by Toll-like receptor (TLR)-2 and TLR4, J Biol Chem 279 (2004) 37227–37230.

57. R. Schwandner, K. Yamaguchi & Z. Cao, Requirement of tumor necrosis factor receptor-associated factor (TRAF)6 in interleukin 17 signal transduction, J Exp Med 191 (2000) 1233–1239.

58. S. Sato, M. Sugiyama & M. Yamamoto, et al., Toll/IL-1 receptor domain-containing adaptor inducing IFN-beta (TRIF) associates with TNF receptor-associated factor 6 and TANK-binding kinase 1, and activates two distinct transcription factors, NF-kappaB and IFN-regulatory factor-3, in the toll-like receptor signaling, J Immunol 171 (2003) 4304–4310.

59. M. Pang, A.F. Martinez & J. Jacobs, et al., RANK ligand and interferon gamma differentially regulate cathepsin gene expression in pre-osteoclastic cells, Biochem Biophys Res Com 328 (2005) 756–763.

60. E. Seminari, A. Castagna & A. Soldarini, et al., Osteoprotegerin and bone turnover markers in heavily pretreated HIV-infected patients, HIV Med 6 (2005) 145–150.

61. S. Kotake, Y. Nanke & M. Mogi, et al., IFN-gamma-producing human T cells directly induce osteoclastogenesis from human monocytes via the expression of RANKL, Eur J Immunol 35 (2005) 3353–3363.

62. P.P. Geusens, R.B. Landewe & P. Garnero, et al., The ratio of circulating osteoprotegerin to RANKL in early rheumatoid arthritis predicts later joint destruction, Arthr Rheum 54 (2006) 1772–1777.

63. M.E. Miranda-Carus, M. Benito-Miguel & A. Balsa, et al., Peripheral blood T lymphocytes from patients with early rheumatoid arthritis express RANKL and interleukin-15 on the cell surface and promote osteoclastogenesis in autologous monocytes, Arthr Rheum 54 (2006) 1154–1164.

64. P. Boissy, O. Destaing & P. Jurdic, RANKL induces formation of avian osteoclasts from macrophages but not from macrophage polykaryons, Biochem Biophys Res Com 288 (2001) 340–346.

65. D. Cappellen, N.H. Luong-Nguyen & S. Bongiovanni, et al., Transcriptional program of mouse osteoclast differentiation governed by the macrophage colony-stimulating factor and the ligand for the receptor activator of NFkappaB, J Biol Chem 277 (2002) 21971–21982.

66. M. Ishii & Y. Saeki, Osteoclast cell fusion: mechanisms and molecules, Mod Rheumatol 18 (2008) 220–227.

67. Z. Li, K. Kong & W. Qi, Osteoclast and its roles in calcium metabolism and bone development and remodeling, Biochem Biophys Res Com 342 (2006) 345–350.

68. H.H. Malluche, N. Koszewski & M.C. Monier-Faugere, et al., Influence of the parathyroid glands on bone metabolism, Eur J Clin Invest 36 (suppl. 2) (2006) 23–33.

69. H.K. Väänänen, H. Zhao & M. Mulari, et al., The cell biology of osteoclast function, J Cell Sci 113 (2000) 377–381.

70. T. Akisaka, H. Yoshida & S. Inoue, et al., Organization of cytoskeletal F-actin, G-actin, and gelsolin in the adhesion structures in cultured osteoclast, J Bone Min Res 16 (2001) 1248–1255.

71. M.A. Chellaiah, Regulation of actin ring formation by Rho GTPases in osteoclasts, J Biol Chem 280 (2005) 32930–32943.

72. L.S. Holliday, M.R. Bubb & J. Jiang, et al., Interactions between vacuolar H^+-ATPases and microfilaments in osteoclasts, J Bioenerg Biomembr 37 (2005) 419–423.

73. T. Toyomura, T. Oka & C. Yamaguchi, et al., Three subunit a isoforms of mouse vacuolar H^+-ATPase. Preferential expression of the alpha3 isoform during osteoclast differentiation, J Biol Chem 275 (2000) 8760–8765.

74. T. Sahara & T. Sasaki, Effects of brefeldin-A: Potent inhibitor of intracellular protein transport on ultrastructure and resorptive function of cultured osteoclasts, Anat Rec 263 (2001) 127–138.

75. K. Henriksen, M.G. Sorensen & R.H. Nielsen, et al., Degradation of the organic phase of bone by osteoclasts: a secondary role for lysosomal acidification, J Bone Min Res 21 (2006) 58–66.

76. B.R. Troen, The role of cathepsin K in normal bone resorption, Drug News Persp 17 (2004) 19–28.

77. G. Stenbeck & M.A. Horton, Endocytic trafficking in actively resorbing osteoclasts, J Cell Sci 117 (2004) 827–836.

78. J. Meagher, R. Zellweger & L. Filgueira, Functional dissociation of the basolateral transcytotic compartment from the apical phago-lysosomal compartment in human osteoclasts, J Histochem Cytochem 53 (2005) 665–670.

79. E. Sakai, H. Miyamoto & K. Okamoto, et al., Characterization of phagosomal subpopulations along endocytic routes in osteoclasts and macrophages, J Biochem 130 (2001) 823–831.

80. S.A. Nesbitt & M.A. Horton, Trafficking of matrix collagens through bone-resorbing osteoclasts, Science 276 (1997) 266–269.

81. J. Salo, P. Lehenkari & M. Mulari, et al., Removal of osteoclast bone resorption products by transcytosis, Science 276 (1997) 270–273.

82. M. Arabmotlagh, R. Sabljic & M. Rittmeister, Changes of the biochemical markers of bone turnover and periprosthetic bone remodeling after cemented hip arthroplasty, J Orthoplasty 21 (2006) 129–134.

83. T. von Schewelov, A. Carlsson & L. Dahlberg, Cross-linked N-telopeptide of type I collagen (NTx) in urine as a predictor of periprosthetic osteolysis, J Orth Res 24 (2006) 1342–1348.

84. A.L.J.J. Bronckers, K. Sasaguri & M.A. Engelse, Transcription and immunolocalization of Runx2/Cbfa1/Pebp2aalphaA in developing rodent and human craniofacial tissues: further evidence suggesting osteoclasts phagocytose osteocytes, Mic Res Tech 61 (2003) 540–548.

85. F. Elefteriou, J.D. Ahn & S. Takeda, et al., Leptin regulation of bone resorption by the sympathetic nervous system and CART, Nature 434 (2005) 514–520.

86. K.O. Han, J.T. Choi & H.A. Choi, et al., The changes in circulating osteoprotegerin after hormone therapy in postmenopausal women and their relationship with oestrogen responsiveness on bone, Clin Endocrinol 62 (2005) 349–353.

87. P. Sambrook & C. Cooper, Osteoporosis, Lancet 367 (2006) 2010–2018.

88. A. Grey & I.R. Reid, Differences between the bisphosphonates for the prevention and treatment of osteoporosis, Ther Clin Risk Man 2 (2006) 77–86.

89. B.K. Han, D. Yang & H. Ha, et al., Tanshinone IIA inhibits osteoclast differentiation through down-regulation of c-Fos and NFATc1, Exp. Mol Med 38 (2006) 256–264.

90. S. Uchiyama & M. Yamaguchi, beta-cryptoxanthin stimulates apoptotic cell death and suppresses cell function in osteoclastic cells: change in their related gene expression, J Biol Chem 98 (2006) 1185–1195.

91. E.M. Lewiecki, Denosumab: A promising drug for the prevention and treatment of osteoporosis, Women's Health 2 (2006) 517–525.

92. S.A. Doggrell, Inhibition of RANKL: a new approach to the treatment of osteoporosis, Exp Opin Pharm 7 (2006) 1097–1100.

93. D.R. Clohisy & M.L. Ramnaraine, Osteoclasts are required for bone tumors to grow and destroy bone, J Orth Res 16 (1998) 660–666.

94. A.H. Gordon, R.J. O'Keefe & E.M. Schwarz, et al., Nuclear factor-kappaB-dependent mechanisms in breast cancer cells regulate tumor burden and osteolysis in bone, Cancer Res 65 (2005) 3209–3217.

95. D.J. Leeming, M. Koizumi & I. Byrjalsen, et al., The relative use of eight collagenous and noncollagenous markers for diagnosis of skeletal metastases in breast, prostate, or lung cancer patients, Cancer Epidem Biom Prev 15 (2006) 32–38.

96. Y.S. Lau, A. Sabokbar & H. Giele, et al., Malignant melanoma and bone resorption, Brit J Cancer 94 (2006) 1496–1503.

97. G. Brunetti, S. Colucci & R. Rizzi, et al., The role of OPG/TRAIL complex in multiple myeloma, Ann NY Acad Sci 1068 (2006) 334–340.

98. T. Matsumoto & M. Abe, Bone destruction in multiple myeloma, Ann NY Acad Sci 1068 (2006) 319–326.

99. S. Bezares, M.L. Amador & D. Castellano, et al., Combined treatment with biphosphonates, low-dose chemotherapy, and trastuzumab in receptor-negative breast cancer patients with bone marrow involvement, Eur J Intern Med 12 (2001) 462–463.

100. D. Melisi, R. Caputo & V. Damiano, et al., Zoledronic acid cooperates with a cyclooxygenase-2 inhibitor and gefitinib in inhibiting breast and prostate cancer, Endocr Rel Cancer 12 (2005) 1051–1058.

101. H. Asahi, A. Mizokami & S. Miwa, et al., Bisphosphonate induces apoptosis and inhibits pro-osteoclastic gene expression in prostate cancer cells, Int J Urol 13 (2006) 593–600.

102. J. Hirata, Y. Kikuchi & K. Kudoh, et al., Inhibitory effects of bisphosphonates on the proliferation of human ovarian cancer cell lines and the mechanism, Med Chem 2 (2006) 223–226.

103. C.E. Hoesl & J.E. Altwein, Biphosphonates in advanced prostate and renal cell cancer: current status and potential applications, Urol Int 76 (2006) 97–105.

104. P.P. Geusens, R.B.M. Landewe & P. Garnero, et al., The ratio of circulating osteoprotegerin to RANKL in early rheumatoid arthritis predicts later joint destruction, Arthr Rheumat 54 (2006) 1772–1777.

105. C.N. Bernstein, Osteoporosis in patients with inflammatory bowel disease, Clin Gastro Hep 4 (2006) 152–156.

106. D.M. Kearney & R.F. Lockey, Osteoporosis and asthma, Ann All Asthm Immunol 96 (2006) 769–774.

107. T.P. Millard, L. Antoniades & A.V. Evans, et al., Bone mineral density of patients with chronic plaque psoriasis, Clin Exp Dermatol 26 (2001) 446–448.

108. B. Frediani, F. Baldi & P. Falsetti, et al., Clinical determinants of bone mass and bone ultrasonometry in patients with systemic sclerosis, Clin Exp Rheumatol 22 (2004) 313–318.

109. M. Bongiovanni & C. Tincati, Bone diseases associated with human immunodeficiency virus infection: pathogenesis, risk factors and clinical management, Cur Mol Med 6 (2006) 395–400.

110. I.E. Adamopoulos, L. Danks & I. Itonaga, et al., Stimulation of osteoclast formation by inflammatory synovial fluid, Virch Arch 449 (2006) 69–77.

111. A.R. Moschen, A. Kaser & B. Enrich, et al., RANKL/OPG system is activated in inflammatory bowel diseases and relates to the state or bone loss, Gut 54 (2005) 479–487.

CHAPTER **6**

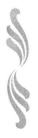

Immunoregulation of Osteoclast Differentiation in Multiple Myeloma Bone Disease

MARIA GRANO[1], GIACOMINA BRUNETTI[1] AND SILVIA COLUCCI[1]

[1]Department of Human Anatomy and Histology, University of Bari, Italy.

Contents

I. INTRODUCTION

Cancer adversely affects bone and mineral metabolism through a broad spectrum of mechanisms. Primary bone tumors make up a small minority of bone-related malignancy. Destructive lesions in the skeleton are a common feature of breast, prostate, lung, kidney, and thyroid carcinomas, as well as multiple myeloma (MM). MM accounts for 10% of malignant hematological diseases. It is characterized by the clonal proliferation of malignant plasma cells in the bone marrow compartment, secretion of monoclonal immunoglobulins, and suppression of normal immunoglobulin production and hematopoiesis. Myeloma patients often have extensive skeletal destruction with osteolytic lesions, osteopenia, pathological fractures, intractable bone pain, and hypercalcemia. These osteolytic lesions are the major cause of morbidity and possible mortality in MM patients [1]. The malignant plasma cells, present in the bone marrow (BM), originate from lymph nodes and then migrate across the endothelium of bone marrow sinuses to the BM microenvironment and localize in contact with stromal cells [2,3]. The interaction of plasma cells with BM stromal cells is crucial to the homing and growth of MM cells in the BM microenvironment. In areas adjacent to myeloma cells

osteoclastic activity increases, resulting in increased bone resorption, while osteoblast activity declines with consequent reduced bone formation [4]. Insight into the interaction of marrow stromal cells of osteoblastic lineage with osteoclasts has provided a better understanding of the mechanisms regulating osteoclast activation and bone resorption. Osteoclastogenesis is a stromal cell and osteoblast-dependent process that is mediated by the receptor activator of the nuclear factor kB (RANK)/RANK ligand (RANKL)/osteoprotegerin (OPG) system. RANKL binds RANK, expressed by osteoclast precursors, and induces osteoclast formation in the presence of Macrophage (M)-colony stimulating factor (M-CSF) [5]. OPG, a member of the tumor necrosis factor (TNF) receptor superfamily, is a secreted RANKL decoy receptor of osteoblastic-lineage cells [6,7]. OPG achieves its effect on osteoclasts indirectly by binding to and blocking the effect of RANKL [8]. It therefore appears that OPG competes with RANK for association with RANKL and that the ratio of OPG/RANKL is critical for osteoclast development and its unbalance is associated with bone disease. RANKL and OPG are also produced by activated T cells, being a crucial paracrine link between bone metabolism and the immune system [9,10]. T lymphocytes and their products are now recognized as key regulators of osteoclast and osteoblast formation, lifespan, and activity [11,12]. The hematopoietic system is a key source of cytokines and growth factors essential for bone cell renewal. T cells are members of the lymphoid lineage that contributes to bone modeling and remodeling in health and disease. T cells have the capacity to secrete a wide repertoire of cytokines, some pro-osteoclastogenic and some anti-osteoclastogenic. In the absence of strong activation signals, T cells appear to repress osteoclast formation [13], but the relevance of this phenomenon *in vivo* has not been established. In contrast, activated T cells play a key role in the regulation of osteoclast formation through increased production of RANKL, TNFα [13–17], and OPG [13]. Activated T cells also produce IFN-α and -γ [18]. The net effect of T cells on OC formation may consequently represent the prevailing balance of anti- and pro-osteoclastogenic T cell cytokine secretion. However, it appears that during stimulated conditions, such as inflammation [16], pro-osteoclastogenic cytokines prevail. In particular, the key role of T lymphocytes, as cells involved in bone loss, has been demonstrated in rheumatoid arthritis [16], as well as in osteoporosis [19], solid tumors [20] and MM [10]. This chapter reviews the main pathogenetic mechanisms and the clinical assessment of myeloma bone disease in the light of our own studies and the literature. In particular, several studies have focused on the molecular events connected with the development of myeloma bone disease, with particular regard to enhanced osteoclast function.

II. OSTEOCLASTOGENESIS IN MULTIPLE MYELOMA: ROLE OF CYTOKINES AND CELLS OF IMMUNE SYSTEM

A. RANK/RANKL/OPG

Physiologically osteoclast formation and activity are regulated by the key osteoclastogenic cytokines MCSF and RANKL. A dysregulated production of additional pro- and anti-osteoclastogenic factors takes place under pathological conditions, such as those occurring in malignant bone diseases, including MM. Most of the molecules able to stimulate osteoclast formation and activity are produced by cells in the immune system. A close relationship between the immune and skeletal systems has attracted much attention due to an observation that bone destruction is caused by abnormal activation of the immune system in pathological conditions with bone involvement. In 1997, Choi and colleagues greatly contributed to the initiation of osteoimmunology study by identifying RANKL in T cells [21,22]. In addition, Penninger and colleagues contributed to the development of osteoimmunology by generating a series of knockout mice and establishing the role of the RANK/RANKL system in the pathogenesis of bone diseases [16, 23,24]. The linkage between cells of the immune system and bone loss is becoming more evident in MM and other bone loss-associated diseases through different mechanisms mainly due to the alteration of RANKL/OPG axis [9,15, 16,18,23,25–28]. Some authors have demonstrated that human MM cells induce RANKL expression in stromal cells and decrease OPG secretion [28–30]. Furthermore, Standal *et al.* demonstrated that syndecan-1, a transmembrane proteoglycan expressed by myeloma cells, binds and sequestrates OPG through interaction with the heparin-binding domain of the OPG protein [31]. Following binding to syndecan-1, OPG was internalized and degraded within the lysosomal compartment of myeloma cells [31]. On the other hand, RANKL expression by MM cells appears to be controversial. Although several studies reported RANKL expression by myeloma cells, using either human myeloma cells from patients [32–34], human myeloma cell lines, or a murine myeloma cell line [35], other studies could not detect RANKL expression in human myeloma cell lines or primary myeloma cells [10,28,29,36].

Moreover, we proposed a new mechanism affecting the RANKL/OPG unbalance in MM bone disease through the involvement of OPG/TRAIL interaction [10]. The TNF-related apoptosis-inducing ligand (TRAIL) is a cytotoxic protein inducing apoptosis upon binding to death-domain-containing receptors. However, its activity can be modulated by association with two membrane-bound decoy receptors which lack functional death domains and conferring TRAIL resistance on expressing cells [10]. Furthermore, it has been shown that TRAIL may regulate OPG activity through the OPG/TRAIL interaction, which can induce a cross regulatory mechanism between the two molecules [37]. In our study [10] into the assessment of biologic mechanisms involved in the pathogenesis of MM bone disease, by using an *in vitro* osteoclastogenesis model, as a paradigm of *in vivo* bone resorption, we demonstrated that in MM patients T cells supported the elevated formation of osteoclasts displaying a long-life span in culture (Figure 6.1). In particular, we found that T cells from the patients overexpressed RANKL (Figure 6.2). This finding is in agreement with data obtained by Giuliani *et al.* who demonstrated that activated T cells, co-cultured with malignant plasma cells, overexpressed RANKL [27]. Additionally, we found that T cells from MM patients surprisingly overexpressed OPG (Figure 6.2). This finding, apparently in contrast with the persistence of osteoclastogenesis in our system, could be explained by the OPG binding to TRAIL. The OPG/TRAIL interaction was demonstrated by the presence of the OPG/TRAIL immunocomplex in both T cells and media of our culture models [10]. The binding between these two molecules prevented the antiosteoclastogenic role of OPG and blocked the apoptosis-inducing TRAIL activity. These results were consistent with the literature data. They demonstrated that the overexpression of OPG, resulting in a protective cell strategy against apoptosis in the presence of high TRAIL levels, is of major relevance as indicated by *in vitro* studies prospecting OPG as a survival factor for human prostate cancer and human MM cells [38,39]. Thus, we proposed that in MM bone disease T cells contributed to the well-documented disruption of the RANKL/OPG *ratio*, through the overproduction of RANKL, OPG and TRAIL, and the formation of the OPG/TRAIL complex (Figure 6.3). In addition, we demonstrated that T cells could contribute to the prolonged lifespan of osteoclasts in MM bone disease by inducing an unbalanced *ratio* between death and decoy TRAIL receptors expressed by

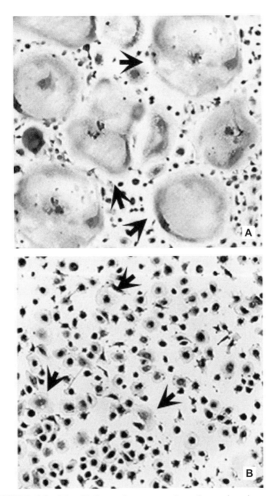

FIGURE 6.1 T cell-dependent osteoclast formation in peripheral blood mononuclear cells (PBMCs) of multiple myeloma bone disease patients. (A) Numerous and large osteoclasts (arrows) were obtained from unfractionated PBMCs. (B) Osteoclastogenesis did not occur in T-cell-depleted PBMCs in which only binucleated cells (arrows) can be observed. Multinucleated (>3 nuclei per cell) and tartrate resistent acid phosphatase positive cells were identified as osteoclasts (magnification ×200).

mature osteoclasts [10]. The TRAIL receptor unbalance conferred osteoclast resistance to TRAIL-induced apoptosis thereby favoring the longer osteoclast survival.

Besides RANKL and OPG, other cytokines, either pro-osteoclastogenic (IL-6, IL-7, IL-3, MIP-1α) or anti-osteoclastogenic (IFN-γ), can stimulate bone destruction in MM.

B. RANKL/IFN-γ/IL-7

It has been found that activated T cells can also negatively affect osteoclastogenesis through IFN-γ production [40]. It is likely that the balance between the actions of RANKL and IFN-γ may regulate osteoclast formation. For example, during acute immune reactions, an enhanced production of IFN-γ counterbalances the augmentation of RANKL

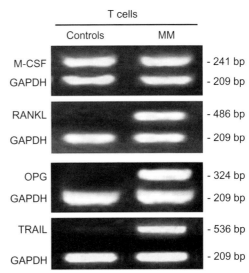

FIGURE 6.2 Cytokine expression by fresh T cells from peripheral blood mononuclear cells (PBMCs) of multiple myeloma bone disease patients. Fresh T cells purified from PBMCs of multiple myeloma bone disease patients as well as from controls were analyzed for MCSF, RANKL, OPG and TRAIL expression, by RT-PCR. The results show the overexpression of RANKL, OPG and TRAIL compared with controls. No change in MCSF expression was found. The housekeeping genes glyceraldehyde phosphate dehydrogenase (GAPDH) was utilized as control.

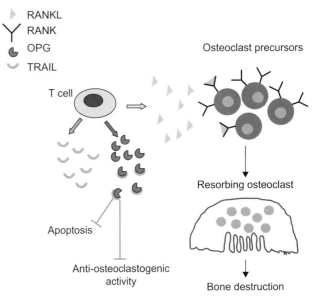

FIGURE 6.3 Model for cytokine-induced osteoclast formation through RANKL and OPG/TRAIL interaction in multiple myeloma bone disease patients. T cells release high levels of RANKL, OPG and TRAIL. The anti-osteoclastogenic activity of OPG is neutralized by TRAIL, thus the binding between TRAIL and OPG could contribute to the unbalance of RANKL/OPG ratio responsible of the increased osteoclast activity in MM.

expression and reduces aberrant formation of osteoclasts. On the other hand, in chronic synovitis of rheumatoid arthritis, this balance may be skewed in favor of RANKL expression. In this context, it is noteworthy that expression of IFN-γ is suppressed in the arthritic joints in which RANKL expression is enhanced, despite a significant infiltration of T cells [41,42]. A similar mechanism has been demonstrated in MM by Giuliani and colleagues showing that MM cells are able to induce an upregulation of RANKL and a downregulation of INF-γ secretion by T lymphocytes [27]. It is likely that the inhibitory effect, shown by MM cells on IFN-γ secretion by T cells, may explain the increased osteoclastogenic activity. The upregulation of RANKL in T lymphocytes by MM cells seems to be mediated by the release of soluble factors. Among the molecules that could be responsible for the stimulation of RANKL, the authors focused their attention on IL-7. It has been postulated that IL-7 might be involved in osteoclast activation because IL-7 stimulates RANKL production by T cells *in vitro* [43] and induces bone loss *in vivo* by induction of RANKL [44]. At this purpose Giuliani *et al.* demonstrated that MM cells expressed IL-7 mRNA and that IL-7 secretion was upregulated in the presence of IL-6 [27]. On the other hand, other authors have demonstrated that IL-7 stimulates IL-6 secretion by bone marrow stromal cells [45]. Thus, a vicious loop between IL-6 and IL-7 in MM can be hypothesized. High levels of IL-6 in the BM environment could induce IL-7 production by MM cells, which in turn contribute to maintain high IL-6 levels and stimulate RANKL expression by T cells. The potential involvement of IL-7 is supported by the *in vivo* findings of higher IL-7 levels in peripheral blood serum and bone marrow plasma of MM patients [27].

C. IL-6

IL-6 is a growth and survival factor for MM cells and is present in marrow plasma samples from patients with myeloma. IL-6 can stimulate human osteoclast formation *in vitro* [46] and *in vivo* [47] and enhance the effects of other osteoclastogenic factors such as PTH and PTHrP [48]. IL-6 mediates the effects of other inflammatory cytokines on osteoclast formation, such as IL-1 and TNFα [49]. IL-6 production can be detected in approximately 40% of freshly isolated MM cells [50]. However, the role of IL-6 in MM bone disease is controversial [51]. Some investigators correlate IL-6 levels with the presence of bone lesions and disease severity [52], while others do not find a correlation between IL-6 and bone disease [53]. Moreover, the source of IL-6 production is also controversial. Although some studies have reported that MM cells express IL-6 [54], others have shown that IL-6 is produced by cells (marrow stromal cells, osteoblasts, and osteoclasts) in the bone marrow microenvironment in response to contact with MM cells. Cell–cell interaction between marrow stromal cells

and myeloma cells results in increased secretion of IL-6 [55]. In addition, Thomas *et al.* have demonstrated that TNFα and IL-1β, produced by myeloma cells, were able to stimulate IL-6 production by marrow stromal cells [56]. Karadag *et al.* showed that primary human osteoblasts increase IL-6 production when co-cultured with MM cell lines [57]. The increase in IL-6 was greatest when MM cells were in contact with osteoblasts, but it could also occur when conditioned medium from myeloma cultures was added to osteoblasts, indicating that a soluble factor may be responsible for the effect [57]. Osteoclasts also express IL-6 when co-cultured with MM cells [58]. Abe *et al.* used peripheral blood mononuclear cell-derived osteoclast cultures that lacked stromal cells and found that IL-6 was also expressed by osteoclasts when in contact with myeloma cells [58]. Because IL-6 is a growth and anti-apoptotic cytokine for MM cells [59], this study suggested that osteoclasts promote the growth and survival of myeloma cells *in vitro*. This effect requires cell–cell contact between osteoclasts and MM cells, because transwell cultures abolish the growth stimulatory effects on MM cells. IL-6 may enhance osteoclast formation in MM by acting on preosteoclasts or simply increasing MM tumor burden, which in turn increases osteoclast formation. IL-6 can induce osteoclastogenesis *in vitro* [60], but it is unclear whether sufficient levels of IL-6 are produced to induce osteoclast formation in MM.

D. IL-3

Studies have demonstrated that IL-3 plays a role in MM bone disease. IL-3 levels are increased in the marrow and blood of patients with MM. Merico *et al.* [61] reported an increase in IL-3 protein levels in peripheral blood serum samples in 40% of patients with MM. Interestingly, Giuliani *et al.* demonstrated that T lymphocytes, and not MM cells or MM cell lines, produced IL-3 in the myeloma bone microenvironment [62]. On the contrary, Lee *et al.* demonstrated that IL-3 is overexpressed in purified MM cells from patients at both the mRNA and the protein levels [63]. They reported increased IL-3 mRNA expression in 75% of bone marrow samples from MM patients and an increase in protein levels in bone marrow plasma samples [63]. Furthermore, they found that bone marrow plasma samples from MM patients stimulated osteoclast formation *in vitro*, and the effect was reversed by the addition of a neutralizing antibody to IL-3 [63]. Barton and Mayer also reported that IL-3 increased the number of preosteoclasts and increased fusion into mature osteoclasts [64]. These studies confirm the potential role of IL-3 as an osteoclast stimulatory factor in MM bone disease.

E. Dendritic Cells and MIP-1α

Dendritic cells (DCs) are specialized antigen-presenting cells able to initiate immune responses [65]. DCs derive from myeloid or lymphoid progenitors. Their functions are determined by their origin as well as by their maturation stage, which depends on the signals received from pathogens and T cells. Myeloid DCs are classified into different subsets. The relationship between the different subsets is still not clearly understood. However, the current paradigm is that most human DCs are derived from blood monocytic precursors under the control of granulocyte-macrophage colony-stimulating factor (GM-CSF) associated with either IL-4 or IL-3 or TNFα [65–67]. It has been shown that in the mouse myeloid DCs share a common progenitor with osteoclasts. Although it has long been assumed that monocyte/macrophage lineage can differentiate either in DCs or in osteoclasts following two separate pathways [68], Rivollier *et al.* have demonstrated that immature DCs transdifferentiate into functional osteoclasts in the presence of MCSF and RANKL [69]. Consistently, Hashimoto *et al.* [70] have suggested that the reduced DC differentiation in MM was mediated by macrophage inflammatory protein-1α (MIP-1α), which induces OC differentiation and blocks DC differentiation of a common precursor in the monocyte lineage. Immature DCs can transdifferentiate into osteoclasts [69], and this reciprocal effect on DC and osteoclast differentiation further contributes to the immunosuppression and bone destruction in MM. MIP-1α is a low-molecular-weight chemokine, which can interact with its receptors, CCR1, CCR5, or CCR9. MIP-1α primarily acts as a chemoattractant and an activator of monocytes and monocyte-like cells [71], and has a role in hematopoiesis and osteoclast recruitment and differentiation in bone marrow [72, 73]. Both CCR1 and CCR5 are expressed by human bone marrow stromal cells and osteoclast precursors [74–76]. MIP-1α acts directly on human osteoclast progenitors at the later stages of differentiation [74]. MIP-1β is a highly homologous chemokine of MIP-1α, and both are constitutively secreted by MM cells and induce the development of osteolytic bone lesions [72–74,77,78]. Levels of MIP-1α are elevated in the majority of bone marrow samples from patients with active myeloma as well as in marrow plasma from MM patients. Increased levels of MIP-1α have been reported in the plasma of MM patients with severe bone disease. Patients with higher serum MIP-1α levels had a significantly lower 3-year survival, indicating that a high MIP-1α level portends a poor prognosis [79]. Gene expression profiling studies have shown that MIP-1α expression was highly correlated with the extent of bone disease in MM patients [80,81]. *In vivo* studies have shown that the growth of MM cells and bone lesions decreases in SCID mice transplanted with ARH-77, human B-lymphoblastoid cells which lacked MIP-1α [82]. Further studies into murine 5TGM1(radl) myeloma-bearing mice, demonstrated that administration of neutralizing anti-MIP-1α antibodies reduced tumor load, prevented splenomegaly, limited development of osteolytic lesions, and concomitantly reduced tumor growth in bone [83]. The same authors concluded that MIP-1α exerts a dual effect in myeloma on osteoclasts and tumor cells.

III. NEW THERAPEUTIC APPROACHES FOR TREATMENT OF MULTIPLE MYELOMA BONE DISEASE PATIENTS

Multiple myeloma cannot be cured by standard chemotherapeutic approaches, and the high morbidity and mortality associated with this malignancy are mainly due to a complication of osteoclast-mediated bone distruction [84]. Although progress has been made in the therapeutic use of bisphosphonates for cancer-induced osteolysis [85], this has not resulted in significantly improved clinical outcomes in MM patients. Understanding the pathophysiology of myeloma progression and associated bone destruction is the key to identifying new interventions that may concomitantly impact tumor burden and reduce bone loss, thereby improving the quality of life of patients. The data discussed in this chapter highlight that the unbalance of the RANKL/OPG system, which could occur with different mechanisms, is crucial in the development of osteolytic bone disease in MM. Systemic RANKL blockade has been evaluated in animal models and clinical trials. The first preclinical study on the impact of RANKL antagonists using severe combined immunodeficient-human (SCID-hu) mice showed that treatment with RANK-Fc results in a markedly reduced bone disease compared to animals receiving controls [29]. Later studies evaluated the effects of RANKL blockade on myeloma tumor burden. Treatment of myelomatous SCID-hu hosts with RANK-Fc not only reduced myeloma-induced bone resorption, but also resulted in a sustained suppression of paraprotein levels by more than 80% [86]. The treatment was associated with a decreased number of osteoclasts but had no effect on apoptosis and proliferation of myeloma cells, indicating that the antimyeloma effect of RANKL inhibitors is related to inhibition of osteoclast activity. Further studies with recombinant OPG, which similarly blocks RANKL/RANK interaction, were effective in decreasing the development of osteolytic bone disease in animal models of MM [87,88]. In humans, the effects of RANKL blockade were evaluated in 28 patients with MM with lytic bone lesions by using AMGN-0007, a recombinant osteoprotegerin construct. OPG suppressed bone resorption rapidly and significantly. The effects were comparable to those with pamidronate and therapy was well tolerated [89]. Denosumab (AMG162), a fully human monoclonal antibody to RANKL that has high affinity and specificity to RANKL, was utilized in 25 MM patients with radiologically confirmed bone lesions, and the treatment was effective in decreasing bone resorption [90]. However, longer studies on a larger number of patients need to be performed in order to reach statistical significance on the efficacy of therapy in MM bone disease patients. Preclinical studies performed in animal models of MM showed that functional blockade of MIP-1α bioactivity by systematically administered neutralizing anti-MIP-1α antibodies not only blocked osteoclastic bone destruction but also reduced overall tumor burden [83]. This confirms previous studies which showed that inhibiting MIP-1α production, using an antisense approach, also impaired development and progression of bone disease in a model in which ARH-77 human B-lymphoblastoid cells inoculated into irradiated SCID mice induced osteolysis and extensive extramedullary disease [72]. Although the use of neutralizing antibodies in patients is not likely to be feasible, non-peptidic small molecule MIP-1α receptor antagonists could be used readily to disrupt MIP-1α-initiated signaling. Of the two well-established signaling receptors for MIP-1α, CCR5 but not CCR1 also mediates the effects of MIP1β, a highly homologous but distinct CC chemokyne [91,92]. Because the neutralizing anti-MIP1α neutralizing antibody did not completely block myeloma growth and osteolysis, a role for MIP1β in myeloma development cannot be excluded. Although it is presently unclear which receptor mediates the osteoclastogenic effects of MIP1α *in vivo*, it is likely that CCR5 is involved. This is consistent with reports that neutralizing antibodies against CCR5 blocked osteoclast formation. Importantly, neutralizing antibodies directed against MIP1α or MIP1β mimicked this effect of anti-CCR5 antibodies [75]. Although not yet clinically used, targeting MIP-1α could provide an additional approach in the treatment of myeloma bone disease.

IV. CONCLUSIONS AND PERSPECTIVES

Studies have given new insights into the pathogenesis of myeloma bone disease and demonstrated a strong interdependence between the immune and skeletal system as well as tumor growth and osteoclast activity. Discovery of the RANK-RANKL system brought a rapid progress in the understanding of the regulatory mechanism of osteoclast differentiation in physiological and pathological conditions. However, numerous connections have been discovered in osteoimmunology beyond merely the actions of RANKL. These include both cells and cytokines participating in osteoclast development and bone destruction. The resulting bone destruction releases several cytokines which in turn promote myeloma cell growth, thus maintaining a vicious circle between the bone destructive process and tumor progression. Therefore, the inhibition of bone resorption could not only decrease myeloma bone disease, but also the tumor progression. Furthermore, research into osteoimmunology promises the discovery of new strategies and the development of innovative therapeutics to cure or alleviate bone loss in MM bone disease.

Acknowledgements

We thank to Dr. Luigi Branca for expert technical support.

References

1. R.E. Coleman, Skeletal complications of malignancy, Cancer 80 (1997) 1588–1594.
2. D. Billadeau, G. Ahmann & P. Greipp, et al., The bone marrow of MM patients contains B cell populations at different stages of differentiation that are clonally related to the malignant plasma cell, J Exp Med 178 (1993) 1023–1031.
3. W. Matsui, C.A. Huff & Q. Wang, et al., Characterization of clonogenic multiple myeloma cells, Blood 103 (2004) 2332–2336.
4. K.C. Anderson, J.D. Shaughnessy Jr. & B. Barlogie, et al., Multiple myeloma, Hematology (Am Soc Hematol Educ Program) (2002) 214–240.
5. D.L. Lacey, H.L. Tan & J. Lu, et al., Osteoprotegerin ligand modulates murine osteoclast survival *in vitro* and *in vivo*, Am J Pathol 157 (2000) 435–448.
6. W.S. Simonet, D.L. Lacey & C.R. Dunstan, et al., Osteoprotegerin: a novel secreted protein involved in the regulation of bone density, Cell 89 (1997) 309–319.
7. H. Yasuda, N. Shima & N. Nakagawa, et al., Identity of osteoclastogenesis inhibitory factor (OCIF) and osteoprotegerin (OPG): a mechanism by which OPG/OCIF inhibits osteoclastogenesis *in vitro*, Endocrinology 139 (1998) 1329–1337.
8. D.L. Lacey, E. Timms & H.L. Tan, et al., Osteoprotegerin ligand is a cytokine that regulates osteoclast differentiation and activation, Cell 93 (1998) 165–176.
9. Y. Choi, K.M. Woo & S.H. Ko, et al., Osteoclastogenesis is enhanced by activated B cells but suppressed by activated CD8(+) T cells, Eur J Immunol 31 (2001) 2179–2188.
10. S. Colucci, G. Brunetti & R. Rizzi, et al., T cells support osteoclastogenesis in an *in vitro* model derived from human multiple myeloma bone disease: the role of the OPG/TRAIL interaction, Blood 104 (2004) 3722–3730.
11. S.L. Teitelbaum, Postmenopausal osteoporosis, T cells, and immune dysfunction, Proc Natl Acad Sci USA 101 (2004) 16711–16712.
12. L. Rifas & S. Arackal, T cells regulate the expression of matrix metalloproteinase in human osteoblasts via a dual mitogen-activated protein kinase mechanism, Arthritis Rheum 48 (2003) 993–1001.
13. D. Grcevic, S.K. Lee & A. Marusic, et al., Depletion of CD4 and CD8T lymphocytes in mice *in vivo* enhances 1,25-dihydroxyvitamin D3-stimulated osteoclast-like cell formation *in vitro* by a mechanism that is dependent on prostaglandin synthesis, J Immunol 165 (2000) 4231–4238.
14. N.J. Horwood, V. Kartsogiannis & J.M. Quinn, et al., Activated T lymphocytes support osteoclast formation *in vitro*, Biochem Biophys Res Commun 265 (1999) 144–150.
15. M.N. Weitzmann, S. Cenci & L. Rifas, et al., T cell activation induces human osteoclast formation via receptor activator of nuclear factor kappaB ligand-dependent and -independent mechanisms, J Bone Miner Res 16 (2001) 328–337.
16. Y.Y. Kong, U. Feige & I. Sarosi, et al., Activated T cells regulate bone loss and joint destruction in adjuvant arthritis through osteoprotegerin ligand, Nature 402 (1999) 304–309.

17. Y.T. Teng, H. Nguyen & X. Gao, et al., Functional human T-cell immunity and osteoprotegerin ligand control alveolar bone destruction in periodontal infection, J Clin Invest 106 (2000) R59–R67.

18. H. Takayanagi, K. Ogasawara & S. Hida, et al., T-cell-mediated regulation of osteoclastogenesis by signalling cross-talk between RANKL and IFN-γ, Nature 408 (2000) 600–605.

19. P. D'Amelio, A. Grimaldi & G.P. Pescarmona, et al., Spontaneous osteoclast formation from peripheral blood mononuclear cells in postmenopausal osteoporosis, FASEB J 19 (2005) 410–412.

20. I. Roato, M. Grano & G. Brunetti, et al., Mechanisms of spontaneous osteoclastogenesis in cancer with bone involvement, FASEB J 19 (2005) 228–230.

21. B.R. Wong, J. Rho & J. Arron, et al., TRANCE is a novel ligand of the tumor necrosis factor receptor family that activates c-Jun N-terminal kinase in T cells, J Biol Chem 272 (1997) 25190–25194.

22. N. Kim, M. Takami & J. Rho, et al., A novel member of the leukocyte receptor complex regulates osteoclast differentiation, J Exp Med 195 (2002) 201–209.

23. Y.Y. Kong, H. Yoshida & I. Sarosi, et al., OPGL is a key regulator of osteoclastogenesis, lymphocyte development and lymph-node organogenesis, Nature 397 (1999) 315–323.

24. M.A. Lomaga, W.C. Yeh & I. Sarosi, et al., TRAF6 deficiency results in osteopetrosis and defective interleukin-1, CD40, and LPS signaling, Genes Dev 13 (1999) 1015–1024.

25. H. Takayanagi, S. Kim & T. Taniguchi, Signaling crosstalk between RANKL and interferons in osteoclast differentiation, Arthritis Res 4 (2002) S227–S232.

26. K. Nosaka, T. Miyamoto & T. Sakai, et al., Mechanism of hypercalcemia in adult T-cell leukemia: overexpression of receptor activator of nuclear factor kappaB ligand on adult T-cell leukemia cells, Blood 99 (2002) 634–640.

27. N. Giuliani, S. Colla & R. Sala, et al., Human myeloma cells stimulate the receptor activator of nuclear factor-kappa B ligand (RANKL) in T lymphocytes: a potential role in multiple myeloma bone disease, Blood 100 (2002) 4615–4621.

28. N. Giuliani, R. Bataille & C. Mancini, et al., Myeloma cells induce imbalance in the osteoprotegerin/osteoprotegerin ligand system in the human bone marrow environment, Blood 98 (2001) 3527–3533.

29. R.N. Pearse, E.M. Sordillo & S. Yaccoby, et al., Multiple myeloma disrupts the TRANCE/osteoprotegerin cytokine axis to trigger bone destruction and promote tumor progression, Proc Natl Acad Sci USA 98 (2001) 11581–11586.

30. Y.W. Qiang, Y. Chen & O. Stephens, et al., Myeloma-derived Dickkopf-1 disrupts Wnt-regulated osteoprotegerin and RANKL production by osteoblasts: a potential mechanism underlying osteolytic bone lesions in multiple myeloma, Blood 112 (2008) 196–207.

31. T. Standal, C. Seidel & O. Hjertner, et al., Osteoprotegerin is bound, internalized, and degraded by multiple myeloma cells, Blood 100 (2002) 3002–3007.

32. U. Heider, C. Langelotz & C. Jakob, et al., Expression of receptor activator of nuclear factor kappaB ligand on bone marrow plasma cells correlates with osteolytic bone disease in patients with multiple myeloma, Clin Cancer Res 9 (2003) 1436–1440.

33. O. Sezer, U. Heider & C. Jakob, et al., Human bone marrow myeloma cells express RANKL, J Clin Oncol 20 (2002) 353–354.

34. O. Sezer, U. Heider & C. Jakob, et al., Immunocytochemistry reveals RANKL expression of myeloma cells, Blood 99 (2002) 4646–4647.

35. P.I. Croucher, C.M. Shipman & J. Lippitt, et al., Osteoprotegerin inhibits the development of osteolytic bone disease in multiple myeloma, Blood 98 (2001) 3534–3540.

36. S. Roux, V. Meignin & J. Quillard, et al., RANK (receptor activator of nuclear factor-kappaB) and RANKL expression in multiple myeloma, Br J Haematol 117 (2002) 86–92.

37. J.G. Emery, P. McDonnell & M.B. Burke, et al., Osteoprotegerin is a receptor for the cytotoxic ligand TRAIL, J Biol Chem 273 (1998) 14363–14367.

38. I. Holen, P.I. Croucher & F.C. Hamdy, et al., Osteoprotegerin is a survival factor for human prostate cancer cell, Cancer Res 62 (2002) 1619–1623.

39. C.M. Shipman & P.I. Croucher, Osteoprotegerin is a soluble decoy receptor for tumor necrosis factor-related apoptosis-inducing ligand/Apo2 ligand and can function as a paracrine survival factor for human myeloma cells, Cancer Res 63 (2003) 912–916.

40. H. Takayanagi, K. Ogasawara & S. Hida, et al., T-cell-mediated regulation of osteoclastogenesis by signalling cross-talk between RANKL and IFN-γ, Nature 408 (2000) 600–605.

41. G.S. Firestein & N.J. Zvaifler, How important are T cells in chronic rheumatoid synovitis?, Arthritis Rheum 33 (1990) 768–773.

42. R.W. Kinne, E. Palombo-Kinne & F. Emmrich, T-cells in the pathogenesis of rheumatoid arthritis villains or accomplices?, Biochim Biophys Acta 1360 (1997) 109–141.

43. M.N. Weitzmann, S. Cenci & L. Rifas, et al., Interleukin-7 stimulates osteoclast formation by up-regulating the T-cell production of soluble osteoclastogenic cytokines, Blood 96 (2000) 1873–1878.

44. G. Toraldo, C. Roggia & W.P. Qian, et al., IL-7 induces bone loss *in vivo* by induction of receptor activator of nuclear factor kappa B ligand and tumor necrosis factor alpha from T cells, Proc Natl Acad Sci USA 100 (2003) 125–130.

45. M. Iwata, L. Graf & N. Awaya, et al., Functional interleukin-7 receptors (IL-7Rs) are expressed by marrow stromal cells: binding of IL-7 increases levels of IL-6 mRNA and secreted protein, Blood 100 (2002) 1318–1325.

46. M. Iwata, L. Graf & N. Awaya, et al., IL-6 stimulates osteoclast-like multinucleated cell formation in long term human marrow cultures by inducing IL-1 release, J Immunol 144 (1990) 4226–4230.

47. K. Black, I.R. Garrett & G.R. Mundy, Chinese hamster ovarian cells transfected with the murine interleukin-6 gene cause hypercalcemia as well as cachexia, leukocytosis and thrombocytosis in tumor-bearing nude mice, Endocrinology 128 (1991) 2657–2659.

48. J. De La Mata, H.L. Uy & T.A. Guise, et al., Interleukin-6 enhances hypercalcemia and bone resorption mediated by parathyroid hormone-related protein *in vivo*, J Clin Invest 95 (1995) 2846–2852.

49. R.D. Devlin, S.V. Reddy & R. Savano, et al., IL-6 mediates the effects of IL-1 or TNF, but not PTHrP or 1,25(OH)2D3, on osteoclast-like cell formation in normal human bone marrow cultures, J Bone Miner Res 13 (1998) 393–399.

50. R. Bataille, D. Chappard & B. Klein, Mechanisms of bone lesions in multiple myeloma, Hematol Oncol Clin North Am 6 (1992) 285–295.

51. J. Epstein, Myeloma phenotype: clues to disease origin and manifestation, Hematol Oncol Clin North Am 6 (1992) 249–256.

52. T. Iwasaki, T. Hamano & A. Ogata, et al., Clinical significance of interleukin-6 gene expression in the bone marrow of patients with multiple myeloma, Int J Hematol 70 (1999) 163–168.

53. O.F. Ballester, L.C. Moscinski & G.H. Lyman, et al., High levels of interleukin-6 are associated with low tumor burden and low growth fraction in multiple myeloma, Blood 83 (1994) 1903–1908.

54. H.I. Sati, J.F. Apperley & M. Greaves, et al., Interleukin-6 is expressed by plasma cells from patients with multiple myeloma and monoclonal gammopathy of undetermined significance, Br J Haematol 101 (1998) 287–295.

55. G. Teoh & K.C. Anderson, Interaction of tumor and host cells with adhesion and extracellular matrix molecules in the development of multiple myeloma, Hematol Oncol Clin North Am 11 (1997) 27–42.

56. X. Thomas, B. Anglaret, J.P. Magaud & J. Epstein, et al., Interdependence between cytokines and cell adhesion molecules to induce interleukin-6 production by stromal cells in myeloma, Leuk Lymphoma 32 (1998) 107–119.

57. A. Karadag, B.O. Oyajobi & J.F. Apperley, et al., Human myeloma cells promote the production of interleukin 6 by primary human osteoblasts, Br J Haematol 108 (2000) 383–390.

58. M. Abe, K. Hiura & J. Wilde, et al., Osteoclasts enhance myeloma cell growth and survival via cell-cell contact: a vicious cycle between bone destruction and myeloma expansion, Blood 104 (2004) 2484–2491.

59. K. Anderson, R.M. Jones & C. Morimoto, et al., Response patterns of purified myeloma cells to hematopoietic growth factors, Blood 73 (1989) 1915–1924.

60. N. Kurihara, D. Bertolini & T. Suda, et al., IL-6 stimulates osteoclast-like multinucleated cell formation in long term human marrow cultures by inducing IL-1 release, J Immunol 144 (1990) 4226–4230.

61. F. Merico, L. Bergui & M.G. Gregoretti, et al., Cytokines involved in the progression of multiple myeloma, Clin Exp Immunol 92 (1993) 27–31.

62. N. Giuliani, F. Morandi & S. Tagliaferri, et al., Interleukin-3 (IL-3) is overexpressed by T lymphocytes in multiple myeloma patients, Blood 107 (2006) 841–842.

63. J.W. Lee, H.Y. Chung & L.A. Ehrlich, et al., IL-3 expression by myeloma cells increases both osteoclast formation and growth of myeloma cells, Blood 103 (2004) 2308–2315.

64. B.E. Barton & R. Mayer, IL-3 induces differentiation of bone marrow precursor cells to osteoclast-like cells, J Immunol 143 (1989) 3211–3216.

65. J. Banchereau, F. Briere & C. Caux, et al., Immunobiology of dendritic cells, Annu Rev Immunol 18 (2000) 767–811.

66. G.J. Randolph, K. Inaba & D.F. Robbiani, et al., Differentiation of phagocytic monocytes into lymph node dendritic cells *in vivo*, Immunity 11 (1999) 753–761.

67. G.J. Randolph, G. Sanchez-Schmitz & R.M. Liebman, et al., The CD16(+) (FcgammaRIII(+)) subset of human monocytes preferentially becomes migratory dendritic cells in a model tissue setting, J Exp Med 196 (2002) 517–527.

68. T. Miyamoto, O. Ohneda & F. Arai, et al., Bifurcation of osteoclasts and dendritic cells from common progenitors, Blood 98 (2001) 2544–2554.

69. A. Rivollier, M. Mazzorana & J. Tebib, et al., Immature dendritic cell transdifferentiation into osteoclasts: a novel pathway sustained by the rheumatoid arthritis microenvironment, Blood 104 (2004) 4029–4037.

70. T. Hashimoto, M. Abe & Y. Tanaka, et al., Macrophage inflammatory protein-1 may cause reciprocal regulation of osteoclast and dendritic cell differentiation from monocytes in myeloma (abstract), Haematologica J 90 (2005) 46.

71. S.D. Wolpe, G. Davatelis & B. Sherry, et al., Macrophages secrete a novel heparin-binding protein with inflammatory and neutrophil chemokinetic properties, J Exp Med 167 (1988) 570–581.

72. T. Kukita, H. Nomiyama & Y. Ohmoto, et al., Macrophage inflammatory protein-1α (LD78) expressed in human bone marrow: its role in regulation of hematopoiesis and osteoclast recruitment, Lab Invest 76 (1997) 399–406.

73. B.A. Scheven, J.S. Milne & I. Hunter, et al., Macrophage-inflammatory protein-1α regulates preosteoclast differentiation *in vitro*, Biochem Biophys Res Commun 254 (1999) 773–778.

74. J.H. Han, S.J. Choi & N. Kurihara, et al., Macrophage inflammatory protein-1α is an osteoclastogenic factor in myeloma that is independent of receptor activator of nuclear factor kappaB ligand, Blood 97 (2001) 3349–3353.

75. M. Abe, K. Hiura & J. Wilde, et al., Role for macrophage inflammatory protein (MIP)-1α and MIP-1β in the development of osteolytic lesions in multiple myeloma, Blood 100 (2002) 2195–2202.

76. S.J. Choi, J.C. Cruz & F. Craig, et al., Macrophage inflammatory protein-1α is a potential osteoclast stimulatory factor in multiple myeloma, Blood 96 (2000) 671–675.

77. G.D. Roodman, Mechanisms of bone lesions in multiple myeloma and lymphoma, Cancer 80 (1997) 1557–1563.

78. S. Uneda, H. Hata & F. Matsuno, et al., Macrophage inflammatory protein-1α is produced by human multiple myeloma (MM) cells and its expression correlates with bone lesions in patients with MM, Br J Haematol 120 (2003) 53–55.

79. E. Terpos, M. Politou & R. Szydlo, et al., Serum levels of macrophage inflammatory protein-1α (MIP-1α) correlate with the extent of bone disease and survival in patients with multiple myeloma, Br J Haematol 123 (2003) 106–109.

80. F. Magrangeas, V. Nasser & H. Avet-Loiseau, et al., Gene expression profiling of multiple myeloma reveals molecular portraits in relation to the pathogenesis of the disease, Blood 101 (2003) 4998–5006.

81. T. Hashimoto, M. Abe & T. Oshima, et al., Ability of myeloma cells to secrete macrophage inflammatory protein (MIP)-1α and MIP-1β correlates with lytic bone lesions in patients with multiple myeloma, Br J Haematol 125 (2004) 38–41.

82. S.J. Choi, Y. Oba & Y. Gazitt, et al., Antisense inhibition of macrophage inflammatory protein 1-α blocks bone destruction in a model of myeloma bone disease, J Clin Invest 108 (2001) 1833–1841.

83. B.O. Oyajobi, G. Franchin & P.J. Williams, et al., Dual effects of macrophage inflammatory protein-1α on osteolysis and tumor burden in the murine 5TGM1 model of myeloma bone disease, Blood 102 (2003) 311–319.

84. G.R. Mundy & B.O. Oyajobi, Pathophysiology of myeloma bone disease, in: G.R. Mundy & R.D. Rubens (Eds.). Cancer and the Skeleton, Martin Dunitz, London, 2000, pp. 21–32.

85. J.R. Green, Bisphosphonates in cancer therapy, Curr Opin Oncol 14 (2002) 609–615.

86. S. Yaccoby, R.N. Pearse & C.L. Johnson, et al., Myeloma interacts with the bone marrow microenvironment to induce osteoclastogenesis and is dependent on osteoclast activity, Br J Haematol 116 (2002) 278–290.

87. K. Vanderkerken, E. De Leenheer & C. Shipman, et al., Recombinant osteoprotegerin decreases tumor burden and increases survival in a murine model of multiple myeloma, Cancer Res 63 (2003) 287–289.

88. P.I. Croucher, C.M. Shipman & J. Lippitt, et al., Osteoprotegerin inhibits the development of osteolytic bone disease in multiple myeloma, Blood 98 (2001) 3534–3540.

89. J.J. Body, P. Greipp & R.E. Coleman, et al., A phase I study of AMGN-0007, a recombinant osteoprotegerin construct, in patients with multiple myeloma or breast carcinoma related bone metastases, Cancer 97 (2003) 887–992.

90. J.J. Body, T. Facon & R.E. Coleman, et al., A study of the biological receptor activator of nuclear factor-kappaB ligand inhibitor, denosumab, in patients with multiple myeloma or bone metastases from breast cancer, Clin Cancer Res 12 (2006) 1221–1228.

91. P. Menten, A. Wuyts & J. Van Damme, Macrophage inflammatory protein-1, Cytokine Growth Factor Rev 13 (2002) 455–481.

92. B. Sherry, P. Tekamp-Olson & C. Gallegos, et al., Resolution of the two components of macrophage inflammatory protein 1, and cloning and characterization of one of those components, macrophage inflammatory protein-1β, J Exp Med 168 (1988) 2251–2259.

CHAPTER 7

Facts and Hypothesis on Osteolytic Lesions Related to Normal and Tumoral Epithelial Dental Cell Differentiation

BLANDINE RUHIN[1,2], FRÉDÉRIC LÉZOT[1], AYMANN BOUATTOUR[1,3], SONIA GHOUL-MAZGAR[4], ARIANE BERDAL[1,5] AND VIANNEY DESCROIX[1,3]

[1]Centre de Recherche des Cordeliers, Oral Facial Biology and Pathology, Paris, France, Inserm UMRS 872.

[2]Stomatology and Maxillofacial Surgery Department, Pitié-Salpêtrière University Hospital, Pierre et Marie Curie University, Paris, France.

[3]Odontology Department, Pitié-Salpêtrière Hospital, Paris cedex 13, France.

[4]Laboratoire d'Histologie-Embryologie, Faculté de Médecine Dentaire de Monastir, Tunisia.

[5]Odontology Department Hôtel-Dieu Hospital, Paris, France.

Contents

I. INTRODUCTION

The maxilla and mandible constitute skeletal structures of the middle and low face. Jaw physiopathology shows distinct features when compared to the one of axial and appendicular bone. First, the oral area contains additional mineralized tissues of teeth: crown-covering enamel, central core dentin and root-lining cementum [1]. Anchoring of teeth within the jaw is ensured by a dedicated anatomical structure: the alveolar bone which is connected to root cementum by the periodontal ligament. The tooth and alveolar bones are directly involved in mastication. Maxillo-facial bone cell physiology is unique *per se*. Some physiopathological features discriminate the maxillo-facial region from the axial and appendicular bone. A unique lability characterizes the alveolar bone which appears and disappears with tooth loss. Its biomechanical plasticity, intimately related to dental movement, enables orthodontic tooth displacement. Jaw osteonecrosis [2] has emerged as a public health problem. It appears to be an adverse effect of antiresorptive agents used for osteoporosis and tumor metastasis, without such an observation on axial and appendicular bone. Therefore, oral facial bone specificity is becoming a physiopathological question raised not only in dentistry and periodontology but also in oncology and maxillofacial surgery.

At present, a molecular specificity for oral facial bone cells is not delineated. This bone specificity could be indirect (i.e., related to tooth and its peculiar situation within buccal medium). A tooth crown is exposed to oral microorganisms and masticatory biomechanics. Tooth decay and periodontal diseases may destroy mineralized tissues; infectious and inflammatory processes then affect dental pulp and periodontium and extend within maxillary bone. In a physiological context, matrix proteins produced by dental cells may enrich the alveolar bone microenvironment [3]. These dental proteins are proposed to determine the singular homeostasis of alveolar bone. They would intervene in addition to the occurring stromal cells/osteoblast-osteoclast communications, which are identical to the ones unraveled in long bones. The physiopathological singularity of alveolar bone cells could also be relied on an intrinsic cell specificity. Data on early development show that oral-facial bone and tooth cells differ from axial bone in their embryology and early signaling processes. Oral facial mineralized tissues originate from neural and epithelial cells while axial bones come from the mesoderm [4]. Initial genetic networks for patterning, morphogenesis and cell differentiation also diverge in the cranial facial (Hox-free) and axial and appendicular (Hox-dependent) skeleton [4]. As mentioned above, biphosphonate-induced maxillary osteonecrosis indicates that there are, in adults, some physiopathological pathways proper to the maxillo-facial bone [2] which are presently not understood.

Bone osteolysis associated with tumoral and cystic odontogenic lesions is presented here. They constitute an exemplary model for the molecular analysis of dental cell impact on their bone microenvironment. This chapter studies squamous cell carcinomas which constitute more than 90% of the malignant tumors in the oral cavity and oropharynx [5] (Figure 7.1). Indeed, the related physiopathological pathways of epithelial cell transformation in relation to bone microenvironment are non-specific. As such, they are reviewed elsewhere in the book. Odontogenic epithelial tumors and cysts regarding their specificity and aggressivity on the bone structure are studied here. They grow in the jaw by active bone resorption (Figure 7.2). They can also expand in the surrounding tissues (masseterian muscles, infratemporalis fossa, orbital structures, the skull basis) and generate metastasis in distant organs such as the lung or liver. Consequently, they may result in the death of the patient. Therefore, a pluridisciplinary approach of these odontogenic tumors is essential, involving odontology, maxillofacial surgery, neurosurgery, ophthalmology, histopathology, molecular biology, genetics and medical oncology. Such a transversal approach will be overviewed in this chapter.

Several maxillofacial osteolytic lesions are easily diagnosed. This is based on their clinical and radiographical characteristics as well as pathological and biological profiles. They will be briefly summarized in this chapter. Positive and differential diagnosis may lead to confusion and result in a problematic therapeutic decision for optimal prognosis concerning some of them. Thus, this chapter will provide a detailed analysis of epithelial-derived lesions called 'ameloblastomas' and 'keratocystic odontogenic tumors (KOT)'. Their effective diagnosis is problematical. They raise theoretical difficulties for their physiopathology

and therefore prognosis. Finally, the actual treatment of osseous maxillofacial lesions is restricted to surgical removal. And these osteolytic lesions may result in partial and even complete jaw destruction (Figure 7.2). These acute situations require extensive surgery, involving the use of large autografts and heavy surgical devices for bone reconstruction [6]. This therapeutic state of the art contrasts with the pharmacological panel used for epithelial metastasis in long bones. These last pathologies benefit by treatment with anti-resorptive agents which impair bone-tumor interactions which lead to tumor growth and expansion. A molecular understanding of the relationships between epithelial odontogenic tumoral/cystic cells and bone microenvironment is a prerequisite to implementing alternative pharmacological rationales for their treatment and eventual prevention.

II. DEVELOPMENTAL STAGES OF MAXILLA AND TOOTH FORMATION

The cranial facial skeleton originates essentially from two tissues—the neurectoderm, which provides ectomesenchymal components (dentin, cementum and bone) and the ectoderm, which gives rise to oral and dental epithelium [1,7]. This contrasts with the axial and appendicular bone which comes exclusively from the mesoderm [3,4]. In human embryogenesis [1], at 3 weeks, neural crest cells leave their original cephalic neural fold and migrate laterally into the mesenchyme of nasal and maxillar buds, first and second branchial arches. At 5 to 6 weeks, during their migration, neural crest cells are actively dividing, inducing facial bud and branchial arch growth [7]. A step called the ectomesenchymal transition is essential for the process of maxillofacial morphogenesis. The formed ectomesenchyme contributes not only to osteogenesis, but also to dental formation [8]. Odontogenesis *per se* results from a defined interaction between dental ectomesenchyme and epithelium [9]. Several steps of dental morphogenesis are morphologically evidenced: bud, cap and, finally, the bell stage, which displays the distinct crown morphology of each tooth germ (incisor, canine, premolar and molar) (Figure 7.3). Tooth

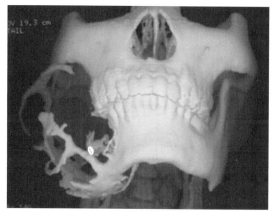

FIGURE 7.1   Major jawbone osteolysis in the context of mandibular giant ameloblastoma, visualized on a tridimentional cephalic scanography.

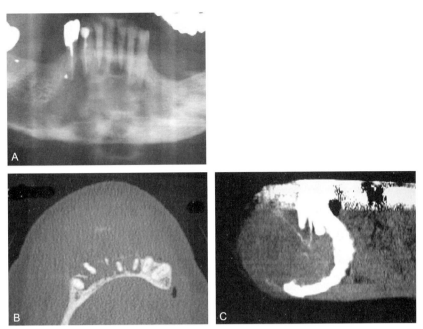

FIGURE 7.2 Mandibular metastasis of an epithelial breast carcinoma visualized on panoramic X-ray (A), axial (B), and sagital (C) scanographic slides.

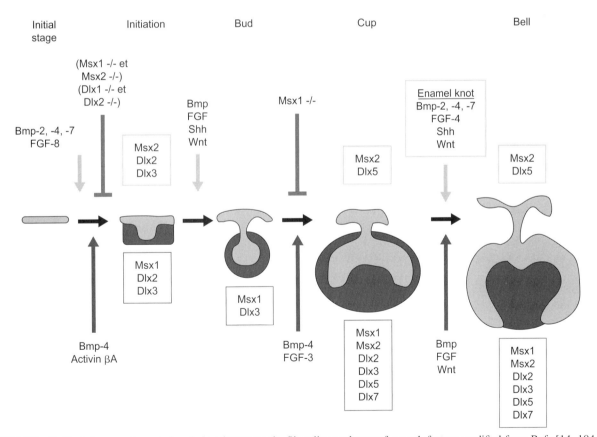

FIGURE 7.3 Epithelial-mesenchymal signals in odontogenesis. Signaling pathway of growth factors modified from Refs [14, 104 (with additional references)]. Evolution (horizontal arrows) is represented in gray for the epithelial compartment and in black for the mesenchymal compartment. Vertical arrows indicate epithelial (gray) and mesenchymal (black) growth factor signals which trigger the expression of Msx and Dlx transcription factors and enable tooth morphogenesis. Composite vertical and horizontal line indicates the stage of arrest of odontogenesis associated with the mutation of specific genes in the first mandibular molar. BMPs: Bone; Morphogenetic Proteins; FGFs: Fibroblast Growth Factors; Shh: Sonic hedgehog; Wnt: Wint; Msx: Muscle segment homeobox gene-encoding proteins; Dlx: Distal-less homeobox gene-encoding proteins; S: Sense RNA; AS: Antisense RNA.

morphogenesis proceeds through a continuing epithelial invagination, which prefigures the future root shape. Ultimately, dental histogenesis is performed by specialized differentiated cell-types. Epithelium-derived ameloblasts form an enamel matrix which contains numerous non-collagenous proteins such as amelogenins, ameloblastin/amelin/sheathlin and enamclin [10]. Odontoblasts (forming dentin) and cementoblasts (forming cementum) secrete various matrix proteins which are also found in the bone [11]. These molecular species include type I collagen and a set of non-collagenous proteins (osteocalcin, osteopontin, bone sialoprotein, osteonectin, MEPE, DMP1...). Other proteins are more specific for dental cells. The DSPP gene is over-expressed by dentin-forming odontoblasts [12]. CAP-protein characterizes cementum [13].

Dental anomalies show that alveolar bone formation and modeling [14] are intimately associated with the odontogenesis process. When tooth agenesis occurs, alveolar bone is lacking [15]. Conversely, when bone cells are affected, tooth formation is affected [16]. Experimental studies show that periodental osteoclast differentiation and activity are spatially and timely coordinated with tooth development and allometric growth [17]. The involved pathways include established bone cell communications such as RANK/RANK ligand/osteoprotegerin and PTHrp/PTH receptor pathways. In the other hand, human genetics has identified more than 300 genes related to tooth development and dental defects [9]. Interestingly, some of them lead to aberrant epithelial growth in association with maxillary bone lesions. This is exemplified in Gorlin's syndrome where Shh signals are altered [18] and in Msx2 homeogene mutations where abnormal tooth eruption is associated with the formation of an odontogenic tumor [14].

When dental development is achieved, teeth are anchored within the alveolar bone and surrounded by gingiva. Remnants of dental epithelium are still found in the periodontal ligament (Malassez rests) and gingiva (Serres pearls) [1]. Comparisons between the osteolytic maxillofacial lesions and tooth development stages are the theoretical basis underlying their histopathological classification [5]. All of the morphological and molecular studies led to the proposal that the lesions arise from a distinct epithelial stage and site depending on their pathological sub-category. Therefore, epithelial cell dysfunctions would be the main actor for the apparition and extension of osteolytic lesions. Other tissues and cells are additionally instrumental in these signaling cascades, such as the ectomesenchymal follicular sac during normal development and its tumoral counterpart, the stroma. As established in tooth development (Figure 7.3), epithelial-mesenchymal cross-talks and their alterations are based on a reciprocal activation/repression of growth factor and transcription factor expression. In this regard, a detailed knowledge of tumoral epithelial phenotype could be useful as a landmark for their physiopathological understanding.

III. EPITHELIAL CELL FATE AND DIFFERENTIATION IN THE ODONTOGENIC AND NON-ODONTOGENIC PATHWAYS DURING NORMAL DEVELOPMENT AND IN ODONTOGENIC OSTEOLYTIC TUMORS AND CYSTS

In order to analyze the epithelial lesions in maxilla, a brief summary of normal epithelial cell fate and morphology is necessary (Figure 7.4). Morphological criteria enable the identification of different stages of oral epithelium evolution, from early development when epithelium forms the dental lamina, to the adult stage when the tooth is anchored within the alveolar bone.

A. Epithelial Odontogenic and Non-odontogenic Cells in the Normal Situation

Embryonic oral epithelium provides two categories of epithelial cells: (1) odontogenic cells which are involved in dental and periodontal formation; and (2) non-odontogenic cells which form the oral mucosa. It covers the jawbone, providing a barrier against aggressive buccal medium [1]. Gingiva constitutes the anatomical junction between these two categories of cells, pertaining to the periodontium, on the one hand, and in physical continuity with oral mucosa, on the other.

The follow-up of epithelial cell fate has been performed by morphological analysis [1]. The processes of ameloblast differentiation and enamel formation have been investigated in depth [1,19]. Some stages are described sparsely at the molecular level. This is the case for the formation of Hertwig's root sheath, reduction of enamel organ and formation of junction epithelium [20]. In fact, few studies have been dedicated to epithelial cell fate and lineage(s) *per se*. Consequently, there are important theoretical gaps in the epithelial cell pathway. Some matters of debate persist on the origin of epithelial root sheath. Textbooks provide a widely accepted scheme: root sheath is formed by the most external layers of odontogenic epithelium, the inner and outer dental epithelium [1]. Alternatively, recent studies propose that the epithelial root sheath would originate from the outer dental epithelium and other odontogenic epithelial cells [21]. A second matter of debate is the ultimate fate of root sheath which would be fragmented either exclusively by cell apoptosis or additionally via an epithelial-mesenchymal transformation. This last process would generate a cementoblastic sub-population [10]. The origin of stratum intermedium cells and their relationships with enamel knots is also unclear (Figure 7.4). Finally, physiology and physiopathology of residual epithelial cells in adult periodontium, the Malassez rests, have been actively studied. They produce enamel-related proteins in the vicinity of root cementum and alveolar bone in the normal situation [22]. When the tooth is triggered by inflammatory/biomechanical stimulation and during the repair process, the levels of

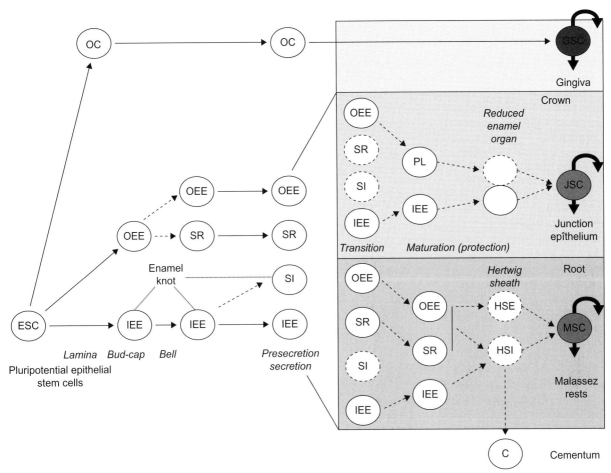

FIGURE 7.4   Normal and tumoral epithelial cell fate and lineages. Black arrows indicate established cell lineages. Dotted arrows indicate proposed cell lineage. Lines indicate suspected lineage relationships between different cells. Non-odontogenic and odontogenic epithelial cells derive from the primitive buccal epithelium where stem cells are present (ESC). The first classification for epithelial cells is their distinct pathways toward non-odontogenic and odontogenic cells. The dental lamina invaginates and gives rise to several buds of the lacteal and permanent dentition. At that cap stage, an internal layer called internal enamel epithelium (IEE) is in contact with the dental papilla mesenchyme. It is distinct from the external enamel epithelium counterpart (OEE) bordered by the follicular sac mesenchyme. The organization of the epithelium gives rise to the enamel knot which is an organizing center for tooth morphogenesis. When bell stage is reached, additional layers appear; that is the stellate reticulum (SR) and the stratum intermedium (SI). Cell differentiation progresses during the presecretion stage. During the secretion stage, ameloblasts secrete an extracellular matrix. During the post-secretion stage, secretion abruptly slows down, a pulse of apoptosis occurs and hypermineralization of enamel intervenes. In the crown aspect of enamel organ, meanwhile, amelogeneis proceeds, the other cells of the enamel organ are transformed in a unique layer called the papillary layer (PL). A transformation of enamel organ epithelial cells accompanies root formation. Only two layers form the invaginating root sheath: its external Hertwig's root sheath epithelium (HSE) and the internal counterpart (HSI). This root sheath is fragmented and provides the Malassez rest cells which are present all through the life of the tooth. Therefore, a contingent of Malassez rest cells constitutes the stem compartment (MSC). This crown enamel organ and root sheath are used to classify the odontogenic tumors, by comparing their cellular and molecular features. Crown epithelium is proposed to give rise to ameloblastoma, while root epithelium would give rise to KOT.

enamel protein expression appear to be upregulated [22]. These molecular species are able to control bone cell behavior. Inhibition of osteoclast differentiation and activity [3] and, conversely, a stimulatory effect on osteoblast differentiation has been reported. *In vitro* [23] and *in vivo* [24] experiments of amelogenin addition were performed for osteoblast cells. In transgenic mice, alveolar bone and tooth resorption were induced by amelogenin gene null mutation, in relation with the activation of RANK/RANK ligand pathway [3]. This field currently attracts much attention and financial support

by industries as they pave the way for promising tools in periodontal regeneration.

B. Epithelial Odontogenic and Non-odontogenic Cells in Odontogenic Tumors

Odontogenic tumors have been classified depending on the presence of epithelial and/or mesenchymal cells (Table 7.1). The second WHO criterion is the differentiation stage of tumoral cells based on their analogy with morphological

TABLE 7.1   Who histological classification of odontogenic tumors

Malignant tumors
- *Odontogenic carcinomas*
  Metastasizing (malignant) ameloblastoma
  Ameloblastic carcinoma–primary type
  Ameloblastic carcinoma–secondary type (differentiated), intraosseous
  Ameloblastic carcinoma–secondary type (differentiated), peripheral
  Primary intraosseous squamous cell carcinoma–solid type
  Primary intraosseous squamous cell carcinoma derived from keratocysticodontogenic tumor
  Primary intraosseous squamous cell carcinoma derived from odontogenic cysts
  Clear cell odontogenic carcinoma
  Ghost cell odontogenic carcinoma
- *Odontogenic sarcoma*
  Ameloblastic fibrosarcoma
  Ameloblastic fibrodentino and fibro-odontosarcoma.

Benign tumors
- *Odontogenic epithelium with mature, fibrous stroma without odontogenic ectomesenchyme*
  Ameloblastoma solid/multicystic type
  Ameloblastoma, extraosseous/peripheral type
  Ameloblastoma, desmoplastic type
  Ameloblastoma, unicystic type
  Squamous odontogenic tumor
  Calcifying epithelial odontogenic tumor
  Adenomatoid odontogenic tumor
  Keratocystic odontogenic tumor
- *Odontogenic epithelium with odontogenic ectomesenchyme with or without hard tissue formation*:
  Ameloblastic fibroma
  Ameloblastic fibrodentinoma
  Ameloblastic fibro-odontoma
  Odontoma (complex or compound type)
  Odontoameloblastoma
  Calcifying cystic odontogenic tumor
  Dentinogenic ghost cell tumor
- *Mesenchyme and/or odontogenic ectomesenchyme, with or without odontogenic epithelium*
  Odontogenic fibroma
  Odontogenic myxoma/myxofibroma
  Cementoblastoma
- *Bone related lesions*
  Ossifying fibroma
  Fibrous dysplasia
  Osseous dysplasia
  Central giant cell lesion (granuloma)
  Cherubism
  Aneurismal bone cyst
  Simple bone cyst

Other tumors
  Melanotic neuroectodermal tumor of infancy

and molecular stages of normal tooth development. The majority of these maxillofacial lesions induce osteolytic phenomena. A differential diagnosis between tumors, on the one hand, and developmental disorders and inflammatory processes, on the other, are crucial. Developmental disorders correspond to osteochondrodysplasia, dysostosis, idiopathic osteolysis and primitive metabolic anomalies. Others belong to dysplasia and dystrophic processes (histiocytosis X

(Figure 7.5), osteoporosis, osteomalacia, rachitism, osteosclerosis, hyperparathyroidism, Gorham-Stout syndrome, osteoradionecrosis, fibrous dysplasia, cherubism, Paget's disease, hemoglobinopathies and sclerodermia). Their diagnoses become easier with progress in the understanding of their genetic, biologic and histologic characteristics. Other entities have infectious and inflammatory origins (osteitis, osteomyelitis, swelling granuloma). Their clinical, radiological

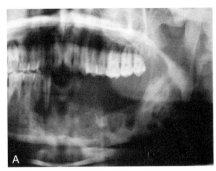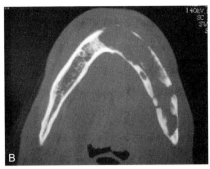

FIGURE 7.5 (A) Panoramic X-ray showing a large osteolytic lesion involving radicular dental processes according to a severe left mandibular histiocytosis (symphysis, left parasymphysis and left mandibular corpus); (B) the same lesion visualized on an axial scanographic slide.

and biological signs generally enable diagnosis. The last categories of bone pathologies are osteolytic cysts and tumors. Their clinical and radiological similarities retained our attention and we have decided to concentrate on the epithelial cysts and tumors. They appeared to constitute interesting natural models for understanding the osteolytic property of the odontogenic and non-odontogenic epithelium within the maxillary and mandibular frame.

1. OSTEOLYTIC EPITHELIAL CYSTS

Clinically, these lesions are found in diverse buccal areas. A pathologic cavity containing a fluid or semi-fluid medium appears to be surrounded by an epithelial wall [5]. These lesions are classified as non-odontogenic and odontogenic cysts depending on their anatomical and histological profile. Osteolytic epithelial non-odontogenic cysts, also called fissural cysts, were proposed to be reliant on an abnormal embryonic tissue fusion. Odontogenic entities are proposed to be secondary to abnormal growth of tissues involved in odontogenesis. A myriad of specific entities (lateral, gingival, eruptive and calcifying odontogenic cysts) are also recorded. The two major lesions are odontogenic keratocysts and follicular cysts. Recent WHO classification includes odontogenic keratocyst into odontogenic tumors (Table 7.1). This is known as keratocyst odontogenic tumor (KOT). Both KOT (Figure 7.6) and follicular cysts may expand distally within the mandible. Interestingly, this area corresponds to the progression zone of odontogenic tissues during development. Their positive and differential diagnosis is established from their clinical and radiographical signs. However, they require a histopathological diagnosis (Figure 7.6E). They may show extensive destruction of bone structures. KOT may form buccal fistulas in association with inflammation, swelling and white secretion. Follicular cysts are also dentigerous (Figure 7.7), showing resorbed teeth whose roots are not edified. The last category of osteolytic epithelial lesions, radicular cysts, represents a circumstancial inflammatory sign of tooth and/or periodontal infections. Produced cytokines would trigger odontogenic cells and modify their homeostasis. These radicular cysts represent 59% of jaw cysts. They show all the grades of inflammatory

stages within desmodontal, periapical and lateroradicular spaces. This leads to the formation of a granuloma and, to a variable extent, in epithelial proliferation from vestigial Malassez rests. In contrast to other epithelial osteolytic lesions, resolution of the dental and/or periodontal infection and inflammation processes will be the appropriate therapeutic strategy. This is usually successful and failures will orientate toward a differential diagnosis.

2. OSTEOLYTIC EPITHELIAL ODONTOGENIC TUMORS

Odontogenic tumors are rare. Some of them are even extremely rare. They sometimes raise a significant diagnosis and therapeutic challenge, comparatively with previously described lesions. The large majority of odontogenic tumors occur within the maxillofacial skeleton. Clinical features of most benign odontogenic tumors are non-specific. They have either a slow expansive pain, or painless growth. In contrast, in nearly all malignant odontogenic tumors, pain is the first and most common symptom followed by rapidly developing swelling related to the erosion affecting the jawbone cortex. Most odontogenic tumors are benign. This chapter will focus on epithelial tumors without inductive power on mesenchymal tissue because of their exemplary osteolytic capacities.

Malignant epithelial odontogenic tumors are extremely rare and aggressive. Several types of tumors are reported: ameloblastic carcinoma, primary squamous cell carcinoma, malignant transformation of KOT. Several benign tumors are discerned: the squamous odontogenic tumor (Figure 7.8), calcifying epithelial odontogenic tumor (Figure 7.9) and clear cell odontogenic tumor. The most frequent ameloblastoma (either solid and multicystic, desmoplastic, unicystic or peripheral) are associated with dental epithelium remnants. They appear to grow and form a follicular or plexiform network into a fibrous stroma (Figure 7.10; see Plate 1). As mentioned for KOT and follicular cysts, their location involves the mandible in 80% of cases. Furthermore, 70% of these cases extend from the angle toward the ramus. This location corresponds, as a

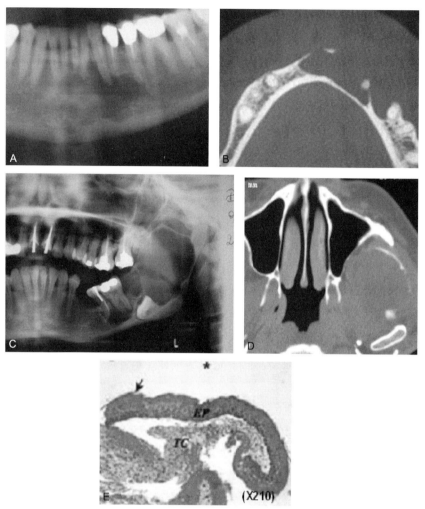

FIGURE 7.6   Two examples of keratocystic lesions. (1) Left parasymphyseal and mandibular corpus KOT: panoramic view (A) and axial scanographic slide (B); (2) voluminous left mandibular corpus and ramus KOT: panoramic view (C) and axial scanographic slide (D). Histologic analysis of this lesion (E): EP (epithelium), TC (mesenchymal tissue), *(cystic luminar), black arrow (keratin layer).

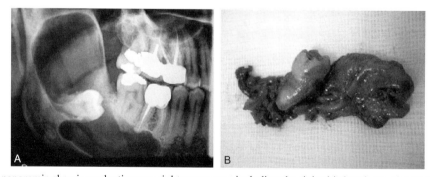

FIGURE 7.7   X-Ray panoramic showing a dentigerous right ramus cyst including the right third molar teeth (A). The macroscopic sample showing the cyst surrounding its crown on its cervical part.

reiterative motif of these osteolytic lesions, to the very distal site of dental lamina extension. Within cancellous bone, they form one or several geodes which are limited by a thin compact bone layer (Plate 1). They do not affect certain bone compartments such as periosteal surfaces and condyle.

In contrast, they may resorb tooth tissues. Tumor extension is often morphologically complex with microgeodes whose identification is crucial. Surgical procedures have to ensure the overall resection of this complex tumor in order to prevent their recurrence.

IV. MOLECULAR STUDIES ON JAW TUMORS AND KOT

At the time of writing, a molecular deciphering of odontogenic tumors is still elusive [25,26]. The development and progression of odontogenic tumors have been associated with some alterations involving non-specific determinants (i.e. the ones known to play a role in cell transformation and tumorigenesis). Additionally, these odontogenic tumors and KOT have been related to modifications in genes identified for their expression and/or role in the process of odontogenesis. The vast majority of the studies compare components of one signaling pathway in human development and odontogenic tumors (for review see Ref. [26]). Several global transcriptome studies have also been performed. Few analyses of gene mutations are available. Finally, animal models provide some experimental robustness to physiopathological hypothesis derived from circumstantial observations in human tumors. Actually, the most promising issues appear to be: (1) enamel proteins ameloblastin/amelin/sheathlin and more recently amelogenins; (2) affected Shh cascade which was initially identified in the context of nevoid basal cell carcinoma (NBCC) or Gorlin's syndrome and secondarily shown in isolated forms of KOT; and finally, (3) the specific pathway of osteoclast differentiation which impairment is associated with development switches toward odontogenic tumor profiles with time, notably in Msx2−/−

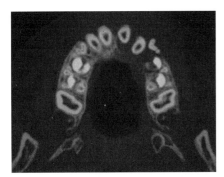

FIGURE 7.8 Axial scanographic slide showing a squamous odontogenic tumor. The radiographic picture is triangular in the alveola process of the concerned root (white arrow).

mouse line. Conversely, tumor growth is associated with osteoclast activation in its bone microenvironment. Further investigations are necessary to delineate molecular physiopathological pathway(s) and their eventual specificity for each pathological entity. This would subsequently help in designing alternative and tumor-type targeted approaches and minimize their surgical treatment which actually dominates the therapeutic strategies.

A. Genetic Changes Underlying Odontogenic Tumorigenesis

Classifying tumors require a description of the genetic changes underlying tumorigenesis [27]. In odontogenic tumors, most studies have been devoted to gene expression pattern analysis. Genetic expression profiling evidenced a molecular identity of the most common ameloblastoma in comparison with normal human teeth [28a]. Other studies provided information on additional tumors: malignant odontogenic tumors, clear cell odontogenic carcinoma [29], malignant granular cell odontogenic tumor [30], ameloblastic carcinoma [31] and dentigerous cyst [32]. In transcriptome analysis of ameloblastoma, one of the mostly overexpressed genes was the proto-oncogene *FOS* [28b]. C-Fos is important for osteoclast differentiation [33]). Elegant mouse studies identified a key role of this proto-oncogene in the control of osteoclast differentiation. In the relied osteopetrosis, dental alterations evoking odontogenic tumors are documented [16]. These defects were proposed to be related either to the action of C-fos within dental cells or to an indirect role on tooth growth via the regulation of osteoclast activity (for review on dental alterations and osteoclast see [16]). This ambiguity on the molecular impact in dental cells (either direct, indirect via bone microenvironment or both) is a recurrent matter of debate for dental genetics. In the alveolar bone, cell–cell communication deals with a second level of complexity when compared to other bone sites, the additional intervention of neighboring dental cells. Microdissecting signaling cascades has been performed in tissues and cells during timely-defined developmental windows: odontogenic

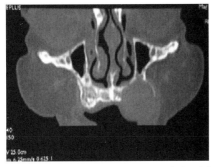 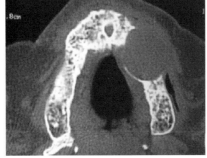

FIGURE 7.9 Axial scanographic slide showing an epithelial calcifying odontogenic tumor with an osteolytic irregular picture and thin opacities in it.

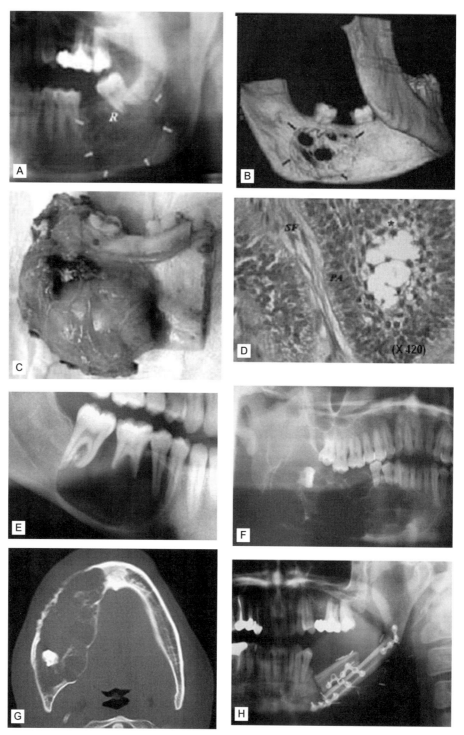

FIGURE 7.10   Three examples of ameloblastoma. Left mandibular corpus ameloblastoma: panoramic view (A); and tridimensional cephalic scanography (B); macroscopic sample showing a soft tissue invasion (C); and the follicular histologic aspect of the same lesion (D): PA (ameloblastic cellular type), SF (mesenchymal tissue); right mandibular corpus unicystic ameloblastoma: panoramic view (E); voluminous left parasymphyseal, mandibular corpus and ramus multicystic ameloblastoma: panoramic view (F); and axial scanographic slide (G); radical resection of a mandibular ameloblastoma (in the left molar, angular and ramus mandibular regions): dental panoramic after a left mandibular reconstruction by a double barrel fibula-free flap (H).

epithelium/mesenchyme during early morphogenesis [9], crown enamel organ/follicular sac/alveolar bone during dental eruption [17], adult periodontal ligament/cementum/alveolar bone in periodontal modeling [34]. The networks and their potential impact on dental tumorigenesis is discussed in Chapter 2.

Very few studies have been devoted to the identification of somatic mutations in odontogenic tumoral cells, presumably in relation with the heterogeneity of these rare pathological entities [25,35]. Frequent loss of chromosome 22 was recorded (8 upon 9 ameloblastomas—[36]). In another study, chromosomal imbalance was found uncommon [37]. In a cohort of ameloblastomas and ameloblastic carcinomas with graded aggressivity, a systematic screening was performed. It evidenced allelic losses of key tumor suppressor genes and intratumoral cell heterogeneity. However, their overall frequency was not correlated with a recurrence and malignant behavior of the tumors. In two other entities, the dentinogenetic ghost cell tumors [38] and calcifying odontogenic cysts [39], different mutations were recorded in the β-catenin gene. One k-ras mutation upon 27 ameloblastomas was evidenced [40] and two p53 mutations, upon 29 ameloblastomas [41]. Some evidence demonstrating loss of heterozygosis of p53 and p16 tumor suppressor genes in KOT supports their neoplastic nature [42]. In conclusion, all of these studies show that somatic DNA damage occurs in odontogenic tumors and KOT. The data suggest that these genetic events would be sporadic and cumulative. So far, attempts to identify a somatic mutation profile predicting aggressiveness of these tumors and KOT have been frustrating. Additional genetic or epigenetic mechanisms might be instrumental in cell transformation, which are not presently evidenced. Along this line, an interesting physiopathological mechanism was proposed for KOT [42]: germ-line mutation of Patched (PTCH) is associated with the NBCC syndrome where numerous KOT appear. On the other hand, sporadic KOT cases show somatic PTCH gene mutations [43]. In NBCC, precursor cells containing a first hereditary 'hit': (1) would develop and form KOT based on a PTCH haploinsufficiency model; or (2) be submitted to a second 'hit' via a somatic mutation of the second PTCH allele based on the alternative two allele models. With a similar scenario, sporadic KOT cases would require one or two somatic 'hits'.

B. Comparative Expression Patterns of Tumor-related Factors in Odontogenesis and Tumors

Misimpression of tumor-related factors may affect cells, modulating cell cycle, differentiation and apoptosis. Several markers for cell cycle phase/cell proliferation have been tested. In ameloblastomas, data on cyclin D1, p16INK4a, p21(WAF1/Cip1), and p27Kip1 suggest that proliferation of odontogenic epithelial cells is similarly controlled in normal development and tumorigenesis [44].

In some epithelial odontogenic tumors, apoptotic cells have been detected by TdT-mediated dUTP-biotin nick end-labeling (TUNEL) and immunohistochemistry using single-stranded DNA (ssDNA) antibody. These data suggest that apoptotic cell death plays an important role in oncogenesis and normal odontogenic epithelium during development [44,45]. In principle, there are two alternative apoptotic pathways: one mediated by death receptors on the cell surface (extrinsic pathway) and the other by mitochondria (intrinsic pathway) [46]. Numerous components of the apoptotic extrinsic pathway have been recognized in ameloblastoma and KOT, notably death receptors as TRAIL receptors 1 and 2, TNFR or Fas. Paradoxically, initiator caspase expression (i.e. caspase 8 and 10) seems to be very limited in these lesions suggesting that TNFα and TRAIL signaling minimally affects the biological properties of odontogenic epithelial components. Concerning the intrinsic pathway, the expression of APAF-1, caspase 9, cytochrome c and AIF were detected in normal and neoplastic odontogenic tissues. Expression of cytochrome c and AIF was evident in odontogenic epithelial cells neighboring the basement membrane, and APAF-1 and caspase 9 were detected in most odontogenic epithelial cells. Immunoreactivity for cytochrome c in tooth germs was slightly weaker than that in benign and malignant ameloblastomas. Keratinizing cells in acanthomatous ameloblastomas and granular cells in granular cell ameloblastomas showed a decrease or loss of immunoreactivity for these mitochondria-mediated apoptosis signaling molecules. Expression of AIF was obviously low in ameloblastic carcinomas [47].

In parallel, some of the mechanisms of apoptosis resistance have been investigated in odontogenic tumors. For example, investigation on Bcl-2 and IAP family protein (Bcl-2, BCL-X, survivin) in ameloblastoma evidenced that ameloblastoma shows increased levels of apoptosis-inhibiting protein than the apoptosis-modulating protein, suggesting that ameloblastoma has a high survival activity [48]. In fact, the expression pattern of pro-apoptotic and anti-apoptotic proteins seems to be complex. Some authors (see Refs [48] and [49]) proposed that ameloblastoma had two relatively distinct patterns: an anti-apoptotic (Bcl2) proliferating site in the peripheral layer and a pro-apoptotic (Fas/FasL; caspase 3) site in the central layer of the tumor islands.

Expression level and patterns of tumor-related factors have been individually investigated in odontogenic tumors. Protocongenes k-Ras, c-fos and c-myc are over-expressed in ameloblastoma and other odontogenic tumors (for review see Ref. [35]). In relation with the c-myc importance in cell immortalization, ameloblastoma cells expressing c-myc also showed increased telomerase activity. Consistently, experimental overexpression of myc (or ras) in mice leads to the development of odontogenic tumors [50]. Several tumor-suppressor genes have been analyzed showing either more (Carvalhais *et al.* [51], p. 53) or less (APC; reviewed in Ref. [35]) elevated expression levels in tumoral versus normal dental cells. Other tumor-related factors influence cell communications between the tumor and its microenvironment. VEGF upregulation and increased micro vessel density have been associated with tumorigenesis or malignant transformation of odontogenic epithelium (for review see Ref. [35]). These effectors are known to control osteoclast differentiation and be instrumental in the specific context of tumor growth and subsequent bone resorption [21]. Dental growth, eruption and odontogenic tumorigenesis show important similarities with the physiopathology of epithelial metastasis within a bone frame (Figure 7.11).

C. Development and Hard-tissue Related Factors

1. GROWTH FACTORS AND TRANSCRIPTION FACTORS

Tooth development and differentiation are controlled by highly conserved growth factor families (FGF, BMP, SHH, WNT, TNF, see Figure 7.3) (for review, see Ref. [9]) during distinct epithelial-mesenchymal interactions. They induce the expression of transcription factors (Msx, Dlx, Runx, Lhx, Pax,)

which in turn triggers growth factor expression (Figure 7.3). These events have been analyzed in detail over the past twenty years. Research include *in vitro* studies such as the organotypic tooth germ culture, epithelial-mesenchymal dissociation and reassociation (or addition of recombinant proteins produced by one tissue), and RNA interference. Specific gene impact is exemplified in transgenic mouse models and human diseases.

The expression patterns and relative levels of the same effectors have been compared in normal development and odontogenic tumors. Epidermal growth factor (EGF) receptors [52] and its two potential ligands, EGF and transforming growth factor α (TGFα), were studied in tooth development. Both these ligands of EGF receptors would be instrumental in normal development and play a role in odontogenic tumors as well. This pathway is essential for the control of epithelial and mesenchymal cell proliferation and may play a role in tumorigenesis through enhanced receptor expression levels in epithelial tumoral cells. The TGFβ superfamily is composed of multifunctional growth factors which are instrumental in embryonic development and cellular functions in postnatal and adults, notably in bone formation. TGFβs, BMPs, their receptors and Smad signal relays would differ depending on the tumor type [53].

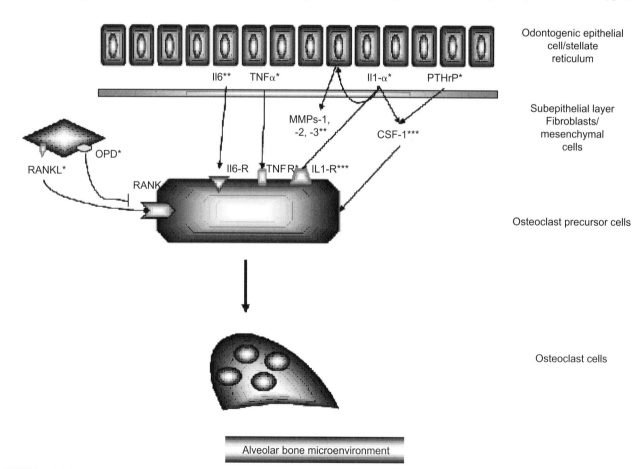

FIGURE 7.11   Possible signaling osteolysis cascade that may explain the activation and differentiation of preosteoclast in tooth eruption and odontogenic tumors in the alveolar bone microenvironment modified from [105]. *Genes implicated in tooth eruption and odontogenic tumor; **genes described in odontogenic tumors only; ***genes described in tooth eruption only.

KOTs are found in the nevoid basal cell carcinoma syndrome or in sporadic cases involve the germ-line or somatic mutations of different genes. Their mutation results in a constitutive activation of the Shh pathway (notably by the triggered expression of Shh target genes, Gli1). Gain of function of the Ptch1 repressor and loss of function of the SMO effector have been reported. An overexpression of the target gene Gli1 mimics this physiopathological mechanism in transgenic mice where odontogenic keratocysts are produced [54]. Based on this animal model, it was shown that KOT emerges from triggered proliferation, stratification and terminal differentiation of normal quiescent Malassez rest cells.

Interestingly, a follow-up study of the Msx2−/− mouse dental phenotype evidenced a late transformation of the third mandibular molar into an odontogenic tumor [14]. The epithelial cells of reducing enamel organ and Malassez rests are hyperabundant when compared to the normal situation, while enamel formation and ameloblast differentiation are impaired. These defects are accompanied by a reduction of peridental osteoclast activity, similar to the situation found in genetic bone disorders, the osteopetrosis. This regional osteoclast inhibition in Msx2−/− mice is associated with RANK ligand expression level downregulation, specifically in the alveolar bone and less clearly in the rest of the skeleton. The analysis of growth factors and transcription factors in the context of odontogenic tumors and KOT would enable a definition of their similarities with Msx2−/− mouse phenotype. Such a comparison between tumors and animal models is also relevant for enamel matrix proteins (Figure 7.12; see Plate 2).

2. HARD TISSUE MATRIX PROTEINS

Enamel matrix is made up of non-collagenous proteins, such as amelogenin, enamelin, ameloblastin (amelin or sheathlin), and tuftelin, and enzymes, such as matrix metalloproteinase (MMP)-20 (enamelysin) and enamel matrix serine proteinase 1 [1]. Expression of amelogenin, enamelin, ameloblastin, and MMP-20 has been recognized in epithelial components of various types of odontogenic tumors [55–58]. In addition, bone sialoprotein is found in many types of odontogenic tumors, suggesting that these proteins play a role in pathologic mineralization and/or tumor formation [12].

In experimental studies, soft epithelial tumors develop in ameloblastin homozygous null mutant mice [59]. Tumoral cells express enamel proteins amelogenin, enamelin and tuftelin, and show unregulated cell proliferation. Interestingly, ameloblastin gene mutations were reported in several clinical reports of ameloblastomas [60,61]. However, the analysis of natural polymorphism of the ameloblastin gene has to be re-evaluated in order to really define the significance of such observations. Gibson *et al.* [62] showed that the expression of a mutated P70T version of the amelogenin gene in amelogenin gene null mutants induces the appearance of a hyperplastic stratum intermedium. The dental structures were evocating calcifying epithelial odontogenic tumors (see the Classification Table 7.1). Proliferative cells formed cords and unevenly expressed amelogenin proteins. A small amount of the abnormal protein enabled this epithelial transformation, suggesting an important role for amelogenin in the control of odontogenic epithelial cell

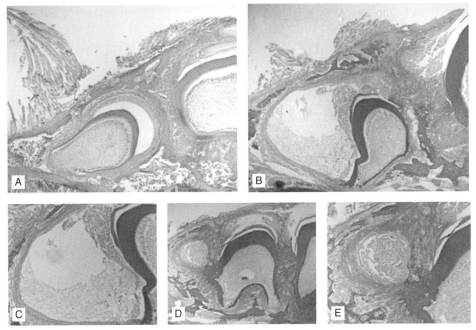

FIGURE 7.12   Molar structures in wild-type and Msx2−/− mice at 21 days. The second (M2) and third (M3) molars are evidenced in the mandible of Msx2+/+ (A) and Msx2−/− (B) mice. In Msx2−/−mice, the enamel organ is not formed properly and gives raise to epithelial cystic structures (B–E). In the distal area of the third molar, epithelial cells delaminate (C). In the distal area of crown-root junction in the second molar, an epithelial cyst is visible (D and enlargement in E).

behavior. Molecular studies on amelogenin gene mutations in human tumors are lacking.

3. OSTEOLYSIS-RELATED FACTORS

A physiologic example of alveolar bone osteolysis is represented by tooth eruption. This phenomenon is a complex and tightly regulated process that involves cells of the tooth organ, dental follicle (DF: connective tissue sac surrounding the enamel organ) and stellate reticulum (SR), and the surrounding alveolar bone. Prior to the onset of eruption and for this resorption to occur, there is an influx of mononuclear cells into the dental follicle, with a concurrent increase in the number of osteoclasts within the alveolar bony crypt. Different studies have demonstrated that the 'eruption gene' and its product are localized primarily in either the dental follicle or stellate reticulum. In fact, it is possible that DF acts as a target tissue to attract the mononuclear cells, to serve as a repository for the cells, and to provide a milieu whereby these cells can fuse and form osteoclasts [17]. In this way, osteoclastogenesis is needed for bone resorption and may involve inhibition of osteoprotegerin gene transcription and synthesis in the follicle, as well as enhancement of receptor activator of NF_{k_B} ligand (RANKL), in the adjacent alveolar bone. Paracrine signaling by parathyroid-hormone-related protein and interleukin-1α, produced in the stellate reticulum adjacent to the follicle, may also play a role in regulating eruption. Thus the mechanism of tooth eruption can be considered as a continuous interrelation between alveolar bone, mesenchymal (DF) and epithelial (SR) tissues.

Tooth eruption appears to constitute a relevant model regarding osteolytic capacity of odontogenic cells. Some analogies in the two contexts of induced resorption may be proposed. Ameloblastomas and other odontogenetic tumors of facial bone are locally invasive tumors. To expand, osteolytic lesions might have different mechanisms for the promotion of bone resorption. Thus, like tooth eruption, the tumor osteolytic mechanism also involves odontogenic epithelium and ectomesenchyme in a neighboring bone microenvironment (Figure 7.11). Therefore, a parallel may be made, on the one hand, between SR and the odontogenic epithelium and, on the other, between DF and tumor stroma. In line with this proposal, the same molecular determinants have been found in tooth eruption and tumor expansion.

The first studies were devoted to the canonic RANK/RANKL/OPG pathway and its possible deregulation [33] (Figure 7.11). The Receptor activator of NF-kappaB ligand (RANKL) is a tumor necrosis factor (TNF) family cytokine which binds membranous receptor RANK and controls osteoclast differentiation and activity. A decoy receptor osteoprotegerin (OPG) modulates the system.

RANKL is strongly expressed in DF and it is probable that interaction between it, CSF-1 and OPG locally regulates the osteoclastogenesis needed for tooth eruption. Regulation of RANKL action appears to be essential for tooth eruption,

because, in null mice devoid of the RANKL gene, the teeth are not erupted [63]. Ameloblastomas express RANKL and OPG predominantly in stromal cells [64]. In KOT, this expression is more important in epithelium.

Besides RANKL, other pro-resorptive cytokines such as TNFα or interleukin-1, were found in tooth eruption and osteolytic lesions. They are expressed in SR where they enhance CSF-1 and NFkB to stimulate the mononuclear cell fusion present in dental folliculè and then the formation of osteoclasts in the alveolar bone microenvironment (Figure 7.11).

In ameloblastomas and KOT, they are also present in the epithelium component and will increase RANKL expression in the stroma and/or stimulate osteoclast precursor differentiation. Both interleukin-1 and -6, have been jointly identified in ameloblastomas and KOT [40,65]. Some studies suggest that odontogenic keratocyst fibroblasts may support osteoclast differentiation in the presence of IL-1.

Finally, expression of parathyroid hormone-related protein (PTHrP) has been detected in neoplastic cells of ameloblastomas and KOT as in SR.

Like RANKL, PTHrP plays a role in eruption because in skeletal-rescued PTHrP knock-out mice the teeth do not erupt [66], although the osteoclasts appear normal. In double rescued knock-outs (both skeleton and epithelium are rescued), the teeth do erupt, suggesting that PTHrP is needed for eruption. More precisely, PTHrP may enhance CSF-1 expression in dental follicle to recruit and stimulate mononuclear cells.

The exact role of PTHrP in progression of osteolytic lesion is not understood. In KOT and ameloblastoma, PTHrP is expressed in epithelial tissue. It is possible that PTHrP modulates growth and bone resorption in odontogenic tumors. PTHrP may act synergistically with interleukin-1 to increase bone resorption. These different observations suggest an important correlation between the signaling pathway of tooth eruption and osteolytic tumors.

It's now clear that osteolytic cytokines have a role in local bone resorption during the progression of odontogenic tumors. More precisely, all of the inflammatory cytokines produced by the tumor and/or by the above bone-resorbing lesion are jointly efficient in RANKL upregulation in tumor stroma, adjoining osteoblast and bone stromal cells.

Even if the mechanism for bone resorption is poorly understood in odontogenic tumors and KOT, RANKL appears to be the main mediator of osteoclastogenesis and therefore extension with jaw structures.

4. MATRIX-DEGRADING PROTEINASES

A second route for a local invasiveness of odontogenic tumors is the activity of matrix-degrading proteinases in the microenvironment of the tumors. Several studies have established the presence of MMP-1, -2 and -9, and TIMP-1 and -2 in ameloblastomas [67,68]. Expression of heparanase, which cleaves proteoglycans, has also been detected

[69]. These matrix-degrading enzymes are proposed to contribute to the local invasiveness of odontogenic tumors by providing the space to expand and/or release mitogenic factors which might secondarily increase the tumor cell rate.

Consecutively to bone resorption by osteoclasts, growth factors, which are normally entrapped within the mineralized bone compartment, are released. This is the case for transforming growth factors β (TGF-β), insulin-like growth factors (IGFs), fibroblast growth factors (FGFs), platelet-derived growth factors (PDGFs), and bone morphogenetic proteins (BMPs). These factors were shown to increase the production of parathyroid hormone-related peptide (PTHrp) by tumor cells as well as growth factors that increase tumor growth. This reciprocal interaction between tumor cells and the bone microenvironment results in a vicious circle that increases both bone destruction and tumor burden [70].

V. THERAPEUTIC STATEMENT IN ODONTOGENIC TUMORS AND CYSTS

Although they are very different with regard to their etiopathogeny and evolution, benign odontogenic tumors and KOT both require surgical treatment [71]. If not, they grow, impair the oral function, may be infected, induce acute dysmorphosis, and result in a significant risk of jaw fracture (Figure 7.2). The discovery and identification of such benign lesions requires a delicate approach, taking care of all clinical and radiographical signs (age of the patient, evolutivity of the pathology, anatomical relationships with surrounding elements—especially with the cortical bone) in order to establish an argued diagnosis [72–74]. In these cases, an initial surgical biopsy is always dangerous because it would lead to histological contamination and a swelling reaction. Such techniques can impair a final diagnosis and future surgical treatment. Treatment of odontogenic tumors and KOTs must be either a bone-conservative enucleation (Figure 7.13), a peripherical osseous resection (Figure 7.14) or a radical resection of the concerned bone (Figure 7.15) [75–82].

If possible, enucleation remains the best conservative treatment for benign tumoral and KOT. This treatment allows for the conservation of teeth, bone, adjacent nerves or other surrounding anatomic elements in the case of orbital or skull localization [83–85]. As the bone corticals are conserved, even if the KOT size appears to be very important, enucleation has to be tried (Figure 7.10; see Plate 1) [86]. Several teams consider that marsupialization is interesting as it reduces the volume of the initial lesion; consensus does not exist on this subject [75,87,88]. A complementary curettage is done to eliminate epidermal remnants, stuck on the cystic adjacent osseous wall. Enucleation orders a regular post-surgery clinical and radiographical following. This will enable a diagnosis of a potential recurrence which occurs at a rate ranging from 17% to 56% [89] and also check that osseous consolidation occurs

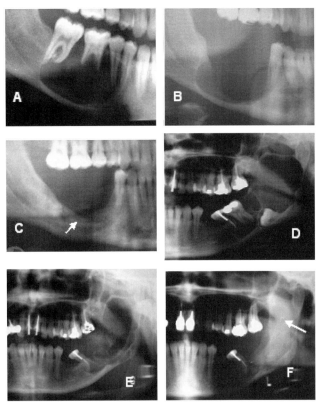

FIGURE 7.13 An example of radiographic bone evolution before and after enucleation procedure for the treatment of mandibular benign lesions. (A) Dental panoramic radiograph: osteolytic lesion regarding right inferior molars and premolars; (B) radiographic control two weeks after a mandibular conservative treatment by lesional enucleation; (C) bone consolidation (arrow) on a radiographic control four months after enucleation (histological diagnosis was follicular ameloblastoma); (D) large KOT lesion concerning the left mandible on a panoramic radiograph; (E) conservative excision of the keratocyst by enucleation and molar removing (radiographic control one day after surgery); (F) radiographic control of bone spontaneous reconstruction one year after surgery (arrow).

properly (Figure 7.10; see Plate 1). Enucleation associated with Carnoy's solution application or after decompression was reported to show lower recurrence rates ([89,90).

Bone resection allows a complete excision of the tumor; it is also retained in case of voluminous KOT with cortical resorption and tissular invasion. At each step of its realization, the surgeon must have perfect visual control of excision limits. Resection may be partial, concerning only a maxillar or mandibular segment (Figure 7.13), or complete when both mandibular cortical and basilar portions are concerned, or when extension occurs in the anterior skull base, the temporal fossae or the pterygomaxilla area [12,91b]. Resection was found to have the lowest recurrence rates (0%) but the highest morbidity [89]. In this case, reconstruction of the jaw is necessary. If bone resection is less than 5–6 cm long, a bone grafting is possible; if resection is longer than 6 cm, then a free flap reconstruction

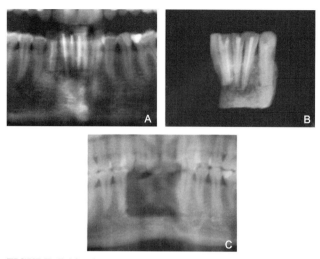

FIGURE 7.14 Conservative mandibular treatment of a symphyseal ameloblastoma by a partial bone resection. (A) Osteolytic lesion surrounding the mandibular incisive roots; (B) excision of the lesion by bone segmental resection; (C) radiographic control by panoramic one week after surgery: this treatment has conserved the mandibular continuity.

will be retained (fibula or iliac free flaps) (Figure 7.14) [6,90,91a] allowing subsequent placement of dental implants for oral prosthetic rehabilitation [92–95].

In the case of treatment, several points should be discussed in order to define the real problems. As regard to enucleation, the result can be macroscopically satisfying, but the main problem is the risk of recurrence, because the microscopic cellular cystic remnants can grow quickly or slowly over a period of years. Reflexion could be enterprised concerning the way we could improve its effect: benefit was noted by several authors after water washing the cavity, liquid nitrogen cryotherapy or chemical treatment (Carnoy's solution, H_2O_2 or acetic acid) [89,96]. This combination to enucleation should offer patients a lower recurrence rate and an avoidance of ostectomy [97].

Philosophically, as regard to resection, a surgeon should be led to consider that the nevertheless elegant therapeutic operation is only an unsatisfying destruction–reparation procedure. Furthermore, this kind of surgical operation is a real physical and psychological challenge for both patient and clinician surgeon: technical difficulties, anesthesic risks, the possibility of vascular ischemia losing the free flap, morbidity, the remains of facial asymmetry, etc. Also, whatever the curative choice, a recurrent rate still remains: while more important in conservative surgery, it is lower in radical tecnics but recurrent lesions have been observed even in the graft or the free flap in place of the jaw reconstruction [98–100].

Work concerning molecular understanding and treatment possibilities shows that no modification of expression of p53, Ki-67, and EGFR was noticed in odontogenic keratocysts before and after decompression [101], and

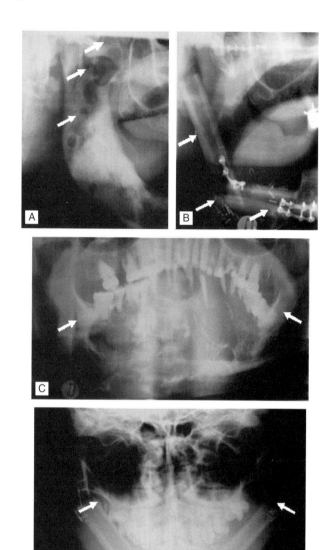

FIGURE 7.15 Radical mandibular resection with fibula free flap reconstruction in recurrent invasive or giant ameloblastoma. (A, B) Multilocular recurrence of a follicular ameloblastoma (thin arrows) with invasion of the coronoid process (thick arrow) in (A); necessity of a radical resection with right mandibular disarticulation. Panoramic radiographic control one week after surgery showing the fibula free flap reconstructing the resected right mandible (arrows) in (B). (C, D) Panoramic radiographs of a giant mandibular ameloblastoma on C (arrows); large anguloangular mandibular resection with reconstruction by a long fibula free flap (arrows on D).

suppression of the SHH signaling pathway can be an effective treatment for odontogen keratocysts [102].

If the sonic hedgehog (SHH) signaling pathway plays a critical role in tooth development [4], Patched (PTCH) is the receptor for the SHH signal, which is thought to combine with smoothened (SMO) to form a transmembrane receptor complex for SHH ligand [102]. The truncated

PTCH protein could not function as an inhibitor of the SMO receptor. This would result in the aberrant activation of the SHH signaling pathway which sequentially increases cell proliferation and inhibits cell death, thus triggering the formation of KOT [103]. Therefore, inhibitors of the SHH pathway can be regarded as possible candidates to be used by oral surgeons in the treatment of KOT.

Although reconstruction is these days very professional and efficient, the future should bring more progress and a good molecular understanding of these cysts and tumors. These would help both the clinician and the surgeon in their therapeutic behavior when faced with surgical or molecular choices.

VI. CONCLUSION

The development and progression of odontogenic tumors are affected by alterations of many kinds of genes and molecules. In particular, the characteristics of odontogenic tumors appear to depend on the molecular mechanisms associated with: (1) tooth development; (2) bone metabolism; and (3) malignant potential of tumors.

Many genes involved in tooth development have now been identified, providing a new basis for studies in oral pathology. A better understanding of underlying molecular mechanisms will help to predict the course of odontogenic tumors and lead to the development of new therapeutic applications, such as molecular-targeted treatment and patient-tailored therapy.

References

1. A. Nanci, Oral Histology, Philadelphia, USA: Mosby (2003) pp. 176–180.
2. C. Dannemann, K.W. Gratz & M.O. Riener, et al., Jaw osteonecrosis related to bisphosphonate therapy: a severe secondary disorder, Bone 40 (4) (2007) 828–834.
3. J. Hatakeyama, T. Sreenath & Y. Hatakeyama, et al., The receptor activator of nuclear factor-kappa B ligand-mediated osteoclastogenic pathway is elevated in amelogenin-null mice, J Biol Chem 278 (37) (2003) 35743–35748.
4. M.T. Cobourne & P.T. Sharpe, Tooth and jaw: molecular mechanisms of patterning in the first branchial arch, Arch Oral Biol 48 (1) (2003) 1–14.
5. R.E. Marx, and D.S. Stern, Oral and Maxillofacial Pathology: A Rationale for Diagnosis and Treatment. Chicago, USA. Quintessence books (2003), 908.
6. W. Zemann, M. Feichtinger & E. Kowatsch, et al., Extensive ameloblastoma of the jaws: surgical management and immediate reconstruction using microvascular flaps, Oral Surg Oral Med Oral Pathol Oral Radiol Endod 103 (2) (2007) 190–196.
7. N.M. Le Douarin & C. Kalcheim, The Neural Crest, 2nd edn., Cambridge University Press (1999).
8. A.G.S. Lumsden, Spatial organization of the epithelium and the role of the neural crest cells in the intiation of the mammalian tooth germ, Development 103 (1988) 155–170.
9. I. Thesleff, Genetic basis of tooth development and dental defects, Acta Odontol Scand 58 (2000) 191–194.
10. M. Zeichner-David, K. Oishi & Z. Su, et al., Role of Hertwig's epithelial root sheath cells in tooth root development, Dev Dyn 228 (4) (2003) 651–663.
11. M. Miura, S. Gronthos & M. Zhao, et al., SHED: stem cells from human exfoliated deciduous teeth, Proc Natl Acad Sci USA 100 (10) (2003) 5807–5812.
12. J. Chen, T.B. Aufdemorte & H. Jiang, et al., Neoplastic odontogenic epithelial cells express bone sialoprotein, Histochem J 30 (1998) 1–6.
13. I. Barkana, A.S. Narayanan & A. Grosskop, et al., Cementum attachment protein enriches putative cementoblastic populations on root surfaces in vitro, J Dent Res 79 (7) (2000) 1482–1488.
14. M. Aïoub, F. Lézot & M. Molla, et al., MSx2 −/− transgenic mice develop compound amelogenesis imperfecta, dentinogenesis imperfecta and periodental osteopetrosis, Bone 41(5) (2007) 851–859.
15. M. J. van den Boogaard, M. Dorland & F. A. Beemer, et al., MSx1 mutation is associated with orofacial clefting and tooth agenesis in humans, Nat Genet 24(4) (2000) 342–343.
16. M.H. Helfrich, et al., Osteoclast diseases and dental abnormalities, Arch Oral Biol 50 (2) (2005) 115–122.
17. G.E. Wise, S. Frazier-Bowers & R.N. D'Souza, Cellular, molecular, and genetic determinants of tooth eruption, Crit Rev Oral Biol Med Review 13 (4) (2002) 323–334.
18. R.J. Gorlin, et al., Related Nevoid basal cell carcinoma (Gorlin) syndrome, Genet Med Review 6 (6) (2004) 530–539.
19. C.E. Smith & A. Nanci, Overview of morphological changes in enamel organ cells associated with major events in amelogenesis, Int J Dev Biol 39 (1) (1995) 153–161.
20. D.D. Bosshardt & N.P. Lang, The junctional epithelium: From health to disease, J Dent Res 84 (1) (2005) 9–20.
21. H. Harada, Y. Ichimori & T. Yokohama-Tamaki, et al., Stratum intermedium lineage diverges from ameloblast lineage via Notch signaling, Biochem Biophys Res Commun 340 (2) (2006) 611–616.
22. N. Hasegawa, H. Kawaguchi & T. Ogawa, et al., Immunohistochemical characteristics of epithelial cell rests of Malassez during cementum repair, J Periodontal Res 38 (1) (2003) 51–56.
23. A. Veis, K. Tompkins & K. Alvares, et al., Specific amelogenin gene splice products have signaling effects on cells in culture and in implants *in vivo*, J Biol Chem 275 (52) (2000) 41263–41272.
24. A. Veis, Amelogenin gene splice products: potential signaling molecules, Cell Mol Life Sci 60 (1) (2003) 38–55.
25. L. Nodit, L. Barnes & E. Childers, et al., Allelic loss of tumor suppressor genes in ameloblastic tumors, Mod Pathol 17 (9) (2004) 1062–1067.
26. H. Kumamoto & K. Ooya, Expression of tumor necrosis factor a, TNF-related apoptosis-inducing ligand, and their associated molecules in ameloblastomas, J Oral Pathol Med 34 (2005) 287–294.
27. A. Dutt & R. Beroukhim, Single nucleotide polymorphism array analysis of cancer, Curr Opin Oncol 19 (1) (2007) 43–49.
28. K. Heikinheimo, R. Voutilainen, & R.P. Happonen, et al., EGF receptor and its ligands, EGF and TGF-alpha, in developing

and neoplastic human odontogenic tissues, Int J Dev Biol 37 (3) (1993) 387–396.

29. F. Carinci, S. Volinia & C. Rubini, et al., Genetic profile of clear cell odontogenic carcinoma, J Craniofac Surg 14 (3) (2003) 356–362.

30. F. Carinci, F. Francioso & C. Rubini, et al., Genetic portrait of malignant granular cell odontogenic tumor, Oral Oncol 39 (1) (2003) 69–77.

31. F. Carinci, A. Palmieri & G. Delaiti, et al., Expression profiling of ameloblastic carcinoma, J Craniofac Surg 15 (2) (2004) 264–269.

32. J. Lim, H. Ahn & S. Min, et al., Oligonucleotide microarray analysis of ameloblastoma compared with dentigerous cyst, J Oral Pathol Med 35 (5) (2006) 278–285.

33. M. Asagiri & H. Takayanagi, The molecular understanding of osteoclast differentiation, Bone 40 (2) (2007) 251–264.

34. T. Popowics, B.L. Foster & E.C. Swanson, et al., Defining the roots of cementum formation, Cells Tissues Organs 181 (3–4) (2005) 248–257.

35. H. Kumamoto, Molecular pathology of odontogenic tumors, J Oral Pathol Med Review 35 (2) (2006) 65–74.

36. M. Toida, M. Balazs & A. Treszl, et al., Analysis of ameloblastomas by comparative genomic hybridization and fluorescence *in situ* hybridization, Cancer Genet Cytogenet 159 (2) (2005) 99–104.

37. K. Jaaskelainen, K.J. Jee & I. Leivo, et al., Cell proliferation and chromosomal changes in human ameloblastoma, Cancer Genet Cytogenet 16 (1) (2002) 31–37.

38. S.A. Kim, S.G. Ahn & S.G. Kim, et al., Investigation of the beta-catenin gene in a case of dentinogenic ghost cell tumor, Oral Surg Oral Med Oral Pathol Oral Radiol Endod 103 (1) (2007) 97–101.

39. S. Sekine, S. Sato & T. Takata, et al., Beta-catenin mutations are frequent in calcifying odontogenic cysts, but rare in ameloblastomas, Am J Pathol 163 (5) (2003) 1707–1712.

40. H. Kumamoto, N. Takahashi & K. Ooya, K-Ras gene status and expression of Ras/mitogen-activated protein kinase (MAPK) signaling molecules in ameloblastomas, J Oral Pathol Med 33 (6) (2004) 360–367.

41. T. Appel, R. Gath & N. Wernert, et al., Molecular biological and immunohistochemical analysis of tp53 in human ameloblastomas, Mund Kiefer Gesichtschir 8 (3) (2004) 167–172.

42. C.C. Gomes & R.S. Gomez, Odontogenic keratocyst: A benign cystic neoplasm?, Oral Oncol 13 (2006) (Epub ahead of print).

43. D.C. Barreto & R.S. Gomez, et al., PTCH gene mutations in odontogenic keratocysts, J Dent Res 79 (6) (2000) 1418–1422.

44. H. Kumamoto, K. Kimi & K. Ooya, Detection of cell cycle related factors in ameloblastomas, J Oral Pathol Med 30 (2001) 309–315.

45. J. Kim, E.H. Lee & J.I. Yook, et al., Odontogenic ghost cell carcinoma: a case report with reference to the relation between apoptosis and ghost cells, Oral Surg Oral Med Oral Pathol Oral Radiol Endod 90 (2000) 630–635.

46. A. Strasser, L. O'Connor & V.M. Dixit, Apoptosis signaling, Annu Rev Biochem 69 (2000) 217–245.

47. H. Kumamoto & K. Ooya, Detection of mitochondria-mediated apoptosis signaling molecules in ameloblastomas, J Oral Pathol Med 34 (9) (2005) 565–572.

48. F. Sandra, N. Nakamura & T. Mitsuyasu, et al., Two relatively distinct patterns of ameloblastoma: an anti-apoptotic proliferating site in the outer layer (periphery) and a pro-apoptotic differentiating site in the inner layer (centre), Histopathology 39 (2001) 93–98.

49. H.Y. Luo, S.F. Yu & T.J. Li, Differential expression of apoptosis-related proteins in various cellular components of ameloblastomas, Int J Oral Maxillofac Surg 35 (8) (2006) 750–755.

50. C.W. Gibson, E. Lally & R.C. Herold, et al., Odontogenic tumors in mice carrying albumin-myc and albumin-rats transgenes, Calcif Tissue Int 51 (2) (1992) 162–167.

51. J. Carvalhais, M. Aguiar & V. Araujo, et al., p53 and MDM2 expression in odontogenic cysts and tumors, Oral Dis 5 (3) (1999) 218–222.

52. J.L. Davideau, C. Sahlberg & C. Blin, et al., Differential expression of the full-length and secreted truncated forms of EGF receptor during formation of dental tissues Int J Dev Biol 39(4) (1995) 605–615.

53. M. Yamamoto, H. Yanaga, & H. Nishina, et al., Fibrin stimulates the proliferation of human keratinocytes through the autocrine mechanism of tranforming growth factor-alpha and epidermal growth factor receptor. Tohoku J Exp Med 207 (2005) 33–40.

54. M. Grachtchouk, J. Liu & A. Wang, et al., Odontogenic keratocysts arise from quiescent epithelial rests and are associated with deregulated hedgehog signaling in mice and humans, Am J Pathol 169 (3) (2006) 806–814.

55. M. Mori, K. Yamada & T. Kasai, et al., Immunohistochemical expression of amelogenins in odontogenic epithelial tumors and cysts, Virchows Arch A Pathol Anat Histopathol 418 (1991) 319–325.

56. M.L. Snead, W. Luo & D.D. Hsu, et al., Human ameloblastoma tumors express the amelogenin gene, Oral Surg Oral Med Oral Pathol 74 (1992) 64–72.

57. T. Takata, M. Zhao & T. Uchida, et al., Immunohistochemical detection and distribution of enamelysin (MMP-20) in human odontogenic tumors, J Dent Res 79 (2000) 1608–1613.

58. P. Papagerakis, M. Peuchmaur & D. Hotton, et al., Aberrant gene expression in epithelial cells of mixed odontogenic tumors, J Dent Res 78 (1) (1999) 20–30.

59. S. Fukumoto, T. Kiba & B. Hall, et al., Ameloblastin is a cell adhesion molecule required for maintaining the differentiation state of ameloblasts, J Cell Biol 167 (5) (2004) 973–983.

60. P.F. Perdigao, F.J. Pimenta & W.H. Castro, et al., Investigation of the GSalpha gene in the diagnosis of fibrous dysplasia, Int J Oral Maxillofac Surg 33 (5) (2004) 498–501.

61. S. Toyosawa, T. Fujiwara & T. Ooshima, Cloning and characterization of the human ameloblastin gene, Gene 256 (1–2) (2000) 1–11.

62. C.W. Gibson, Z.A. Yuan & Y. Li, et al., Transgenic mice that express normal and mutated amelogenins, J Dent Res 86 (4) (2007) 331–335.

63. Y.Y. Kong, H. Yoshida & I. Sarosi, et al., OPGL is a key regulator of osteoclastogenesis, lymphocyte development and lymph-node organogenesis, Nature 397 (6717) (1999) 315–323.

64. J.Y. Tay, B.H. Bay & J.F. Yeo, Identification of RANKL in osteolytic lesions of the facial skeleton, J Dent Res 83 (4) (2004) 349–353.

65. Y. Kubota, S. Nitta & S. Oka, et al., Discrimination of ameloblastomas from odontogenic keratocysts by cytokine levels and gelatinase species of the intracystic fluids, J Oral Pathol Med 30 (2001) 421–427.

66. W.M. Philbrick, B.E. Dreyer & I.A. Nakchbandi, et al., Parathyroid hormone-related protein is required for tooth eruption, Proc Natl Acad Sci USA 95 (1998) 11846–11851.

67. B.T. Bast, M.A. Pogrel & J.A. Regezi, The expression of apoptotic proteins and matrix metalloproteinases in odontogenic myxomas, J Oral Maxillofac Surg 61 (2003) 1463–1466.

68. J.J. Pinheiro, V.M. Freitas & A.I. Moretti, et al., Local invasiveness of ameloblastoma. Role played by matrix metalloproteinases and proliferative activity, Histopathology 45 (2004) 65–72.

69. H. Nagatsuka, P.P. Han & H. Tsujigiwa, et al., Heparanase gene and protein expression in ameloblastoma: Possible role in local invasion of tumor cells, Oral Oncol 41 (2005) 542–548.

70. J.M. Chirgwin & T.A. Guise, Molecular mechanisms of tumor-bone interactions in osteolytic metastases, Crit Rev Eukaryot Gene Expr Review 10 (2) (2000) 159–178.

71. B. Ruhin, S. Creuzet & C. Vincent, et al., Patterning of the hyoid cartilage depends upon signals arising from the ventral foregut endoderm, Developmental Dynamics (IF 3,16) 228 (2003) 239–246.

72. R. Becelli, A. Carboni & G. Cerilli, et al., Mandibular ameloblastoma: analysis of surgical treatment carried out in 60 patients between 1977 and 1998, J Craniofac Surg 13 (3) (2002) 395–400.

73. W. Edgin, R. Simmons & G.T. Terezhalmy, et al., Ameloblastoma, Quintessence Int 34 (5) (2003) 394–395.

74. G. Sammartino, C. Zarrelli, V. Urciuolo, et al. (2006). Effectiveness of a new decisional algorithm in managing mandibular ameloblastomas: A 10-years experience. Br J Oral Maxillofac Surg, Oct 20.

75. Y.F. Zhao, B. Liu & Z.Q. Jiang, Marsupialization or decompression of the cystic lesions of the jaws, Shanghai Kou Qiang Yi Xue 14 (4) (2005) 325–329.

76. H.O. Olasoji & O.N. Enwere, Treatment of ameloblastoma—a review, Niger J Med 12 (1) (2003) 7–11.

77. K.A. Chapelle, P.J. Stoelinga & P.C. de Wilde, et al., Rational approach to diagnosis and treatment of ameloblastomas and odontogenic keratocysts, Br J Oral Maxillofac Surg 42 (5) (2004) 381–390.

78. E.R. Carlson & R.E. Marx, The ameloblastoma: primary curative surgical management, J Oral Maxillofac Surg 64 (3) (2006) 484–494.

79. D. Ghandhi, A.F. Ayoub & M.A. Pogrel, et al., Ameloblastoma: a surgeon's dilemma, J Oral Maxillofac Surg 64 (7) (2006) 1010–1014.

80. R.A. Gortzak, B.S. Latief & C. Lekkas, et al., Growth characteristics of large mandibular ameloblastomas: report of 5 cases with implications for the approach to surgery, Int J Oral Maxillofac Surg 35 (8) (2006) 691–695.

81. P. Bouletreau, A.R. Paranque & M. Steve, et al., Management of mandibular ameloblastoma, Rev Stomatol Chir Maxillofac 107 (1) (2006) 52–56.

82. S.A. Sachs, Surgical excision with peripheral ostectomy: a definitive, yet conservative, approach to the surgical management of ameloblastoma, J Oral Maxillofac Surg 64 (3) (2006) 476–483.

83. S. Ozlugedik, M. Ozcan & O. Basturk, et al., Ameloblastic carcinoma arising from anterior skull base, Skull Base 15 (4) (2005) 269–272.

84. I. Leibovitch, R.M. Schwarcz & S. Modjtahedi, et al., Orbital invasion by recurrent maxillary ameloblastoma, Ophthalmology 113 (7) (2006) 1227–1230.

85. P.E. Maurette, J. Jorge & M. de Moraes, Conservative treatment protocol of odontogenic keratocyst: a preliminary study, J Oral Maxillofac Surg 64 (3) (2006) 379–383.

86. M. Giuliani, G.B. Grossi & C. Lajolo, et al., Conservative management of a large odontogenic keratocyst: report of a case and review of the literature, J Oral Maxillofac Surg 64 (2) (2006) 308–316.

87. A. Kolokythas, R.P. Fernandes & A. Pazoki, et al., Odontogenic keratocyst: to decompress or not to decompress? A comparative study of decompression and enucleation versus resection/peripheral ostectomy, J Oral Maxillofac Surg 65 (4) (2007) 640–644.

88. M.A. Pogrel, Decompression and marsupialization as definitive treatment for keratocysts—a partial retraction, J Oral Maxillofac Surg 65 (2) (2007) 362–363.

89. N. Blanas, B. Freund & M. Schwartz, et al., Systematic review of the treatment and prognosis of the odontogenic keratocyst, Oral Surg Oral Med Oral Pathol Oral Radiol Endod 90 (5) (2000) 553–558.

90. U. Bilkay, C. Tokat, E. Helvaci, P.K. Lee, N. Samman & I. O. Ng, et al., Free fibula flap mandible reconstruction in benign mandibular lesions. Unicystic ameloblastoma—use of Carnoy's solution after enucleation, J Craniofac Surg Int J Oral Maxillofac Surg 15 33 (6) (3) (2004) (2004) 1002– 263–1009267.

91a. H. Vayvada, F. Mola & A. Menderes, et al., Surgical management of ameloblastoma in the mandible: segmental mandibulectomy and immediate reconstruction with free fibula or deep circumflex iliac artery flap (evaluation of the long-term esthetic and functional results), J Oral Maxillofac Surg 64(10) (2006) 1532–1539.

91b. E.W. To, W.M. Tsang, & P.C. Pang, Recurrent ameloblastoma presenting in the temporal fossa, Am J Otolaryngol 23(2) (2002) 105–107.

92. J.A. Feledy Jr., L.H. Hollier Jr. & M. Klebuc, et al., Iliac crest osteocutaneous flap reconstruction for ameloblastoma of the mandible in a patient with bilateral peronea artery magna: case report, J Craniofac Surg 14 (5) (2003) 809–814.

93. J.S. Chana, Y.M. Chang & F.C. Wei, et al., Segmental mandibulectomy and immediate free fibula osteoseptocutaneous flap reconstruction with endosteal implants: an ideal treatment method for mandibular ameloblastoma, Plast Reconstr Surg 113 (1) (2004) 80–87.

94. C.P. Kelly, A. Moreira-Gonzalez & M.A. Ali, et al., Vascular iliac crest with inner table of the ilium as an option in maxillary reconstruction, J Craniofac Surg 15 (1) (2004) 23–28.

95. B. Ruhin, Ph. Menard, J. Ceccaldi, et al. Mandibular reconstruction by double-barrel fibula free flap for dental implanted prosthesis, Rev Sto Chir Maxillofac (2006) 338–4.

96. P.J. Stoelinga, The treatment of odontogenic keratocysts by excision of the overlying, attached mucosa, enucleation, and

treatment of the bony defect with carnoy solution, J Oral Maxillofac Surg 63 (11) (2005) 1662–1666.

97. J.L. Zhou, S.L. Jiao & X.H. Chen, et al., Treatment of recurrent odontogenic keratocyst with enucleation and cryosurgery: a retrospective study of 10 cases, Shanghai Kou Qiang Yi Xue (Chinese) 14 (5) (2005) 476–478.

98. W.D. Martins & D.M. Favaro, Recurrence of an ameloblastoma in an autogenous iliac bone graft, Oral Surg Oral Med Oral Pathol Oral Radiol Endod 98 (6) (2004) 657–659.

99. Y.S. Choi, J. Asaumi & Y. Yanagi, et al., A case of recurrent ameloblastoma developing in an autogenous iliac bone graft 20 years after the initial treatment, Dentomaxillofac Radiol 35 (1) (2006) 43–46.

100. S.L. Lau & N. Samman, Recurrence related to treatment modalities of unicystic ameloblastoma: a systematic review, Int J Oral Maxillofac Surg 35 (8) (2006) 681–690.

101. P. Clark, P. Marker & H.L. Bastian, et al., Expression of p53, Ki-67, and EGFR in odontogenic keratocysts before and after decompression, J Oral Pathol Med 35 (9) (2006) 568–572.

102. L. Zhang, Z.J. Sun & Y.F. Zhao, et al., Inhibition of SHH signaling pathway: Molecular treatment strategy of odontogenic keratocyst, Med Hypotheses 67 (5) (2006) 1242–1244.

103. Y.D Zhang, Z. Chen & Y.Q. Song, et al., Making a tooth: growth factors, transcription factors, and stem cells, Cell Res 15(5) (2005) 301–306.

104. I. Thesleff, The genetic basis of tooth development and dental defects, Am J Med Genet A 140 (23) (2006) 2530–2535.

105. G.E. Wise, S. Yao & P.R. Odgren, et al., CSF-1 regulation of osteoclastogenesis for tooth eruption, J Dent Res 84 (9) (2005) 837–841.

CHAPTER **8**

The Role of the Interleukin-6 Family of Cytokines in Bone Remodeling and Bone Cancer

FRÉDÉRIC BLANCHARD[1,2]*, EMMANUELLE DAVID[1,2] AND BÉNÉDICTE BROUNAIS[1,2]

[1]INSERM, U957, Nantes, France.
[2]Université de Nantes, Nantes Atlantique Universités, Laboratoire de Physiopathologie de la Résorption Osseuse et Thérapie des Tumeurs Osseuses Primitives, EA3822, Nantes, France.

Contents

I. INTRODUCTION

Cytokines of the interleukin (IL)-6 family are recognized as pleiotropic factors influencing many biological events in several organs, especially bone [1–4]. Since its discovery some 25 years ago, the list of IL-6 effects is still growing and recent *in vivo* and genetic data have challenged our concept saying that IL-6 was a major positive regulator of bone resorption [4]. Adding to our confusion, other IL-6-type cytokines can have opposite effects on bone pathophysiology, despite their overlapping biological effects. Not surprisingly, these cytokines are also implicated in various bone cancers. However, clinical trials have been performed either using these cytokines as anti-cancer adjuvants [5] or neutralizing their unwanted effects on tumor growth and osteolysis [6]. This review describes the dual effects of IL-6-type cytokines in bone remodeling and cancer and discusses recent data on IL-6 signaling, which may have therapeutic implications.

II. THE IL-6-TYPE CYTOKINES

The ever growing IL-6 family of cytokines actually comprises 10 members: the founding member IL-6, as well as IL-11, IL-27, IL-31, leukemia inhibitory factor (LIF), oncostatin M (OSM), ciliary neurotrophic factor (CNTF), cardiotrophin-1 (CT-1), cardiotrophin-like cytokine (CLC) and neuropoietin (NP) [1–3,7–10]. They share similarities in their gene organization, protein structure, receptor recruitment and therefore in their biological effects. In addition to their redundancy, these cytokines have a plethora of functions in various, apparently unrelated tissues or situations. They are implicated in embryonic development, organogenesis, differentiation, inflammation and regeneration of the liver, bone, and the central nervous and hematopoietic systems [11–15]. As pointed out by D. Metcalf 'there is no situation in developmental biology or in disease where such a disparate collection of tissues needs to be coordinated or simultaneously regulated' [13]. Therefore, and not surprisingly, several studies indicated that some effects are specific to individual IL-6-type cytokines and that each of these cytokines could have a predominant role in a particular situation. In principle, this specificity could be given by the restricted production of one cytokine or its receptor and/or by the particular signaling pathways that are activated. Not exclusively, IL-6 seems to have a major role in acute phase protein production by the liver [16], in postmenopausal osteoporosis [17] and rheumatoid arthritis [18]. IL-11 possesses striking anti-inflammatory activities in gastrointestinal diseases such as Crohn's disease [19,20],

Bone Cancer
ISBN: 978-0-12-374895-9

whereas LIF is necessary for embryo implantation [21]. OSM drives differentiation of foetal hepatocytes [22] and is the most potent growth suppressor of a variety of carcinoma/sarcoma cell lines [15,23]. Major roles of CNTF, NP and CLC seem to be in the central nervous system [9,10,24,25] whereas CT-1 has an important role in cardiac repair [26]. IL-27 has a unique role in innate and adaptive immune responses [27], whereas IL-31 is implicated in skin inflammation [8].

Whereas IL-6, IL-11 and LIF can be produced by numerous cell types such as T lymphocytes, monocytes, epithelial cells, fibroblasts, osteoblasts and various cancer cells, secretion of OSM seems to be restricted to activated monocytes, neutrophils, mast cells and lymphocytes [1,13,15,28]. The secretion of CNTF and CLC is striking because it depends on the co-production of specific receptor chains and/or is believed to occur only after cell damage [9,24]. Production of IL-6-type cytokines is mainly inducible (for example, by lipopolysaccharides, tumor necrosis factor-α, IL-1, parathyroid hormone related protein) and depends on various signaling pathways such as Mitogen Activated Protein Kinase (MAPK), Protein Kinase C (PKC), activator protein 1 (AP-1) and Nuclear Factor-kB (NFkB) [28–30].

III. SIGNALING THROUGH THE IL-6-TYPE RECEPTORS

All IL-6-type cytokines utilize the receptor β-subunit gp130 as part of a multimeric receptor complex, except IL-31 which uses the gp130-like (GPL) subunit [8–12] (Figure 8.1). IL-6 binds to a specific receptor α-subunit (IL-6R) that lacks intrinsic signaling properties. The IL-6/IL-6R complex then interacts with two gp130 subunits to form a hexameric

complex [12]. Similarly, other IL-6-type cytokines are recognized by a specific receptor subunit (IL-11R, LIFR, CNTFR, cytokine-like factor-1 (CLF) for CLC, WSX-1 for IL-27), and in combination with gp130, they form high affinity, signaling-competent receptor complexes (Figure 8.1). In the case of CT-1 and NP, a specific receptor subunit has not yet been identified. In humans, OSM is exceptional because it interacts with gp130 and with either LIFR or OSMR to form the signaling-competent receptor complex I or II [15]. IL-31 also binds to OSMR but in combination to GPL [8]. It was also shown that highly glycosylated LIF is able to bind to and is internalized/degraded via the receptor for Man-6-P/IGF-II [31].

Naturally occurring soluble versions of receptor chains enable cells to respond to IL-6-type cytokine in the absence of specific membrane-associated subunits. This 'trans-activation' is especially well demonstrated by the agonistic activity of soluble IL-6R (sIL-6R; Figure 8.1), and also exists with sIL-11R and sCNTFR [32]. CLF is a receptor that is only found soluble [9]. In contrast, naturally occurring soluble gp130 [32], LIFR [33] and OSMR [34] antagonize cytokine activity by preventing the formation of homo- or hetero-dimeric signaling-competent receptors.

Ligand-induced oligomerization of receptor subunits activates Janus protein-tyrosine kinases (JAKs; mainly JAK1, JAK2 and TYK2), which, in turn, phosphorylate tyrosine residues in the receptor cytoplasmic domain [12,15] (Figure 8.2). These phosphorylated tyrosine residues on the receptor act as docking sites for SH2 (Src homology 2)-domain-containing signaling molecules such as SHP2 (SH2 domain-containing tyrosine phosphatase 2), SHC (SH2 domain-containing transforming protein 1) and the transcription factors known as STATs (Signal Transducer and Activator of transcription; mainly STAT1, STAT3 and

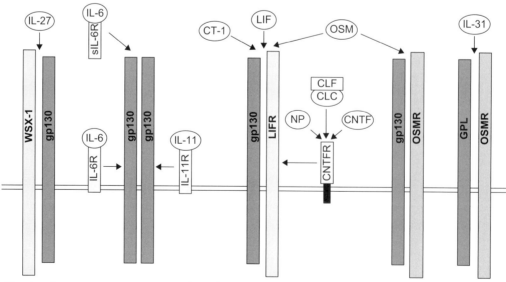

FIGURE 8.1   The signaling-competent receptor complexes for IL-6-type cytokines.

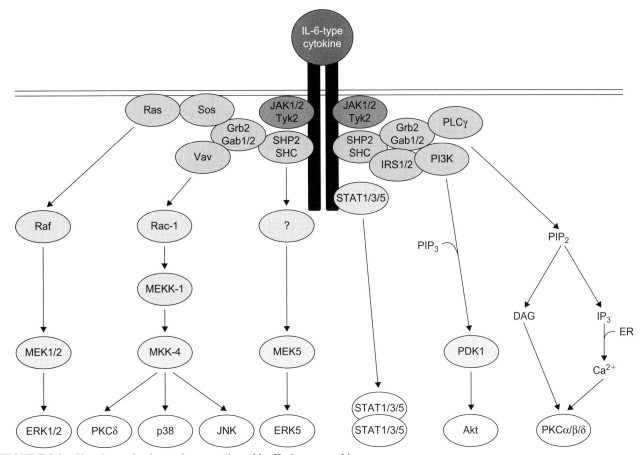

FIGURE 8.2 Signal transduction pathways activated by IL-6-type cytokines.

STAT5a/b). In the absence of receptor activation, STAT proteins mainly exist as latent, cytoplasmic monomers. They become activated when phosphorylated by JAKs, inducing their dimerization and nuclear translocation where they regulate the transcription of target genes. In contrast, cytoplasmic SHP2 mediates activation of the MAPKs (mainly Extracellular Regulated Kinase (ERK) 1/2, p38 and jun kinase (JNK)) via the adaptor proteins Grb2 (Growth factor receptor-bound 2) and/or Gab1/2 (GRB2-associated binding protein 1) [12]. Other signaling cascades known to be activated by IL-6-type cytokines comprise the PI3K (Phosphoinositide 3-kinase)/AKT (protein kinase B) [12], MEK5 (MAPK/ERK kinase 5)/ERK5 [35] and PKC pathways, the latter being induced either by MKK4 (MAPK kinase 4) [36], PI3K [37] or PLCγ (phospholipase Cγ) (Figure 8.2). For OSMR, the adaptor molecule SHC replaces SHP2 and mediates a higher MAPKs signaling than with gp130 or LIFR [12].

Signaling by IL-6-type cytokines is transient, restricted temporally and in magnitude by the action of negative regulators [12]. The tyrosine phosphatases SHP1 and -2, through their catalytic function, attenuate the activity of receptor-associated JAKs. The suppressor of cytokine signaling (SOCS)-1 and -3 are rapidly induced by IL-6-type cytokines

and interact/deactivate JAKs or receptor subunits. The protein inhibitors of activated STATs (PIAS) associate with activated STATs, leading to their inactivation. Finally, receptor subunits are subjected to complex ligand-induced degradation processes, implicating serine phosphorylation by ERK1/2, internalization, endosomal/lysosomal degradation, ubiquitination and proteosomal degradation [39].

In various cell systems, it was shown that the MAPK pathway can antagonize the STAT pathway and that the balance between these two pathways dictates the cellular outcome. First, mutated receptor subunits that are unable to activate the MAPK pathway show an enhanced and long lasting activation of STATs, whereas mutation of the STATs' docking sites leads to improved MAPK activation [4,40,41]. Second, STATs and MAPKs can have inverse effects on cell proliferation, apoptosis and differentiation. In general, STATs are associated with reduced proliferation and induced differentiation, whereas ERK1/2 is linked to enhanced proliferation and survival [40–42]. However, opposite effects were also observed depending on the cell type and the transformation status [43,44]. Interestingly, it has been shown that in SOCS3-deficient fibroblasts where STAT3 is activated in a prolonged manner, this anti-apoptotic transcription factor becomes pro-apoptotic [45]. Therefore, it appears that the STAT and MAPK pathways regulate each other's activity in amplitude and time, this balance being specific to a given cytokine and cell type.

IV. EFFECTS ON BONE CELLS

Bone tissue remodeling results from the coordinate activities of osteoblasts, the 'bone-forming' cells, and osteoclasts, the multinucleated cells that are uniquely capable of bone resorption. IL-6-type cytokines influence both osteoblast and osteoclast activities through a variety of complex, often contradictory mechanisms.

Osteoblasts express low levels of IL-6R and therefore presence of sIL-6R is required for maximum IL-6 effects on these cells [4,28,46,47]. Thus, numerous reports indicate that IL-6+sIL-6R, IL-11, LIF, CNTF and OSM enhance *in vitro* differentiation on osteoblasts or osteoblast precursors isolated from the calvaria or bone marrow [1–4,46–49]. These cytokines are able to increase osteoblast marker expression such as alkaline phosphatase (ALP), osteocalcine or bone sialoprotein and to enhance bone nodule formation and extracellular matrix mineralization. Activation of STAT3 is necessary for osteoblast differentiation and bone formation induced by IL-6-type cytokines [48,50]. Similarly, they can reduce proliferation of various osteoblastic cells through activation of STAT3 and enhanced expression of the cell cycle inhibitor p21^{WAF1}, this protein being also necessary for induction of ALP by IL-6-type cytokines [51]. Finally, they can protect certain osteoblastic cells from apoptosis induced by serum depletion or TNFα [52]. However, other reports have shown an inhibitory effect of IL-6-type cytokines on bone formation and marker expression *in vitro*, as well as a potent pro-apoptotic effect [53–58]. Kinases such as PKCδ and ERK1/2 are implicated in these inhibitory effects on bone formation [56] whereas the transcription factors STAT5a/b and p53 act in concert to enhance the Bax (Bcl-2–associated X)/Bcl2 (B-cell CLL/lymphoma 2) ratio and thus sensitize osteoblastic cells to the mitochondrial apoptotic pathway [59,60]. It is possible that these dual effects depend on the differentiation stage of the osteoblast: on precursor cells, they would stimulate the first stages of differentiation but on more mature cells, they would prevent further stimulation [56–58]. However, considering that the terminal differentiation of osteoblasts into osteocytes is characterized by reduced marker expression/bone formation/proliferation and enhanced apoptosis, these cytokines could in fact induced an osteocytic phenotype [56]. Further experiments are needed to test this intriguing hypothesis.

IL-6-type cytokines can stimulate osteoclast activity and bone resorption by an indirect mechanism, increasing interaction between osteoblasts and osteoclasts. In co-cultures containing both osteoblasts/stromal cells and osteoclasts, they clearly stimulate osteoclast differentiation and activity

[61–65]. In fact, these cytokines induce osteoblastic production of various downstream effectors that activate osteoclast differentiation or activity, such as RANKL (receptor activator of NFkB ligand), IL-1, PTHrP and PGE2 (prostaglandin E2) [2,28,64–69]. Inversely TNFα, IL-1, PTH/PTHrP and PGE2 stimulate IL-6, IL-11 and LIF production by osteoblasts to further amplify the production of factors that activate osteoclasts [1,2,28–30,69,70]. Some data have indicated that induction of RANKL by IL-6-type cytokines is necessary for their pro-resorption action, and that STAT3 was implicated in RANKL induction [64,65,71,72]. However, in other reports on purified osteoclasts or other models, IL-6-type cytokines could have an inhibitory role [54,73]. Indeed, IL-6 and IL-27 reduced the RANKL-induced osteoclast formation and bone resorption obtained from purified osteoclast precursors, such as mouse bone marrow CD11b$^+$ monocytes, human circulating CD14$^+$ monocytes or the macrophage cell line RAW264.7 [74–76]. This direct inhibitory effect is associated with reduced expression of several osteoclastic markers (TRAP (acid phosphatase 5, tartrate resistant), cathepsin K, calicitonin receptor) and inhibition of RANKL signaling pathways such as activation of NF-kB and the MAPKs JNK and p38 [74,75]. On RAW264.7 cells, we observed that IL-6 inhibits RANKL-induced osteoclastogenesis by diverting cells into the macrophage lineage [74]. Moreover STAT3, and its relative phosphorylation on tyrosine or serine residues, appeared to be necessary for macrophage and osteoclast differentiation respectively [74].

Various transgenic and knockout mice have been developed to determine the real involvement of IL-6-type cytokine in bone remodeling. IL-6 deficient mice showed an increase in bone formation [17] whereas transgenic mice overexpressing IL-6 showed a decrease in osteoblast and osteoid, as well as a decrease in osteoclast and bone resorption [77]. In contrast, IL-11 transgenic mice had increased osteoblasts and bone formation, whereas osteoclastogenesis and bone resorption were not modified [49]. Transgenic mice for OSM also had impressive osteopetrotic bones [78]. Gp130 or LIFR knockout mice had a decreased trabecular bone volume and increased osteoclast number [79,80]. OSMRβ$^{-/-}$ mice had normal bones but bone marrow stromal cells did not support hematopoiesis as their wild-type counterparts [81]. Altogether, these results suggested that IL-6-type cytokines could have opposite and unexpected effects on bone formation and resorption. A genetic approach (knock-in mutations in mice) confirmed the ying/yang effects of the STAT versus MAPK pathways. These reports indicated that the gp130/STAT pathway is important to sustain osteoblast formation whereas the gp130/MAPK pathway has an inhibitory role on osteoclastogenesis [3,4,41,82].

In other words, it appears that: (1) the activity of a given receptor complex is the result of the antagonistic role of the STAT versus MAPK pathways; and (2) IL-6-type cytokines have a non-redundant role on bone remodeling because they are not produced at the same site and time—and because their receptor complex does not induce the same level of activated STAT versus activated MAPK. Additional studies then established that IL-6 has a major role in various osteo-articular pathologies. IL-6$^{-/-}$ mice were significantly protected from joint inflammation and destruction in mouse models of arthritis and were also protected from bone loss caused by oestrogen depletion, as observed in postmenopausal osteoporosis (reviewed in Refs [2–4]). Moreover, clinical trials indicated that inhibition of IL-6 or IL-6R improves the clinical response of patients with rheumatoid arthritis [2–5]. In contrast, systemic administration of IL-11 reduced joint inflammation and destruction in murine arthritis [3], whereas overexpression of OSM induced inflammation and destruction in mouse joints [83].

V. IMPLICATIONS IN BONE TUMOR DEVELOPMENT

Bones are the sites of various primary cancers arising from bone cells, as well as a privileged environment for metastatic development. Proliferation of cancer cells in bones is coupled to inflammation, osteolysis and abnormal new bone formation, and a vicious cycle is established between tumor proliferation and bone resorption, mainly through enhanced RANKL expression [28,84,85]. Consequently, antiresorption agents such as bisphosphonates or OPG (osteoprotegerin) are particularly active in not only the management of cancer-associated bone resorption but also in inhibition of tumor growth in bones [84,85]. As observed on normal bone cells, IL-6-type cytokines have both pro- or anti-tumoral effects on cancer cells growing in the bone environment.

From the beginning, IL-6-type cytokines were known as potent growth inhibitors or stimulators depending on the cancer cell type. For example, IL-6+sIL-6R, OSM and to a lesser extent LIF and IL-11 inhibit the proliferation and block in the G1 phase of the cell cycle various cell lines obtained from melanoma [42,44,86], breast cancer [15], osteosarcoma [48,51,56] and neuroblastoma [23,24]. All of these cancer cells have a propensity to form osteolytic bone lesions. This growth suppression is believed to occur through STATs activation and induction of cell cycle inhibitors such as p21^{WAF1} and/or p27^{KIP1} [40,42,48,51]. *In vivo*, recombinant IL-6 and OSM also mediates tumor regression of various sarcomas and carcinomas that form lung or liver metastases [87,88]. In a rat model of osteosarcoma engrafted on the bone surface, we described that OSM alone does not modify the tumor burden, but in association with the kinases inhibitor Midostaurin this cytokine induces tumor apoptosis and necrosis, thus reducing the primary bone tumor development and the incidence of lung metastasis [60]. In contrast, IL-6-type cytokines are able to induce or sustain proliferation of various myeloma [89], melanoma [44], chondrosarcoma [90] and prostate cancer [91] cell lines for which osteolysis participates to tumor development. For

melanoma, it is clear that primary cancer cells are growth inhibited by IL-6-type cytokines but that during the metastatic process, these cells become resistant or even growth stimulated by these cytokines [44,86]. They can lose expression of OSMRβ [86], produce IL-6 as an autocrine growth factor [44] and modify the transduction pathways in such a way that growth inhibition mediated by STATs is shifted to growth promotion [92,93]. Thus, constitutively active STATs have been observed in numerous cancers and targeting this pathway appears as a potent new anti-cancer therapy [93,94]. Similarly, myeloma [89], giant cell tumors of bone [95], squamous carcinoma [96,97] as well as breast [98] and prostate [99] cancer can produce IL-6, IL-11 and LIF but not OSM [1,28]. Finally, patients with osteosarcoma, chondrosarcoma, Ewing's sarcoma, giant cell tumor of bone [100], melanoma [101] and breast cancer [98] have significant elevated levels of serum IL-6, in correlation with a poor overall survival.

These protumoral effects of IL-6-type cytokines could be related to their ability to enhance tumor cell motility, invasion and angiogenesis (through vascular endothelial growth factor production) [14,93,94,98]. However, several lines of evidence indicate that these cytokines could also be implicated in tumor growth in bone. Firstly, it was demonstrated that cancer cells produce high amounts of IL-6 induced bone resorption. Thus, IL-6 enhances hypercalcemia mediated by PTHrP in mice engrafted with CHO cells engineered to produce these proresorption agents [102]. Similarly, a neutralizing antibody against IL-6 prevents bone loss in a model of squamous carcinoma associated with hypercalcemia [96,97]. Secondly, various cancer cells induce production of IL-6, IL-11 and LIF by osteoblasts or bone marrow stromal cells and these cytokines then induce bone resorption. For example, breast cancer cells induce osteoclast formation by stimulating IL-11 production by osteoblasts [103]. Similarly, metastatic A375 melanoma cells induce osteolysis by activating TGFβ (transforming growth factor β), which leads IL-11 production by osteoblasts to promote bone resorption [104]. A similar situation occurs with myeloma, metastatic neuroblastoma or mammary tumors which produce or induce the production of IL-6/LIF by bone marrow stromal cells to sustain bone resorption and tumor growth [89,105–108]. In all of these cases, a synergy exists between the IL-6-type cytokines and other proresorption agents such as PTHrP, PGE2, IL-1 and RANKL. Therefore, it is quite possible that despite their potent direct growth inhibitory effect, IL-6-type cytokines that are produced in the bone-tumor environment, mainly IL-6, IL-11 and LIF, participate in bone resorption and thus in tumor proliferation in bone.

So what about the other IL-6-type cytokines? OSM is the major growth inhibitor in the IL-6 family, especially for osteosarcoma, breast cancer and melanoma, and is not produced by cancer cells or osteoblasts [1,15,56]. However, OSM also induces severe side effects such as bone loss, generalized inflammation and cachexia, leading to death if the doses are too high [60]. This feature is not specific, as IL-6 and LIF also induce significant weight loss, together with fever and flu-like symptoms [5,13,102,109]. IL-27 is able to limit cancer progression and pulmonary metastasis by activating the antitumor immune response and by inhibiting angiogenesis [110]. *In vitro*, CNTF induces differentiation of various neuroblastoma cell lines [24] whereas CLC is a growth factor for myeloma [111]. IL-31 is able to inhibit proliferation of some epithelial cancer cells [112]. No data are available regarding CT-1 and NP effects on cancer cells.

VI. CONCLUSION

There is no doubt that IL-6-type cytokines are important regulators of bone pathophysiology. However, their exact role is still an enigma because they appear as double-edged swords. They have both positive and negative effects on osteoblast and osteoclast differentiation, they can drive encouraging anti-cancer effects, but in the bone environment they appear to participate in bone resorption and tumor growth. Moreover, IL-6-type cytokines are not redundant and can have opposite effects. Thus, IL-6 has a key destructive role in rheumatoid arthritis, osteoporosis and bone cancers, whereas IL-11 possesses striking anti-inflammatory effects in arthritis and bowel/Crohn's disease. We have to admit that our knowledge of the role of other IL-6-type cytokines on bone and cancer is limited and future experiments will certainly reveal important new clues, especially with OSM and IL-27 that possess intriguing anticancer properties. Similarly, a better comprehension of the dual signaling pathways activated by IL-6-type cytokines will allow the design of new reagents that block the unwanted effect but keep the best side of these dual cytokines.

References

1. D. Heymann & A.V. Rousselle, gp130 Cytokine family and bone cells, Cytokine 12 (2000) 1455–1468.
2. X.H. Liu, A. Kirschenbaum & S. Yao, et al., The role of the interleukin-6/gp130 signaling pathway in bone metabolism, Vitam Horm 74 (2006) 341–355.
3. P.K. Wong, I.K. Campbell & P.J. Egan, et al., The role of the interleukin-6 family of cytokines in inflammatory arthritis and bone turnover, Arthritis Rheum 48 (2003) 1177–1189.
4. N. Franchimont, S. Wertz & M. Malaise, Interleukin-6: An osteotropic factor influencing bone formation?, Bone 37 (2005) 601–606.
5. J.A. Sosman, F.R. Aronson & M. Sznol, et al., Concurrent phase I trials of intravenous interleukin 6 in solid tumor patients: reversible dose-limiting neurological toxicity, Clin Cancer Res 3 (1997) 39–46.
6. C. Ding & G. Jones, Technology evaluation: MRA, Chugai, Curr Opin Mol Ther 5 (2003) 64–69.
7. S. Pflanz, L. Hibbert & J. Mattson, et al., WSX-1 and glycoprotein 130 constitute a signal-transducing receptor for IL-27, J Immunol 172 (2004) 2225–2231.
8. S.R. Dillon, C. Sprecher & A. Hammond, et al., Interleukin 31, a cytokine produced by activated T cells, induces dermatitis in mice, Nat Immunol 5 (2004) 752–760.
9. G.C. Elson, E. Lelievre & C. Guillet, et al., CLF associates with CLC to form a functional heteromeric ligand for the CNTF receptor complex, Nat Neurosci 3 (2000) 867–872.
10. D. Derouet, F. Rousseau & F. Alfonsi, et al., Neuropoietin, a new IL-6-related cytokine signaling through the ciliary neurotrophic factor receptor, Proc Natl Acad Sci USA 101 (2004) 4827–4832.
11. R.A. Gadient & P.H. Patterson, Leukemia inhibitory factor, interleukin 6, and other cytokines using the GP130 transducing receptor: roles in inflammation and injury, Stem Cells 17 (1999) 127–137.
12. P.C. Heinrich, I. Behrmann & S. Haan, et al., Principles of interleukin (IL)-6-type cytokine signalling and its regulation, Biochem J 374 (Pt 1) (2003) 1–20.
13. D. Metcalf, The unsolved enigmas of leukemia inhibitory factor, Stem Cells 21 (2003) 5–14.
14. T. Hirano, K. Ishihara & M. Hibi, Roles of STAT3 in mediating the cell growth, differentiation and survival signals relayed through the IL-6 family of cytokine receptors, Oncogene 19 (2000) 2548–2556.
15. S.L. Grant & C.G. Begley, The oncostatin M signalling pathway: reversing the neoplastic phenotype?, Mol Med Today 5 (1999) 406–412.
16. M. Kopf, H. Baumann & G. Freer, et al., Impaired immune and acute-phase responses in interleukin-6-deficient mice, Nature 368 (1994) 339–342.
17. V. Poli, R. Balena & E. Fattori, et al., Interleukin-6 deficient mice are protected from bone loss caused by estrogen depletion, EMBO J 13 (1994) 1189–1196.
18. T. Alonzi, E. Fattori & D. Lazzaro, et al., Interleukin 6 is required for the development of collagen-induced arthritis, J Exp Med 187 (1998) 461–468.
19. W.L. Trepicchio & A.J. Dorner, Interleukin-11. A gp130 cytokine, Ann NY Acad Sci 856 (1998) 12–21.
20. K.R. Herrlinger, T. Witthoeft & A. Raedler, et al., Randomized, double blind controlled trial of subcutaneous recombinant human interleukin-11 versus prednisolone in active Crohn's disease, Am J Gastroenterol 101 (2006) 793–797.
21. C.L. Stewart, P. Kaspar & L.J. Brunet, et al., Blastocyst implantation depends on maternal expression of leukaemia inhibitory factor, Nature 359 (1992) 76–79.
22. A. Kamiya, T. Kinoshita & Y. Ito, et al., Fetal liver development requires a paracrine action of oncostatin M through the gp130 signal transducer, EMBO J 18 (1999) 2127–2136.
23. D. Horn, W.C. Fitzpatrick & P.T. Gompper, et al., Regulation of cell growth by recombinant oncostatin M, Growth Factors 2 (1990) 157–165.
24. M.W. Sleeman, K.D. Anderson & P.D. Lambert, et al., The ciliary neurotrophic factor and its receptor, CNTFR alpha, Pharm Acta Helv 74 (2000) 265–272.
25. N.G. Forger, D. Prevette & O. deLapeyriere, et al., Cardiotrophin-like cytokine/cytokine-like factor 1 is an essential trophic

factor for lumbar and facial motoneurons in vivo, J Neurosci 23 (2003) 8854–8858.

26. D.H. Freed, R.H. Cunnington & A.L. Dangerfield, et al., Emerging evidence for the role of cardiotrophin-1 in cardiac repair in the infarcted heart, Cardiovasc Res 65 (2005) 782–792.

27. A.V. Villarino, E. Huang & C.A. Hunter, Understanding the pro- and anti-inflammatory properties of IL-27, J Immunol 173 (2004) 715–720.

28. S. Kwan Tat, M. Padrines & S. Theoleyre, et al., IL-6, RANKL, TNF-alpha/IL-1: interrelations in bone resorption pathophysiology, Cytokine Growth Factor Rev 15 (2004) 49–60.

29. J.L. Sanders & P.H. Stern, Protein kinase C involvement in interleukin-6 production by parathyroid hormone and tumor necrosis factor-alpha in UMR-106 osteoblastic cells, J Bone Miner Res 15 (2000) 885–893.

30. K. Kurokouchi, F. Kambe & K. Yasukawa, et al., TNF-alpha increases expression of IL-6 and ICAM-1 genes through activation of NF-kappaB in osteoblast-like ROS17/2.8 cells, J Bone Miner Res 13 (1998) 1290–1299.

31. F. Blanchard, L. Duplomb & S. Raher, et al., Mannose 6-phosphate/insulin-like growth factor II receptor mediates internalization and degradation of leukemia inhibitory factor but not signal transduction, J Biol Chem 274 (1999) 24685–24693.

32. S. Rose-John, J. Scheller & G. Elson, et al., Interleukin-6 biology is coordinated by membrane-bound and soluble receptors: role in inflammation and cancer, J Leukoc Biol 80 (2006) 227–2236.

33. V. Pitard, V. Lorgeot & J.L. Taupin, et al., The presence in human serum of a circulating soluble leukemia inhibitory factor receptor (sgp190) and its evolution during pregnancy, Eur Cytokine Netw 9 (1998) 599–605.

34. C. Diveu, E. Venereau & J. Froger, et al., Molecular and functional characterization of a soluble form of oncostatin m/interleukin-31 shared receptor, J Biol Chem 281 (2006) 36673–36682.

35. Y. Nakaoka, K. Nishida & Y. Fujio, et al., Activation of gp130 transduces hypertrophic signal through interaction of scaffolding/docking protein Gab1 with tyrosine phosphatase SHP2 in cardiomyocytes, Circ Res 93 (2003) 221–229.

36. J.J. Schuringa, L.V. Dekker & E. Vellenga, et al., Sequential activation of Rac-1, SEK-1/MKK-4, and protein kinase Cdelta is required for interleukin-6-induced STAT3 Ser-727 phosphorylation and transactivation, J Biol Chem 276 (2001) 27709–27715.

37. D.C. Smyth, C. Kerr & C.D. Richards, Oncostatin M-induced IL-6 expression in murine fibroblasts requires the activation of protein kinase Cdelta, J Immunol 177 (2006) 8740–8747.

38. Y.H. Lee, S.S. Bae & J.K. Seo, et al., Interleukin-6-induced tyrosine phosphorylation of phospholipase C-gamma1 in PC12 cells, Mol Cells 10 (2000) 469–474.

39. F. Blanchard, Y. Wang & E. Kinzie, et al., Oncostatin M regulates the synthesis and turnover of gp130, leukemia inhibitory factor receptor alpha, and oncostatin M receptor beta by distinct mechanisms, J Biol Chem 276 (2001) 47038–47045.

40. H. Kim & H. Baumann, Dual signaling role of the protein tyrosine phosphatase SHP-2 in regulating expression of acute-phase plasma proteins by interleukin-6 cytokine receptors in hepatic cells, Mol Cell Biol 19 (1999) 5326–5338.

41. N.C. Tebbutt, A.S. Giraud & M. Inglese, et al., Reciprocal regulation of gastrointestinal homeostasis by SHP2 and STAT-mediated trefoil gene activation in gp130 mutant mice, Nat Med 8 (2002) 1089–1097.

42. M. Kortylewski, P.C. Heinrich & A. Mackiewicz, et al., Interleukin-6 and oncostatin M-induced growth inhibition of human A375 melanoma cells is STAT-dependent and involves upregulation of the cyclin-dependent kinase inhibitor p27/Kip1, Oncogene 18 (1999) 3742–3753.

43. L. Duplomb, B. Chaigne-Delalande & P. Vusio, et al., Soluble mannose 6-phosphate/insulin-like growth factor II (IGF-II) receptor inhibits interleukin-6-type cytokine-dependent proliferation by neutralization of IGF-II, Endocrinology 144 (2003) 5381–5389.

44. C. Lu, C. Sheehan & J.W. Rak, et al., Endogenous interleukin 6 can function as an in vivo growth-stimulatory factor for advanced-stage human melanoma cells, Clin Cancer Res 2 (1996) 1417–1425.

45. Y. Lu, S. Fukuyama & R. Yoshida, et al., Loss of SOCS3 gene expression converts STAT3 function from anti-apoptotic to pro-apoptotic, J Biol Chem 281 (2006) 36683–36690.

46. Y. Taguchi, M. Yamamoto & T. Yamate, et al., Interleukin-6-type cytokines stimulate mesenchymal progenitor differentiation toward the osteoblastic lineage, Proc Assoc Am Physicians 110 (1998) 559–574.

47. A. Erices, P. Conget & C. Rojas, et al., Gp130 activation by soluble interleukin-6 receptor/interleukin-6 enhances osteoblastic differentiation of human bone marrow-derived mesenchymal stem cells, Exp Cell Res 280 (2002) 24–32.

48. T. Bellido, V.Z. Borba & P. Roberson, et al., Activation of the Janus kinase/STAT (signal transducer and activator of transcription) signal transduction pathway by interleukin-6-type cytokines promotes osteoblast differentiation, Endocrinology 138 (1997) 3666–3676.

49. Y. Takeuchi, S. Watanabe & G. Ishii, et al., Interleukin-11 as a stimulatory factor for bone formation prevents bone loss with advancing age in mice, J Biol Chem 277 (2002) 49011–49018.

50. S. Itoh, N. Udagawa & N. Takahashi, et al., A critical role for interleukin-6 family-mediated Stat3 activation in osteoblast differentiation and bone formation, Bone 39 (2006) 505–512.

51. T. Bellido, C.A. O'Brien & P.K. Roberson, et al., Transcriptional activation of the p21(WAF1,CIP1,SDI1) gene by interleukin-6 type cytokines. A prerequisite for their pro-differentiating and anti-apoptotic effects on human osteoblastic cells, J Biol Chem 273 (1998) 21137–21144.

52. R.L. Jilka, R.S. Weinstein & T. Bellido, et al., Osteoblast programmed cell death (apoptosis): modulation by growth factors and cytokines, J Bone Miner Res 13 (1998) 793–802.

53. F.J. Hughes & G.L. Howells, Interleukin-11 inhibits bone formation in vitro, Calcif Tissue Int 53 (1993) 362–364.

54. P.R. Jay, M. Centrella & J. Lorenzo, et al., Oncostatin-M: a new bone active cytokine that activates osteoblasts and inhibits bone resorption, Endocrinology 137 (1996) 1151–1158.

55. L. Malaval, A.K. Gupta & J.E. Aubin, Leukemia inhibitory factor inhibits osteogenic differentiation in rat calvaria cell cultures, Endocrinology 136 (1995) 1411–1418.

56. C. Chipoy, M. Berreur & S. Couillaud, et al., Downregulation of osteoblast markers and induction of the glial fibrillary

acidic protein by oncostatin M in osteosarcoma cells require PKCdelta and STAT3, J Bone Miner Res 19 (2004) 1850–1861.

57. L. Malaval & J.E. Aubin, Biphasic effects of leukemia inhibitory factor on osteoblastic differentiation, J Cell Biochem 81 (2001) 63–70.

58. L. Malaval, F. Liu & A.B. Vernallis, et al., GP130/OSMR is the only LIF/IL-6 family receptor complex to promote osteoblast differentiation of calvaria progenitors, J Cell Physiol 204 (2005) 585–593.

59. C. Chipoy, B. Brounais & V. Trichet, et al., Sensitization of osteosarcoma cells to apoptosis by Oncostatin M depends on STAT5 and p53, Oncogene 26 (2007) 6653–6664.

60. B. Brounais, C. Chipoy & K. Mori, et al., Oncostatin M induces bone loss and sensitizes rat osteosarcoma to the antitumor effect of Midostaurin in vivo, Clin Cancer Research 14 (2008) 5400–5409.

61. G. Girasole, G. Passeri & R.L. Jilka, et al., Interleukin-11: a new cytokine critical for osteoclast development, J Clin Invest 93 (1994) 1516–1524.

62. C.D. Richards, C. Langdon & P. Deschamps, et al., Stimulation of osteoclast differentiation in vitro by mouse oncostatin M, leukaemia inhibitory factor, cardiotrophin-1 and interleukin 6: synergy with dexamethasone, Cytokine 12 (2000) 613–621.

63. C.A. O'Brien, S.C. Lin & T. Bellido, et al., Expression levels of gp130 in bone marrow stromal cells determine the magnitude of osteoclastogenic signals generated by IL-6-type cytokines, J Cell Biochem 79 (2000) 532–541.

64. J. Ahlen, S. Andersson & H. Mukohyama, et al., Characterization of the bone-resorptive effect of interleukin-11 in cultured mouse calvarial bones, Bone 31 (2002) 242–251.

65. P. Palmqvist, E. Persson & H.H. Conaway, et al., IL-6, leukemia inhibitory factor, and oncostatin M stimulate bone resorption and regulate the expression of receptor activator of NF-kappa B ligand, osteoprotegerin, and receptor activator of NF-kappa B in mouse calvariae, J Immunol 169 (2002) 3353–3362.

66. N. Kurihara, D. Bertolini & T. Suda, et al., IL-6 stimulates osteoclast-like multinucleated cell formation in long term human marrow cultures by inducing IL-1 release, J Immunol 144 (1990) 4226–4230.

67. C. Guillen, A.R. de Gortazar & P. Esbrit, The interleukin-6/soluble interleukin-6 receptor system induces parathyroid hormone-related protein in human osteoblastic cells, Calcif Tissue Int 75 (2004) 153–159.

68. C. Guillen, P. Martinez & A.R. de Gortazar, et al., Both N- and C-terminal domains of parathyroid hormone-related protein increase interleukin-6 by nuclear factor-kappa B activation in osteoblastic cells, J Biol Chem 277 (2002) 28109–28117.

69. X.H. Liu, A. Kirschenbaum & S. Yao, et al., Cross-talk between the interleukin-6 and prostaglandin E(2) signaling systems results in enhancement of osteoclastogenesis through effects on the osteoprotegerin/receptor activator of nuclear factor-{kappa}B (RANK) ligand/RANK system, Endocrinology 146 (2005) 1991–1998.

70. R.D. Devlin, S.V. Reddy & R. Savino, et al., IL-6 mediates the effects of IL-1 or TNF, but not PTHrP or 1,25(OH)2D3, on osteoclast-like cell formation in normal human bone marrow cultures, J Bone Miner Res 13 (1998) 393–399.

71. C.A. O'Brien, I. Gubrij & S.C. Lin, et al., STAT3 activation in stromal/osteoblastic cells is required for induction of the receptor activator of NF-kappaB ligand and stimulation of osteoclastogenesis by gp130-utilizing cytokines or interleukin-1 but not 1,25-dihydroxyvitamin D3 or parathyroid hormone, J Biol Chem 274 (1999) 19301–19308.

72. S. Kim, M. Yamazaki & N.K. Shevde, et al., Transcriptional control of receptor activator of nuclear factor-kappaB ligand by the protein kinase A activator forskolin and the transmembrane glycoprotein 130-activating cytokine, oncostatin M, is exerted through multiple distal enhancers, Mol Endocrinol 21 (2007) 197–214.

73. E. Van Beek, L. Van der Wee-Pals & M. van de Ruit, et al., Leukemia inhibitory factor inhibits osteoclastic resorption, growth, mineralization, and alkaline phosphatase activity in fetal mouse metacarpal bones in culture, J Bone Miner Res 8 (1993) 191–198.

74. L. Duplomb, M. Baud'huin & C. Charrier, et al., IL-6 inhibits RANKL-induced osteoclastogenesis by diverting cells into the macrophage lineage: key role of Serine727 phosphorylation of STAT3, Endocrinology 149 (2008) 3688–3697.

75. F. Yoshitake, S. Itoh & H. Narita, et al., IL-6 directly inhibits osteoclast differentiation by suppressing rank signaling pathways, J Biol Chem 283 (2008) 11535–11540.

76. S. Kamiya, C. Nakamura & T. Fukawa, et al., Effects of IL-23 and IL-27 on osteoblasts and osteoclasts: inhibitory effects on osteoclast differentiation, J Bone Miner Metab 25 (2007) 277–285.

77. H. Kitamura, H. Kawata & F. Takahashi, et al., Bone marrow neutrophilia and suppressed bone turnover in human interleukin-6 transgenic mice. A cellular relationship among hematopoietic cells, osteoblasts, and osteoclasts mediated by stromal cells in bone marrow, Am J Pathol 147 (1995) 1682–1692.

78. N. Malik, H.S. Haugen & B. Modrell, et al., Developmental abnormalities in mice transgenic for bovine oncostatin M, Mol Cell Biol 15 (1995) 2349–2358.

79. K. Kawasaki, Y.H. Gao & S. Yokose, et al., Osteoclasts are present in gp130-deficient mice, Endocrinology 138 (1997) 4959–4965.

80. C.B. Ware, M.C. Horowitz & B.R. Renshaw, et al., Targeted disruption of the low-affinity leukemia inhibitory factor receptor gene causes placental, skeletal, neural and metabolic defects and results in perinatal death, Development 121 (1995) 1283–1299.

81. M. Tanaka, Y. Hirabayashi & T. Sekiguchi, et al., Targeted disruption of oncostatin M receptor results in altered hematopoiesis, Blood 102 (2003) 3154–3162.

82. N.A. Sims, B.J. Jenkins & J.M. Quinn, et al., Glycoprotein 130 regulates bone turnover and bone size by distinct downstream signaling pathways, J Clin Invest 113 (2004) 379–389.

83. C.D. Richards, Matrix catabolism in arthritis: priming the guns with oncostatin M, J Rheumatol 31 (2004) 2326–2328.

84. D.H. Jones, T. Nakashima & O.H. Sanchez, et al., Regulation of cancer cell migration and bone metastasis by RANKL, Nature 440 (2006) 692–696.

85. T.A. Guise, K.S. Mohammad & G. Clines, et al., Basic mechanisms responsible for osteolytic and osteoblastic bone metastases, Clin Cancer Res 12 (2006) 6213s–6216s.

86. A. Lacreusette, J.M. Nguyen & M.C. Pandolfino, et al., Loss of oncostatin M receptor beta in metastatic melanoma cells, Oncogene 26 (2007) 881–892.

87. J.J. Mule, J.K. McIntosh & D.M. Jablons, et al., Antitumor activity of recombinant interleukin 6 in mice, J Exp Med 171 (1990) 629–636.

88. L. Ouyang, L.Y. Shen & T. Li, et al., Inhibition effect of oncostatin M on metastatic human lung cancer cells 95-D in vitro and on murine melanoma cells B16BL6 in vivo, Biomed Res 27 (2006) 197–202.

89. S.P. Treon & K.C. Anderson, Interleukin-6 in multiple myeloma and related plasma cell dyscrasias, Curr Opin Hematol 5 (1998) 42–48.

90. P.A. Guerne & M. Lotz, Interleukin-6 and transforming growth factor-beta synergistically stimulate chondrosarcoma cell proliferation, J Cell Physiol 149 (1991) 117–124.

91. Y. Lu, J. Zhang & J. Dai, et al., Osteoblasts induce prostate cancer proliferation and PSA expression through interleukin-6-mediated activation of the androgen receptor, Clin Exp Metastasis 21 (2004) 399–408.

92. V.A. Florenes, C. Lu & N. Bhattacharya, et al., Interleukin-6 dependent induction of the cyclin dependent kinase inhibitor p21WAF1/CIP1 is lost during progression of human malignant melanoma, Oncogene 18 (1999) 1023–1032.

93. M. Kortylewski, R. Jove & H. Yu, Targeting STAT3 affects melanoma on multiple fronts, Cancer Metastasis Rev 24 (2005) 315–327.

94. J. Bromberg & J.E. Darnell Jr., The role of STATs in transcriptional control and their impact on cellular function, Oncogene 19 (2000) 2468–2473.

95. Y. Ohsaki, S. Takahashi & T. Scarcez, et al., Evidence for an autocrine/paracrine role for interleukin-6 in bone resorption by giant cells from giant cell tumors of bone, Endocrinology 131 (1992) 2229–2234.

96. T. Yoneda, M. Nakai & K. Moriyama, et al., Neutralizing antibodies to human interleukin 6 reverse hypercalcemia associated with a human squamous carcinoma, Cancer Res 53 (1993) 737–740.

97. Y. Nagai, H. Yamato & K. Akaogi, et al., Role of interleukin-6 in uncoupling of bone in vivo in a human squamous carcinoma coproducing parathyroid hormone-related peptide and interleukin-6, J Bone Miner Res 13 (1998) 664–672.

98. H. Knupfer & R. Preiss, Significance of interleukin-6 (IL-6) in breast cancer (review), Breast Cancer Res Treat 102 (2007) 129–135.

99. P.C. Smith, A. Hobisch & D.L. Lin, et al., Interleukin-6 and prostate cancer progression, Cytokine Growth Factor Rev 12 (2001) 33–40.

100. P. Rutkowski, J. Kaminska & M. Kowalska, et al., Cytokine and cytokine receptor serum levels in adult bone sarcoma patients: correlations with local tumor extent and prognosis, J Surg Oncol 84 (2003) 151–159.

101. C. Soubrane, O. Rixe & J.B. Meric, et al., Pretreatment serum interleukin-6 concentration as a prognostic factor of overall survival in metastatic malignant melanoma patients treated with biochemotherapy: a retrospective study, Melanoma Res 15 (2005) 199–204.

102. J. de la Mata, H.L. Uy & T.A. Guise, et al., Interleukin-6 enhances hypercalcemia and bone resorption mediated by parathyroid hormone-related protein in vivo, J Clin Invest 95 (1995) 2846–2852.

103. H. Morgan, A. Tumber & P.A. Hill, Breast cancer cells induce osteoclast formation by stimulating host IL-11 production and downregulating granulocyte/macrophage colony-stimulating factor, Int J Cancer 109 (2004) 653–660.

104. Y. Morinaga, N. Fujita & K. Ohishi, et al., Stimulation of interleukin-11 production from osteoblast-like cells by transforming growth factor-beta and tumor cell factors, Int J Cancer 71 (1997) 422–428.

105. Y. Sohara, H. Shimada & C. Minkin, et al., Bone marrow mesenchymal stem cells provide an alternate pathway of osteoclast activation and bone destruction by cancer cells, Cancer Res 65 (2005) 1129–1135.

106. M. Chatterjee, T. Stuhmer & P. Herrmann, et al., Combined disruption of both the MEK/ERK and the IL-6R/STAT3 pathways is required to induce apoptosis of multiple myeloma cells in the presence of bone marrow stromal cells, Blood 104 (2004) 3712–3721.

107. T. Akatsu, K. Ono & Y. Katayama, et al., The mouse mammary tumor cell line, MMT060562, produces prostaglandin E2 and leukemia inhibitory factor and supports osteoclast formation in vitro via a stromal cell-dependent pathway, J Bone Miner Res 13 (1998) 400–408.

108. R. Bataille, D. Chappard & B. Klein, The critical role of interleukin-6, interleukin-1B and macrophage colony-stimulating factor in the pathogenesis of bone lesions in multiple myeloma, Int J Clin Lab Res 21 (1992) 283–287.

109. B.E. Barton & T.F. Murphy, Cancer cachexia is mediated in part by the induction of IL-6-like cytokines from the spleen, Cytokine 16 (2001) 251–257.

110. M. Shimizu, M. Shimamura & T. Owaki, et al., Antiangiogenic and antitumor activities of IL-27, J Immunol 176 (2006) 7317–7324.

111. R. Burger, F. Bakker & A. Guenther, et al., Functional significance of novel neurotrophin-1/B cell-stimulating factor-3 (cardiotrophin-like cytokine) for human myeloma cell growth and survival, Br J Haematol 123 (2003) 869–878.

112. S. Chattopadhyay, E. Tracy & P. Liang, et al., Interleukin-31 and oncostatin-M mediate distinct signaling reactions and response patterns in lung epithelial cells, J Biol Chem 282 (2007) 3014–3026.

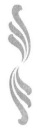

CHAPTER 9

Proteases and Therapeutic Approaches of Bone Tumors

VELASCO C. RUIZ[1,2], Y. FORTUN[1,2,3], D. HEYMANN[1,2,4] AND M. PADRINES[1,2]*

[1]INSERM, U957, Nantes, F-44035, France.

[2]Université de Nantes, Nantes Atlantique Universités, Laboratoire de Physiopathologie de la Résorption Osseuse et Thérapie des Tumeurs Osseuses Primitives, EA3822, Nantes, F-44035 France.

[3]Université d'Angers, IUT, France.

[4]Centre Hospitalier Universitaire de Nantes, France.

*Corresponding author: Dr Marc Padrines, INSERM U957, EA3822, Faculté de Médeciùe, 1 rue G. Veil 44033 Nantes, France.

Contents

I. INTRODUCTION

Bone-forming and bone-resorbing cells are closely associated in time and space. Indeed, following a bone stimulus (mechanical load, hormones, growth factors), osteoclastic cells are recruited at the bone surface and thus degrade bone mineral components by an acid extra-cellular mechanism called resorption phase [1]. The osteogenic cells (osteoclasts, osteoblasts) contribute individually to the bone remodeling whereas their interactions control their cellular activities as well as the intensity of bone remodeling. These interactions can be established either through a cell-to-cell contact with the involvement of molecules from the integrin family or by the release of many polypeptidic factors and/or their soluble receptor chains. These factors can act directly on osteogenic cells and their precursors to control differentiation, formation and functions (matrix formation, mineralization, resorption...) [2]. Any disturbance between these effectors leads to the development of skeletal abnormalities, characterized by decreased (osteoporosis) or increased (osteopetrosis) bone mass. Increased osteoclast activity is observed in many osteopathic disorders, including postmenopausal osteoporosis, Paget's disease, primary bone tumors, lytic bone metastases, multiple myeloma, or rheumatoid arthritis, leading to an increased bone resorption and a loss of bone mass.

Bone is a highly hospitable environment for the colonization and growth of metastatic tumors. Tumor cells in the bone microenvironment initiate an inflammatory response that leads to recruitment of activated osteoclasts and then to bone resorption [3]. Moreover, tumor cells create a favorable environment for their own growth [4]. The inflammatory response and the tumor environment lead to a vicious cycle establishment between bone and tumor cells. Evidences suggest that the established vicious cycle acts by co-opting the physiological mechanisms that normally favor bone resorption. Tumor cells release agents (growth factors, cytokines, etc.) into the bone microenvironment, which, in turn, act on osteoblastic stromal cells to enhance the production of osteoclast activating factors such as Receptor Activator of Nuclear Factor-κB Ligand (RANKL) [5].

Bone resorption depends on the concord action of specific proteases able to remove the organic matrix and the formation of an acidic microenvironment necessary for solubilization of the hydroxyapatite. Fibrillar collagen is highly resistant to proteolytic degradation and the only proteases that have been shown to cleave the native triple helical region of fibrillar collagen are the collagenases of the matrix metalloproteinase (MMP) family and members of the cysteine protease family.

II. CATHEPSIN K

Following tight attachment to the bone surface, osteoclasts secrete protons into a closed extracellular compartment surrounded by a sealing zone. This local acidification (about pH 4) solubilizes the mineral bone and renders the organic matrix, which consists of 90% type I collagen, available to proteases. Osteoclasts also secrete proteases that digest the matrix components. Among these proteases is cathepsin K, a member of the papain cystein protease family. Cathepsin K is abundantly and predominantly expressed (about 98% of the total cystein protease) in osteoclasts where it is localized in lysosomes, in the ruffled border and in the resorption lacunae on the bone surface [6–10]. However, a cathepsin K expression has been shown in osteoblastic cells [11]. The localization in osteoclastic cells, and the ability to degrade type I collagen both within and outside the helical regions, and to act as an acidic and neutral pH, make cathepsin K a unique mammalian protease [12]. Thus cathepsin K is considered to be the principal protease responsible for the degradation of most of the bone matrix.

The cysteine protease implication in osteoclast-mediated bone resorption was initially demonstrated by the use of E64 and leupeptin. Indeed, these two papain-like cathepsin inhibitors are able to inhibit bone resorption *in vitro* [13]. The particular importance of cathepsin K is observed in pycnodysostosis, an autosomal recessive bone sclerosing disorder due to a cathepsin K mutation and so to a deficiency in cathepsin K activity resulting in a strong osteotropic phenotype [14,15]. A strong accumulation of demineralized collagen fibers in the subosteoclastic resorption zone and an intracellular accumulation of collagen fibrils in fibroblasts are observed [16]. These phenotype parameters are reproduced in cathepsin K deficient mice [17] and cathepsin K knockout mice [18]. On the contrary,

an overexpression of cathepsin K in mice results in an acceleration of the turnover of metaphyseal trabecular bone which is an indication for an osteoporosis phenotype [19].

The mature form of cathepsin K contains 215 amino acids that are processed intracellularly and subsequently excreted into the resorption lacuna [20]. The collagenolytic activity of cathepsin K is related to a specific complex of the enzyme with chondroitin sulfate. The complex is an oligomer constituted of five cathepsin K and five chondroitin sulfate molecules. Only this complex has a triple helical collagen-degrading activity, whereas the monomeric form of cathepsin K can degrade non-collagenous substrates [21]. Many of the factors that induce osteoclast formation and activation or inhibit osteoclast activity, respectively, enhance or suppress cathepsin K gene expression. Thus RANKL, a member of the tumor necrosis factor superfamily, stimulates cathepsin K mRNA and protein expression in human osteoclasts after binding to its osteoclastic receptor RANK [22] (Figure 9.1). All of the agents that stimulate (vitamin D, parathyroid hormone...) or inhibit (estrogen, transforming growth factor-β, osteoprotegerin...) RANKL, indirectly exert corresponding stimulatory or inhibitory effects on cathepsin K expression.

As an early and proximal event, the RANKL stimulating effect on the transcription of the cathepsin K gene occurs via a number of mechanisms. An overexpression of TRAF6 (TNF receptor-associated factor 6), which is a critical adaptor molecule for the cognate receptor of RANKL, stimulates the cathepsin K promotor activity. On the contrary, the RANKL stimulation of cathepsin K promotor activity is inhibited by the overexpression of dominant negative

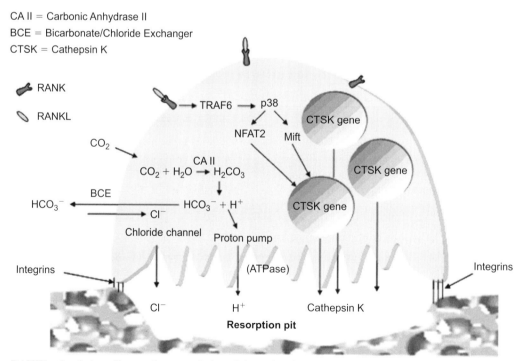

FIGURE 9.1   RANKL stimulating effect on the transcription of the cathepsin K.

TRAF6 [23]. More distally in the signaling pathway, RANKL leads to the phosphorylation by p38 of NFAT2, a calcineurin-dependent transcription factor belonging to the nuclear factor of activated T cell family of transcription factors. This phosphorylation induces NFAT2 translocation into the nucleus and the subsequent transactivation of the cathepsin K promotor [24]. It has been shown that RANKL induces NFAT2 mRNA expression in pre-osteoclasts [25] and that cyclosporine, which inhibits the phosphatase activity of calcineurin and thus NFAT activation, suppresses RANKL induced cathepsin K expression [23]. In addition, RANKL induces phosphorylation of the microphthalmia transcription factor (Mift) by p38 [26]. Mift is a member of the helix-loop-helix (HLH) leucine zipper family and directly regulates cathepsin K gene transcription. Dominant negative mutations of Mift exhibit osteopetrosis and lack cathepsin K mRNA and protein [27] whereas an overexpression of wild-type Mift in cultured osteoclasts enhances cathepsin K expression.

Thus, cathepsin K inhibitors represent a novel therapeutic target for diseases marked by excessive bone resorption. The inhibition of this enzyme slows down or corrects pathological conditions due to an imbalance in bone resorption, such as osteoporosis and rheumatoid arthritis. The development of a primary bone tumor, such as osteosarcoma or a metastatic bone tumor, is always associated with local enhancement of cathepsin K expression and excretion resulting in pathological excessive bone resorption. This enhancement follows osteoclast differentiation and activation by cytokines, such as RANKL, produced by tumor cells or activated osteoblasts. As for the non-tumoral osteolytic pathologies, cathepsin K inhibitors could therefore represent a therapeutic target to reduce the vicious circle between tumor development and bone resorption. Natural inhibitors of cysteine proteases (including cathepsin K), such as cystatins [28] and prodomains of the zymogens [29] have been well studied. Thus, cystatin B is effective in inhibiting bone resorption by downregulating cathepsin K activity [30] and cathepsin C decreases osteoclast formation in mouse bone marrow cultures [31]. Numerous cysteine protease inhibitors of low molecular weight have been synthesized and investigated extensively in the past as novel drugs candidates [32–36]. The design of these compounds is based on the nucleophilic thiol residue (cysteine) of the active site. This residue can be targeted by an electrophilic center placed in a peptide, or any structure that will be recognized by the substrate binding region of the protease, and thus will give its specificity to the final drug. According to the electrophilic moiety nature, the inhibitor acts in a reversible or irreversible manner [37,38]. Whatever inhibitor is used, a therapeutic application involves a good specificity and also a good ability of the compound to reach its target enzyme in a specific cell and an appropriate cellular compartment (for example, the resorption lacuna in the case of cathepsin K). If the synthetic cathepsin K inhibitors have

demonstrated their efficacy to prevent an excessive osteolysis essentially in non tumoral pathologies [39], it clearly appears that the development of new cathepsin K inhibitors with an improved specificity to osteoclastic cells could be an important research axis to stop or reduce the pathological bone resorption observed in the presence of bone metastasis or primitive bone tumor like osteosarcoma [40–41]. Inhibitors of cathepsin K effectively suppress bone resorption in animal tumor models [42]. All of the results indicate that cathepsin K inhibitors are very promising anti-resorptive therapeutic agents, and may be beneficial for the treatment of osteoporosis and breast cancer metastasis-induced osteolysis. Moreover, several inhibitors seem to possess good oral availability [43].

III. MATRIX METALLOPROTEINASES

Matrix Metalloproteinases (MMPs) are secreted proteins belonging to a family of zinc metalloendopeptidases that have the capacity to cleave extracellular matrix (ECM). Because MMPs can degrade ECM molecules, their main function has been presumed to be remodeling of the ECM [44]. *In vitro* studies suggest that MMPs can affect fundamental cellular processes such as proliferation, survival, migration, and morphogenesis. Discovering the roles of the MMPs in physiological processes has not been simple. Many processes that are affected *in vitro* by alteration of MMP activity do not seem to be affected by the lack of the relevant MMP *in vivo* [45]. Inactivating individual MMPs may show defects in processes in which the MMP play an indispensable function, but may not reveal minor functions.

The MMP family consists of at least 26 members, which are produced as zymogens, with a signal sequence and propeptide segment that must be proteolytically processed to be activated. The propeptide domain contains a conserved cysteine residue, which chelates the active zinc site [46]. An exception is MMP-23 which lacks this conserved cysteine, and has a very different propeptide domain [47]. A subset of MMPs, including the membrane bound MMPs (MT-MMPs), as well as MMP-11, MMP-21, MMP-23, and MMP-28, contains a furin recognition sequence between their propeptide and catalytic domains, allowing cleavage and activation by furin convertase enzymes in the Golgi apparatus [48]. The MT-MMPs are bound to the cell surface via a C-terminal transmembrane domain or glycosylphosphatidylinositol anchor [49]. Except for the MMPs activated intracellularly by furin proteases, the other MMPs are secreted as inactive zymogens and must be activated in the extracellular space by proteolytic cleavage of the N-terminal propeptide domain [46]. Thus, plasmin can initiate MMP activation cascade [50,51]. MMPs, themselves, are implicated in a complex cascade of activation (Figure 9.2). Thus, activated MMP-3 can in turn activate proMMP-1 and proMMP-9 [52]. MT1-MMP activates proMMP-2 as

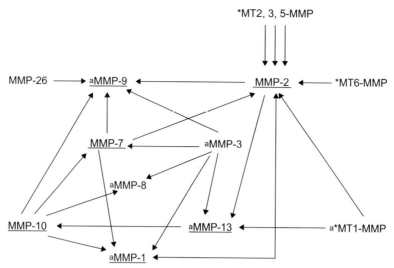

FIGURE 9.2 Cascade of MMPs activation, ($\rightarrow$) by the MMPs, ([a]) by the plasmin, ([*]) by the furin and (–) autocatalytically.

well as proMMP-13 at the cell surface [53,54]. Activated MMP-2 and MMP-13 can both in turn activate proMMP-9 [55,56]. Tissue Inhibitor of MetalloProteinase-2 (TIMP-2) has a specialized role in the activation of proMMP-2 by MT1-MMP. The N-terminal domain of TIMP-2 forms an inhibitory complex with the active site of MT1-MMP, while the C-terminal domain interacts with the hemopexin domain of MMP-2. A second non-inhibited MT1-MMP molecule is recruited to the complex and activates the MMP-2 [57]. Similar pericellular activation is also shown to play a role in the activation of pro-MMP-7 where this soluble zymogen is captured and activated on the cell membrane through interaction with CD151 [58].

In addition to degrading ECM components and activating other MMPs, several other physiological substrates for MMPs have been described. Thus, using oriented peptide libraries to identify potential MMP cleavage sites, several integrins, proteoglycans and chemokines or their receptors have been identified as MMP substrates. Thus, MMPs can release growth factors from the ECM or the cell surface. They can modify both cell-cell and cell-ECM interactions by the proteolysis of cell surface growth factors and adhesion receptors, and they are key regulators of inflammatory responses, which can be pro-inflammatory or anti-inflammatory [59]. Thus, this activity makes available active growth factors and cytokines. MMPs can be either free in the cytosol or bound to the surface of a cell. The cell surface-bound forms are thought to enhance inflammatory cell functions. Thus, MMP-1, MMP-2, and MMP-9 have been found to bind to specific cell surface proteins such as $\alpha_v\beta_3$-integrin, $\alpha_2\beta_1$, and CD44 [60–64]. Their localization on the cell surface confers resistance to TIMP inhibition [65] and may be responsible for the increase in pericellular proteolytic activity. Together with the cell surface activation of MMP-2 and MMP-7, these

experiments suggest that localization of MMPs to the cell surface is a general means of regulating MMP activity.

IV. MATRIX METALLOPROTEINASES AND BONE

MMPs play an important role in bone physiology. By using proteinase inhibitors, several studies have demonstrated that the relative importance of MMPs varies depending on the bone type and/or the stage of the resorption cycle [66,67]. In addition, reports on MMP knockout mice and human genetic diseases have drawn attention to the importance of MMPs for skeletal development [68]. Thus, MMP-13, an interstitial collagenase, participates in the removal of collagen in the resorption pit at the end of the resorption cycle. This removal is a prerequisite for the deposition of a new matrix in the resorption lacuna. An early indication that MMPs might be required for this recruitment process came from experiments showing that the development of the marrow cavity is impaired in primitive long bones treated with MMP inhibitors [69].

MMPs have also been implicated in osteoclast migration. The most probable candidate for this function is MT1-MMP, an interstitial collagenase expressed on the plasma membrane of osteoclasts [70]. Its collagenase activity may assist with the movement of osteoclasts through the collagen network. Interestingly, it has been observed that MT1-MMP is located either at the leading edge of migrating osteoclast or concentrated at the sealing zone of the polarized resorbing osteoclast [71]. MMP-9 also plays a role in osteoclastic bone resorption by facilitating the migration of osteoclastic cells toward bone surfaces through proteoglycan-rich matrices [72] without any apparent affect on the osteoclast resorptive activity itself. The molecular mode of action of

MMP-9 in this invasion remains to be determined. With respect to growth plate invasion, it may be speculated that MMP-9 releases VEGF from the matrix [73], or contributes to the degradation of type II collagen [74].

A null mutation in the MMP-9 gene results in a very specific defect in endochondral bone formation [75]. Mice with this defect accumulate hypertrophic cartilage at the skeletal growth plates. The simplest model for the action of MMP-9 in this process is the regulation of a release of an angiogenic factor from hypertrophic cartilage ECM stores. Thus, lack of MMP-9 leads to a decrease in vascular invasion with its attendant processes. Alternatively, MMP-9 may have other functions and the decrease in angiogenic activity of MMP-9-null hypertrophic cartilage may be an indirect consequence. The relevant angiogenic factor at the growth plate is VEGF, which is expressed by hypertrophic cartilage. However, VEGF appears to do more than regulating angiogenesis at the growth plate [76].

Inactivation of MT1-MMP results in several skeletal defects that are different from those in the MMP-9-null mice [77]. MT1-MMP deficiency causes craniofacial dysmorphism, arthritis, osteopenia, dwarfism, and fibrosis of soft tissues due to ablation of a collagenolytic activity that is essential for modeling of skeletal and extraskeletal connective tissues. In the MT1-MMP-deficient mice, no vascular canal is formed. Similar defects have been observed in mice with a mutation in the collagenase cleavage site of type I collagen [78]. This demonstrates the pivotal function of MT1-MMP in connective tissue metabolism, and illustrates that modeling of the soft connective tissue matrix by resident cells is essential for the development and maintenance of the hard tissues of the skeleton.

V. REGULATING MATRIX METALLOPROTEINASE PRODUCTION BY OPG/RANK/RANKL

Distinctive inductive and suppressive factors regulate the expression of each of the members of the MMP family [79]. Interestingly, most of the same factors that regulate the expression of MMPs can also act as their substrates, providing a built-in and, most likely, essential component of the regulatory cascades. This coordination between MMP and substrate ensures efficient activation and control of MMPs *in vivo* [80,81].

Thus, *in vitro*, the proinflammatory cytokines interleukin-1 (IL-1), IL-6, and TNF-α upregulate MMPs [82]. More importantly, this is also observed *in vivo*. IL-1β is produced in a biologically inactive form and can be activated by cleavage with MMP9 [83]. IL-1 is a potent stimulator of bone resorption and an inhibitor of bone formation, whereas RANKL is essential and sufficient for osteoclast differentiation. IL-1α affects mineralized nodule formation *in vitro* and halts bone matrix turnover. IL-1α also stimulates osteoclast formation via the interaction of RANKL with RANK by increasing M-CSF and prostaglandin E2 and decreasing osteoprotegerin (OPG). Recently, Fujisaki *et al.* showed that the expression of carbonic anhydrase II, cathepsin K, and MMP-9 in osteoclastic precursor cells (RAW264.7) is induced by RANKL in the presence of IL-1α [84].

RANKL is a transmembrane glycoprotein that has an essential role in the development of osteoclasts. The extracellular portion of RANKL is cleaved proteolytically to produce soluble RANKL. MMP-7 has been reported to cleave RANKL *in vitro* or under overexpressing conditions and has an important role in prostate cancer-induced osteolysis [85]. However, MMP-7 does not cleave full-length RANKL in other systems [86]. Blobel and co-workers [87] demonstrated that ADAM17 (TNF-α converting enzyme) cleaves a partial fragment of RANKL protein, but not full-length RANKL [88]. Suppression of MT1-MMP in primary osteoblasts increases membrane-bound RANKL and promotes osteoclastogenesis in co-cultures with macrophages. Soluble RANKL produced by osteoblasts from MT1-MMP-deficient mice is markedly reduced, and their osteoclastogenic activity is promoted, consistent with the findings of increased osteoclastogenesis *in vivo*. RANKL shedding is an important process that downregulates local osteoclastogenesis [86].

OPG/RANK and RANKL have been identified as members of a ligand-receptor system that directly regulates osteoclast differentiation and osteolysis. Whether RANKL is a powerful inducer of bone resorption through its interaction with RANK, OPG is a soluble decoy receptor and acts as a strong inhibitor of osteoclastic differentiation. OPG and RANKL exert differential effects on protease activities in osteoclast cultures [89–91]. Thus, OPG stimulated pro-MMP-9 activities and MMP-9 expression, and concomitantly upregulated TIMP-1 expression in purified osteoclast cultures [89]. In a similar model, RANKL increased pro-MMP-9 activities and MMP-9 expression, and simultaneously decreased TIMP-1 expression. In this context, OPG is an inhibitor of bone resorption, and RANKL is a pro-resorptive mediator via the control of protease activities [90]. Indeed, OPG-induced pro-MMP-9 activity is abolished by ras/MAPK inhibitors in purified osteoclasts via the phosphorylation of p38 and ERK1/2 in RAW264.7 murine osteoclastic progenitors. This signal transduction is partly dependent on RANKL, as p38 activation is totally abolished by a blocking anti-RANKL antibody whereas ERK1/2 is only weakly inhibited. Moreover, OPG/RANK/RANKL can form a hetero-molecular complex as demonstrated by surface plasmon resonance analyses [92]. Whether OPG binds to RANKL, it can also strongly interact with proteoglycans [93,94], which mediate its internalization [95]. Thus, OPG exerts a direct biological effect in osteoclasts suggesting a more complex regulation of bone resorption by this factor than originally described.

The RANKL-RANK signaling promotes the binding of TNF receptor associated factor (TRAF) family proteins such as TRAF6 to RANK receptor resulting in activation of NF-κB and Jun N-terminal kinase (JNK) pathways [5]. With siRNA interference, Sundaram *et al.* show that, like cathepsin K (Figure 9.1), RANKL signals through TRAF6, but not TRAF2, to enhance MMP 9 gene expression in osteoclast precursor cells [96]. In addition, RANKL differently regulates MMP-9 expression through p38 and ERK signaling pathways during osteoclast differentiation. Besides, the calcitonin receptor, mouse tartrate-resistant acid phosphatase and human beta-3 integrin gene promoters during osteoclast differentiation are regulated by NFAT2 [97–99]. Furthermore, NFAT2 expression is auto-regulated during osteoclastogenesis [100]. Inhibition of NFAT2 using siRNA decreases RANKL stimulation of MMP-9 activity. These results suggest that NFAT2 is a downstream effector of RANKL signaling to modulate MMP-9 gene expression during osteoclast differentiation.

VI. MATRIX METALLOPROTEINASES AND BONE TUMOR

Tumor cells can produce enzymes that destroy the matrix barriers, permitting invasion into surrounding connective tissues and metastasis to distant organs. The tumor cells are not the only source of MMPs. Thus, many other MMPs, like MMP-2 and -9, are predominantly produced by stromal cells (for review, see Ref. [101]). MMPs secreted by stromal cells can still be recruited to the cancer-cell membrane [102]. The evidence for MMPs as active contributors to cancer progression comes from animal studies. For example, overexpression of TIMPs reduces experimental metastasis [45], and mouse 3T3 cells become tumorigenic after antisense depletion of TIMP-1 [103]. The expression and activity of MMPs are increased in almost every type of human cancer, and this correlates with the advanced tumor stage, increased invasion and metastasis, and shortened survival. These results suggest that MMPs are important contributors to tumor progression. MMPs promote tumor progression not only through ECM degradation, but also by countering apoptosis, orchestrating angiogenesis, and regulating innate immunity.

In osteolytic metastases, the destruction of bone is mediated by osteoclasts [104]. However, the factors responsible for the activation of osteoclasts depend on the tumor. For instance, conditioned medium (CM) from prostate cancer cell lines enhances expression of RANKL mRNA in a mouse osteoblast cell line, and has no effect on expression of OPG mRNA. Co-culture of MC3T3-E1 with prostate cancer cells yields similar results. The number of mature osteoclasts induced by soluble RANKL increases significantly when osteoclast precursor cells are cultured with CM from LNCaP and DU145 prostate cancer cells. CM from LNCaP and DU145 cells also induces maturation from precursor in the absence of soluble RANKL, and this effect is not blocked by OPG. Addition of CM from DU145 cells increases expression of MMP-9 mRNA by osteoclast precursors. These results indicate that prostate cancer mediates osteoclastogenesis through induction of RANKL expression by osteoblasts and through direct action on osteoclast precursors mediated by some factors other than RANKL [105].

Osteosarcoma is the most frequent primary bone tumor. It develops mainly in the young, the median age of diagnosis being 18 years [106]. The fact that two different MMP-inhibitors significantly reduce osteosarcoma cell invasion suggests that MMPs are important factors for the invasion of human osteosarcoma cells [107]. In addition, a disturbance of the MMP/TIMP balance in favor of enhanced proteolytic activity has been suspected in osteosarcoma since osteosarcoma growth is accompanied by bone formation and bone destruction. Overexpression of MMPs in malignant tissue compared to corresponding normal tissue has been demonstrated and confers a poor clinical prognosis in several of these tumor types. In general, the gelatinases (MMP-2 and -9) are the two MMPs most consistently overexpressed in malignant tissues and, thus, are associated with tumor aggressiveness, metastatic potential, and poor prognosis [108]. Thus, a correlation between MMP-9 and invasiveness has been observed in rat osteosarcoma cells [109]. In addition, immunohistochemical analysis on human osteosarcoma biopsies suggests a more evident role for MMP-9 than MMP-2 in tumor progression [110]. Besides, among 55 patients with stage-IIB osteosarcoma around the knee, the only factor strongly associated with disease-free survival is the immunohistochemical status of tumor cells for MMP-9 in the resection specimens [111]. Uchibori *et al.* have also demonstrated that increased expression of MT1-MMP is correlated with poor prognosis in patients with osteosarcoma [112]. Thus, in cases of an overexpression of both MMP-2 and MT1-MMP, there is a tendency for poor prognosis and an increased gelatinase activity is observed. In 36 cases that underwent neoadjuvant chemotherapy, wide resection of the tumors and postoperative adjuvant chemotherapy, increased expression of MT1-MMP resulted in a significant negative prognostic factor for disease-free survival.

VII. MMP AND THERAPEUTIC APPROACHES

Several MMP inhibitors have been identified [113]. Thus, α2-macroglobulin, a general natural inhibitor, is a plasma protein that irreversibly inhibits MMPs. Four TIMPs have been identified and characterized in mammals. Each TIMP inhibits specific MMPs, and the molar ratio of MMP to TIMP correlates significantly with disease outcome and/or severity in several model systems and human diseases. The important role of MMPs in the process of tumor growth and metastasis has led to the development of synthetic inhibitors of these enzymes. Several of these inhibitors have entered clinical trials, and results of these studies have been presented [114, Table 9.1]. The catalytic domains of most MMPs have a high degree of homology and therefore many of the early MMP inhibitors exhibit a broad spectrum inhibition profile. Thus, these inhibitors interfere with numerous MMPs and may have deleterious affects due to the multiplicity of the MMP system. Inhibition of MMP activity has been effective in various animal tumor models, including bone metastasis models [115]. However, results from clinical trials with synthetic MMP inhibitors have been disappointing. MMP inhibitors have been relatively effective in preventing development and progression of early disease, but have had little effect on advanced disease [114]. In clinical trials, MMP inhibitors have been administered to patients with advanced cancer. In contrast, in the mouse models, MMP inhibition is observed at early stages of disease and maintained throughout tumor progression, with size or number of tumors as the endpoint. Of these results, one can predict that MMP inhibition would decrease the rate of tumor progression and that the therapeutic benefit of this decrease would be minimized at late stages of the disease. Other possibilities may be that the inhibitor concentration reached *in vivo* was insufficient to inhibit target enzymes in the tissue or that non-target enzymes were inhibited. Currently, 23 MMPs and 30 ADAMs (a disintegrin and metalloproteases) are known in humans, but their biological functions are not clearly understood [115]. Thus, a better understanding of the regulatory mechanisms that control MMP transcription in cancer cells could provide new ways for therapeutic intervention that are more specific and effective. Besides, to elucidate the *in vivo* roles of proteases in cellular pathways, and thereby identify protease drug targets, it is essential to determine their degradome [114]. The term 'degradomics' has been introduced to partly illustrate the large substrate specificity of MMPs [118,119], as well as to depict our ignorance, in most cases, concerning the target substrate of a given member of that family for a given cancer type and for the different stages of tumor progression. The design of specific inhibitors for these metalloproteinases is an important future challenge. Such inhibitors are useful not only for gaining insight into the biological roles of MMPs but also for the identification of the MMP target and anti-target substrates that are a

TABLE 9.1 Clinical trials with MMPIs

MMPI	Tumor type	Result	References
s-3304	Patients with advanced and refractory solid tumors	Phase I clinical trial, s-3304 inhibits gelatinase activity in tumor biopsies. Four of eight patients with renal cell carcinoma had stable disease.	146
MMI270 (CGS27023A)	Colorectal	Phase I clinical trial, six patients had a partial response and seven had stable disease.	147
BMS-275291 (Neovastat)	Patients with advanced and refractory solid tumors	Phase I clinical trial, well tolerated	148
	Non-small cell lung or hormone refractory prostate cancer with bone metastases	Phase II clinical trial, well tolerated and no dose-limiting arthritis	149, 150
	Non-small cell lung	Phase III clinical trial, does not improve survival in advanced NSCLC.	151
BAY 12-9566 (Tanomastat)	Patients with solid tumors	Phase I clinical trial, no consistent effects on the plasma concentrations of MMP-2 and MMP-9, well tolerated	152–154
	Patients with advanced ovarian cancer	Phase III clinical trial, no evidence of an impact on progression-free survival or overall survival.	155
COL-3 (Metastat)	Patients with refractory metastatic cancer	Phase I clinical trial, disease stabilization in several patients who had a non-epithelial type of malignancy	156–157
	Patients with advanced soft tissue sarcomas	Phase II clinical trial, no objective responses and 33% patients experienced disease progression	158
AG 3340 (Prinomastat)	Advanced non-small cell lung cancer	Phase III clinical trial, no survival benefit	159–160
BB-2516 (Marimastat)	Pancreatic, breast cancer	Phase III clinical trial, no survival benefit	161–162

matter for developing better, and newer, MMP inhibitors for cancer treatment [120]. These new approaches are adaptable to other classes of protease for exploring proteolytic function in complex dynamic biological contexts.

Bisphosphonates (BPs) have been used successfully for many years to reduce the skeletal complications associated with benign and malignant bone diseases that are characterized by enhanced osteoclastic bone resorption. Studies have demonstrated that BPs inhibit the growth, attachment and invasion of cancer cells in culture and promote their apoptosis. These results suggest that BPs are also anti-cancer agents, raising the possibility that BPs could inhibit cancer-cell colonization in visceral organs. However, results from clinical trials are conflicting, and whether BPs possess anti-cancer effects or not remains controversial [121]. One contributory mechanism may be the inhibition of MMP activity, which is necessary for tumor cell invasion of the extracellular matrix. Bisphosphonates have been shown to inhibit the activity of MMPs produced by tumor cell lines, and this seems to be correlated by reduced invasiveness in the Matrigel™ assay [122]. Bisphosphonates (clodronate, alendronate, pamidronate and zoledronate), at therapeutically attainable non-cytotoxic concentrations, inhibited MMP-1, -2, -3, -7, -8, -9, -12, -13, and -14, but not urokinase-type plasminogen activator (uPA), a serine proteinase and a pro-MMP activator [122–124]. Bisphosphonates are broad-spectrum MMP inhibitors and this inhibition involves cation chelation [123]. Besides, clodronate interferes with the prognostic value of serum MMP-2. Clodronate has a negative impact on the outcome among patients with low serum MMP-2 and MMP-9 levels, while no such influence is observed among patients with high MMP-2 and MMP-9 levels. In addition, MMP-9 is differently regulated at mRNA and enzyme protein levels by BPs, which affect ATP-dependent intracellular enzymes (clodronate) or post-translational modification of GTPases (pamidronate) [125]. Interestingly, there are also indications that MMP inhibition may potentiate the effects of conventional chemotherapy [126–128]. Another important characteristic of MMP inhibitors is their potential inhibitory effect on angiogenesis. Thus, zoledronate could exert an anti-angiogenic activity and inhibition of tumor cell bone invasiveness by a transient reduction of VEGF, βFGF and MMP-2 circulating levels after infusion [129,130]. Besides, bisphosphonates have been demonstrated to act on OPG and RANKL production by human osteoblast-like cells. Pamidronate and zoledronate stimulate OPG production by primary human osteoblasts [131], and zoledronate influences soluble RANKL expression in human osteoblast-like cells by activating TNF-α-converting enzyme [132]. These findings show that bisphosphonates, in addition to exerting a direct effect on bone and tumor cells, act on bone resorption through the modulation of the OPG/RANK/RANKL equilibrium.

TIMPs, endogen inhibitors of MMPs, are secreted proteins, but may be found at the cell surface in association with membrane-bound proteins [133]. In addition to MMP-inhibiting activities, TIMPs have other biological functions [134]. Thus, Sobue *et al.* showed that both TIMP-1 and TIMP-2 stimulate the bone-resorbing activity of osteoclasts through tyrosine kinase and MAP kinase pathways, and that synthetic MMP inhibitors do not have this affect [135]. In addition, TIMP-1 and TIMP-2 have erythroid-potentiating activity [136,137] and cell growth-promoting activities [138,139]. For example, high levels of TIMP-1 mRNA as well as TIMP-1 protein have been demonstrated in several types of cancer and this has been associated with poor prognoses of the patients [133,140]. In the same way, in osteosarcoma, high levels of plasma TIMP-1, but not tumor tissue TIMP-1, have been found in patients with advanced disease [110]. Paradoxically, overexpression of TIMP-1, TIMP-2, and TIMP-3 reduces tumor growth [141]. This paradox points to TIMPs as multifunctional proteins, which, in addition to the MMP-inhibitory effect, has distinct tumor-promoting functions. Besides, TIMP-3 has proapoptotic activity whereas TIMP-1 and TIMP-2 have antiapoptotic activity. TIMPs promote the proliferation of some cell types, and their antiapoptotic affects may favor tumor expansion during the onset and early growth of the primary tumor [142–144]. In addition, the expression of MT1-MMP by tumor cells has been shown to mediate internalization and intracellular degradation of TIMP-2, thereby altering the balance between active MMPs and TIMPs [145]. TIMPs do contain domains with specific functions that need to be characterized with the aim of developing engineered TIMPs as therapeutic tools in cancer.

Acknowledgement

Thanks to Laurence Duplomb, INSERM, INSERM, U957, Nantes, Nantes Atlantique Universités, Laboratoire de Physiopathologie de la Résorption Osseuse et Thérapie des Tumeurs Osseuses Primitives, EA3822, for proofreading and helpful discussions.

References

1. A.V. Rousselle & D. Heymann, Osteoclastic acidification pathways during bone resorption, Bone 30 (2002) 533–540.
2. T. Théoleyre, Y. Wittrant & S. Kwan Tat, et al., The molecular triad OPG/RANK/RANKL: involvement in the orchestration of pathophysiological bone remodeling, Cyt Growth Fact Rev 15 (2004) 457–475.
3. D. Goltzman, Osteolysis and cancer, J Clin Invest 107 (2001) 1219–1220.
4. G.D. Roodman, Mechanisms of bone metastasis, N Engl J Med 350 (2004) 1655–1664.
5. M. Baud'huin, L. Duplomb & C. Ruiz Velasco, et al., Key roles of the OPG-RANK-RANKL system in bone oncology, Expert Rev Anticancer Ther 7 (2007) 221–232.
6. F.H. Drake, R.A. Dodds & I.E. James, et al., Cathepsin K, but not cathepsins B, L, or S, is abundantly expressed in human osteoclasts, J Biol Chem 271 (1996) 12511–12516.

7. J. Rantakokko, H.T. Aro & M. Savontaus, et al., Mouse cathepsin K: cDNA cloning and predominant expression of the gene in osteoclasts, and in some hypertrophying chondrocytes during mouse development, FEBS Lett 393 (1996) 307–313.

8. K. Tezuka, Y. Tezuka & A. Maejima, et al., Molecular cloning of a possible cysteine proteinase predominantly expressed in osteoclasts, J Biol Chem 269 (1994) 1106–1109.

9. T. Kamaya, Y. Kobayashi & K. Kanaoka, et al., Fluorescence microscopic demonstration of cathepsin K activity as the major lysosomal cysteine proteinase in osteoclasts, J Biochem 123 (1998) 752–759.

10. A. Littlewood-Evans, T. Kokubo & O. Ishibashi, et al., Localization of cathepsin K in human osteoclasts by *in situ* hybridization and immunohistochemistry, Bone 20 (1997) 81–86.

11. J. Mandelin, M. Hukkanen & T.F. Li, et al., Human osteoblasts produce cathepsin K, Bone 38 (2006) 769–777.

12. P. Garnero, O. Borel & I. Byrjalsen, et al., The collagenolytic activity of cathepsin K is unique among mammalian proteinases, J Biol Chem 273 (1998) 32347–32352.

13. V. Everts, W. Beertsen & R. Schroder, Effects of the proteinase inhibitors leupeptin and E–64 on osteoclastic bone resorption, Calcif Tissue Int 43 (1988) 172–178.

14. B.D. Gelb, G.P. Shi & H.A. Chapman, et al., Pycnodysostosis, a lysosomal disease caused by cathepsin K deficiency, Science 273 (1996) 1236–1238.

15. W.S. Hou, D. Bromme & Y. Zhao, et al., Characterization of novel cathepsin K mutations in the pro and mature polypeptide regions causing pycnodysostosis, J Clin Invest 103 (1999) 731–738.

16. V. Everts, W.S. Hou & X. Rialland, et al., Cathepsin K deficiency in pycnodysostosis results in accumulation of non-digested phagocytosed collagen in fibroblasts, Calcif Tissue Int 73 (2003) 380–386.

17. P. Saftig, E. Hunziker & O. Wehmeyer, et al., Impaired osteoclastic bone resorption leads to osteopetrosis in cathepsin-K-deficient mice, Proc Natl Acad Sci USA 95 (1998) 13453–13458.

18. M. Gowen, F. Lazner & R. Dodds, et al., Cathepsin K knockout mice develop osteopetrosis due to a deficit in matrix degradation but not demineralization, J Bone Miner Res 14 (1999) 1654–1663.

19. R. Kiviranta, J. Morko & H. Uusitalo, et al., Accelerated turnover of metaphyseal trabecular bone in mice overexpressing cathepsin K, J Bone Miner Res 16 (2001) 1444–1452.

20. R.A. Dodds, I.E. James & D. Rieman, et al., Human osteoclast cathepsin K is processed intracellularly prior to attachment and bone resorption, J Bone Miner Res 16 (2001) 478–486.

21. Z. Li, W.S. Hou & C.R. Escalante-Torres, et al., Collagenase activity of cathepsin K depends on complex formation with chondroitin sulfate, J Biol Chem 277 (2002) 28669–28676.

22. V. Shalhoub, J. Faust & W.J. Boyle, et al., Osteoprotegerin and osteoprotegerin ligand effects on osteoclast formation from human peripheral blood mononuclear cell precursors, J Cell Biochem 72 (1999) 251–261.

23. B.R. Troen, The regulation of cathepsin K gene expression, Ann NY Acad Sci 1068 (2006) 165–172.

24. M. Matsumoto, M. Kogawa & S. Wada, et al., Essential role of p38 mitogen-activated protein kinase in cathepsin K gene expression during osteoclastogenesis through association of NFATc1 and PU.1, J Biol Chem 279 (2004) 45969–45979.

25. L.L. Zhu, S. Zaidi & B.S. Moong, et al., RANK-L induces the expression of NFATc1, but not of NFkappaB subunits during osteoclast formation, Biochem Biophys Res Commun 326 (2005) 131–135.

26. K.C. Mansky, U. Sankar & J. Han, et al., Microphthalmia transcription factor is a target of the p38 MAPK pathway in response to receptor activator of NF-kappa B ligand signaling, J Biol Chem 277 (2002) 11077–11083.

27. G. Motyckova, K.N. Weilbaecher & M. Horstmann, et al., Linking osteopetrosis and pycnodysostosis: regulation of cathepsin K expression by the microphthalmia transcription factor family, Proc Natl Acad Sci USA 98 (2001) 5798–5803.

28. D. Keppler, Towards novel anti-cancer strategies based on cystatin function, Cancer Lett 235 (2006) 159.

29. J. Guay, J.P. Falgueyret & A. Ducret, et al., Potency and selectivity of inhibition of cathepsin K, L and S by their respective propeptides, Eur J Biochem 267 (2000) 6311–6318.

30. T. Laitala-Leinonen, R. Rinne & P. Saukko, et al., Cystatin B as an intracellular modulator of bone resorption, Matrix Biol 25 (2006) 149–157.

31. M. Brage, A. Lie & M. Ransjö, et al., Osteoclastogenesis is decreased by cysteine proteinase inhibitors, Bone 34 (2004) 412–420.

32. D.S. Yamashita & R.A. Dodds, Cathepsin K and the design of inhibitors of cathepsin K, Curr Pharm Des 6 (2000) 1–24.

33. D.G. Barrett, D.N. Deaton & A.M. Hassell, et al., Acyclic cyanamide-based inhibitors of cathepsin K, Bioorg Med Chem Lett 15 (2005) 3039–3043.

34. D.G. Barrett, J.G. Catalano & D.N. Deaton, et al., Orally bioavailable small molecule ketoamide-based inhibitors of cathepsin K, Bioorg Med Chem Lett 14 (2004) 2543–2546.

35. J.G. Catalano, D.N. Deaton & E.S. Furfine, et al., Exploration of the P1 SAR of aldehyde cathepsin K inhibitors, Bioorg Med Chem Lett 14 (2004) 275–278.

36. J.G. Catalano, D.N. Deaton & S.T. Long, et al., Design of small molecule ketoamide-based inhibitors of cathepsin K, Bioorg Med Chem Lett 14 (2004) 719–722.

37. F. Lecaille, J. Kaleta & D. Brömme, Human and parasitic papain-like cysteine proteases: their role in physiology and pathology and recent developments in inhibitor design, Chem Rev 102 (2002) 4459–4488.

38. Y. Yasuda, J. Kaleta & D. Brömme, The role of cathepsins in osteoporosis and arthritis: rationale for the design of new therapeutics, Adv Drug Deliv Rev 57 (2005) 973–993.

39. C. Le Gall, A. Bellahcène & E. Bonnelye, et al., A cathepsin K inhibitor reduces breast cancer induced osteolysis and skeletal tumor burden, Cancer Res 67 (2007) 9894–9902.

40. K. Husmann, R. Muff & M.E. Bolander, et al., Cathepsins and osteosarcoma: Expression analysis identifies cathepsin K as an indicator of metastasis, Mol Carcinog 47 (2008) 66–73.

41. K. Fuller, K.M. Lawrence & J.L. Ross, et al., Cathepsin K inhibitors prevent matrix-derived growth factor degradation by human osteoclasts, Bone 42 (2008) 200–211.

42. G.B. Stroup, M.W. Lark & D.F. Veber, et al., Potent and selective inhibition of human cathepsin K leads to inhibition of bone resorption *in vivo* in a nonhuman primate, J Bone Miner Res 16 (2001) 1739–1746.

43. D. Wang, S.C. Miller & P. Kopeckova, et al., Bone-targeting macromolecular therapeutics, Adv Drug Deliv Rev 57 (2005) 1049–1076.

44. R. Visse & H. Nagase, Matrix metalloproteinases and tissue inhibitors of metalloproteinases: structure, function, and biochemistry, Circ Res 92 (2003) 827–839.

45. L.M. Coussens, B. Fingleton & L.M. Matrisian, Matrix metalloproteinase inhibitors and cancer: trials and tribulations, Science 295 (2002) 2387–2392.

46. H. Nagase & J.F. Woessner Jr., Matrix metalloproteinases, J Biol Chem 274 (1999) 21491–21494.

47. G. Velasco, A.M. Pendas & A. Fueyo, et al., Cloning and characterization of human MMP-23, a new matrix metalloproteinase predominantly expressed in reproductive tissues and lacking conserved domains in other family members, J Biol Chem 274 (1999) 4570–4576.

48. C.J. Malemud, Matrix metalloproteinases (MMPs) in health and disease: an overview, Front Biosci 11 (2006) 1696–1701.

49. S. Kojima, Y. Itoh & S. Matsumoto, et al., Membrane-type 6 matrix metalloproteinase (MT6-MMP, MMP-25) is the second glycosyl-phosphatidyl inositol (GPI)-anchored MMP, FEBS Lett 480 (2000) 142–146.

50. C.N. Rao, S. Mohanam & A. Puppala, et al., Regulation of ProMMP-1 and ProMMP-3 activation by tissue factor pathway inhibitor-2/matrix-associated serine protease inhibitor, Biochem Biophys Res Commun 255 (1999) 94–98.

51. G.E. Davis, K.A. Pintar Allen & R. Salazar, et al., Matrix metalloproteinase-1 and -9 activation by plasmin regulates a novel endothelial cell-mediated mechanism of collagen gel contraction and capillary tube regression in three-dimensional collagen matrices, J Cell Sci 114 (2001) 917–930.

52. H. Nagase, Stromelysins 1 and 2, in: W.C. Parks & R.P. Mecham (Eds.) Matrix Metalloproteinases, Academic Press, San Diego, 1998, pp. 43–84.

53. V. Knauper, H. Will & C. Lopez-Otin, et al., Cellular mechanisms for human procollagenase-3 (MMP-13) activation. Evidence that MT1-MMP (MMP-14) and gelatinase a (MMP-2) are able to generate active enzyme, J Biol Chem 271 (1996) 17124–17131.

54. A.Y. Strongin, I. Collier & G. Bannikov, et al., Mechanism of cell surface activation of 72-kDa type IV collagenase. Isolation of the activated form of the membrane metalloprotease, J Biol Chem 270 (1995) 5331–5338.

55. R. Fridman, M. Toth & D. Pena, et al., Activation of progelatinase B (MMP-9) by gelatinase A (MMP-2), Cancer Res 55 (1995) 2548–2555.

56. R. Dreier, S. Grassel & S. Fuchs, et al., Pro-MMP-9 is a specific macrophage product and is activated by osteoarthritic chondrocytes via MMP-3 or a MT1-MMP/MMP-13 cascade, Exp Cell Res 297 (2004) 303–312.

57. Y.P. Han, C. Yan & L. Zhou, et al., A matrix metalloproteinase-9 activation cascade by hepatic stellate cells in transdifferentiation in the three-dimensional extracellular matrix, J Biol Chem 282 (2007) 12928–12939.

58. H. Nagase, Cell surface activation of progelatinase A (proMMP-2) and cell migration, Cell Res 8 (1998) 179–186.

59. T. Shiomi, I. Inoki & F. Kataoka, et al., Pericellular activation of proMMP-7 (promatrilysin-1) through interaction with CD151, Lab Invest 85 (2005) 1489–1506.

60. F.F. Mohammed, D.S. Smookler & R. Khokha, Metalloproteinases, inflammation, and rheumatoid arthritis, Ann Rheum Dis 62 (suppl 2) (2003) ii43–ii47.

61. J.A. Dumin, S.K. Dickeson & T.P. Stricker, et al., Procollagenase-1 (matrix metalloproteinase-1) binds the alpha(2)beta(1) integrin upon release from keratinocytes migrating on type I collagen, J Biol Chem 276 (2001) 29368–29374.

62. T.P. Stricker, J.A. Dumin & S.K. Dickeson, et al., Structural analysis of the alpha(2) integrin I domain/procollagenase-1 (matrix metalloproteinase-1) interaction, J Biol Chem 276 (2001) 29375–29381.

63. P.C. Brooks, S. Stromblad & L.C. Sanders, et al., Localization of matrix metalloproteinase MMP-2 to the surface of invasive cells by interaction with integrin alpha v beta 3, Cell 85 (1996) 683–693.

64. Q. Yu & I. Stamenkovic, Cell surface-localized matrix metalloproteinase-9 proteolytically activates TGF-beta and promotes tumor invasion and angiogenesis, Genes Dev 14 (2000) 163–176.

65. C.A. Owen, Z. Hu & C. Lopez-Otin, et al., Membrane-bound matrix metalloproteinase-8 on activated polymorphonuclear cells is a potent, tissue inhibitor of metalloproteinase-resistant collagenase and serpinase, J Immunol 172 (2004) 7791–7803.

66. V. Everts, J.M. Delaisse & W. Korper, et al., The bone lining cell: its role in cleaning Howship's lacunae and initiating bone formation, J Bone Miner Res 17 (2002) 77–90.

67. V. Everts, W. Korper & K.A. Hoeben, et al., Osteoclastic bone degradation and the role of different cysteine proteinases and matrix metalloproteinases: differences between calvaria and long bone, J Bone Miner Res 21 (2006) 1399–1408.

68. J.M. Delaisse, T.L. Andersen & M.T. Engsig, et al., Matrix metalloproteinases (MMP) and cathepsin K contribute differently to osteoclastic activities, Microsc Res Tech 61 (2003) 504–513.

69. L. Blavier & J.M. Delaisse, Matrix metalloproteinases are obligatory for the migration of preosteoclasts to the developing marrow cavity of primitive long bones, J Cell Sci 108 (1995) 3649–3659.

70. Y. Itoh, MT1-MMP: a key regulator of cell migration in tissue, IUBMB Life 58 (2006) 589–596.

71. K. Irie, E. Tsuruga & Y. Sakakura, et al., Immunohistochemical localization of membrane type 1-matrix metalloproteinase (MT1-MMP) in osteoclasts *in vivo*, Tissue Cell 33 (2001) 478–482.

72. O. Ishibashi, S. Niwa & K. Kadoyama, et al., MMP-9 antisense oligodeoxynucleotide exerts an inhibitory effect on osteoclastic bone resorption by suppressing cell migration, Life Sci 79 (2006) 1657–1660.

73. H.P. Gerber, T.H. Vu & A.M. Ryan, et al., VEGF couples hypertrophic cartilage remodeling, ossification and angiogenesis during endochondral bone formation, Nat Med 5 (1999) 623–628.

74. E.R. Lee, G. Murphy & M. El-Alfy, et al., Active gelatinase B is identified by histozymography in the cartilage resorption sites of developing long bones, Dev Dyn 215 (1999) 190–205.

75. T.H. Vu, J.M. Shipley & G. Bergers, et al., MMP-9/gelatinase B is a key regulator of growth plate angiogenesis and apoptosis of hypertrophic chondrocytes, Cell 93 (1998) 411–422.

76. J.E. Rundhaug, Matrix metalloproteinases and angiogenesis, J Cell Mol Med 9 (2005) 267–285.

77. K. Holmbeck, P. Bianco & J. Caterina, et al., MT1-MMP-deficient mice develop dwarfism, osteopenia, arthritis, and connective tissue disease due to inadequate collagen turnover, Cell 99 (1999) 81–92.

78. X. Liu, H. Wu & M. Byrne, et al., A targeted mutation at the known collagenase cleavage site in mouse type I collagen impairs tissue remodeling, J Cell Biol 130 (1995) 227–237.

79. S. Varghese, Matrix metalloproteinases and their inhibitors in bone: an overview of regulation and functions, Front Biosci 11 (2006) 2949–2966.

80. G.A. McQuibban, J.H. Gong & J.P. Wong, et al., Matrix metalloproteinase processing of monocyte chemoattractant proteins generates CC chemokine receptor antagonists with anti-inflammatory properties *in vivo*, Blood 100 (2002) 1160–1167.

81. P.E. Van den Steen, P. Proost & A. Wuyts, et al., Neutrophil gelatinase B potentiates interleukin–8 tenfold by aminoterminal processing, whereas it degrades CTAP-III, PF-4, and GRO-alpha and leaves RANTES and MCP-2 intact, Blood 96 (2000) 2673–2681.

82. K.J. Greenlee, Z. Werb & F. Kheradmand, Matrix metalloproteinases in lung: multiple, multifarious, and multifaceted, Physiol Rev 87 (2007) 69–98.

83. U. Schonbeck, F. Mach & P. Libby, Generation of biologically active IL-1 beta by matrix metalloproteinases: a novel caspase-1-independent pathway of IL-1 beta processing, J Immunol 161 (1998) 3340–3346.

84. K. Fujisaki, N. Tanabe & N. Suzuki, et al., Receptor activator of NF-kappaB ligand induces the expression of carbonic anhydrase II, cathepsin K, and matrix metalloproteinase-9 in osteoclast precursor RAW264.7 cells, Life Sci 80 (2007) 1311–1318.

85. C.C. Lynch, A. Hikosaka & H.B. Acuff, et al., MMP-7 promotes prostate cancer-induced osteolysis via the solubilization of RANKL, Cancer Cell 7 (2005) 485–496.

86. A. Hikita, I. Yana & H. Wakeyama, et al., Negative regulation of osteoclastogenesis by ectodomain shedding of receptor activator of NF-kappaB ligand, J Biol Chem 281 (2006) 36846–36855.

87. L. Lum, B.R. Wong & R. Josien, et al., Evidence for a role of a tumor necrosis factor-alpha (TNF-alpha)-converting enzyme-like protease in shedding of TRANCE, a TNF family member involved in osteoclastogenesis and dendritic cell survival, J Biol Chem 274 (1999) 13613–13618.

88. J. Schlondorff, L. Lum & C.P. Blobel, Biochemical and pharmacological criteria define two shedding activities for TRANCE/OPGL that are distinct from the tumor necrosis factor alpha convertase, J Biol Chem 276 (2001) 14665–14674.

89. Y. Wittrant, S. Couillaud & S. Théoleyre, et al., Osteoprotegerin differentially regulates protease expression in osteoclast cultures, Biochem Biophys Res Commun 293 (2002) 38–44.

90. Y. Wittrant, S. Théoleyre & S. Couillaud, et al., Regulation of osteoclast protease expression by RANKL, Biochem Biophys Res Commun 310 (2003) 774–778.

91. Y. Wittrant, S. Théoleyre & S. Couillaud, et al., Relevance of an *in vitro* osteoclastogenesis system to study receptor activator of NF-kB ligand and osteoprotegerin biological activities, Exp Cell Res 293 (2004) 292–301.

92. S. Théoleyre, Y. Wittrant & S. Couillaud, et al., Cellular activity and signaling induced by osteoprotegerin in osteoclasts: involvement of receptor activator of nuclear factor kappaB ligand and MAPK, Biochim Biophys Acta 1644 (2004) 1–7.

93. T. Standal, C. Seidel & O. Hjertner, et al., Osteoprotegerin is bound, internalized, and degraded by multiple myeloma cells, Blood 100 (2002) 3002–3007.

94. S. Théoleyre, S. Kwan Tat & P. Vusio, et al., Characterization of osteoprotegerin binding to glycosaminoglycans by surface plasmon resonance: role in the interactions with receptor activator of nuclear factor kappaB ligand (RANKL) and RANK, Biochem Biophys Res Commun 347 (2006) 460–467.

95. S. Kwan Tat, M. Padrines & S. Théoleyre, et al., OPG/membranous-RANKL complex is internalized via the clathrin pathway before a lysosomal and a proteasomal degradation, Bone 39 (2006) 706–715.

96. K. Sundaram, R. Nishimura & J. Senn, et al., RANK ligand signaling modulates the matrix metalloproteinase-9 gene expression during osteoclast differentiation, Exp Cell Res 313 (2007) 168–178.

97. F. Ikeda, R. Nishimura & T. Matsubara, et al., Critical roles of c-Jun signaling in regulation of NFAT family and RANKL-regulated osteoclast differentiation, J Clin Invest 114 (2004) 475–484.

98. K. Matsuo, D.L. Galson & C. Zhao, et al., Nuclear factor of activated T-cells (NFAT) rescues osteoclastogenesis in precursors lacking c-Fos, J Biol Chem 279 (2004) 26475–26480.

99. T.N. Crotti, M. Flannery & N.C. Walsh, et al., NFATc1 regulation of the human beta3 integrin promoter in osteoclast differentiation, Gene 372 (2006) 92–102.

100. M. Asagiri, K. Sato & T. Usami, et al., Autoamplification of NFATc1 expression determines its essential role in bone homeostasis, J Exp Med 202 (2005) 1261–1269.

101. M. Egeblad & Z. Werb, New functions for the matrix metalloproteinases in cancer progression, Nature Rev Cancer 2 (2002) 161–174.

102. M. Polette, N. Gilbert & I. Stas, et al., Gelatinase A expression and localization in human breast cancers. An *in situ* hybridization study and immunohistochemical detection using confocal microscopy, Virchows Arch 424 (1994) 641–645.

103. R. Khokha, P. Waterhouse & S. Yagel, et al., Antisense RNA-induced reduction in murine TIMP levels confers oncogenicity on Swiss 3T3 cells, Science 244 (1989) 947–950.

104. K.G. Halvorson, M.A. Sevcik & J.R. Ghilardi, et al., Similarities and differences in tumor growth, skeletal

remodeling and pain in an osteolytic and osteoblastic model of bone cancer, Clin J Pain 22 (2006) 587–600.

105. H. Inoue, K. Nishimura & D. Oka, et al., Prostate cancer mediates osteoclastogenesis through two different pathways, Cancer Lett 223 (2005) 121–128.

106. R.C. Thompson, E.Y. Cheng & D.R. Clohisy, et al., Results of treatment for metastatic osteosarcoma with neoadjuvant chemotherapy and surgery, Clin Orthop Realt Res 397 (2002) 240–247.

107. A. Kido, M. Tsutsumi & K. Iki, et al., Inhibition of spontaneous rat osteosarcoma lung metastasis by 3S-[4-(N-hydroxyamino)-2R-isobutylsuccinyl]amino-1-methoxy-3,4-dihydroc arbostyril, a novel matrix metalloproteinase inhibitor, Jpn J Cancer Res 90 (1999) 333–341.

108. K. Bjornland, K. Flatmark & S. Pettersen, et al., Matrix metalloproteinases participate in osteosarcoma invasion, J Surg Res 127 (2005) 151–156.

109. A. Kawashima, I. Nakanishi & H. Tsuchiya, et al., Expression of matrix metalloproteinase 9 (92-kDa gelatinase/type IV collagenase) induced by tumour necrosis factor alpha correlates with metastatic ability in a human osteosarcoma cell line, Virchows Arch 424 (1994) 547–552.

110. C. Ferrari, S. Benassi & F. Ponticelli, et al., Role of MMP-9 and its tissue inhibitor TIMP-1 in human osteosarcoma: findings in 42 patients followed for 1–16 years, Acta Orthop Scand 75 (2004) 487–491.

111. A.F. Foukas, N.S. Deshmukh & R.J. Grimer, et al., Stage-IIB osteosarcomas around the knee. A study of MMP-9 in surviving tumour cells, J Bone Joint Surg Br 84 (2002) 706–711.

112. M. Uchibori, Y. Nishida & T. Nagasaka, et al., Increased expression of membrane-type matrix metalloproteinase-1 is correlated with poor prognosis in patients with osteosarcoma, Int J Oncol 28 (2006) 33–42.

113. R. Hoekstra, F.A. Eskens & J. Verweij, Matrix metalloproteinase inhibitors: current developments and future perspectives, Oncologist 6 (2001) 415–427.

114. C.M. Overall & O. Kleifeld, Tumour microenvironment—opinion: Validating matrix metalloproteinases as drug targets and anti-targets for cancer therapy, Nature Rev Cancer 6 (2006) 227–239.

115. G.W. Sledge, M. Qulali & R. Goulet, et al., Effect of matrix metalloproteinase inhibitor batimastat on breast cancer regrowth and metastasis in athymic mice, J Natl Cancer Inst 87 (1995) 1546–1550.

116. G. Bergers, K. Javaherian & K.M. Lo, et al., Effects of angiogenesis inhibitors on multistage carcinogenesis in mice, Science 284 (1999) 808–812.

117. C.R. Flannery, MMPs and ADAMTSs: functional studies, Front Biosci 11 (2006) 544–569.

118. C.M. Overall & R.A. Dean, Degradomics: systems biology of the protease web. Pleiotropic roles of MMPs in cancer, Cancer Metastasis Rev 25 (2006) 69–75.

119. O. Schilling & C.M. Overall, Proteome-derived, database-searchable peptide libraries for identifying protease cleavage sites, Nat Biotechnol 26 (2008) 685–694.

120. C.M. Overall & O. Kleifeld, Towards third generation matrix metalloproteinase inhibitors for cancer therapy, Br J Cancer 94 (2006) 941–946.

121. F. Lamoureux, V. Trichet & C. Chipoy, et al., Recent advances in the management of osteosarcoma and forthcoming therapeutic strategies, Expert Rev Anticancer Ther 7 (2007) 169–181.

122. O. Teronen, P. Heikkila & Y.T. Konttinen, et al., MMP inhibition and down-regulation by bisphosphonates, Ann NY Acad Sci 878 (1999) 453–465.

123. P. Heikkila, O. Teronen & M. Moilanen, et al., Bisphosphonates inhibit stromelysin-1 (MMP-3), matrix metalloelastase (MMP-12), collagenase-3 (MMP-13) and enamelysin (MMP-20), but not urokinase-type plasminogen activator, and diminish invasion and migration of human malignant and endothelial cell lines, Anticancer Drugs 13 (2002) 245–254.

124. P. Heikkila, O. Teronen & M.Y. Hirn, et al., Inhibition of matrix metalloproteinase-14 in osteosarcoma cells by clodronate, J Surg Res 111 (2003) 45–52.

125. H. Valleala, R. Hanemaaijer & J. Mandelin, et al., Regulation of MMP-9 (gelatinase B) in activated human monocyte/macrophages by two different types of bisphosphonates, Life Sci 73 (2003) 2413–2420.

126. R. Montague, C.A. Hart & N.J. George, et al., Differential inhibition of invasion and proliferation by bisphosphonates: anti-metastatic potential of Zoledronic acid in prostate cancer, Eur Urol 46 (2004) 389–401.

127. J.K. Woodward, H.L. Neville-Webbe & R.E. Coleman, et al., Combined effects of zoledronic acid and doxorubicin on breast cancer cell invasion *in vitro*, Anticancer Drugs 16 (2005) 845–854.

128. D. Heymann, B. Ory & F. Blanchard, et al., Enhanced tumor regression and tissue repair when zoledronic acid is combined with ifosfamide in rat osteosarcoma, Bone 37 (2005) 74–86.

129. G. Ferretti, A. Fabi & P. Carlini, et al., Zoledronic-acid-induced circulating level modifications of angiogenic factors, metalloproteinases and proinflammatory cytokines in metastatic breast cancer patients, Oncology 69 (2005) 35–43.

130. G. Leto, G. Badalamenti & C. Arcara, et al., Effects of zoledronic acid on proteinase plasma levels in patients with bone metastases, Anticancer Res 26 (2006) 23–26.

131. V. Viereck, G. Emons & V. Lauck, et al., Bisphosphonates pamidronate and zoledronic acid stimulate osteoprotegerin production by primary human osteoblasts, Biochem Biophys Res Commun 291 (2002) 680–686.

132. B. Pan, A.N. Farrugia & L.B. To, et al., The nitrogen-containing bisphosphonate, zoledronic acid, influences RANKL expression in human osteoblast-like cells by activating TNF-alpha converting enzyme (TACE), J Bone Miner Res 19 (2004) 147–154.

133. W. Hornebeck, E. Lambert & E. Petitfrere, et al., Beneficial and detrimental influences of tissue inhibitor of metalloproteinase-1 (TIMP-1) in tumor progression, Biochimie 87 (2005) 377–383.

134. Y. Jiang, I.D. Goldberg & Y.E. Shi, Complex roles of tissue inhibitors of metalloproteinases in cancer, Oncogene 21 (2002) 2245–2252.

135. T. Sobue, Y. Hakeda & Y. Kobayashi, et al., Tissue inhibitor of metalloproteinases 1 and 2 directly stimulate the bone-resorbing activity of isolated mature osteoclasts, J Bone Miner Res 16 (2001) 2205–2214.

136. L. Chesler, D.W. Golde & N. Bersch, et al., Metalloproteinase inhibition and erythroid potentiation are independent activities of tissue inhibitor of metalloproteinases-1, Blood 86 (1995) 4506–4515.

137. W.G. Stetler-Stevenson, N. Bersch & D.W. Golde, Tissue inhibitor of metalloproteinase-2 (TIMP-2) has erythroid-potentiating activity, FEBS Lett 296 (1992) 231–234.

138. T. Hayakawa, K. Yamashita & K. Tanzawa, et al., Growth-promoting activity of tissue inhibitor of metalloproteinases-1 (TIMP-1) for a wide range of cells. A possible new growth factor in serum, FEBS Lett 298 (1992) 29–32.

139. J.A. Nemeth, A. Rafe & M. Steiner, et al., TIMP-2 growth-stimulatory activity: a concentration- and cell type-specific response in the presence of insulin, Exp Cell Res 224 (1996) 110–115.

140. S.O. Wurtz, A.S. Schrohl & N.M. Sorensen, et al., Tissue inhibitor of metalloproteinases-1 in breast cancer, Endocr Relat Cancer 12 (2005) 215–227.

141. P. Henriet, L. Blavier & Y.A. Declerck, Tissue inhibitors of metalloproteinases (TIMP) in invasion and proliferation, APMIS 107 (1999) 111–119.

142. G. Li, R. Fridman & H.R. Kim, Tissue inhibitor of metalloproteinase-1 inhibits apoptosis of human breast epithelial cells, Cancer Res 59 (1999) 6267–6275.

143. Y. Jiang, M. Wang & M.Y. Celiker, et al., Stimulation of mammary tumorigenesis by systemic tissue inhibitor of matrix metalloproteinase 4 gene delivery, Cancer Res 61 (2001) 2365–2370.

144. M.L. Davidsen, S.O. Wurtz & M.U. Romer, et al., TIMP-1 gene deficiency increases tumour cell sensitivity to chemotherapy-induced apoptosis, Br J Cancer 95 (2006) 1114–1120.

145. A. Noel, C. Maillard & N. Rocks, et al., Membrane associated proteases and their inhibitors in tumour angiogenesis, J Clin Pathol 57 (2004) 577–584.

146. A.A. Chiappori, S.G. Eckhardt & R. Bukowski, et al., A phase I pharmacokinetic and pharmacodynamic study of s-3304, a novel matrix metalloproteinase inhibitor, in patients with advanced and refractory solid tumors, Clin Cancer Res 13 (2007) 2091–2099.

147. M. Eatock, J. Cassidy & J. Johnson, et al., A dose-finding and pharmacokinetic study of the matrix metalloproteinase inhibitor MMI270 (previously termed CGS27023A) with 5-FU and folinic acid, Cancer Chemother Pharmacol 55 (2005) 39–46.

148. N.A. Rizvi, J.S. Humphrey & E.A. Ness, et al., A phase I study of oral BMS-275291, a novel nonhydroxamate sheddase-sparing matrix metalloproteinase inhibitor, in patients with advanced or metastatic cancer, Clin Cancer Res 10 (2004) 1963–1970.

149. J.Y. Douillard, C. Peschel & F. Shepherd, et al., Randomized phase II feasibility study of combining the matrix metalloproteinase inhibitor BMS-275291 with paclitaxel plus carboplatin in advanced non-small cell lung cancer, Lung Cancer 46 (2004) 361–368.

150. P.N. Lara Jr., W.M. Stadler & J. Longmate, et al., A randomized phase II trial of the matrix metalloproteinase inhibitor BMS-275291 in hormone-refractory prostate cancer patients with bone metastases, Clin Cancer Res 12 (2006) 1556–1563.

151. N.B. Leighl, L. Paz-Ares & J.Y. Douillard, et al., Randomized phase III study of matrix metalloproteinase inhibitor BMS-275291 in combination with paclitaxel and carboplatin in advanced non-small-cell lung cancer: National Cancer Institute of Canada-Clinical Trials Group Study BR.18, J Clin Oncol 23 (2005) 2831–2839.

152. E.K. Rowinsky, R. Humphrey & L.A. Hammond, et al., Phase I and pharmacologic study of the specific matrix metalloproteinase inhibitor BAY 12-9566 on a protracted oral daily dosing schedule in patients with solid malignancies, J Clin Oncol 18 (2000) 178–186.

153. C. Erlichman, A.A. Adjei & S.R. Alberts, et al., Phase I study of the matrix metalloproteinase inhibitor, BAY 12-9566, Ann Oncol 12 (2001) 389–395.

154. E.I. Heath, S. O'Reilly & R. Humphrey, et al., Phase I trial of the matrix metalloproteinase inhibitor BAY12-9566 in patients with advanced solid tumors, Cancer Chemother Pharmacol 48 (2001) 269–274.

155. H. Hirte, I.B. Vergote & J.R. Jeffrey, et al., A phase III randomized trial of BAY 12-9566 (tanomastat) as maintenance therapy in patients with advanced ovarian cancer responsive to primary surgery and paclitaxel/platinum containing chemotherapy: a National Cancer Institute of Canada Clinical Trials Group Study, Gynecol Oncol 102 (2006) 300–308.

156. M.A. Rudek, W.D. Figg, V. Dyer, W. Dahut, M.L. Turner, S.M. Steinberg, D.J. Liewehr, D.R. Kohler, J.M. Pluda & E. Reed, Phase I clinical trial of oral COL-3, a matrix metalloproteinase inhibitor, in patients with refractory metastatic cancer, J Clin Oncol 19 (2001) 584–592.

157. S. Syed, C. Takimoto & M. Hidalgo, et al., A phase I and pharmacokinetic study of CoL-3 (Metastat), an oral tetracycline derivative with potent matrix metalloproteinase and antitumor properties, Clin Cancer Res 10 (2004) 6512–6521.

158. Q.S. Chu, B. Forouzesh & S. Syed, et al., A phase II and pharmacological study of the matrix metalloproteinase inhibitor (MMPI) COL-3 in patients with advanced soft tissue sarcomas, Invest New Drugs 25 (2007) 359–367.

159. M. Smylie, R. Mercier & D. Aboulafia, et al., Phase III study of the matrix metalloprotease inhibitor Prinomastat in patients having advanced non-small cell lung cancer, Proc Am Soc Clin Oncol 20 (2001) 307.

160. D. Bissett, K.J. O'Byrne & J. von Pawel, et al., Phase III study of matrix metalloproteinase inhibitor prinomastat in non-small-cell lung cancer, J Clin Oncol 23 (2005) 842–849.

161. S.R. Bramhall, A. Rosemurgy & P.D. Brown, et al., Marimastat as first-line therapy for patients with unresectable pancreatic cancer: a randomized trial, J Clin Oncol 19 (2001) 3447–3455.

162. J.A. Sparano, P. Bernardo & P. Stephenson, et al., Randomized phase III trial of marimastat versus placebo in patients with metastatic breast cancer who have responding or stable disease after first-line chemotherapy: Eastern Cooperative Oncology Group trial E2196, J Clin Oncol 22 (2004) 4683–4690.

Section III. Bone Markers of Cancer (Genes and Proteins)

CHAPTER 10

Bone Remodeling Markers and Bone Cancer

MARKUS J. SEIBEL[1]

[1]Bone Research Program, ANZAC Research Institute, University of Sydney, and Department of Endocrinology & Metabolism, Concord Hospital, Concord, Sydney, Australia.

Contents

DEDICATION

This chapter is dedicated to the memory of the late Pierre D. Delmas, who died so untimely amidst productive work.

I. INTRODUCTION

Bone metastases are frequent and seen in many malignancies, but preferentially occur in patients with breast, prostate, thyroid, kidney, bladder and lung cancers. Although usually not lethal in themselves, bone metastases often cause refractory pain, hypercalcemia, fractures, neurological symptoms and, as a result, profound morbidity and a reduction in quality of life [1]. In one follow-up series, over 60% of breast cancer patients with skeletal metastasis had skeletal complications, averaging at four such events per year of follow-up [2]. Of note, newer bisphosphonates (BP) are able to significantly reduce the rate of skeletal events in cancer patients, particularly when used early in the disease process [3]. Consequently, there is a clear clinical requirement to identify patients with bone metastases as early as possible, and to develop sensitive and specific means to monitor treatment efficacy and predict outcomes.

The diagnostic approach to metastatic bone disease traditionally focuses on the localization and characterization of the lesion, employing an array of different imaging techniques such as radiographs, CT, MRI, (quantitative) ^{99}Tc bone scans, and positron-emission tomography (PET). All of these procedures are of value in case finding studies,

where the goal is to identify patients with established metastatic spread. At earlier stages of the disease process, however, changes in skeletal morphology or radionuclide uptake may be discrete, non-specific or completely absent. Also, not all imaging techniques are equally well suited for the monitoring of skeletal disease progression or therapeutic response, particularly in patients with short survival times. Tumor markers such as PSA have been found to closely correlate with the extent of neoplastic tissue and may therefore be useful in the clinical monitoring of tumor behavior and treatment response [4]. With scant exceptions, however, these markers do not provide information specific to the skeleton's involvement.

Under normal conditions, the bone remodeling process is a balanced, life-long continuum of resorbing old bone (through the action of osteoclasts) and replacing the removed tissue by an equal amount of newly formed bone (through the action of osteoblasts). The presence of bone metastases greatly perturbs this balance. Driven by a number of tumor-derived factors, the osteoclasts surrounding cancer metastases become activated to resorb bone. In contrast, bone formation may be increased or decreased, but is usually inadequate to compensate for the escalation in bone resorption. Radiographically, this results in predominantly lytic or mixed lytic-sclerotic lesions, as typically seen in breast cancer metastases to bone. In contrast, prostate cancers usually cause sclerotic lesions characterized at the cellular level by a relative excess of bone formation compared to bone resorption. However, even the skeletal metastases of prostate cancer are characterized by an increase in the rate of both bone resorption and formation. High bone turnover with excess bone resorption therefore is an archetypal feature of most, if not all bone metastases. (The pathophysiology of this process is beyond the scope of this chapter, but has recently been reviewed in Yoneda *et al.* [5] and Chung *et al.* [6].)

Biochemical markers of bone turnover (Figure 10.1) are non-invasive and relatively inexpensive tools that, if applied and interpreted correctly, can be effectively used in assessing changes in bone remodeling associated with metastatic bone

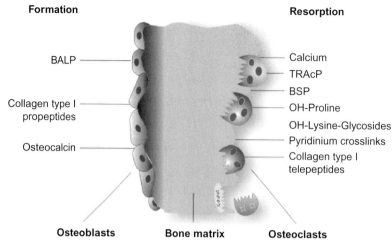

FIGURE 10.1   Biochemical markers of bone remodeling.

disease. Table 10.1 summarizes the biological and technical details of the currently used bone markers. For an in-depth review of the basic biochemistry of bone markers, please refer to Ref. [7]. The present review focuses on the clinical application of biochemical markers of bone turnover in metastatic bone disease, with specific emphasis on the clinically important topics of diagnosis, prognosis and monitoring.

II. DIAGNOSTIC USE

Most studies in this area have compared biochemical markers of bone turnover between groups of cancer patients with and without established bone metastases. While this is a sensible and straightforward approach, its validity largely depends on a correct diagnosis in the 'negative' group (i.e. the group of cancer patients declared to be free of skeletal disease). Given the different techniques employed to prove the absence of malignant bone lesions in the more than 100 studies reported so far, and their specific limitations particularly in early stage bone disease, the assumption of a 'negative status' may not always be correct. In addition, many studies have investigated different types of cancers in a heterogeneous mix of subjects, and almost as a rule, data on estimates of tumor burden are missing. Not surprisingly, the available information on the diagnostic use of bone markers in metastatic bone disease is heterogeneous and often incongruent. The picture becomes more consistent when comparisons are made between a marker of bone turnover and specific imaging techniques, namely bone radioisotope scans, or surgical outcomes in well-defined groups of patients [8–11].

Of the available bone *formation* markers (Table 10.1), serum total (TAP) and bone specific alkaline phosphatase (BAP) usually exhibit the most pronounced changes in response to metastatic bone involvement. In most cases of advanced cancers metastatic to bone, serum TAP and BAP levels are elevated, pointing either to a strong osteoblastic

component or, in lytic lesions, to active repair [12–14]. However, a number of studies reported no differences in serum TAP or BAP levels when patients with and without cancer metastases to bone were compared (e.g., Ref. [15]). In patients with prostate cancer, the combined measurement of PSA and BAP in serum appears to increase the diagnostic sensitivity for bone lesions, compared to healthy subjects or patients with benign prostate hyperplasia [16–18].

In general, serum OC levels are more variable compared to other bone formation markers, and in advanced, untreated metastatic bone disease, serum OC levels may be low in the presence of high BAP levels [19]. The reasons for this dissociation are unclear, but possibilities include proteolytic cleavage of OC, changes in gene expression or disturbed osteoid maturation in the presence of active tumor osteopathy. In patients with multiple myeloma (MM), a number of studies have reported low serum OC values in the presence of high bone resorption markers. Suppressed serum OC concentrations are believed to reflect impaired osteoblast activity and have been associated with poor survival [20]. Consequently, some authors postulated a myeloma cell derived factor that would specifically inhibit osteoblast activity. Tian *et al.* [21] demonstrated increased expression of dickkopf1 (Dkk1), an inhibitor of osteoblast differentiation, in myeloma cells from lytic tumors. Myeloma cells express the receptor activator of nuclear factor kappa ligand (RANKL), a major driver of osteoclastogenesis. Thus, simultaneous overexpression of RANKL and Dkk1 by myeloma cells would increase bone resorption while inhibiting osteoblast differentiation and bone formation, that is, repair. Other factors involved in this process come to light as research progresses [22].

The serum concentrations of both the carboxyterminal (PICP) and the aminoterminal propeptide of type I procollagen (PINP) levels have been found elevated in patients with breast, prostate or lung cancer metastatic to bone [23–25]. In patients with breast cancer, a decreased PICP/PINP ratio appears to signify a more aggressive phenotype with a higher propensity to metastasize to bone [23].

TABLE 10.1   Markers of bone turnover

Marker (abbreviation)	Tissue	Specimen	Method	Remarks
Markers of bone formation				
Bone-specific alkaline phosphatise (BAP)	Bone	Serum	Electrophoresis, Precipitation, IRMA, EIA	Specific product of osteoblasts. Some assays show up to 20% cross-reactivity with liver isoenzyme (LAP).
Osteocalcin (OC)	Bone, platelets	Serum	RIA, IRMA, ELISA	Specific product of osteoblasts; many immunoreactive forms in blood; some may be derived from bone resorption.
C-terminal propeptide of type I procollagen (PICP)	Bone, soft tissue, skin	Serum	RIA, ELISA	Specific product of proliferating osteoblasts and fibroblasts.
N-terminal propeptide of type I procollagen (PINP)	Bone, soft tissue, skin	Serum	RIA, ELISA	Specific product of proliferating osteoblast and fibroblasts; partly incorporated into bone extracellular matrix.
Markers of bone resorption				
Collagen related markers				
Hydroxyproline, total and dialyzable (Hyp)	Bone, cartilage, soft tissue, skin	Urine	Colorimetry, HPLC	Present in all fibrillar collagens and partly collagenous proteins, including C1q and elastin. Present in newly synthesized and mature collagen, i.e. both collagen synthesis and tissue breakdown contribute to urinary hydroxyproline.
Hydroxylysine-glycosides	Bone, soft tissue, skin, serum complement	Urine (serum)	HPLC, ELISA	Hydroxylysine in collagen is glycosylated to varying degrees, depending on tissue type. Glycosylgalactosyl-OHLys in high proportion in collagens of soft tissues, and C1q; Galyctosyl-OHLys in high proportion in skeletal collagens.
Pyridinoline (PYD)	Bone, cartilage, tendon, blood vessels	Urine, serum	HPLC, ELISA	Collagens, with highest concentrations in cartilage and bone; absent from skin; present in mature collagen only.
Deoxypyridinoline (DPD)	Bone, dentin	Urine, serum	HPLC, ELISA	Collagens, with highest concentration in bone; absent from cartilage or skin; present in mature collagen only.
Carboxyterminal cross-linked telopeptide of type I collagen(ICTP, CTX-MMP)	Bone, skin	Serum	RIA	Collagen type I, with highest contribution probably from bone; may be derived from newly synthesized collagen.
Carboxyterminal cross-linked telopeptide of type I collagen (CTX-I)	All tissues containing type I collagen	Urine (a-/β), serum ($\alpha\alpha$/$\beta\beta$)	ELISA, RIA	Collagen type I, with highest contribution probably from bone. Isomerization of aspartyl to β-aspartyl occurs with ageing of collagen molecule.
Aminoterminal cross-linked telopeptide of type I collagen (NTX-I)	All tissues containing type I collagen	Urine, serum	ELISA, CLIA, RIA	Collagen type I, with highest contribution from bone.
Collagen I alpha 1 helicoidal peptide (HELP)	All tissues containing type I collagen	Urine	ELISA	Degradation fragment derived from the helical part of type I collagen (α1 chain, AA 620-633). Correlates highly with other markers of collagen degradation, no specific advantage or difference in regards to clinical outcomes.

(Continued)

TABLE 10.1   *(Continued)*

Marker (abbreviation)	Tissue	Specimen	Method	Remarks
Non-collagenous proteins				
Bone Sialoprotein (BSP)	Bone, dentin, hypertrophic cartilage	Serum	RIA, ELISA	Acidic, phosphorylated glycoprotein, synthesized by osteoblasts and osteoclastic-like cells, laid down in bone extracellular matrix. Appears to be associated with osteoclast function.
Osteocalcin fragments (ufOC, U-Mid-OC, U-LongOC)	Bone	Urine	ELISA	Certain age-modified OC fragments are released during osteoclastic bone resorption and may be considered an index of bone resorption.
Osteopontin (OPN)	Bone, kidney, placenta, dentin, cartilage, brain, muscle, blood vessels	Serum	ELISA	Synthesized by a variety of tissue types. Synthesis in bone is stimulated by 1,25-dihydroxy-vitamin D3.
Osteoclast enzymes				
Tartrate-resistant acid phosphatase (TRAcP)	Bone, blood	Plasma, serum	Colorimetry, RIA, ELISA	Six isoenzymes found in human tissues (osteoclasts, platelets, erythrocytes). Band 5b predominant in bone (osteoclasts). Enzyme identified in both the ruffled border of the osteoclast membrane and the secretions in the resorptive space.
Cathepsins (e.g., K, L) (CathK, Cath L)	K: Primarily in osteoclasts L: Macrophage, osteoclasts	Plasma, serum	ELISA	Cathepsin K, cysteine protease, plays an essential role in osteoclast-mediated bone matrix degradation by cleaving helical and telopeptide regions of collagen type I. Cathepsin K and L cleave the loop domain of TRACP and activate the latent enzyme. Cathepsin L has a similar function in macrophages. Tests for measurement of cathepsins in blood are presently under evaluation.

Once established in the bone microenvironment, viable cancer cells are believed to initiate bone resorption through the activation of resident osteoclasts. This process rapidly creates space for further growth of the new settlement, and ultimately leads to widespread destruction of skeletal structures [5,6]. Hence, it is not surprising that bone resorption markers are considered prime candidates for the diagnosis of such lesions.

The majority of patients with breast, prostate, lung or oral squamous cell cancers metastatic to bone exhibited abnormally high urinary levels of the collagen crosslink, deoxypyridinoline (DPD) [11,26–29]. In some studies (e.g., Ref. [27]), a significant proportion of cancer patients without evidence for malignant bone involvement also had elevated urinary crosslink levels (Figure 10.2). This observation may be attributable to the presence of undiagnosed bone metastases in the 'negative' control group, and may point to

an inherent problem in study design (see above). On the other side, these observations may reflect systemic, cytokine-mediated acceleration of bone turnover [30].

Pecherstorfer *et al.* [31] reported significantly higher levels of urinary DPD in patients with MM as compared to healthy adults, patients with monoclonal gammopathy of undetermined significance (MGUS) or patients with postmenopausal osteoporosis. While urinary DPD correctly identified patients with advanced MM (stage III), the test did not discriminate between patients with MGUS, patients with early (stage I) MM or osteoporosis. While disappointing from a clinical point of view, this result is not surprising at all; in fact, it reiterates that bone markers reflect bone turnover, not underlying pathologies. As bone resorption rates are similarly low in MGUS and early stage MM, bone markers would not be expected to discriminate between these entities.

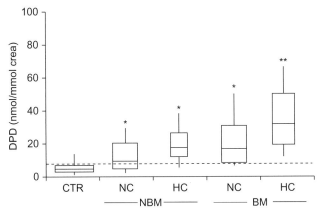

FIGURE 10.2 Urinary deoxypyridinoline (DPD) in patients with and without bone metastases. A normal range was established by measuring urinary DPD in healthy young adults (dashed line: upper limit of normal). Cancer patients were then stratified by calcaemic status (HC, hypercalcemic patients; sCa > 2.6 mmol/l; NC, normocalcemic patients) and by the presence or absence of neoplastic bone involvement (BM, Patients with bone metastases; NBM, patients without bone metastases). Box and whisker plot; horizontal lines depict the medians. $^{*}p < 0.001$, $^{**}p < 0.0001$(from Pecherstorfer *et al.* [27] with permission).

The higher molecular weight ('telopeptide') markers of collagen type I degradation (ICTP, CTX-I, NTX-I) (Table 10.1) have also been used in the evaluation of metastatic bone disease, although with varying results. For example, one study compared urinary NTX-I, serum ICTP and serum BAP in 106 breast cancer patients with and without bone metastases. With a clinical specificity of 91%, serum ICTP was found to be the marker with the highest sensitivity for established bone metastases [32]. Similar results were reported for a comparison of serum ICTP, TRAcP, urinary NTX-I and serum BAP in a study of 156 breast cancer patients [33]. Other studies indicate that urinary NTX-I has a higher predictive value for the diagnosis of bone metastatic progression than serum ICTP and BAP [34]. While there is no general agreement on which telopeptide marker yields the best results, most studies indicate that these peptide markers are sensitive tools in patients with skeletal lesions attributable to breast [14,35–36] and prostate cancer [37–40].

The CTX-I telopeptide is present in two isoforms, namely α and β CTX-I. The α form is found in newly synthesized collagen, while the epitope associated with β-CTX-I is believed to represent older, more mature collagen. More recently, a new assay for the measurement of the α-CTX-I isoforms in serum (termed $\alpha\alpha$CTX) and its use in cancer patients has been described [41]. It has been suggested that the separate measurement of these isoforms, and calculation of the $\tilde{\alpha}/\beta$-CTX-I ratio, may help to identify patients with benign or malignant bone diseases [36]. While intriguing as an idea, the clinical relevance of this concept

remains unclear and further studies are warranted before definitive recommendations can be made.

Serum levels of tartrate-resistant acid phosphatase (TRAcP), an enzyme released by active osteoclasts, have been found elevated in patients with established bone metastases [42–44]. A study comparing serum TRAcP, urinary calcium, PYD and DPD levels found that PYD in urine had the highest diagnostic validity to distinguish between patients with and without bone metastases [27]. However, the assay used in this study measured total TRAcP instead of the osteoclast specific isoenzyme, TRAcP 5b. Newer studies, employing assays specific for the 5b band of TRAcP in serum, found this marker to be highly sensitive to the presence of metastatic bone disease [42–44]. Furthermore, a study in patients with renal cell cancer reported no differences in serum TRAcP 5b levels when comparing patients with and without bone metastases [15]. In contrast, a recent study by Klepzig found serum PINP levels to be of significant diagnostic and monitoring value in regards to the development of bone metastases in patients with renal cell cancers [45].

More recently, bone sialoprotein (BSP) has emerged as a new marker of bone resorption in metastatic bone disease. The glycoprotein is a product of active osteoblasts, is incorporated into the bone matrix during bone formation, and released from bone during osteoclastic bone resorption. Importantly, BSP is also synthesized and secreted by breast, prostate and thyroid cancer cells. Expression of BSP in these tumors has been proposed to play a role in the homing of tumor cells to bone, and enhanced survival of tumor cells in the bone microenvironment [46]. We demonstrated that serum BSP levels correlate with markers of bone resorption in metabolic or malignant bone disease and are often elevated in patients with tumors metastatic to bone [47]. Interestingly, highest levels seemed to occur in patients with bone metastases from cancers that are known to ectopically express BSP, such as breast, prostate or thyroid cancers [48]. In another study, serum BSP levels were closely related to serum PSA levels [49]. High serum BSP values are also found in patients with untreated MM, and measurement of the protein's serum concentration seems to distinguish between patients with MM and benign osteoporosis [50]. In general, patients with osteolytic lesions often have higher levels than individuals diagnosed with non-lytic bone disease.

In summary, most markers of bone remodeling, and particularly those of bone resorption, are elevated in patients with established bone metastases. The newer serum assays may be more sensitive to malignancy-induced changes in bone turnover than the older urine based assays [51]. While evidence suggests that bone markers may be useful diagnostic tools in cancer patients, the currently available data do not allow final conclusions regarding the accuracy and validity of any of the presently used markers in the early diagnosis of bone metastases.

III. PROGNOSTIC USE

Whether or not bone markers are useful for the prediction of skeletal events in cancer patients with or without prevalent malignant spread is a controversial question. The results of studies seem to favor such an association.

Brown *et al.* [52] reported on the association between baseline serum BAP and urinary NTX-I levels and subsequent skeletal event rate in 203 patients with prostate cancer and 238 patients with NSCLC followed in the placebo arms of two phase-III bisphosphonate trials. High levels of both bone markers were associated with poor prognosis as defined by greater rates of skeletal events and shorter survival times. In patients with prostate cancer, for example, elevated NTX-I levels carried a relative risk of 3.25 (95% CI: 2.26–4.68) for skeletal events (Figure 10.3). The authors conclude that in cancer patients, a rise in urinary NTX-I values should prompt more aggressive treatment to prevent skeletal-related morbidity. Costa *et al.* [34] and Vinholes [53] demonstrated that an increase of 130–150% in urinary NTX-I or serum ICTP was a valid indicator of clinical disease progression.

Studies on breast cancer patients indicate that postoperative serum PINP [54,55] and NTX-I [50,52,94] levels are predictive of poor survival and shorter time to progression (Figure 10.4). In lung cancer patients, only markers of bone resorption, but not markers of bone formation, were associated with survival time [24]. Similarly, higher urinary [58] and serum (ICTP) [59] crosslink concentrations were associated with the incidence of skeletal-related events and poor survival in patients with prostate cancer. However, other

studies have not confirmed these finding [60,61], possibly due to the high variability of the bone markers studied [62], and the small number of cancer patients developing bone metastases.

Using a retrospective study design, Bellahcène *et al.* demonstrated that the amount of BSP expressed in breast cancer tissues (as assessed by semi-quantitative immunohistochemistry) was found to correlate with the propensity of the cancer to metastasize to bone [48]. Similarly, tissue expression of bone sialoprotein in prostate cancer may enable the identification of subgroups of patients that are at risk of bone metastasis or recurrence [63]. Our clinical 2-year prospective study demonstrated that in women with newly diagnosed breast cancer, serum BSP concentrations were highly predictive of future bone metastases [64]. Women with breast cancer and elevated serum BSP levels at baseline (i.e., before the operation) had a significantly increased risk of developing bone metastases than similar patients with normal baseline BSP concentrations.

A recent study in patients with NSCLC, who subsequently developed BM, showed that expression of BSP protein in the primary cancer was associated with progression of distant bone metastases in the same patient. The authors suggest that determination of the BSP expression level in lung cancers may be helpful identifying patients at risk of developing bone metastases [65].

Ramankulov *et al.* suggested that the plasma concentrations of another non-collagenous bone protein, osteopontin, alone or in combination with other bone markers, may be useful as a diagnostic and prognostic marker in the detection of bone metastases in patients with prostate cancer [18].

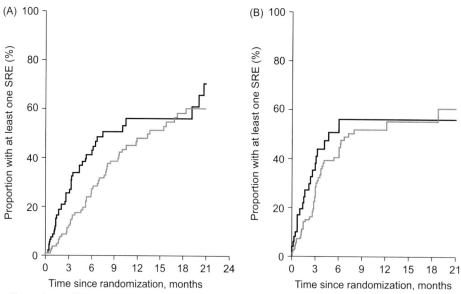

FIGURE 10.3 Baseline urinary NTX-I levels predict future skeletal related events. Cumulative proportion of skeletal-related events in patients with prostate cancer (A) and other malignancies (including NSCLC; B) according to urinary NTX-I concentrations at baseline (dashed line: urinray NTX < 100 nmol/mmolCr; solid line: urinary NTX > 100 nmol/mmolCr (from Brown *et al.* 2005 [52], with permission).

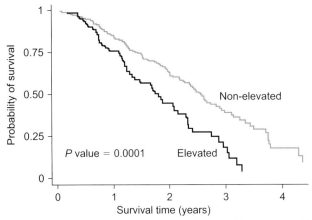

FIGURE 10.4 Serum NTX-I levels and survival in patients with breast cancer bone metastases after commencement of hormonal therapy according to serum NTX-I concentrations (from Ali *et al.* 2004 [56], with permission).

In MM, reduced serum OC levels seem to be associated with rapid disease progression and poor survival [20]. However, this association was not confirmed in other studies [66,67] and more recent studies indicate that serum ICTP levels are a better prognostic marker in MM than most other biochemical indices [68,69]. In patients with MM, serum BSP concentrations increase with disease progression and higher levels of the protein are associated with shorter survival time. A recent study by Jakob and colleagues [70] investigated the prognostic impact of serum ICTP in combination with other, more established parameters of prognosis (such as beta2microglobulin) in 100 patients with newly diagnosed symptomatic multiple myeloma. Much like beta2microglobuline or albumin, the serum ICTP level was a significant prognostic factor for overall survival in these patients. Moreover, in multivariate analyses, individual serum ICTP levels were the most powerful prognostic factor, which was able to separate the study population into subgroups with good and worse prognosis. Hence, inclusion of serum ICTP added to the prognostic value of the international staging system (ISS) for myeloma [70].

IV. MONITORING OF ANTI-TUMOR THERAPY

In addition to newer antineoplastic therapies, BPs have evolved as first line agents in the treatment of patients with bone metastases. BPs have been demonstrated to alleviate pain and to decrease the incidence of skeletal-related events such as fractures [3,71,72]. However, the introduction of these expensive agents has not only improved clinical outcomes in patients with bone metastases, but has also precipitated the requirement for clinically useful, simple to use, and inexpensive tools to determine therapeutic efficacy and monitor response in individual patients. Today, there is little

doubt that markers of bone remodeling are useful in assessing the effect of BP on bone, as they have been shown to reflect therapy induced changes earlier than most other techniques currently used in clinical practice.

In general, bone markers respond to BP with a rapid and pronounced fall in circulating and urinary concentrations. In most patients, markers of bone resorption will react first (often within days) while markers of bone formation follow suit several weeks or months later [47,69,71,72–76] (Figure 10.5). This sequence is not unexpected, as osteoclasts are the primary target of BP. The later reduction in osteoblast activity is considered an effect of the normal coupling between anabolic and catabolic actions in bone. However, as this balance may be perturbed in metastatic bone disease, 'paradoxical' effects are often observed. For example, in patients with MM or metastatic breast cancer, chemotherapy-induced remissions [20,77] or treatment with BP [78] may lead to a normalization or even increase of serum OC or BAP levels. In this context, it has been suggested that calculating the ratio of two bone markers may be more useful for identifying therapeutic responders than following changes in individual markers [23,37,79]. The timing of bisphosphonate administration does not seem to affect its overall effect on bone turnover, at least when zoledronate acid is being used [80].

Blomqvist *et al.* [81] were the first to demonstrate that after 6 months of therapy the percent change in bone markers versus baseline was a good predictor of therapeutic outcome. Later studies indicate that pre-therapeutic bone resorption rates predict the response to BP treatment. In the short term, a double blind study on the effects of pamidronate on bone turnover and clinical outcomes [82] observed that cancer patients with high urinary NTX-I levels were less likely to respond to treatment than patients with a normal result. Furthermore, normalization of urinary NTX-I excretion was associated with better clinical outcomes [82]. The best currently available data in this regard was published by Lipton and colleagues [75] who retrospectively analyzed the relationship between normalization of urinary NTX after 3 months of treatment with either placebo, pamidronate or zoledronate, and clinical outcomes in three phase III cancer trials. The advantage of this study is that data were available on a large number of patients with bone metastases from a number of different cancers, including breast cancer (*n* = 578), hormone-refractory prostate cancer (*n* = 472), non-small-cell lung cancer and other solid tumors (*n* = 291). Hence, the data appear to be applicable to a wider range of clinical situations. The authors found that normalized urinary NTX levels, as compared to persistently elevated NTX levels, were associated with improved overall survival and a reduced risk of skeletal complications. Lüftner *et al.* [83] reported similar results for serum BAP and PINP. In yet another study, measuring the post-therapeutic changes in collagen telopeptide markers and urinary calcium achieved the best results when monitoring

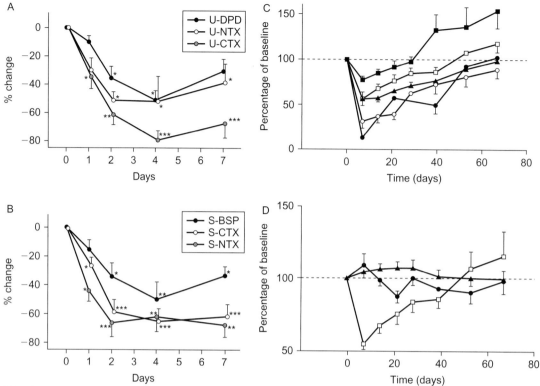

FIGURE 10.5   Changes in markers of bone turnover after treatment with IV pamidronate. (A) Short-term changes in *urinary* bone resorption markers: deoxypyridinoline (U-DPD), C-terminal (U-CTX), N-terminal (U-NTX) telopeptide of type I collagen; (B) short-term changes in serum markers of bone resorption: bone sialoprotein (S-BSP), C-terminal (S-CTX), N-terminal (S-NTX) telopeptides of type I collagen. $^{*}p < 0.05$, $^{**}p < 0.01$, $^{***}p < 0.001$ versus healthy controls (A and B from Woitge *et al*. 1999 [51], with permission); (C) long-term changes in urinary markers of bone resorption (□, DPD; ■, PYD; ●, CTX-I; ▲, hydroxyproline; ○, calcium); (D) long-term changes in serum markers of bone formation (▲, total alkaline phosphatase; ●, osteocalcin). Changes in urinary DPD (□) are shown again for comparison (C and D from Body *et al*. 1997 [99], with permission).

cancer patients treated with zoledronate [84]. Brown *et al*. demonstrated that the number needed to treat (NNT) to avoid one skeletal-related event equaled 2 when baseline urinary NTX-I concentrations were clearly abnormal (above 200 nmol/mmol creatinine), whereas the NNT was 31 with normal urinary NTX-I values [85]. In patients with breast cancer, serum concentrations of TRAcP 5b fall significantly in response to BP treatment when no progression is detectable, but rise again with disease progression [42].

In a post-hoc exploratory analysis of three large, randomized clinical trials, Coleman and co-workers [86] confirmed that bone turnover markers might prove valuable prognostic tools in patients with bone metastases receiving bisphosphonates. Specifically, the authors demonstrated that compared to subjects with normal bone turnover, cancer patients with high levels of urinary NTX (and to a lesser extent, serum BAP) had a significantly increased risk of skeletal complications, disease progression and death. This was particularly true for values measured during therapy with zoledronate, supporting the notion that the goal of

bisphosphonate therapy in cancer patients with metastatic bone disease should be to suppress bone resorption. However, this clinical concept is still awaiting final proof in appropriately designed, prospective studies (which are under way).

The effects of anti-oestrogens such as tamoxifen on markers of bone remodeling are quite different to those of the BP. Given as an adjuvant therapy in patients with breast cancer metastatic to bone, tamoxifen induced an increase in pyridinium crosslinks [87], and either a suppression [88] or no change [89] in bone formation markers. Noguchi *et al*. [90] found that in patients with prostate cancer metastatic to bone, serial measurements of serum ICTP and PINP were superior to the measurement of PSA in monitoring the effects of hormonal treatment (median follow-up: 29 months). More recently, Johansen and colleagues demonstrated that serial monitoring of serum PINP, BAP and CTX-I provides prognostic information in 106 patients with prostate cancer metastatic to bone who undergo hormonal treatment (i.e., total androgen ablation or parenteral estrogen) [57].

The effect of chemotherapy on bone markers appears to vary depending on the type of chemotherapy and whether or not glucocorticoids are being used. It seems that most markers of bone formation change slowly following several cycles of chemotherapy as long as no glucocorticoids are involved. In contrast, serum levels of OC suppress profoundly and rapidly once cortisone is introduced [91]. In patients with breast cancer the progression of bone metastases after chemotherapy appears to be closer associated with changes in serum TAP than with CEA or CA 15-3. In this study, however, measurements of serum TAP were unable to distinguish between responders and non-responders to chemotherapy [12]. In patients with breast cancer and osteolytic bone lesions, a rise in serum OC or TAP/ BAP following chemotherapy has, in some studies, been associated with focal recalcification and therefore interpreted as a sign of therapeutic success [92]. Therapeutic responders exhibited a significant fall in both serum TRACP5b activity and NTX levels, while in non-responding patients, serum NTX significantly increased over time. In this recent study, serum TRACP5b activity appeared to be a valuable tool to monitor post-therapeutic changes in breast cancer patients with bone metastasis [93]. However, the significance of these observations needs to be shown in further and larger studies.

In patients with MM, high-dose chemotherapy with autografting normalized bone turnover, although these effects were slow to appear [94]. Serum BSP seems to reflect the response to chemotherapy in patients with MM, as the treatment-induced changes in serum BSP values correlate with the changes in the monoclonal protein [50]. However, markers of bone turnover may also be used to show non-effects or even harmful effects of ceratin agents in myeloma and other conditions (e.g., Ref. [95]).

It should be noted that absolute changes in marker values are often misleading if the respective marker's analytical and biological variability are not taken into account. Numerous biological factors affect bone turnover and therefore bone marker levels [96,97]. As a rule, markers demonstrating large changes in response to disease processes or interventions also exhibit substantial degrees of non-specific variability. A comparison of two widely used resorption markers, urinary CTX-I and DPD, best illustrate this fact: therapy-induced changes in CTX-I are always more pronounced than those seen with DPD, a fact that is often misinterpreted as a sign of greater sensitivity on the side of CTX-I. However, the short- and long-term variability of CTX-I is also by far greater than that of DPD [62]. In the clinical setting, variability of bone markers should be of particular concern when it comes to serial measurements (for example, during therapeutic monitoring). Often, a moderate reduction in a bone resorption marker is believed to be the effect of anti-resorptive treatment, when it really should be attributed to non-specific variability or to a regression to the mean (RTM)

[96]. However, a true response can only be assumed when, within a single individual, the change in signal is greater than the imprecision of the measurement. Based upon the available evidence, a change in bone formation markers of greater than 40% is likely to be significant. In contrast, changes below 60–80% in most bone resorption markers are within the range of non-specific variation ('background noise').

In summary, markers of bone resorption respond promptly and profoundly to BP and antineoplastic therapy, and this response appears to be associated with a favorable clinical outcome in patients with bone metastases. While the available evidence suggests that the aim of BP therapy should be to normalize increased rates of bone remodeling, it is presently unknown whether the use of bone markers in the routine clinical setting has any defined beneficial effects on overall outcome in cancer patients.

V. CONCLUSIONS AND PERSPECTIVES

At present, it seems clear that most bone turnover markers are abnormal in patients with active bone metastases. In these unfortunate patients, the diagnostic validity of bone markers seems at last equal to that of other diagnostic tools, including radioisotope bone scans, CT and MRI techniques. Further studies are required, however, to determine the diagnostic accuracy and validity of these markers in patients at *early* or uncertain stages of the disease. The critical point in this undertaking will be to overcome the notorious variability of present day bone markers [97] and worldwide efforts will be required to reduce technical variability and to standardize the available assays [98].

Further data will become available on the prognostic use of bone markers. While the available information is indeed promising, larger and longer-term studies are required to strengthen the observed associations between high levels of bone turnover markers and future skeletal events and/or poor survival in cancer patients. It will be of interest to see whether such associations are a general biological phenomenon, or a feature typical for some but not for other tumors, patients or situations. Again, overcoming the problem of variability will be critical.

Finally, bone turnover markers will increasingly be used to monitor chemo and other therapies. Already, it appears that high bone turnover markers following treatment are indicative of an unfavorable therapeutic response and prognosis. Vice versa, a reduction in bone markers after anti-resorptive treatment is often associated with reduced pain, fewer fractures and slower tumor progression. However, all of the supportive evidence is short term and we need longer-term studies. Nevertheless, in five years' time, it may be standard procedure to attempt normalization of bone turnover markers in order to achieve better clinical outcomes for our cancer patients.

References

1. R.D. Rubens, Clinical aspects of bone metastases, in: J.-J. Body (Ed.), Tumor Bone Diseases and Osteoporosis in Cancer Patients, Marcel Dekker Inc, New York, 2000, pp. 85–96.
2. A. Lipton, R.L. Theriault & G.N. Hortobagyi, et al., Pamidronate prevents skeletal complications and is effective palliative treatment in women with breast carcinoma and osteolytic bone metastases: long term follow-up of two randomised placebo-controlled trials, Cancer 88 (2000) 1082–1090.
3. J.R. Ross, Y. Saunders & P.M. Edmonds, et al., Systematic review of role of bisphosphonates on skeletal morbidity in metastatic cancer, BMJ 327 (2003) 469–472.
4. G.J. Bubley, M. Carducci & W. Dahut, et al., Eligibility and response guidelines for phase II clinical trials in androgen-independent prostate cancer: recommendations from the Prostate Specific Antigen Working Group, J Clin Oncol 18 (1999) 3461–3477.
5. T. Yoneda & T. Hiraga, Crosstalk between cancer cells and bone microenvironment in bone metastasis, Biochem Biophys Res Commun 328 (2005) 679–687.
6. L.W. Chung, A. Baseman & V. Assikis, et al., Molecular insights into prostate cancer progression: the missing link of tumor microenvironment, J Urol 173 (2005) 10–20.
7. M.J. Seibel, Biochemical markers of bone remodeling, Endocrinol Metab Clin North Am 32 (2003) 83–113 vi–vii.
8. N. Fukumitsu, M. Uchiyama & Y. Mori, et al., Correlation of urine type I collagen-cross-linked N telopeptide levels with bone scintigraphic results in prostate cancer patients, Metabolism 51 (2002) 814–818.
9. W.G. Meijer, E. van der Veer & P.L. Jager, et al., Bone metastases in carcinoid tumors: clinical features, imaging characteristics, and markers of bone metabolism, J Nucl Med 44 (2003) 184–191.
10. W. Ebert, T. Muley & K.P. Herb, et al., Comparison of bone scintigraphy with bone markers in the diagnosis of bone metastasis in lung carcinoma patients, Anticancer Res 24 (2004) 3193–3201.
11. I.N. Springer, H. Terheyden & M.A. Suhr, et al., Follow-up of collagen crosslink excretion in patients with oral squamous cell carcinoma and analysis of tissue samples, Br J Cancer 89 (2003) 1722–1728.
12. A. Berruti, L. Dogliotti & G. Gorzegno, et al., Differential patterns of bone turnover in relation to bone pain and disease extent in bone in cancer patients with skeletal metastases, Clin Chem 45 (1999) 1240–1247.
13. I. Kanakis, M. Nikolaou & D. Pectasides, et al., Determination and biological relevance of serum cross-linked type I collagen N-telopeptide and bone-specific alkaline phosphatase in breast metastatic cancer, Pharm Biomed Anal 34 (2004) 827–832.
14. G.M. Oremek, A. Weis & N. Sapoutzis, et al., Diagnostic value of bone and tumour markers in patients with malignant diseases, Anticancer Res 23 (2003) 987–990.
15. K. Jung, M. Lein & M. Ringsdorf, et al., Diagnostic and prognostic validity of serum bone turnover markers in metastatic renal cell carcinoma, J Urol 176 (2006) 1326–1331.
16. J.A. Lorente, H. Valenzuela & J. Morote, et al., Serum bone alkaline phosphatase levels enhance the clinical utility of prostate specific antigen in the staging of newly diagnosed prostate cancer patients, Eur J Nucl Med 26 (1999) 625–632.

17. L.F. Wymenga, K. Groenier & J. Schuurman, et al., Pretreatment levels of urinary deoxypyridinoline as a potential marker in patients with prostate cancer with or without bone metastasis, Br J Urol 88 (2001) 231–235.
18. A. Ramankulov, M. Lein & G. Kristiansen, et al., Plasma osteopontin in comparison with bone markers as indicator of bone metastasis and survival outcome in patients with prostate cancer, Prostate 67 (2007) 330–340.
19. S. Wada, Y. Katayama & Y. Yasutomo, et al., Changes of bone metabolic markers in patients with bone metastases: clinical significance in assessing bone response to chemotherapy, Int Med 32 (1993) 611–618.
20. R. Bataille, P.D. Delmas & D. Chappard, et al., Abnormal serum bone Gla protein levels in multiple myeloma, Crucial role of bone formation and prognostic implications, Cancer 66 (1990) 167–172.
21. E. Tian, F. Zhan & R. Walker, et al., The role of the Wnt-signaling antagonist DKK1 in the development of osteolytic lesions in multiple myeloma, N Engl J Med 349 (2003) 2483–2494.
22. F. Silvestris, P. Cafforio & M. De Matteo, et al., Negative regulation of the osteoblast function in multiple myeloma through the repressor gene E4BP4 activated by malignant plasma cells, Clin Cancer Res 14 (2008) 6081–6091.
23. A. Jukkola, R. Tähtelä & E. Thölix, et al., Aggressive breast cancer leads to discrepant serum levels of the type I procollagen propeptides PINP and PICP, Cancer Res 57 (1997) 5517–5520.
24. G. Oremek, H. Sauer-Eppel & M. Klepzig, Total procollagen type 1 amino-terminal propeptide (total P1NP) as a bone metastasis marker in gynecological carcinomas, Anticancer Res 27 (2007) 1961–1962.
25. M. Koizumi, S. Takahashi & E. Ogata, Comparison of serum bone resorption markers in the diagnosis of skeletal metastasis, Anticancer Res 23 (2003) 4095–4099.
26. C.R. Paterson, S.P. Robins & J.M. Horobin, et al., Pyridinium crosslinks as markers of bone resorption in patients with breast cancer, Br J Cancer 64 (1991) 884–886.
27. M. Pecherstorfer, I. Zimmer-Roth & T. Schilling, et al., The diagnostic value of urinary pyridinium cross-links of collagen, serum total alkaline phosphatase, and urinary calcium excretion in neoplastic bone disease, J Clin Endocrinol Metab 80 (1995) 97–103.
28. F. Alata , O. Alata & M. Metinta , et al., Usefulness of bone markers for detection of bone metastases in lung cancer patients, Clin Biochem 35 (2002) 293–296.
29. P. Behrens, J. Bruns & K.P. Ullrich, et al., Pyridinoline crosslinks as markers for primary and secondary bone tumors, Scand J Clin Lab Invest 63 (2003) 37–44.
30. J.L. Motellón, F.J. Jiménez & F. de Miguel, et al., Relationship of plasma bone cytokines with hypercalcemia in cancer patients, Clin Chim Acta 302 (2000) 59–68.
31. M. Pecherstorfer, M.J. Seibel & H.W. Woitge, et al., Bone resorption in multiple myeloma and in monoclonal gammopathy of undetermined significance: quantification by urinary pyridinium cross-links of collagen, Blood 90 (1997) 3743–3750.
32. U. Ulrich, K. Rhiem & J. Schmolling, et al., Cross-linked type I collagen C- and N-telopeptides in women with bone metastases from breast cancer, Arch Gynecol Obstet 264 (2001) 186–190.

33. N. Wada, M. Fujisaki & S. Ishii, et al., Evaluation of bone metabolic markers in breast cancer with bone metastasis, Breast Cancer 8 (2001) 131–137.

34. L. Costa, L.M. Demers & A. Gouveia-Oliveira, et al., Prospective evaluation of the peptide-bound collagen type I crosslinks N-telopeptide and C-telopeptide in predicting bone metastases status, J Clin Oncol 20 (2002) 850–856.

35. K. Kiuchi, T. Ishikawa & Y. Hamaguchi, et al., Cross-linked collagen C- and N-telopeptides for an early diagnosis of bone metastasis from breast cancer, Oncol Rep 9 (2002) 595–598.

36. P.A. Cloos, N. Lyubimova & H. Solberg, et al., An immuno-assay for measuring fragments of newly synthesized collagen type I produced during metastatic invasion of bone, Clin Lab 50 (2004) 279–289.

37. M. Koizumi, J. Yonese & I. Fukui, et al., Metabolic gaps in bone formation may be a novel marker to monitor the osseous metastasis of prostate cancer, J Urol 167 (2002) 1863–1866.

38. M. Noguchi & S. Noda, Pyridinoline cross-linked carboxy-terminal telopeptide of type I collagen as a useful marker for monitoring metastatic bone activity in men with prostate cancer, J Urol 166 (2001) 1106–1110.

39. C. de la Piedra, N.A. Castro-Errecaborde & M.L. Traba, et al., Bone remodeling markers in the detection of bone metastases in prostate cancer, Clin Chim Acta 331 (2003) 45–53.

40. M. Lein, M. Wirth & K. Miller, et al., Serial markers of bone turnover in men with metastatic prostate cancer treated with zoledronic acid for detection of bone metastases progression, Eur Urol 52 (5) (2007) 1381–1387.

41. J. Leeming, M. Koizumi & I. Byrjalsen, et al., The relative use of eight collagenous and noncollagenous markers for diagnosis of skeletal metastases in breast, prostate, or lung cancer patients, Cancer Epidemiol Biomarkers Prev 15 (2006) 32–38.

42. B. Capeller, H. Caffier & M.W. Sütterlin, et al., Evaluation of tartrate-resistant acid phosphatase (TRAP) 5b as serum marker of bone metastases in human breast cancer, Anticancer Res 23 (2003) 1011–1015.

43. T.Y. Chao, C.L. Ho & S.H. Lee, et al., Tartrate-resistant acid phosphatase 5b as a serum marker of bone metastasis in breast cancer patients, J Biomed Sci 11 (2004) 511–516.

44. J. Korpela, S.L. Tiitinen & H. Hiekkanen, et al., Serum TRACP 5b and ICTP as markers of bone metastases in breast cancer, Anticancer Res 26 (2006) 3127–3132.

45. M. Klepzig, H. Sauer-Eppel & D. Jonas, et al., Value of pro-collagen type 1 amino-terminal propeptide in patients with renal cell carcinoma, Anticancer Res 28 (2008) 2443–2446.

46. A. Jain, A. Karadag & B. Fohr, et al., Three SIBLINGs enhance Factor H's cofactor activity enabling MCP-like cellular evasion of complement-mediated attack, J Biol Chem 277 (2002) 13700–13708.

47. M.J. Seibel, H.W. Woitge & M. Pecherstorfer, et al., Serum immunoreactive bone sialoprotein as a new marker of bone turnover in metabolic and malignant bone disease, J Clin Endocrinol Metab 81 (1996) 3289–3294.

48. A. Bellahcène, S. Menard & R. Bufalino, et al., Expression of bone sialoprotein in primary human breast cancer is associated with poor survival, Int J Cancer 69 (1996) 350–353.

49. N.S. Fedarko, A. Jain & A. Karadag, et al., Elevated serum bone sialoprotein and osteopontin in colon, breast, prostate, and lung cancer, Clin Cancer Res 7 (2001) 4060–4066.

50. H.W. Woitge, M. Pecherstorfer & E. Horn, et al., Serum bone sialoprotein as a marker of tumour burden and neoplastic bone involvement and as a prognostic factor in multiple myeloma, Br J Cancer 84 (2001) 344–351.

51. H.W. Woitge, M. Pecherstorfer & Y. Li, et al., Novel serum markers of bone resorption: clinical assessment and comparison with established urinary indices, J Bone Miner Res 14 (1999) 792–801.

52. J.E. Brown, R.J. Cook & P. Major, et al., Bone turnover markers as predictors of skeletal complications in prostate cancer, lung cancer, and other solid tumors, J Natl Cancer Inst 97 (2005) 59–69.

53. J. Vinholes, R. Coleman & D. Lacombe, et al., Assessment of bone response to systemic therapy in an EORTC trial: preliminary experience with the use of collagen cross-link excretion. European Organization for Research and Treatment of Cancer, Br J Cancer 80 (1999) 221–228.

54. A. Jukkola, R. Bloigu & K. Holli, et al., Postoperative PINP in serum reflects metastatic potential and poor survival in node-positive breast cancer, Anticancer Res 21 (2001) 2873–2876.

55. R. Thurairaja, R.K. Iles & K. Jefferson, et al., Serum amino-terminal propeptide of type 1 procollagen (P1NP) in prostate cancer: a potential predictor of bone metastases and prognosticator for disease progression and survival, Urol Int 76 (2006) 67–71.

56. S.M. Ali, L.M. Demers & K. Leitzel, et al., Baseline serum NTx levels are prognostic in metastatic breast cancer patients with bone-only metastasis, Ann Oncol 15 (2004) 455–459.

57. J.S. Johansen, K. Brasso & P. Iversen, et al., Changes of biochemical markers of bone turnover and YKL-40 following hormonal treatment for metastatic prostate cancer are related to survival, Clin Cancer Res 13 (2007) 3244–3249.

58. A. Berruti, L. Dogliotti & M. Tucci, et al., Metabolic effects of single-dosepamidronate administration in prostate cancer patients with bone metastases, Int J Biol Markers 17 (2002) 244–252.

59. T. Kylmälä, T.L. Tammela & L. Risteli, et al., Type I collagen degradation product (ICTP) gives information about the nature of bone metastases and has prognostic value in prostate cancer, Br J Cancer 71 (1995) 1061–1064.

60. R. Petrioli, S. Rossi & M. Caniggia, et al., Analysis of biochemical bone markers as prognostic factors for survival in patients with hormone-resistant prostate cancer and bone metastases, Urology 63 (2004) 321–326.

61. M.J. Seibel, M. Koehler & B. Auler, Markers of bone turnover do not predict bone metastases in breast cancer, Clin Lab 48 (2002) 583–588.

62. M.J. Seibel, B. Auler & M. Koehler, Long-term variability of markers of bone turnover in patients with breast cancer, Clin Lab 48 (2002) 576–582.

63. G. De Pinieux, T. Flam & M. Zerbib, et al., Bone sialoprotein, bone morphogenetic protein 6 and thymidine phosphorylase expression in localized human prostatic adenocarcinoma as predictors of clinical outcome: a clinicopathological and immunohistochemical study of 43 cases, J Urol 166 (2001) 1924–1930.

64. I.J. Diel, E.F. Solomayer & M.J. Seibel, et al., Serum bone sialoprotein in patients with primary breast cancer as a prognostic marker for subsequent bone metastasis, Clin Cancer Res 5 (1999) 3914–3919.

65. M. Mauro-Papotti, T. Kalebic & M. Volante, et al., Bone sialoprotein is predictive of bone metastases in resectable non-small-cell lung cancer: a retrospective case-control study, Clin Oncol 24 (2006) 4818–4824.

66. O. Mejjad, X. Le Loët & J.P. Basuyau, et al., Osteocalcin is not a marker of progress in multiple myeloma, Eur J Haematol 56 (1996) 30–34.

67. K. Carlson, A. Larsson & B. Simonsson, et al., Evaluation of bone disease in multiple myeloma: a comparison between the resorption markers urinary deoxypyridinoline/creatinine (DPD) and serum ICTP, and an evaluation of the DPD/osteocalcin and ICTP/osteocalcin ratios, Eur J Haematol 62 (1999) 300–306.

68. R. Fonseca, M.C. Trendle & T. Leong, et al., Prognostic value of serum markers of bone metabolism in untreated multiple myeloma patients, Br J Haematol 109 (2000) 24–29.

69. N. Abildgaard, J. Rungby & H. Glerup, et al., Long-term oral pamidronate treatment inhibits osteoclastic bone resorption and bone turnover without affecting osteoblastic function in multiple myeloma, Eur J Haematol 61 (1998) 128–134.

70. C. Jakob, J. Sterz & P. Liebisch, et al., Incorporation of the bone marker carboxy-terminal telopeptide of type-1 collagen improves prognostic information of the International Staging System in newly diagnosed symptomatic multiple myeloma, Leukemia 22 (2008) 1767–1772.

71. S.P. Jagdev, P. Purohit & S. Heatley, et al., Comparison of the effects of intravenous pamidronate and oral clodronate on symptoms and bone resorption in patients with metastatic bone disease, Ann Oncol 12 (2001) 1433–1438.

72. J.R. Berenson, R.A. Vescio & L.S. Rosen, et al., A phase I dose-ranging trial of monthly infusions of zoledronic acid for the treatment of osteolytic bone metastases, Clin Cancer Res 7 (2001) 478–485.

73. E. Terpos, J. Palermos & K. Tsionos, et al., Effect of pamidronate administration on markers of bone turnover and disease activity in multiple myeloma, Eur J Haematol 65 (2000) 331–336.

74. D. Santini, B. Vincenzi & R.A. Hannon, et al., Changes in bone resorption and vascular endothelial growth factor after a single zoledronic acid infusion in cancer patients with bone metastases from solid tumours, Oncol Rep 15 (2006) 1351–1357.

75. A. Lipton, R. Cook & F. Saad, et al., Normalization of bone markers is associated with improved survival in patients with bone metastases from solid tumors and elevated bone resorption receiving zoledronic acid, Cancer 113 (2008) 193–201 [*Subset analyses of this larger study have previously been published by:* A. Lipton, R.J. Cook, P. Major, et al., Zoledronic acid and survival in breast cancer patients with bone metastases and elevated markers of osteoclast activity. Oncologist 12 (2007) 1035–1043. V. Hirsh, P.P. Major, A. Lipton, et al., Zoledronic acid and survival in patients with metastatic bone disease from lung cancer and elevated markers of osteoclast activity. J Thorac Oncol 3 (2008) 228–236.].

76. A. Martinetti, E. Seregni & C. Ripamonti, et al., Serum levels of tartrate-resistant acid phosphatase-5b in breast cancer patients treated with pamidronate, Int J Biol Markers 17 (2002) 253–258.

77. K. Carlson, S. Ljunghall & B. Simonsson, et al., Serum osteocalcin concentrations in patients with multiple myeloma—correlation with disease stage and survival, J Intern Med 231 (1992) 133–137.

78. P. Magnusson, L. Larsson & G. Englund, et al., Differences of bone alkaline phosphatase isoforms in metastatic bone disease and discrepant effects of clodronate on different skeletal sites indicated by the location of pain, Clin Chem 44 (1998) 1621–1628.

79. M. Koizumi, J. Yonese & I. Fukui, et al., The serum level of the amino-terminal propeptide of type I procollagen is a sensitive marker for prostate cancer metastasis to bone, BJU Int 87 (2001) 348–351.

80. D. Generali, A. Dovio & M. Tampellini, et al., Changes of bone turnover markers and serum PTH after night or morning administration of zoledronic acid in breast cancer patients with bone metastases, Br J Cancer 98 (2008) 1753–1758.

81. C. Blomqvist, I. Elomaa & P. Virkkunen, et al., The response evaluation of bone metastases in mammary carcinoma, the value of radiology, scintigraphy, and biochemical markers of bone metabolism, Cancer 60 (1987) 2907–2912.

82. J.J. Vinholes, O.P. Purohit & M.E. Abbey, et al., Relationships between biochemical and symptomatic response in a double-blind randomised trial of pamidronate for metastatic bone disease, Ann Oncol 8 (1997) 1243–1250.

83. D. Lüftner, A. Richter & R. Geppert, et al., Normalisation of biochemical markers of bone formation correlates with clinical benefit from therapy in metastatic breast cancer, Anticancer Res 23 (2003) 1017–1026.

84. T. Chen, J. Berenson & R. Vescio, et al., Pharmacokinetics and pharmacodynamics of zoledronic acid in cancer patients with bone metastases, J Clin Pharmacol 42 (2002) 1228–1236.

85. J.E. Brown, C.S. Thomson & S.P. Ellis, et al., Bone resorption predicts for skeletal complications in metastatic bone disease, Br J Cancer 89 (2003) 2031–2037.

86. R.E. Coleman, P. Major & A. Lipton, et al., Predictive value of bone resorption and formation markers in cancer patients with bone metastases receiving the bisphosphonate zoledronic acid, J Clin Oncol 23 (2005) 4925–4935.

87. M.B. Marttunen, P. Hietanen & A. Titinen, et al., Effects of tamoxifen and toremifene on urinary excretion of pyridinoline and deoxypyridinoline and bone density in postmenopausal patients with breast cancer, Calcif Tissue Int 65 (1999) 365–368.

88. A.M. Kenny, K.M. Prestwood & C.C. Pilbeam, et al., The short term effects of tamoxifen on bone turnover in older women, J Clin Endocrinol Metab 80 (1995) 3287–3291.

89. F. Li, P.I. Pitt & R. Sherwood, et al., Biochemical markers of bone turnover in women with surgically treated carcinoma of the breast, Eur J Clin Invest 23 (1993) 566–571.

90. M. Noguchi, J. Yahara & S. Noda, Serum levels of bone turnover markers parallel the results of bone scintigraphy in monitoring bone activity of prostate cancer, Urology 61 (2003) 993–998.

91. T. Diamond, S. Levy & P. Day, et al., Biochemical, histomorphometric and densitometric changes in patients with multiple myeloma: effects of glucocorticoid therapy and disease activity, Br J Haematol 97 (1997) 641–648.

92. A. Piovesan, A. Berruti & M. Torta, et al., Comparison of assay of total and bone-specific alkaline phosphatase in the assessment of osteoblast activity in patients with metastatic bone disease, Calcif Tissue Int 61 (1997) 362–369.

93. Y.C. Chung, C.H. Ku & T.Y. Chao, et al., Tartrate-resistant acid phosphatase 5b activity is a useful bone marker for monitoring bone metastases in breast cancer patients after treatment, Cancer Epidemiol Biomarkers Prev 15 (2006) 424–428.

94. R.E. Clark, A.J. Flory & E.M. Ion, et al., Biochemical markers of bone turnover following high-dose chemotherapy and auto-grafting in multiple myeloma, Blood 96 (2000) 2697–2702.

95. T. Sondergaard, P. Pedersen, T. Andersen, et al., A phase II clinical trial does not show that high dose simvastatin has beneficial effect on markers of bone turnover in multiple myeloma, Hematol Oncol Jul 31 (2008).

96. T. Nguyen, C. Meier, and M.J. Seibel, Variability of bone marker measurements, in: Dynamics of Bone and Cartilage Metabolism. 2nd edn, M.J. Seibel, S.P. Robins & J.P. Bilezikian, (eds.), Elsevier/Academic Press, San Diego, 2006, pp. 565–582.

97. C. Meier, T. Nguyen, and M.J. Seibel. Monitoring of anti-resorptive treatment, in: Dynamics of Bone and Cartilage Metabolism. 2nd edn, M.J. Seibel, S.P. Robins & J.P. Bilezikian, (eds.), Elsevier/Academic Press, San Diego, 2006, pp. 649–670.

98. M.J. Seibel, M. Lang & W.J. Geilenkeuser, Interlaboratory variation of biochemical markers of bone turnover, Clin Chem 47 (2001) 1443–1450.

99. J.J. Body, J.C. Dumon & E. Gineyts, et al., Comparative evaluation of markers of bone resorption in patients with breast cancer-induced osteolysis before and after bisphosphonate therapy, Br J Cancer 75 (1997) 408–412.

CHAPTER 11

Cytogenetic and Molecular Genetic Alterations in Bone Tumors

SUVI SAVOLA[1], TOM BÖHLING[1] AND SAKARI KNUUTILA[1]

[1]*Department of Pathology, Haartman Institute and HUSLAB, University of Helsinki and Helsinki University Central Hospital, Helsinki, Finland.*

Contents

I. INTRODUCTION

Bone tumors are a relatively uncommon and heterogeneous group of neoplasms of the skeleton, accounting for approximately 0.2% of all tumors. In comparison to soft tissue tumors, the incidence of bone tumors is low (0.8–1 per 100,000 individuals) [1] and their age specific frequencies are bicentric. The median age at diagnosis for malignant bone tumors is 38 years according to SEER [1]. However, certain bone tumors, like osteosarcoma and Ewing's sarcoma, occur predominantly during the second decade of life and therefore comprise a remarkable share of pediatric oncology practice, while others (e.g., chondrosarcoma) show gradual mounting up to the age of 80. Due to their rareness and variability by histopathology, the unambiguous classification of bone tumors is often challenging. Further epidemiology, pathogenesis and etiology of specific bone tumors are still largely unknown. However, remarkable progress has taken place in the genetic typing of bone tumors, as shown by a myriad of published articles. The identification of many tumor specific alterations, including tumor specific translocations, cytogenetic changes and mutations in different bone tumors, has shown that the genetic analysis is a valuable and important adjunct to standard histopathological and morphological diagnostics in this entity. Moreover, rapid development over the past decades in molecular genetics and laboratory techniques has led to more sophisticated analyses (e.g. microarray CGH and expression array techniques) that can be used to find novel tumor specific aberrations and naturally to be used for more accurate differential diagnosis of these lesions [2].

II. TECHNIQUES FOR DETECTING GENETIC ALTERATIONS IN BONE TUMORS

A growing number of different techniques are becoming available for detecting genomic abnormalities and rearrangements in oncologic research. Conventional cytogenetic analysis by G-banding has been utilized extensively to detect genetic alterations in bone tumors. The major drawback of this method is low resolution and poor results when metaphase cells are scarce, as usually in the case of solid tumors. Instead, molecular genetic techniques can be utilized in detection of genetic aberrations when only a minimal amount of tissue is available and in the absence of metaphase cells. Fluorescent *in situ* hybridization (FISH) and polymerase chain reaction (PCR) in different applications are targeted to analyze one or few specific loci and they are also broadly used in clinical diagnostics of bone tumors. These locus specific analyses can be applied if the target locus responsible for the precise pathologic condition is known. In comparison, some assays are designed to scan aberrations on whole genome scale, like conventional comparative genomic hybridization (CGH) [3] and array-based CGH [4] (see Figure 11.1 for more details of this technique). These array-based techniques can give considerably higher resolution when compared to conventional cytogenetics, especially if oligo-based applications with 60–100 bp probes are utilized. Array CGH can detect, with high resolution and sensitivity, recurrent amplified chromosomal

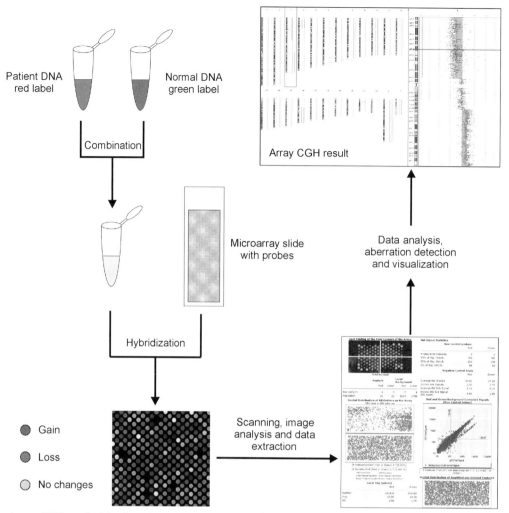

FIGURE 11.1 Array CGH method in detection of gene copy number aberrations. Genomic DNA is extracted from both patient and normal sample and they are labeled with fluorescent dyes, red (Cy5) and green (Cy3), respectively. The labeled samples are combined in equal amounts and hybridized on microarray slides, which can contain oligo-, BAC- or cDNA-probes. Samples hybridize to probe spots in relation to the amount of labeled DNA of the test and control samples. When the tumor sample has a higher copy number than the normal sample the probe spot is red. When lower, then the spot is green. When no copy number changes are detected, the spot is yellow. Following the hybridization microarray slides are washed and scanned with a confocal laser scanner. The image analysis, data extraction, analysis, visualization and, finally, aberration detection are done with appropriate software. The final result of array CGH interprets which genomic regions in the patient sample are gained and which are lost.

regions, small homozygous deletions, pinpointing the putative locations for oncogenes and tumor suppressor genes [5]. A notable disadvantage of this method is that only changes related to gene copy numbers are detected, not balanced rearrangements, e.g. inversions, translocations or whole-genome ploidy changes. Expression profiling with microarray platforms holds a great promise for supplying additional information about bone tumors. These array applications have the potential to be applied to bone tumor classification [6,7] and, in addition, to predict tumor metastasis [8], response to chemotherapy [9] and prognosis [10]. Moreover, combination of multiple approaches to study genetic alterations (e.g., integration of RNA and DNA level data) can enhance the reliability of genetic analysis in understanding

relevant changes for tumorigenesis and subsequent tumor progression.

III. MOLECULAR CYTOGENETIC ABERRATIONS IN BONE TUMORS

Bone tumor classification (see Table 11.1) and the text below follows the 2002 WHO Classification [11].

A. Benign Cartilage Tumors of Bone

Osteochondroma, which usually arises sporadically as a single lesion, is the most common benign bone tumor

TABLE 11.1 Summary of genetic changes in bone tumors according to WHO classification

Bone tumor	Tumor type	Genetic abnormality	Putative gene involved or fusion gene	Prevalence	Reference
Osteochondroma	Cartilage—benign	Loss or rearrangement of 8q24.1, Deletion of 11p11-13, 1p alterations	EXT1, EXT2	~80%	12–15,22
• Multiple osteochondroma	Cartilage—benign	Germline mutations of 8q24.1	EXT1	41–70%	16
		Germline mutations of 11p11-12	EXT2	19–33%	17,132
		Germline mutations of 19p?	EXT3?	Rare	18
Chondroma	Cartilage—benign	Rearrangements of chromosome 6 and 12q13-15	NA	NA	21,22,24
			HMGA2	NA	
• Multiple chondromatosis	Cartilage—benign	Mutations of 3p22-21.1?	PTHR1?	NA	25,26,28
Chondroblastoma	Cartilage—benign	Typically diploid, no specific cytogenetic abnormality	NA	NA	29,30
Chondromyxoid fibroma	Cartilage—benign	Rearrangements of chromosome 6 and 12q13	NA	NA	22,32–35
Chondrosarcoma	Cartilage—malignant	Complex*	NA	NA	133,134
		Gain or amplification of 8q24,	C-MYC	NA	38,44
		LOH, loss or deletion of 9p21.3.	CDKN2A	NA	47,48,50
		Gain of chromosome 12 (especially p11, p13 and q13)	CDK4, MDM2, FGF23, FGF6	NA	40
• Dedifferentiated, mesenchymal and clear cell		No recurrent or specific genetic aberrations	NA	NA	133
Osteoblastoma	Osteogenic—benign	Generally absence of genetic alterations, no specific cytogenetic aberrations	NA	NA	61,133
Osteosarcoma • Conventional	Osteogenic—malignant	Complex*	NA	>70%	66
		Gains and amplifications of 6p	CDC5L	35%	69,72,73
		Loss or deletion of 9p21.3	CDKN2A	5–26%	77
		Amplifications of 8q (especially 8q24)	MYC	7–12%	74
		Gain or amplification of 12q13	MDM2, CDK4	5–36%	70
		LOH, rearrangements or point mutations of 13q14	RB1	10–70%	76
		LOH, point mutations and rearrangements of 17p13	TP53	10–80%	75
• Small cell		No recurrent or specific genetic aberration	NA	NA	78,79
• Low grade central		Gain or amplification of 12q13-14, 12p and 6p21.1-21.3	MDM2, CDK4, SAS	NA	80–82

(Continued)

TABLE 11.1 (*Continued*)

Bone tumor	Tumor type	Genetic abnormality	Putative gene involved or fusion gene	Prevalence	Reference
• Parosteal		Gain or amplification of 12q13 due to ring chromosomes	MDM2, CDK4, SAS	NA	66,83–85
Fibrosarcoma	Fibrogenic—malignant	No recurrent or specific genetic aberration		NA	
		Gain of 22q, ring chromosome 6	PDGF-B		86,87
Malignant fibrous histiocytoma	Fibrohistiocytic—malignant	Complex*		NA	
		Gain or amplification of 8q24	MYC		88
Ewing's sarcoma family of tumors	Small blue round cell—malignant	t(11;22)(q24:q12)	EWSR1-FLI1	85–95%	90
		t(21;22)(q22:q12)	EWSR1-ERG	5–10%	91
		t(7;22)(p22:q12)	EWSR1-ETV1	Rare	92
		t(17;22)(q12:q12)	EWSR1-ETV4	Rare	93
		t(2;22)(q33:q12)	EWSR1-FEV	Rare	94
		t(16;21)(p11:q22)	FUS-ERG	Rare	96
		t(1;22)(p36:q12)	EWSR1-ZNF278	Rare	95
		Secondary genetic alterations:	NA	NA	98–100
		Gains of 1q, 8, 12 and losses of 9p21.2 and 16q			
Chordoma	Notochordal—malignant	Complex*			
		Deletion of 9p21.3	CDKN2A	~75%	114
		Losses of 1p, 3p, 10, 22	NA	>50%	22,113,114
		Gains of chromosome 7			
Adamantinoma	Miscellaneous—malignant	Gains of chromosomes 7, 8, 12, 19 and 21	NA	NA	115,116,136
Fibrous dysplasia	Miscellaneous—benign	Point mutations in 20q13.3	GNAS	73–93%	117–119,137
		Rearrangements of 12p13 and trisomy of 2			

*Complex karyotypes with multiple numerical and structural aberrations.

comprising 35% of all benign bone tumors. Clonal rearrangements or losses of 8q24.1 and 11p11-13 (harboring genes *EXT1* and *EXT2*, respectively) are characteristic for osteochondroma [12–14]. Additionally, 1p13-22 alterations have been reported as being non-randomly involved in osteochondroma [15]. Similarly in multiple osteochondroma, which is an autosomal dominant disorder with nearly complete penetrance, germline mutations in 8q24 and 11p11-12 (*EXT1* and *EXT2*, respectively) are found [16,17]. In rare cases of multiple osteochondroma, the linkage to chromosome 19p is also found [18]. However, it should be noted that the existence of putative *EXT3* gene has not yet been confirmed in 19p. The data implies that the inactivation of both copies for *EXT* gene leading to absent IHH/PTHLH signaling is required for the development of osteochondroma both in sporadic and familial cases [19].

Chondromas are a group of tumors, which can be divided into **enchondromas, periosteal chondroma** and **enchondromatosis**. So far, no distinctive cytogenetic finding has been discovered to distinguish these various types of chondromas. Enchondromas and periosteal chondromas show non-random rearrangements of chromosome 6 and 12q13-15 [20–23]. Chromosomal band 12q15 harbors *HMGA2* gene, which seems to be the common target for 12q13-15 rearrangements in chondroma leading to transcriptional activation and increased expression of *HMGA2* [24]. Enchondromatosis (also known as multiple chondromatosis) includes two sporadic developmental disorders, Ollier disease and Maffucci syndrome. A study by Hopyan *et al.* reported that two cases of enchondromatosis showed mutations in parathyroid hormone receptor type 1 (*PTHR1*) gene (3p22-p21.1) resulting in upregulation of IHH/PTHrP-signaling pathways [25]. A later study was not able to show any mutations in *PHTR1* [26]. Besides, an immunohistochemical study suggested that IHH signaling is absent in enchondromas and chondrosarcomas, while parathyroid hormone related peptide (PTHrP) signaling remains active [27]. A more recent study suggests that heterozygous missense mutations in *PTHR1* impair receptor function contributing to the development of enchondromatosis in some patients [28]. In order to untangle the molecular defect in enchondromatosis confirmatory studies with larger sample sets are warranted.

Chondroblastomas are tumors with typically diploid or near-diploid karyotypes and no consistent abnormalities [29]. Some reports suggest that rearrangements of chromosomes 5 and 8 [30] and others that formation of ring chromosome 4 [31] could be characteristic for chondroblastomas.

Chondromyxoid fibroma cases studied with cytogenetic methods suggest that clonal rearrangement of chromosome 6 (particularly 6p23-25, 6q12-15 and 6q23-27) are non-random [22,32–35]. Rearrangements involving chromosomal band 6q13 seems to be absent in other cartilage tumors and therefore it could be used as a comparatively specific chromosomal marker of chondromyxoid fibroma

[32]. Among all the benign cartilage tumors, chromosome aberrations in the region of 6q12-21 seem to be associated with locally aggressive behavior and harbor genes associated with the pathogenesis of cartilage tumors [34].

B. Malignant Cartilage Tumors of Bone

Chondrosarcomas are a group of malignant cartilage forming tumors with heterogeneous clinical and histopathological subtypes. Conventional chondrosarcomas consist of 90% of all chondrosarcomas and can be further divided into **central chondrosarcoma** and **peripheral chondrosarcoma** according to their location in the bone. Other variants of chondrosarcoma (dedifferentiated, mesenchymal and clear cell chondrosarcoma) are rare. Both central and peripheral chondrosarcoma can arise secondary to their benign precursor (enchondroma and osteochondroma, respectively) and they seem to differ at both molecular and genetic level [36,37]. Numerous reports on the cytogenetic alterations in chondrosarcomas have been published using conventional cytogenetic methods and higher resolution array CGH, showing that karyotypes in chondrosarcoma can range from simple karyotypes to extremely complex karyotypes containing both numerical and structural rearrangements [22,38–40]. Aneuploidy and karyotypic complexity are associated with higher histological grade [41,42], but so far no recurrent or specific cytogenetic aberration has been described. Consistent chromosomal aberrations are gains or amplifications of 12q13 and deletion of 9p21.3 [40,43]. Gains or amplifications of 8q24 harboring *MYC* oncogene are frequent especially in high-grade chondrosarcoma and associated with poor overall survival [44]. Consequently, *MYC* amplification or polysomy of chromosome 8 could be employed as a prognostic marker. Loss of 13q has been proposed as an independent factor for metastasis [39]. Nevertheless, histological grading seems to be the best prognostic predictor hitherto [45]. However, one study proposed that expression profiles could be used as prognostic markers [46]. Losses of 9p21.3 and gains of chromosome 22 are more frequent in central chondrosarcomas in comparison to peripheral ones [47]. In addition, molecular studies have shown that alterations in retinoblastoma (*RB1*) pathway (including *CDKN2A*, *CDKN2B* and *CDK4* genes) are common especially in high-grade chondrosarcoma [48–50]. Cytogenetic studies have not been able to pinpoint any specific or recurrent aberration in **dedifferentiated** [51–53], **mesenchymal** [54,55] or **clear cell chondrosarcoma** [56,57] mainly because of the rarity of these lesions. Additionally, although three specific translocations and their fusion products (*EWS-CHN*, *TFA2-CHN* and *TCF12-CHN*) have been described for extraskeletal chondrosarcoma [58–60], no translocation has been found in chondrosarcomas of bone. To better understand the molecular events behind chondrosarcoma development, histological subtype and grade should be carefully determined, since these various chondrosarcoma subtypes seem to have different genetic characteristics.

C. Benign and Malignant Osteogenic Tumors of Bone

Osteoblastoma is often difficult to separate from osteosarcoma due to similarities in their clinical and pathologic appearance. Moreover, no consistent cytogenetic or molecular genetic aberration has been discovered in osteoblastoma, which could distinguish it from osteosarcoma. However, the total number of genetic alterations is lower in osteoblastomas in comparison to osteosarcoma [61]. Isolated cases of osteoblastoma have shown unbalanced translocations of chromosomes 15, 17 and 20 [62], *p53* gene mutations [63] and balanced translocations involving chromosomes 4, 7 and 14 [64].

As with chondrosarcomas, the majority of **osteosarcomas** contain complex karyotypes, including an abundance of both structural and numerical aberrations with considerable heterogeneity and cell-to-cell variation [65–67]. Moreover, high frequencies of gene amplification (e.g. double minutes, ring chromosomes, homogenously staining regions) have been shown by cytogenetic methods [68] and in studies by array CGH, when the most frequently amplified chromosomal regions were 1p36.32, 6p21-22, 8q24, 12q14.3, 16p13 and 17p11.2-12 [69–71]. Gains and amplifications of 6p have been described in more than one-third of all osteosarcomas and the putative target gene in the region is a cell cycle regulator *CDC5L* (6p21) [72,73]. Other frequent amplifications are found at 8q24 harboring *MYC* locus [74] and at 12q13-15 harboring *MDM2* and *CDK4* loci [72]. Molecular studies have shown that *RB1* and *p53* are frequently rearranged, harboring point mutations or LOH in osteosarcoma [75,76]. Additionally, in osteosarcomas lacking *RB1* alterations, loss or deletion of 9p21.3 harboring tumor suppressor gene *CDKN2A* is frequently found [77].

Small cell osteosarcoma resembles histologically small round cells of Ewing's sarcoma, but *EWS*-translocation t(11;22) is not detected in this entity. Only a few genetic studies have been published and yet no consistent abnormality has been identified [78,79]. In **low grade central osteosarcoma**, p53 gene alterations are less frequent than in conventional osteosarcoma [80] and recurrent gains are 12q13-14, 12p and 6p21.1-21.3 [81]. Strong expression by immunohistochemistry has been shown for MDM2 and CDK4 proteins [80,82]. Karyotypes in **parosteal osteosarcoma** differ from conventional osteosarcoma by presenting a simple karyotype and the presence of a ring chromosome as a sole cytogenetic aberration [66,83]. CGH studies have shown that ring chromosomes contain 12q13-15 sequences [84] and target genes in this chromosomal region seem to be *CDK4, SAS* and *MDM2* [85]. Interestingly, both low grade central osteosarcoma and parosteal osteosarcoma show gains of 12q13-15 and same target genes in this area (*CDK4, SAS* and *MDM2*), which can reflect their similarities in morphology.

D. Other Bone Tumors

Genetic studies of **fibrosarcoma of bone** are very limited, but two reports present data claiming that this tumor is characterized by gains of 22q (*PDGF-B* gene most frequently imbalanced) and ring chromosome 6 [86,87]. However, so far no recurrent genetic abnormality has been identified in fibrosarcoma of bone that could distinguish it from malignant fibrous histiocytoma (MFH).

Malignant fibrous histiocytoma (MFH) is a rare and very aggressive fibrohistiocytic tumor of bone. Genetic changes appear to be very complex with high incidence of gene copy number changes reflecting the high aggressivity of MHF [88]. Most recurrent aberrations are gains of 7q22-q31, 8q21.3-qter, 9q32-qter and losses of 13q21-q22 and positivity for *MYC* expression shown by immunohistochemistry [88]. Sequencing studies on MFH of bone have indicated that p16 mutations are absent and p53 mutations occur in low frequency, suggesting that p53 pathway takes part in the tumorigenesis of MHF of bone rather than p16 [89].

Ewing's sarcoma is the only tumor of bone, which has a tumor specific translocation charactised so far. More than 85% of Ewing's sarcoma tumors contain translocation of t(11;22)(q24;12) leading to *EWSR1-FLI1* gene fusion [90]. Variant gene fusions between *EWSR1* and other partners (*ERG, ETV1, ETV4, FEV* and *ZNF278*) [91–95] and fusion of *FUS-ERG* [96] account for the rest of patients. *EWS-FLI1* fusion type 1 is shown to be associated with a better prognosis than other variants [97]. Although Ewing's sarcoma tumor cells often present a simple karyotype with translocation as a sole cytogenetic abnormality, secondary genetic alterations have been described in 60–80% of tumors. The most prominent gains are 1q, 8 and 12, while losses are detected in 9p21.3 and 16q [98–100]. The overall number of chromosomal imbalances [101,102], while also gains of 1q, 8 and 12 as well as losses of 9p21.3 and 16q, correlate with poor overall survival [99,103–105]. Ewing's sarcoma tumors frequently have the *CDKN2A* gene (9p21.3) homozygously deleted [106,107] (see Figure 11.2) and patients with both p53 mutations and homozygous *CDKN2A* deletions show decreased survival with poor chemoresponse [105].

Giant cell tumors of bone (GCTB) are benign but locally aggressive tumors. Telomeric fusions of chromosomes have been reported [42,108,109] and in these fusions chromosomes 11p, 13p, 15p, 18p, 19p and 21p are regularly involved [110]. It is somewhat surprising that telomeric fusions are present in benign tumors like GCTB, since telomeric association is usually seen exclusively in high-grade malignant tumors. Amplification of 20q11.1 was shown to be present in giant cell tumors of bone leading to *TPX2* overexpression and this was shown to have prognostic value in GCTB [111]. One study demonstrated that GCTBs activate telomerase enzyme leading to telomere maintenance, which can play an important role in the pathogenesis of GCTB [112].

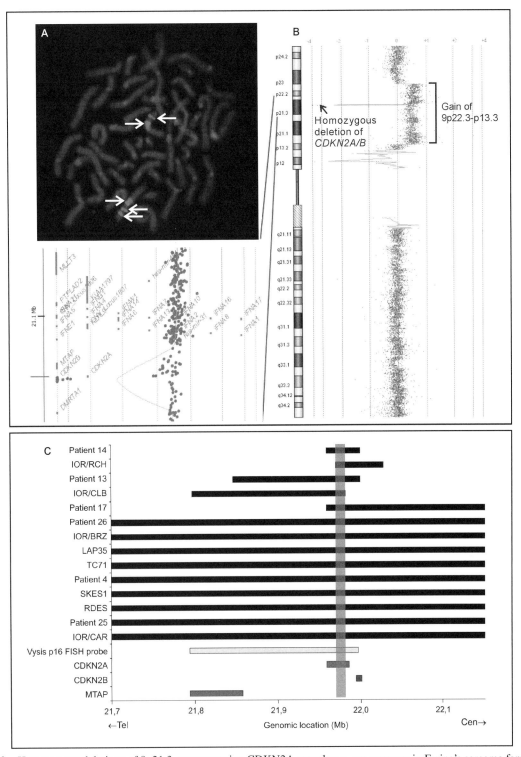

FIGURE 11.2 Homozygous deletions of 9p21.3, encompassing CDKN2A gene locus, are common in Ewing's sarcoma family of tumors. Homozygous 9p21.3 deletions, harboring *CDKN2A* locus coding for p16 and p14 tumor suppressor proteins, are frequent in the Ewing's sarcoma patient and cell line samples. Inactivation of *CDKN2A* by deletions, point mutations or by promoter methylation is also a common and early event in other bone tumors like chondrosarcoma, osteosarcoma and chordoma. (A) Narrowest microdeletions (<190 kb) in 9p21.3 can create false negative results by using commercial FISH probes, as shown in FISH analysis on Ewing's sarcoma cell lines (IOR/RCH). FISH results show that one *CDKN2A* locus is gained as indicated by three red signals (arrows to left) in the sample. For experimental details see Ref. [107]. (B) Array CGH analysis with high-resolution oligo-microarray (244,000 probes) on the same IOR/RCH Ewing's sarcoma cell line shows that within the gain of 9p22.3-p13.3, there is a homozygous deletion of 9p21.3. The size of homozygous deletion is 58 kb and it harbors only genes *CDKN2A* and *CDKN2B*. (C) Genomic locations of 9p deletions in Ewing's sarcoma patients and cell line samples arranged by their size. Genes *CDKN2A* (yellow), *CDKN2B* (red) and *MTAP* (green), their sizes and locations are also indicated in the figure. The smallest overlapping region of deletion (12,2 kb), which is indicated by purple bar, is much smaller than the size of the most commonly used commercial FISH probe (Vysis p16 FISH probe). This commercial FISH probe is ~190 kb in size and it covers genes *CDKN2A*, *CDKN2B* and *MTAP*, explaining the false negative results seen in FISH analysis (see A). (A) and (B) reproduced from *Cytogenetic Genome Research* (2007), **119**, 21–26, by permission of S. Karger AG, Basel.

Chordomas are notochordal tumors, which can be described by near-diploid but complex karyotypes with several structural and numerical aberrations. However, no consistent or tumor specific cytogenetic abnormality has been detected. Characteristic chromosomal changes are primarily losses of whole chromosomes or chromosome arms, including losses of 1p, 3, 9p, 10, 22, but also gains of 1q, 7q and 19 were detected [22,113,114]. High-level amplifications are not detected, but *CDKN2A/B* loci was homozygously or heterozygously deleted in 70% of tumors, suggesting that p16 pathway is pivotal for the pathogenesis of chordomas [114].

Adamantinoma of long bones is a rare tumor, which closely resembles osteofibrous dysplasia. Cytogenetic analysis has shown recurrent numerical chromosome imbalances, predominantly trisomies of chromosomes 7, 8, 12, 19 and 21 [115,116].

Fibrous dysplasia of bones is a benign neoplasm, which is caused by activating mutations of *GNAS* (20q13.3) [117]. Clonal chromosomal aberrations have been reported in 12p13 (structural) and chromosome 2 (trisomy) [118,119].

IV. GENETIC ALTERATIONS IN BONE TUMOR DIAGNOSTICS

Of all the different types of bone tumors, only the Ewing's sarcoma family of tumors has shown tumor specific translocations that can be efficiently used in molecular and differential diagnostics (see Figure 11.3). In the case of a Ewing's sarcoma, *EWS*-gene is translocated to a member of *ETS* gene family creating a chimeric fusion gene, which leads to transcriptional deregulation and aberrant signaling [90]. These gene fusions can serve as powerful diagnostic markers and also monitor residual disease, because they can be easily detected by FISH or RT-PCR techniques [2,120]. Unlike the Ewing's sarcoma family of tumors, most malignant bone tumors do not have specific translocations, but instead they can have complex, sometimes even chaotic, karyotypes. This poses a true challenge for their differential diagnosis. An example of this kind is high-grade chondrosarcoma, which is often characterized by chromosomal instability resulting in gains and losses, telomere dysfunction and alterations in cell-cycle genes. Bone tumors, which have no tumor specific translocations, can have nonreciprocal and non-specific translocations often causing gene copy number changes; but the tumor specific genetic aberration remains to be discovered in most bone tumors. However, chromosomal imbalances seem to be diagnostically and prognostically important as shown, e.g., in chondrosarcoma [39], osteosarcoma [74], Ewing's sarcoma [102,103,105] and in giant cell-tumors of bone [111]. By using CGH, FISH or array CGH techniques, chromosomal imbalances can be used in differential diagnosis of these bone tumors and to better define treatment protocols and optimize clinical management of patients.

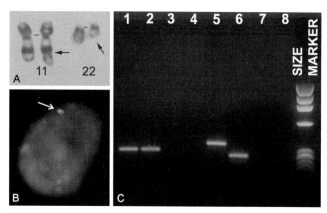

FIGURE 11.3 EWSR1-FLI1 translocation in Ewing's sarcoma family of tumors can be detected by (A) G-banding, (B) FISH or by (C) RT-PCR. (A) Conventional karyotype analysis on Ewing's sarcoma patient sample shows a translocation between chromosomes 11 and 22 (indicated by arrows). (B) *EWSR1-FLI1* translocation detection with fusion signal FISH analysis. In fusion FISH strategy a red probe flanks one breakpoint and the other green probe flanks the other breakpoint. If the signals are brought together by translocation, the fusion signal is yellow. The fusion signal is indicated by a white arrow here. (C) RT-PCR analysis on Ewing's sarcoma patient samples shows an *EWSR1-FLI1* gene fusion on gel lanes 1, 2, 5 and 6. *EWSR1-FLI1* type 1 fusion (328 bp) is detected on gel lines 1 and 2. Samples 5 and 6 show variant *EWSR1-FLI1* gene fusion types. Samples on lines 3, 4, 7 and 8 are negative for *EWSR1-FLI1* fusions. (A) and (C) are reproduced from *Current Diagnostic Pathology* (2002) 8, 338–348, by permission of Elsevier Ltd.

V. NOVEL APPROACHES FOR BONE TUMOR GENETICS AND BEYOND

Advances in DNA sequencing techniques, together with the growing amount of available human genome sequencing data, have enabled further studies into the cancer genome in ultra high resolution. Massively parallel paired-end sequencing methods can gather simultaneously high resolution data from point mutations, copy number changes and chromosomal rearrangements at base-pair level in the cancer genome of interest [121]. *A priori* knowledge of target mutations and chromosomal imbalances is not needed for performing this analysis. Previously unrecognized fusion genes and other rearrangements, which are implicated in the tumorigenesis of bone tumors, could be identified with this method and used in differential diagnosis as future therapeutic targets.

Since the discovery of the first microRNAs in *C. elegans* [122,123] and miRNA the field has expanded outstandingly and, at the moment, 695 miRNA sequences in human genomes have been annotated in miRBase (http://microrna. sanger.ac.uk). MicroRNAs have been shown to play an important role in various cell functions including cell fate determination, proliferation and apoptosis. In addition, they are aberrantly expressed in a variety of tumor types, including sarcomas, and contribute to various steps in tumor progression (e.g. angiogenesis, invasion and metastasis) [124]. In a study by Subramanian *et al.*, miRNA expression profiles of 27 sarcoma samples were analyzed by microarray and small RNA sequencing methods [125]. The miRNA expression signatures clearly differed between tumor types analyzed and, most interestingly, miRNA expression signatures suggested that initial diagnosis of two sarcomas was incorrect, which was further confirmed by histopathologic and molecular analysis [125]. This highlights the potential of using miRNAs as a diagnostic tool in differential diagnosis and in pinpointing novel genetic markers in bone tumors, since miRNA expression signatures reflect tumor origin and other clinical variables [124].

Epigenetic changes—including hypomethylation, hypermethylation, loss of imprinting and chromatin modifications—are fundamentally linked to the development of cancer, leading to, e.g., deregulation of gene expression, chromosomal instability, loss of apoptosis and production of spontaneous mutations in cancer cells [126,127]. Epigenetic changes are reversible, since they do not alter the DNA sequence. Instead, they are heritable, since they are inherited from the dividing mother to daughter cells. Methylation profiles of two osteosarcoma cell lines were studied by combining methylation-, CGH- and expression arrays. This analysis identified several genes that had aberrant DNA methylation pattern and also that some oncogenes, like *MYC*, were both hypomethylated, gained and overexpressed in osteosarcoma [128]. Another study deciphered genomic imprinting events in the transformation process of osteosarcoma and the results suggested that epigenetic changes are one of the earliest events in the neoplastic progression of bone [129]. By studying promoter hypermethylation of several genes associated with carcinogenesis, osteosarcoma patient samples were shown to harbor significantly higher levels of hypermethylation in comparison to normal tissue. In addition, metastatic tumors had higher degrees of hypermethylation than non-metastatic tumors, implying that hypermethylation could be exploited in a prognostic sense using it as a biomarker in predicting patient outcome [130]. Epigenetic changes in other bone tumors remain to be investigated in order to validate these results in bone tumors generally.

Development in molecular genetics with high-throughput applications has revolutionized bone tumor research. However, it should be noted that aberrations in genome or transcriptome are not invariably able to explain the whole picture of neoplastic development and tumorigenesis in bone. Changes that are post-translational, e.g. modifications in protein phosphorylation or degradation, are also characteristic of tumor cells. Global protein expression of bone tumors with two-dimensional difference gel electrophoresis (2D-DIGE) and mass spectrometry has been used to untangle the tumor biology behind this phenomenon [131]. This approach can provide information on novel biomarkers and therapeutic targets in different bone tumors, which cannot be discovered using merely genetic methods. Furthermore, integration of genomic, transcriptomic, epigenomic and proteomic studies can provide us with novel and more thorough insights into the etiology of bone tumors.

VI. CONCLUSIONS AND PERSPECTIVES

Genetic changes are detected in most bone tumors and these rearrangements are recognized as playing a pathogenic role in an increasing number of bone tumors. Cytogenetic and molecular genetic changes have also refined and clarified the classification of bone tumors. Moreover, some of these genetic imbalances have shown to be clinically and prognostically relevant. However, especially in malignant bone tumors, there is a need for a wider and better knowledge of genetic changes on the whole genome scale, since most of these tumors lack a recurrent and specific genetic rearrangement that could be used as a biomarker in the diagnostic or prognostic sense. Since a remarkable share of bone tumor patients—particularly with osteosarcoma and Ewing's sarcoma—are children, continuous research is especially significant for this group of pediatric patients. Therefore, screening for genomic rearrangements is a fundamental task in finding novel biomarkers in malignant bone tumors for more accurate diagnosis, prognostication and, most importantly, in identifying targets for novel therapeutic approaches. New molecular genetic techniques with higher resolutions, specificity and accuracy continue to emerge and these new techniques may prove useful both in bone tumor research and clinical diagnostics. Genome-wide analysis of aberrations in gene expression, copy number, miRNA expression and methylation in array-based or other high-throughput applications holds great promise for understanding the underlying events in neoplastic development of bone tumors. However, due to the complexity of these alterations in cancer cells, it is extremely demanding to recognize the key events leading to tumorigenesis. Additionally, the effect of polymorphisms and structural variation in the genome for susceptibility to bone tumors remains to be untangled in this entity. It therefore appears that extensive research is still needed to elucidate the complete picture of the genetic changes and molecular pathways leading to the development of bone tumors, to confirm these results in the context of model organisms and to unravel their functional relevance.

References

1. L.A.G. Ries, D. Melbert & M. Krapcho, et al., SEER Cancer Statistics Review (2007) 1975–2005.
2. H. Vauhkonen, S. Savola & S. Kaur, et al., Molecular karyotyping in sarcoma diagnostics and research, Adv Exp Med Biol 587 (2006) 53–63.
3. A. Kallioniemi, O.P. Kallioniemi & D. Sudar, et al., Comparative genomic hybridization for molecular cytogenetic analysis of solid tumors, Science 258 (1992) 818–821.

4. D. Pinkel, R. Segraves & D. Sudar, et al., High resolution analysis of DNA copy number variation using comparative genomic hybridization to microarrays, Nat Genet 20 (1998) 207–211.

5. A. Kallioniemi, CGH microarrays and cancer, Curr Opin Biotechnol 19 (2008) 36–40.

6. K. Baird, S. Davis & C.R. Antonescu, et al., Gene expression profiling of human sarcomas: insights into sarcoma biology, Cancer Res 65 (2005) 9226–9235.

7. K. Tschoep, A. Kohlmann & M. Schlemmer, et al., Gene expression profiling in sarcomas, Crit Rev Oncol Hematol 63 (2007) 111–124.

8. C. Khanna, J. Khan & P. Nguyen, et al., Metastasis-associated differences in gene expression in a murine model of osteosarcoma, Cancer Res 61 (2001) 3750–3759.

9. K. Ochi, Y. Daigo & T. Katagiri, et al., Prediction of response to neoadjuvant chemotherapy for osteosarcoma by gene-expression profiles, Int J Oncol 24 (2004) 647–655.

10. A. Ohali, S. Avigad & R. Zaizov, et al., Prediction of high risk Ewing's sarcoma by gene expression profiling, Oncogene 23 (2004) 8997–9006.

11. C.D.M. Flecher, K. Unni & F. Mertens, World Health Organization Classification of Tumors, Pathology & Genetics of Tumours of Soft Tissue and Bone (2002) 430.

12. F. Mertens, A. Rydholm & A. Kreicbergs, et al., Loss of chromosome band 8q24 in sporadic osteocartilaginous exostoses, Genes Chromosomes Cancer 9 (1994) 8–12.

13. J.A. Bridge, M. Nelson & C. Orndal, et al., Clonal karyotypic abnormalities of the hereditary multiple exostoses chromosomal loci 8q24.1 (EXT1) and 11p11-12 (EXT2) in patients with sporadic and hereditary osteochondromas, Cancer 82 (1998) 1657–1663.

14. M.G. Feely, A.K. Boehm & R.S. Bridge, et al., Cytogenetic and molecular cytogenetic evidence of recurrent 8q24.1 loss in osteochondroma, Cancer Genet Cytogenet 137 (2002) 102–107.

15. J.R. Sawyer, E.L. Thomas & J.L. Lukacs, et al., Recurring breakpoints of 1p13 approximately p22 in osteochondroma, Cancer Genet Cytogenet 138 (2002) 102–106.

16. A. Cook, W. Raskind & S.H. Blanton, et al., Genetic heterogeneity in families with hereditary multiple exostoses, Am J Hum Genet 53 (1993) 71–79.

17. Y.Q. Wu, P. Heutink & B.B. de Vries, et al., Assignment of a second locus for multiple exostoses to the pericentromeric region of chromosome 11, Hum Mol Genet 3 (1994) 167–171.

18. M. Le Merrer, L. Legeai-Mallet & P.M. Jeannin, et al., A gene for hereditary multiple exostoses maps to chromosome 19p, Hum Mol Genet 3 (1994) 717–722.

19. J.V. Bovee, A.M. Cleton-Jansen & A.H. Taminiau, et al., Emerging pathways in the development of chondrosarcoma of bone and implications for targeted treatment, Lancet Oncol 6 (2005) 599–607.

20. J.A. Bridge, D.L. Persons & J.R. Neff, et al., Clonal karyotypic aberrations in enchondromas, Cancer Detect Prev 16 (1992) 215–219.

21. N. Mandahl, H. Willen & A. Rydholm, et al., Rearrangement of band q13 on both chromosomes 12 in a periosteal chondroma, Genes Chromosomes Cancer 6 (1993) 121–123.

22. G. Tallini, H. Dorfman & P. Brys, et al., Correlation between clinicopathological features and karyotype in 100 cartilaginous and chordoid tumours. A report from the Chromosomes and Morphology (CHAMP) Collaborative Study Group, J Pathol 196 (2002) 194–203.

23. E.P. Buddingh, S. Naumann & M. Nelson, et al., Cytogenetic findings in benign cartilaginous neoplasms, Cancer Genet Cytogenet 141 (2003) 164–168.

24. A. Dahlen, F. Mertens & A. Rydholm, et al., Fusion, disruption, and expression of HMGA2 in bone and soft tissue chondromas, Mod Pathol 16 (2003) 1132–1140.

25. S. Hopyan, N. Gokgoz & R. Poon, et al., A mutant PTH/PTHrP type I receptor in enchondromatosis, Nat Genet 30 (2002) 306–310.

26. L.B. Rozeman, L. Sangiorgi & I.H. Briaire-deBruijn, et al., Enchondromatosis (Ollier disease, Maffucci syndrome) is not caused by the PTHR1 mutation p.R150C, Hum Mutat 24 (2004) 466–473.

27. L.B. Rozeman, L. Hameetman & A.M. Cleton-Jansen, et al., Absence of IHH and retention of PTHrP signalling in enchondromas and central chondrosarcomas, J Pathol 205 (2005) 476–482.

28. A. Couvineau, V. Wouters & G. Bertrand, et al., PTHR1 mutations associated with Ollier disease result in receptor loss of function, Hum Mol Genet 17 (2008) 2766–2775.

29. H. Sjogren, C. Orndal & O. Tingby, et al., Cytogenetic and spectral karyotype analyses of benign and malignant cartilage tumours, Int J Oncol 24 (2004) 1385–1391.

30. S.J. Swarts, J.R. Neff & S.L. Johansson, et al., Significance of abnormalities of chromosomes 5 and 8 in chondroblastoma, Clin Orthop Relat Res (349) (1998) 189–193.

31. S.L. van Zelderen-Bhola, J.V. Bovee & H.W. Wessels, et al., Ring chromosome 4 as the sole cytogenetic anomaly in a chondroblastoma: a case report and review of the literature, Cancer Genet Cytogenet 105 (1998) 109–112.

32. S.R. Granter, A.A. Renshaw & H.P. Kozakewich, et al., The pericentromeric inversion, inv (6)(p25q13), is a novel diagnostic marker in chondromyxoid fibroma, Mod Pathol 11 (1998) 1071–1074.

33. A.R. Halbert, W.R. Harrison & M.J. Hicks, et al., Cytogenetic analysis of a scapular chondromyxoid fibroma, Cancer Genet Cytogenet 104 (1998) 52–56.

34. J.R. Sawyer, C.M. Swanson & J.L. Lukacs, et al., Evidence of an association between 6q13-21 chromosome aberrations and locally aggressive behavior in patients with cartilage tumors, Cancer 82 (1998) 474–483.

35. A. Safar, M. Nelson & J.R. Neff, et al., Recurrent anomalies of 6q25 in chondromyxoid fibroma, Hum Pathol 31 (2000) 306–311.

36. J.V. Bovee, A.M. Cleton-Jansen & N.J. Kuipers-Dijkshoorn, et al., Loss of heterozygosity and DNA ploidy point to a diverging genetic mechanism in the origin of peripheral and central chondrosarcoma, Genes Chromosomes Cancer 26 (1999) 237–246.

37. J.V. Bovee, A.M. Cleton-Jansen & W. Wuyts, et al., EXT-mutation analysis and loss of heterozygosity in sporadic and hereditary osteochondromas and secondary chondrosarcomas, Am J Hum Genet 65 (1999) 689–698.

38. M.L. Larramendy, M. Tarkkanen & J. Valle, et al., Gains, losses, and amplifications of DNA sequences evaluated by comparative genomic hybridization in chondrosarcomas, Am J Pathol 150 (1997) 685–691.

39. N. Mandahl, P. Gustafson & F. Mertens, et al., Cytogenetic aberrations and their prognostic impact in chondrosarcoma, Genes Chromosomes Cancer 33 (2002) 188–200.
40. L.B. Rozeman, K. Szuhai & Y.M. Schrage, et al., Array-comparative genomic hybridization of central chondrosarcoma: identification of ribosomal protein S6 and cyclin-dependent kinase 4 as candidate target genes for genomic aberrations, Cancer 107 (2006) 380–388.
41. J.A. Bridge, P.S. Bhatia & J.R. Anderson, et al., Biologic and clinical significance of cytogenetic and molecular cytogenetic abnormalities in benign and malignant cartilaginous lesions, Cancer Genet Cytogenet 69 (1993) 79–90.
42. M. Tarkkanen, A. Kaipainen & E. Karaharju, et al., Cytogenetic study of 249 consecutive patients examined for a bone tumor, Cancer Genet Cytogenet 68 (1993) 1–21.
43. J. Asp, L. Sangiorgi & S.E. Inerot, et al., Changes of the p16 gene but not the p53 gene in human chondrosarcoma tissues, Int J Cancer 85 (2000) 782–786.
44. C. Morrison, M. Radmacher & N. Mohammed, et al., MYC amplification and polysomy 8 in chondrosarcoma: array comparative genomic hybridization, fluorescent in situ hybridization, and association with outcome, J Clin Oncol 23 (2005) 9369–9376.
45. F.Y. Lee, H.J. Mankin & G. Fondren, et al., Chondrosarcoma of bone: an assessment of outcome, J Bone Joint Surg Am 81 (1999) 326–338.
46. S. Boeuf, P. Kunz, T. Hennig, B. Lehner, P. Hogendoorn, J. Bovee & W. Richter, A chondrogenic gene expression signature in mesenchymal stem cells is a classifier of conventional central chondrosarcoma, J. Pathol. 216 (2008) 158–166.
47. J.V. Bovee, R. Sciot & P.D. Cin, et al., Chromosome 9 alterations and trisomy 22 in central chondrosarcoma: a cytogenetic and DNA flow cytometric analysis of chondrosarcoma subtypes, Diagn Mol Pathol 10 (2001) 228–235.
48. J. Asp, S. Inerot & J.A. Block, et al., Alterations in the regulatory pathway involving p16, pRb and cdk4 in human chondrosarcoma, J Orthop Res 19 (2001) 149–154.
49. H.M. van Beerendonk, L.B. Rozeman & A.H. Taminiau, et al., Molecular analysis of the INK4A/INK4A-ARF gene locus in conventional (central) chondrosarcomas and enchondromas: indication of an important gene for tumour progression, J Pathol 202 (2004) 359–366.
50. Y.M. Schrage, S. Lam, A.G. Jochemsen, et al., Central chondrosarcoma progression is associated with pRb pathway alterations; CDK4 downregulation and p16 overexpression inhibit cell growth in vitro, J Cell Mol Med (2008) (Epub ahead of print).
51. M. Tarkkanen, T. Wiklund & M. Virolainen, et al., Dedifferentiated chondrosarcoma with t(9;22)(q34;q11-12), Genes Chromosomes Cancer 9 (1994) 136–140.
52. S.J. Swarts, J.R. Neff & S.L. Johansson, et al., Cytogenetic analysis of dedifferentiated chondrosarcoma, Cancer Genet Cytogenet 89 (1996) 49–51.
53. M. Ropke, C. Boltze & H.W. Neumann, et al., Genetic and epigenetic alterations in tumor progression in a dedifferentiated chondrosarcoma, Pathol Res Pract 199 (2003) 437–444.
54. L. Sainati, A. Scapinello & A. Montaldi, et al., A mesenchymal chondrosarcoma of a child with the reciprocal translocation (11;22)(q24;q12), Cancer Genet Cytogenet 71 (1993) 144–147.
55. S. Naumann, P.A. Krallman & K.K. Unni, et al., Translocation der(13;21)(q10;q10) in skeletal and extraskeletal mesenchymal chondrosarcoma, Mod Pathol 15 (2002) 572–576.
56. C. Sreekantaiah, S.P. Leong & J.R. Davis, et al., Cytogenetic and flow cytometric analysis of a clear cell chondrosarcoma, Cancer Genet Cytogenet 52 (1991) 193–199.
57. J. Nishio, J.D. Reith & A. Ogose, et al., Cytogenetic findings in clear cell chondrosarcoma, Cancer Genet Cytogenet 162 (2005) 74–77.
58. J. Clark, H. Benjamin & S. Gill, et al., Fusion of the EWS gene to CHN, a member of the steroid/thyroid receptor gene superfamily, in a human myxoid chondrosarcoma, Oncogene 12 (1996) 229–235.
59. H. Sjogren, J.M. Meis-Kindblom & C. Orndal, et al., Studies on the molecular pathogenesis of extraskeletal myxoid chondrosarcoma-cytogenetic, molecular genetic, and cDNA microarray analyses, Am J Pathol 162 (2003) 781–792.
60. M. Hisaoka, T. Ishida & T. Imamura, et al., TFG is a novel fusion partner of NOR1 in extraskeletal myxoid chondrosarcoma, Genes Chromosomes Cancer 40 (2004) 325–328.
61. K. Radig, R. Schneider-Stock & U. Mittler, et al., Genetic instability in osteoblastic tumors of the skeletal system, Pathol Res Pract 194 (1998) 669–677.
62. J.T. Mascarello, H.F. Krous & P.M. Carpenter, Unbalanced translocation resulting in the loss of the chromosome 17 short arm in an osteoblastoma, Cancer Genet Cytogenet 69 (1993) 65–67.
63. E. Kunze, A. Enderle & K. Radig, et al., Aggressive osteoblastoma with focal malignant transformation and development of pulmonary metastases. A case report with a review of literature, Gen Diagn Pathol 141 (1996) 377–392.
64. A.C. Baker, L. Rezeanu, M.J. Klein, et al., aggressive osteoblastoma: a case report involving a unique chromosomal aberration, Int J Surg Pathol July 8, (2008) (Epub ahead of print).
65. J.A. Biegel, R.B. Womer & B.S. Emanuel, Complex karyotypes in a series of pediatric osteosarcomas, Cancer Genet Cytogenet 38 (1989) 89–100.
66. F. Mertens, N. Mandahl & C. Orndal, et al., Cytogenetic findings in 33 osteosarcomas, Int J Cancer 55 (1993) 44–50.
67. J.A. Fletcher, M.C. Gebhardt & H.P. Kozakewich, Cytogenetic aberrations in osteosarcomas. Nonrandom deletions, rings, and double-minute chromosomes, Cancer Genet Cytogenet 77 (1994) 81–88.
68. J.A. Bridge, M. Nelson & E. McComb, et al., Cytogenetic findings in 73 osteosarcoma specimens and a review of the literature, Cancer Genet Cytogenet 95 (1997) 74–87.
69. T.K. Man, X.Y. Lu & K. Jaeweon, et al., Genome-wide array comparative genomic hybridization analysis reveals distinct amplifications in osteosarcoma, BMC Cancer 4 (2004) 45.
70. J. Atiye, M. Wolf & S. Kaur, et al., Gene amplifications in osteosarcoma-CGH microarray analysis, Genes Chromosomes Cancer 42 (2005) 158–163.
71. S. Selvarajah, M. Yoshimoto & O. Ludkovski, et al., Genomic signatures of chromosomal instability and osteosarcoma progression detected by high resolution array CGH and interphase FISH, Cytogenet Genome Res 122 (2008) 5–15.
72. A. Forus, D.O. Weghuis & D. Smeets, et al., Comparative genomic hybridization analysis of human sarcomas: II. Identification of novel amplicons at 6p and 17p in osteosarcomas, Genes Chromosomes Cancer 14 (1995) 15–21.

73. X.Y. Lu, Y. Lu & Y.J. Zhao, et al., Cell cycle regulator gene CDC5L, a potential target for 6p12-p21 amplicon in osteosarcoma, Mol Cancer Res 6 (2008) 937–946.

74. M. Tarkkanen, I. Elomaa & C. Blomqvist, et al., DNA sequence copy number increase at 8q: a potential new prognostic marker in high-grade osteosarcoma, Int J Cancer 84 (1999) 114–121.

75. C.W. Miller, A. Aslo & C. Tsay, et al., Frequency and structure of p53 rearrangements in human osteosarcoma, Cancer Res 50 (1990) 7950–7954.

76. M.S. Benassi, L. Molendini & G. Gamberi, et al., Alteration of pRb/p16/cdk4 regulation in human osteosarcoma, Int J Cancer 84 (1999) 489–493.

77. G.P. Nielsen, K.L. Burns & A.E. Rosenberg, et al., CDKN2A gene deletions and loss of p16 expression occur in osteosarcomas that lack RB alterations, Am J Pathol 153 (1998) 159–163.

78. R. Noguera, S. Navarro & T.J. Triche, Translocation (11;22) in small cell osteosarcoma, Cancer Genet Cytogenet 45 (1990) 121–124.

79. J. Nishio, J.D. Gentry & J.R. Neff, et al., Monoallelic deletion of the p53 gene through chromosomal translocation in a small cell osteosarcoma, Virchows Arch 448 (2006) 852–856.

80. H.R. Park, W.W. Jung & F. Bertoni, et al., Molecular analysis of p53, MDM2 and H-ras genes in low-grade central osteosarcoma, Pathol Res Pract 200 (2004) 439–445.

81. M. Tarkkanen, T. Bohling & G. Gamberi, et al., Comparative genomic hybridization of low-grade central osteosarcoma, Mod Pathol 11 (1998) 421–426.

82. P. Ragazzini, G. Gamberi & M.S. Benassi, et al., Analysis of SAS gene and CDK4 and MDM2 proteins in low-grade osteosarcoma, Cancer Detect Prev 23 (1999) 129–136.

83. J.F. Sinovic, J.A. Bridge & J.R. Neff, Ring chromosome in parosteal osteosarcoma. Clinical and diagnostic significance, Cancer Genet Cytogenet 62 (1992) 50–52.

84. J. Szymanska, N. Mandahl & F. Mertens, et al., Ring chromosomes in parosteal osteosarcoma contain sequences from 12q13-15: a combined cytogenetic and comparative genomic hybridization study, Genes Chromosomes Cancer 16 (1996) 31–34.

85. J.S. Wunder, K. Eppert & S.R. Burrow, et al., Co-amplification and overexpression of CDK4, SAS and MDM2 occurs frequently in human parosteal osteosarcomas, Oncogene 18 (1999) 783–788.

86. C.M. Hattinger, M. Tarkkanen & S. Benini, et al., Genetic analysis of fibrosarcoma of bone, a rare tumour entity closely related to osteosarcoma and malignant fibrous histiocytoma of bone, Eur J Cell Biol 83 (2004) 483–491.

87. K.H. Hallor, M. Heidenblad & O. Brosjo, et al., Tiling resolution array comparative genomic hybridization analysis of a fibrosarcoma of bone, Cancer Genet Cytogenet 172 (2007) 80–83.

88. M. Tarkkanen, M.L. Larramendy & T. Bohling, et al., Malignant fibrous histiocytoma of bone: analysis of genomic imbalances by comparative genomic hybridisation and C-MYC expression by immunohistochemistry, Eur J Cancer 42 (2006) 1172–1180.

89. H. Taubert, D. Berger & R. Hinze, et al., How is the mutational status for tumor suppressors p53 and p16(INK4A) in MFH of the bone?, Cancer Lett 123 (1998) 147–151.

90. O. Delattre, J. Zucman & B. Plougastel, et al., Gene fusion with an ETS DNA-binding domain caused by chromosome translocation in human tumours, Nature 359 (1992) 162–165.

91. J. Zucman, T. Melot & C. Desmaze, et al., Combinatorial generation of variable fusion proteins in the Ewing family of tumours, EMBO J 12 (1993) 4481–4487.

92. I.S. Jeon, J.N. Davis & B.S. Braun, et al., A variant Ewing's sarcoma translocation (7;22) fuses the EWS gene to the ETS gene ETV1, Oncogene 10 (1995) 1229–1234.

93. Y. Kaneko, K. Yoshida & M. Handa, et al., Fusion of an ETS-family gene, EIAF, to EWS by t(17;22)(q12;q12) chromosome translocation in an undifferentiated sarcoma of infancy, Genes Chromosomes Cancer 15 (1996) 115–121.

94. M. Peter, J. Couturier & H. Pacquement, et al., A new member of the ETS family fused to EWS in Ewing tumors, Oncogene 14 (1997) 1159–1164.

95. T. Mastrangelo, P. Modena & S. Tornielli, et al., A novel zinc finger gene is fused to EWS in small round cell tumor, Oncogene 19 (2000) 3799–3804.

96. D.C. Shing, D.J. McMullan & P. Roberts, et al., FUS/ERG gene fusions in Ewing's tumors, Cancer Res 63 (2003) 4568–4576.

97. E. de Alava, A. Kawai & J.H. Healey, et al., EWS-FLI1 fusion transcript structure is an independent determinant of prognosis in Ewing's sarcoma, J Clin Oncol 16 (1998) 1248–1255.

98. G. Armengol, M. Tarkkanen & M. Virolainen, et al., Recurrent gains of 1q, 8 and 12 in the Ewing family of tumours by comparative genomic hybridization, Br J Cancer 75 (1997) 1403–1409.

99. T. Ozaki, M. Paulussen & C. Poremba, et al., Genetic imbalances revealed by comparative genomic hybridization in Ewing tumors, Genes Chromosomes Cancer 32 (2001) 164–171.

100. B.I. Ferreira, J. Alonso & J. Carrillo, et al., Array CGH and gene-expression profiling reveals distinct genomic instability patterns associated with DNA repair and cell-cycle checkpoint pathways in Ewing's sarcoma, Oncogene 27 (2007) 2084–2090.

101. A.A. Sandberg & J.A. Bridge, Updates on cytogenetics and molecular genetics of bone and soft tissue tumors: Ewing sarcoma and peripheral primitive neuroectodermal tumors, Cancer Genet Cytogenet 123 (2000) 1–26.

102. M. Zielenska, Z.M. Zhang & K. Ng, et al., Acquisition of secondary structural chromosomal changes in pediatric Ewing sarcoma is a probable prognostic factor for tumor response and clinical outcome, Cancer 91 (2001) 2156–2164.

103. C.M. Hattinger, S. Rumpler & S. Strehl, et al., Prognostic impact of deletions at 1p36 and numerical aberrations in Ewing tumors, Genes Chromosomes Cancer 24 (1999) 243–254.

104. C.M. Hattinger, U. Potschger & M. Tarkkanen, et al., Prognostic impact of chromosomal aberrations in Ewing tumours, Br J Cancer 86 (2002) 1763–1769.

105. H.Y. Huang, P.B. Illei & Z. Zhao, et al., Ewing sarcomas with p53 mutation or p16/p14ARF homozygous deletion: a highly lethal subset associated with poor chemoresponse, J Clin Oncol 23 (2005) 548–558.

106. J.A. Lopez-Guerrero, A. Pellin & R. Noguera, et al., Molecular analysis of the 9p21 locus and p53 genes in Ewing family tumors, Lab Invest 81 (2001) 803–814.

107. S. Savola, F. Nardi & K. Scotlandi, et al., Microdeletions in 9p21.3 induce false negative results in CDKN2A FISH analysis of Ewing sarcoma, Cytogenet Genome Res 119 (2007) 21–26.

108. H.S. Schwartz, R.B. Jenkins & R.J. Dahl, et al., Cytogenetic analyses on giant-cell tumors of bone, Clin Orthop Relat Res 240 (1989) 250–260.

109. J.R. Sawyer, L.S. Goosen & R.L. Binz, et al., Evidence for telomeric fusions as a mechanism for recurring structural aberrations of chromosome 11 in giant cell tumor of bone, Cancer Genet Cytogenet 159 (2005) 32–36.

110. J.A. Bridge, J.R. Neff & B.J. Mouron, Giant cell tumor of bone. Chromosomal analysis of 48 specimens and review of the literature, Cancer Genet Cytogenet 58 (1992) 2–13.

111. L.T. Smith, J. Mayerson & N.J. Nowak, et al., 20q11.1 amplification in giant-cell tumor of bone: array CGH, FISH, and association with outcome, Genes Chromosomes Cancer 45 (2006) 957–966.

112. R.G. Forsyth, G. De Boeck & S. Bekaert, et al., Telomere biology in giant cell tumour of bone, J Pathol 214 (2008) 555–563.

113. S. Scheil, S. Bruderlein & T. Liehr, et al., Genome-wide analysis of sixteen chordomas by comparative genomic hybridization and cytogenetics of the first human chordoma cell line, U-CH1, Genes Chromosomes Cancer 32 (2001) 203–211.

114. K.H. Hallor, J. Staaf & G. Jonsson, et al., Frequent deletion of the CDKN2A locus in chordoma: analysis of chromosomal imbalances using array comparative genomic hybridisation, Br J Cancer 98 (2008) 434–442.

115. H.M. Hazelbag, J.W. Wessels & P. Mollevangers, et al., Cytogenetic analysis of adamantinoma of long bones: further indications for a common histogenesis with osteofibrous dysplasia, Cancer Genet Cytogenet 97 (1997) 5–11.

116. M. Kanamori, C.R. Antonescu & M. Scott, et al., Extra copies of chromosomes 7, 8, 12, 19, and 21 are recurrent in adamantinoma, J Mol Diagn 3 (2001) 16–21.

117. L.S. Weinstein, A. Shenker & P.V. Gejman, et al., Activating mutations of the stimulatory G protein in the McCune-Albright syndrome, N Engl J Med 325 (1991) 1688–1695.

118. P. Dal Cin, R. Sciot & F. Speleman, et al., Chromosome aberrations in fibrous dysplasia, Cancer Genet Cytogenet 77 (1994) 114–117.

119. P. Dal Cin, R. Sciot & P. Brys, et al., Recurrent chromosome aberrations in fibrous dysplasia of the bone: a report of the CHAMP study group. Chromosomes and morphology, Cancer Genet Cytogenet 122 (2000) 30–32.

120. S. Knuutila, Cytogenetics and molecular pathology in cancer diagnostics, Ann Med 36 (2004) 162–171.

121. P.J. Campbell, P.J. Stephens & E.D. Pleasance, et al., Identification of somatically acquired rearrangements in cancer using genome-wide massively parallel paired-end sequencing, Nat Genet 40 (2008) 722–729.

122. R.C. Lee, R.L. Feinbaum & V. Ambros, The C. elegans heterochronic gene lin-4 encodes small RNAs with antisense complementarity to lin-14, Cell 75 (1993) 843–854.

123. B. Wightman, I. Ha & G. Ruvkun, Posttranscriptional regulation of the heterochronic gene lin-14 by lin-4 mediates temporal pattern formation in C. elegans, Cell 75 (1993) 855–862.

124. Y.S. Lee, & A. Dutta, MicroRNAs in cancer. Annu Rev Pathol (2008) (Epub ahead of print)

125. S. Subramanian, W.O. Lui & C.H. Lee, et al., MicroRNA expression signature of human sarcomas, Oncogene 27 (2008) 2015–2026.

126. M. Esteller & J.G. Herman, Cancer as an epigenetic disease: DNA methylation and chromatin alterations in human tumours, J Pathol 196 (2002) 1–7.

127. M. Esteller, Cancer epigenomics: DNA methylomes and histone-modification maps, Nat Rev Genet 8 (2007) 286–298.

128. B. Sadikovic, M. Yoshimoto & K. Al-Romaih, et al., *In vitro* analysis of integrated global high-resolution DNA methylation profiling with genomic imbalance and gene expression in osteosarcoma, PLoS ONE 3 (2008) e2834.

129. Y. Li, G. Meng & Q.N. Guo, Changes in genomic imprinting and gene expression associated with transformation in a model of human osteosarcoma, Exp Mol Pathol 84 (2008) 234–239.

130. P. Hou, M. Ji & B. Yang, et al., Quantitative analysis of promoter hypermethylation in multiple genes in osteosarcoma, Cancer 106 (2006) 1602–1609.

131. A. Kawai, T. Kondo & Y. Suehara, et al., Global protein-expression analysis of bone and soft tissue sarcomas, Clin Orthop Relat Res 466 (2008) 2099–2106.

132. M. Wolf, A. Hemminki & A. Kivioja, et al., A novel splice site mutation of the EXT2 gene in a Finnish hereditary multiple exostoses family. Mutations in brief no. 197. Online, Hum Mutat 12 (1998) 362.

133. A.A. Sandberg & J.A. Bridge, Updates on the cytogenetics and molecular genetics of bone and soft tissue tumors: osteosarcoma and related tumors, Cancer Genet Cytogenet 145 (2003) 1–30.

134. A.A. Sandberg & J.A. Bridge, Updates on the cytogenetics and molecular genetics of bone and soft tissue tumors: chondrosarcoma and other cartilaginous neoplasms, Cancer Genet Cytogenet 143 (2003) 1–31.

135. N. Mandahl, F. Mertens & H. Willen, et al., Nonrandom pattern of telomeric associations in atypical lipomatous tumors with ring and giant marker chromosomes, Cancer Genet Cytogenet 103 (1998) 25–34.

136. N. Mandahl, S. Heim & A. Rydholm, et al., Structural chromosome aberrations in an adamantinoma, Cancer Genet Cytogenet 42 (1989) 187–190.

137. B.D. Idowu, M. Al-Adnani & P. O'Donnell, et al., A sensitive mutation-specific screening technique for GNAS1 mutations in cases of fibrous dysplasia: the first report of a codon 227 mutation in bone, Histopathology 50 (2007) 691–704.

CHAPTER **12**

Cytogenetics of Bone Tumors

JIYUN LEE[1], MALLORY MARTIN[1] AND SHIBO LI[1]

[1]*Genetics Laboratory, Department of Pediatrics at the University of Oklahoma Health Sciences Center, Oklahoma City, OK 73104.*

Contents

I. INTRODUCTION

After the discovery of the Philadelphia chromosome in patients with chronic myeloid leukemia [1], investigators in the cancer field tried to find other associations between chromosomes and cancer, including bone tumors [2]. The cytogenetic findings of bone tumors have shown findings of very extreme heterogeneity including loss or gain of chromosomes, deletion or duplication of chromosomal segments, and double minutes or homogeneously stained regions. The majority of these changes are not specific enough to provide clinical diagnostic values. The most common recurrent structural changes are rearrangements of 8q24 in osteochondroma, t(9;22)(q22;q12) in extra-skeletal myxoid chondrosarcoma, t(11;22)(q24;q12) in Ewing's sarcoma and t(16;17)(q22;p13) in aneurysmal bone cysts. Molecular cytogenetics, such as fluorescence *in situ* hybridization (FISH) and the recent newly-advanced array comparative genomic hybridization (CGH) assay and their findings, will be covered in other chapters.

II. CARTILAGE TUMORS

A. Osteochondroma

Osteochondroma is the most common benign bone tumor, often found in patients under the age of 20 years. The majority of cases (85%) of osteochondroma present as sporadic, solitary, non-hereditary lesions. The rest occur as multiple lesions in the context of hereditary multiple osteochondromas (HMOs) which are inherited in an autosomal dominant manner and as part of the contiguous gene syndrome Langer-Giedion and DEFECT-11 syndromes [3]. Linkage analysis has pinpointed three different chromosomal locations: 8q24.1 (*EXT1*), 11p11-p12 (*EXT2*) and 19p (*EXT3*) (Figure 12.1) [4–6]. The first two gene loci, *EXT1* on 8q24.1 and *EXT2* on 11p11-p12 have subsequently been cloned. The third gene, *EXT3* on 19p, has not been cloned yet. Almost 90% of patients with HMOs have *EXT1* or *EXT2* mutations [7]. Approximately 0.5–2% of patients with osteochondromas have malignant transformation in adulthood but these rarely metastasize [8,9].

Cytogenetic investigations of limited samples obtained from sporadic osteochondroma showed that loss or rearrangement of 8q were the most consistent findings, especially at the breakpoint 8q24.1. One sporadic tumor also had a deletion of the 11p11-p12 region, while one

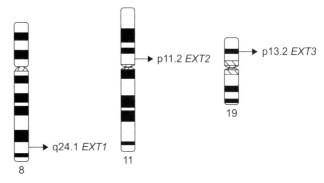

FIGURE 12.1 Ideograms of chromosomes 8, 11 and 19, showing the locations of the *EXT* genes.

Bone Cancer
ISBN: 978-0-12-374895-9

hereditary tumor was found to have a cytogenetic change at the 8q24.1 region [3,10,11]. Feely *et al.* [10] reported that 10 out of 37 (27%) osteochondroma samples (including both sporadic and hereditary lesions) had a loss or structural change of 8q24.1. The same samples were further investigated by FISH analysis using the DNA probe specific for the 8q24.1 region and showed that 27 out of 34 (79%) had a loss of one hybridization signal in the 8q24.1 region [10]. Sawyer *et al.* [12] reported cytogenetic data on eight osteochondroma tumors and demonstrated not only that chromosome 8q24 was involved, but that five out of seven abnormal tumor samples also had rearrangements of chromosome 1, which clustered in the 1p13-p22 region, including inversions, insertions or translocations. Hameetman *et al.* [13] studied eight non-heriditary osteochondromas using array-CGH assay, and found that all eight oestochondromas had a large deletion of 8q; seven of them had an additional small deletion of the other allele of 8q that contained the *EXT1* gene. This finding proved that the *EXT1* is a classical tumor suppressor gene in the non-hereditary osteochondromas.

B. Chondroma

Based on the location of the lesions, chondromas are classified as: (1) enchondroma (within the medullary cavity); (2) perosteal chondroma (on the surface of the bone); and (3) soft tissue chondroma (in the soft tissue). Cytogenetic analysis of the tumors has been attempted and so far no consistent, specific structural or numerical chromosomal changes have been identified. However, Dahlén *et al.* [14] reported their cytogenetic findings in 14 chondroma samples (eight soft tissue chondromas and six skeletal chondromas). Seven of 14 cases showed chromosomal rearrangements of the 12q13-q15 region. The *HMGA2* gene was mapped to the 12q15 region and *HMGA2* gene expression was detected in chondromas with and without cytogenetically visible 12q rearrangements. In addition to 12q, a gain of chromosome 5 and loss of chromosomes 6, 13, 19 and 22 were also detected [15,16].

C. Chondroblastoma

No consistent structural or numerical changes in the chondroblastomas were found in limited sporadic case studies [16].

D. Chondromyxoid Fibroma

Chondromyxoid fibroma is a rare benign bone tumor most commonly arising in the metaphysis of long bones in young adults [17]. Cytogenetic analysis from less than two dozen cases showed non-random chromosomal rearrangements of chromosome 6 (reviewed by Armah *et al.* [18] and Safar *et al.* [19]). Twelve out of 16 reported cases had rearrangements on the long arm of chromosome 6 at breakpoints of 6q13 and 6q25; four of these cases had pericentric inversion of chromosome 6, inv(6)(p25q13), and one case also had a pericentric inversion of chromosome 6, but at a different breakpoint on the long arm,

inv(6)(p25q23). However, no candidate gene within these candidate regions has been identified.

E. Chondrosarcoma

Chondrosarcoma is a malignant tumor with pure hyaline cartilage differentiation. Based on the histology, it can be further classified into subtypes including dedifferentiated, mesenchymal, clear cell and periosteal. The majority of patients tested had very complex chromosomal changes. However, all of these changes were non-specific (i.e., they were different from cell to cell and in heterogeneity). Approximately 5% of chondrosarcomas are classified as extra-skeletal myxoid chondrosarcoma.

Dedifferentiated chondrosarcoma is a tumor in which a low-grade chondrosarcoma transforms into a high-grade sarcoma, most frequently exhibiting features of osteosarcoma, fibrosarcoma, or malignant fibrous histiocytoma. The dedifferentiated chondromsarcoma has no specific detectable cytogenetic aberrations. However, both structural and numerical changes of chromosomes 1 and 9 have been found to be common [20–23].

Mesenchymal chondrosarcoma is a very rare, low-grade variant of chondrosarcoma. A recurrent chromosomal anomaly, the Robertsonian translocation between chromosomes 13 and 21, was identified in two patients [24].

Clear cell and periosteal chondrosarcomas have not been associated with any specific cytogenetic anomalies. Clear cell chondrosarcoma is a low-grade variant of chondrosarcoma, whereas periosteal chondrosarcoma is a malignant hyaline cartilage tumor on the surface of the bone.

Extra-skeletal myxoid chondrosarcoma is a malignant soft tissue tumor. Recurrent structural chromosomal changes were found in more than 70% of cases studied [25,26]. These structural changes were mainly one specific change: the reciprocal translocation between chromosomes 9 and 22 at breakpoints of 9q22 and 22q12 [24–27]. The nuclear receptor gene, *NOR1* (also known as *CHN* or *TEC*) mapped to the 9q22 region, was fused to the N-terminal of the *EWS* gene on chromosome 22q12, which resulted in a fusion protein with oncogenic properties [28]. The remaining 25% of cases are due to two chromosomal variants, t(9;17)(q22;q11) and t(9;15)(q22;q21). The partner genes for the *NOR1* fusion gene product are *RBP56* on chromosome 17q11 and *TCF12* on chromosome 15q21. It is clearly indicated that the *NOR1* gene fusion plays a very important role in this subgroup of chondrosarcomas (Figure 12.2).

III. OSTEOGENIC TUMORS

Osteoid osteoma is a benign bone-forming tumor characterized by small size, limited growth potential and disproportionate pain. Two of the three reported cases

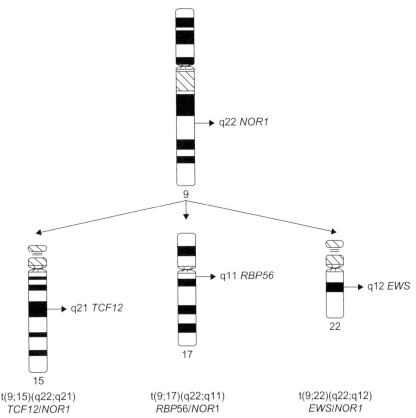

q22 *NOR1*

9

q21 *TCF12*

q11 *RBP56*

q12 *EWS*

17

22

15

t(9;15)(q22;q21)
TCF12/NOR1

t(9;17)(q22;q11)
RBP56/NOR1

t(9;22)(q22;q12)
EWS/NOR1

FIGURE 12.2   Schematic presentation of translocations in extraskeletal myxoid chondrosarcoma involving 9q22 (*NOR1*) with a number of different partner chromosomes.

had cytogenetics changes involving chromosome 22 at 22q13 and loss of the distal part of chromosome arm 17q. However, no candidate gene(s) have been mapped [29].

Osteoblastoma is a rare benign bone-forming neoplasm which produces woven bone spicules, which are bordered by prominent osteoblasts. Cytogenetic analysis was done in limited cases and no recurrent chromosomal changes were identified [30].

Osteosarcoma is a malignant neoplasm of bone. Approximately 75% of osteosarcomas arise in the intramedullary cavity and are referred to as classical or conventional osteosarcoma. Conventional osteosarcoma is further divided into various subtypes based on histological origin. The cytogenetics of osteosarcoma was recently reviewed by Sandberg and Bridge [26]. The majority of osteosarcomas analyzed had clonal, complex chromosomal changes, either structural or numerical. Multiple clones can be detected in a tumor and chromosomal changes can also vary from cell to cell in the same tumor. The regions commonly involved in structural changes include 1q11-q12, 1q21-q22, 11p14-p15, 14p11-p13, 15p11-p13, 17p and 19q13. Ring chromosomes, homogeneously stained regions (HSR) or double minutes (dmin) are frequently seen in conventional osteosarcoma. Some of the complex structural changes cannot be assigned due to complexity. The ploidy number in osteosarcoma has ranged from

haploidy to near-hexaploidy. Gain of chromosome 1 and loss of chromosomes 9, 10, 13, and 17 was the most common overall.

Conventional osteosarcoma is a primary intramedullary high-grade malignant tumor in which the neoplastic cells produce osteoid structures, even if only in small amounts. The majority of these tumors have chromosomal changes, both numerical and structural. Trisomy 1, loss of the long arm of chromosome 6, monosomies of chromosomes 9, 10, 13 and 17 were considered to be common chromosomal imbalances. Chromosomal regions 1p11-p13, 1q21-q22, 11p14-p15, 14p11-p13, 15p11-p13, 17p and 19q13 were the common regions involved in rearrangements. Also in this type of tumor, double minutes and homogeneously stained regions were observed [26].

Telangiectatic osteosarcoma is a malignant bone-forming tumor characterized by large spaces filled with blood with or without septa. Only four cases of telangiectatic osteosarcoma have been reported; one case had trisomy 3 and the other three had very complex chromosomal changes [31–33].

Small cell osteosarcoma is an osteosarcoma composed of small cells with variable degrees of osteoid production. No cytogenetic data are available.

Low-grade central osteosarcoma is a low-grade osteosarcoma that arises from the medullary cavity of bone. Amplification of 12q13-q15, which was also present in the parosteal osteosarcoma, may share a similar mechanism due to ring formation [34].

Secondary osteosarcoma is a bone-forming sarcoma occurring in bones that are affected by pre-existing abnormalities, the most common being Paget's disease and radiation-associated tumors. Loss of heterozygosity (LOH) of the long arm of chromosome 18 was found to be involved.

Parosteal osteosarcoma has very unique chromosome changes compared to others; a ring chromosome derived from chromosome 12 was the common finding. This ring chromosome is amplified in the region of 12q13-q15. The genes *SAS*, *CDK4* and *MDM2* were mapped to this amplified region and seem to have a role in parosteal osteosarcoma [34].

Periosteal osteosarcoma is an intermediate-grade chondroblastic osteosarcoma arising on the surface of bone. So far, only four cases have been investigated; one case had trisomy 17 and the rest had unspecified complex chromosomal changes [33,35,36].

High-grade surface osteosarcoma had no cytogenetic data available.

IV. FIBROGENIC TUMORS

Desmoplastic fibroma of bone and fibrosarcoma of bone had no cytogenetic data available.

V. FIBROHISTIOCYTIC TUMORS

Benign fibrous histiocytoma of bone is a benign lesion of bone composed of spindle-shaped fibroblasts, arranged in a storiform pattern. It has no cytogenetic data available. However, the malignant form of fibrous histiocytoma of bone does have cytogenetic changes by LOH only (i.e., the loss of the 9p21-22 region) [37].

VI. EWING'S SARCOMA/PRIMITIVE NEUROECTODERMAL TUMOR

Ewing's sarcoma and primitive neuroectodermal tumor (PNET) are defined as round cell sarcomas that show varying degrees of neuroectodermal differentiation. The term 'Ewing's sarcoma' has been used for tumors that lack evidence of neuroectodermal differentiation as assessed by light microscopy, immunohistochemistry, and electron microscopy, whereas the term 'PNET' has been used for tumors that demonstrate neuroectodermal features as evaluated by one or more of these modalities. The characteristic chromosomal translocation, t(11;22)(q24;q12), was found in 80–85% of patients with Ewing's sarcoma [38,39]. The remaining patients with Ewing's sarcoma have t(21;22)(q22;q12), t(7;22)(p22;q12), t(17;22)(q21;q12), or t(2;11;22)(q33;q24;q12) [40–43] (Figure 12.3). The t(21;22) was the second most common translocation in Ewing's sarcoma, accounting for about 5 to 10% of all Ewing's sarcoma [44]. As a result of those

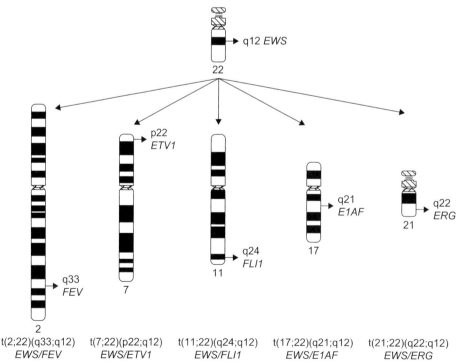

FIGURE 12.3 Schematic presentation of chromosomal rearrangements in Ewing's sarcoma involving 22q12 (*EWS*) with a number of different chromosomes.

chromosomal rearrangements, the 5′ portion of the *EWS* gene (22q12) is fused to the 3′ portion of the *ETS*-family genes: *FLI1*(11q24), *ERG* (21q22), *ETV1* (7p22), *FEV* (2q33) and *E1AF*(17q21), resulting in the formation of oncogenic chimeric proteins [45]. Unusual variant translocations involve a third chromosome, such as 4q21, 5q31, 6p21, 7q12, 10p11.2, 12q14, 14q11, 18p23, or 19q13.2 [46,47]. In addition to those specific pathogenic chromosomal changes, secondary chromosomal changes are also found in up to 80% of patients with Ewing's sarcoma: a gain of whole chromosomes 8 (40%) or 12 (20%), an unbalanced translocation involving chromosomes 1 and 16 (11%), or deletions of the short arm of chromosome 1 are the most common. Ewing's sarcoma patients with either complex chromosomal changes or a chromosome number above 50 had the poorest survival rate overall. Trisomy 20 is considered as a marker of a more aggressive subset of this group [48].

VII. GIANT CELL TUMORS

The giant cell tumor is a benign, locally aggressive neoplasm composed of sheets of neoplastic ovoid mononuclear cells interspersed with uniformly distributed osteoclast-like giant cells. Cytogenetics revealed telomeric association or telomeric fusion in more than 75% of patients with a giant cell tumor of bone. A higher frequency was observed in giant cell tumors occurring in the long bones, such as the tibia, femur, fibula, humerus and radius compared to giant cell tumors in the hands and feet [49].

VIII. NOTOCHORDAL TUMORS

A. Chordoma

Chordoma is rare and arises from remnants of the fetal notochord. It commonly occurs along the axial skeleton, especially in the sacrococcygeal region (50%) and sphenooccipital (35%), the rest are found in the vertebral region (15%) [50,51]. The majority of the cases reported are sporadic; however, a few familial cases have also been reported (dominant pattern) [52–54]. So far, cytogenetically there have been no consistent specific numerical or structural rearrangements associated with chordoma identified. The only consistent findings have shown that there is a tendency of a near-diploid or moderately hypodiploid karyotype. Loss of chromosomes X, Y, 1, 3, 4, 6, 9, 10, 11, 13, 14, 18, 20 and 22, and gain of chromosomes 2 and 7 were among those common recurrent chromosomal changes. The deletions of 1p and 9p have been investigated by different methodologies, including routine cytogenetics, FISH and LOH. Through this investigation, three genes in the 1p36 region (*TNFRSF8*, *TNFRSF9*, and *TNFRSF14*), and two genes in 9p21 region (*CDKN2A* and *CDKN2B*), are thought to play a role in chordoma development [55,56].

IX. VASCULAR TUMORS

Haemangioma is a benign vasoformative neoplasm of developmental condition of endothelial origin. So far, no consistent chromosomal changes have been identified.

Angiosarcoma has tumor cells showing endothelial differentiation. Mendlick *et al.* [57] reported two cases with a translocation between chromosomes 1 and 3, t(1;3)(p36.3;q25).

X. MYOGENIC, LIPOGENIC, NEURONAL AND EPITHELIAL TUMORS

Leiomyosarcoma of the bone is a very rare malignant spindle-cell sarcoma which shows smooth muscle features. Leiomyosarcoma of the bone does not have consistent, specific recurrent chromosomal changes. However, most of the reported cases have very complex chromosomal changes including the loss of 3p21-p23, 8p21-pter, 13q12-q13, 13q32-qter, and the gain of 1q21-q31 [58].

Lipoma of the bone is a benign neoplasm of adipocytes that arises within the medullary cavity, cortex or on the surface of bone. Cytogenetic analysis revealed that a lipoma is very heterogeneous in chromosome changes, but translocation or rearrangement of the long arm of chromosome 12 at the 12q13-q15 region is a very common, consistent structural change. Among these changes, t(3;12)(q27-q28;q13-q15) is the most common. Rearrangement of chromosome 13, mainly deletion of the 13q14 region, is the next most common chromosome change in a lipoma. These changes are easily detected by FISH. Changes in chromosomes 6p21-p23 and 7 were also present in a percentage of patients with lipoma, which may represent a subgroup of lipomas. The translocation between chromosomes 3 and 12 generates a fusion gene *HMGIC/LPP*. A germ line mutation due to a *de novo* pericentric inversion of chromosome 12, inv(12)(p11.22-q14.3), was found in a patient who had postnatal onset of extreme somatic overgrowth, advanced endochondral bone and dental ages with megaepiphyseal dysplasia, and multiple subcutaneous lipomas. This unique case demonstrated the clear role of the *HMGA2* gene in the development of lipomas and other general growth control [16].

Adamantinoma is a low-grade, malignant biphasic tumor characterized by a variety of morphological patterns, most commonly epithelial cells, surrounded by a relatively bland spindle-cell osteofibrous component. Adamantinomas have chromosomal changes similar to those of osteofibrous dysplasia, including gain of extra chromosomes 7, 8, 12 and 19. Some of the 'atypical' cases called 'Ewing-like' adamantinomas have shown a t(11;22) by FISH and molecular methods. One adamantinoma case report showed that the patient had chromosomal changes overlapping with those of osteofibrous dysplasia, but the chromosomal changes were more complex. This led them to hypothesize that these additional complex chromosomal changes are due to the progression from osteofibrous dysplasia to adamantinoma [59].

XI. TUMORS OF AN UNDEFINED NEOPLASTIC NATURE

Aneurysmal bone cysts are benign cyst lesions of bone composed of blood-filled spaces separated by connective tissue septa containing fibroblasts, osteoclast-type giant cells and reactive woven bone. The initial cytogenetic investigation of three patients with aneurysmal bone cysts showed that two of the three cases had a translocation between chromosomes 16 and 17 at breakpoints of 16q22 and 17p13; one case had a deletion of chromosome 16q22. Subsequently, it turned out that t(16;17) is the most common cytogenetic change for aneurysmal bone cysts. This translocation led to the fusion gene *CDH11/USP6*; the strong promoter of the *CDH11* gene at 16q22, is fused to the entire *USP6* coding sequence at 17p13. This fusion gene (*CDH11/USP6*) causes the *USP6* to be upregulated. Rearrangements of the *USP6* with several other partner genes have been reported; these include t(1;17)(p34;p13), t(3;17)(q21;p13), t(9;17)(q22;p13) and t(17;17)(q21;p13) [60]. The corresponding partner genes for each of these translocations are *THRAP3* on 1p34, *CNBP* on 3q21, *OMD* at 9q22 and *COL1A1* on 17q21 (Figure 12.4).

A **simple bone cyst** is an intramedullary, usually unilocular bone cyst filled with serous or seo-sanguineous fluid.

Cytogenetic findings were only reported in a single case and very complex clonal structural changes were found, including chromosomes 4, 6, 8, 16, 21 and both copies of chromosome 12 [61].

Osteofibrous dysplasia is a self-limited benign fibroosseous bone lesion characteristically involving cortical bone of the anterior mid-shaft of the tibia during infancy and childhood. So far, only four cases of osteofibrous dysplasia with cytogenetic findings have been reported. Of these four, two patients had trisomies of 7 and 8, and one of these two patients also had two extra copies of chromosome 21. One patient had trisomy 12 and one patient had a rearrangement of chromosome 2 at the breakpoint of the long arm at 2q11.2 [62]. Those changes were also found in patients with adamantinoma, which has similar histological features of osteofibrous dysplasia [63,64].

Langerhans cell histiocytosis is a neoplastic proliferation of Langerhans cells. A single case with t(7;12) translocation was described by Betts *et al.* [65]. LOH utilizing selected microsatellite markers combined with CGH assay showed an increased incidence of chromosomal imbalances at chromosomes 1, 5, 6, 7, 9, 16, 17 and 22 [66].

XII. CONCLUSION

The mechanism of bone tumor development is complex and largely unknown. We have summarized the current status of cytogenetic changes in bone tumors (Table 12.1). However

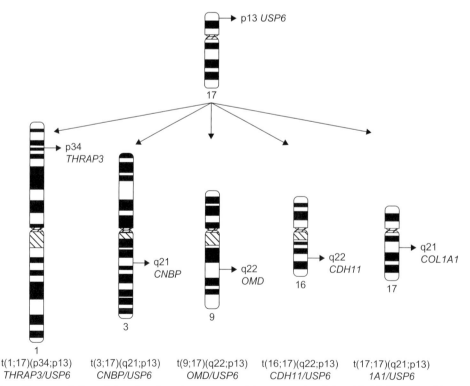

FIGURE 12.4 Schematic presentation of translocations in aneurysmal bone cyst involving 17p13 (*USP6*) with a number of different partner chromosomes.

TABLE 12.1 Selected recurrent cytogenetic changes in bone tumors

Origin	Tumor type	Recurrent numerical abnormality	Recurrent structural rearrangements	Gene
Cartilage tumors	Chondroma[b]		12q13-15	
	Chondroblastoma[b]	low proliferative diploid neoplasm, with minor aneuploid near-diploidy	No consistent abnormality	
	Chondromyxoid fibroma[b]		6p25, 6q13 and 6q23	
	Chondrosarcoma[m]	hyperhaploidy—near pentaplooidy: −6, +7, +10, +13, +14, −19 and −20	Heterogeneous/Complex. 1q21, 5q13, 7q22, 12q13, 19p13 and 19q13	
	Extraskeletal myxoid chondrosarcoma[m]		t(9;22)(q22;q12) t(9;17)(q22;q11) t(9;15)(q22;q21)	*EWS/NOR1(CHN)* *RBP56/NOR1(CHN)* *TCF12/NOR1(CHN)*
	Osteochondroma[b] (osteocartilaginous exostosis)		8q24, 11p11-p12	*EXT1* *EXT2*
	Multiple osteochondromatosis (Hereditary multiple exostosis)		8q24 11p11-12 19p	*EXT1* *EXT2* *EXT3*
Osteogenic tumors	Osteoid osteoma[b] (2 cases)		del(22)(q13)	
	Osteoblastoma[b]		No consistent abnormality	
	Osteosarcoma[m]	haploidy to near-hexaploidy +1, −9, −10, −13, and −17	Heterogeneous/Complex. 1p11-13, 1q11-q12, 1q21-q22, 11p14-p15, 14p11-p13, 15p11-p13, 17p and 19q13.	
Ewing's sarcoma and peripheral primitive neuroectodermal tumors	Ewing's sarcoma and peripheral primitive neuroectodermal tumors[m]		t(11;22)(q24;q12) t(21;22)(q22;q12) t(7;22)(p22;q12) t(17;22)(q21;q12) t(2;22)(q33;q12)	*EWS/FLI1* *EWS/ERG* *EWS/ETV1* *EWS/E1AF* *EWS/FEV*
Giant cell tumor	Giant cell tumor[b/m] (Osteoclastoma)	+7, −13	Telomeric association. 11p15, 19q13	
Notochordal tumors	Chordoma[m]	hypodiploidy +7, −3, −4, −10, −13	9p24, 14q11, i(1q)	
Myogenic, lipogenic, neural and epithelial tumors	Lipoma of bone		12q13-q15	
	Adamantinoma[m]	+7, +8, +12, +19, +21		
Tumor of undefined neoplastic nature	Aneurysmal bone cyst[b]		t(16;17)(q22;p13) t(1;17)(p34;p13) t(3;17)(q21;p13) t(9;17)(q22;p13) t(17;17)(q21;p13)	*CDH11/USP6* *THRAP3/USP6* *CNBP/USP6* *OMD/USP6* COL1A1/*USP6*

[b]Benign; [m]Malignant.

routine, traditional cytogenetics has its limitations in identifying chromosomal changes in bone tumors. As an adjunct tool, array CGH technology should be used to identify subtle deletions and duplications that reveal gene(s) responsible for some of these bone tumors.

References

1. P.C. Nowell & D.A. Hungerford, A minute chromosome in human granulocytic leukemia, Science 132 (1960) 1497–1501.
2. F. Mitelman, B. Johansson, and F. Mertens (eds.) (2008). Mitelman Database of Chromosome Aberrations in Cancer. Accessed at: http://cgap.nci.nih.gov/Chromosomes/Mitelman.
3. J.A. Bridge, M. Nelson & C. Orndal, et al., Clonal karyotypic abnormalities of the hereditary multiple exostoses chromosomal loci 8q24.1 (*EXT1*) and 11p11-12 (*EXT2*) in patients with sporadic and hereditary osteochondromas, Cancer 82 (9) (1998) 1657–1663.
4. A. Cook, W. Raskind, S.H. Blanton & R.M. Pauli, et al., Genetic heterogeneity in families with hereditary multiple exostoses, Am J Hum Genet 53 (1) (1993) 71–79.
5. Y.Q. Wu, P. Heutink & B.B. de Vries, et al., Assignment of a second locus for multiple exostoses to the pericentromeric region of chromosome 11, Hum Mol Genet 3 (1) (1994) 167–171.
6. M. Le Merrer, L. Legeai-Mallet & P.M. Jeannin, et al., A gene for hereditary multiple exostoses maps to chromosome 19p, Hum Mol Genet 3 (5) (1994) 717–722.
7. J.V. Bovée, Multiple osteochondromas, Orphanet J Rare Dis 13 (3) (2008) 3.
8. R.C. Hennekam, Hereditary multiple exostoses, J Med Genet 28 (4) (1991) 262–266.
9. N.C. Leone, J.L. Shupe & E.J. Gardner, et al., Hereditary multiple exostosis. A comparative human-equine-epidemiologic study, J Hered 78 (3) (1987) 171–177.
10. M.G. Feely, A.K. Boehm & R.S. Bridge, et al., Cytogenetic and molecular cytogenetic evidence of recurrent 8q24.1 loss in osteochondroma, Cancer Genet Cytogenet 137 (2) (2002) 102–107.
11. F. Mertens, A. Rydholm & A. Kreicbergs, et al., Loss of chromosome band 8q24 in sporadic osteocartilaginous exostoses, Genes Chromosomes Cancer 9 (1) (1994) 8–12.
12. J.R. Sawyer, E.L. Thomas & J.L. Lukacs, et al., Recurring breakpoints of 1p13 approximately p22 in osteochondroma, Cancer Genet Cytogenet 138 (2) (2002) 102–106.
13. L. Hameetman, K. Szuhai & A. Yavas, et al., The role of EXT1 in nonhereditary osteochondroma: identification of homozygous deletions, J Natl Cancer Inst 99 (2007) 396–406.
14. A. Dahlén, F. Mertens & A. Rydholm, et al., Fusion, disruption, and expression of *HMGA2* in bone and soft tissue chondromas, Mod Pathol 16 (11) (2003) 1132–1140.
15. E.P. Buddingh, S. Naumann & M. Nelson, et al., Cytogenetic findings in benign cartilaginous neoplasms, Cancer Genet Cytogenet 141 (2) (2003) 164–168.
16. A.A. Sandberg, Genetics of chondrosarcoma and related tumors, Curr Opin Oncol 16 (4) (2004) 342–354.
17. C.T. Wu, C.Y. Inwards & S. O'Laughlin, et al., Chondromyxoid fibroma of bone: a clinicopathologic review of 278 cases, Hum Pathol 29 (5) (1998) 438–446.
18. H.B. Armah, R.L. McGough & M.A. Goodman, et al., Chondromyxoid fibroma of rib with a novel chromosomal translocation: a report of four additional cases at unusual sites, Diagn Pathol 242 (2007) 44.
19. A. Safar, M. Nelson & J.R. Neff, et al., Recurrent anomalies of 6q25 in chondromyxoid fibroma, Hum Pathol 31 (3) (2000) 306–311.
20. J.A. Bridge, J. DeBoer & J. Travis, et al., Simultaneous interphase cytogenetic analysis and fluorescence immunophenotyping of dedifferentiated chondrosarcoma. Implications for histopathogenesis, Am J Pathol 144 (2) (1994) 215–220.
21. S.J. Swarts, J.R. Neff & S.L. Johansson, et al., Cytogenetic analysis of dedifferentiated chondrosarcoma, Cancer Genet Cytogenet 89 (1996) 49–51.
22. D.P. O'Malley, K.E. Opheim & T.S. Barry, et al., Chromosomal changes in a dedifferentiated chondrosarcoma: a case report and review of the literature, Cancer Genet Cytogenet 124 (2001) 105–111.
23. M.M. Zalupski, J.F. Ensley & J. Ryan, et al., A common cytogenetic abnormality and DNA content alterations in dedifferentiated chondrosarcoma, Cancer 66 (1990) 1176–1182.
24. S. Naumann, P.A. Krallman & K.K. Unni, et al., Translocation der(13;21)(q10;q10) in skeletal and extraskeletal mesenchymal chondrosarcoma, Mod Pathol 15 (2002) 572–576.
25. A.A. Sandberg, Updates on the cytogenetics and molecular genetics of bone and soft tissue tumors: lipoma, Cancer Genet Cytogenet 150 (2004) 93–115.
26. A.A. Sandberg & J.A. Bridge, Updates on the cytogenetics and molecular genetics of bone and soft tissue tumors: chondrosarcoma and other cartilaginous neoplasms, Cancer Genet Cytogenet 143 (1) (2003) 1–31.
27. G. Stenman, H. Andersson & N. Mandahl, et al., Translocation t(9;22) is a primary cytogenetic abnormality in extraskeletal myxooid chondrosarcoma, Int J Cancer 62 (1995) 398–402.
28. J. Clark, H. Benjamin & S. Gill, et al., Fusion of the *EWS* gene to *CHN*, a member of the steroid/thyroid receptor gene superfamily, in a human myxoid chondrosarcoma, Oncogene 12 (2) (1996) 229–235.
29. M.R. Baruffi, J.B. Volpon & J.B. Neto, et al., Osteoid osteomas with chromosome alterations involving 22q, Cancer Genet Cytogenet 124 (2) (2001) 127–131.
30. K. Radig, R. Schneider-Stock & U. Mittler, et al., Genetic instability in osteoblastic tumors of the skeletal system, Pathol Res Pract 194 (1998) 669–677.
31. J.A. Bridge, M. Nelson & E. McComb, et al., Cytogenetic findings in 73 osteosarcoma specimens and a review of the literature, Cancer Genet Cytogenet 95 (1) (1997) 74–87.
32. J.A. Fletcher, M.C. Gebhardt & H.P. Kozakewich, Cytogenetic aberrations in osteosarcomas. Nonrandom deletions, rings, and double-minute chromosomes, Cancer Genet Cytogenet 77 (1994) 81–88.
33. W. Hoogerwerf, A.L. Hawkins & E.J. Perlman, et al., Chromosome analysis of nine osteosarcomas, Genes Chromosomes Cancer 9 (1994) 88–92.
34. F. Mertens, N. Mandahl & C. Orndal, et al., Cytogenetic findings in 33 osteosarcomas, Int J Cancer 55 (1993) 44–50.
35. D. Gisselsson, M. Hoglund & F. Mertens, et al., Chromosomal organization of amplified chromosome 12 sequences in mesenchymal tumors detected by fluorescence *in situ* hybridization, Genes Chromosomes Cancer 23 (1998) 203–212.

36. M. Tarkkanen, A. Kaipainen & E. Karaharju, et al., Cytogenetic study of 249 consecutive patients examined for a bone tumor, Cancer Genet Cytogenet 68 (1993) 1–21.

37. J.A. Martignetti, B.D. Gelb & H. Pierce, et al., Malignant fibrous histocytoma: inherited and sporadic forms have loss of heterozygosity at chromosome bands 9p21-22 evidence for a common genetic defect, Genes Chromosomes Cancer 27 (2000) 191–195.

38. A. Aurias, C. Rimbaut & D. Buffe, et al., Translocations of chromosome 22 in Ewing's sarcoma. An analysis of 4 fresh tumors, N Engl J Med 309 (1983) 496–497.

39. C. Turc-Carel, I. Philip & M.P. Berger, et al., Translocation (11;22) (q24;q12) in Ewing's sarcoma cell lines, N Engl J Med 309 (1983) 497–498.

40. O. Delattre, J. Zucman & B. Plougastel, et al., Gene fusion with an ETS DNA-binding domain caused by chromosome translocation in tumors, Nature 359 (1992) 162–165.

41. I.S. Jeon, J.N. Davis & B.S. Braun, et al., A variant Ewing's sarcoma translocation (7;22) fuses the *EWS* gene to the ETS gene *ETV1*, Oncogene 10 (6) (1995) 1229–1234.

42. Y. Kaneko, H. Kobayashi & M. Handa, et al., *EWS-ERG* fusion transcript produced by chromosomal insertion in a Ewing sarcoma, Genes Chromosomes Cancer 18 (1997) 228–231.

43. M. Peter, J. Couturier & H. Pacquement, et al., A new member of the ETS family fused to EWS in Ewing tumors, Oncogene 14 (1994) 1159–1164.

44. P.H. Sorensen, S.L. Lessnick & D. Lopez-Terrada, et al., A second Ewing's sarcoma translocation, t(21;22), fuses the EWS gene to another ETS-family transcription factor, ERG, Nat Genet 6 (2) (1994) 146–151.

45. W.A. May, S.L. Lessnick & B.S. Braun, et al., The Ewing's sarcoma *EWS/FLI-1* fusion gene encodes a more potent transcriptional activator and is a more powerful transforming gene than *FLI-1*, Mol Cell Biol 13 (1993) 7393–7398.

46. J. Lee, D.J. Hopcus-Niccum & J.J. Mulvihill, et al., Cytogenetic and molecular cytogenetic studies of a variant of t(21;22), ins(22;21)(q12;q21q22), with a deletion of the 3′ *EWSR1* gene in a patient with Ewing sarcoma, Cancer Genet Cytogenet 159 (2) (2005) 177–180.

47. G. Maire, C.W. Brown & J. Bayani, et al., Complex rearrangement of chromosomes 19, 21, and 22 in Ewing sarcoma involving a novel reciprocal inversion-insertion mechanism of *EWS-ERG* fusion gene formation: a case analysis and literature review, Cancer Genet Cytogenet 181 (2) (2008) 81–92.

48. P. Roberts, S.A. Burchill & S. Brownhill, et al., Ploidy and karyotype complexity are powerful prognostic indicators in the Ewing's sarcoma family of tumors: a study by the United Kingdom Cancer Cytogenetics and the Children's Cancer and Leukaemia Group, Genes Chromosomes Cancer 47 (3) (2008) 207–220.

49. J.A. Bridge, J.R. Neff & B.J. Mouron, Giant cell tumor of bone. Chromosomal analysis of 48 specimens and review of the literature, Cancer Genet Cytogenet 58 (1) (1992) 2–13.

50. J. Mirra, S. Nelson, C. Della Roca, C.D. Fletcher, K. Unni & F. Mertens (Eds.), et al., Pathology and Genetics of Tumors of Soft Tissue and Bone, Lyon, France: IARC Press, 2002, pp. 316–317.

51. J. Bjornsson, L.E. Wold & M.J. Ebersold, et al., Chordoma of the mobile spine. A clinicopathologic analysis of 40 patients, Cancer 71 (3) (1993) 735–740.

52. A.K. Bhadra & A.T. Casey, Familial chordoma. A report of two cases, J Bone Joint Surg Br 88 (5) (2006) 634–636.

53. M.J. Kelley, J.F. Korczak & E. Sheridan, et al., Familial chordoma, a tumor of notochordal remnants, is linked to chromosome 7q33, Am J Hum Genet 69 (2) (2001) 454–460.

54. J. Stepanek, S.A. Cataldo, M.J. Ebersold, et al., Familial chordoma with probable autosomal dominant inheritance, Am J Med Genet 23 75(3) (1998) 335–336.

55. M. Longoni, F. Orzan & M. Stroppi, et al., Evaluation of 1p36 markers and outcome in a skull base chordoma study, Neuro Oncol 10 (1) (2008) 52–60.

56. K.H. Hallor, J. Staaf & G. Jönsson, et al., Frequent deletion of the CDKN2A locus in chordoma: analysis of chromosomal imbalances using array comparative genomic hybridization, Br J Cancer 98 (2) (2008) 434–442.

57. M.R. Mendlick, M. Nelson & D. Pickering, et al., Translocation t(1;3)(p36.3;q25) is a nonrandom aberration in epithelioid hemangioendothelioma, Am J Surg Pathol 25 (2001) 684–687.

58. A.A. Sandberg, Updates on the cytogenetics and molecular genetics of bone and soft tissue tumors: leiomyosarcoma, Cancer Genet Cytogenet 161 (2005) 1–19.

59. M.D. Camp, R.K. Tompkins & S.S. Spanier, et al., Best cases from the AFIP: adamantinoma of the tibia and fibula with cytogenetic analysis, Radiographics 28 (4) (2008) 1215–1220.

60. A.M. Oliveira, A.R. Perez-Atayde & P. Dal Cin, et al., Aneurysmal bone cyst variant translocations upregulate USP6 transcription by promoter swapping with the ZNF9, COL1A1, TRAP150, and OMD genes, Oncogene 24 (21) (2005) 3419–3426.

61. S.A. Vayego, O.J. De Conti & M. Varella-Garcia, Complex cytogenetic rearrangement in a case of unicameral bone cyst, Cancer Genet Cytogenet 86 (1996) 46–49.

62. D.M. Parham, J.A. Bridge & J.L. Lukacs, et al., Cytogenetic distinction among benign fibro-osseous lesions of bone in children and adolescents: value of karyotypic findings in differential diagnosis, Pediatr Dev Pathol 7 (2) (2004) 148–158.

63. M.S. Benassi, L. Campanacci & G. Gamberi, et al., Cytokeratin expression and distribution in adamantinoma of the long bones and osteofibrous dysplasia of tibia and fibula. An immunohistochemical study correlated to histogenesis, Histopathology 25 (1) (1994) 71–76.

64. M. Kanamori, C.R. Antonescu & M. Scott, et al., Extra copies of chromosomes 7, 8, 12, 19, 21 are recurrent in adamantinoma, J Mol Diag 3 (2001) 16–21.

65. D.R. Betts, K.E. Leibundgut & A. Feldges, et al., Cytogenetic abnormalities in Langerhans cell histiocytosis, Br J Cancer 77 (4) (1998) 552–555.

66. I. Murakami, J. Gogusev & J.C. Fournet, et al., Detection of molecular cytogenetic aberrations in Langerhans cell histiocytosis of bone, Hum Pathol 33 (2002) 555–560.

CHAPTER **13**

Genetic Aspects of Bone Tumors

SHAMINI SELVARAJAH[1], MARIA ZIELENSKA[2,3], JEREMY A. SQUIRE[4] AND PAUL C. PARK[4]

[1]Center for Medical Oncologic Pathology, Dana-Farber Cancer Institute, Jimmy Fund Building 215G, Boston, MA 02115, USA.
[2]Department of Pediatric Laboratory, Medicine and Pathobiology, The Hospital for Sick Children, Toronto, Ontario, Canada.
[3]Genetics and Genome Biology, The Hospital for Sick Children, Toronto, Ontario, Canada.
[4]Department of Pathology and Molecular Medicine, Richardson Labs, Queen's University, Kingston, Ontario, Canada.

Contents

I. INTRODUCTION

Primary neoplasms of the skeleton are relatively rare, comprising only 0.2% of human tumors. Despite this low frequency, this group of lesions poses a significant challenge in clinical management, with 2100 newly diagnosed cases and 1300 deaths in the US each year. This clinical challenge is due in part, to the heterogeneity of this group, as the lesions vary widely in their morphology, making histopathological diagnosis difficult. Moreover, there is wide diversity in the biological behavior, ranging from innocuous to rapidly progressive, including many of intermediate malignancy, behaving as locally aggressive but non-metastatic tumors. In the face of this diversity, accurate diagnoses and staging is critical in the treatment strategy, and ultimately in determining morbidity and mortality.

With advancements in molecular genetics, the critical events associated with the development of several bone cancers are now being unraveled. The growing catalog of new molecular information promises an effective adjunct to the histological diagnosis and prognostication, much as they have played a role in the management of hematological and soft tissue malignancies. In addition, our evolving insight of the biological mechanisms and signaling pathways underlying tumor progression offers possibilities for novel, targeted therapeutic options in the future.

Under the WHO classification system, the majority of bone tumors are classified according to the tissue of origin.

Overall, matrix-producing and fibrous tumors are the most common. Of the benign tumors, osteochondroma and fibrous cortical defects have the highest incidences, while osteosarcoma, chondrosarcoma and Ewing's sarcoma are the most frequent primary bone malignancy excluding those of marrow origin (myeloma, lymphoma, and leukemia). This review aims to provide a brief overview of the genetics of some of the more common bone tumors, both benign and malignant. It will focus on well-known genetic and cytogenetic lesions that are considered in the molecular diagnoses of these tumors. This chapter is by no means an exhaustive survey of the genetics of all bone malignancies, and readers are referred to other resources for a more comprehensive listing [1,2].

II. CARTILAGINOUS NEOPLASMS

A. Benign

Benign tumors of cartilages are the most common primary bone tumors that arise in the pediatric population.

1. OSTEOCHONDROMA

Osteochondroma is the most common benign neoplasm of the bone. The lesions present as cartilage-capped bony protuberances at the metaphyses of long bones, either as solitary or multiple lesions. The latter condition characterizes the hereditary multiple exostoses syndrome (HME), an autosomal dominant skeletal disorder that is associated with excessive bony growths. In 10% of osteochondroma associated with HME, malignant transformation occurs within the cartilaginous cap, leading to a secondary peripheral chondrosarcoma (CS). Conversely, about 15% of all CS arise secondarily to osteochondroma [3]. Two genes, EXT1 and EXT2 located at 8q24 and 11p11-p12, have been isolated to cause HME. They encode type II transmembrane glycoproteins localized to the endoplasmic reticulum and are required for heparin sulfate polymerization. In osteochondromas resulting from HME, the expression of EXT1 and/or EXT2 is decreased, corresponding to their frequently observed mutations [4,5]. In non-hereditary lesions, 85% exhibit loss of heterozygosity (LOH) and clonal rearrangement at the chromosomal locus of EXT1 [6]. Inactivation of EXT results in altered heparin sulfate expression at the cell surface of chondrocytes and adversely affects the Indian hedgehog (IHh), parathyroid hormone related peptide (PTHrP) and fibroblast growth factor (FGF) signaling pathways. Diminished levels of the EXT1 and EXT2 protein and their putative downstream effectors have been found in both sporadic and hereditary osteochondromas [4,7].

Cytogenetically, osteochondromas generally present with normal karyotypes, whether sporadic or associated with HME. However, molecular cytogenetic studies of the EXT1 locus have revealed recurrent, submicroscopic loss of this region in karyotypes of hereditary and sporadic osteochondromas, further reinforcing the role of EXT1 in the pathogenesis [7].

2. CHONDROMA

Chondromas can occur in the bone (enchondroma), the periosteum (periosteal chondroma), and in soft tissues (soft-part chondroma), typically affecting the proximal phalanges of the hands and feet. The chromosomal changes observed in chondroma do not differentiate the enchondroma from lesions arising in the periosteum or soft tissues. The genetics of chondroma is not extensively defined. However, data from a few genomic hybridization (CGH) studies indicate an uncomplicated profile, including gains of 13q21 and losses on chromosomes 19 and 22q [8]. Early studies also implicate recurrent rearrangements of chromosome 6, including an isochromosome of the short arm of chromosome 6(p10), as well as t(12;15)(q13;q26) [7,9]. The non-random translocation of the 12q13-15 segment has been shown to involve the HMGA2 (HMGI-C) locus as the critical site [10].

Approximately 30% of the chondromas present as multiple lesions [11]. These cases are typically syndromic in nature, overlapping with spindle cell hemangioendotheliomas in Mafucci's syndrome, or with ovarian sex-cord stromal tumors in Ollier's disease [12,13]. As such, chondromas have a significantly higher risk of malignant transformation into chondrosarcoma [14]. The genetic basis for these syndromes remains to be elucidated.

3. CHONDROBLASTOMA

Chondroblastoma is a rare benign bone tumor, usually affecting the epiphysis of long bones such as the femur, tibia and humerus. Few chromosomal studies have been performed, with no specific cytogenetic findings in most studies. Some authors have reported abnormalities of chromosomes 5 and 8 [15], while another group reported a ring chromosome 4 in approximately 1/3 of cells from a single case of chondroblastoma [16]. SKY and fluorescence *in situ*

hybridization studies show typically diploid or near-diploid karyotypes [17]. Further analyses have shown recurrent breakpoints at 2q35, 3q21-23, and 18q21 [10].

B. Malignant

1. CONVENTIONAL CHONDROSARCOMA

Chondrosarcomas (CS) are a heterogeneous group of tumors with various clinical and histopathological patterns. Most CS are skeletal lesions; however, extraskeletal lesions do occur infrequently. Progression of an indolent, locally aggressive, low-grade cartilaginous lesion to a metastasizing high-grade CS (dedifferentiation) is associated with the loss of cartilaginous phenotype, genomic instability and aneuploidy [7].

With the exception of extraskeletal myxoid CS (EMC), cytogenetic studies of CS have revealed considerable karyotypic heterogeneity. Karyotypes may range from simple numerical changes to abundant, complex numerical and structural abnormalities. To date, cytogenetic studies have revealed the following imbalances: loss of chromosomes or regions 1p36, 1p13~p22, 4, 5q13~q31, 6q22~qter, 9p22~pter, 10p, 10q24~qter, 11p13~pter, 11q25, 13q21~qter, 14q24~qter, 18p, 18q22~qter, and 22q13, and gain of 7p13~pter, 12q15~qter, 19, 20pter~q11, and 21q. Certain chromosomal regions show recurrent involvement, and appear to be phenotype specific. For example, abnormalities of 9p and extra copies of chromosome 22 distinguish the central CS from the peripheral CS. Furthermore, in primary tumors, CGH studies have identified frequent gains of 20q12~qter, 20q whole arm, 8q24~qter, 20p and 14q24~qter, and losses of Xcen~q21, 6cen~q22 and 18cen~q11.2. In contrast, recurrent and metastatic tumors showed gains of chromosome 7, 5q14~q32, 6p and 12q, while losses were much less frequent [7]. In general, the tumor grade seems to increase in proportion to its degree of aneuploidy [18].

Overexpression, structural alterations (i.e., mutations), and/or LOH of the TP53 gene have been observed in a minority of CS, predominantly in high-grade tumors associated with aggressive behavior [19]. Some studies have also reported LOH of 13q14 in a subset of chondrosarcoma [20,21]. However, pRb mutations have not been found [22]. Deletions of the p16 (CDKN2A) gene also occur in a small subset of primary CS and CS cell lines, consistent with the genomic loss of its locus at 9p21, as detected by CGH analysis [7].

Matrix metalloproteinases (MMP) are zinc proteinases responsible for the degradation of extracellular matrix macromolecules in embryonic development, angiogenesis, and tumor invasion. In studies on benign and malignant cartilaginous neoplasms, a pattern of increased expression of MMP-1, MMP-2, and MMP-13 and decreased expression of MMP-3 and MMP-8 have corresponded with the malignant phenotype [7]. A high ratio of MMP-1 to TIMP-1 (tissue inhibitor of MMP-1) may also correspond with a more aggressive clinical course and poor prognosis for patients with CS [7].

The MYC oncogene has also been shown to play a possible role in the clinical course of the tumor. In an array CGH-based study of 15 tumors, MYC was shown to be amplified and overexpressed in approximately 15 to 20% of high-grade CS. This is in keeping with the observation that the presence of polysomy 8 and MYC amplification in higher grade CS were prognostic markers of poor outcome [23].

2. DEDIFFERENTIATED CS

Dedifferentiated CS is comprised of two distinct histologic components: a low-grade CS adjacent to a high-grade sarcoma with varying features (malignant fibrous histiocytoma, osteosarcoma, or rhabdomyosarcoma). The dedifferentiated component is almost exclusively seen in metastases [7]. The presence of shared genetic anomalies between both components lends support to the theory of a common primitive mesenchymal progenitor with divergent differentiation. At the same time, there are distinct genetic alterations in each component, corresponding to the late changes that occur as late events, in the histogenesis of dedifferentiated CS [24].

One of the genes implicated in the development of dedifferentiated CS is the STK15 gene, which encodes a centrosome-associated, serine/threonine kinase, the normal function of which is to ensure accurate segregation of chromosomes during mitosis and prevent aneuploidy [25]. Overexpression of the STK15 gene may play a role in tumor progression, and can be used as a prognostic factor for identifying patients who are at high risk for the development of local recurrence or distant metastases [7]. Similarly, H-ras mutation has also been associated with recurrence and poor prognosis [26].

III. BONE FORMING TUMORS

Osteoid osteoma and osteoblastoma are the most common benign bone forming tumors, especially in the pediatric population. Osteomas, however, rarely occur in children [27].

A. Benign

1. OSTEOID OSTEOMA

Osteoid osteoma is an osteoblastic lesion that is thought to arise secondary to an inflammatory reaction or to represent an unusual healing and reparative process. Though it is one of the most frequent benign primary bone tumors, little is known about the genetics and cytogenetics of this tumor. In one study, two osteoid osteomas showed del(22)(q13.1) as a clonal alteration in one tumor, and as non-clonal in another [28]. Chromosomal alterations involving 22q13 have also been described in malignant fibrous histiocytoma and fibrosarcoma [29,30]. This region harbors the YWHAH gene, which may be involved in cell proliferation regulation,

specifically in signal transduction and checkpoint control pathways, and functions in inhibiting apoptosis in mammals. Another gene mapped in this region is the platelet-derived growth factor (PDGF) which is a potent mitogen for cells of mesenchymal origin, and is involved in the transformation process [28]. Whereas these alterations seem necessary for tumor initiation, cytogenetics of recurrent osteoid osteomas have been reported to be more complex [31].

2. OSTEOBLASTOMA

This is an uncommon benign bone forming tumor that arises more often in children and adolescents. A subset of this entity which exhibits local invasion and a tendency for recurrence, without distal metastasis, is often termed an 'aggressive osteoblastoma' [27]. The aggressive osteoblastomas exhibit p53 and proliferation cell nuclear antigen immunoexpression that mimic osteosarcoma rather than classical osteoblastoma [32]. There is a relative paucity of cytogenetics information on osteoblastoma, with, notably, alterations on chromsomes 15, 17 and 20 [33].

B. Malignant

1. OSTEOSARCOMA

Of primary bone tumors, osteosarcoma (OS) is the most frequent. It is a malignant mesenchymal sarcoma characterized by the formation of bone or osteoid by malignant tumor cells. The peak incidence of OS is in the second decade of life, corresponding to the peak period of skeletal growth, with a gradual decline in incidences thereafter. OS tends to develop in areas of rapid bone growth or turnover, such as in the metaphyseal regions of long bones of a developing adolescent [34]. OS in patients over 40 years of age is usually secondary since it can occur after exposure to radiation, chemical agents, or viruses, or arise in areas of pre-existing Paget's disease of the bone [35]. It should, therefore, be considered as a disease which differs from OS in young patients with regard to histology, although its clinical course is comparable [36].

As well as the conventional high-grade OS, other subtypes are known. The telangiectatic OS is characterized by the occurrence of large spaces filled with blood with or without septa. Survival indications are similar to conventional high-grade OS. Small cell OS has a slightly worse prognosis compared to conventional OS and is composed of small cells with variable degrees of osteoid production [36].

The etiology of sporadic OS is unclear. These tumors may have arisen from osteoblasts or cells driven towards the osteoblastic lineage, compliant with their capacity to produce osteoid, alkaline phosphatase, osteocalcin, osterix and bone sialoprotein [36]. The development of OS is likely to be a multistep process that arises from the accumulation of critical genetic changes. The molecular changes leading to the development of OS have been shown to occur in several of the cell cycle regulatory genes [37–40]. An association between retinoblastoma (RB1) and OS has long been recognized. Individuals with hereditary RB are at increased risk of developing OS and exhibit up to 1000 times the incidence of OS as the general population. Loss of heterozygosity (LOH) of the RB1 locus is present in 60 to 70% of OS tumors [41], and has been suggested as a poor prognostic indicator [42]. Structural rearrangements and point mutations occur less commonly (30 and 10%, respectively). The RB1 gene functions as a tumor suppressor gene and is located on the q14 band of chromosome 13. The gene product participates in a cell-cycle regulatory pathway that functions to inhibit entry of cells into the S phase. Other proteins in the cell-cycle regulatory pathway in which the RB1 protein functions include p16 protein, a cyclin dependent kinase 4 (CDK4) inhibitor and encoded by INK4A. Loss of p16 expression has been reported in some OS lacking RB mutations, which may allow phosphorylation and inactivation of the RB protein [43].

The second gene significantly associated with OS is the TP53 tumor suppressor gene, which is commonly mutated in sporadic OS [44]. As a central player in the cell's many anti-cancer mechanisms, p53 can induce growth arrest, apoptosis and cell senescence. It functions as a cell-cycle checkpoint after DNA damage following irradiation with cells appearing to enter a sustained arrest in the G2 phase of the cell cycle. Thus, alterations of TP53 may alter cellular resistance to DNA damage sensing and response mechanisms [45]. Alterations in TP53 in OS consist of point mutations (20–30%, mostly missense mutations), gross gene rearrangements (10–20%), and allelic loss (75–80%) [41].

As with RB1, mutations in genes that regulate p53 have been identified in OS. The MDM2 gene, located on chromosome 12q13 along with CDK4, encodes a protein that binds p53 and blocks the activity of the p53 by directing it to the ubiquitination pathway. Overexpression of MDM2 in OS provides an alternative means to disrupt the normal p53 pathway [44]. Ladanyi *et al.* reported that amplification of MDM2 is more frequent in metastatic or recurrent tumors and suggest that amplification may be associated with tumor progression [46]. Another protein involved in this pathway is the p14 product of the INK4A gene, which is produced through bicistronic transcription involving the use of an alternative reading frame [41,47]. Whereas p16 indirectly regulates RB1 function, p14 regulates the TP53 function by binding MDM2 and sequestering it in the nucleolus. This protective role prevents MDM2 from shuttling p53 to the cytoplasm for proteasomal degradation. Alterations consistent with inactivation of p14 have been found in OS tumors and cell lines [44,48], with approximately 10% of OS showing deletions of INK4A which would knock out p14 expression [49].

Genes other than p53 and RB1 have also been associated with OS. High frequencies of allelic loss have been detected at 3q, suggesting that other tumor suppressor genes important in OS may exist [50]. HER2/neu (c-erbB-2) overexpression has been observed in several cases and has been associated with early pulmonary metastases and decreased survival [51,52]. However, results for HER2 expression in OS remain controversial, with some studies reporting up to 61% positive cases and others reporting only negative results. Furthermore, expression of HER2 has been reported to be a favorable prognostic indicator by some groups and unfavorable by others [53]. Bone morphogenetic proteins (BMPs) are important in the induction of cartilage and bone formation and patterning of skeletal elements. Expression of BMP type II receptor was found to correlate with metastasis in OS [54]. High-copy number gain of the MYC-C oncogene at 8q24 is also frequently demonstrated in OS and observed to be associated with poor outcome [55]. Significantly, this same cytoband is also the location of two genes: RecQL4 and EXT1. RecQL4 helicase protein inactivating mutations lead to the Rothmund-Thomson syndrome [56,57]. Patients with this syndrome have frequent chromosome aberrations in their lymphocytes, and a strong predisposition to OS. Increased RecQL4 expression in OS has been shown to correlate with elevated rates of structural chromosomal alterations in OS tumors [58]. As discussed above, the EXT1 gene leads to multiple exostoses, and the predisposition to OS in this syndrome may be mechanistically similar to the occurrence of osteochondromas in multiple exostoses.

One of the first oncogenes to be implicated in OS is c-fos. Functionally, c-fos dimerizes with Jun family members forming the AP-1 transcription complex and it is involved in the regulation of cell proliferation, differentiation and transformation. Overexpression of c-fos was found in over half of the cases in one study, particularly from patients who developed metastatic disease [48,59]. Studies have shown a number of growth factors to be elevated in OS.

High levels of TGF beta-1 in high-grade OS and low or absent mRNA in low-grade tumors suggest a role for TGF beta-1 in tumor progression [60]. In a study analyzing 62 cases of OS for P-glycoprotein expression, 27 of the cases exhibited overexpression. The patients with elevated expression had a significantly higher recurrence rate than those without increased expression [61], and such patients may benefit from additional chemotherapeutic modalities [62]. Studies have identified an association between the differential gene expression pattern of three genes with a phenotypic role in OS metastasis and invasion. THBS3 was expressed at significantly high levels in patients with metastasis at diagnosis, which is a predictor of overall survival, event-free survival, and relapse-free survival at diagnosis. High SPARC expression was found in 96.3% of OS samples and correlated with worse event-free survival and relapse-free survival. Overexpression of SPP1 was found in 89% of the samples and correlated with better overall survival, event-free survival and relapse-free survival at diagnosis. Interestingly, all encode for proteins involved in extracellular remodeling suggest potential roles in the OS progression [63]. In another study, OS samples from surgery showed a correlation between the expression of a major vault protein (MVP), metastatic disease at diagnosis and event-free survival. MVP gene expression was found to correlate with metastatic disease at diagnosis after neoadjuvant chemotherapy, and was also associated with worse event-free survival. These findings suggest that MVP expression is involved in one of the mechanisms of drug resistance in OS and is induced by chemotherapy [64]. Aberrant functions of some of the above-mentioned genes impair cell-cycle checkpoints that normally ensure proper replication, repair and segregation of the genome. Replication errors that occur during DNA synthesis will not be detected and corrected by DNA repair machinery [65], and these chromosomal aberrations will be propagated to daughter chromosomes. Moreover, inadequate mitotic checkpoints will lead to abnormal spindle formation, and subsequent mis-segregation of chromosomes, further promoting genomic instability—one of the hallmarks of cancer [66].

Most members of the sarcoma family have well-defined chromosomal aberrations, usually consisting of recurrent chromosomal translocations that result in fusion genes with oncogenic fusion protein products. However, no recurrent translocations have been identified so far in OS. Cytogenetic studies reveal that the majority of OS are characterized by elevated ploidy and heterogeneous complex chromosomal abnormalities that often vary widely from cell to cell [67]. They exhibit a high degree of aneusomies, gene amplifications, and multiple unbalanced chromosomal structural rearrangements that have precluded definitive identification of any recurrent cytogenetic aberrations [68]. Despite the complex pattern of genetic changes in OS, certain discrete chromosomal regions appear to be affected more often than others, and may highlight locations of genes involved in the development and progression of these tumors. Conventional cytogenetic techniques have shown that the most common chromosomal abnormalities were gain of $+1$ and loss of -9, -10, -13, and -17. Partial or complete loss of the long arm of chromosome 6 was also observed [69]. Common chromosomal rearrangements were found in 1p11-13, 1q10-12, 1q11, 1q21-22, 4q27-33, 6p23-25, 7p13-22, 7q11-36, 11p10-5, 11p14-15, 12p13, 15p11-13, 17p12-13, 19q13, and 22q11-13 [69,70]. Metaphase comparative genomic hybridization (CGH) has been systematically applied and has identified numerous regions of copy number change, including high-level gain or amplification at chromosomal regions 1p, 1q21~q31, 3q26, 6p, 6p12.1, 6p12-21, 8p, 8q12.21.3, 8q22-q23, 8q24.2, 12q12-13, 12q13-q14, 14q24-qter, 17p11-12, Xp11.2-21, and Xq12 [55,70–76]. The improved mapping resolution of array CGH has shown that 1p36, 6p21, 8q24, 16p13, 17p11 and 19p13 are recurrently gained/amplified [77–81]. In addition, DNA sequence loss has also been observed at 2q, 3q, 6p, 8p, 10p, and 17p13 [75,80]. Spectral karyotyping (SKY) demonstrated that OS has a complex pattern of clonal and non-clonal rearrangements and helped confirm the structural basis for the imbalances detected by CGH. SKY analysis of primary OS and cell lines identified a high frequency of structural instability present as translocations, inversions, deletions and amplifications, often superimposed on near tetraploid karyotypes (Figure 13.1; see Plate 3). In addition, centromeric rearrangements were often observed involving chromosomes 1, 6, 13, 14, 17 and 10 [82]. These data suggest that numerical as well as structural instability are important features of OS, and implicate pathways that normally maintain genomic integrity [83].

IV. SMALL ROUND CELL TUMORS OF BONE

Primary small round cell tumors of the bone are a heterogeneous group of malignant neoplasm presenting predominantly in children and adolescents. They include Ewing's sarcoma/peripheral neuroectodermal tumors or the Ewing's family of tumors (ESFT), lymphoma, mesenchymal chondrosarcoma, and small cell OS. Their unique biological and

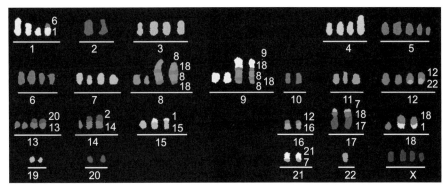

FIGURE 13.1 Typical osteosarcoma karyotype as analyzed by spectral karyotyping (SKY) derived from short-term culture of patient tumor (reported in Ref. [82]). Of note is the high frequency of duplicated complex structural chromosome aberrations such as translocations t(8;18), t(7;17;18) present in this near tetraploid karyotype. These findings indicate that multiple chromosomal translocations in this tumor occurred at high frequency and took place in a diploid progenitor prior to tetraploidization. This process is likely ongoing as alterations such as t(1;6) and t(12;22) are present singly in the tetraploid cells.

genetic characteristics have provided substantial insights into the pathology of these diverse tumors, though they share many morphological similarities.

A. Ewing's Sarcoma

The Ewing's family of tumors (ESFT), which includes Ewing's Sarcoma (ES), extraosseous ES, Askin tumor and primitive peripheral neuroectodermal tumors (PNET), is the second most common primary malignancy of bone in children and adolescents after OS, accounting for 10% of primary malignant bone tumors in children. Although ES can also occur in soft tissue, this review will be limited to the osseous subtype. ES primarily occurs in the first two decades of life [84]. However, incidences have even been reported in adults well into their 80s. The biological course and the outcomes of adults with ES is unclear [34].

ES, along with PNET, was the first sarcoma to be defined by a specific chromosomal change [84]. The unique and specific translocation that it shares along with the rest of the ESFT family is the t(11;22)(q24;q12), seen in about 85 to 95% of ES tumors. This translocation leads to the fusion of the 5′ portion of the *EWS* gene, located at 22q12, and the 3′ portion of a *FLI-1* gene from the *ETS* family of transcription factors at 11q24. The second most common translocation is t(21;22)(q22;q12) leading to a fusion between *EWS* and the *ERG* gene at 21q22 [85]. To date, 14 different EWS fusion partners have been described, including 2q31.1, 2q33.3, 2q36, 6p21.33, 7p21.2, 9q31.1, 11p13, 12p12, 12q13.13, 17q12, and 22q12. Most are extremely rare, representing altogether <1% of the cases. Some studies report the presence of complex and often cryptic rearrangements of *EWS-ERG*, as exemplified by a report on the three-chromosome rearrangement involving chromosomes 19, 21 and 22 that carried a cytogenetically cryptic *EWS-ERG* fusion gene [86].

The *EWS* gene belongs to a family of RNA binding proteins, whose amino terminal has the capacity to bind to DNA-binding domains of various transcription factors, thus providing a strong transcriptional activating domain to the resulting chimeric protein [87]. The partner genes of EWS in ES such as *FLI-1, ERG, ETV1, EIAF,* and *FEV* belong to the *ETS* family of transcription factors. Though *EWS* is ubiquitously expressed in all tissues, *FLI-1* expression is seen in high levels in hematopoietic cells, endothelial cells and mesenchyme derived from the neural crest cells [87–90]. The product of EWS-ETS translocation results in fusion proteins, where the ETS component is brought under the transactivating domain of EWS. These fusion products modulate multiple target genes resulting in malignant transformation [87].

Type 1 (exon 7 of *EWS* to exon 6 of *FLI-1*) and type II (exon 7 of *EWS* to exon 5 of *FLI-1*) are the most common (>85%) fusion transcripts [91]. In patients with localized diseases, *EWS-FLI-1* type 1 fusion transcript has been reported as being associated with improved outcomes compared to other fusion transcript types. This has been attributed to the transcript encoding a less active chimeric protein and is associated with a lower proliferative index [92,93].

Additionally reported secondary karyotypic changes include gains of chromosomes 8, 12, and 18, deletion of the short arm of chromosome 1, unbalanced translocation t(1;16)(q12;q11), and other rare structural abnormalities [94,95]. The unbalanced translocation der(16)t(1;16) with variable breaks on both chromosomes is considered the most common secondary abnormality in ES. Der(16) has been detected by cytogenetic analysis in a number of conditions such as leukemia, breast cancer, Wilms' tumor, retinoblastoma, alveolar rhabdomyosarcoma, extraskeletal myxoid chondrosarcoma [85,96]. In a 13-year study that evaluated secondary chromosome changes in relation to clinical outcome, the most frequent secondary change was +8, followed by +12, +2, +5, +9, +15 and a gain of material from the long and short arms of chromosome 1. The only recurrent secondary change restricted to tumors from the patients who died was a gain of 1q material. In addition, poor outcome was also correlated to tumors that exhibited a modal chromosome number greater than 50. Although relatively uncommon in ES, deletions of 1p have also been associated with an unfavorable outcome in patients with localized diseases [97].

In studies examining the significance of trisomy 8 in ES, this cytogenetic anomaly appeared to occur in higher frequencies in relapsed than in primary tumors. Also, in cell line models, populations with tetrasomy 8 exhibit a proliferative advantage over those with other chromosome changes [98,99].

Comparative genomic hybridization (CGH) has been used to detect genomic imbalances in ES. In a study examining 20 samples, gains of DNA sequences were much more frequent than losses, most of them affecting whole chromosomes or whole chromosome arms. Recurrent findings included copy number increases for chromosome 8, 1q and 12. The minimal common regions of these gains were whole chromosomes 8 and 12 and 1q21-q22, with high-level amplifications affecting 8q13-24, 1q and 1q21-q22 [100]. Another CGH study examining 17 ES specimens also reported gains at 1q31-q41 and 8q [101]. These copy number changes correlate with certain parameters. For example, copy number increases at 1q21-q22 and of chromosomes 8 and 12 tend to be associated with a worse overall outcome, while an increase in 6p copy number correlates with worse disease-free interval and overall survival [102].

Up to one-third of patients have metastatic disease at the time of presentation, and their outcome remains poor in spite of aggressive chemotherapy. Multiple biological factors such as fusion transcript type, mutations and deletions of *p16INK4, p14ARF* and *TP53,* telomerase, *IGF-1* and aneuploidy have been implicated in playing a role in the prognosis of EW [103–105].

In a mouse transgenic model, EWS-FLI1 oncoprotein was not a strong initiator of sarcoma formation. However, it accelerated the formation of sarcomas and strongly favored the generation of poorly differentiated sarcomas when expressed in cells with a *TP53* null mutation [106]. The fact that *TP53* was found to have synergistic effects with *EWS-FLI1* is consistent with clinical observations where *TP53* mutation has been shown to be associated with highly aggressive behavior and poor chemoresponses [107]. Homozygous deletion and alterations of *p14ARF* and *p16INK4* have been detected in approximately 20% of ES/PNET tumor samples [108], and have been associated with shorter event-free and overall survival [105,108]. A role for the Wnt pathway in EWS has also been suggested. In a study that profiled the global gene expression of 27 ESFT to compare metastatic and localized ESFT, most differently regulated genes were linked to the Wnt-signaling pathway. This pathway plays a key role in cell migration, tissue architecture, and embryonic development. Its activation blocks β-catenin phosphorylation and degradation in the proteasome, enabling β-catenin to accumulate and enter the nucleus to activate gene transcription [109]. Wnt-3a induces stabilization of β-catenin in ESFT *in vitro*, which in turn leads to a dramatic increase in chemotactic cell migration [110].

B. Giant Cell Tumors of the Bone

The giant cell tumor of the bone (osteoclastoma) is a benign, primary skeletal neoplasm with variable biologic aggressiveness. Usually arising in the epiphysis of the long bone in skeletally mature patients [27], these tumors have been shown to demonstrate telomeric associations of chromosomes 11, 16, 19, 20 and 21, reduction of telomere length, marker chromosomes, double minutes, chromosome fragments, ring chromosomes and polyploidy [111].

V. CONCLUSION AND PERSPECTIVES

Over the past few years, the molecular genetic changes underlying cartilaginous and bone tumor development and progression have been increasingly elucidated. However, the development of optimal treatment strategies for some of these entities has been greatly complicated by the large number of subtypes, the heterogeneity in their genetics and biological behavior, and the rarity of these tumors. In addition, inconsistencies have emerged from different studies examining prognostic factors, probably as a result of different study designs and treatment protocols, confounding variables associated with retrospective analyses and the use of diverse molecular methods. In order to resolve these issues, prognostic factors should be validated using uniform and multiple methods in both retrospective investigations and prospective multi-center studies. The advent of the human genome map and molecular techniques, such

as microarray-based copy number and gene expression profiling, provide a new approach to classifying tumors and promise to improve our ability to predict both the probability of metastasis and overall clinical course. In addition, an understanding of the molecular biology of these tumors is leading to the identification of targets for novel therapeutic approaches.

Acknowledgement

We are grateful for the support of Canadian Cancer Society grant 016215.

References

1. C.D. Fletcher, U.K. Unni & F. Mertens, Pathology and Genetics of Soft Tissue and Bone, IRC Press, Lyon, (2002).
2. Y.M. Schrage, Bone Tumors, An Overview (2005).
3. D.S. Springfield, M.C. Gebhardt & M.H. McGuire, Chondrosarcoma, a review, Instr Course Lect 45 (1996) 417–424.
4. L. Hameetman, et al., Decreased EXT expression and intracellular accumulation of heparan sulphate proteoglycan in osteochondromas and peripheral chondrosarcomas, J Pathol 211 (4) (2007) 399–409.
5. J.V. Bovee, Multiple osteochondromas, Orphanet J Rare Dis 3 (2008) 3.
6. L. Hameetman, et al., The role of EXT1 in nonhereditary osteochondroma, identification of homozygous deletions, J Natl Cancer Inst 99 (5) (2007) 396–406.
7. A.A. Sandberg & J.A. Bridge, Updates on the cytogenetics and molecular genetics of bone and soft tissue tumors, chondrosarcoma and other cartilaginous neoplasms, Cancer Genet Cytogenet 143 (1) (2003) 1–31.
8. T. Ozaki, et al., Comparative genomic hybridization in cartilaginous tumors, Anticancer Res 24 (3a) (2004) 1721–1725.
9. J.A. Bridge, et al., Clonal karyotypic aberrations in enchondromas, Cancer Detect Prev 16 (4) (1992) 215–219.
10. W.C. Bell, et al., Molecular pathology of chondroid neoplasms, part 1, benign lesions, Skeletal Radiol 35 (11) (2006) 805–813.
11. K. Takigawa, Chondroma of the bones of the hand. A review of 110 cases, J Bone Joint Surg Am 53 (8) (1971) 1591–1600.
12. R.J. Lewis & A.S. Ketcham, Maffucci's syndrome, functional and neoplastic significance. Case report and review of the literature, J Bone Joint Surg Am 55 (7) (1973) 1465–1479.
13. H.K. Tamimi & J.W. Bolen, Enchondromatosis (Ollier's disease) and ovarian juvenile granulosa cell tumor, Cancer 53 (7) (1984) 1605–1608.
14. J.V. Bovee, et al., Malignant progression in multiple enchondromatosis (Ollier's disease), an autopsy-based molecular genetic study, Hum Pathol 31 (10) (2000) 1299–12303.
15. S.J. Swarts, et al., Significance of abnormalities of chromosomes 5 and 8 in chondroblastoma, Clin Orthop Relat Res 349 (1988) 189–193.
16. S.L. van Zelderen-Bhola, et al., Ring chromosome 4 as the sole cytogenetic anomaly in a chondroblastoma, a case

report and review of the literature, Cancer Genet Cytogenet 105 (2) (1998) 109–112.

17. H. Sjogren, et al., Cytogenetic and spectral karyotype analyses of benign and malignant cartilage tumours, Int J Oncol 24 (6) (2004) 1385–1391.

18. H.J. Mankin, et al., The use of flow cytometry in assessing malignancy in bone and soft tissue tumors, Clin Orthop Relat Res 397 (2002) 95–105.

19. L.B. Rozeman, et al., Absence of IHH and retention of PTHrP signalling in enchondromas and central chondrosarcomas, J Pathol 205 (4) (2005) 476–482.

20. J.V. Bovee, et al., Loss of heterozygosity and DNA ploidy point to a diverging genetic mechanism in the origin of peripheral and central chondrosarcoma, Genes Chromosomes Cancer 26 (3) (1999) 237–246.

21. M. Ropke, et al., Rb-loss is associated with high malignancy in chondrosarcoma, Oncol Rep 15 (1) (2006) 89–95.

22. T. Yamaguchi, et al., Loss of heterozygosity and tumor suppressor gene mutations in chondrosarcomas, Anticancer Res 16 (4A) (1996) 2009–2015.

23. C. Morrison, et al., MYC amplification and polysomy 8 in chondrosarcoma, array comparative genomic hybridization, fluorescent in situ hybridization, and association with outcome, J Clin Oncol 23 (36) (2005) 9369–9376.

24. J.V. Bovee, et al., Molecular genetic characterization of both components of a dedifferentiated chondrosarcoma, with implications for its histogenesis, J Pathol 189 (4) (1999) 454–462.

25. L. Lentini, et al., Simultaneous Aurora-A/STK15 overexpression and centrosome amplification induce chromosomal instability in tumour cells with a MIN phenotype, BMC Cancer 7 (2007) 212.

26. M.K. McAfee, et al., Chondrosarcoma of the chest wall, factors affecting survival, Ann Thorac Surg 40 (6) (1985) 535–541.

27. M. Vlychou & N.A. Athanasou, Radiological and pathological diagnosis of paediatric bone tumours and tumour-like lesions, Pathology 40 (2) (2008) 196–216.

28. M.R. Baruffi, et al., Osteoid osteomas with chromosome alterations involving 22q, Cancer Genet Cytogenet 124 (2) (2001) 127–131.

29. N. Mandahl, et al., Separate karyotypic features in a local recurrence and a metastasis of a fibrosarcoma, Cancer Genet Cytogenet 37 (1) (1989) 139–140.

30. N. Mandahl, et al., Characteristic karyotypic anomalies identify subtypes of malignant fibrous histiocytoma, Genes Chromosomes Cancer 1 (1) (1989) 9–14.

31. P. Dal Cin, et al., Osteoid osteoma and osteoblastoma with clonal chromosome changes, Br J Cancer 78 (3) (1998) 344–348.

32. C.R. Oliveira, et al., Classical osteoblastoma, atypical osteoblastoma, and osteosarcoma, a comparative study based on clinical, histological, and biological parameters, Clinics 62 (2) (2007) 167–174.

33. J.T. Mascarello, H.F. Krous & P.M. Carpenter, Unbalanced translocation resulting in the loss of the chromosome 17 short arm in an osteoblastoma, Cancer Genet Cytogenet 69 (1) (1993) 65–67.

34. K.M. Skubitz & D.R. D'Adamo, Sarcoma, Mayo Clin Proc 82 (11) (2997) 1409–1432.

35. B. Fuchs & D.J. Pritchard, Etiology of osteosarcoma, Clin Orthop Relat Res 397 (2002) 40–52.

36. L.B. Rozeman, A.M. Cleton-Jansen & P.C. Hogendoorn, Pathology of primary malignant bone and cartilage tumours, Int Orthop 30 (6) (2006) 437–444.

37. M.S. Benassi, et al., Alteration of pRb/p16/cdk4 regulation in human osteosarcoma, Int J Cancer 84 (5) (1999) 489–493.

38. L. Molendini, et al., Prognostic significance of cyclin expression in human osteosarcoma, Int J Oncol 12 (5) (1998) 1007–1011.

39. K. Radig, et al., Genetic instability in osteoblastic tumors of the skeletal system, Pathol Res Pract 194 (10) (1998) 669–677.

40. K. Radig, et al., Mutation spectrum of p53 gene in highly malignant human osteosarcomas, Gen Diagn Pathol 142 (1) (1996) 25–32.

41. N. Tang, et al., Osteosarcoma development and stem cell differentiation, Clin Orthop Relat Res 466 (9) (2008) 2114–2130.

42. O. Feugeas, et al., Loss of heterozygosity of the RB gene is a poor prognostic factor in patients with osteosarcoma, J Clin Oncol 14 (2) (1996) 467–472.

43. G.P. Nielsen, et al., CDKN2A gene deletions and loss of p16 expression occur in osteosarcomas that lack RB alterations, Am J Pathol 153 (1) (1998) 159–163.

44. M.F. Hansen, Genetic and molecular aspects of osteosarcoma, J Musculoskelet Neuronal Interact 2 (6) (2002) 554–560.

45. A.J. Levine, p53, the cellular gatekeeper for growth and division, Cell 88 (3) (1997) 323–331.

46. M. Ladanyi, et al., MDM2 gene amplification in metastatic osteosarcoma, Cancer Res 53 (1) (1993) 16–18.

47. A. Maitra, et al., Loss of p16(INK4a) expression correlates with decreased survival in pediatric osteosarcomas, Int J Cancer 95 (1) (2001) 34–38.

48. M. Kansara & D.M. Thomas, Molecular pathogenesis of osteosarcoma, DNA Cell Biol 26 (1) (2007) 1–18.

49. C.R. Walkley, et al., Conditional mouse osteosarcoma, dependent on p53 loss and potentiated by loss of Rb, mimics the human disease, Genes Dev 22 (12) (2008) 1662–1676.

50. R.P. Kruzelock, et al., Localization of a novel tumor suppressor locus on human chromosome 3q important in osteosarcoma tumorigenesis, Cancer Res 57 (1) (1997) 106–109.

51. R. Gorlick, et al., Expression of HER2/erbB-2 correlates with survival in osteosarcoma, J Clin Oncol 17 (9) (1999) 2781–2788.

52. M. Onda, et al., ErbB-2 expression is correlated with poor prognosis for patients with osteosarcoma, Cancer 77 (1) (1996) 71–78.

53. G.R. Somers, et al., HER2 amplification and overexpression is not present in pediatric osteosarcoma, a tissue microarray study, Pediatr Dev Pathol 8 (5) (2005) 525–532.

54. W. Guo, et al., Expression of bone morphogenetic proteins and receptors in sarcomas, Clin Orthop Relat Res 365 (1999) 175–183.

55. C. Stock, et al., Chromosomal regions involved in the pathogenesis of osteosarcomas, Genes Chromosomes Cancer 28 (3) (2000) 329–336.

56. P. Mohaghegh & I.D. Hickson, DNA helicase deficiencies associated with cancer predisposition and premature ageing disorders, Hum Mol Genet 10 (7) (2001) 741–746.

57. L.L. Wang, et al., Association between osteosarcoma and deleterious mutations in the RECQL4 gene in Rothmund-Thomson syndrome, J Natl Cancer Inst 95 (9) (2003) 669–674.

58. G. Maire, M. Yosdhimoto & S. Chilton-MacNeill, et al., Increased gene expression levels are associated with structural chromosomal instability in sporadic osteosarcoma, Neoplasia 11 (3) (2009) 260–268.

59. J.X. Wu, et al., The proto-oncogene c-fos is over-expressed in the majority of human osteosarcomas, Oncogene 5 (7) (1990) 989–1000.

60. A. Franchi, et al., Expression of transforming growth factor beta isoforms in osteosarcoma variants, association of TGF beta 1 with high-grade osteosarcomas, J Pathol 185 (3) (1998) 284–289.

61. H.S. Chan, et al., P-glycoprotein expression, critical determinant in the response to osteosarcoma chemotherapy, J Natl Cancer Inst 89 (22) (1997) 1706–1715.

62. N. Baldini, et al., P-glycoprotein expression in osteosarcoma, a basis for risk-adapted adjuvant chemotherapy, J Orthop Res 17 (5) (1999) 629–632.

63. C.A. Dalla-Torre, et al., Effects of THBS3, SPARC and SPP1 expression on biological behavior and survival in patients with osteosarcoma, BMC Cancer 6 (2006) 237.

64. C.A. Dalla-Torre, et al., Expression of major vault protein gene in osteosarcoma patients, J Orthop Res 25 (7) (2007) 958–963.

65. K.A. Cimprich & D. Cortez, ATR, an essential regulator of genome integrity, Nat Rev Mol Cell Biol 9 (8) (2008) 616–627.

66. D. Hanahan & R.A. Weinberg, The hallmarks of cancer, Cell 100 (1) (2000) 57–70.

67. B.D. Ragland, et al., Cytogenetics and molecular biology of osteosarcoma, Lab Invest 82 (4) (2002) 365–373.

68. A.A. Sandberg & J.A. Bridge, Updates on the cytogenetics and molecular genetics of bone and soft tissue tumors, osteosarcoma and related tumors, Cancer Genet Cytogenet 145 (1) (2003) 1–30.

69. J.A. Bridge, et al., Cytogenetic findings in 73 osteosarcoma specimens and a review of the literature, Cancer Genet Cytogenet 95 (1) (1997) 74–87.

70. J.R. Batanian, et al., Evaluation of paediatric osteosarcomas by classic cytogenetic and CGH analyses, Mol Pathol 55 (6) (2002) 389–393.

71. A. Forus, et al., Comparative genomic hybridization analysis of human sarcomas, II. Identification of novel amplicons at 6p and 17p in osteosarcomas, Genes Chromosomes Cancer 14 (1) (1995) 15–21.

72. T.J. Hulsebos, et al., Malignant astrocytoma-derived region of common amplification in chromosomal band 17p12 is frequently amplified in high-grade osteosarcomas, Genes Chromosomes Cancer 18 (4) (1997) 279–285.

73. T. Ozaki, et al., Genetic imbalances revealed by comparative genomic hybridization in osteosarcomas, Int J Cancer 102 (4) (2002) 355–365.

74. M. Tarkkanen, et al., DNA sequence copy number increase at 8q, a potential new prognostic marker in high-grade osteosarcoma, Int J Cancer 84 (2) (1999) 114–121.

75. M. Tarkkanen, et al., Gains and losses of DNA sequences in osteosarcomas by comparative genomic hybridization, Cancer Res 55 (6) (1995) 1334–1338.

76. M. Zielenska, et al., Comparative genomic hybridization analysis identifies gains of 1p35 approximately p36 and chromosome 19 in osteosarcoma, Cancer Genet Cytogenet 130 (1) (2001) 14–21.

77. J. Atiye, et al., Gene amplifications in osteosarcoma-CGH microarray analysis, Genes Chromosomes Cancer 42 (2) (2005) 158–163.

78. C.C. Lau, et al., Frequent amplification and rearrangement of chromosomal bands 6p12-p21 and 17p11.2 in osteosarcoma, Genes Chromosomes Cancer 39 (1) (2004) 11–21.

79. T.K. Man, et al., Genome-wide array comparative genomic hybridization analysis reveals distinct amplifications in osteosarcoma, BMC Cancer 4 (2004) 45.

80. J.A. Squire, et al., High-resolution mapping of amplifications and deletions in pediatric osteosarcoma by use of CGH analysis of cDNA microarrays, Genes Chromosomes Cancer 38 (3) (2003) 215–225.

81. M. Zielenska, et al., High-resolution cDNA microarray CGH mapping of genomic imbalances in osteosarcoma using formalin-fixed paraffin-embedded tissue, Cytogenet Genome Res 107 (1–2) (2004) 77–82.

82. J. Bayani, et al., Spectral karyotyping identifies recurrent complex rearrangements of chromosomes 8, 17, and 20 in osteosarcomas, Genes Chromosomes Cancer 36 (1) (2003) 7–16.

83. J. Bayani, et al., Genomic mechanisms and measurement of structural and numerical instability in cancer cells, Semin Cancer Biol 17 (1) (2007) 5–18.

84. R. Carvajal & P. Meyers, Ewing's sarcoma and primitive neuroectodermal family of tumors, Hematol Oncol Clin North Am 19 (3) (2005) 501–525 vi–vii.

85. A.A. Sandberg & J.A. Bridge, Updates on cytogenetics and molecular genetics of bone and soft tissue tumors, Ewing sarcoma and peripheral primitive neuroectodermal tumors, Cancer Genet Cytogenet 123 (1) (2000) 1–26.

86. G. Maire, et al., Complex rearrangement of chromosomes 19, 21, and 22 in Ewing sarcoma involving a novel reciprocal inversion-insertion mechanism of EWS-ERG fusion gene formation, a case analysis and literature review, Cancer Genet Cytogenet 181 (2) (2008) 81–92.

87. M. Hameed, Small round cell tumors of bone, Arch Pathol Lab Med 131 (2) (2007) 192–204.

88. H. Kovar, Context matters, the hen or egg problem in Ewing's sarcoma, Semin Cancer Biol 15 (3) (2005) 189–196.

89. V.I. Sementchenko & D.K. Watson, Ets target genes, past, present and future, Oncogene 19 (55) (2000) 6533–6548.

90. C. Siligan, et al., EWS-FLI1 target genes recovered from Ewing's sarcoma chromatin, Oncogene 24 (15) (2005) 2512–2524.

91. H. Kovar, Ewing tumor biology, perspectives for innovative treatment approaches, Adv Exp Med Biol 532 (2003) 27–37.

92. P.P. Lin, et al., Differential transactivation by alternative EWS-FLI1 fusion proteins correlates with clinical heterogeneity in Ewing's sarcoma, Cancer Res 59 (7) (1999) 1428–1432.

93. O. Slater & J. Shipley, Clinical relevance of molecular genetics to paediatric sarcomas, J Clin Pathol 60 (11) (2007) 1187–1194.

94. A.M. Udayakumar & T.S. Sundareshan, Cytogenetic characterization of Ewing tumors, further update on 20 cases, Cancer Genet Cytogenet 133 (1) (2002) 102–103.

95. A.M. Udayakumar, et al., Cytogenetic characterization of Ewing tumors using fine needle aspiration samples: a 10-year experience and review of the literature, Cancer Genet Cytogenet 127 (1) (2001) 42–48.

96. C.M. Hattinger, et al., Demonstration of the translocation der (16)t(1;16)(q12;q11.2) in interphase nuclei of Ewing tumors, Genes Chromosomes Cancer 17 (3) (1996) 141–150.

97. C.M. Hattinger, et al., Prognostic impact of deletions at 1p36 and numerical aberrations in Ewing tumors, Genes Chromosomes Cancer 24 (3) (1999) 243–254.

98. D. Maurici, et al., Frequency and implications of chromosome 8 and 12 gains in Ewing sarcoma, Cancer Genet Cytogenet 100 (2) (1998) 106–110.

99. L. Trakhtenbrot, et al., *In vitro* proliferative advantage of bone marrow cells with tetrasomy 8 in Ewing sarcoma, Cancer Genet Cytogenet 90 (2) (1996) 176–178.

100. G. Armengol, et al., Recurrent gains of 1q, 8 and 12 in the Ewing family of tumours by comparative genomic hybridization, Br J Cancer 75 (10) (1997) 1403–1409.

101. S. Knuutila, et al., Comparative genomic hybridization study on pooled DNAs from tumors of one clinical-pathological entity, Cancer Genet Cytogenet 100 (1) (1998) 25–30.

102. M. Tarkkanen, et al., Clinical correlations of genetic changes by comparative genomic hybridization in Ewing sarcoma and related tumors, Cancer Genet Cytogenet 114 (1) (1999) 35–41.

103. A. Amiel, et al., Molecular cytogenetic parameters in Ewing sarcoma, Cancer Genet Cytogenet 140 (2) (2003) 107–112.

104. S.A. Burchill, Ewing's sarcoma, diagnostic, prognostic, and therapeutic implications of molecular abnormalities, J Clin Pathol 56 (2) (2003) 96–102.

105. T. Tsuchiya, et al., Analysis of the p16INK4, p14ARF, p15, TP53, and MDM2 genes and their prognostic implications in osteosarcoma and Ewing sarcoma, Cancer Genet Cytogenet 120 (2) (2000) 91–98.

106. P.P. Lin, et al., EWS-FLI1 induces developmental abnormalities and accelerates sarcoma formation in a transgenic mouse model, Cancer Res 68 (21) (2008) 8968–8975.

107. H.Y. Huang, et al., Ewing sarcomas with p53 mutation or p16/p14ARF homozygous deletion, a highly lethal subset associated with poor chemoresponse, J Clin Oncol 23 (3) (2005) 548–558.

108. H. Kovar, et al., Among genes involved in the RB dependent cell cycle regulatory cascade, the p16 tumor suppressor gene is frequently lost in the Ewing family of tumors, Oncogene 15 (18) (1997) 2225–2232.

109. M. Peifer, Cell biology. Travel bulletin – traffic jams cause tumors, Science 289 (5476) (2000) 67–69.

110. A. Uren, et al., Wnt/Frizzled signaling in Ewing sarcoma, Pediatr Blood Cancer 43 (3) (2004) 243–249.

111. G.D. Letson & C.A. Muro-Cacho, Genetic and molecular abnormalities in tumors of the bone and soft tissues, Cancer Control 8 (3) (2001) 239–251.

CHAPTER **14**

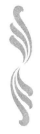

Proteomics of Bone Cancer

STEPHANIE BYRUM[1,3], ERIC R. SIEGEL[2,3], SUDEEPA BHATTACHARYYA[1,3] AND LARRY J. SUVA[1,3]

[1]*Department of Orthopaedic Surgery.*

[2]*Department of Biostatistics.*

[3]*Center for Orthopaedic Research, Barton Research Institute, University of Arkansas for Medical Sciences, Little Rock, AR 72205, USA.*

Contents

I. INTRODUCTION

Ongoing advances in proteomic technology offer great promise and have begun to contribute to the increased understanding of the molecular basis of cancer. Clearly genomic, proteomic and other 'omics' are the primary discovery research tool for biomarker and target discovery. Innovations in the application of high-throughput proteomic profiling, particularly using surface-enhanced laser desorption/ionization time-of-flight (SELDI-TOF) MS have become best practice for biomarker discovery. As such, the identified protein profiles are powerful diagnostic markers that can predict treatment efficacy, disease progression and possibly even cancer risk. From a proteomics perspective, the bone cancer field seems to be amongst the most understudied diseases [1].

The proclivity of many tumors (e.g., breast and prostate) for bone is frequently associated with intractable bone pain, pathological fractures, nerve compression, and hypercalcemia due to osteolysis [2] and is a feature often distinct from locoregional and visceral spread. In addition, for primary skeletal tumors such as multiple myeloma, or osteosarcoma, the associated extensive bone destruction denotes a dramatic

change in the prognosis for the patient that significantly increases morbidity [3]. As a result, the pattern of disease progression, response to therapy and ultimately patient survival following diagnosis is subject to extremely wide variation [4].

Tumor metastasis (to bone or any other tissue) involves progression through a complex series of steps [5], which includes tumor growth at the primary site; the release of tumor cells into lymphatic and systemic circulation; the survival of the tumor cells within the circulation; tumor cell arrest in the microvasculature of the target organ, extravasation of tumor cells; tumor cell invasion of target organs; and, ultimately, growth of the tumor at the distant metastatic site [5,6].

Metastasis to any site, including the skeleton is a non-random process [7]. The selectivity of tumors for a specific target site is determined by the ability of the tumor cells to accomplish all of the steps of the complex metastatic cascade [5]. Although anatomical and mechanical effects such as blood flow influence the sites of tumor metastasis to some degree [8], it is the microenvironment that not only promotes tumor proliferation at the distant site, but determines which metastatic site(s) is preferred. Similarly, the growth in bone of primary tumors such as osteosarcoma and myeloma also relies on the intimate relationship between the tumor and the host microenvironment.

For growth in the skeleton, tumor cells in bone must first stimulate bone resorption (mediated by specialized bone resorbing osteoclasts [9]) via the secretion of potent osteolytic agents [2,10,11]. The increased bone resorption that follows releases bone-derived growth factors into the extracellular milieu and systemic circulation [2], thereby promoting increased bone resorption, and promoting tumor growth, at least in animal models. This feed-forward process likely also modifies the local microenvironment (and the tumor cells) supporting subsequent tumor progression [12] at either the primary or metastatic site (Figure 14.1).

Although the investigation of tumor development in bone as well as the metastasis of tumors to bone has been the focus of intensive investigation, relatively little is known

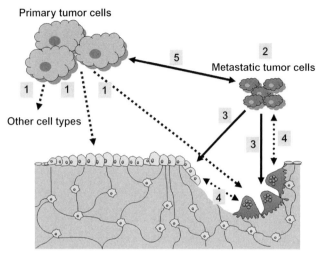

Primary tumor cells

Metastatic tumor cells

Other cell types

FIGURE 14.1 Schematic representation of the progression of tumors in bone. Primary tumors (1) secrete factors that activate (directly or indirectly) a variety of cell types, such as osteoblasts and osteoclasts on the bone surface as well as other cells locally and within the bone marrow microenvironment. Primary tumors also release cells into the lymph and/or systemic circulation that become metastatic (2). Metastatic tumor cells secrete factors that activate osteoblasts and/or osteoclasts (3), thereby enhancing bone turnover. Once activated, osteoclasts and osteoblasts (4) increase metastatic tumor growth. Metastatic cells stimulated by the increased bone turnover may also re-seed the primary tumor site, and/or secrete factors that impact the primary tumor (5).

about the molecular mechanisms that control the process, even though widespread skeletal dissemination is an important step in the progression of many tumors [7,10,13,14]. Despite the well-characterized clinical issues associated with skeletal tumors, such as the presence of concurrent visceral metastases, skeletal tumor load and the expression of relevant tumor therapeutic targets, detailed investigation of the molecular mechanisms involved has been hindered by a lack of appropriate clinical specimens [7]. As a result, the majority of the studies investigating tumor progression in bone have been performed using xenograft models in immune-compromised mice, or genetic murine models of tumor development and almost exclusively focused on the potential of the tumor transcriptome [13,15].

Histological examination and gene expression profiling of primary human tumors has revealed a remarkable cellular heterogeneity [7,14,16]. For example, morphologically diverse areas can occur within a tumor such as foci of ductal carcinoma *in situ* within a primary breast carcinoma [17] or the different bone metastases of a single patient with metastatic prostate cancer [18]. Similarly, estrogen receptor, Her2/neu, or p53 expression varies between and within tumors and metastases, ranging from 1% to >90% of cells [19]. As such, it is not surprising that gene expression profiling of primary tumors has not provided clinically relevant prognostic or diagnostic markers, with the widespread utility necessary for clinical practice.

II. WHY USE A PROTEOMIC APPROACH?

As outlined above, the analysis of the tumor transcriptome by gene expression profiling has proven extremely useful in the sub-classification and outcome assessment for a variety of invasive bone cancers [13,14,20–23]. However, many of the identified classifiers and target genes in the various studies are largely non-overlapping, raising questions about their biologic significance and their clinical implications [15]. Moreover, it is increasingly evident that genes do not act as individual units but collaborate in a series of overlapping and interrelated networks, the deregulation of which is a classic hallmark of cancer [24]. Current gene expression profiling technology provides the ability to identify large numbers of differentially expressed genes, but excludes the role of multiple protein products from individual genes and neglects their functional significance. The obvious implication from these collective observations is that other approaches such as proteomics-based assays are required to validate and/or define those pathways and targets identified by gene expression profiling as predictive of tumor development and progression [1].

The currently used postoperative treatment guidelines for breast cancer use consensus criteria to determine if a patient is at risk for a distant metastasis. The guidelines include age, histological tumor grade and immunohistochemical characterization of particular cell markers, such as estrogen or progesterone receptor, expressed in tumor biopsy material. Although useful, these criteria (also used in many other tumor types) have low specificity and have been considered insufficient for predicting metastatic behavior. As a result, more accurate prognostic and diagnostic markers are urgently needed [25].

A number of specific protein markers of multiple cancers (such as estrogen receptor, and Her2/neu in breast cancer [26] and syndecan 1 and dkk in multiple myeloma [23,27]) have been individually identified and tested, yet none have significantly improved disease stratification or predict outcome. It is becoming increasingly apparent that the presence or absence of an individual biomarker aiding prognosis is not reasonable [1]. If this is the case (and it likely is) then it is incumbent on (bone) cancer researchers to move away from single marker/single pathway approaches and embrace a more global assessment of bone cancer.

III. PROTEOMIC TECHNOLOGY

In contrast to gene expression profiling, proteomic approaches can identify changes in a wide variety of dynamic cellular processes including protein expression, protein–protein interactions, critical post-translational modifications (not observed in any transcriptional analyses), specific cellular and sub-cellular localization, and even the temporal patterns of protein expression suggesting disease status [7]. An appreciation of how the complex series of molecular interactions contribute to the unique ability of certain tumor types to colonize and alter the skeleton is essential for the development of more effective therapies.

Without a doubt, amongst the most important challenges is to identify the components of the bone cancer proteome that support and define the ability of tumor cells to colonize the bone marrow microenvironment and eventually even bone itself. The identification of the specific protein signatures (and of the specific proteins by the signatures) that characterize bone cancer and its progression is of utmost importance. From a therapeutic perspective, these molecules represent potential disease biomarkers and/or novel therapeutic targets, since the majority of drug targets are proteins and not genes.

Proteomics is more than just the identification of proteins that are altered in expression as a consequence of pathophysiology; it is a term that also encompasses the search for biomarkers, an important and necessary tool for the detection, treatment, and monitoring of cancer [12,28,29]. The development of new methodologies to reliably identify and validate protein biomarker expression and improve disease diagnosis is underscored by the increased survival of bone cancer patients who are diagnosed early [30,31].

An ever-increasing number of proteomic techniques are now available for the analytical separation and identification of proteins from complex mixtures of fluids or tissues [32,33]. One- and two-dimensional gel electrophoresis and high-performance liquid chromatography (HPLC) are the most common protein separation methods used by cancer biologists, while mass spectrometry (MS) remains the gold standard for protein detection and identification. With the ever increasing focus of the global research community on cancer biology, MS is beginning to be demystified and is now within the reach of the majority of cancer biologists. Fortunately, MS technology is being removed from specialized and highly technical spectroscopy settings and is accessible to all. This is due in part to the simplified operation and automation of the new instrumentation and the fact that MS is assuming a relatively routine position in many research laboratories. The increasing access to MS technology is facilitating multidisciplinary approaches and producing unique collaborations across the cancer research arena.

With increased sophistication in technology, protein mixtures of increasing complexity can be analyzed. Samples are combined with an acidic matrix and applied to a stainless steel plate (matrix assisted laser desorption/ionization, MALDI), or introduced in liquid form (electrospray, ES), before ionization and the peptide masses detected by MS. The instrumentation routinely achieves sensitivity down to the sub-femtomole level.

Different mass spectrometers determine peptide mass in a variety of ways. In time-of-flight (TOF) instruments, desorbed proteins/peptides 'fly' down an evacuated flight tube, where the TOF is directly proportional to the peptide mass [34]. Other mass spectrometers employing quadropoles, ion traps, chemical tagging of proteins on cysteine residues or amine groups, Fourier transform ion cyclotron resonance (FTICR) to analyze the components of the sample [35] and Multidimensional Protein Identification Technology (Mud-PIT), protein array technology are the proteomics strategies that have been most widely used for cancer research [36].

Mud-PIT is a particularly interesting and novel proteomic technique in which two liquid chromatographic steps are interfaced back to back in a fused silica capillary to permit two-dimensional high performance liquid chromatography. This technique incorporates high-pressure liquid chromatography (HPLC, LC/LC), tandem mass spectrometry (MS/MS) and database-searching algorithms to rapidly analyze complex protein mixtures [37]. Mud-PIT has become widely accepted as the proteomic strategy to help alleviate some of the concerns associated other proteomics technologies, as it permits a rapid separation and simultaneous identification of constituents in complex protein mixtures without the need for pre- or post-separation labeling [36].

The resulting mass spectrum from any of the above technologies is converted to a list of peptide masses that are searched against extensive protein databases, trypsin digested and identified *in silico*. All identified proteins have a unique peptide mass fingerprint that is the result of its unique amino acid sequence. As a result, the peptide masses resolved by MS can reliably and accurately identify the protein from the thousands of proteins in the database.

A critical addition to conventional MS approaches is the ability to subject peptides to complete fragmentation, down to the constituent individual amino acids, with technology referred to as tandem mass spectrometry (MS/MS). In this case the specific sequence of peptides can be identified, which when combined with the peptide mass fingerprint unambiguously identifies the protein. The development of specialized algorithms to rapidly search MS databases with MS-derived datasets and the application of statistical tools for data analysis and interpretation [38] ensure high throughput analysis from specimen collection to sequence identification [39].

MS-based serum protein profiling methods are increasingly being used to detect, validate and characterize disease biomarkers [1]. In general, the utility of these methods to identify specific biomarker profiles is, in part, dependent on the selection of the correct analysis of the data obtained from the experiments. Important decisions have to be made with respect to the correct handling of the data, implementation of appropriate analytical procedures and statistical principles applicable to high dimensional data. In addition, a fundamental knowledge of the statistical and data mining tools for complex pattern recognition are required. These bioinformatic requirements, in addition to an understanding of the particular biological question, underscore the critical nature of the interactions between biologists, technologists and informaticists that are required for successful proteomic analyses. Based on sensitivity, high throughput capability and ease of operation, SELDI-TOF MS has emerged as the primary modality for biomarker discovery of early-stage cancers (reviewed in Ref. [29]).

IV. SELDI-TOF MS PROTEOMICS WORKFLOW

In SELDI-TOF MS signal output is a time-dependent current generated by the detector upon impact by the charged particles, which is then converted to a time-dependent voltage and digitized by a high-speed analog-to-digital converter. The m/z values are determined by calibrating the machine by measuring the TOF for a number of well-characterized samples and correlating the observed TOF with known m/z values. The peak amplitudes at any particular m/z are presumed to represent that peptide/protein's relative intensity within the particular specimen.

Once spectra are collected, the next step is data preprocessing, which generates a peak list that can be used for downstream data mining. The data preprocessing step involves background correction, filtering, noise estimation, peak detection, normalization and standardizations especially when data is collected over a period of time and compiled together for pattern recognition [40–43] (Figure 14.2).

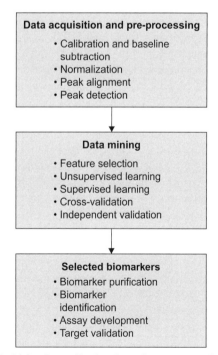

FIGURE 14.2 Generalized schematic representation of the work flow process for SELDI-TOF MS-based proteomic profiling of biological samples.

To identify peaks of interest, some investigators prefer to use the raw m/z values from the instrument [44,45]. Peak detection algorithms allow users to adjust parameters to filter peaks based on height, signal-to-noise etc. However, this approach is prone to introducing human bias into the biomarker discovery process [45]. Usually, some amount of measurement error is associated with the reported mass of any peak, therefore, methods to cluster peaks together for comparison across spectra are frequently employed [45].

Normalization of the spectra is performed to compensate for variations in sample concentrations, or slight shifts in mass due to technical imperfections. Normalization can be applied to peak intensities based on total ion current or peak height or area or mass [45]. The choice of the particular method depends on the type of experiment performed and the biological context of the question. However, the most commonly used and validated normalization method in SELDI-TOF MS is by total ion current [46]. The method calculates the total ion current (sum of all data points) for all the sample spectra, averages the intensity and adjusts the intensity scales for all the spectra. No data are lost; they are just displayed on the same scale for efficient comparison and subsequent analyses.

In a typical SELDI-TOF MS workflow (Figure 14.2) after the collected data have been pre-processed, the data require feature selection before submission to additional data mining algorithms. This is essential in order to overcome the asymmetry that exists between the number of input features (or peaks) and the number of samples (or individual specimens) analyzed [47]. Any MS spectrum contains tens of thousands of data points, and a given patient sample may generate dozens of spectra, depending on the design of the particular experiment. The currently available data mining algorithms are unable to handle such large and skewed datasets; they contain too many features and too few samples [47].

In all MS approaches (including SELDI-TOF MS) an extremely useful feature selection modality is peak detection. Further feature selection is performed using t-tests of the identified peaks to identify basic differences. Many unsupervised as well as supervised learning algorithms also incorporate feature selection. Another optional step, prior to data mining, is data transformation. For clinical and/or analytical reasons, a specific feature in a sample set may be highly variable, which may artificially improve its chance of being selected as a classifying feature. In this case, data transformation approaches such as log or square-root transformations and linear or logarithmic scaling can be performed. These data transformations reduce the impact of the high variability by restricting the values within a more defined range [47]. However, some other data analysis techniques such as classification trees do not require transformations, as the underlying algorithms ignore feature variance.

Data mining approaches can be considered to be of two major types: unsupervised and supervised. Unsupervised learning techniques are analogous to clustering in gene expression analyses and do not require knowledge of class labels. In contrast, supervised approaches require knowledge of class labels and are analogous to classification systems [47].

Commonly used unsupervised learning algorithms have been used to identify biomarkers in bone cancers include k-means clustering, hierarchal clustering, principal component analysis, and discriminant analysis [45,48]. In contrast, classification and regression trees (CART) [49], neural networks [50] and genetic algorithms [51] comprise the remaining repertoire of commonly used supervised learning techniques in SELDI-TOF MS. The choice of data mining technique is not simple, and in fact there is no ideal single method that can be applied to every dataset. In addition, each algorithm has its own strengths and weaknesses that must be considered before applying any approach to a particular statistical problem [47]. As such, we (and others) routinely analyze single datasets using multiple analytical algorithms, in parallel and/or sequentially [1,52,53] (Figure 14.2).

V. PROTEOMIC PROFILING OF BONE TUMORS

Given the multi-gene and multi-protein nature of human disease, there is greater diagnostic and prognostic power in the combined application of the proteome technologies to the analysis of complex biological samples, resulting in the deciphering of specific proteomic signatures [54–56]. Collectively, these analyses have the potential to provide a better understanding of the molecular basis of cancer and to identify novel biomarkers [57]. The power of the systems-based approach is best represented by its successful application to the field of cancer biology.

Of particular interest is the rapidly expanding development of serum proteomic pattern diagnostics using SELDI-TOF MS [58, 59]. This technology identifies patterns of ion signatures generated from high-dimensional mass spectrometry data as diagnostic tumor classifiers [60]. Numerous SELDI-TOF MS-derived protein signatures have been identified, characterized, and modeled and are now moving into validation in extensive and expanding cancer patient cohorts [40, 46, 61–69], including several bone cancers [42, 43, 70–72]. The characterization and sequencing of these and other key protein features should provide new insights into cancer etiology and presumably provide unique opportunities for intervention [73]. We have recently reported the identification of the specific protein components of a protein signature indicative of post-menopausal patients with high bone turnover and osteoporosis, further validating the diagnostic potential of the technology in other non-cancer bone diseases [53].

Clinically, there is currently no method to reliably detect or predict which patients are at risk of developing bone

cancer. It is only possible to detect the existence of disease and at that time, the extent of bone involvement. The identification, usually via X-ray, bone scan, CT (computed tomography) scan or PET (positron emission tomography) scan, identifies tumor already resident in bone. The survival from the time of diagnosis varies among different tumor types, whereas the prognosis after the development of bone metastases in breast cancer is considerably better than that after a recurrence at visceral sites [74]. Thus, the discovery of biomarkers that could distinguish patients with early local disease from those with advanced and/or metastatic disease would be of great clinical value.

Using SELDI-TOF MS, we (and others) have tested the hypothesis that unique serum biomarker patterns exist that can diagnose tumor progression [63,69,75–77], as well as other skeletal disorders, such as post-menopausal osteoporosis [53] and arthritis [78]. Serum, plasma and other biological fluids (including nipple aspirate fluid and urine) from patients with breast cancer, prostate cancer, osteosarcoma, osteochondroma, and multiple myeloma have also been profiled to identify protein patterns indicative of bone disease status [42,43,71,72].

VI. BREAST CANCER

Both breast and prostate cancer have a well-described enhanced proclivity to metastasize to the skeleton [2,12], the mechanisms of which are far from completely understood [7,12]. The diagnosis of a metastatic breast tumor mandates systemic treatment, along with local intervention targeting the primary tumor. Although there has been progress resulting from early detection and improved adjuvant therapy, the prognosis of breast cancer patients is still limited by the occurrence of distant metastases largely due to clinically occult micrometastases that remain undetected.

Breast cancer is the most common malignancy in women in the United States and the most life-threatening aspect of breast cancer lies in the ability of cancer cells to spread from the primary tumor to form distant metastases. In particular, greater than 80% of women dying with breast cancer have bony metastases [12]. Although studies of breast cancer constitute the major proportion of bone cancer investigation, few have studied bone metastasis using proteomic technologies, but instead focused on gene expression profiling of primary tumors and/or human cell lines (reviewed in Ref. [15]). This focus is presumably related to the paucity of matched primary tumor and bone metastasis samples and the relative ease of acquisition of primary breast tumor specimens or patient serum.

In an interesting proteomic study, Willipinski-Stapelfeldt and colleagues [79] examined protein expression patterns characteristic for micrometastatic cells, using cell lines derived from the bone marrow of breast cancer patients. These cell lines were profiled against three standard human breast cancer cell lines using two-dimensional gel electro-phoresis followed by MALDI-TOF analysis. Interestingly, the micrometastatic cancer cell lines universally displayed a loss of epithelial cytokeratins (CK8, CK18, and CK19) as well as the ectopic expression of vimentin, a cytoskeleton filament protein commonly expressed in mesenchymal cells. The specific protein expression changes are indicative of an epithelial-mesenchymal transition. In critical cross validation studies, these authors also demonstrated that the loss of cytokeratin and ectopic vimentin expression was a common feature that was significantly associated with a higher tumor grade, high mitotic index, and negative estro-gen/progesterone-receptor status [79]. However, and reflec-tive of the complex phenotype of human breast cancer [12], by univariate analyses none of the specific cytokeratins identified and analyzed were independently associated with either overall or cancer-specific survival.

More recently, another group has been able to demon-strate concordance between clinical classifiers and SELDI-TOF MS protein signatures. In order to identify relevant molecular signatures of breast cancer Brozkova and col-leagues evaluated whole tissue lysates of 105 breast carci-nomas [80]. Their classification approaches identified subgroups of patients with differential co-expression of selected protein peaks in diverse tumor subclasses. The analysis demonstrated distinct clinically-relevant character-istics such as tumor type, nuclear grade, hormonal status, mucin 1, and cytokeratin 5/6 or 14 expression between the groups. Perhaps most importantly, the patient subgroups identified by hierarchical clustering of SELDI-TOF MS peak data were analogous (for the first time) to breast can-cer classifications based on gene expression profiling and capable of classifying the tumors into luminal, basal and HER2 subtypes. A major extension of the fundamental part of the study conducted by Brozokova was the progression from the initial descriptive knowledge of the protein bio-marker signature to the identification of two potential bio-markers. This is the critical next step that is required for all ongoing SELDI analyses, and that we too have recently accomplished [53]. Together, these important studies repre-sent the initial steps into the dissection of the bone/bone cancer proteome.

VII. PROSTATE CANCER

Clinically, prostate cancer progression from hormone-sensitive to hormone-refractory is recognized biochemically by repeated elevation in the level of serum prostate-specific antigen (PSA) [42]. The biochemical change is accompa-nied by the appearance of symptoms of progressive disease and/or radiographic evidence of relapse. As such, the period of biochemical failure precedes clinical hormone refractori-ness and has been reported to last for a median of 6 months [81].

Le and colleagues [82] used SELDI-TOF MS to profile sera from prostate cancer patients with and without bone metastases. The biomarker signature obtained was able to distinguish prostate cancer patients with bone metastasis with a sensitivity and specificity of 89.5% [82]. Using two-dimensional gel electrophoresis, in-gel trypsin diges-tion, and tandem MS, a cluster of unique proteins in the profile of patients with bone metastases was identified as discrete isoforms of serum amyloid A. The potential clinical significance of this finding in prostate cancer or osteosar-coma [72] is as yet unclear. It is interesting to consider that two tumor types whose primary skeletal activity is to increase bone formation may be characterized by altered expression or activity of the same protein, serum amyloid protein A, whereas the identification of amyloid A in the serum of lytic cancer patients has not been described.

Prostate cancer also has a well-documented propensity to metastasize to bone and in the absence of curative treat-ments for this stage of the disease, sensitive serum biomark-ers indicative of the presence or development of bony involvement are lacking. With this clinically important sce-nario in mind, the serum proteome of advanced prostate cancer patients undergoing androgen ablation therapy who presented with a rising PSA level was profiled using SELDI-TOF MS and compared with the serum profile of patients with advanced prostate cancer and a stable PSA response, actively undergoing androgen ablation therapy [42].

Using the determined discriminating biomarker profile as the primary classifier, seven individual peaks were identified that showed statistically significant ($p < 0.05$) differences between both prostate cancer patient treatment groups. In addition, several of the peaks showed significant associations with overall survival, independent of the measured PSA status.

These interesting observations were further interrogated using multiple machine-based learning approaches. Specifically, patients with both clinical risk factors (a rising PSA level and greater-than-median SELDI peak intensity) had the shortest survival, whereas patients with only one risk factor (rising PSA level or greater-than-median SELDI peak intensity) had comparable and considerably longer survivals. Importantly, patients with neither risk factor had no deaths after 33 months of follow-up. These data suggest that the measurement of these particular biomarkers have the potential to identify patients with advanced prostate cancer and potentially even metastasis to bone [42]. Interestingly, the biomarker profile was similar to that reported by others seeking to discriminate prostate cancer patients from non-cancer patients [83].

VIII. OSTEOSARCOMA

Li and colleagues provided one of the first examples of the characterization and validation of the protein biomarker signature of primary bone cancer [72]. Plasma from osteosarcoma patients (the most common malignant bone tumor in children) was profiled and compared to osteochondroma patients. Using the determined 19 protein peak biomarker signature as a classifier, the authors were able to distinguish osteosarcoma from osteochondroma patients with a respectable 97% sensitivity and 80% specificity. Significantly, one of the component proteins in the biomarker signature (m/z 11,704) was identified as serum amyloid protein A (SAA). The increased level observed in the plasma of patients was independently confirmed and validated. As a result, the unique plasma proteomic signature has utility for the discrimination of malignant bone cancer from benign bone tumors and for the early detection of osteosarcoma in at-risk patients.

IX. MULTIPLE MYELOMA

Multiple myeloma is a B-cell neoplasia characterized by clonal expansion of plasma cells locally in the bone marrow. The disease represents only approximately 1% of all hematologic malignancies in the United States, yet is one of the most malignant plasma cell dyscrasias [84]. The progression of multiple myeloma clinically is dependent on the development of an aggressive bone destructive phenotype, which is critical for the support of tumor cell survival [23]. These observations are indicative of an intimate relationship between the skeleton and multiple myeloma progression. Increased tumor-induced osteloysis absent during early disease stages, and limited and often asymptomatic when present in indolent myeloma, is virtually universally associated with advanced stages of the disease [23]. Consequently, the osteolytic bone destruction characteristic of late stage multiple myeloma is one of the most debilitating manifestations of the disease process.

Using serum samples from multiple myeloma patients, with more than three osteolytic bone lesions or with no clinical evidence of bone disease, we identified and validated a diagnostic fingerprint [43]. The biomarker profile has the potential to augment existing approaches for the diagnosis and treatment of the progression of multiple myeloma [43].

The identified peptide peaks were analyzed using a variety of classification algorithms and the biomarker signature was able to discriminate multiple myeloma patients with bone disease from multiple myeloma patients with no evidence of disease with specificity and sensitivity between 96 and 100%. In particular, a set of four peaks were identified as the most discriminating between the two cohorts [43]. One of the major discriminatory classifiers (m/z 8.928 kDa) is similar to the molecular weight of intact human IL-8 [76, 85], a chemokine shown to have potent osteolytic activity [87] and linked with increased osteoclastogenesis and poor prognosis in a variety of bone cancers [12,88,89].

X. WHAT ABOUT THE FUTURE?

The ongoing advances in proteomics that the bone cancer field is experiencing offer great promise for the discovery of novel tumor biomarkers that may provide new understanding of the molecular mechanisms associated with the skeletal consequences of malignancy (Figure 14.1). However, many challenges remain before these new discoveries can be translated into the clinic and the care of patients.

Optimistically, it is highly likely that this enabling technology (proteomic analysis and profiling) will provide the foundation for the development of new therapies to target tumor-specific pathways, as well as diagnostic and prognostic assays to monitor treatment efficacy. Likewise, the specific bone cancer biomarker profiles and bone-tumor proteins reviewed here represent vital first steps in the discovery of new bone cancer targets. The extent to which the identified proteins can serve as potential biomarkers of bone cancers must be investigated rigorously.

Although serum proteomics using SELDI-TOF MS has made invaluable contributions to biology, its continued use is likely limited, even in the face of direct tissue-SELDI techniques [90] and new generation SELDI-TOF MS instrumentation [91]. The evolution of user-friendly high resolution MS technologies with the sensitivity and resolution necessary for the examination of the low molecular weight proteome [58], supported by spectroscopists intent on understanding biology may signal the demise of SELDI instruments, as is the risk for all first-generation technologies. Nevertheless, the approaches, analyses and data described here indicate the existence of a repertoire of proteomic profiles that can accurately identify patients at risk of bone cancer.

The overwhelming outcome of the application of proteomic technology to bone cancer biology is that the molecules controlling the key biologic processes in the colonization of bone by tumor cells will be uncovered. Further proteomic-based studies using improved study design, sample collection and processing with appropriate bioinformatic analyses in larger patient cohorts are warranted and ongoing. The continued application of state-of-the-art proteomic technologies is rapidly advancing our understanding of bone cancer at the molecular level, and has the potential to provide new directions for the diagnosis and treatment of the skeletal complications of cancer.

Acknowledgements

Our research into the proteomics of bone cancer is supported by grants from the Virginia Clinton Kelley/FFANY Cancer Research Fund, the Arkansas Breast Cancer Research Endowment, the Department of Orthopaedic Surgery and the Carl L. Nelson Chair of Orthopaedic Creativity.

References

1. S. Bhattacharyya, S. Byrum & E.R. Siegel, et al., Proteomic analysis of bone cancer: a review of current and future developments, Expert Rev Proteomics 4 (2007) 371–378.
2. G.R. Mundy, Metastasis to bone: causes, consequences and therapeutic opportunities, Nat Rev Cancer 2 (2002) 584–593.
3. G.D. Roodman, Mechanisms of bone metastasis, N Engl J Med 350 (2004) 1655–1664.
4. K.J. Sweeney, P.J. Boland & T. King, The management of asymptomatic skeletal breast cancer: a paradigm shift, Ann Surg Oncol 14 (2007) 2430–2431.
5. I.J. Fidler, The pathogenesis of cancer metastasis: the 'seed and soil' hypothesis revisited, Nat Rev Cancer 3 (2003) 453–458.
6. I. Fidler & G. Poste, The pathogenesis of cancer metastasis, Nature 283 (1979) 139–146.
7. G.P. Gupta & J. Massague, Cancer metastasis: building a framework, Cell 127 (2006) 679–695.
8. B. Boyce, T. Yoneda & T. Guise, Factors regulating the growth of metastatic cancer in bone, Endocrine-Related Cancer 6 (1999) 333–347.
9. T.J. Martin & N.A. Sims, Osteoclast-derived activity in the coupling of bone formation to resorption, Trends Mol Med 11 (2005) 76–81.
10. M. Bendre, D. Gaddy & R.W. Nicholas, et al., Breast cancer metastasis to bone: it is not all about PTHrP, Clin Orthop (2003) S39–S45.
11. L.A. Kingsley, P.G. Fournier & J.M. Chirgwin, et al., Molecular biology of bone metastasis, Mol Cancer Ther 6 (2007) 2609–2617.
12. A.G. Marguiles, V.S. Klimberg & S. Bhattacharrya, et al., Genomics and proteomics of bone cancer, Clin Cancer Res 12 (2006) 6217s–6221s.
13. A.J. Minn, Y. Kang & I. Serganova, et al., Distinct organ-specific metastatic potential of individual breast cancer cells and primary tumors, J Clin Invest 115 (2005) 44–55.
14. Y. Kang, P.M. Siegel & W. Shu, et al., A multigenic program mediating breast cancer metastasis to bone, Cancer Cell 3 (2003) 537–549.
15. J. Massague, Sorting out breast-cancer gene signatures, N Engl J Med 356 (2007) 294–297.
16. L.D. Wood, D.W. Parsons & S. Jones, et al., The genomic landscapes of human breast and colorectal cancers, Science 318 (2007) 1108–1113.
17. G.D. Leonard & S.M. Swain, Ductal carcinoma *in situ*, complexities and challenges, J Natl Cancer Inst 96 (2004) 906–920.
18. M.P. Roudier, L.D. True & C.S. Higano, et al., Phenotypic heterogeneity of end-stage prostate carcinoma metastatic to bone, Hum Pathol 34 (2003) 646–653.
19. J.E. Talmadge, Clonal selection of metastasis within the life history of a tumor, Cancer Res 67 (2007) 11471–11475.
20. O. Peyruchaud, B. Winding & I. Pecheur, et al., Early detection of bone metastases in a murine model using fluorescent human breast cancer cells: application to the use of the bisphosphonate zoledronic acid in the treatment of osteolytic lesions, J Bone Miner Res 16 (2001) 2027–2034.
21. T. Yoneda, P. Williams & T. Hiraga, et al., A bone-seeking clone exhibits different biological properties from the MDA-MB-231 parental breast cancer cells and a brain-seeking clone in vivo and in vitro, J Bone Miner Res 16 (2001) 1486–1495.
22. M.S. Bendre, D. Gaddy-Kurten & T. Mon-Foote, et al., Expression of interleukin 8 and not parathyroid hormone-related protein by human breast cancer cells correlates with bone metastasis in vivo, Cancer Res 62 (2002) 5571–5579.
23. E. Tian, F. Zhan & R. Walker, et al., The role of the Wnt-signaling antagonist DKK1 in the development of osteolytic lesions in multiple myeloma, N Engl J Med 349 (2003) 2483–2494.
24. D. Hanahan & R.A. Weinberg, The hallmarks of cancer, Cell 100 (2000) 57–70.
25. L.A. Liotta & E.F. Petricoin, Serum peptidome for cancer detection: spinning biologic trash into diagnostic gold, J Clin Invest 116 (2006) 26–30.
26. D. Gancberg, A. Di Leo & F. Cardoso, et al., Comparison of HER-2 status between primary breast cancer and corresponding distant metastatic sites, Ann Oncol 13 (2002) 1036–1043.
27. M. Dhodapkar, E. Abe & A. Theus, et al., Syndecan-1 is a multifunctional regulator of myeloma pathobiology: control of tumor cell survival, growth, and bone cell differentiation, Blood 91 (1998) 2679–2688.
28. F. Simpkins, J.A. Czechowicz & L. Liotta, et al., SELDI-TOF mass spectrometry for cancer biomarker discovery and serum proteomic diagnostics, Pharmacogenomics 6 (2005) 647–653.
29. G.L. Hortin, S.A. Jortani & J.C. Ritchie Jr., et al., Proteomics: a new diagnostic frontier, Clin Chem 52 (2006) 1218–1222.
30. G. Selvaggi & G.V. Scagliotti, Management of bone metastases in cancer: a review, Crit Rev Oncol Hematol 56 (2005) 365–378.
31. A. Lipton, Management of bone metastases in breast cancer, Curr Treat Options Oncol 6 (2005) 161–171.
32. N.M. Verrills, Clinical proteomics: present and future prospects, Clinical Biochemistry Reviews 27 (2007) 99–116.
33. S. Goodison & V. Urquidi, Breast tumor metastasis: analysis via proteomic profiling, Expert Rev Proteomics 5 (2008) 457–467.
34. G.L. Hortin, The MALDI-TOF mass spectrometric view of the plasma proteome and peptidome, Clin Chem 52 (2006) 1223–1237.
35. M.S. Lim & K.S. Elenitoba-Johnson, Proteomics in pathology research, Lab Invest 84 (2004) 1227–1244.
36. R.I. Somiari, S. Somiari & S. Russell, et al., Proteomics of breast carcinoma, J Chromatogr B Analyt Technol Biomed Life Sci 815 (2005) 215–225.
37. C.C. Wu & M.J. MacCoss, Shotgun proteomics: tools for the analysis of complex biological systems, Curr Opin Mol Ther 4 (2002) 242–250.
38. L. Li, H. Tang & Z. Wu, et al., Data mining techniques for cancer detection using serum proteomic profiling, Artif Intell Med 32 (2004) 71–83.
39. P.D. von Haller, E. Yi & S. Donohoe, et al., The application of new software tools to quantitative protein profiling via isotope-coded affinity tag (ICAT) and tandem mass spectrometry: II. Evaluation of tandem mass spectrometry methodologies for large-scale protein analysis, and the application of statistical tools for data analysis and interpretation, Mol Cell Proteomics 2 (2003) 428–442.
40. E.F. Petricoin, A.M. Ardekani & B.A. Hitt, et al., Use of proteomic patterns in serum to identify ovarian cancer, Lancet 359 (2002) 572–577.
41. K.R. Kozak, M.W. Amneus & S.M. Pusey, et al., Identification of biomarkers for ovarian cancer using strong anion-exchange

ProteinChips: potential use in diagnosis and prognosis, Proc Natl Acad Sci USA 100 (2003) 12343–12348.

42. M. Kohli, E. Siegel & S. Bhattacharya, et al., Surface-enhanced laser desorption/ionization time-of-flight mass spectrometry (SELDI-TOF MS) for determining prognosis in advanced stage hormone relapsing prostate cancer, Cancer Biomark 2 (2006) 249–258.

43. S. Bhattacharyya, J. Epstein & L.J. Suva, Biomarkers that discriminate multiple myeloma patients with or without skeletal involvement detected using SELDI-TOF mass spectrometry and statistical and machine learning tools, Dis Markers 22 (2006) 245–255.

44. E.T. Fung & C. Enderwick, ProteinChip clinical proteomics: computational challenges and solutions, Biotechniques (Suppl) (2002) 34–38 40–41.

45. E.T. Fung, S.R. Weinberger & E. Gavin, et al., Bioinformatics approaches in clinical proteomics, Expert Rev Proteomics 2 (2005) 847–862.

46. D.A. Cairns, D. Thompson & D.N. Perkins, et al., Proteomic profiling using mass spectrometry—does normalising by total ion current potentially mask some biological differences?, Proteomics 8 (2008) 21–27.

47. R.L. Somorjai, B. Dolenko & R. Baumgartner, Class prediction and discovery using gene microarray and proteomics mass spectroscopy data: curses, caveats, cautions, Bioinformatics 19 (2003) 1484–1491.

48. I.T. Joliffe & B.J. Morgan, Principal component analysis and exploratory factor analysis, Stat Methods Med Res 1 (1992) 69–95.

49. K.A. Grajski, L. Breiman & G. Viana Di Prisco, et al., Classification of EEG spatial patterns with a tree-structured methodology: CART, IEEE Trans Biomed Eng 33 (1986) 1076–1086.

50. C.M. Bishop, Curvature-driven smoothing: a learning algorithm for feedforward networks, IEEE Trans Neural Netw 4 (1993) 882–884.

51. P. Willett, Genetic algorithms in molecular recognition and design, Trends Biotechnol 13 (1995) 516–521.

52. S.M. Carlson, A. Najmi & H.J. Cohen, Biomarker clustering to address correlations in proteomic data, Proteomics 7 (2007) 1037–1046.

53. S. Bhattacharyya, E.R. Siegel & S.J. Achenbach, et al., Serum biomarker profile associated with high bone turnover and BMD in postmenopausal women, J Bone Miner Res 23 (2008) 1106–1117.

54. Y.K. Paik, S.K. Jeong & E.Y. Lee, et al., C. elegans: an invaluable model organism for the proteomics studies of the cholesterol-mediated signaling pathway, Expert Rev Proteomics 3 (2006) 439–453.

55. B. Wittmann-Liebold, H.R. Graack & T. Pohl, Two-dimensional gel electrophoresis as tool for proteomics studies in combination with protein identification by mass spectrometry, Proteomics 6 (2006) 4688–4703.

56. K.R. Calvo, L.A. Liotta & E.F. Petricoin, Clinical proteomics: from biomarker discovery and cell signaling profiles to individualized personal therapy, Biosci Rep 25 (2005) 107–125.

57. C. Gulmann, K.M. Sheehan & E.W. Kay, et al., Array-based proteomics: mapping of protein circuitries for diagnostics, prognostics, and therapy guidance in cancer, J Pathol 208 (2006) 595–606.

58. E.F. Petricoin & L.A. Liotta, Mass spectrometry-based diagnostics: the upcoming revolution in disease detection, Clin Chem 49 (2003) 533–534.

59. O. Chertov, J.T. Simpson & A. Biragyn, et al., Enrichment of low-molecular-weight proteins from biofluids for biomarker discovery, Expert Rev Proteomics 2 (2005) 139–145.

60. L.A. Liotta & E.C. Kohn, Cancer's deadly signature, Nat Genet 33 (2003) 10–11.

61. J.D. Wulfkuhle, L.A. Liotta & E.F. Petricoin, Early detection: proteomic applications for the early detection of cancer, Nat Rev Cancer 3 (2003) 267–275.

62. C. Rosty, L. Christa & S. Kuzdzal, et al., Identification of hepatocarcinoma-intestine-pancreas/pancreatitis-associated protein I as a biomarker for pancreatic ductal adenocarcinoma by protein biochip technology, Cancer Res 62 (2002) 1868–1875.

63. S. Bhattacharyya, E.R. Siegel & G.M. Petersen, et al., Diagnosis of pancreatic cancer using serum proteomic profiling, Neoplasia 6 (2004) 674–686.

64. Z. Xiao, D. Prieto & T.P. Conrads, et al., Proteomic patterns: their potential for disease diagnosis, Mol Cell Endocrinol 230 (2005) 95–106.

65. Y. Su, J. Shen & H. Qian, et al., Diagnosis of gastric cancer using decision tree classification of mass spectral data, Cancer Sc 98 (2007) 37–43.

66. M. Roesch-Ely, M. Nees & S. Karsai, et al., Proteomic analysis reveals successive aberrations in protein expression from healthy mucosa to invasive head and neck cancer, Oncogene 26 (2007) 54–64.

67. S. Kanmura, H. Uto & K. Kusumoto, et al., Early diagnostic potential for hepatocellular carcinoma using the SELDI ProteinChip system, Hepatology 45 (2007) 948–956.

68. C.M. Hegedus, C.F. Skibola & P. Bracci, et al., Screening the human serum proteome for genotype-phenotype associations: an analysis of the IL6 -174G>C polymorphism, Proteomics 7 (2007) 548–557.

69. K.Q. Han, G. Huang & C.F. Gao, et al., Identification of lung cancer patients by serum protein profiling using surface-enhanced laser desorption/ionization time-of-flight mass spectrometry, Am J Clin Oncol 31 (2008) 133–139.

70. R.E. Brown & J.L. Boyle, Mesenchymal chondrosarcoma: molecular characterization by a proteomic approach, with morphogenic and therapeutic implications, Ann Clin Lab Sci 33 (2003) 131–141.

71. E. Izbicka, D. Campos & J. Marty, et al., Molecular determinants of differential sensitivity to docetaxel and paclitaxel in human pediatric cancer models, Anticancer Res 26 (2006) 1983–1988.

72. Y. Li, T.A. Dang & J. Shen, et al., Identification of a plasma proteomic signature to distinguish pediatric osteosarcoma from benign osteochondroma, Proteomics 6 (2006) 3426–3435.

73. E.F. Petricoin & L.A. Liotta, SELDI-TOF-based serum proteomic pattern diagnostics for early detection of cancer, Curr Opin Biotechnol 15 (2004) 24–30.

74. R.E. Coleman & R.D. Rubens, The clinical course of bone metastases from breast cancer, Br J Cancer 55 (1987) 61–66.

75. S. Liu, C. Ginestier & E. Charafe-Jauffret, et al., BRCA1 regulates human mammary stem/progenitor cell fate, Proc Natl Acad Sci USA 105 (2008) 1680–1685.

76. Y. Wang, J.G. Klijn & Y. Zhang, et al., Gene-expression profiles to predict distant metastasis of lymph-node-negative primary breast cancer, Lancet 365 (2005) 671–679.

77. J. Holcakova, L. Hernychova & P. Bouchal, et al., Identification of alphaB-crystallin, a biomarker of renal cell carcinoma by SELDI-TOF MS, Int J Biol Markers 23 (2008) 48–53.

78. D. de Seny, M. Fillet & C. Ribbens, et al., Monomeric calgranulins measured by SELDI-TOF mass spectrometry and calprotectin measured by ELISA as biomarkers in arthritis, Clin Chem 54 (2008) 1066–1075.

79. B. Willipinski-Stapelfeldt, S. Riethdorf & V. Assmann, et al., Changes in cytoskeletal protein composition indicative of an epithelial-mesenchymal transition in human micrometastatic and primary breast carcinoma cells, Clin Cancer Res 11 (2005) 8006–8014.

80. K. Brozkova, E. Budinska & P. Bouchal, et al., Surface-enhanced laser desorption/ionization time-of-flight proteomic profiling of breast carcinomas identifies clinicopathologically relevant groups of patients similar to previously defined clusters from cDNA expression, Breast Cancer Res 10 (2008) R48.

81. D.W. Newling, L. Denis & K. Vermeylen, Orchiectomy versus goserelin and flutamide in the treatment of newly diagnosed metastatic prostate cancer. Analysis of the criteria of evaluation used in the European Organization for Research and Treatment of Cancer—Genitourinary Group Study 30853, Cancer 72 (1993) 3793–3798.

82. L. Le, K. Chi & S. Tyldesley, et al., Identification of serum amyloid A as a biomarker to distinguish prostate cancer patients with bone lesions, Clin Chem 51 (2005) 695–707.

83. S. Lehrer, J. Roboz & H. Ding, et al., Putative protein markers in the sera of men with prostatic neoplasms, BJU Int 92 (2003) 223–225.

84. G.D. Roodman, Biology of osteoclast activation in cancer, J Clin Oncol 19 (2001) 3562–3571.

85. M.S. Bendre, A.G. Margulies & B. Walser, et al., Tumor-derived interleukin-8 stimulates osteolysis independent of the receptor activator of nuclear factor-kappaB ligand pathway, Cancer Res 65 (2005) 11001–11009.

86. Y. Lu, Z. Cai & G. Xiao, et al., Monocyte chemotactic protein-1 mediates prostate cancer-induced bone resorption, Cancer Res 67 (2007) 3646–3653.

87. M.S. Bendre, D.C. Montague & T. Peery, et al., Interleukin-8 stimulation of osteoclastogenesis and bone resorption is a mechanism for the increased osteolysis of metastatic bone disease, Bone 33 (2003) 28–37.

88. I.H. Benoy, R. Salgado & P. Van Dam, et al., Increased serum interleukin-8 in patients with early and metastatic breast cancer correlates with early dissemination and survival, Clin Cancer Res 10 (2004) 7157–7162.

89. H. Uehara, P. Troncoso & D. Johnston, et al., Expression of interleukin-8 gene in radical prostatectomy specimens is associated with advanced pathologic stage, Prostate 64 (2005) 40–49.

90. A. Bouamrani, J. Ternier & D. Ratel, et al., Direct-tissue SELDI-TOF mass spectrometry analysis: a new application for clinical proteomics, Clin Chem 52 (2006) 2103–2106.

91. M.C. Gast, J.Y. Engwegen & J.H. Schellens, et al., Comparing the old and new generation SELDI-TOF MS: implications for serum protein profiling, BMC Med Genomics 1 (2008) 4.

CHAPTER **15**

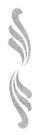

Genomic and Proteomic Profiling of Osteosarcoma

TSZ-KWONG MAN[1], PULIVARTHI H. RAO[1] AND CHING C. LAU[1]

[1] *Texas Children's Cancer Center, Baylor College of Medicine, Houston, TX, USA.*

Contents

I. INTRODUCTION

The primary treatment of osteosarcoma (OS) uses high dose chemotherapy in both the neoadjuvant and adjuvant settings in association with surgery. Despite such aggressive treatment, up to 40% of osteosarcoma patients eventually succumb to their disease. Many of the survivors also suffer from significant acute and long-term side effects from their therapy. Thus, there is a need to identify biomarkers that could predict the therapeutic response of an individual osteosarcoma prior to the initiation of therapy. This would potentially lead to the customization of therapy for each patient; thus allowing the reduction of therapy and their side effects for patients who have more responsive tumors, while choosing a more aggressive or targeted therapy for the more resistant cases. One strategy to determine such biomarkers is to identify the underlying genetic changes of each tumor, which could then be used to predict biological behavior of the tumor cells and the clinical course of the disease. In the past, this type of approach was considered unpractical because of the limited ability to decipher the complexity of the cancer genome, especially that of

osteosarcoma. However, with the advent of high throughput genomic and proteomic technologies, it is now possible to generate comprehensive molecular profiles of tumors by using small quantities of tissue or blood samples. This chapter summarizes the different strategies of molecular profiling and illustrates results of genomic and proteomic characterization of osteosarcoma, how these strategies can refine prognostic assessments, and impact the design of future clinical trials.

II. CHROMOSOME ABERRATIONS IN OSTEOSARCOMA

Malignant transformation of a cell requires the accumulation of multiple genetic changes during the process of tumor initiation and progression. In order to understand the underlying biology of cancer, one has to identify as many of the genetic alterations during cancer development as possible. Theodor Boveri's evaluation that chromosome abnormalities play a central role in the malignant transformation of a normal cell laid the foundation for our current understanding of chromosomal basis of cancer. These chromosomal aberrations can be analyzed using a number of genomic technologies, such as chromosomal banding, multicolor spectral kayotyping (SKY/m-FISH), comparative genomic hybridization (CGH), array based-CGH and fluorescence *in situ* hybridization (FISH). Several investigators, including our group, have used these technologies to decipher the chromosomal complexity in osteosarcoma (OS).

III. DNA PLOIDY

The DNA content in tumor cells has been reported as a useful way to define the malignant potential of human cancers. Earlier studies showed a correlation between DNA ploidy and histologic grading in OS [1–4]. This was particularly true in the case of high-grade tumors, of which 96% of them were hyperploid, whereas all low-grade parosteal osteosarcomas were diploid [1]. Others have examined the association between the degree of aneuploidy and prognosis and response to chemotherapy [4–6]. One study demonstrated that, among hyperploid tumors, the presence of neardiploid stem lines was associated with a better prognosis, including both a lower incidence of pulmonary metastasis and an improved disease-free survival after treatment [6]. The study by Bosing *et al.* showed a higher frequency of aneuploidy after preoperative chemotherapy among tumors exhibiting a poor response [5]. However, contrary to these earlier reports, a later study reported that patients whose tumors showing non-diploid DNA content had a longer event-free survival after surgical resection and chemotherapy than did those with diploid tumors, suggesting a better response to chemotherapy in the former [4]. Thus, the exact role of aneuploid DNA content in relation to prognosis and response to therapy remains unclear.

Serra *et al.* compared results from DNA ploidy and conventional cytogenetics/FISH studies on the same OS cell lines and found that the ploidy determined by cytogenetics/FISH analysis was frequently lower than those evaluated by cytometric methods [7]. They concluded that this discrepancy might be due to the presence of unbalanced chromosomal aberrations, including high-level focal amplifications, which may significantly affect the total DNA content with no effect on the total chromosome numbers.

IV. CONVENTIONAL CYTOGENETICS AND SKY

With the exception of osteosarcoma and leiomysarcoma, all other sarcomas are cytogenetically simple and exhibit reciprocal translocations resulting in the formation of fusion genes. These translocations not only serve as diagnostic markers but also hold the key to insights into the biology of these sarcomas. On the other hand, osteosarcomas often show complex chromosomal rearrangements and numerous gene amplifications and deletions, suggesting that genomic instability is linked to the development of this tumor (Figures 15.1 and 15.2; see also Plate 4). Although several reciprocal translocations were reported in OS, none of them were present more than once (Table 15.1). Cytogenetic evidence of gene amplification (~21%) in the form of homogeneously staining regions (hsr) and double minutes (dmin) was reported in 5 and 16% of the cases, respectively [8]. Ring chromosomes, hsrs and dmins are more frequently seen in conventional OS than in parosteal OS. The ring chromosomes in parosteal OS are usually accompanied by numerous complex chromosomal abnormalities.

Based on G-banding analysis of previously published clonally abnormal karyotypes of 168 specimens of OS, a number of recurrent breakpoints have been identified at 1p11-13,1q12-12,11p15,12p13,17p12-p13,19q13 and 20q11-13 and trisomy for chromosome 1 and total or partial monosomy for chromosomes 6q, 9, 10, 13, and 17 (8; http://cgap.nci.nih.gov/Chromosomes/Mitelman). Because of the high

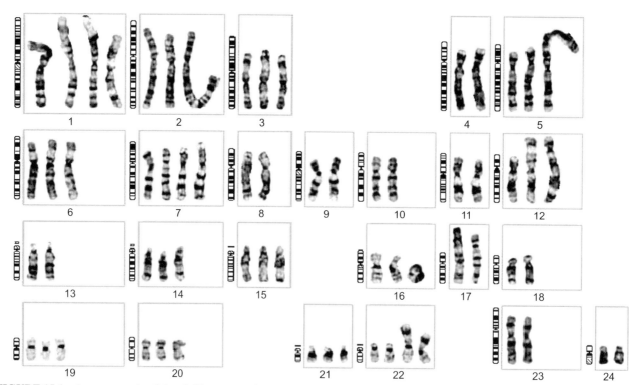

FIGURE 15.1   A representative G-banded karyotype obtained from short-term culture derived from a patient with osteosarcoma.

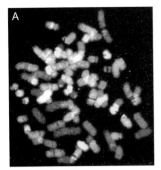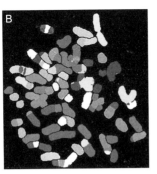

FIGURE 15.2 An example of metaphase chromosomes from osteosarcoma after hybridization with 24 differently labeled whole-chromosome painting probes. (A) Spectra-based display colors; (B) spectral classification from the same metaphase.

percentage of unidentified marker chromosomes, the accurate identification of these markers is extremely difficult in OS. A combined approach of G-banding, spectral karyotyping/m-FISH, CGH/arrayCGH and FISH would enhance the sensitivity of detection of chromosomal aberrations in OS. We and others used a similar approach and identified several novel sites of chromosomal rearrangements at Xp11, Xp22, Xq22, 1q11, 1q32, 2p11, 2p13, 3p11, 3p13, 4q12, 4q21, 4q27, 6p12, 6p21, 8p11, 8q11, 8q22, 8q23, 8q24, 9p10, 9p13, 9q11, 9q22, 10p11, 10q11, 11q23, 12p11, 12q24, 13q11, 13q14, 13q32, 14p11, 14q24, 15p11, 15q15, 16p11.2, 17q11, 17q21, 17q25, 18q21, 20p13, 20p11, 21q22 and 22q11 [9–10].

Telomere maintenance is a key mechanism in overcoming cellular senescence in tumor cells and, in most cases, is achieved by the activation of telomerase. However, there is at least one alternative mechanism of telomere lengthening (ALT) which is characterized by heterogeneous and elongated telomeres in the absence of telomerase activity (TA). A comprehensive study of telomere maintenance mechanisms in 62 OS specimens found that a subset of cases which lacked both telomerase activity and evidence of ALT had the most favorable prognosis [11]. Scheel *et al.* evaluated the prevalence of TA, gene expression of telomerase subunits and ALT in relation to telomere morphology and function in matrix producing bone tumors and in osteosarcoma cell lines [12]. They presented evidence of a direct association of ALT with telomere dysfunction and chromosomal instability. They concluded that ALT in association with telomere dysfunction and chromosomal instability might have major implications for tumor progression. Gisselsson *et al.* generated chromosomal breakpoint profiles of 140 OS specimens to investigate the role of breakpoints in genomic instability. Based on their study, they concluded that the cases with few chromosomal alterations tend to have alterations clustering to the terminal chromosomal bands whereas tumors with many changes showed abnormalities preferentially clustering to the interstitial or centromeric regions [13]. Furthermore, they showed that the terminal breakpoint frequency was negatively correlated to

TABLE 15.1 Reciprocal translocations identified in osteosarcoma[*]

Translocation
t(1;5)(q21; p15.3)
t(1;9)(p32;q22)
t(1;11)(p31;q23-q25)
t(1;11)(q44;q12)
t(1;12)(p11;p11)
t(1;14)(q21;q32)
t(1;19)(p22;p13-3)
t(1;19)(q21;q13)
t(2;4)(p23;q21)
t(2;12)(q13;q13)
t(2;16)(q24;q23)
t(3;13;19)(p22;q22;q13.1)
t(4;6)(q27;q21)
t(4;20)(p13;p11-2)
t(5;9)(q22;q21)
t(5;10)(p13;p14-p15)
t(5;17)(q11;p11)
t(5;18)(q13;q22)
t(6;7)(q15;q22)
t(6;13)(p21;q33)
t(7;15)(q32;24)
t(7;20)(p13;p11-2)
t(8;11)(q11;q11)
t(8;12)(q24;q13)
t(8;21)(q12;q11)
t(9;15)(q34;q22)
t(10;17)(p11-2;q21.3)
t(11;16)(q13;p13-3)
t(11;17)(q21;q24)
t(12;12)(q10:q24.3)
t(12;21)(p11;q11)
t(16; 19)(q12;q13.2)
t(16;19)(q12;q13.2)
t(X;7)(p22.3;q11)

[*]These translocations are based on the review of 168 published G-banded karyotypes.
Source: http://cgap.nci.nih.gov/Chromosomes/Mitelman;[8].

telomeric TTAGGG repeat length. This is consistent with the theory of breakage-fusion-bridge (BFB) cycle, in which cycles are initiated by teleomeric fusion, followed by a gradual shift of breakpoints from the chromosomal ends towards central regions as recurring anaphase breakage erodes the chromosomal arms [14]. Previous studies have shown that these BFB events contribute to genetic heterogeneity in a number of aggressive epithelial and mesenchymal tumors [15].

Similar to some other primary human tumors, the mutation of p53 correlates significantly with the presence of high levels of genomic instability in osteosarcomas. Overholtzer *et al.* examined the relationship between p53 mutation and genomic instability in human osteosarcomas [16] using genomic instability index scores based on the total genomic imbalances identified by CGH. Osteosarcomas harboring an amplification of the HDM2 oncogene, which inhibits the tumor-suppressive properties of p53, do not display high levels of genomic instability. They concluded that the inactivation of p53 in osteosarcomas directly by mutation versus indirectly by HDM2 amplification might have different cellular consequences with respect to the stability of the genome.

V. GENOMIC PROFILING BY CGH AND ARRAY CGH

CGH is one of the most powerful global assays for detecting losses and gains in a given genomic complement. This method involves competitive hybridization of differently labeled test DNA (tumor) and reference DNA (green) to normal human metaphase chromosome spreads. Based on the relative intensity of the two fluorescent colors, chromosomal regions with gain or loss can be identified in a single

hybridization. One of the advantages of CGH is that it can make use of archival materials when frozen tissues are not available, thus greatly expanding the number of cases that can be analyzed. Several groups have used this technique to identify genomic imbalances in OS [16–24]. Increased DNA copy numbers have been reported on every autosome and the X chromosome in OS by CGH. Regions most frequently involved in chromosomal losses are 2q34-qter, 3p, 3qcen-q22, 5q, 6q16-qter, 8p12-pter, 9p13-pter, 10p12, 10q23, 11p12-pter, 13qcen-q21, 14q, 15qcen-q21, 16p, 17p and 18q. The most common chromosomal gains have been detected at 1p21-p31, 1p35-p36, 1q21-q31, 2p, 2q31-32, 3q25-qter, 4q12-q13, 4q27-q32, 5p13-p15.2, 5q, 7q31-q32, 8q21.3-q22, 8qcen-q13, 9q21-22, 11q14, 14q24-qter, 16p, 17p, 19(p), 20q, 21q, Xpcen-p21 and Xq25-qter. The most frequently gained or amplified chromosomal regions were 1p22, 1p31, 1q21, 1q23, 2q24, 3p25, 3q26, 6q24.3, 4q12, 5p14-p15, 5q33, 6p12-p21, 6q24.3, 7p21-p22, 8q12-q23, 10p21, 10q11.1, 10q22, 11q13, 11q23, 12p13, 12q12-q15, 17p11.2, 17q21, 18q22, 19p13.1 and 20p11.2 (Figure 15.3; see Plate 5). Of these, amplification of 6p12-p21 (15–26%) and 17p11.2 (13–29%) appeared to be an early event in pathogenesis of OS because it was observed in all specimen types, including those from biopsies, definitive surgery, and metastatic lesions [10]. These chromosomal bands are also

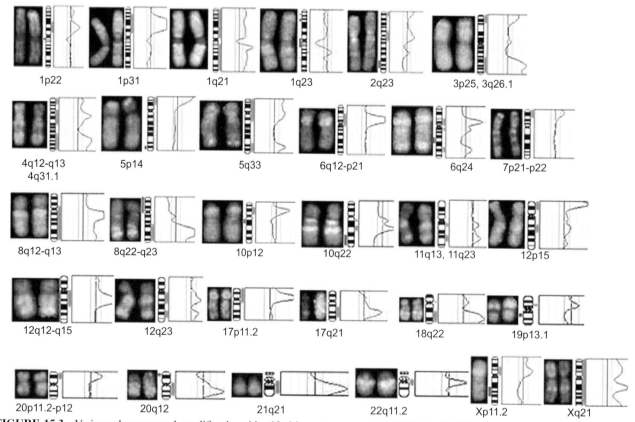

FIGURE 15.3 Various chromosomal amplifications identified in osteosarcoma by CGH. Partial CGH karyotype for individual chromosomes (left) and corresponding ratio profiles showing high-level amplifications. The vertical red and green bars on the right of the ideogram indicate the threshold values of 0.80 and 1.20 for loss and gain, respectively.

shown to be involved in chromosomal rearrangements [10]. This high frequency of increased copy numbers at these regions suggests the selection for oncogenes that remain uncharacterized. In addition, DNA sequence loss has also been observed at 2q, 6p, 8p, 10p, and 17p13 [16–24].

In the first genome-wide array comparative genomic hybridization on osteosarcoma, we reported frequent deletions at the chromosomal regions 2q31.1, 3p14.1, 4p16.2, 6q12, 6q21, 7q35, 10p15.1, 10q22-q23, 10q25-q26, 11q25, 13q12.2, 13q14.3, 13q22.1, 17p13.3 and 17q12 and seven recurrent homozygous deletions at 1q25.1, 3p14.1, 4p15.1, 6q12, 6q13 and 13q12.22 [25]. The chromosomal regions that represented gains were mapped to 1p36, 4p16, 6p12-p21, 8q21, 8q23-24, 12q14.3, 16p13.3, 17p11-p12, 19p13.3 and 21q22.3. This study also refined the 6p amplicon to 9.4 Mb with amplification peak for clone RP11-81F7. Previous study by the same group demonstrated the origin of 6p amplicon as a consequence of tandem duplication of clones RP11-81F7 and RP11-79F13 [10]. Based on combined array CGH and FISH analysis we identified *CDC5L, HSPCB, NFKBIE, HGNC* and *MRPL14* as candidate genes from the 6p12-p21 amplicon [25]. A more recent study established the correlation between amplification of 6p12-p21 and the overexpression of *CDC5L,* a G2-M transition regulatory gene. We further corroborated this observation using a functional assay, demonstrating that CDC5L possesses oncogenic properties [26].

The 17p amplicon identified by CGH and microsatellite marker analysis [10,17,18,20,23,27,28] is also a common structural abnormality identified by cytogenetic techniques [10,29]. Several candidate genes were suggested from the 17p amplicon in OS. Man *et al.* have identified by array CGH three clones with high-level amplifications that spans ~3.7 Mb region on 17p11.2 [25]. Several candidate genes were identified within these clones (*TPP3A, SMCR5, DRG2, FL11, MYCD, SOX 17, ELAC2,* and *PMP22*). Other studies have shown the amplification of *PMP22* and *TOP3A* from 17p11.2-p12 in high-grade OS by semi-quantitative PCR and cDNA microarrays [23,30]. We note that, despite its overall amplification, segments of DNA loss have been identified within the 17p amplicon [27,31], indicating that not just gene amplification, but also loss of genetic material, may be an important factor within this amplicon for the development of OS. Using a different method (representational difference analysis (RDA)) to isolate DNA fragments deleted, amplified, or rearranged in tumor cells, Simons *et al.* identified in conjunction with CGII, two regions of amplification, 17p11.2-p12 and 19q12-q13 (32). Yan *et al.* identified *COPS3* as a putative oncogene from the 17p amplicon in OS and reported amplification of this gene in 31% of the osteosarcomas [33]. Amplification of *COPS3* was strongly associated with a large tumor size, but was not associated with age at diagnosis, site, gender, and tumor necrosis. A genome-wide high-resolution gene copy number analysis of 22 osteosarcoma samples using comparative genomic hybridization

on a cDNA microarray that contained cDNA clones of about 13,000 genes had amplifications that on average spanned more than 1 Mb and contained more than 10 genes [34]. The study identified two candidate genes—*TOM1L2* and *CYP27B1* from 17p and 12q amplicons, respectively.

Tarkkanen *et al.* reported that the increased copy number at 8q13 and/or 8q21.3-q22 was associated with statistically significant poorer distant disease-free survival and a trend towards short overall survival [18]. The same group reported that patients with a copy number increase at 1q21 also showed a trend towards shorter overall survival. In contrast, Stock *et al.* [21] found that copy number increases at 8q and 1q21 did not have an unfavorable impact on prognosis.

VI. MOLECULAR SIGNATURE OF METASTASIS BASED ON EXPRESSION PROFILING

The most common cause of death among osteosarcoma patients is pulmonary metastasis. Thus, understanding the genetic determinants of metastasis in osteosarcoma and therapeutically modulating these factors should improve the outcome of these patients. Several genomics studies have implicated the involvement of pathways in cell motility, adherence, angiogenesis and bone differentiation in osteosarcoma metastasis. Using cDNA microarrays, Khanna *et al.* compared the expression profiles of two orthotopic ostoesarcoma xenograft mouse models [35]. One was developed from a less aggressive K12 cell line originating from a spontaneous BALB/c osteosarcoma which is primarily non-metastatic. The other model was derived from a clonally related K7M2 cell line, which is much more aggressive and highly metastatic. Fifty-three unique genes were differently expressed between these two types of tumors. These differently expressed genes were divided into six functional categories, including proliferation and apoptosis, motility and cytoskeleton, invasion, immune surveillance, adherence and angiogenesis. Based on several criteria, such as previously identified functions in several metastasis-associated processes, novelty to osteosarcoma, and not previously described in mesenchymal tumors, they selected a membrane-cytoskeleton organizer protein, Ezrin, for further analysis and confirmed its increased expressions in metastatic osteosarcoma at both the RNA and protein levels. The same group later reported that Ezrin expression provided an early survival advantage for cancer cells that reach the lung [36]. This early survival characteristic was partially dependent on the activation of MAPK, but not AKT. They also found that Ezrin expression was associated with an early development of metastases in a canine model as well as a poor outcome in human osteosarcoma patients. By examining over 5000 human cancers and normal tissue of various types, it was shown that Ezrin was expressed higher in sarcomas than in carcinomas [37]. Ezrin expression was shown to have a significant association with advanced histological grade in sarcomas and poor outcome in breast cancer. A similar study using tissue microarrays and immunohisto chemical staining has also shown that Ezrin expression predicted disease-free survival in osteosarcoma [38].

Instead of mouse models, Nakano *et al.* used a more focused microarray containing 637 cancer-related genes to compare the expression profiles of the highly metastatic sublines and less metastatic sublines from a human osteosarcoma cell line, HuO9 [39]. From their analysis, only seven genes were differently expressed between the highly metastatic and less metastatic sublines. Four genes (*AXL, TGFA, COLLA7A* and *WNT5A*) were upregulated and three genes (*IL-16, MKK6,* and *BRAG*) were down-regulated in the highly metastatic osteosarcoma sublines. Some of these genes are associated with adherence, motility, and invasiveness pathways.

Other than the cDNA microarray approach, representational difference analysis has also been used by Gillette *et al.* to analyze human primary osteosarcomas and metastatic lung lesions [40]. Several genes were identified as differently expressed between the two types of tumors. L-Ferritin and *ANXA2* were downregulated while *MDM2* was up-regulated in the metastatic lesions. Further functional assays suggested that *ANXA2* did not affect motility, adhesion, or proliferation. Instead, it was hypothesized that since anxA2 affects the mineralization process of osteoblastic cells *in vitro*, the higher expression of *ANXA2* in the less metastatic tumors might indicate a more differentiated osteoblastic pheotype in osteosarcoma with less aggressiveness.

VII. MOLECULAR SIGNATURE OF CHEMORESISTANCE BY EXPRESSION PROFILING

More than 40% of osteosarcomas showed relative chemoresistance in various clinical trials. After diagnosis is made by an initial biopsy, treatment typically consists of pre-operative chemotherapy followed by definitive surgery when the tumor is removed and evaluated for histologic responses to pre-operative chemotherapy. The degree of necrosis in the tumor specimen in response to pre-operative chemotherapy is a reliable prognostic factor for localized osteosarcoma. Patients with tumors which show at least 90% necrosis are considered to be good responders who have an excellent prognosis (80% overall survival), while those with less than 90% necrosis are considered as poor responders who have a significantly poorer outcome (40% overall survival). Previous attempts to improve the outcome of the poor responders by modifying the postoperative chemotherapy have not been successful. We attribute the failure of such therapeutic strategies partly to the fact that the degree of necrosis is known only after 8–10 weeks of pre-operative therapy. It is possible that resistant tumor cells have additional time either to

metastasize to the lungs or to evolve further during the period when ineffective pre-operative chemotherapy is given. Therefore, we believe there is a need to identify, at the time of initial diagnosis, the patients who are likely to have a poor response to standard pre-operative therapy and therefore a poor outcome eventually. Therapies tailored to improve the outcome for those patients identified, at the time of diagnosis, to have a poor outcome can then be instituted at the outset when the chance for success is potentially higher. To achieve this goal, we used cDNA microarrays to analyze a series of osteosarcomas from patients enrolled in a single treatment protocol and identified a molecular signature that can predict chemoresistance of osteosarcoma [41]. In our study, we hypothesized that the definitive surgery (post-treatment) samples from the poor responders should be enriched for resistant tumor cells. Therefore, using expression profiles from these post-treatment samples would enhance the sensitivity and likelihood of detecting the difference between sensitive and resistant cell populations; as opposed to using initial biopsy (pre-treatment) samples, because resistant cells may only constitute a small fraction in the pre-treatment tumors. To test this hypothesis, we used various classification algorithms to develop classifiers that could distinguish good and poor responders using post-treatment tumors as the training set. Based on a leave-one-out cross-validation method, Support Vector Machine (SVM) algorithm was one of the best performing algorithms (70% correct classification). The predictive power of the SVM classifier was tested on 14 initial biopsy (IB) samples that consisted of paired and independent samples. The patients of the paired samples had corresponding definitive surgery specimens used in the training of the classifier. The independent samples did not have corresponding samples included in the training set. The SVM classifier misclassified one sample out of six in the paired samples, with a correct classification rate of 83%. In the independent group, the classifier correctly predicted eight out of eight samples (100% correct). These results further indicated that the gene expression signature of the resistant cells in the post-treatment samples was already present in the pre-treatment samples at the time of diagnosis, which is consistent with the notion proposed by Ramaswamy *et al.* that the metastatic signature of metastatic tumors is already present in the primary tumor [42]. The high accuracy of the multigene classifier to identify poor responders from two separate groups of pre-treatment samples suggests that response to chemotherapy can potentially be predicted at the time of diagnosis.

The SVM classifier consisted of 45 predictor genes and most of them (91%) were upregulated in tumors from the poor responders (Table 15.2). Based on gene ontology classification, the majority of these genes belong to pathways of nucleobase, nucleoside, nucleotide and nucleic acid metabolism, protein metabolism, and cell proliferation. Many of the predictor genes in the classifier are related to bone development, cell cycle, or drug resistance. For instance, TWIST1

TABLE 15.2 Forty-five predictor genes in the chemoresistance prediction model

Ubiquitin specific protease 32

CHK1 checkpoint homolog (*S. pombe*)

Ras homolog gene family, member Q

Twist homolog 1 (acrocephalosyndactyly 3; Saethre-Chotzen syndrome) (Drosophila)

Cell division cycle 2-like 2 (PITSLRE proteins)

Sec1 family domain containing 1

Zinc finger protein 184 (Kruppel-like)

Matrin 3

Thymopoietin

LIM domain only 6

Ligase I, DNA, ATP-dependent

SWI/SNF related, matrix associated, actin dependent regulator of chromatin, subfamily a, member 1

RNA binding motif protein 25

CDC-like kinase 3

Ubiquitin-conjugating enzyme E2D 2 (UBC4/5 homolog, yeast)

Hydroxyacyl-coenzyme A dehydrogenase, type II

Adenosine monophosphate deaminase 2 (isoform L)

Interleukin-6 signal transducer (gp130, oncostatin M receptor)

Chromosome 6 open reading frame 68

Dimethylarginine dimethylaminohydrolase 1

Succinate dehydrogenase complex, subunit B, iron sulfur (Ip)

Transmembrane protein 1

Programmed cell death 5

MCM2 minichromosome maintenance deficient 2, mitotin (*S. cerevisiae*)

GDP dissociation inhibitor 1

SMC4 structural maintenance of chromosomes 4-like 1 (yeast)

Chromosome 10 open reading frame 7

CDC20 cell division cycle 20 homolog (*S. cerevisiae*)

Praja 2, RING-H2 motif containing

PTD008 protein

3-oxoacid CoA transferase 1

SNRPN upstream reading frame

Centromere protein A, 17 kDa

Heat shock 70 kDa protein 4

SWI/SNF related, matrix associated, actin dependent regulator of chromatin, subfamily e, member 1

NADH dehydrogenase (ubiquinone) Fe-S protein 5, 15 kDa (NADH-coenzyme Q reductase)

Ubiquitin-conjugating enzyme E2A (RAD6 homolog)

Fetal Alzheimer antigen

Mature T-cell proliferation 1

RNA binding motif protein, X-linked

Tubulin tyrosine ligase

Transcribed locus, moderately similar to XP_509796.1 similar to CGI-145 protein [Pan troglodytes]

Ephrin-B2

Triggering receptor expressed on myeloid cells 2

Membrane-spanning 4-domains, subfamily A, member 3 (hematopoietic cell-specific)

encodes a helix-loop-helix transcription factor [43] and has been implicated in the Saethre-Chotzen syndrome, radial aplasia, Robinow-Sorauf syndrome and craniosynostosis [44–47]. Mice with heterozygous TWIST1 mutation showed defects in craniofacial and limb development [48], which resemble those found in Saethre-Chotzen syndrome patients. It has been reported that TWIST1 affects CBFA1/RUNX2 expression [49] and DNA binding ability of RUNX2 [50], suggesting that TWIST1 is important for osteoblast differentiation and bone formation. Thus, dysregulation of TWIST1 expression may play a role in the pathogenesis of osteosarcoma [51,52]. In addition, several studies indicated the function of TWIST1 as a potential oncogene in c-myc- and N-myc-induced, p53-dependent apoptotsis pathways [53,54]. Other findings have also shown that TWIST1 was involved in Taxol resistance and metastasis [55,56], further implicating the important role of this gene in chemoresistance and tumor invasion. Another predictor gene in the chemoresistance signature is PDCD5 which has been implicated in the regulation of apoptosis [57]. The expression of PDCD5 was higher in cells undergoing apoptosis as compared to normal cells. During apoptosis, PDCD5 was shown to translocate rapidly from cytoplasm to nucleus [58]. PDCD5 is upregulated in pancreatic ductal carcinoma cells treated with trichostain-A, suggesting that PDCD5 may play a role in drug response [59]. CDC2L2 is involved in cell cycle progression, RNA processing and apoptosis [60]. It is a part of CDK11 protein kinases and may have tumor suppression function as demonstrated in melanoma [61]. TMPO belongs to a group of ubiquitously expressed nuclear proteins, which play an important role in nuclear envelope organization and cell cycle control. Upregulation of TMPO was seen in medulloblastoma when compared to normal cerebellum [62]. TMPO-beta transcript was expressed highly in human neuroblastoma cell lines, which may correlate with the occurrence of the cancer [63]. UBE2D2 encodes a member of the E2 ubiquitin-conjugating enzyme family. Inhibition of UBE2D2 (UBC4) inhibits E6-stimulated p53 [64]. MCM2 is a member of the family of mini-chromosome maintenance proteins (MCM) involved in the initiation of eukaryotic genome replication. The function of MCM2 is to regulate the helicase activity of the complex. A high expression of MCM2 has been shown to be associated with poor survival in prostate cancer [65].

Using a similar cDNA microarray approach, Ochi *et al.* employed a drug response scoring system to distinguish the good and poor responders in osteosarcoma [66]. The scoring system was based on the expression values of 60 genes that were significantly associated with the response to preoperative chemotherapy. The results of cross validation in the training set of 19 samples and five additional independent test samples showed that the scoring system classified the good and poor responders perfectly. However, the small sample size used in the test set [5] diminished the confidence of the results. Among the 60 genes used in the scoring system, several of them have been previously implicated in the resistance of chemotherapy. For example, ALR1C4 is a member of the aldo-keto reductase family, which may be involved in multi-drug resistance [67]. GPX1 can protect cells from oxidative stress [68] while GSTTLp28 belongs to the family of glutathione-S-transferase, which plays an important role in cellular detoxification and drug resistance [69,70].

In addition to cDNA microarrays, oligonucleotide arrays were also used for genomic analyses of osterosarcomas. Mintz *et al.* used Affymetrix oligonucleotide arrays (U95Av2) to identify a prognostic signature that was based on a histologic response in osteosarcoma [71]. Using both *p*-value and fold change criteria, they identified 104 genes that were differently expressed between Huvos Grade I/II and Grade III/IV osteosarcomas. In the Huvos system, Grade I/II tumors show a poor response, whereas Grade III/IV tumors show a good response towards the pre-operative chemotherapy. Different from the other two studies, Mintz *et al.* directly used the expressions of these differently expressed genes to perform hierarchical clustering on the original tumors that were used to derive the significant genes and three additional xenograft samples. These xenograft tumors were derived from aggressively growing and chemoresistant primary tumor cells. The clustering result showed that the xenograft tumors were clustered together with tumors from poor responders. Based on the functions of the 104 genes, they suggested that the poor prognosis tumors are associated with osteoclastogenesis and bone resorption, ECM remodeling, tumor progression, and resistance to apoptosis.

Despite addressing a similar question using comparable approaches, genes identified from these three microarray studies shared very little in common. While such discordance could be partly explained by the potential differences in microarray platforms and analytical strategies, one of the most important issues that ultimately needs to be addressed is the small sample size used in each of these studies. Although genes used in different classifiers need not be the same as long as they are accurate in classifying samples in different datasets, small sample sizes may pose a serious bias in the results given the high dimensionality in the data [72]. Given the relatively low incidence rate of osteosarcoma and differences in treatment protocol at different institutions, a large-scale, multi-institutional collaborative effort using the same treatment protocol is needed to evaluate the validity of these signatures and classifiers. Such a study will be carried out with the ongoing joint European/North American Osteosarcoma Study (EURAMOS).

VIII. PROTEOMIC PROFILING OF PLASMA

Although transcriptomic profiling is the most common platform used in the molecular classification of human cancers,

it is less suitable than proteomic profiling for analyzing cell-free body fluids, such as plasma due to very limited quantities of intact RNA present in such fluids. Because of post-transcriptional and post-translational regulations and modifications, RNA and protein expression measurements for the same gene may not correlate. In addition, plasma is much easier to access than a tumor biopsy, thus providing a means to monitor the disease progression and perform early detection of cancer. Individuals with retinoblastoma and RB mutation [73], Li-Fraumeni syndrome and p53 mutation [74], Werner syndrome [75], or Rothmund-Thomson syndrome and REQL4 mutation [76] have a higher risk of developing osteosarcoma. Therefore, an accurate but minimally invasive assay will be useful to monitor these patients for the development of osteosarcoma. We have previously used proteomic profiles generated from patients' plasma to test if we could develop a classifier that can distinguish osteosarcoma from benign osteochondroma [77]. The proteomic profiles were generated by the Surface Enhanced Laser Desorption/Ionization (SELDI) technique. SELDI is a high-throughput proteomic platform that combines solid phase chromatography with time-of-flight(TOF) mass spectrometry to detect protein peaks in many samples simultaneously. Solid phase chromatography is accomplished using microliter quantities of samples on protein chips with various surface chemistries to capture different types of proteins. Based on these plasma-based proteomic profiles, we developed a 3-nearest neighbor classifier to distinguish malignant osteosarcomas from benign osteochondromas. The ultimate goal is to develop a proteomic signature in plasma that could be used to screen the high risk population for early detection of osteosarcoma. In the pilot study, however, we chose to use the plasma of osteochondroma patients, to control for non-specific host reactions that might manifest as plasma protein changes in response to bone lesions. The classifier achieved 97% specificity and 80% sensitivity to classify osteosarcoma using an external leave-one-out cross validation. The classifier consisted of 19 protein peaks of various m/z ratios. One of the protein peaks was identified by peptide mass fingerprinting to be serum amyloid protein A (SAA), which is a known biomarker in various cancers [78–81].

Consistent with our proteomic analysis, Song *et al.* has independently shown that SAA was increased in the sera of osteosarcoma patients when compared to sera from normal individuals [82]. They first performed two-dimensional fluorescence difference gel electrophoresis (2-D DIGE) on sera from four osteosarcoma patients and four age- and sex-matched healthy controls. 2-D DIGE is a modification of 2-D gel electrophoresis, which can analyze multiple samples at the same time [83]. From this analysis, they identified the increase of 18 and decrease of 25 proteins in osteosarcoma sera relative to normal sera using matrix-assisted laser deadsorption/ionization (MALDI)-TOF mass spectrometry. Topping the list of proteins increased in osteosarcoma sera were SAA, ceruloplasmin, DGKG protein, and human complement component C3. Proteins that were decreased in osteosarcoma sera included fibronectin 1 isoform 6 preprotein, MTA2 protein, inter-alpha-trypsin inhibitor heavy chain H4 precursor, and fibrinogen gamma. Most interesting, when these investigators tested the abundance of SAA in another set of patients' sera, they found that the abundance of SAA was lower in the samples after chemotherapy and after surgical removal of primary tumors, but its level was higher in the samples from relapsed patients. Therefore, they suggested that serum SAA might be a relapse biomarker for osteosarcoma. The consistency of these two proteomic studies suggests that SAA may be useful for detecting the occurrence of osteosarcoma in high-risk individuals and recurrence in previously diagnosed osteosarcoma patients.

IX. CONCLUSIONS

Genomic profiling approaches should advance our knowledge of the pathogenesis of osteosarcoma and refine the management of this disease, although the optimal application of these data requires that several conditions be met. First and foremost is that these clinically relevant profiles need to be validated with independent data sets by multiple institutions. Although the currently available microarray platforms are proving to be technically robust and reliable, subtle differences in sample collection and preparation can have a profound impact on the final data. This is evidenced by the often discordant results by different investigators in the published literature. Moreover, the bioinformatic and statistical methods used in analyzing these data sets are far from uniform or adequate, making it difficult to perform comparisons between data sets. Another important step in the utilization of these profiles to guide clinical decision-making involves translating these technologies from the research setting into clinically applicable diagnostic studies that can be performed rapidly and reliably on surgically obtained tumor specimens. It is questionable whether it is practical or necessary to perform genome-wide profiling of every tumor in a clinical laboratory setting. The requirement of standardized laboratories with standardized procedures for performance and analysis of genomic profiling is far too cumbersome. Alternatively, it is possible to narrow down the number of clinically relevant genes from a genome-wide profile into a more manageable number, which can then be assayed using more conventional methods such as immunohistochemistry and quantitative PCR that are already established and employed in clinical laboratories. Thirdly, the validity of these prognostic correlates must be confirmed in an independent, preferably prospective, cohort of patients. Studies designed to address these challenges for osteosarcoma are currently either in progress or under development within the Children's Oncology Group and several European cooperative groups. The ultimate challenge involves demonstrating that biologic stratification can support risk-based therapeutic stratification that will improve the outcome of osteosarcoma patients. The realization of this long-range goal will also require the identification of novel therapeutic strategies that promise to improve the outcome in tumor subgroups that have been resistant to conventional therapies. We believe that molecular profiling will provide important clues regarding critical pathways that the tumor cells depend on to maintain their malignant phenotype. Such pathways will be ideal therapeutic targets for tumor-specific therapies. An equally important aspect of this goal will involve the continuation of ongoing efforts to cautiously decrease the intensity of potentially toxic therapies in order to reduce the morbidity of treatment in tumors that have particularly favorable risk factors based on genomic and proteomic profiling. In conclusion, despite all the limitations described, genomic and proteomic profiling offers an exciting possibility for refining the diagnosis, stratification and therapy of osteosarcoma. It is not too hard to imagine that in the near future predictive individualized care based on molecular classification and targeted therapy will become a reality for this type of cancer.

References

1. H.C. Bauer, A. Kreicbergs & C. Silfversward, et al., DNA analysis in the differential diagnosis of osteosarcoma, Cancer 61 (1988) 2532–2540.
2. W. Hiddemann, A. Roessner & B. Wormann, et al., Tumor heterogeneity in osteosarcoma as identified by flow cytometry, Cancer 59 (1987) 324–328.
3. A. Kreicbergs, C. Silfversward & B. Tribukait, Flow DNA analysis of primary bone tumors: relationship between cellular DNA content and histopathologic classification, Cancer 53 (1984) 129–136.
4. K. Kusuzaki, H. Takeshita & H. Murata, et al., Prognostic significance of DNA ploidy pattern in osteosarcomas in association with chemotherapy, Cancer Lett 137 (1999) 27–33.
5. T. Bosing, A. Roessner & W. Hiddemann, et al., Cytostatic effects in osteosarcomas as detected by flow cytometric DNA analysis after preoperative chemotherapy according to the COSS 80/82 protocol, J Cancer Res Clin Oncol 113 (1987) 369–375.
6. A.T. Look, E.C. Douglass & W.H. Meyer, Clinical importance of near-diploid tumor stem lines in patients with osteosarcoma of an extremity, N Engl J Med 318 (1988) 1567–1572.
7. M. Serra, M. Tarkkanen & N. Baldini, et al., Simultaneous paired analysis of numerical chromosomal aberrations and DNA content in osteosarcoma, Mod Pathol 14 (7) (2001) 710–716.
8. A.A. Sandberg & J.A. Bridge, Updates on the cytogenetics and molecular genetics of bone and soft tissue tumors: osteosarcoma and related tumors, Cancer Genet Cytogenet 145 (1) (2003) 1–30.
9. J. Bayani, M. Zielenska & A. Pandita, et al., Spectral karyotyping identifies recurrent complex rearrangements of chromosomes 8, 17, and 20 in osteosarcomas, Genes Chromosomes Cancer 36 (2003) 7–16.

10. C.C. Lau, C.P. Harris & X.Y. Lu, et al., Frequent amplification and rearrangement of chromosomal bands 6p12-p21 and 17p11.2 in osteosarcoma, Genes Chromosomes Cancer 39 (2004) 11–21.

11. G.A. Ulaner, H.-Y. Huang & J. Otero, et al., Absence of a telomere maintenance mechanism as a favorable prognostic factor in patients with osteosarcoma, Cancer Res 63 (2003) 1759–1763.

12. C. Scheel, K.L. Schaefer & A. Jauch, et al., Alternative lengthening of telomeres is associated with chromosomal instability in osteosarcomas, Oncogene 20 (2001) 3835–3844.

13. D. Gisselsson, T. Jonson & A. Petersen, et al., Telomere dysfunction triggers extensive DNA fragmentation and evolution of complex chromosome abnormalities in human malignant tumors, Proc Natl Acad Sci USA 98 (2001) 12683–12688.

14. B. McClintock, The fusion of broken ends of sister half-chromatids following chromatid breakage at meiotic anaphases, Missouri Agric Exp Sta Res Bull 290 (1938) 48.

15. D. Gisselsson, L. Pettersson & M. Hoglund, et al., Chromosomal breakage-fusion-bridge events cause genetic intratumor heterogeneity, Proc Natl Acad Sci USA 97 (2000) 5357–5362.

16. M. Overholtzer, P.H. Rao & R. Favis, et al., The presence of p53 mutations in human osteosarcomas correlates with high levels of genomic instability, Proc Natl Acad Sci USA 100 (2003) 11547–11552.

17. M. Tarkkanen, R. Karhu & A. Kallioniemi, et al., Gains and losses of DNA sequences in osteosarcomas by comparative genome hybridization, Cancer Res 55 (1995) 1334–1338.

18. M. Tarkkanen, I. Elomaa & C. Blomqvist, et al., DNA sequence copy number increase at 8q: a potential new prognostic marker in high-grade osteosarcoma, Int J Cancer 84 (1999) 114–121.

19. A. Forus, D.O. Weghuis & D. Smeets, et al., Comparative genomic hybridization analysis of human sarcomas: I. Occurrence of genomic imbalances and identification of a novel major amplicon at 1q21-q22 in soft tissue sarcomas, Genes Chromosomes Cancer 14 (1995) 8–14.

20. A. Forus, D.O. Weghuis & D. Smeets, et al., Comparative genomic hybridization analysis of human sarcomas: II. Identification of novel amplicons at 6p and 17p in osteosarcomas, Genes Chromosomes Cancer 14 (1995) 15–21.

21. C. Stock, L. Kager & F-M. Fink, et al., Chromosomal regions involved in the pathogenesis of osteosarcoma, Genes Chromosomes Cancer 28 (2000) 329–336.

22. M. Zielenska, J. Bayani & A. Pandira, et al., Comparative genomic hybridization analysis identifies gains of 1p35-36 and chromosome 19 in osteosarcoma, Cancer Genet Cytogenet 130 (2001) 14–21.

23. M. van Dartel, P.W. Cornelissen & S. Redeker, et al., Amplification of 17p11.2 approximately p12, including PMP22, TOP3A, and MAPK7, in high-grade osteosarcoma, Cancer Genet Cytogenet 139 (2002) 91–96.

24. S. dos Santos Aguiar, L. de Jesus Girotto Zambaldi & A.M. dos Santos, et al., Comparative genomic hybridization analysis of abnormalities in chromosome 21 in childhood osteosarcoma, Cancer Genet Cytogenet 175 (2007) 35–40.

25. T.K. Man, X.Y. Lu & K. Jaeweon, et al., Genome-wide array comparative genomic hybridization analysis reveals distinct amplifications in osteosarcoma, BMC Cancer 4 (2004) 45.

26. X.Y. Lu, Y. Lu & Y.J. Zhao, et al., Cell Cycle Regulator Gene CDC5L, a potential target for 6p12-p21 amplicon in osteosarcoma, Mol Cancer Res 6 (2008) 937–946.

27. T.J.M. Hulsebos, E.H. Bijleveld & N.T. Oskam, et al., Malignant astrocytoma-derived region of common amplification in chromosomal band 17p12 is frequently amplified in high-grade osteosarcomas, Genes Chromosomes Cancer 18 (1997) 279–285.

28. C. Brinkschmidt, S. Blasius & H. Burger, et al., Comparative genomic hybridization (CGH) for detecting a heretofore undescribed amplified chromosomal segment in high-grade medullary osteosarcoma, Verh Dtsch Ges Pathol 82 (1998) 184–188.

29. A.K. Boehm, J.R. Neff & J.A. Squire, et al., Cytogenetic findings in 36 osteosarcoma specimens and a review of the literature, Pediatr Pathol Mol Med 19 (2000) 359–376.

30. J.A. Squire, J. Pei & P. Marrano, et al., High-resolution mapping of amplifications and deletions in pediatric osteosarcoma by use of CGH analysis of cDNA microarrays, Genes Chromosomes Cancer 38 (2003) 215–225.

31. M. Wolf, M. Tarkkanen & T. Hulsebos, et al., Characterization of the 17p amplicon in human sarcomas: microsatellite marker analysis, Int J Cancer 82 (1999) 329–333.

32. A. Simons, I.M. Janssen & R.F. Suijkerbuijk, et al., Isolation of osteosarcoma-associated amplified DNA sequences using representational difference analysis, Genes Chromosomes Cancer 20 (1997) 196–200.

33. T. Yan, J.S. Wunder, N. Gokgoz & M. Gill, et al., COPS3 amplification and clinical outcome in osteosarcoma, Cancer 109 (2007) 1870–1876.

34. J. Atiye, M. Wolf & S. Kaur, et al., Gene amplifications in osteosarcoma-CGH microarray analysis, Genes Chromosomes Cancer 42 (2005) b158–b163.

35. C. Khanna, J. Khan & P. Nguyen, et al., Metastasis-associated differences in gene expression in a murine model of osteosarcoma, Cancer Res 61 (2001) 3750–3759.

36. C. Khanna, X. Wan & S. Bose, et al., The membrane-cytoskeleton linker ezrin is necessary for osteosarcoma metastasis, Nat Med 10 (2004) 182–186.

37. B. Bruce, G. Khanna & L. Ren, et al., Expression of the cytoskeleton linker protein ezrin in human cancers, Clin Exp Metastasis 24 (2007) 69–78.

38. M.S. Kim, W.S. Song & W.H. Cho, et al., Ezrin expression predicts survival in stage IIB osteosarcomas, Clin Orthop Relat Res 459 (2007) 229–236.

39. T. Nakano, M. Tani & Y. Ishibashi, et al., Biological properties and gene expression associated with metastatic potential of human osteosarcoma, Clin Exp Metastasis 20 (2003) 665–674.

40. J.M. Gillette, D.C. Chan & S.M. Nielsen-Preiss, Annexin 2 expression is reduced in human osteosarcoma metastases, J Cell Biochem 92 (2004) 820–832.

41. T.K. Man, M. Chintagumpala & J. Visvanathan, et al., Expression profiles of osteosarcoma that can predict response to chemotherapy, Cancer Res 65 (2005) 8142–8150.

42. S. Ramaswamy, K.N. Ross & E.S. Lander, et al., A molecular signature of metastasis in primary solid tumors, Nat Genet 33 (2003) 49–54.

43. P. Bourgeois, A.L. Bolcato-Bellemin & J.M. Danse, et al., The variable expressivity and incomplete penetrance of the twist-null heterozygous mouse phenotype resemble those of human Saethre-Chotzen syndrome, Hum Mol Genet 7 (1998) 945–957.

44. T.D. Howard, W.A. Paznekas & E.D. Green, et al., Mutations in TWIST, a basic helix-loop-helix transcription factor, in Saethre-Chotzen syndrome, Nat Genet 15 (1997) 36–41.

45. M. Yousfi, F. Lasmoles & G.V. El, et al., Twist haploinsufficiency in Saethre-Chotzen syndrome induces calvarial osteoblast apoptosis due to increased TNFalpha expression and caspase-2 activation, Hum Mol Genet 11 (2002) 359–369.

46. K.W. Gripp, C.A. Stolle & L. Celle, et al., TWIST gene mutation in a patient with radial aplasia and craniosynostosis: further evidence for heterogeneity of Baller-Gerold syndrome, Am J Med Genet 82 (1999) 170–176.

47. J. Kunz, M. Hudler & B. Fritz, Identification of a frameshift mutation in the gene TWIST in a family affected with Robinow-Sorauf syndrome, J Med Genet 36 (1999) 650–652.

48. P. Bourgeois, A.L. Bolcato-Bellemin & J.M. Danse, et al., The variable expressivity and incomplete penetrance of the twist-null heterozygous mouse phenotype resemble those of human Saethre-Chotzen syndrome, Hum Mol Genet 7 (1998) 945–957.

49. P. Bialek, B. Kern & X. Yang, et al., A twist code determines the onset of osteoblast differentiation, Dev Cell 6 (2004) 423–435.

50. M. Yousfi, F. Lasmoles & P.J. Marie, TWIST inactivation reduces CBFA1/RUNX2 expression and DNA binding to the osteocalcin promoter in osteoblasts, Biochem Biophys Res Commun 297 (2002) 641–644.

51. N. Entz-Werle, T. Lavaux & N. Metzger, et al., Involvement of MET/TWIST/APC combination or the potential role of ossification factors in pediatric high-grade osteosarcoma oncogenesis, Neoplasia 9 (2007) 678–688.

52. N. Entz-Werle, C. Stoetzel & P. Berard-Marec, et al., Frequent genomic abnormalities at TWIST in human pediatric osteosarcomas, Int J Cancer 117 (2005) 349–355.

53. R. Maestro, A.P. Dei Tos & Y. Hamamori, et al., Twist is a potential oncogene that inhibits apoptosis, Genes Dev 13 (1999) 2207–2217.

54. S. Valsesia-Wittmann, M. Magdeleine & S. Dupasquier, et al., Oncogenic cooperation between H-Twist and N-Myc overrides failsafe programs in cancer cells, Cancer Cell 6 (2004) 625–630.

55. X. Wang, M.T. Ling & X.Y. Guan, et al., Identification of a novel function of TWIST, a bHLH protein, in the development of acquired taxol resistance in human cancer cells, Oncogene 23 (2004) 474–482.

56. J. Yang, S.A. Mani & J.L. Donaher, et al., Twist, a master regulator of morphogenesis, plays an essential role in tumor metastasis, Cell 117 (2004) 927–939.

57. H. Liu, Y. Wang & Y. Zhang, et al., TFAR19, a novel apoptosis-related gene cloned from human leukemia cell line TF-1, could enhance apoptosis of some tumor cells induced by growth factor withdrawal, Biochem Biophys Res Commun 254 (1999) 203–210.

58. Y. Chen, R. Sun & W. Han, et al., Nuclear translocation of PDCD5 (TFAR19): an early signal for apoptosis?, FEBS Lett 509 (2001) 191–196.

59. D. Cecconi, A. Scarpa & M. Donadelli, et al., Proteomic profiling of pancreatic ductal carcinoma cell lines treated with trichostatin-A, Electrophoresis 24 (2003) 1871–1878.

60. Y. Feng, A.C. Goulet & M.A. Nelson, Identification and characterization of the human Cdc2l2 gene promoter, Gene 330 (2004) 75–84.

61. M.A. Nelson, M.E. Ariza & J.M. Yang, et al., Abnormalities in the p34cdc2-related PITSLRE protein kinase gene complex (CDC2L) on chromosome band 1p36 in melanoma, Cancer Genet Cytogenet 108 (1999) 91–99.

62. N. Yokota, T.G. Mainprize & M.D. Taylor, et al., Identification of differentially expressed and developmentally regulated genes in medulloblastoma using suppression subtraction hybridization, Oncogene 23 (2004) 3444–3453.

63. P.J. Weber, C.P. Eckhard & S. Gonser, et al., On the role of thymopoietins in cell proliferation. Immunochemical evidence for new members of the human thymopoietin family, Biol Chem 380 (1999) 653–660.

64. M. Rolfe, P. Beer-Romero & S. Glass, et al., Reconstitution of p53-ubiquitinylation reactions from purified components: the role of human ubiquitin-conjugating enzyme UBC4 and E6-associated protein (E6AP), Proc Natl Acad Sci USA 92 (1995) 3264–3268.

65. M.V. Meng, G.D. Grossfeld & G.H. Williams, et al., Minichromosome maintenance protein 2 expression in prostate: characterization and association with outcome after therapy for cancer, Clin Cancer Res 7 (2001) 2712–2718.

66. K. Ochi, Y. Daigo & T. Katagiri, et al., Prediction of response to neoadjuvant chemotherapy for osteosarcoma by gene-expression profiles, Int J Oncol 24 (2004) 647–655.

67. S. Dan, T. Tsunoda & O. Kitahara, et al., An integrated database of chemosensitivity to 55 anticancer drugs and gene expression profiles of 39 human cancer cell lines, Cancer Res 62 (2002) 1139–1147.

68. J.B. de Haan, C. Bladier & P. Griffiths, et al., Mice with a homozygous null mutation for the most abundant glutathione peroxidase, Gpx1, show increased susceptibility to the oxidative stress-inducing agents paraquat and hydrogen peroxide, J Biol Chem 273 (1998) 22528–22536.

69. A.K. Godwin, A. Meister & P.J. O'Dwyer, et al., High resistance to cisplatin in human ovarian cancer cell lines is associated with marked increase of glutathione synthesis, Proc Natl Acad Sci USA 89 (1992) 3070–3074.

70. A.L. Wang & K.D. Tew, Increased glutathione-S-transferase activity in a cell line with acquired resistance to nitrogen mustards, Cancer Treat Rep 69 (1985) 677–682.

71. M.B. Mintz, R. Sowers & K.M. Brown, et al., An expression signature classifies chemotherapy-resistant pediatric osteosarcoma, Cancer Res 65 (2005) 1748–1754.

72. T.A. Dang & T.K. Man, Classification of sarcomas using bioinformatics and molecular profiling, Curr Pharm Biotechnol 8 (2007) 83–91.

73. E. Matsunaga, Hereditary retinoblastoma: host resistance and second primary tumors, J Natl Cancer Inst 65 (1980) 47–51.

74. F.P. Li, J.F., Fraumeni, Jr. & J.J. Mulvihill, et al., A cancer family syndrome in twenty-four kindreds, Cancer Res 48 (1988) 5358–5362.

75. M. Goto, R.W. Miller & Y. Ishikawa, et al., Excess of rare cancers in Werner syndrome (adult progeria), Cancer Epidemiol Biomarkers Prev 5 (1996) 239–246.

76. L.L. Wang, A. Gannavarapu & C.A. Kozinetz, et al., Association between osteosarcoma and deleterious mutations in the RECQL4 gene in Rothmund-Thomson syndrome, J Natl Cancer Inst 95 (2003) 669–674.

77. Y. Li, T.A. Dang & J. Shen, et al., Identification of a plasma proteomic signature to distinguish pediatric osteosarcoma

from benign osteochondroma, Proteomics 6 (2006) 3426–3435.

78. M. Kimura, Y. Tomita & T. Imai, et al., Significance of serum amyloid A on the prognosis in patients with renal cell carcinoma, Cancer 92 (2001) 2072–2075.

79. I. Glojnaric, M.T. Casl & D. Simic, et al., Serum amyloid A protein (SAA) in colorectal carcinoma, Clin Chem Lab Med 39 (2001) 129–133.

80. H. Biran, N. Friedman & L. Neumann, et al., Serum amyloid A (SAA) variations in patients with cancer: correlation with disease activity, stage, primary site, and prognosis, J Clin Pathol 39 (1986) 794–797.

81. W.C. Cho, T.T. Yip & C. Yip, et al., Identification of serum amyloid a protein as a potentially useful biomarker to monitor relapse of nasopharyngeal cancer by serum proteomic profiling, Clin Cancer Res 10 (2004) 43–52.

82. S. Jin, J-N. Shen & Q-C. Guo, et al., 2-D DIGE and MALDI-TOF-MS analysis of the serum proteome in human osteosarcoma, Proteomics Clin Appl 1 (2007) 272–285.

83. M. Unlu, M.E. Morgan & J.S. Minden, Difference gel electrophoresis: a single gel method for detecting changes in protein extracts, Electrophoresis 18 (1997) 2071–2077.

CHAPTER **16**

Molecular Pathology of Osteosarcoma

WALTER C. BELL[1] AND GENE P. SIEGAL[2]

[1]University of Alabama at Birmingham, Birmingham, AL 35249, USA.
[2]University of Alabama at Birmingham, Birmingham, AL 35233, USA.

Contents

I. INTRODUCTION

Although osteosarcoma is a relatively rare neoplasm, it does represent the most common bone malignancy of childhood with an incidence of 4–5 per million population [1]. Diagnosis and classification of osteosarcoma relies on correlation of biopsy findings with imaging studies [2]. While molecular findings continue to be of limited value in the diagnosis of osteosarcoma, our understanding of the molecular pathogenesis of this neoplasm and the molecular pathways involved has increased significantly in recent years. These findings do contribute to our understanding of tumor prognosis, and may in the future yield important information for directed therapy. Our understanding of these processes has been enhanced through the study of syndromes associated with an increased risk of osteosarcoma, with studies of sporadic osteosarcoma, and with research involving animal models. In this chapter, we will review specific tumor suppressor genes, oncogenes, and molecular pathways which have been implicated in the development and progression of osteosarcoma.

II. TUMOR SUPPRESSOR GENES

As discussed in our previous review, the association of alterations of p53 and the retinoblastoma gene (RB) have long been well established [3]. These tumor suppressor pathways remain the most clearly established in terms of

osteosarcoma development, but our understanding of their role has increased, and a number of other tumor suppressor pathways have now also shown an association with osteosarcoma pathogenesis.

A. Retinoblastoma Pathway

The role of the retinoblastoma gene (RB) as a tumor suppressor has long been recognized in retinoblastoma of the eye in children. Study of the epidemiology of retinoblastoma led to the development of Knudson's 'two hit hypothesis' which is now understood in the context of biallelic mutations resulting in loss of suppressor gene function [4,5].

RB is a member of the 'pocket protein' family of cell cycle regulators which serve to control cell cycle progression from G1 to S through regulation of the E2F transcription factors [6]. The retinoblastoma protein (pRB) is localized to the cell nucleus. In its hypophosphorylated state, pRB binds E2F. Phosphorylation of pRB allows the release of E2F and progression of the cell into the S phase of the cell cycle. Phosphorylation of pRB is driven by cyclin D in conjunction with cdk4 and cdk6 and by cyclin E in conjunction with cdk2.

Patients with retinoblastoma have an incidence of osteosarcoma up to 1000 times that of the general population suggesting that RB alterations might also be seen in sporadic osteosarcoma [7]. RB is located at chromosome 13 q14 and a number of studies have shown loss of heterozygosity (LOH) at this locus in osteosarcomas [8–11]. LOH at 13q14 furthermore is associated with high grade osteosarcomas and poor prognosis [12]. Wadayama *et al.* examined 63 cases of osteosarcoma and demonstrated LOH at the RB locus in 63% of cases, with structural abnormalities (rearrangements or point mutations) identified in approximately 35% of these tumors. Expression of pRB has also been investigated by immunohistochemistry with loss of expression in 54% of cases. Interestingly, this loss of protein expression occurred in a similar percentage among cases with LOH for RB (54.5%) as compared to cases without LOH (50%). This suggests that other proteins in the retinoblastoma regulatory pathway must be altered in some cases of osteosarcoma [13].

As described, CDK4 plays an important role in phosphorylation of pRB, and increased expression of CDK4 has been described in osteosarcoma [14–16]. The cyclin dependent kinase inhibitors (CDKI) play a role in regulation of pRB phosphorylation by inhibiting phosphorylation of pRB by cyclin D/CDK4-6. Loss of p16^{INK4a} expression has been described in osteosarcomas lacking RB mutations [17,18]. This loss of p16's inhibitory function, would allow for phosphorylation of pRB and progression of the cell cycle from G1 to S. Similarly, alteration of p19, another CDKI in this pathway, has been shown to be altered in a small number of osteosarcoma cases [19]. The pRB pathway in cell cycle regulation is illustrated in Figure 16.1.

B. p53

The p53 protein is involved in cell cycle arrest and induction of apoptosis as part of the cell's response to DNA damage. The gene is located on chromosome 17 at position 31.1 and mutations have been observed in many tumor types. In response to DNA damage, p53 induces an upregulation of p21(formerly known as WAF1), a CDKI, which inhibits cell division through binding of the cyclinD/CDK4-6 complex, preventing phosphorylation of pRB [20–22]. In response to severe DNA damage, cell cycle arrest is prolonged and p53 induces increased transcription of BAX leading to apoptosis of the cell [23].

Germline mutations of p53 result in Li Fraumeni syndrome. Patients with this syndrome are at high risk of developing many types of malignancies including carcinomas of the breast, leukemias, brain tumors, soft tissue sarcomas, and osteosarcomas [24]. In mouse models of Li Fraumeni syndrome up to 60% of mice develop osteosarcoma [25]. Osteosarcoma occurs in up to 12% of Li Fraumeni patients [26]. Biallelic inactivating mutations of the p53 gene have been reported in up to 50% of sporadic osteosarcomas with the frequency of p53 mutations increased in higher grade tumors [27].

Alterations in genes involved in the regulation of p53 have also been described in osteosarcoma. The mouse double minute 2 gene (MDM2) is located on chromosome 12q and its protein has the ability to bind and inactivate p53 as well as inhibit transcription of p53 and has also been shown to be involved in p53 degradation [28,29]. MDM2 also affects the RB pathway by directly binding pRB, causing effective activation through the release of E2F [30]. Thus, oncogenic activation of MDM2 plays a dual role in that it effectively activates pRB, driving cell division, while at the same time crippling the cellular mechanisms of DNA repair by inhibiting the transcription and function of p53. MDM2 has been shown to be amplified in up to 17% of osteosarcomas [31–35]. Overexpression has been correlated with a poorer prognosis with a higher rate of recurrence and metastasis [32,33,36].

Other regulatory proteins in the p53 pathway include p14^{ARF} and checkpoint kinase 2 (CHK2). The gene for the p14^{ARF} protein is located on chromosome 9p21 and in an alternate reading frame also encodes p16^{INK4}. p14^{ARF} inhibits MDM2 function preventing degradation of p53 [37,38]. Based on this function in stabilizing p53, the role of p14^{ARF} as a tumor suppressor gene is suggested. Biallelic loss of p14^{ARF} has been reported in up to 10% of osteosarcomas [39]. CHK2 is involved in repair of DNA damage and is thought to play

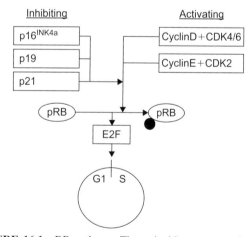

FIGURE 16.1 RB pathway. The retinoblastoma protein (pRB) plays a central role in regulating progression of the cell cycle from G1 to S phase through binding of E2F transcription factor in its hypophosphorylated form and release of E2F when hyperphosphorylated. Phosphorylation of pRB is driven by cyclins D and E in conjunction with cyclin dependent kinases (CDK). Phosphorylation is inhibited by the cyclin dependent kinase inhibitors, including p16^{INK4a}, p19, and p21. Alterations in each of these steps have been identified in osteosarcomas.

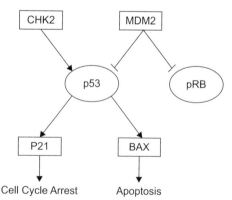

FIGURE 16.2 p53 Pathway. P53 plays an important role in cellular repair mechanisms. In response to DNA damage, p53 induces p21, a cyclin dependent kinase inhibitor, inhibiting phosphorylation of pRB, leading to cell cycle arrest. Induction of BAX by p53 in response to extensive damage or repair failure leads to apoptosis. P53 is stabilized by CHK2. MDM2 enhances degradation of p53 and also binds to pRB, so that E2F is released. Alterations in each of these p53 associated pathways have been identified in osteosarcomas.

a role in degradation of p53. One study reports mutations of CHK2 in 7% of osteosarcomas [40]. The role of the p53 pathway in response to DNA damage and regulatory pathways associated with p53 are illustrated in Figure 16.2.

C. DCC

Horstmann *et al.* evaluated 19 high grade osteosarcomas and six low grade osteosarcomas and found absent or decreased expression of the deleted in colon cancer (DCC) gene on 18q21.1 in 14 of the high grade tumors and three of the low grade tumors [41].

III. ONCOGENES IN OSTEOSARCOMA

Oncogenes are derived from proto-oncogenes, genes which encode proteins involved in cell cycle progression. Oncogenic transformation takes place through activating mutations or translocations, by amplification, or by dysregulation leading to increased gene transcription. Numerous oncogenes have been reported to play a role in the development and progression of osteosarcoma.

We have previously described the role of MDM2 as an oncogene with frequent amplification in osteosarcoma and the interaction of the MDM2 protein with p53. Ladanyi *et al.* suggest that MDM2 amplification is more common in metastatic or recurrent tumors [32].

MYC, FOS, and RAF alterations are frequently observed in osteosarcoma and may occur singly, in combination, and with or without accompanying deletions in p53 and RB [42–44]. Wu *et al.* report FOS amplification in 61% of osteosarcomas evaluated [45]. Osteosarcomatous transformation has been described in fibrous dysplasia as well as in McCune-Albright syndrome and Mazabraud syndrome, both of which have fibrous dysplasia as a component [46–49]. Interestingly, Weisstein *et al.* evaluated expression of FOS in benign and malignant tumors of bone using *in situ* hybridization. They report high FOS expression levels in all fibrous lesions evaluated, including six cases of fibrous dysplasia, and in three of eight osteosarcomas, suggesting that FOS overexpression may be important in the development of fibrous dysplasia and some osteosarcomas [50].

Amplification of erbB2 has been reported by some groups in osteosarcoma and has been linked to an increased risk for pulmonary metastasis [51–53]. Others have reported that amplification of erbB2 is uncommon in osteosarcoma and found no association with its presence and tumor grade [54–57]. Fellenberg *et al.* performed real time RT-PCR for erbB2 on samples obtained by laser capture microdissection from archival osteosarcoma biopsies. They found expression of erbB2 to correlate with sensitivity to chemotherapy, suggesting that erbB2 might be used as a prognostic marker predicting chemotherapy response [58].

IV. RECQ HELICASES

The RECQ helicase family of proteins is involved in DNA unwinding, and members serve important roles in replication, transcription and repair. Three of the RECQ helicases (RECQL4, WRN, and BLM) are associated with autosomal recessive syndromes with increased risk of osteosarcoma [59–63].

Bloom syndrome, associated with BLM mutations, results in growth retardation and a predilection for development of cancers of all types including osteosarcoma. This high prevalence of cancer is due to overall genetic instability with a high frequency of somatic mutation [64–66].

Werner syndrome is associated with premature aging. It occurs most frequently in the Japanese population. Mutations in the WRN gene cause truncation of WRN helicase preventing nuclear localization. WRN appears to have a role in maintenance of telomeric structure [67–70].

Rothmund-Thompson syndrome (RTS) causes skin lesions, small stature, and skeletal dysplasias. Patients with RTS, which results from RECQ4 mutations, have a predisposition to developing cancer, particularly osteosarcoma [59,71]. Other syndromes with defects in the RECQ4 gene have also been described (i.e., Baller-Gerold syndrome and RAPADININO syndrome, which have no known increased cancer risk [72–74]).

V. GENES INVOLVED IN OSTEOSARCOMA METASTASIS

The presence of metastatic disease at the time of clinical presentation is a major predictor of poor clinical outcome in osteosarcoma, and the majority of deaths associated with osteosarcoma are due to metastases. We are beginning to gain a greater understanding of the molecular biology of metastasis, and recently, genes have been identified which play a role in the metastasis of osteosarcoma.

A. Ezrin

Ezrin is a membrane bound cytoskeleton linker protein which has been associated with poor outcome in a number of cancers [75,76]. High levels of ezrin expression have been shown to correlate with higher grade tumors, decreased disease-free survival rate in pediatric patients, and had a greater risk of metastatic relapse [77–80]. Ferrari *et al.* examined ezrin expression in non-metastatic osteosarcoma and found a significant difference in disease-free survival based on the pattern of staining. Patients with tumors demonstrating only cytoplasmic expression had a >80% 3-year disease-free survival, while those with cytoplasmic and membrane reactivity had a 54% 3-year disease-free survival [81].

B. Annexin 2

Annexin 2 is a phospholipid binding protein which has been shown in studies of differential expression of proteins between primary osteosarcomas and subsequent metastases to be downregulated in the metastases [82]. The role of annexin 2 in osteosarcoma metastasis is currently uncertain but suspected.

C. CXCR4

CXCR4 is a chemokine receptor with expression levels which correlate with metastasis in many types of cancer. Laverdiere *et al.* demonstrated a correlation between increased CXCR4 mRNA, reduced survival, and the presence of metastases at diagnosis [83]. Mouse studies using treatment directed at inhibition of CXCR4 have shown promising results in treatment of lung metastases from osteosarcoma [84].

VI. OTHER GENES ASSOCIATED WITH CHEMORESISTANCE AND TUMOR PROGRESSION

P-glycoprotein is encoded by the multiple drug resistant-1 (MDR-1) gene and has been shown to confer multidrug chemoresistance in many cancers. The MDR-1 gene is regulated by p53 which inhibits transcription [85]. Chan *et al.* examined expression levels of P-glycoprotein in 62 cases of osteosarcoma and found overexpression in 27 cases. In patients with overexpression of P-glycoprotein, higher tumor recurrence rates were found [86]. Others have also reported a higher relapse rate in these patients and found that there was benefit in adding additional chemotherapeutic agents [87]. Park *et al.* report a reduced survival time in patients with both mutant p53 and P-glycoprotein expression as compared to patients with wild-type p53 and without P-glycoprotein expression [85]. A meta-analysis of 14 studies on P-glycoprotein and osteosarcoma, demonstrates a correlation between immunohistochemistry for P-glycoprotein and osteosarcoma progression [88], but a recent Children's Oncology Group study failed to find an association between immunohistochemical expression of P-glycoprotein and outcome [89]. Heat shock protein 72 expression has been shown to predict a better response to induction chemotherapy in one study [90].

Survivin is a protein involved in the inhibition of apoptosis through binding of procaspases and is generally expressed in cancer but not normal tissue [91]. In a study of survivin, RNA was extracted from 16 paraffin-embedded osteosarcoma samples. Reduced survival time was noted for patients with high surviving levels (using the median as the cutoff between high and low) [92]. An inverse correlation has also been reported between survivin expression and

tumor differentiation [93]. One conflicting study by Trieb *et al.* reports increased survival with nuclear reactivity for survivin by immunohistochemistry [94].

VII. CONCLUSION

Our understanding of the molecular pathology of osteosarcoma continues to progress. The role of p53 and RB pathways are well established as are the contributions of a variety of oncogenes in the pathogenesis of this highly lethal neoplasm. The frontier is now moving toward a better understanding of tumor progression, metastasis, and therapeutic response for this tumor. We expect that as our knowledge of the basic molecular events involved in osteosarcoma development and progression increases, treatment modalities directed at these basic molecular pathways will be developed and further refined. These include, but are not limited to, gene therapy strategies [95].

References

1. A.K. Raymond, A.G. Ayala & S. Knuutila, Conventional osteosarcoma, in: C.D.M. Fletcher, K.K. Unni & F. Mertens (Eds.) Pathology and Genetics of Tumours of Soft Tissue and Bone, IARC Press, Lyon, 2002, pp. 264–270.
2. M.J. Klein & G.P. Siegal, Osteosarcoma: anatomic and histologic variants, Am J Clin Path 125 (2006) 555–581.
3. B.D. Ragland, W.C. Bell & R.R. Lopez, et al., Cytogenetics and molecular biology of osteosarcoma, Laboratory Investigation; a Journal of Technical Methods and Pathology 82 (2002) 365–373.
4. A.G. Knudson Jr., Mutation and cancer: statistical study of retinoblastoma, Proceedings of the National Academy of Sciences of the United States of America 68 (1971) 820–823.
5. A.G. Knudson Jr., H.W. Hethcote & B.W. Brown, Mutation and childhood cancer: a probabilistic model for the incidence of retinoblastoma, Proceedings of the National Academy of Sciences of the United States of America 72 (1975) 5116–5120.
6. D. Cobrinik, Pocket proteins and cell cycle control, Oncogene 24 (2005) 2796–2809.
7. F.D. Kitchin & R.M. Ellsworth, Pleiotropic effects of the gene for retinoblastoma, J Med Genet 11 (1974) 244–246.
8. M.F. Hansen, A. Koufos & B.L. Gallie, et al., Osteosarcoma and retinoblastoma: a shared chromosomal mechanism revealing recessive predisposition, Proceedings of the National Academy of Sciences of the United States of America 82 (1985) 6216–6220.
9. T.P. Dryja, J.M. Rapaport & J. Epstein, et al., Chromosome 13 homozygosity in osteosarcoma without retinoblastoma, A Hum Genet 38 (1986) 59–66.
10. H. Scheffer, Y.C. Kruize & J. Osinga, et al., Complete association of loss of heterozygosity of chromosomes 13 and 17 in osteosarcoma, Cancer Genet Cytogen 53 (1991) 45–55.
11. D.A. Belchis, C.A. Meece & F.A. Benko, et al., Loss of heterozygosity and microsatellite instability at the retinoblastoma locus in osteosarcomas, Diagn Mol Pathol 5 (1996) 214–219.

12. O. Feugeas, N. Guriec & A. Babin-Boilletot, et al., Loss of heterozygosity of the RB gene is a poor prognostic factor in patients with osteosarcoma, J Clin Oncol 14 (1996) 467–472.
13. B. Wadayama, J. Toguchida & T. Shimizu, et al., Mutation spectrum of the retinoblastoma gene in osteosarcomas, Cancer Res 54 (1994) 3042–3048.
14. M.S. Benassi, L. Molendini & G. Gamberi, et al., Alteration of pRb/p16/cdk4 regulation in human osteosarcoma, Int J Cancer 84 (1999) 489–493.
15. G. Wei, F. Lonardo & T. Ueda, et al., CDK4 gene amplification in osteosarcoma: reciprocal relationship with INK4A gene alterations and mapping of 12q13 amplicons, Int J Cancer 80 (1999) 199–204.
16. G.M. Maelandsmo, J.M. Berner & V.A. Florenes, et al., Homozygous deletion frequency and expression levels of the CDKN2 gene in human sarcomas—relationship to amplification and mRNA levels of CDK4 and CCND1, Brit J Cancer 72 (1995) 393–398.
17. T. Tsuchiya, K. Sekine & S. Hinohara, et al., Analysis of the p16INK4, p14ARF, p15, TP53, and MDM2 genes and their prognostic implications in osteosarcoma and Ewing sarcoma, Cancer Genet Cytogen 120 (2000) 91–98.
18. C.W. Miller, A. Aslo & M.J. Campbell, et al., Alterations of the p15, p16, and p18 genes in osteosarcoma, Cancer Genet Cytogen 86 (1996) 136–142.
19. C.W. Miller, C. Yeon & A. Aslo, et al., The p19INK4D cyclin dependent kinase inhibitor gene is altered in osteosarcoma, Oncogene 15 (1997) 231–235.
20. J. Mitra, C.Y. Dai & K. Somasundaram, et al., Induction of p21(WAF1/CIP1) and inhibition of Cdk2 mediated by the tumor suppressor p16(INK4a, Mol Cell Biol 19 (1999) 3916–3928.
21. W.S. el-Deiry, J.W. Harper & P.M. O'Connor, et al., WAF1/CIP1 is induced in p53-mediated G1 arrest and apoptosis, Cancer Res 54 (1994) 1169–1174.
22. W.S. el-Deiry, T. Tokino & V.E. Velculescu, et al., WAF1, a potential mediator of p53 tumor suppression, Cell 75 (1993) 817–825.
23. A.J. Levine, p53, the cellular gatekeeper for growth and division, Cell 88 (1997) 323–331.
24. F.P. Li, J.F. Fraumeni Jr. & J.J. Mulvihill, et al. A cancer family syndrome in twenty-four kindreds, Cancer Res 48 (1988) 5358–5362.
25. T. Jacks, L. Remington & B.O. Williams, et al., Tumor spectrum analysis in p53-mutant mice, Curr Biol 4 (1994) 1–7.
26. R. Siddiqui, K. Onel & F. Facio, et al., The TP53 mutational spectrum and frequency of CHEK2*1100delC in Li-Fraumeni-like kindreds, Familial Cancer 4 (2005) 177–181.
27. N. Gokgoz, J.S. Wunder & S. Mousses, et al., Comparison of p53 mutations in patients with localized osteosarcoma and metastatic osteosarcoma, Cancer 92 (2001) 2181–2189.
28. C.Y. Chen, J.D. Oliner & Q. Zhan, et al., Interactions between p53 and MDM2 in a mammalian cell cycle checkpoint pathway, Proceedings of the National Academy of Sciences of the United States of America 91 (1994) 2684–2688.
29. J.D. Oliner, J.A. Pietenpol & S. Thiagalingam, et al., Oncoprotein MDM2 conceals the activation domain of tumour suppressor p53, Nature 362 (1993) 857–860.
30. D.S. Haines, The mdm2 proto-oncogene, Leukemia Lymphoma 26 (1997) 227–238.
31. M. Berger, N. Stahl & G. Del Sal, et al., Mutations in proline 82 of p53 impair its activation by Pin1 and Chk2 in response to DNA damage, Mol Cell Biol 25 (2005) 5380–5388.
32. M. Ladanyi, C. Cha & R. Lewis, et al., MDM2 gene amplification in metastatic osteosarcoma, Cancer Res 53 (1993) 16–18.
33. F. Lonardo, T. Ueda & A.G. Huvos, et al., p53 and MDM2 alterations in osteosarcomas: correlation with clinicopathologic features and proliferative rate, Cancer 79 (1997) 1541–1547.
34. H.R. Park, W.W. Jung & F. Bertoni, et al., Molecular analysis of p53, MDM2 and H-ras genes in low-grade central osteosarcoma, Pathol Res Pract 200 (2004) 439–445.
35. P. Ragazzini, G. Gamberi & M.S. Benassi, et al., Analysis of SAS gene and CDK4 and MDM2 proteins in low-grade osteosarcoma, Cancer Detect Prev 23 (1999) 129–136.
36. R. Yokoyama, R. Schneider-Stock & K. Radig, et al., Clinicopathologic implications of MDM2, p53 and K-ras gene alterations in osteosarcomas: MDM2 amplification and p53 mutations found in progressive tumors, Pathol Res Pract 194 (1998) 615–621.
37. M.A. Lohrum, M. Ashcroft & M.H. Kubbutat, et al., Contribution of two independent MDM2-binding domains in p14(ARF) to p53 stabilization, Curr Biol 10 (2000) 539–542.
38. F.J. Stott, S. Bates & M.C. James, et al., The alternative product from the human CDKN2A locus, p14(ARF), participates in a regulatory feedback loop with p53 and MDM2, EMBO J 17 (1998) 5001–5014.
39. J.A. Lopez-Guerrero, C. Lopez-Gines & A. Pellin, et al., Deregulation of the G1 to S-phase cell cycle checkpoint is involved in the pathogenesis of human osteosarcoma, Diagn Mol Pathol 13 (2004) 81–91.
40. C.W. Miller, T. Ikezoe & U. Krug, et al., Mutations of the CHK2 gene are found in some osteosarcomas, but are rare in breast, lung, and ovarian tumors, Gene Chromosome Canc 33 (2002) 17–21.
41. M.A. Horstmann, M. Posl & R.B. Scholz, et al., Frequent reduction or loss of DCC gene expression in human osteosarcoma, Brit J Cancer 75 (1997) 1309–1317.
42. F. Pompetti, P. Rizzo & R.M. Simon, et al., Oncogene alterations in primary, recurrent, and metastatic human bone tumors, J Cell Biochem 63 (1996) 37–50.
43. M. Ladanyi, C.K. Park & R. Lewis, et al., Sporadic amplification of the MYC gene in human osteosarcomas, Diagn Mol Pathol 2 (1993) 163–167.
44. S. Ikeda, H. Sumii & K. Akiyama, et al., Amplification of both c-myc and c-raf-1 oncogenes in a human osteosarcoma, Jpn J Cancer Res 80 (1989) 6–9.
45. J.X. Wu, P.M. Carpenter & C. Gresens, et al., The proto-oncogene c-fos is over-expressed in the majority of human osteosarcomas, Oncogene 5 (1990) 989–1000.
46. B. Doganavsargil, M. Argin, & B. Kececi, et al. (2008). Secondary osteosarcoma arising in fibrous dysplasia, case report, Arch Orthop Trauma Surg June 17.
47. D.N. Jhala, I. Eltoum & A.J. Carroll, et al., Osteosarcoma in a patient with McCune-Albright syndrome and Mazabraud's syndrome: a case report emphasizing the cytological and cytogenetic findings, Hum Pathol 34 (2003) 1354–1357.
48. R. Lopez-Ben, M.J. Pitt & K.A. Jaffe, et al., Osteosarcoma in a patient with McCune-Albright syndrome and Mazabraud's syndrome, Skeletal Radiol 28 (1999) 522–526.

49. G.B. Witkin, W.B. Guilford & G.P. Siegal, Osteogenic sarcoma and soft tissue myxoma in a patient with fibrous dysplasia and hemoglobins, Clin Orthop Relat R 51 (1986) 245–252.

50. J.S. Weisstein, R.J. Majeska & M.J. Klein, et al., Detection of c-fos expression in benign and malignant musculoskeletal lesions, J Orthop Res 19 (2001) 339–345.

51. H. Zhou, R.L. Randall & A.R. Brothman, et al., Her-2/neu expression in osteosarcoma increases risk of lung metastasis and can be associated with gene amplification, J Pediatr Hematol Oncol 25 (2003) 27–32.

52. M. Onda, S. Matsuda & S. Higaki, et al., ErbB-2 expression is correlated with poor prognosis for patients with osteosarcoma, Cancer 77 (1996) 71–78.

53. R. Gorlick, A.G. Huvos & G. Heller, et al., Expression of HER2/erbB-2 correlates with survival in osteosarcoma, J Clin Oncol 17 (1999) 2781–2788.

54. J.Y. Tsai, H. Aviv & J. Benevenia, et al., HER-2/neu and p53 in osteosarcoma: an immunohistochemical and fluorescence in situ hybridization analysis, Cancer Invest 22 (2004) 16–24.

55. D.G. Thomas, T.J. Giordano & D. Sanders, et al., Absence of HER2/neu gene expression in osteosarcoma and skeletal Ewing's sarcoma, Clin Cancer Res 8 (2002) 788–793.

56. A. Maitra, D. Wanzer & A.G. Weinberg, et al., Amplification of the HER-2/neu oncogene is uncommon in pediatric osteosarcomas, Cancer 92 (2001) 677–683.

57. J.K. Anninga, M.J. van de Vijver & A.M. Cleton-Jansen, et al., Overexpression of the HER-2 oncogene does not play a role in high-grade osteosarcomas, Eur J Cancer 40 (2004) 963–970.

58. J. Fellenberg, A. Krauthoff & K. Pollandt, et al., Evaluation of the predictive value of Her-2/neu gene expression on osteosarcoma therapy in laser-microdissected paraffin-embedded tissue, Laboratory Investigation; a journal of technical methods and pathology 84 (2004) 113–121.

59. A.J. van Brabant, R. Stan & N.A. Ellis, DNA helicases, genomic instability, and human genetic disease, Annual Review of Genomics and Human Genetics 1 (2000) 409–459.

60. J.A. Harrigan & V.A. Bohr, Human diseases deficient in RecQ helicases, Biochimie 85 (2003) 1185–1193.

61. K. Hanada & I.D. Hickson, Molecular genetics of RecQ helicase disorders, Cell Mol Life Sci 64 (2007) 2306–2322.

62. A. Franchitto, RecQ helicases and topoisomerases: implications for genome stability in humans, Ital J Biochem 56 (2007) 115–121.

63. T. Enomoto, Functions of RecQ family helicases: possible involvement of Bloom's and Werner's syndrome gene products in guarding genome integrity during DNA replication, J Biochem 129 (2001) 501–507.

64. R. Rothstein & S. Gangloff, Hyper-recombination and Bloom's syndrome: microbes again provide clues about cancer, Genome Res 5 (1995) 421–426.

65. N.A. Ellis & J. German, Molecular genetics of Bloom's syndrome, Hum Mol Gen 5 (Spec No) (1996) 1457–1463.

66. J.K. Karow, R.K. Chakraverty & I.D. Hickson, The Bloom's syndrome gene product is a 3′-5′ DNA helicase, J Biol Chem 272 (1997) 30611–30614.

67. C.J. Epstein & A.G. Motulsky, Werner syndrome: entering the helicase era, Bioessays 18 (1996) 1025–1027.

68. M.D. Gray, J.C. Shen & A.S. Kamath-Loeb, et al., The Werner syndrome protein is a DNA helicase, Nature Genet 17 (1997) 100–103.

69. L. Crabbe, A. Jauch & C.M. Naeger, et al., Telomere dysfunction as a cause of genomic instability in Werner syndrome, Proceedings of the National Academy of Sciences of the United States of America 104 (2007) 2205–2210.

70. J.M. Sidorova, Roles of the Werner syndrome RecQ helicase in DNA replication, DNA repair 7 (2008) 1776–1786.

71. N.M. Lindor, Y. Furuichi & S. Kitao, et al., Rothmund-Thomson syndrome due to RECQ4 helicase mutations: report and clinical and molecular comparisons with Bloom syndrome and Werner syndrome, Am J Med Genet 90 (2000) 223–228.

72. L. Larizza, I. Magnani & G. Roversi, Rothmund-Thomson syndrome and RECQL4 defect: splitting and lumping, Cancer Letters 232 (2006) 107–120.

73. L. Van Maldergem, H.A. Siitonen & N. Jalkh, et al., Revisiting the craniosynostosis-radial ray hypoplasia association: Baller-Gerold syndrome caused by mutations in the RECQL4 gene, J Med Genet 43 (2006) 148–152.

74. T. Dietschy, I. Shevelev & I. Stagljar, The molecular role of the Rothmund-Thomson-, RAPADILINO- and Baller-Gerold-gene product, RECQL4: recent progress, Cell Mol Life Sci 64 (2007) 796–802.

75. K.W. Hunter, Ezrin, a key component in tumor metastasis, Trends Mol Med 10 (2004) 201–204.

76. M. Curto & A.I. McClatchey, Ezrin…a metastatic detERMinant?, Cancer Cell 5 (2004) 113–114.

77. C. Khanna, J. Khan & P. Nguyen, et al., Metastasis-associated differences in gene expression in a murine model of osteosarcoma, Cancer Res 61 (2001) 3750–3759.

78. C. Khanna, X. Wan & S. Bose, et al., The membrane-cytoskeleton linker ezrin is necessary for osteosarcoma metastasis, Nat Med 10 (2004) 182–186.

79. H.R. Park, W.W. Jung & P. Bacchini, et al., Ezrin in osteosarcoma: comparison between conventional high-grade and central low-grade osteosarcoma, Pathol Res Pract 202 (2006) 509–515.

80. W. Ogino, Y. Takeshima & T. Mori, et al., High level of ezrin mRNA expression in an osteosarcoma biopsy sample with lung metastasis, J Pediatr Hematol Oncol 29 (2007) 435–439.

81. S. Ferrari, L. Zanella & M. Alberghini, et al., Prognostic significance of immunohistochemical expression of ezrin in non-metastatic high-grade osteosarcoma, Pediatr Blood Cancer 50 (2008) 752–756.

82. J.M. Gillette, D.C. Chan & S.M. Nielsen-Preiss, Annexin 2 expression is reduced in human osteosarcoma metastases, J Cell Biochem 92 (2004) 820–832.

83. C. Laverdiere, B.H. Hoang & R. Yang, et al., Messenger RNA expression levels of CXCR4 correlate with metastatic behavior and outcome in patients with osteosarcoma, Clin Cancer Res 11 (2005) 2561–2567.

84. E. Perissinotto, G. Cavalloni & F. Leone, et al., Involvement of chemokine receptor 4/stromal cell-derived factor 1 system during osteosarcoma tumor progression, Clin Cancer Res 11 (2005) 490–497.

85. Y.B. Park, H.S. Kim & J.H. Oh, et al., The co-expression of p53 protein and P-glycoprotein is correlated to a poor prognosis in osteosarcoma, Int Orthop 24 (2001) 307–310.

86. H.S. Chan, T.M. Grogan & G. Haddad, et al., P-glycoprotein expression: critical determinant in the response to osteosarcoma chemotherapy, J Natl Cancer I 89 (1997) 1706–1715.

87. N. Baldini, K. Scotlandi & M. Serra, et al., P-glycoprotein expression in osteosarcoma: a basis for risk-adapted adjuvant chemotherapy, J Orthop Res 17 (1999) 629–632.

88. E.E. Pakos & J.P. Ioannidis, The association of P-glycoprotein with response to chemotherapy and clinical outcome in patients with osteosarcoma. A meta-analysis, Cancer 98 (2003) 581–589.

89. C.L. Schwartz, R. Gorlick & L. Teot, et al., Multiple drug resistance in osteogenic sarcoma: INT0133 from the Children's Oncology Group, J Clin Oncol 25 (2007) 2057–2062.

90. K. Trieb, T. Lechleitner & S. Lang, et al., Heat shock protein 72 expression in osteosarcomas correlates with good response to neoadjuvant chemotherapy, Hum Pathol 29 (1998) 1050–1055.

91. S.K. Chiou, M.K. Jones & A.S. Tarnawski, Surviving an anti-apoptosis protein: its biological roles and implications for cancer and beyond, Med Sci Monit 9 (2003) PI25–PI29.

92. E. Osaka, T. Suzuki & S. Osaka, et al., Survivin expression levels as independent predictors of survival for osteosarcoma patients, J Orthop Res 25 (2007) 116–121.

93. W. Wang, H. Luo & A. Wang, Expression of survivin and correlation with PCNA in osteosarcoma, J Surg Oncol 93 (2006) 578–584.

94. K. Trieb, R. Lehner & T. Stulnig, et al., Survivin expression in human osteosarcoma is a marker for survival, Eur J Surg Oncol 29 (2003) 379–382.

95. B.F. Smith, D.T. Curiel & V.V. Ternovoi, et al., Administration of a conditionally replicative oncolytic canine adenovirus in normal dogs, Cancer Biother Radio 21 (2006) 601–606.

Section IV. Histopathology of Primary Bone Tumors and Bone Metastases

CHAPTER **17**

Technical Aspects: How Do We Best Prepare Bone Samples for Proper Histological Analysis?

DANIEL CHAPPARD[1]

[1]INSERM, U922–LHEA, Faculté de Médecine, 49045 Angers Cédex, France.

Contents

I. INTRODUCTION

Histological analysis of bone is a critical step for the diagnosis of malignancies. It allows a direct identification of malignant cells inside marrow spaces in the case of bone metastases or hematological disorders. Bone biopsy is superior to marrow aspiration because the microarchitecture of the bone marrow is preserved, a parameter that is especially important in hematological disorders. Because marrow cells are in direct contact with bone cells (lining cells, osteoblasts, osteoclasts and their precursors) an abnormal bone remodeling rate has been described in a variety of malignant cell proliferations when developing and expanding inside marrow spaces. Bone cells elaborate and synthesize a variety of cytokines acting on hematological precursors (e.g., M-CSF) [1] and malignant cells release other cytokines active on bone remodeling [2–4]: it is likely that bone changes are almost always associated with bone marrow alterations and vice versa. Histomorphometric analysis is a powerful tool in the evaluation of bone remodeling in metabolic bone diseases and has also been successfully applied to hematological disorders and metastases from solid tumors [5,6]. Bone histomorphometry is a powerful method in the early diagnosis of B-cell malignancies and smoldering myeloma or

lymphomas can be characterized in patients with a monoclonal gammopathy of undetermined significance (MGUS) several years before the tumor has a clinical expression. Bone histomorphometry is also useful in animal models of cancer bone lesions since it permits a precise evaluation of the bone remodeling changes induced by tumor cells [7–9]. However, bone histomorphometry must be done on undecalcified bone sections which allow a perfect identification of osteoid tissue (the unmineralized bone matrix recently synthesized by osteoblasts), a precise identification of osteoclasts (by using histoenzymatic detection) and histodynamic analyses (after a double tetracycline labeling in humans or using a variety of other fluorochromes in animals). These methods cannot be done on decalcified and paraffin embedded bone since decalcification abolishes the osteoid/bone matrix differential staining, removes the fluorochrome labels and hot paraffin embedding destroys enzyme activities. However, decalcification and paraffin remains useful for immunohistochemistry which is difficult and hazardous on plastic sections. The main disadvantage of polymer embedding was formerly the prolonged time for preparing bone specimens (several months were needed when polyester resins were used). With the development of histological techniques, it is now possible to have polymer embedding methods which are as fast as conventional paraffin methods. The following techniques have been developed and improved in our laboratory during the last two decades and used on more than 3000 human bone biopsies and a large number of animal studies performed in a variety of animal species (mouse, rat, chicken, dog, goat, sheep, pig).

II. BONE BIOPSY IN HUMANS (OR LARGE ANIMALS)

As recommended since the 1970s, bone trephines with a large inner diameter must be used: a 7 mm trephine is necessary to preserve bone microarchitecture and to analyze a representative amount of marrow spaces. We have proposed several modifications concerning ergonomics of the Meunier's trephine making it easier to handle and providing better preserved bone cores [10]. The trephine developed in our laboratory is proposed by Commeca (Commeca, Beaucouzé-Angers, France) (website at http://www.commeca.com/anglais/cadresoma.html). Bone biopsy in human patients is painless when done with a double cortical anesthesia. The technique (including video) is described elsewhere (http://www.med.univ-angers.fr/discipline/lab_histo/bone_biopsy.htm).

III. BONE FIXATION

Classically the collagenous bone matrix is said to be better preserved in a 70° ethanol fixative. However, it induces marked cell shrinkage incompatible with cytological examination. Formalin fixation provides very good cell preservation but induces poor staining of the collagen when using a trichrome method. The combination of both ethanol and formalin was proposed by Beebe and works perfectly well [11]. The formula known as BB's fluid is:

• 95° ethanol—900 ml
• 37–40% formaldehyde—100 ml
• Deionized water—150 ml

Bone biopsies are fixed for 24 hours at 4°C in a refrigerator. Then the fixative is discarded and replaced by acetone. BB's allows the preservation of bone cell enzymes and retains the staining properties of collagen. Fixation in the cold (4–8°C in a refrigerator) improves quality. After 24 hours, the fixative is discarded and replaced either by acetone or by the fast dehydrating fluid as above.

IV. MICROCOMPUTED TOMOGRAPHY (MICROCT)

MicroCT is a new microscopic technique developed over the last few decades [12,13]. It is a miniaturized version of computed tomographs commonly used by radiologists and the system now has a resolution in the order of 2 μm. MicroCT is based on a sealed microfocus X-ray source, a CDD camera and a step-by-step platform which receives the bone samples. Bone biopsies or animal bones can be analyzed when still in the fixative. They are transferred into an Eppendorf test tube filled with polyester fibers impregnated with the fixative (which are radiolucent and immobilize the samples). MicroCT scans are obtained within an hour; reconstruction of images, 3D model building and morphometry are done within 2 hours in human or animal samples [6,14]. Examples of microCT images appear on Figure 17.1A, B. They are useful as an early diagnostic method since sclerotic and osteolytic changes can be identified rapidly.

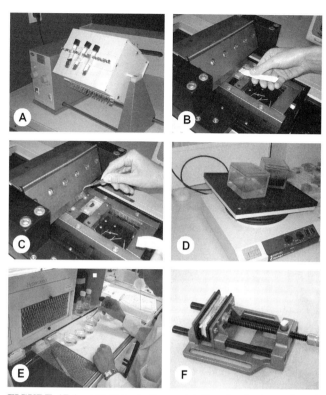

FIGURE 17.1 (A) Dehydration and infiltration in the activated MMA medium are considerably shortened when bone samples are placed in screw-capped vials under constant agitation; (B) sectioning on a Polycut S microtome: a strip of moistened paper is used to facilitate sectioning and avoid rolling of the section; (C) thin sections are picked up with forceps; (D) sections are stained by free floating in the staining solutions under constant agitation on a 'rock and roller'; (E) stained sections are dehydrated in several bathes of 2-propanol and Histolemon® before mounting; (F) mounted sections are gently pressed to reduce the minifolds of the polymer sections.

V. DEHYDRATION AND INFILTRATION

A rapid dehydration and defatting procedure is done by combining acetone and xylene at the same time [11]. Acetone is preferred to ethanol since it does not inactivate bone cell activities. We found that using a rotative device (running at a low speed) considerably shortens the dehydration time (Figure 17.2A). Bone biopsies are transferred in screw-capped test tubes that allow complete infiltration. Dehydration and defatting is accomplished during 3 hours in three consecutive baths (1 hour each). A final bath in pure xylene (1 hour) will ensure complete clearing.

VI. BONE EMBEDDING

Formerly, bones were embedded in polyester resins. Araldite and epoxies have also been proposed. However, the high viscosity of these monomers necessitates prolonged

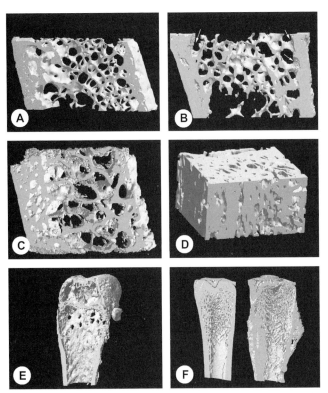

FIGURE 17.2   (A) MicroCT of a control bone biopsy, note the two cortices and the regularity of the 3D network of trabecular bone; (B) microCT of a bone biopsy from a patient with multiple myeloma, note the focal disappearance of trabecular bone due to massive osteolysis and the eroded endosteal surfaces with deep resorption pits (arrows); (C) microCT of a bone biopsy from a patient with an osteosclerotic metastasis due to a prostatic adeno-carcinoma. The trabeculae are covered by thin trabeculae of meta-plastic bone; (D) microCT of a bone biopsy from a patient with a sclerosing myeloma. Note that almost all marrow spaces have dis-appeared; (E) microCT of a mouse with an end-stage myeloma (5T2 model in the C57BL/KaLwRij mouse). Trabecular bone has completely disappeared and cortical perforations are evidenced; (F) microCT of a femur from a control rat (left) and from a rat with osteosclerotic metastases due to Mat-Ly-Lu carcinoma (right). Note the osteosclerotic foci in the primary and secondary spongiosa and under the periosteum.

infiltration times (more than 3 weeks, a time that is not compatible with routine diagnosis in cancer patients). Methylmethacrylate (MMA)-based embedding fluids are now favored because the monomer has the same viscosity as water and diffuses rapidly inside the bony tissues. However, a number of mistakes and handling errors are common in laboratories when working with MMA (and its polymerized form pMMA) and the following simple rules can be recommended.

A. Purification of MMA

Purification of commercial MMA is always necessary when reliable results are needed. The monomer always contains a polymerization inhibitor (usually hydroquinone or 4-methoxyphenol) added by the manufacturers to avoid auto-polymerization. Several methods are available but the simplest consists of using several washes in 1M NaOH as follows [15]: one liter of crude MMA is mixed with 500 ml of 1M NaOH in water by using a separator funnel. The mixture is shaken vigorously for 2 min and then allowed to separate. Because MMA is hydrophobic, two phases sepa-rate: the lower phase contains water, NaOH and brownish oxidized phenolates; the upper is MMA with residual water droplets in suspension. The lower phase is withdrawn and replaced by 500 ml of fresh NaOH and shaken as above. This lower phase is then discarded and replaced by deion-ized water, shaken and the aqueous phase is discarded once more. At that time, the MMA phase is cloudy (due to remaining water droplets in suspension); it is transferred into a screw capped bottle and placed in a freezer at −20°C. By the following day, ice crystals will have formed and are separated from MMA by vacuum filtration using a Büchner funnel with a Whatman no. 3 filtration paper. MMA free of inhibitor is stored at −20°C in screw capped bottles until use.

B. Preparation of the Accelerated MMA Medium for Infiltration and Embedding

The embedding medium is prepared by mixing 12 g of ben-zoyl peroxide BPO with purified MMA 1000 ml using a magnetic stirrer. Since BPO is explosive when dry, it is always stabilized with large amounts of water. These traces of water are eliminated by refreezing at −20°C and elimina-tion of ice crystals by a new vacuum filtration [15]. A plasti-cizer (usually dibutylphthalate) is then added (100 ml for 900 ml of activated MMA) and the infiltration medium is then stored at −20°C to avoid BPO decomposition. An initi-ating mixture (to induce redox polymerization) is prepared by mixing 2 ml of the tertiary amine (N-N-dimethylaniline) with 18 ml of 2-propanol. This initiating solution is kept at +4°C in a refrigerator.

C. Fast Infiltration and Embedding Method

We found that a gentle constant agitation also considerably shortened the infiltration time. The test tubes containing the bone samples (dehydrated and cleared as above) are then filled with 10 ml of the accelerated MMA mixture and placed on the rotative machine for 1 hour. The mixture is then changed and left rotating for an additional hour at room temperature. A third and final bath is then prepared by using an accelerated and initiated MMA bath:

• Accelerated MMA mixture—25 ml
• Initiating solution—400 μl

It is recommended that Gilson Pipetman® with dispos-able polyethylene tips is used for handling MMA and initi-ating mixtures.

The bone samples immersed in the accelerated and initiated MMA are then stored in a freezer at $-20°C$ overnight. This ensures a complete and uniform diffusion of all components inside bone.

D. Embedding

Former authors used embedding in glass vials, a dangerous method since block retrieval necessitates breaking the vial with a hammer. We have found that polyethylene molds (Peel-a-Way® embedding system, Polyscience Inc., Warrington, PA) constitute a well-adapted disposable system. A strip of polyester sponge or a piece of polyester wadding (used in aquarium or kitchen hood filters) is placed at the bottom of the mold to avoid the interface-linked shrinkage during polymerization [16,17]. Air contact is prevented by placing a thin film of Parafilm® (Alcan, Packaging, Neenah, WI) since atmospheric oxygen is a strong polymerization inhibitor [18]. The Peel-a-Way® molds are placed in a water bath at 4°C for 24 hours and polymerization slowly proceeds in the cold. Decomposition of BPO by N-N-dimethylanilin is an exponential function of the temperature (Arrhenius' law): at $-20°C$, polymerization is inhibited (but infiltration is favored); when the temperature is raised at $+4°C$, the redox polymerization starts [19]. The water bath is used to limit the exothermic peak associated with MMA polymerization. This preserves enzyme activities (e.g., tartrate resistant, acid phosphatase—TRAcP). Embedding and polymerization under vacuum is senseless since this increases MMA evaporation, and increases the number of holes inside objects (note that the polymerization defects often referred to by technicians are not gas bubbles but holes created by the shrinkage of the embedding mass during polymerization) [17].

E. Sectioning

Sections are cut at 7 pm using a heavy duty microtome (e.g., Leica, Polycut-S) equipped with 50–60° tungsten carbide knives for histomorphometry. Sections 14 μm in thickness are used for tetracycline (or calcein) histodynamic studies. Flat sections can be obtained with a strip of paper and a forceps (Figure 17.2B and C).

VII. STAINING METHODS

A. Osteoid Tissue and Calcified Bone

Masson, Mallory or Goldner's trichrome are favored for the identification of osteoid/mineralized matrix. However, classical procedures stain osteoid and marrow cells with the same red intensity, making osteoid difficult to analyze accurately. We have designed a special trichromic method which considerably improves the differentiation of osteoid from the bone narrow [20]. Sections are stained by free floating in glass vials containing the staining solutions. A 'rock-and-roller' device allows homogeneous staining and

avoids sections staying in contact with the sides of the vial (Figure 17.2D).

- Stain for 30 min in a saturated picric acid solution (1.2 g in 100 ml of water)
- Wash 30 sec in deionized water
- Stain for 15 min in Meyer's hematoxylin (Merck)
- Rinse in deionized water, bluish in a saturated lithium carbonate aqueous solution (5 g in 1000 ml of water), rinse in deionized water
- Stain for 15 min in the following solution:
    Acid fushine—0.1 g
    Xylidine ponceau—0.4 g
    Deionized water—100 ml
    Glacial acetic acid—1 ml
- Wash in 1% acetic acid for 30 sec
- Differentiate for 1 min in:
    Orange G—1 g
    Deionized water—100 ml
    Phosphomolybdic acid—1.5 g
- Do not wash, counterstain in the following solution:
    Fast green FCF—0.1 g
    Deionized water—200 ml
    Glacial acetic acid—1 ml
- Rinse in 1% acetic acid
- Dehydrate in 2-propanol (2-propanol is a dehydrating solvent that has no effect on pMMA sections; on the contrary mixture of water-ethanol can soften the sections considerably)
- Transfer into three successive baths of methylcyclohexane or Histolemon® (these compounds are non-solvent for pMMA) (Figure 17.2E)
- Mount in a synthetic medium (e.g., Neo Entellan®, Merck)
- Flatten sections by compression between two wood pieces for 12 hours (Figure 17.2F)

The use of picric acid considerably enhances the red staining of osteoid tissue and reduces marrow cell staining; nuclei are faintly stained (Figure 17.3; see Plate 6). Other old methods for the identification of osteoid on undecalcified sections are not described: Von Kossà is known to be less precise than trichromes and is not specific for calcium [21]. Solochrome cyanin has poor lightfastness.

B. Argentophilic Proteins (AgNOR Method)

Argentophilic proteins are found in the nucleoli of all cells (nucleolin, RNA polymerase I, protein B23) where they constitute the Nucleolar Organizing Regions (NOR). We found that osteopontin, a non-collagenic protein of the bone matrix rich in Asp residues, was also stainable by the AgNOR method [23,24]. The following technique can be recommended. Undecalcified sections need to be decalcified for 1 hour in 10% aqueous formic acid before staining to avoid substitution of calcium (of the bone matrix) by silver atoms. Sections are incubated for 55 min at room

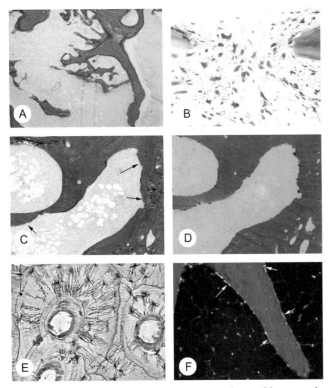

FIGURE 17.3 (A) Bone biopsy in a patient with prostatic adenocarcinoma. The bone marrow is completely invaded by the tumor but cells are lightly stained. On the contrary, osteoid is well demonstrated in red and calcified bone matrix in green. Note the extended bone metaplasia. Modified Goldner's trichrome. Original magnification ×100; (B) TRAcP stained cells in the bone marrow of a patient with metastatic breast cancer. Note the considerable osteoclastogenesis occurring in the tumor stroma with numerous osteoclasts. Original magnification ×200; (C) bone biopsy from a patient with multiple myeloma with extended eroded surfaces (arrowed). Modified Goldner's trichrome. Original magnification ×100; (D) paired section of the same case with histoenzymatic identification of osteoclasts by their TRAcP content; (E) argentophilic proteins (osteopontin) in the resting lines, osteocytes lacunae and canaliculi and NORs of the nuclei. Modified AgNOR method. Original magnification ×100; (F) nuclei of living cells stained with Hoechst 33342 (brilliant green) and bone matrix counterstained in red. Lining cells are arrowed. Fluorescence microscopy. Original magnification ×100.

temperature in the dark, in a staining solution prepared by combining silver nitrate (2 volumes of 50% aqueous solution) with formic acid (1 volume of a 1% solution containing 2% gelatin). After staining, sections are thoroughly washed in deionized water and transferred for 10 min to a 5% aqueous sodium thiosulfate solution prepared extemporaneously. Sections are then rinsed with deionized water dehydrated and mounted as above.

AgNORs appear as black dots in the nucleoli of all cells. The reaction is clearly evidenced in marrow, cancer and bone cells and the number of NORs is known to be increased in cancer cells [25]. On bone sections, dense strips of

argentophilic material are found around the osteocytes and canaliculi and at the periphery of their lacunae (Figure 17.3E Plate 6E). The delicate inter-osteocyte relationships are clearly evidenced. Linear deposits are also observed in the matrix and corresponded to the cement and resting lines.

C. Histoenzymatic Identification of Osteoclast by TRAcP Staining

TRAcP is a thermo-sensitive enzyme which is also destroyed by prolonged fixation in formalin or alcohol. The above-mentioned procedures for fixation and embedding ensure a perfect preservation of TRAcP activity in osteoclasts [15,26]. The following procedure is well adapted to histomorphometry because the naphthol phosphate used tends to provide a homogeneous staining of the osteoclast cytoplasm [27]. Substituted naphthols (AS-BI, AS-TR) can be used but they provide a more precise localization of the enzyme inside intracytoplasmic lysozomes, making identification of osteoclast more difficult at low magnification (Figure 17.3B and D; Plate 6B and D). The staining method is a follows:

Prepare an acetate buffer by mixing:
Sodium acetate, 3H$_2$O—19 g
Glacial acetic acid—4.5 ml
Deionized water—1000 ml
Sodium tartrate—150 mg
- Prepare solution A which is the enzyme substrate:
α-naphthyl phosphate, Na salt—100 mg
Acetate buffer, pH 5—100 ml
- Prepare solution B which contains the dye:
Fast violet B salt—250 mg
Acetate buffer, pH 5—50 ml
- Mix both solutions and filter immediately
- Incubate freshly prepared bone sections by free floating at 37°C for 60 to 90 min
- Rinse in deionized water
- Inactivate the remaining enzymatic molecule by incubation for 60 min in:
Sodium fluoride—4.2 g
Deionized water—1000 ml
- Rinse in deionized water
- Counterstain for 20 min in:
Anilin blue WS—66 mg
Phosphotungstic acid—2 g
Deionized water—200 ml
- Rinse in deionized water and mount in Apathy's syrup.

Because the condensation product between the naphthol and the diazonium is soluble in water, sections must be mounted in an aqueous medium. Synthetic media often contain alcoholic groups or other functions that destroy the colored precipitate. Currently, the best known medium is Apathy's syrup prepared in large quantities using centrifugation to eliminate minute residual air bubbles [28], as follows. Briefly, powder of arabic gum (500 g) and saccharose (500 g) are placed in a bottle containing deionized water (500 ml) and a large thymol crystal. The bottle is then closed with a screwed plug and transferred in a drying oven at 65°C for 48 hours. It is regularly agitated every 4–6 hour period. A viscous brown syrup is obtained and distributed into 25 ml centrifuge tubes. The tubes (containing hot syrup) are then centrifuged at 2000 rpm for 30 min. The very fine residual layer of bubbles which persists at the end of the centrifugation is then eliminated with a spatula. The syrup is then distributed into 20 ml syringes. This syrup can be preserved for more than 1 year in the refrigerator.

D. Mast Cell Identification in Mastocytosis

Mast cells contain granules rich in sulfated GAG (such as heparane sulfate), histamine, cytokines and proteases (tryptase). The sulfated GAGs confer metachromasia to the mast cell granules. In systemic mastocytosis, these cells are increased in number; they can form nodules in the bone marrow and can adhere to osteoblast or lining cells at the surface of bone trabeculae. Because mast cells can contain a few granules in some types of mastocytosis, a sharp contrast is obtained using the following method:

- Stain section by free floating for 15 min in:
  Toluidine blue—0.5 g
  Deionized water—100 ml
  Glacial acetic acid—1 ml
- Rinse in 1% acetic acid until no more blue stain is extracted from the sections
- Dehydrate in 2-propanol and mount as above.

Granules of mast cells appear deep violet and the tint of the cell depends on the number of cytoplasmic granules.

E. Living Osteocytes in the Bone Matrix

Osteocytes are mechanosensitive cells responsible for maintaining bone trophicity. These cells can disappear inside their lacunae and it is thought that bone packets devoid of osteocytes can be removed by osteoclasts. Living osteocytes can by detected inside the bone matrix by using a highly fluorescent nuclear stain associated with a fluorescent counterstain for the bone matrix. The following method works remarkably well.

Stain nuclei during 30 min with Hoescht 33342 prepared as follows:

- Hoescht 33342—2 mg
- Deionized water—1000 ml
- Rinse in deionized water

  Counterstain during 10 min in:

- Nuclear yellow fast R—1 g
- Formalin—100 ml
- Phosphotungstic acid—1 g
- Rinse in deionized water and mount in Apathy's syrup.

Hoescht 33342 has been used widely as a fluorescent dye for staining the nuclei of living cells. It preferentially binds to AT regions of DNA and shows no cytoplasmic staining. Observations and measurements are made under UV fluorescence microscopy with a WU near-ultraviolet fluorescence cube. Osteocytes appear as intensely stained green spots (and only intact nuclei are stained) on a red-stained background corresponding to the calcified bone matrix. Nuclei of bone marrow cells, endothelium and lining cells are also stained.

These staining methods have been developed over the last few decades. The success of many of them depends on the use and quality of the pMMA embedding in the cold. The use of pMMA as an embedding medium allows identification of a large number of details or structures that cannot be identified on decalcified and paraffin embedded bones. However, immunohistochemical studies are difficult and only a few reports have been presented. Undecalcified embedding methods have provided a number of clinically and scientifically reliable reports and have considerably changed the evaluation of benign and malignant bone diseases.

Acknowledgements

The author is indebted to Mrs Nadine Gaborit, Florence Pascaretti, Guénaëlle Brossard and Christine Gaudin for their help in everyday histotechnological assistance.

References

1. M. Karst, G. Gorny & R.J. Galvin, et al., Roles of stromal cell RANKL, OPG, and M-CSF expression in biphasic TGF-beta regulation of osteoclast differentiation, J Cell Physiol 200 (2004) 99–106.
2. R. Bataille, New insights in the clinical biology of multiple myeloma, Semin Hematol 34 (1997) 23–28.
3. T.A. Guise & J.M. Chirgwin, Transforming growth factor-beta in osteolytic breast cancer bone metastases, Clin Orthop Relat Res 415 S (2003) 32–38.
4. T.A. Guise & G.R. Mundy, Cancer and bone, Endocr Rev 19 (1998) 18–54.
5. C. Marcelli, D. Chappard & J.F. Rossi, et al., Histologic evidence of an abnormal bone remodeling in B-cell malignancies other than multiple myeloma, Cancer 62 (1988) 1163–1170.
6. A. Schmidt, O. Blanchet & M. Dib, et al., Bone changes in myelofibrosis with myeloid metaplasia: a histomorphometric and microcomputed tomographic study, Eur J Haematol 78 (2007) 500–509.
7. R. Bataille, D. Chappard & M. Baslé, Excessive bone resorption in human plasmacytomas: direct induction by tumour cells *in vivo*, Br J Haematol 90 (1995) 721–724.
8. R. Bataille, D. Chappard & M. Baslé, Quantifiable excess of bone resorption in monoclonal gammopathy is an early symptom of malignancy: a prospective study of 87 bone biopsies, Blood 87 (1996) 4762–4769.
9. R. Bataille, D. Chappard & C. Marcelli, et al., Mechanisms of bone destruction in multiple myeloma: the importance of an

unbalanced process in determining the severity of lytic bone disease, J Clin Oncol 7 (1989) 1909–1914.

10. D. Chappard, C. Alexandre, G. Bousquet & G. Riffat, New modifications of Bordier's trocar for quantitative bone biopsy, Rev Rhum Mal Osteoartic 50 (1983) 307–308.

11. K. Beebe, Alcohol/xylene: the unlikely fixative/dehydrant/clearant, J Histotechnol 23 (2000) 45–50.

12. R. Muller, H. Van Campenhout & B. Van Damme, et al., Morphometric analysis of human bone biopsies: a quantitative structural comparison of histological sections and micro-computed tomography, Bone 23 (1998) 59–66.

13. A. Sasov & D. Van Dyck, Desktop X-ray microscopy and microtomography, J Microsc 191 (1998) 151–158.

14. H. Libouban, M.F. Moreau & M. Lesourd, et al., Osteolytic bone lesions in the 5T2 multiple myeloma model: radiographic, scanning electron microscopic and microtomographic studies, J Histotechnol 24 (2001) 81–86.

15. D. Chappard, S. Palle & C. Alexandre, et al., Bone embedding in pure methyl methacrylate at low temperature preserves enzyme activities, Acta Histochem 81 (1987) 183–190.

16. D. Chappard, C. Alexandre & S. Palle, et al., Polyester wadding for specimen orientation during embedding in methacrylates, Stain Technol 61 (1986) 93–96.

17. D. Chappard, C. Alexandre & J.P. Monthéard, Polymerization of methacrylates, The 'bubble-hole' artefact reconsidered with a bone morphometric approach, J Histotechnol 15 (1992) 51–55.

18. D. Chappard, F. Vocanson & J.P. Monthéard, Polymerization of methacrylates used as histological embedding mediums: local variations and time course of hardness of methylmethacrylate blocks, J Histotechnol 16 (1993) 65–68.

19. D. Chappard, C. Alexandre & M. Camps, et al., Embedding iliac bone biopsies at low temperature using glycol and methyl methacrylates, Stain Technol 58 (1983) 299–308.

20. D. Chappard, S. Palle & C. Alexandre, et al., Simultaneous identification of calcified cartilage, bone and osteoid tissue on plastic sections. New polychrome procedures specially adapted to image analysor systems, J Histotechnol 9 (1986) 95–97.

21. L.F. Bonewald, S.E. Harris & J. Rosser, et al., von Kossa staining alone is not sufficient to confirm that mineralization *in vitro* represents bone formation, Calcif Tissue Int 72 (2003) 537–547.

22. A.J. Chaplin & S.R. Grace, Calcium oxalate and the von Kossa method with reference to the influence of citric acid, Histochem J 7 (1975) 451–458.

23. C. Gaudin-Audrain, Y. Gallois & F. Pascaretti-Grizon, et al., Osteopontin is histochemically detected by the AgNOR acid-silver staining, Histol Histopathol 23 (2008) 469–478.

24. F. Pascaretti-Grizon, C. Gaudin-Audrain & Y. Gallois, et al., Osteopontin is an argentophilic protein in the bone matrix and in cells of kidney convoluted tubules, Morphologie 91 (2007) 180–185.

25. D. Chappard, N. Retailleau/Gaborit & R. Filmon, et al., Increased nucleolar organizer regions in osteoclast nuclei of Paget's bone disease, Bone 22 (1998) 45–49.

26. D. Chappard, C. Alexandre & G. Riffat, Histochemical identification of osteoclasts. Review of current methods and reappraisal of a simple procedure for routine diagnosis on undecalcified human iliac bone biopsies, Basic Appl Histochem 27 (1983) 75–85.

27. D. Chappard, Osteoclast count on human bone biopsies: why and how?, in: H.E. Takahashi (Ed.), Bone Morphometry, Nishimura-Smith-Gordon, 1990, pp. 248–255.

28. D. Chappard, N. Gaborit-Retailleau & J.P. Monthéard, et al., Photopolymerized 2-hydroxyethylmethacrylate as a mounting medium preserving immunocytochemical reaction and nuclear counterstain, Biotech Histochem 74 (1999) 135–140.

CHAPTER **18**

Osteoclast-rich Lesions of Bone: A Clinical and Molecular Overview

ADRIENNE M. FLANAGAN[1,2,3], ROBERTO TIRABOSCO[2] AND PANAGIOTIS D. GIKAS[4]

[1]Institute of Orthopaedics, University College, London.
[2]Department of Histopathology, Royal National Orthopaedic Hospital, Stanmore, Middlesex, UK.
[3]Cancer Institute, University College, London, UK.
[4]Bone Tumour unit, Royal National Orthopaedic Hospital, Stanmore, Middlesex, UK.

Contents

I. INTRODUCTION

Osteoclast-rich lesions of bone represent morphologically similar entities which behave in a clinically distinct manner. Unlike many other primary bone tumors the lesional cells are not primarily bone- or cartilage-forming. Nevertheless, metaplastic/reactive bone can be found, especially at the periphery of the lesions. Common to all osteoclast-rich lesions is the presence of innumerable osteoclast-like giant cells, which are capable of resorbing bone, uniformly distributed or arranged in clusters among oval to spindle shaped mononuclear cells. Although there are some specific morphological features associated with particular osteoclast-rich lesions, the key to distinguishing the various entities from one another is their distinctive clinical and radiographic characteristics. The pathogenesis by which this group of lesions develops is diverse and includes inherited germline mutations (cherubism, Noonan syndrome and at least some non-ossifying fibromas), neoplasia (giant cell tumor of bone, aneurysmal bone cysts and tenosynovial giant cell tumors/pigmented villonodular synovitis) and metabolic disorders (hyperparathyroidism). Advances in identifying the genetic abnormalities associated with some of these lesions not only allow the provision of robust tissue diagnosis but have also shown that the pathology in some lesions is driven primarily by an abnormality of the osteoclast, whereas in others the primary abnormality is in

the stromal component. To date, the treatment of osteoclast-rich lesions is largely by surgical removal of the tumors, but unraveling the molecular and cellular basis of osteoclast-rich lesions provides the opportunity for the development of novel therapeutic approaches.

II. OSTEOCLAST-RICH NEOPLASMS OF BONE

A. Giant Cell Tumor of Bone

1. DEFINITION

Giant cell tumor of the bone is classified as a primary benign tumor. Nevertheless, it has the ability to metastasize in a small minority of cases [1].

2. DEMOGRAPHICS AND CLINICAL FEATURES

Giant cell tumors occur in all ethnic groups accounting for 4–5% of all primary bone tumors and approximately 18% of non-sarcomatous bone tumors in the Western world, whereas they represent approximately 20% of primary bone tumors in the Chinese population [2,3]. In contrast to most bone tumors, giant cell tumors occur slightly more commonly in females [1].

The histopathological features of giant cell tumors overlap with other osteoclast-rich lesions. Consequently the diagnosis can only be made securely when it occurs in a skeletally mature individual involving the subarticular bone and when hyperparathyroidism has been excluded [1]. However, not everyone adheres to this strict definition and approximately 1–5% of lesions have been reported to occur in the skeletally immature [4–7]. Therefore, it remains unknown whether tumors occurring in children in non-epiphyseal sites develop as a consequence of a disease process different to that of the more typical giant cell tumors.

Bone Cancer
ISBN: 978-0-12-374895-9

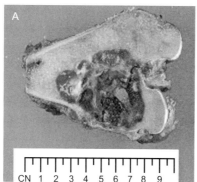
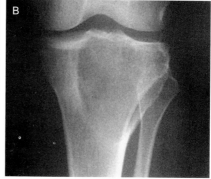

FIGURE 18.1   A distal femoral resection showing the macroscopic appearance of a giant cell tumor of bone. There is extensive hemorrhage and necrosis. Note the subarticular site in a long bone in which the epiphysis is closed (A). The radiographic appearance of a typical giant cell tumor of the proximal tibia: this expansile lytic tumor is sited in the subarticular area in a skeletally mature individual. Also note the absence of a periosteal reaction (B). These tumors generally are without a sclerotic margin (a narrow zone of transition) and, if present, is seldom complete. Septa may be seen in the lesion in 33–57% of patients; these represent non-uniform growth of the tumor rather than true septa.

Giant cell tumors are radiologically expansile, osteolytic, radiolucent lesions without a sclerotic margin and usually without a periosteal reaction (Figure 18.1; see Plate 7) [2]. The tumors are typically large when discovered, with diameters generally in the range of 5–7 cm. Eighty-five percent of giant cell tumors occur in long bones with a remarkable 50% being sited in the distal femur or proximal tibia, and approximately 5% in the bones of the hand and feet. Approximately 5% also involve flat bones, particularly those of the pelvis, with most occurring in the sacrum [8]. Occasionally, the entire sacrum is involved and giant cell tumors may extend across the sacroiliac joint to involve the ilium, and across the L5-S1 disc to involve the posterior elements of the L5 vertebra. The location of giant cell tumors within vertebrae varies but most commonly involve the body, followed by the vertebral arch and as a result there is a risk of extension into the spinal canal, with cord compression and consequent neurological symptoms [9–11].

3. MULTICENTRIC GIANT CELL TUMORS

So-called 'multicentric giant cell tumors' are rare [12–14] and account for approximately 1% of all osteoclast-rich lesions. There is evidence that approximately 60% occur in individuals less than 20 years of age, which contrasts with the natural history of conventional giant cell tumors which occur in the third to fifth decades [6]. These tumors either occur synchronously or metachronously in one or more bones. The average time between the presentation of the first and second lesion is approximately 6 years but has been as long as 23 years [6]. As with solitary variants, the most commonly affected site is around the knee. The small bones of the hand are also commonly involved with between 20 and 40% of cases of multicentric giant cell tumors having at least one focus in the hand [14].

It is not known if multicentric giant cell tumors represent metastatic or multiple independent foci of disease. However,

as only a minority of patients develop disease in the lung (metastatic) which usually occurs following curettage, and the majority of individuals with multicentric disease do not succumb to their disease, it seems that metastatic disease is an unlikely explanation for the multiple lesions. The fact that these tumors occur not infrequently in the immature skeleton and involve non-epiphyseal sites—findings which for some would exclude a diagnosis of giant cell tumor—suggests that multicentric giant cell tumors are biologically different from the solitary/conventional variant [6].

In view of multiple giant cell tumors most commonly occurring at a relatively young age the possibility that this disease is accounted for by mosaicism or a germline mutation should be considered [6,12–14]. Indeed, it is already known that multiple osteoclast-rich lesions, often referred to as non-ossifying fibromas (Figure 18.2; see Plate 8), occur in the skeleton of individuals with neurofibromatosis type 1 [15]. Jaffe-Campanacci syndrome is a term used to classify individuals with osteoclast-rich lesions (non-ossifying fibromas) and multiple café-au-lait spots without clinical evidence of neurofibromatosis [16]. Some consider this to be part of the spectrum of neurofibromatosis [15]. Hence, it is clear that some of the most basic issues regarding multicentric osteoclast-rich lesions remain unknown: for instance, it is not known whether these lesions represent neoplasms or a developmental abnormality. Simple studies to discover whether multicentric and solitary lesions share common pathogenetic mechanisms are needed, and could include loss of heterozygosity analyses and assessment as to whether the multiple tumors have telomeric associations similar to those observed in solitary giant cell tumors.

4. METASTATIC GIANT CELL TUMORS

Between 1 and 10% of solitary giant cell tumors with typical non-sarcomatous morphological features metastasize to the lungs. In many of these cases, there is a history of multiple curettages. The lesions in the lung may be solitary

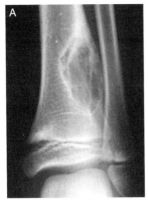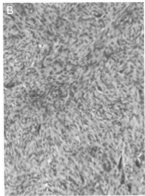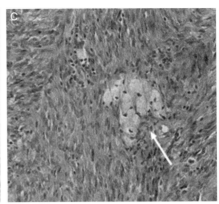

FIGURE 18.2   A non-ossifying fibroma in a young patient with neurofibromatosis type 1. In contrast to a giant cell tumor, the non-ossifying fibroma is sited in the metadiaphysis of the bone, has a sclerotic rim surrounding the central lytic area and most often presents in a growing child (skeletally immature) (A). Microscopic appearance of a non-ossifying fibroma showing bland fibroblastic cells in a storiform arrangement (B) in which clusters of foamy histiocytes are seen (arrow) (C).

or multiple but have identical microscopic appearances to those of the original neoplasm. In many cases, the lung tumors can be resected successfully [17–20]. Extra-tumoral vascular invasion can be detected in up to 23% of giant cell tumors of bone but there is no relationship between this finding and metastatic disease in the lung [21].

5. MALIGNANT TRANSFORMATION OF GIANT CELL TUMORS

A malignant giant cell tumor is an exceptionally rare tumor with one case being reported in a series of 529 giant cell tumors [22]. This tissue diagnosis is made when a giant cell tumor of bone with typical histopathological features is juxtaposed to tumor with an unequivocal sarcomatous growth pattern. If the tumor presents for the first time with both histopathological components, it is classified as 'de novo' or 'primary' whereas it is described as a secondary event if the sarcomatous component develops at the site of a recurrent conventional giant cell tumor. The natural behavior of these neoplasms is similar to other sarcomas, in that they disseminate to the lungs.

Secondary malignant giant cell tumor has been most commonly seen in individuals subjected to radiation therapy as part of their treatment for conventional giant cell tumors of bone. It has been reported that malignant transformation occurred in the era of orthovoltage radiation in as many as 4 of 12 tumors [9]. During the period when giant cell tumors were treated with orthovoltage radiation, patients usually received several courses of treatment, each of which consisted of a modest dose, but often the cumulative dose was high (>70 Gy). There was a median period of 10 years between exposure to the radiation and either malignant transformation of the giant cell tumor or development of a radiation-induced sarcoma in the surrounding tissue. Pooled data from studies in which patients are treated with a single course of megavoltage radiation (approximately 40–70 Gy) have indicated a far lower rate

of malignant transformation—less than 3% (one malignant transformation in 37 patients)—after a mean of 10 years of follow-up [23].

Spontaneous malignant transformation of a conventional giant cell tumor of bone is exceedingly rare and in at least some cases it remains doubtful whether the tumor was not in fact malignant from the onset. However, Hoch *et al.* reported such a case arising in a patient with multicentric disease providing strong evidence that spontaneous malignant transformation does occur. Malignant transformation of a giant cell tumor, whether spontaneous or as a result of radiotherapy, usually occurs within 5 years of the presentation of the primary bone lesion. Prognosis is very poor with a mortality rate of approximately 70% at 5 years [6].

6. CONVENTIONAL TREATMENT OF GIANT CELL TUMORS

If not treated, giant cell tumors of bone destroy bone locally and eventually give rise to a pathological fracture. To date, surgery—either wide local resection or curettage—followed by grafting (bone or polymethylmethacrylate) with or without adjuvant therapy (cryotherapy or a chemical adjuvant phenol, zinc chloride alcohol, and H_2O_2) has proved to be the most effective and safest treatment for appendicular giant cell tumors of bone. If treatment is limited to curettage and bone grafting alone, the tumor may recur in up to 45% of the time. The use of bone cement rather than bone graft results in a lower rate of recurrence. Enhancing the curettage with a high-speed burr or with the use of agents such as liquid nitrogen, hydrogen peroxide, or phenol, followed by placement of bone cement decreases the recurrence rate to 10–30% [2,3,9,24–27].

Radiation therapy, a non-surgical treatment option for giant cell tumors, has also been found to be effective; although, because of the close association of secondary sarcomatous transformation of giant cell tumor or of the surrounding tissue, it is now contra-indicated in most situations

[28]. Nevertheless, radiotherapy still plays a role, albeit a small one, in the treatment of giant cell tumors where complete excision or curettage is impractical for medical or functional reasons. The use of modern-day megavoltage radiation helps to reduce the rate of malignant transformation that was seen during the earlier era of orthovoltage radiation. The currently recommended dose of radiation ranges from 35 to 70 Gy which is reported as being associated with recurrence rates of between 10 and 15%, and rare malignant transformation [29,30]. However, long-term follow-up of these patients is still warranted to determine the long-term risk of developing a sarcoma.

Radiotherapy is now most commonly administered to giant cell tumors of the spine and sacrum, or to locally aggressive tumors which have recurred multiple times [23,28,30,31]. Specifically, giant cell tumors involving the axial skeleton, with the exception of the sacrum, are generally treated with excision and stabilization of the spine including biologic reconstruction of the anterior column and this is followed by radiation of 45 Gy over 4.5 weeks. This adjuvant therapy is given on the assumption that microscopic residual tumor is present and that adjuvant therapy offers the patient the best chance of long-term local control [32].

Giant cell tumors of the sacrum and pelvic bones, which are commonly difficult to excise, may benefit from preoperative embolization. Unresectable tumors can also be embolized. However, as blood flow reconstitution invariably occurs, repeated embolization is required at monthly intervals until significant disease control is achieved. Subsequent embolization can be performed when there is symptomatic or radiographic relapse of the tumor [33].

7. Morphology and Molecular Pathology

The typical giant cell tumor of bone, and other osteoclast-rich lesions, is dominated by two cell types which include the mononuclear stromal cell, and the osteoclast-like giant cell containing between five and several hundred nuclei (Figure 18.3). It was the presence of osteoclast-like cells that led Jaffe *et al.* to describe this tumor as an 'osteoclastoma' and considered it to be a neoplasm of osteoclast lineage [34]. A third less conspicuous cellular component is a mononuclear macrophage population, the nuclei of which show similar morphology to those in the osteoclast-like giant cells [1]. However, in our experience this represents a minority of cells in view of the relative paucity of CD68-positive mononuclear cells in these tumors.

The two major cellular components in giant cell tumors vary in their amount and distribution within and between giant cell tumors: some areas of tumors are composed of solid sheets of osteoclast-like cells with the mononuclear cell population being difficult to identify whereas others contain fibroblast-rich areas, often arranged in a storiform growth pattern, in which only small numbers of osteoclast-like cells are present (Figure 18.4). Giant cell

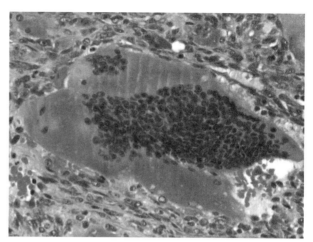

FIGURE 18.3   A high power magnification of a transmitted light photomicrograph showing a haematoxylin and eosin-stained section of an osteoclast in a giant cell tumor of bone. Note the presence of literally hundreds of nuclei.

tumors containing conspicuous areas of fibroblastic overgrowth are not infrequently related to areas of infarction, and are associated with numerous foamy histiocytes, and cyst formation, referred to as secondary aneurysmal bone cyst (see below), which suggests this finding is a secondary event. Cyst formation can be so striking that distinguishing giant cell tumor from a primary aneurysmal bone cyst can be troublesome, although detection of the recurrent non-random translocations in the latter largely resolves this problem (discussed in greater detail below) [35,36]. The term 'benign fibrous histiocytoma' is sometimes used to describe lesions with extensive fibrohistiocytic overgrowth of a conventional giant cell tumor but this nomenclature is now employed infrequently [37].

8. The Stromal Cell Population of Giant Cell Tumors

The two major cellular components in giant cell tumor of bone have been compared to an *in vivo* cellular co-culture and consequently considered to represent a valuable natural model for the study of stromal-hematopoietic cellular interaction. It is now known that osteoclast formation is dependent on Receptor Activator of Nuclear factor-κB (RANK) ligand (L), a member of the Tumor Necrosis Factor (TNF) superfamily, and Macrophage Colony-Stimulating Factor (M-CSF), and absence of either result in an osteopetrotic phenotype [38–40]. RANKL and M-CSF are synthesized by stromal cells in the bone marrow and mediate their osteoclast-inductive effect on osteoclast precursors through receptors RANK and cfms, respectively [41–44] (for review see Refs [45,46]). RANKL is negatively regulated by osteoprotegerin, a soluble receptor for RANK, which acts as a decoy receptor and competes with RANKL [41,47]. Therefore, the current pathogenetic model for this neoplasm holds that the tumor mononuclear cell is analogous

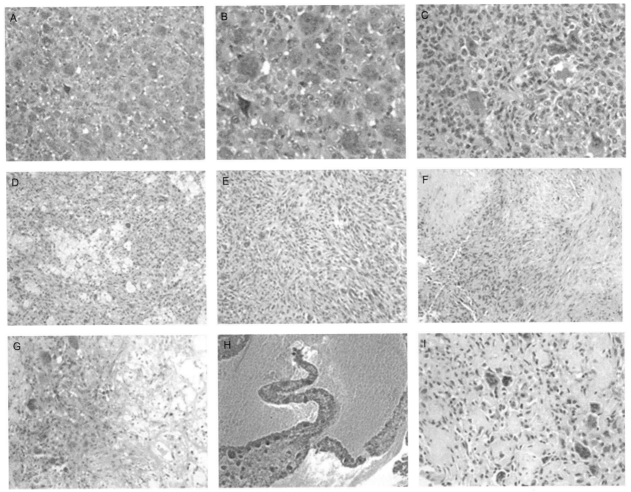

FIGURE 18.4 Transmitted light photomicrographs showing the wide range of appearances found in a giant cell tumor of bone. Predominantly osteoclasts are seen with a much less conspicuous number of mononuclear cells (A, B). In contrast, osteoclasts are present in significantly fewer numbers in C and almost undetectable in D in which collections of foamy histiocytes are noted. A fibroblastic overgrowth is noted in E and there is considerable scarring in F. Focal areas of infarction are present in G. Secondary aneurysmal cyst formation, indistinguishable from that of a primary aneurysmal bone cyst, also occurs in giant cell tumors (H). Focally, there is metaplastic osteoid deposition which makes giant cell tumors difficult to distinguish from osteosarcomas (I).

to the bone marrow stromal cell which supports osteoclast formation under physiological conditions. As the tumor stromal cell component is also thought to represent the neoplastic element of the giant cell tumor [21,48,49] the osteoclasts are considered to be a reactive 'passenger' population [21,50–53].

The stromal cells of giant cell tumor of bone derive from mesenchymal stem cells and are considered to be of osteoblast lineage on the basis of the expression of pre-osteoblastic markers, cbfa1 and osterix [54], being capable of forming bone [50,55] and supporting osteoclast formation through production of the requisite molecules including RANKL and M-CSF [21,48]. It is therefore considered by most, although not by all [56], that the abnormal regulation, by stromal cells, of molecules involved in osteoclastogenesis is likely to explain the large numbers of osteoclasts in these tumors [51,52]. However, to date, no specific

genetic abnormalities have been identified to account for the accumulation of osteoclasts that is characteristic of these tumors.

RANKL is expressed in a variety of cells other than those of the osteoblastic lineage including T lymphocytes and epithelial cells, so the expression of this molecule *per se* in the stromal cells of giant cell tumors is not evidence for the abnormal recruitment and/or survival of osteoclasts [43,57,58]. The accumulation of osteoclasts is likely to result from an imbalance of the molecules involved in osteoclast formation. For example, a genetic event giving rise to absence/reduction of osteoprotegerin, a molecule which inhibits osteoclast formation by preventing the binding of RANKL to its receptor RANK, could theoretically account for the accumulation of osteoclasts in these and other osteoclast-rich lesions. Abnormal expression of osteoprotegerin is of particular interest because homozygous deletions of the gene, *TNFRSF11B*, which encodes this protein cause juvenile Pagetic bone disease, and the incidence of giant cell tumors is increased in patients with Paget's disease of the bone [59,60]. Likewise, excess production of M-CSF or overexpression of its receptor, cfms, must also be considered as a possible explanation for the presence of osteoclasts in these tumors in view of a translocation involving *M-CSF* occurring in a majority of tenosynovial giant cell tumors/pigmented villonodular synovitis [61].

Other molecules that are potentially implicated in the phenotype of giant cell tumors include those molecules involved in osteoclast formation under pathological conditions. Interleukin-1 (IL-1) and Tumor Necrosis Factor-alpha (TNFα) are powerful osteoclast-inducing factors under inflammatory states, particularly in rheumatoid arthritis, and cherubism (See below) [62–65] (for review see Ref. [66]) TNFα mediates its osteoclastogenic effect in many ways. It acts synergistically with RANKL but it remains unclear if it functions independently, or requires permissive levels of RANKL to recruit osteoclasts [67–69]. TNFα also increases expression of macrophage colony-stimulating factor (M-CSF), a factor crucial for osteoclast-formation and induces cfms, the receptor for M-CSF, expression. Interleukin-1 also induces osteoclast formation but requires the presence of RANKL, and mediates many of the effects of TNFα in a pMAP kinase-dependent manner [69–74].

The strongest evidence that the neoplastic component of giant cell tumor is represented by the stromal spindle cells is based on data accrued from cytogenetic studies. Apart from the chromosomal abnormalities described in several reports [48,49,75–80], the most frequent and consistent genetic aberration is the telomeric fusions/association, which are non-covalent interactions at chromosomal ends (telomeric region), mostly affecting the chromosomes 11p, 13p, 14p, 15p, 19q, 20q and 21p [76,81–83]. The other argument for the stromal cell being the neoplastic component is that when a giant cell tumor transforms to a malignant process, the atypical morphological features are found in this population.

9. THE OSTEOCLAST POPULATION IN GIANT CELL TUMORS AND FUTURE THERAPEUTIC APPROACHES

The general consensus is that osteoclasts in giant cell tumors of bone represent a non-neoplastic component (See above). Osteoclasts derive from the monocyte/macrophage lineage under the influence of RANKL and M-CSF in physiological states and are cells that resorb bone [41–44,47]. Prior to development of experimental human model systems that allowed osteoclasts to be generated from bone marrow precursors and peripheral blood mononuclear cells [84–86], osteoclasts were obtained from giant cell tumors for studying the bone resorptive process [87]. Giant cell tumor of bone was the first of the osteoclast-rich neoplasms from which the multinucleate giant cells were isolated and

shown to be capable of excavating the surface of bone. Furthermore, much of our knowledge of the osteoclast phenotype was discovered by studying the multinucleate cells in giant cell tumors and other osteoclast-rich lesions [88–92].

Osteoclasts in giant cell tumors and other osteoclast-rich neoplasms have a similar phenotype to normal osteoclasts which are found along bone surfaces, although they contain far more nuclei, up to several 100s, compared to normal osteoclasts which have between 2 and 5 (Figure 18.3). They express tartrate-resistant acid phosphatase, calcitonin receptors, RANK, and markers of leukocytes including CD45, myeloid markers such as CD11/18, and proteases including cathepsin K [53,55,91–93].

Osteoclasts in giant cell tumors, like normal osteoclasts, employ integrin cell adhesion molecules, particularly $\alpha_v\beta_3$, the principle osteoclast integrin receptor which binds to several non-collagenous protein ligands in an RGD (Arg-Gly-Asp)-dependent manner. $\alpha_2\beta_1$ is also expressed on osteoclasts and recognizes collagen, whereas other integrins, particularly $\alpha_v\beta_5$, have not been found on osteoclasts in a series of analyses of various species [94,95] (for review see Ref. [96]). Consequently, vitronectin inhibitors have been developed with the possibility of introducing them as therapeutic agents to inhibit bone resorption and reduce bone metastases [97,98]. Relevant to the development of such agents as antiresorptive therapy was the report of *in vitro* human studies of osteoclast formation and resorption using osteoclasts generated from peripheral blood mononuclear cells of Iraqi-Jewish individuals with a severe form of Glanzmann thrombasthenia. This revealed that the lack of β_3 integrin results in reduced bone resorption. However, the osteoclasts were found to have increased expression of $\alpha_2\beta_1$, which partly compensated for the lack of $\alpha_v\beta_3$ and allowed the osteoclasts to resorb bone albeit at a submaximal level. This compensatory response might reduce the efficacy of vitronectin receptor antagonists and make these inhibitors inefficient as antiresorptive agents in a tumor setting [99].

Giant cell tumor-derived osteoclasts also exhibit the unique cytoskeleton, F-actin ring structure which surrounds the bone-apposed ruffled membrane seen in normal osteoclasts when attached to mineralized matrix. The ring structure represents a sealing zone with the bone and provides an enclosed subcellular (also extracellular) space into which acid and proteases, for the purpose of bone degradation, are secreted [96]. Once the sealing zone has formed, the bone-apposed plasma membrane develops a villous structure, referred to as a ruffled membrane/border, and protons are secreted into the subcellular/extracellular microenvironment by means of the proton pump (H + ATPase) [100,101]. However, as only the osteoclasts at the periphery of giant cell tumors come into contact with mineralized matrix the vast majority do not demonstrate F-actin rings or ruffled borders.

Whether osteoclasts are required for, or contribute to, the development and progression of giant cell tumors is not known, although there is some evidence that this is the case

[102]. However, as only osteoclasts at the tumor periphery are involved in the bone resorptive process, it is unlikely that purely antiresorptive agents, such as vitronectin receptor antagonists [98] or cathepsin K [103,104], would exert a significant effect on tumor growth or disease control. Although use of antiresorptive agents has been shown to provide clinical benefit in neoplastic disease, such as in myeloma, where extensive bone destruction occurs [105], inhibitors of osteoclast formation rather than inhibitors of bone resorption are theoretically more attractive for the treatment of osteoclast-rich lesions. Nevertheless, agents that inhibit bone resorption are likely to retard the local destruction of host bone in patients with osteoclast-rich lesions. Bisphosponates are good examples of such drugs. In contrast to agents that inhibit osteoclast resorption by interrupting osteoclast formation, bisphosphonates, analogues of endogenous pyrophosphates, exert their antiresorptive action by interfering with osteoclast function [106], and are used effectively in the treatment of osteoporosis, Paget's disease of bone, and as an adjuvant to reduce the bone resorption associated with some types of metastatic carcinoma to bone. They mediate their affect by selective adsorption to hydroxyapatite and subsequent internalization by bone-resorbing osteoclasts in which they interfere with two major biochemical pathways [107]. Of interest are more recent reports which suggest that pamidronate or zoledronate may be a useful adjuvant therapy in the treatment of giant cell tumors [108,109]. However, greater numbers of patients need to be studied for longer periods before the true effect value of such treatment can be assessed.

Drugs that either inhibit osteoclast formation or induce apoptosis independently of resorption, would be more likely to provide clinical benefit if osteoclasts were implicated in survival and/or progression of osteoclast-rich lesions. TNFα inhibitors are one potential group of drugs and these are known to block bone destruction effectively in rheumatoid arthritis [66]. Alternatively, drugs that target the RANK/RANK ligand/osteoprotegerin pathways, such the antibody to RANK ligand, denosumab, which are currently being developed and some of which are in clinical trials may prove useful therapeutic agents [110,111]. In addition, research is also being pursued on other novel classes of bone resorption inhibitors, including biphenylcarboxylic acid derivates [112].

In summary, non-surgical adjuvant therapy is a promising and intriguing alternative for the treatment of GCT and other osteoclast-rich lesions. However, to date there are no reports of long-term follow-up of this new classes of agents in a control trial and this is what is required to test the efficacy of these drugs.

B. Aneurysmal Bone Cyst

The primary aneurysmal bone cyst is a benign, osteoclast-rich, locally destructive, expansile lesion characterized by multiloculated blood-filled cystic spaces. However, it is now recognized that aneurysmal bone cysts can be predominantly solid neoplasms [113] and before this was accepted, extragnathic solid variants of aneurysmal bone cyst were generally referred to as giant cell reparative granulomas. Giant cell reparative granuloma of jaw is still reported as a distinct entity and retains its nomenclature. Aneurysmal bone cysts affect all age groups but generally occur during the first two decades of life and have no sex predominance. The metaphyses of long bones and the posterior segments of vertebral bodies are most frequently affected. The most common signs and symptoms are pain and swelling; rarely patients will present with a pathological fracture. In cases of vertebral involvement nerves may be compressed giving rise to neurological symptoms [114].

Radiographically, an aneurysmal bone cyst is usually an eccentric, expansile lesion with well-defined margins (Figure 18.5; see Plate 9). Most lesions are completely lytic and often contain a thin shell of reactive bone at the periphery. Computer Tomography (CT) and Magnetic Resonance Imaging (MRI) scans demonstrate internal septa and characteristic fluid-filled levels. The macroscopic findings are reflected in the imaging (Figure 18.5; see Plate 9). The lesion can be quite varied microscopically and shares features with other osteoclast-rich lesions. However, the text book findings of an aneurysmal bone cyst are of numerous blood-filled cysts, not lined by endothelial cells, separated

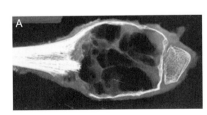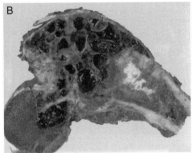

FIGURE 18.5 This radiographic image of a fine cut slab shows the typical appearance of a primary aneurysmal bone cyst (A). The findings consist of a central expansive lytic lesion, appearing cystic as a result of fine septae. The macroscopic appearance of an aneurysmal bone cyst involving the greater trochanter (B).

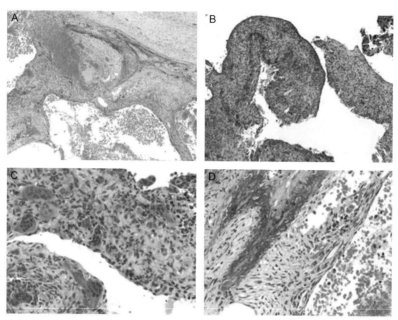

FIGURE 18.6   The typical microscopic features of an aneurysmal bone cyst. Low-power magnification shows the overall architecture of the tumor (A, B). Note, at higher magnification, the blood-filled spaces not lined by endothelial cells, the walls of which are composed of fibroblastic cells in which osteoclasts line up in variable numbers (C). A characteristic feature is the presence of 'blue' bone which represents calcified osteoid which is present in tumor septa (A, D).

by fibrous septa, containing oval-spindle shaped cells, multinucleated osteoclast-type giant cells, and osteoid which often has a characteristic 'blue' hue to it (Figure 18.6).

Further studies have demonstrated the presence of five different recurrent non-random translocations in aneurysmal bone cysts. All of the translocations involve the USP6/TRE17 oncogene which is overexpressed and fused with different gene promoters, 75% of which involve a USP6-Cadherin11 fusion. The other partners include thyroid receptor-associated protein 150, Zinc Finger 9, osteomodulin, and collagen 1A1. All of the rearranged genes have been identified in a small population of stromal cells. Hence, this population represents the neoplastic population and the resident osteoclasts represent a reactive population. The fusion partners collagen 1A1, osteomodulin and cadherin 11 appear well suited to drive USP6 transcription in these bone tumors as they are expressed in cells of the osteoblastic lineage [35,36,115].

Conventional treatment of aneurysmal bone cysts is surgery, usually in the form of curettage ($+/-$ grafting/cementation/use of phenol) although excision is sometimes undertaken [116–118]. The recurrence rate after *en bloc* excision is about 7% [119]. Selective arterial embolization has shown some promise and can be used for the management of tumors which are difficult to resect [119]. Radiotherapy is not generally employed; nevertheless, there are reports in the literature where this has been used to treat patients with incompletely resected, aggressive, and/or recurrent disease. The dose of radiation administered is low (26–30 Gy) and gives local control in approximately

90% of cases [120]. To date, there is no chemotherapeutic agent used for the treatment of these neoplasms, and no targeted treatment against the USP6 gene has been developed. On the basis of the similarities to giant cell tumor of bone, they too could theoretically be treated with antiresorptive agents [119].

Secondary aneurysmal bone cysts are found to be associated with other benign and malignant bone tumors that have undergone secondary cystic change. The giant cell tumor of bone and osteoblastoma are the tumors that most commonly have secondary aneurysmal bone cyst change, but is also not uncommonly seen in fibrous dysplasia and chondroblastoma. It is important to identify the underlying neoplastic condition associated with secondary aneurysmal cyst formation as it is this component of the tumor that will ultimately dictate the behavior, treatment and prognosis of the disease. To date, the translocations identified in primary aneurysmal bone cysts have not been reported in the secondary lesions [121].

C. Tenosynovial Giant-cell Tumor/Pigmented Villonodular Synovitis

Tenosynovial giant-cell tumors/pigmented villonodular synovitis are osteoclast-rich neoplasms which involve the synovium and tendon sheaths and, in a small number of cases, they are extremely destructive of the adjacent bone. They have features not dissimilar to giant cell tumors, although generally they are composed of a more spindled population, and the presence of hemosiderin and reactive

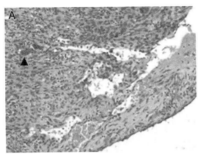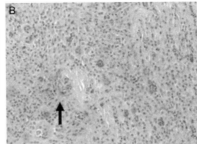

FIGURE 18.7 Hematoxylin and eosin sections of pigmented villonodular synovitis/tenosynovial giant cell tumor. This osteoclast-rich tumor generally contains a more spindled population compared to that seen in giant cell tumors and the osteoclasts (arrow heads) are more scattered throughout the spindled cells (A). Hemosiderin is also a common finding (arrows) (B).

change such as the presence of numerous foamy histiocytes is common (Figure 18.7; see Plate 10). Recurrent non-random translocations causing fusion of chromosome 1p13 to COL6A3 (2q35) results in overexpression of the osteoclast-inductive cytokine M-CSF. The mononuclear stromal cells harbor the translocation and express M-CSF, whereas the osteoclasts express cfms, the M-CSF receptor [61]. This implies that the neoplastic component of the tumor is the stromal cell and that the osteoclasts, which express the receptor to this molecule, are recruited to the tumors as a reactive 'passenger' population.

Radical synovectomy is the recommended current treatment for tenosynovial giant-cell tumor/pigmented villonodular synovitis. However, because of the high recurrence rate, adjuvant radiotherapy has given encouraging results [122]. Experts currently recommend a total dose of 30–50 Gy, which does not appear to be associated with a sarcomatous change of the irradiated field [123]. Using molecules which could interfere with the M-CSF receptor offers a potential approach to treating these lesions as there is experimental evidence that osteoclastic resorption in the inflammatory joint is completely interrupted by blocking the effect of this cytokine [72,124].

III. THE CHERUBISM PHENOTYPE: CHERUBISM, NOONAN-LIKE/MULTIPLE GIANT CELL LESION OF THE JAW AND NEUROFIBROMATOSIS

Cherubism (OMIM 118400), Noonan-like/multiple giant cell lesions of the jaw (OMIM 163955) and neurofibromatosis type 1 (OMIM 162200) are caused by germline mutations involving *SH3BP2* [65,125], *PTPN11* [126,127] and *NF1* [15,128–130], respectively. Individuals with any of these germline mutations may present with symmetric enlargement of the jaw caused by osteoclast-rich lesions and it may be difficult to distinguish these syndromes in the absence of genetic analysis [128,131]. However, we have found that mutations in these genes are not always detected in individuals with a cherubism phenotype, or in individuals with multiple osteoclast-rich lesions with or without involvement of the jaw indicating that genes harboring mutations remain to be discovered to account for osteoclast-rich lesions. Activation of RAS-MAP kinase signaling is the molecular event that unites the genetic mutations in *SH3BP2*, *PTPN11* and *NF1* which cause cherubism, Noonan syndrome and neurofibromatosis type 1, respectively, and therefore provides a link to explain the overlapping phenotype of these clinical syndromes (Figure 18.8).

The osteoclast-rich lesions occurring on a background of the above germline mutations have not been shown to be neoplastic. Furthermore, there are only rare occasions where sarcomatous transformation has occurred, and to our knowledge this has developed subsequent to cherubism lesions being treated with radiotherapy [132].

A. Cherubism

Cherubism, a disease which presents in early childhood, is inherited as an autosomal dominant trait, showing 80% penetrance, and characterized by painless disfiguring multilocular, symmetric enlargement of the mandible and/or maxilla as a result of an osteoclast-rich lesion (Figure 18.9; see Plate 11) [133]. Apart from one deletion in exon 3 in *SH3BP2* [134], all of the reported mutations are limited to a short specific section of the adaptor protein Src Homology-3 Binding Protein-2 (SH3BP2) [125,135–140]. Other evidence shows that the genetic alterations result in a gain of function [65,139].

In all genetically proven cases of cherubism, the abnormality is limited to the mandible and/or maxilla [132] and cervical lymphadenopathy [141]. There are also occasional reports of unilateral cherubism, and some cases of individuals with lesions in ribs and 'cafe-au-lait' spots, in addition to the cherubism facies but all of these reports pre-date the identification of mutations in *SH3BP2* as being the causative genetic defect [142,143].

A mouse model of cherubism provides strong evidence that the osteoclast is the cell that is central to the disease. Research showed that the disease phenotype was transmitted by bone marrow transplantation, that there was increased M-CSF signaling to the MAPK-ERK pathway, that there were increased levels of TNFα produced, and

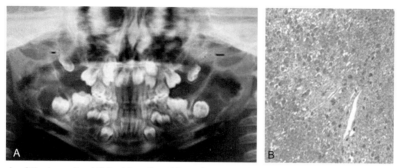

FIGURE 18.8   A radiograph of the jaw of a child with a cherubism phenotype but who has a *PTPN11* mutation (Noonan syndrome). Note the bilateral symmetric radiolucent bubbly appearance of the mandible and maxilla (A). The histology shows an osteoclast-rich lesion with features not dissimilar to that of a non-ossifying fibroma: there is a spindled cell population of cells in which osteoclast-like cells are scattered (B).

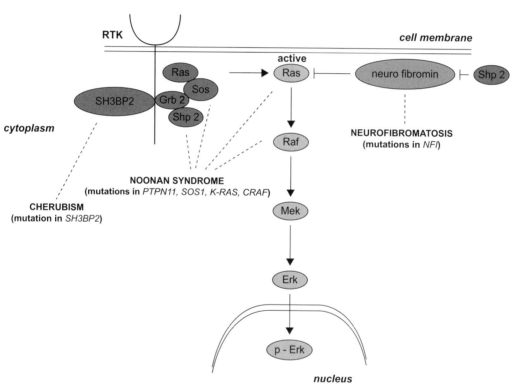

FIGURE 18.9   Activation of Ras-MAP kinase signaling is the molecular event that unites the overlapping phenotype occurring in cherubism, Noonan syndrome and neurofibromatosis type 1. Activation can either occur directly (mutations in *SH3BP2, PTPN11, SOS1, K-RAS, CRAF*) or indirectly by disabling negative regulators of Ras (mutations in *NF1, PTPN11*).

that the phenotype was corrected by crossing the *SH3BP2* mutants into TNFα-null mice [65,144]. Finally, myeloid cells (i.e., osteoclast precursors) from this mutant strain generated more osteoclasts *in vitro* than wild-type mice. The discovery that TNFα is central to the pathogenesis of cherubism using an animal model provides a sound basis on which to test whether TNFα inhibitors could control this disease in humans [144].

B. Noonan Syndrome

Noonan syndrome is an autosomal dominant disorder clinically characterized by a variety of features, which are variable expressed, and includes short stature, sternal deformity, facial dysmorphism, and/or a webbed neck, congenital heart defects, developmental delay and bleeding diathesis. Approximately 40–50% of individuals with Noonan syndrome harbor a missense mutation in the *PTPN11* gene that is transcribed to produce the SHP2 protein [127]. Mutations associated with Noonan syndrome lead to increased activation of SHP2 ultimately leading to an upregulation of RAS activity. SHP2 also activates RAS by downregulating NF1 transcription [145]. A further 20% of Noonan syndrome cases harbor gain-of-function mutations in *SOS1* [146], an activator of RAS, 2% in *K-RAS* [147,148], and 3% in CRAF [149,150] although to date giant cell lesions of the jaw have not been associated with mutations in these three genes.

It has been recognized for some time that a small number of individuals with a Noonan phenotype have multiple giant cell lesions of the jaw resulting in a similar phenotype to that observed in cherubism [151,152], and it has also been shown genetically that this is the case [131]. As with cherubism, extragnathic osteoclast-rich lesions have never been reported to date in individuals with a proven *PTPN11* mutation. Some patients with a typical Noonan phenotype also have multiple café-au-lait spots/lentigines—in which case the phenotype is known as Leopard syndrome (OMIM 151100) [153]. These three entities (classical Noonan syndrome, Noonan syndrome/multiple giant cell tumor of the jaw and Leopard syndrome) are allelic disorders and are associated with mutations in *PTPN11* [127].

C. Neurofibromatosis Type 1

Neurofibromatosis type 1 (OMIM: 162200) has a phenotype that overlaps with Noonan syndrome, including short stature and scoliosis in addition to cardiac abnormalities and leukemia. This syndrome is caused by haploinsufficiency of the neurofibromin protein that acts as a tumor suppressor which negatively regulates RAS activity.

A percentage of patients with neurofibromatosis type 1 have osteoclast-rich lesions of the skeleton, often referred to as non-ossifying fibromas (Figure 18.2; see Plate 8) [16]. In contrast to osteoclast-rich lesions caused by *SH3BP2* and *PTPN11* mutations that are restricted to the jaw, osteoclast-rich lesion associated with *NF1* mutations may be solitary or multiple, and involve gnathic and/or extragnathic sites [128–130,154]. When solitary and involve the jaw, they can present as giant cell reparative granulomas, or can be mistaken for cherubism if the jaw is diffusely involved [128,129].

Further studies are required to determine whether the osteoclast is central to the development of osteoclast-rich lesions of the jaw in Noonan syndrome and neurofibromatosis and other lesions in the same way as it is for cherubism. It is interesting to speculate that this is the case in the light of the evidence that myeloid precursors are hypersensitive to cytokines including GM-CSF in Noonan syndrome [155,156], and granulocyte-macrophage colony-stimulating factor and M-CSF in neurofibromatosis [157,158]. In addition to the existence of antagonists to TNFα, there are also molecules that specifically inhibit the RAS signaling pathway and which could be used for the treatment of the osteoclast-rich lesions in patients.

References

1. R. Reid, S.S. Banerjee, and R. Sciot, (2002). Giant cell tumor: in C.D.M. Fletcher, K.K. Unni, and F. Mertens, (eds) World Health Organization Classification of Tumors. Pathology and Genetics. Tumors of Soft Tissue and Bone. IARC Press, Lyon, 2002, pp. 310–312.
2. M. Campanacci, N. Baldini & S. Boriani, J Bone Joint Surg (Am) 69 (1987) 106.
3. H.W. Sung, D.P. Kuo & W.P. Shu, J Bone Joint Surg (Am) 64 (1982) 755.
4. M.J. Kransdorf, D.E. Sweet & P.C. Buetow, et al., Radiology 184 (1992) 233.
5. P. Picci, M. Manfrini & V. Zucchi, J Bone Joint Surg (Am) 65 (1983) 486.
6. B. Hoch, C. Inwards & M. Sundaram, et al., J Bone Joint Surg (Am) 88 (2006) 1998.
7. J.S. Fain, K.K. Unni & J.W. Beabout, Cancer 71 (1993) 3514.
8. G.S. Bogumill & L.C. Johnson, J Bone Joint Surg (Am) 54 (1972) 1558.
9. R.R. Goldenberg, C. Campbell & M. Bonfiglio, J Bone Joint Surg (Am) 52 (1970) 619.
10. M. Campanacci, A. Giunti & R. Olmi, Italian J Orthop Traumat 1 (1975) 249.
11. D.J. McDonald, F. Sim & R.A. McLeod, et al., J Bone Joint Surg (Am) 68 (1986) 235.
12. F.H. Sim, D.C. Dahlin & J.W. Beabout, J Bone Joint Surg (Am) 59 (1977) 1052.
13. B.W. Hindman, L.L. Seeger & P. Stanley, Skeletal Radiol 23 (1994) 187.
14. C.A. Cummins, M.T. Scarborough & W.F. Enneking, Clin Orthop 322 (1996) 245.
15. R.S. Colby & R.A. Saul, Am J Med Genet 123A (2003) 60.
16. J.M. Mirra, R.H. Gold & F. Rand, Clin Ortho Rel Res 168 (1982) 192.
17. D. Connell, P.L. Munk & M.J. Lee, Skeletal Radiol 27 (1998) 341.
18. W.S. Tubbs, L.R. Brown & J.W. Beabout, Am J Roentgenol 158 (1992) 331.
19. W.J. Maloney, L.M. Vaughan & H.H. Jones, Clin Orthop 243 (1989) 208.
20. J.C. Cheng & J.O. Johnston, Clin Orthop 338 (1997) 205.
21. M. Wulling, C. Engels & N. Jesse, et al., J Cancer Res Clin Oncol 127 (2001) 467.
22. R.J.B. Sakkers, R.O. Van der Heul & H.M. Kroon, et al., J Bone Joint Surg (Am) 79 (1997) 259.
23. A. Chakravarti, I.J. Spiro & E.B. Hug, et al., J Bone Joint Surg (Am) 81 (1999) 1566.
24. A.J. Aboulafia, D.H. Rosenbaum & L. Sicard-Rosenbaum, Clin Orthop 307 (1994) 189.
25. M. Campanacci, R. Capanna & N. Fabbri, Chir Organi Mov 75 (1990) 212.
26. H.R. Durr, M. Maier & V. Jansson, Eur J Surg Oncol 25 (1999) 610.
27. H.J. Mankin, F.S. Fogelson & A.Z. Thrasher, New Engl J Med 294 (1976) 1247.

28. S. Malone, B. O'Sullivan & C. Catton, et al., Int J Radiat Oncol Biol Phys 33 (1995) 689.
29. C.J. Bennett, R.B. Marcus & R.R. Million, Int J Radiat Oncol Biol Phys 26 (1993) 299.
30. M.K. Nair & R. Jyothirmayi, Int J Radiat Oncol Biol Phys 43 (1999) 1065.
31. S.J. Feigenberg, R.B. Marcus & M.T. Scarborough, et al., Clin Ortho Rel Res 411 (2003) 207.
32. M.W. Fidler, Eur Spine J 10 (2001) 69.
33. R.D. Lackman, L.D. Khoury & A. Esmail, et al., J Bone Joint Surg (Br) 84 (2002) 873.
34. H.L. Jaffe, L. Lichtenstein & R. Portis, Arch Pathol 30 (1940) 993.
35. A.M. Oliveira, A.R. Perez-Atayde & C.Y. Inwards, et al., Am J Pathol 165 (2004) 1773.
36. A.M. Oliveira, B.L. Hsi & S. Weremowicz, et al., Cancer Res 64 (2004) 1920.
37. M. Kyriakos, Benign fibrous histiocytoma of bone, in: C.D.M. Fletcher, K.K. Unni, & F. Mertens (eds) World Health Organization Classification of Tumors. Pathology and Genetics. Tumors of Soft Tissue and Bone. IARC Press, Lyon, 2002, pp. 292–293.
38. H. Yoshida, S. Hayashi & T. Kunisada, et al., Nature 345 (1990) 442.
39. Y.Y. Kong, H. Yoshida & I. Sarosi, et al., Nature 397 (1999) 315.
40. C. Sobacchi, A. Frattini & M.M. Guerrini, et al., Nature Genet 39 (2007) 960.
41. H. Hsu, D.L. Lacey & C.R. Dunstan, et al., Proc Natl Acad Sci 96 (1999) 3540.
42. D.L. Lacey, E. Timms & H.L. Tan, et al., Cell 93 (1998) 165.
43. B.R. Wong, R. Josien & S.Y. Lee, et al., J Exp Med 186 (1997) 2075.
44. H. Yasuda, N. Shima & N.Y. Nakagawa, et al., Proc Natl Acad Sci 95 (1998) 3597.
45. W.J. Boyle, W.S. Simonet & D.L. Lacey, Nature 423 (2003) 337.
46. T.J. Chambers, J Pathol 192 (2000) 4.
47. W.S. Simonet, D.L. Lacey & C.R. Dunstan, et al., Cell 89 (1997) 309.
48. A. Murata, T. Fujita & N. Kawahara, et al., J Orthop Sci 10 (2005) 581.
49. R. Sciot, H. Dorfman & P. Brys, et al., Mod Pathol 13 (2000) 1206.
50. I.E. James, R.A. Dodds & D.L. Olivera, et al., J Bone Min Res 11 (1996) 1453.
51. G.J. Atkins, D.R. Haynes & S.E. Graves, et al., J Bone Min Res 15 (2000) 640.
52. L. Huang, J. Xu & D.J. Wood, et al., Am J Pathol 156 (2000) 761.
53. S. Roux, L. Amazit & G. Meduri, et al., Am J Clin Pathol 117 (2002) 210.
54. L. Huang, X.Y. Teng & Y.Y. Cheng, et al., Bone 34 (2004) 393.
55. I.E. James, R.A. Dodds & E. Lee-Rykaczewski, et al., J Bone Min Res 11 (1996) 1608.
56. T. Morgan, G.J. Atkins & M.K. Trivett, et al., Am J Pathol 167 (2005) 117.
57. K. Loser, A. Mehling & S. Loeser, et al., Nat Med 1 (2) (2006) 1372.
58. J.E. Fata, Y.Y. Kong & J. Li, et al., Cell 103 (2000) 41.
59. A.E. Hughes, S.H. Ralston & J. Marken, et al., Nature Genet 24 (2000) 45.
60. M.P. Whyte, S.E. Obrecht & P.M. Finnegan, et al., New Engl J Med 347 (2002) 175.
61. R.B. West, B.P. Rubin & M.A. Miller, et al., Proc Natl Acad Sci 103 (2006) 690.
62. J. Saklatvala, L.M. Pilsworth & S.J. Sarsfield, et al., Biochem J 224 (1984) 461.
63. F.M. Brennan, D. Chantry & A. Jackson, et al., Lancet 2 (1989) 244.
64. R. Maini, E.W. St Clair & F. Breedveld, et al., Lancet 354 (1999) 1932.
65. Y. Ueki, C.Y. Lin & M. Senoo, et al., Cell 128 (2007) 71.
66. M. Feldmann & R.N. Maini, Joint Bone Spine 69 (2002) 12.
67. N. Kim, Y. Kadono & M. Takami, et al., J Exp Med 202 (2005) 589.
68. J. Lam, S. Takeshita & J.E. Barker, et al., J Clin Invest 106 (2000) 1481.
69. K. Fuller, C. Murphy & B. Kirstein, et al., Endocrinology 143 (2002) 1108.
70. J. Zwerina, S. Hayer & K. Redlich, et al., Arthrit Rheum 54 (2006) 463.
71. Z. Yao, P. Li & Q. Zhang, et al., J Biol Chem 281 (2006) 11846.
72. H. Kitaura, P. Zhou & H.J. Kim, et al., J Clin Invest 115 (2005) 3418.
73. A.C. Lovibond, S.J. Haque & T.J. Chambers, et al., Biochem Biophys Res Commun 309 (2003) 762.
74. J. Zwerina, S. Hayer & M. Tohidast-Akrad, et al., Arthrit Rheum 50 (2004) 277.
75. J.A. Bridge, J.R. Neff & B.J. Mouron, Cancer Genet Cytogenet 58 (1992) 2.
76. M. Werner, Int Orthop 30 (2006) 484.
77. J.R. Sawyer, L.S. Goosen & R.L. Binz, et al., Cancer Genet Cytogenet 159 (2005) 32.
78. I. Panagopoulos, F. Mertens & H.A. Domanski, et al., Int J Cancer 93 (2001) 769.
79. G. Bardi, N. Pandis & N. Mandahl, et al., Cancer Genet Cytogenet 57 (1991) 161.
80. H.S. Schwartz, J.D. Eskew & M.G. Butler, J Orthop Res 20 (2002) 387.
81. M.H. Zheng, P. Siu & J.M. Papadimitriou, et al., Pathology 31 (1999) 373.
82. O. Montero, M.T. Salle & R. Guevara, et al., Cancer Genet Cytogenet 146 (2003) 170.
83. M. Tarkkanen, A. Kaipainen & E. Karaharju, et al., Cancer Genet Cytogenet 68 (1993) 1.
84. J.M. Quinn, S. Neale & Y. Fujikawa, et al., Calcif Tissue Int 62 (1998) 527.
85. H.M. Massey & A.M. Flanagan, Br J Haematol 106 (1999) 167.
86. U. Sarma & A.M. Flanagan, Blood 88 (1996) 2531.
87. T.J. Chambers, K. Fuller & J.A. Darby, et al., Bone Miner 1 (1986) 127.
88. M.A. Horton, D. Lewis & K. McNulty, et al., Cancer Res 45 (1985) 5663.

89. M.A. Horton, D. Lewis & K. McNulty, et al., Br J Exp Pathol 66 (1985) 103.

90. M.A. Horton, J.A. Pringle & T.J. Chambers, New Engl J Med 312 (1985) 923.

91. A.M. Flanagan, S.M. Tinkler & M.A. Horton, et al., Cancer 62 (1988) 1139.

92. A.M. Flanagan & T.J. Chambers, J Pathol 159 (1989) 53.

93. C.J. Joyner, J.M. Quinn & J.T. Triffitt, et al., Bone Miner 16 (1992) 37.

94. S. Nesbitt, A. Nesbit & M. Helfrich, et al., J Biol Chem 268 (1993) 16737.

95. M.H. Helfrich, S.A. Nesbitt & P.T. Lakkakorpi, et al., Bone 19 (1996) 317.

96. M.A. Horton, S.A. Nesbitt & J.H. Bennett, et al., Integrins and other cell surface attachment molecules of bone cells, in: J.P. Bilezikian, L.G. Raisz & G.A. Rodan (Eds.) Principles of Bone Biology, Academic Press, San Diego, USA, 2002, pp. 265–286.

97. J.F. Harms, D.R. Welch & R.S. Samant, et al., Clin Exp Metastasis 21 (2004) 119.

98. W.H. Miller, D.P. Alberts & P.K. Bhatnagar, et al., J Med Chem 43 (2000) 22.

99. M.A. Horton, H.M. Massey & N. Rosenberg, et al., Br J Haematol 122 (2003) 950.

100. H.C. Blair, S.L. Teitelbaum & H.L. Tan, et al., Am J Physiol 260 (1991) C1315.

101. R. Baron, L. Neff & W. Brown, et al., J Cell Biol 106 (1988) 1863.

102. D.R. Clohisy, M.L. Ramnaraine & S. Scully, et al., J Orthop Res 18 (2000) 967.

103. P. Saftig, E. Hunziker & O. Wehmeyer, et al., Proc Natl Acad Sci 95 (1998) 13453.

104. O. Vasiljeva, T. Reinheckel & C. Peters, et al., Curr Pharm Des 13 (2007) 385.

105. H.S. Yeh & J.R. Berenson, Eur J Cancer 42 (2006) 1554.

106. A.M. Flanagan & T.J. Chambers, Bone Miner 6 (1989) 33.

107. R.G. Russell, Pediatr 119 (Suppl 2) (2007) S150.

108. S.S. Chang, S.J. Suratwala & K.M. Jung, et al., Clin Ortho Rel Res 426 (2004) 103.

109. N. Fujimoto, K. Nakagawa & A. Seichi, et al., Oncol Rep 8 (2001) 643.

110. N.A. Hamdy, Curr Opin Investig Drugs 8 (2007) 299.

111. P.I. Croucher, C.M. Shipman & J. Lippitt, et al., Blood 98 (2001) 3534.

112. R.J. Van 't Hof, A.I. Idris & S.A. Ridge, et al., J Bone Min Res 19 (2004) 1651.

113. N.G. Sanerkin, M.G. Mott & J. Roylance, Cancer 51 (1983) 2278.

114. K.K. Unni, C.Y. Inwards, & J.A. Bridge, et al. *Tumors of the Bones and Joints.* American Registry of Pathology in collaboration with the AFIP, Washington, DC, 2005.

115. A.M. Oliveira, A.R. Perez-Atayde & P. Dal Cin, et al., Oncogene 24 (2005) 3419.

116. R.C. Marcove, D.S. Sheth & S. Takemoto, et al., Clin Ortho Rel Res 311 (1995) 157.

117. R. Capanna, D.A. Campanacci & M. Manfrini, Orthop Clin North Am 27 (1996) 605.

118. H.W. Schreuder, R.P. Veth & M. Pruszczynski, J Bone Joint Surg (Br) 79 (1997) 20.

119. J. Cottalorda & S. Bourelle, Arch Orthop Trauma Surg 127 (2007) 105.

120. S.J. Feigenberg, R.B. Marcus & R.A. Zlotecki, et al., Int J Radiat Oncol Biol Phys 49 (2001) 1243.

121. G. Panoutsakopoulos, N. Pandis & I. Kyriazoglou, et al., Genes Chromosomes Cancer 26 (1999) 265.

122. B. O'Sullivan, B. Cummings & C. Catton, et al., Int J Radiat Oncol Biol Phys 32 (1995) 777.

123. B. Berger, U. Ganswindt & M. Bamberg, et al., Int J Radiat Oncol Biol Phys 67 (2007) 1130.

124. S. Wei, H. Kitaura & P. Zhou, et al., J Clin Invest 115 (2005) 282.

125. Y. Ueki, V. Tiziani & C. Santanna, et al., Nature Genet 28 (2001) 125.

126. M. Tartaglia, E.L. Mehler & R. Goldberg, et al., Nature Genet 29 (2001) 465.

127. M. Tartaglia, K. Kalidas & A. Shaw, et al., Am J Hum Genet 70 (2002) 1555.

128. C.I. van Capelle, P.H.G. Hogeman & C.J.M. van der Sijs-Bos, et al., Eur J Pediatrs 166 (2006) 905.

129. F.J. Martinez-Tello, P. Manjon-Luengo & M. Martin-Perez, et al., Skeletal Radiol 34 (2005) 793.

130. U. Krammer, K. Wimmer & P. Wiesbauer, et al., J Child Neurol 18 (2003) 371.

131. T. Jafarov, F. N. & R. E., Clin Genet 68 (2005) 190.

132. J. Mangion, N. Rahman & S. Edkins, et al., Am J Hum Genet 65 (1999) 151.

133. W.A. Jones, Cancer 17 (1933) 946.

134. V.M. Carvalho, P.F. Perdigao, F.J. Pimento, et al. Oral Oncol. 44(2) (2008) 153–155.

135. J. de Lange, M.C. van Maarle, H.P. van den Akker, et al, Oral and maxillofacial pathology 103(3) (2007) 378–381.

136. S.M. Miha, T. Hatani & X. Qu, et al., Genes Cells 9 (2004) 993.

137. C.Y. Li & S.F. Yu, Zhonghua Kou Qiang Yi Xue Za Zhi 41 (2006) 368.

138. B. Lo, M. Faiyaz-Ul-Haque & S. Kennedy, et al., Am J Med Genet 121 (2003) 37.

139. S.A. Lietman, N. Kalinchinko & X. Deng, et al., Hum Mutat 27 (2006) 717.

140. Y. Imai, K. Kanno & T. Moriya, et al., Cleft Palate Craniofac J 40 (2003) 632.

141. W.A. Jones, J. Gerrie & J. Pritchard, J Bone Joint Surg (Br) 32B (1950) 334.

142. N. Thompson, Br J Plast Surg 12 (1959) 89.

143. J. Mangion, S. Edkins & A.N. Goss, et al., J Med Genet 37 (2000) E37.

144. D.V. Novack & R. Faccio, Cell 128 (2007) 15.

145. W. Huang, G. Saberwal & E. Horvath, et al., Mol Cell Biol 26 (2006) 6311.

146. M. Tartaglia, L.A. Pennacchio & C. Zhao, et al., Nature Genet 39 (2007) 75.

147. S. Schubert, M. Zenker & S.L. Rowe, et al., Nature Genet 38 (2006) 331.

148. A.E. Roberts, T. Araki & K.D. Swanson, et al., Nat Genet 39 (2007) 70.

149. B. Pandit, A. Sarkozy & L.A. Pennacchio, et al., Nature Genet 39 (2007) 1007.

150. M.A. Razzaque, T. Nishizawa & Y. Komoike, et al., Nature Genet 39 (2007) 1013.

151. C. Dunlap, B. Neville & R.A. Vickers, et al., Oral Pathol 67 (1989) 698.

152. M.M.J. Cohen & R.J. Gorlin, Am J Med Genet 40 (1991) 159.

153. R.J. Gorlin, R.C. Anderson & M. Blaw, Am J Dis Child 117 (6) (1969) 652.

154. M. Ruggieri, V. Pavone & I.A. Polizz, et al., Oral Surg Oral Med Oral Pathol Oral Radiol Endod 87 (1999) 67.

155. T. Araki, M.G. Mohi & F.A. Ismat, et al., Nat Med 10 (2004) 849.

156. S. Schubbert, K. Lieuw & S.L. Rowe, et al., Blood 106 (2005) 311.

157. D.A. Largaespada, C.I. Brannan & J.D. Shaughnessy, et al., Curr Top Microbiol Immunol 211 (1996) 233.

158. F.C. Yang, S. Chen & A.G. Robling, et al., J Clin Invest 116 (2006) 2880.

CHAPTER **19**

Recent Advances in the Biology of Bone Tumors and New Diagnostic Tools

GONZAGUE DE PINIEUX[1,2] AND CORINNE BOUVIER[3,4]

[1]Service d'Anatomie et Cytologie pathologiques, Hôpital Trousseau, CHRU de Tours.
[2]Faculté de Médecine, Université François Rabelais, Tours.
[3]Service d'Anatomie et Cytologie pathologiques, Hôpital La Timone, CHU de Marseille.
[4]UMR 911, Faculté de Médecine de Timone, Marseille.

Contents

I. INTRODUCTION

The diagnosis of bone tumors is still mainly based on histopathological features and on their comparison with radiological and clinical findings.

The advent of new technical approaches to tissue study, such as immunohistochemistry, cytogenetics and molecular biology, now allows better characterization of these tumors and hence progress in the understanding of their pathogenesis. These advances potentially provide pathologists with new diagnostic and prognostic markers, thus improving the diagnostic approach to bone tumors. They also possibly provide the opportunity to reclassify bone tumors following new criteria, or even describe new entities. This has been particularly effective in the field of soft tissue tumors, to which numerous new entities have been added over the last decade. It has been self limiting in bone tumors, probably because of the greater rarity of these tumors and the deleterious effects of decalcification on the quality of bone tumor samples.

The aim of this chapter is not to review all of the histopathological features of all bone tumors. It focuses on advances made in the characterization of bone tumors and on the new diagnostic tools emerging from research that should assist pathologists in their approach to diagnosis.

II. BONE-FORMING TUMORS

A. Benign Bone-forming Tumors: Osteoid Osteoma and Osteoblastoma

Osteoid osteoma and osteoblastoma have a similar histological pattern, consisting of the combination of a network of osteoid and bony trabeculae, systematized peri-trabecular proliferation of regular osteoblasts and loose fibrovascular stroma, but they are two distinct anatomo-clinical entities. Osteoid osteoma is a process of limited growth potential, size usually not exceeding 1 cm, and is characterized by a typical pain pattern, worse at night and relieved with aspirin. This symptom pattern may be related to the production of prostaglandins by the nidus of the osteoid osteoma and the presence of nerve fibers in this nidus [1].

Osteoblastoma is an expansive tumor process with growth potential, which can reach 11 cm at its widest dimension, and which may be locally aggressive and sometimes very difficult to differentiate from an osteosarcoma.

A link between certain histological features observed in osteoblastoma, particularly the epithelioid appearance of osteoblasts, and aggressive tumor behavior has been suggested [2]. However, it has been reported that such epithelioid osteoblasts may also occur in 'non-aggressive' tumors and aggressive osteoblastoma cannot be considered as a well-defined and consistent histopathological entity. On the other hand, osteoblastoma-like osteosarcomas have also been reported. Their diagnosis depends on tumor biopsy sampling and the presence of permeation of pre-existing bone by the tumor. This last feature may be impossible to

Bone Cancer
ISBN: 978-0-12-374895-9

reveal on limited biopsy material. However, molecular and genetic studies on osteoblastomas, particularly on aggressive or 'border-line' osteoblastic lesions, are very few, and there is currently no marker that could be used to classify these tumors more effectively.

B. Malignant Bone-forming Tumors: Osteosarcomas

'Conventional' osteosarcomas represent about 90% of all osteosarcomas and are high-grade tumors. Low-grade osteosarcomas, representing only 5 to 6% of all osteosarcomas, are quite rare. However, it is for the latter that the understanding of the mechanisms of oncogenesis have evolved most.

1. Low-grade Osteosarcomas

Low-grade osteosarcomas may originate from the central medullary cavity or from the bone surface, called central low-grade osteosarcomas and parosteal osteosarcomas, respectively. While high-grade osteosarcomas are genetically complex tumors, with numerous aberrations, low-grade osteosarcomas are characterized by a simple genetic profile, very similar to that of well-differentiated liposarcomas.

Cytogenetic studies performed on these tumors show the presence of ring chromosomes and giant chromosome markers, with amplified sequences of the short arm of chromosome 12 involving the oncogenes MDM2 and CDK4 [3–5]. Expression of the two corresponding proteins can be studied by immunohistochemistry and thus represents an interesting new tool in the positive and differential diagnosis of low-grade osteosarcomas (Figure 19.1A, B), especially with benign fibroosseous lesions which show no expression.

The above findings raise the hypothesis of a link between the histogenesis of well-differentiated liposarcoma and low-grade osteosarcoma. They suggest that both tumors might originate from a single pluripotent stem cell able to differentiate, depending on the tumor micro-environment (growth factors), into an adipocytic or an osseous phenotype, as has been observed in normal cell differentiation, adipocytes and osteoblasts sharing a common cellular origin and originating from the same mesenchymal stem cell [6].

Moreover, it is very interesting to recognize that the two groups of tumors have a fairly similar outcome, mainly characterized by local malignancy, with the risk of recurrence in the case of incomplete resection, and also by the risk of tumor progression or dedifferentiation, resulting in the acquisition of metastatic potential. Dedifferentiation consists of the occurrence of a high-grade homologous or heterologous sarcomatous component within the low-grade tumor (e.g., osteosarcoma, fibrosarcoma, undifferentiated sarcoma, rhabdomyosarcoma). These findings suggest that genotypic classification should sometimes complement

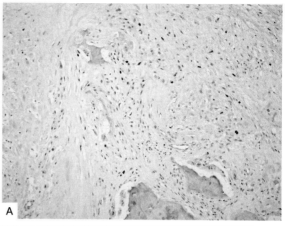

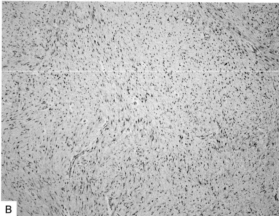

FIGURE 19.1 Immunohistochemistry performed in a case of low-grade osteosarcoma (parosteal type) showing a nuclear staining for MDM2 (1a) and CDK4 (1b) of the tumor spindle cells.

phenotypic classification of sarcomas in terms of evaluation of prognosis.

2. High-grade Osteosarcomas

In contrast to low-grade osteosarcomas, conventional high-grade osteosarcomas are genetically complex tumors. None of the cytogenetic abnormalities have been shown to be valuable in diagnosis, prediction of prognosis or the understanding of the pathogenesis of high-grade osteosarcomas.

Histopathologic evaluation of the post-chemotherapy percentage of tumor necrosis evaluated on the tumor resection specimen according to the method described by Huvos *et al.* is still the main prognostic factor for osteosarcomas. DNA microarray technology has provided interesting approaches to research into new factors predictive of response to chemotherapy by investigating patterns of expression characterizing chemo-resistants tumors. Mintz *et al.* [7] showed in a series of 30 pediatric osteosarcomas that, by reflecting the changes induced by osteosarcoma on the bone tissue micro-environment, the profile of expression of some genes involved in bone remodeling and in osteogenesis and/or osteoclastogenesis might provide characterization to predict the response of the tumor to chemotherapy. One of the candidate markers that emerged from this study is osteoprotegerin, an inhibitor of osteoclastogenesis whose expression is reduced in cases of poor response to chemotherapy. However, further studies on a larger number of tumors are required.

Of the other prognostic markers studied to date in osteosarcoma, HER2 and P-glycoprotein expression appear to be correlated with poor outcome [8]. Morphologically, a rosette pattern in osteosarcoma is also associated with unfavorable prognosis but is very infrequent [9].

Overexpression of ezrin protein has been correlated to the metastatic potential of several cancers especially osteosarcoma. Ezrin belongs to the ERM protein family (ezrin/radixin/moesin) which acts as membrane organizers and linkers between plasma membrane and cytoskeleton. Khanna *et al.*, using sets of cell line variants of osteosarcomas with low or high metastatic properties, found that *vil2* gene coding for ezrin protein was consistently overexpressed in the metastatically capable clones [10]. In a small series of pediatric osteosarcomas (19 cases) the risk of metastatic relapse was 80% greater for patients with high ezrin expression compared to those with low ezrin [11]. More recently, ezrin expression detected by IHC was an independant pronostic factor for disease-free survival and overall survival in multivariate analysis meaning that ezrin expression in biopsy specimens could be one marker that allows identifying high risk group of patients [12,13].

III. CARTILAGINOUS TUMORS

A. Chondroblastoma and Chondromyxoid Fibroma

Chondroblastoma is a rare benign cartilaginous neoplasm with a particular feature of involving the epiphysis of long tubular bones. Histologically, proliferation of mononuclear chondroblasts is intermixed in varying degrees with a population of reactive multinucleated giant cells and an immature cartilaginous matrix [14].

When giant cells are numerous, chondroblastoma may mimic the histological pattern of a giant cell tumor, another benign bone tumor occurring in the epiphysis of long bones. The cytological features of chondroblasts, typically exhibiting a longitudinal nuclear groove, and the presence of chondroid matrix areas distinguish the two entities in most cases.

Immunohistochemistry for S100 protein with positively stained chondroblasts may be helpful in some cases. Chondroblasts have also been shown to stain for cytokeratin and muscle-specific actin [15].

One study [16] has suggested the possible involvement of the CDKN2/p16 gene in the tumorigenesis of both chondroblastoma and primary chondrosarcoma of the bone.

Evaluation of the expression of the corresponding protein by immunohistochemistry may constitute an additional diagnostic marker.

There are some overlapping histological features in chondroblastoma and clear cell chondrosarcoma, another rare cartilaginous tumor with epiphyseal tropism. The cytoplasm of tumor cells of clear cell chondrosarcoma, typically abundant and clear, may in some cases have a more condensed and eosinophilic appearance, then mimicking a chondroblast. Immunohistochemistry for S100 protein is not discriminating and is positive in both tumors. Soder *et al.* [17] suggested the potential value of performing immunostaining for type II collagen to distinguish the two entities. They reported positive staining in all the clear cell chondrosarcomas but none in any of the chondroblastomas studied. Ezrin may also be useful to distinguish clear cell chondrosarcoma from chondroblastoma since it is always negative in this type of chondrosarcoma [18].

Chondromyxoid fibroma is another rare benign cartilaginous tumor, generally involving the metaphysis of long bones. It is characterized histologically by a lobulated growth pattern and proliferation of spindle and stellate cells embedded in a myxoid matrix. Cells with chondroblast-like features can be observed.

S100 protein immunostaining has been shown to be of little help as a positive marker for chondromyxoid fibroma, S100 protein expression being restricted to the chondroid areas. Chondromyxoid fibroma has immunohistochemical and ultrastructural features of partial myofibroblastic differentiation. Romeo *et al.* [19] reported tumor cells exhibiting diffuse immunoreactivity for muscle-specific actin and smooth muscle actin, but not for desmin, h-caldesmon or calponin. The authors hypothesize the role of the TGF-β-1 signaling pathway in the acquisition of this myofibroblastic pattern.

B. Conventional Chondrosarcomas and Differential Diagnosis Between Chondroma and Low-grade Chondrosarcoma

The diagnosis and prognostic evaluation of a chondrosarcoma is still mainly based on morphological, cytological and architectural features, and on their comparison with the radiological and clinical data [20]. Although the molecular pathways involved in the genesis and progression of cartilaginous tumors are still not fully understood, studies have made advances in this field. Chondrosarcomas are divided into conventional chondrosarcomas and the several other rare variants, including dedifferentiated, mesenchymal, clear cell and periosteal chondrosarcomas. Conventional chondrosarcomas may occur in the medullary cavity (central chondrosarcoma) or at the surface of the bone (peripheral chondrosarcoma). These two subtypes of chondrosarcoma, which share similar histopathological features, have seemingly different molecular and cytogenetic bases [21].

1. Central Conventional Chondrosarcomas

The majority of conventional chondrosarcomas (about 85%) are central. Some of them (evaluated between 1 and 40%, or even all of the cases, according to some authors) may result from the transformation of a pre-existing enchondroma. The main difficulty encountered with these tumors is differentiating enchondroma from grade 1 chondrosarcoma, as they exhibit similar cytological features in about 25% of cases.

No genetic abnormality or specific marker has been identified and validated to date. However, some candidate markers appear to be emerging from the greater understanding we have of the tumorogenesis and progression of these tumors. Progression of central chondrosarcoma is a multistage process.

Low-grade central chondrosarcomas are peri-diploid tumors, exhibiting a low percentage of LOH. Among the recurrent abnormalities observed, according to different cytogenetic, LOH and CGH studies, those involving the 9p21 chromosomal region could play an important role in the genesis of these central cartilaginous tumors [21]. Other molecular factors possibly involved in the early development of such chondrosarcomas include the expression of JUNB and COX2. The latter can be revealed by immunohistochemistry and, in both cases, levels of expression are significantly higher in grade 1 chondrosarcomas than in enchondromas [21,22]. These two markers could thus constitute markers of malignancy in a central cartilaginous tumor, but should be validated on larger series of tumors. Study by immunohistochemistry of the expression of tenascin and the proliferation marker KI67 might also constitute a diagnostic tool in the differential diagnosis between grade 1 chondrosarcoma and enchondroma [23]. Immunoreactivity of the tumor cartilaginous matrix with tenascin would indicate a benign cartilaginous tumor.

Progression of chondrosarcoma from low to high grade is characterized by the appearance of aneuploidy and more significant karyotypic abnormalities, with the occurrence of changes in P53 and the increased expression of several metaloproteinases (MMP 1, 2, 9, 12, 13), cathepsins B and L, and PDGFRα [21]. Immunoreactivity for cathepsin B and PDGFRα within a chondrosarcoma appears to be linked to poor outcome, high risk of recurrence and increased metastatic potential.

Loss of INK4A/p16 protein expression, assessed by immunohistochemistry, has been shown to probably be involved in the pathogenesis of chondrosarcoma, correlated with higher histological grade [24]. Papachristou *et al.* showed that the JNK/ERK-AP1/-RUNX2 signaling pathway was associated with the development of chondrosarcoma [25]. The levels of expression of the different constituents of this pathway revealed by immunohistochemistry were found to be significantly higher in low-grade chondrosarcomas compared with enchondromas and rose with grade of malignancy. A similar pattern of expression was also found simultaneously for VEGF.

The expression of gene coding for different types of collagen of the cartilaginous matrix (particularly COL9 and COL2) is decreased in high-grade chondrosarcomas, reflecting the histopathological appearance of these tumors. A study by Mandahl *et al.* [26] suggested that the loss of chromosome 13q, observed in cases of grades 2 and 3 chondrosarcoma but not occurring in cases of grade 1 chondrosarcoma, might constitute a prognostic marker of metastatic dissemination in chondrosarcoma. Rozeman *et al.* [27] identified two candidate genes linked to tumor progression and to the prognosis of central chondrosarcomas in a CGH-array study, i.e. RPS6, located on the short arm of chromosome 9, and CDK4, located on the long arm of chromosome 12.

The PTHLH (parathyroid hormone-like hormone) signaling pathway that has an essential role in the physiological chondrocytic proliferation and differentiation arising in the growth plate, is active in central conventional chondrosarcomas, both benign and malignant. This activity increases with grade of chondrosarcoma, resulting in increased expression of BCL2 and PTHR1.

2. Peripheral Chondrosarcomas

Peripheral chondrosarcomas are much less frequent, accounting for about 15% of conventional chondrosarcomas, and may be secondary to the malignant transformation of an osteochondroma. Activation of the PTHLH signaling pathway and the resulting expression of BCL2 are also observed in peripheral chondrosarcomas but in this case, and notably in that of malignant transformation of osteochondroma, may have diagnostic relevance. This signaling pathway is inactivated in osteochondroma. Its reactivation in the case of malignant transformation results in the expression of BCL2, revealed by immunohistochemistry (Figure 19.2). Moderate to strong or diffuse nuclear immunoreactivity strongly indicates malignancy [28]. However, such immunostaining lacks sensitivity in this author's experience.

In a study performed on osteochondromas and peripheral chondrosarcomas, Hammeetman *et al.* demonstrated a

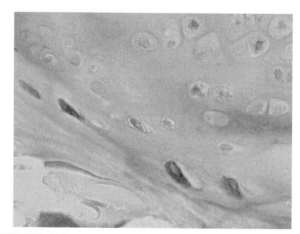

FIGURE 19.2 Positive immunostaining for BCL2 in a case of malignant transformation of an osteochondroma.

significant positive correlation between increased histological grade and expression of CD44 isoforms at the mRNA level, but this correlation was not confirmed at the protein level by immunohistochemistry [29].

Peripheral chondrosarcomas appear to be characterized by greater genetic instability and complexity. They are highly aneuploid tumors, exhibiting a high percentage of LOH and numerous non-specific chromosomal aberrations.

C. Mesenchymal Chondrosarcoma

Mesenchymal chondrosarcoma exhibits complex and unspecific cytogenetic changes [30]. The mesenchymal chondrosarcoma is a small blue round cell tumor consisting of the juxtaposition of a proliferation of small round cells and islands of hyaline cartilage in varying proportions. Wehrli *et al.* [31] showed that the small cell component expressed transcription factor Sox9, which plays a major role in the early stages of chondrocytic differentiation. Expression of this marker may be helpful in differentiating mesenchymal chondrosarcoma from other small blue cell tumors such as the Ewing's tumor, particularly when the cartilaginous hyaline component of the tumor has not been sampled by the biopsy.

IV. FIBROGENIC AND FIBRO-HISTIOCYTIC BONE TUMORS

A. Desmoplastic Fibroma

Desmoplastic fibroma of the bone is a rare benign primary bone tumor, considered to be the bony counterpart of the desmoid-type fibromatosis of soft tissue. It should be histologically distinguished from low-grade central osteosarcoma which may exhibit prominent fibromatosis-like areas. The finding of foci of tumoral bone formation, even small, would indicate osteosarcoma. Immunostaining for MDM2 and CDK4, positive in most low-grade osteosarcomas, might be useful in limited biopsy samples. Such staining is negative in desmoplastic fibroma (author's unpublished data). The β-catenin pathway is known to play an essential role in desmoid-type fibromatosis of soft tissue. Nuclear and cytoplasmic expression can be revealed in these cases by immunohistochemistry and helps to exclude other differential diagnoses. According to the results of a study performed by Hauben *et al.*, this diagnostic tool seems to be useless in the case of desmoplastic fibroma of the bone, as no β-catenin mutation was detected in six cases studied, and positive cytoplasmic and nuclear immunostaining was observed in only one case of the 13 studied [32].

B. Benign Fibrous Histiocytoma

The denomination 'fibrous histiocytoma' should be restricted to symptomatic bone tumors exhibiting the histological features of non-ossifying fibroma, occurring in older patients

and in different locations, particularly the iliac wing. When it occurs within an epiphysis, the giant cell tumor with extensive fibrohistiocytic changes should be excluded [33].

C. Malignant Fibrous Histiocytoma and Fibrosarcoma of the Bone

Malignant fibrous histiocytoma (MFH) and fibrosarcoma of the bone are rare primary non-osteosarcomatous malignant bone tumors. MFH is a high-grade sarcoma, whereas fibrosarcomas are classified in three grades of malignancy. They are diagnosed on their histological appearance and pattern (storiform and herringbone patterns for MFH and fibrosarcoma, respectively) and, in principle, by the absence of an osseous or cartilaginous tumor matrix. In contrast to soft tissue MFH, the entity bone MFH has not been broken down. Immunohistochemically, MFH of the bone frequently expresses smooth muscle markers such as α smooth muscle actin and calponin. Such expression is not specific and is also found in most cases of osteosarcoma.

In a study performed on 26 cases of bone MFH, Tarkannen *et al.* compared CGH findings in MFH with those of osteosarcoma and fibrosarcoma of the bone and found some distinct differences between these three tumors, suggesting they are individual bone tumor entities [34]. In the same study, overexpression of C-MYC protein, correlated with amplification at 8p24, was desmonstrated by immunohistochemistry in 33% of the bone MFHs studied.

V. EWING'S FAMILY TUMORS

Results of cytogenetic studies have made it possible to group together several entities originally regarded as totally separate in a same tumor family, including Ewing's sarcoma, initially described in the bone, PNETs, soft tissue tumors and Askin's tumor, mainly characterized by its thoracopulmonary location. These Ewing's family tumors share a similar cytogenetic abnormality, i.e. balanced t(11; 22)(q24; q12) translocation or one of its variants. Ewing's sarcoma and PNET thus constitute the two extremes of this morphological spectrum known as Ewing's family tumors. As the immunohistochemical markers expressed by these tumors (particularly CD99 and Fli1) lack specificity, demonstration of one of these translocations has increasingly emerged as the 'gold standard' for the diagnosis of Ewing's family tumors. The use of this new diagnostic tool then led to broadening of the morphologic and immunohistochemical spectrum of Ewing's family tumors, with inclusion of non-small blue round cell tumors exhibiting the same specific cytogenetic signature [35]. Adamantinoma-like (Figure 19.3), spindle cell, sclerosing, clear cell or cytokeratin-positive variants of Ewing's sarcoma have thus been described.

There are no specific immunohistochemical markers of Ewing's family tumors. Anti-CD99 (MIC2) and anti-Fli1

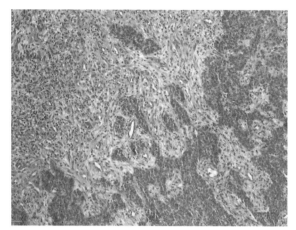

FIGURE 19.3 Ewing's sarcoma mimicking the features of adamantinoma, characterized by cords and sheets of tumor cells in a desmoplastic stroma.

antibodies are expressed by other round cell tumors, particularly lymphoblastic lymphoma. One goal would be to develop monoclonal or polyclonal antibodies recognizing the fusion proteins resulting from the specific balanced translocations characterizing the Ewing's family tumors.

The cellular origin of Ewing's tumor is highly debated. Tirode *et al.* showed that the profiles of gene expression of different EWS-FLI1-silenced Ewing's cell lines converged towards that of mesenchymal stem cells suggesting that Ewing's sarcoma cells could originate from them [36].

VI. NOTOCHORDAL TUMORS

A chordoma is the malignant tumor derived from notochordal remnants. The recognition of a possible benign counterpart (i.e., a 'benign notochordal cell tumor, precursor of chordoma') has been suggested [37]. The histological differential diagnosis of chordoma is mainly chondrosarcoma. Most of the difficulties of diagnosis may be resolved with a simple panel of antibodies, including cytokeratin, the expression of which is present in chordoma and absent in chondrosarcoma. However, some difficulties remain with chondroid chordomas, a particular histological variant of chordoma, mainly encountered at the base of the skull and showing prominent areas of chondroid differentiation. Cytokeratin expression is not always present in these chondroid areas and distinction from chondrosarcoma of the skull base may sometimes be impossible, particularly with needle core biopsy. New markers specific for chordomas have been sought for some years. Tau protein expression has been shown in chordomas by immunohistochemistry (Figure 19.4A) [38], but this immunostaining lacks sensitivity. Tau protein is not expressed by chondrosarcomas (Figure 19.4B). Immunohistochemistry for CAMs was also found to be of diagnostic value for discriminating chordoma from chondrosarcoma especially NCAM which was found

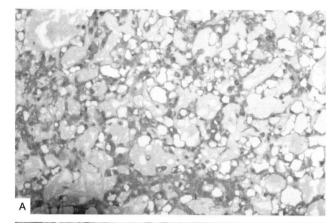

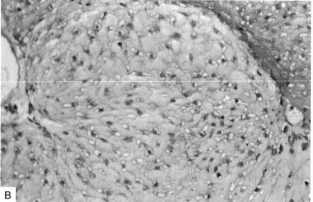

FIGURE 19.4 Differential diagnosis between chordoma and chondrosarcoma: immunohistochemistry for Tau protein: positive in chordoma (A), negative in chondrosarcoma (B).

in more than 90% of chordomas while chondrosarcomas were usually negative [39].

Brachyury, a very promising novel marker emerging from microarray data analysis, has also been identified. Brachyury is a T-box transcription factor involved in notochordal development. Its nuclear expression may be revealed by immunohistochemistry and appears to be a specific and sensitive marker of the notochord and of all notochord-derived tumors, including the different variants of chordoma (classical, chondroid and dedifferentiated). In the latter variant, brachyury expression is absent in undifferentiated areas [40,41]. No brachyury expression has been shown to date in neoplasms that may be mistaken for a chordoma, particularly cartilaginous neoplasms.

VII. GIANT CELL TUMOR

The giant cell tumor of bone is composed of three cell types: mononuclear stromal cells, representing the true proliferative neoplastic component, mononuclear histiocytic cells and multinuclear osteoclast-like giant cells. The last two are recruited by the neoplastic stromal cells by means of factors including key regulators of osteoclastic

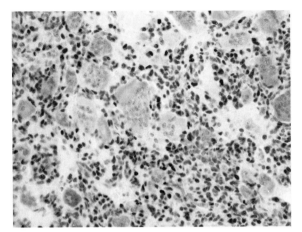

FIGURE 19.5 Immunostaining for P63 in a case of giant cell tumor of bone: nuclear expression in the mononuclear tumor component.

differentiation and function such as the receptor activator of nuclear factor-κB (RANK) and its ligand (RANKL), osteoprotegerin and M-CSF.

Several studies have shown that the mononuclear stromal tumor cells express several osteoblastic markers, including alkaline phosphatase, collagen type I, bone sialoprotein and osteocalcin [41,43]. These markers should be tested in other giant cell-rich lesions, including entities such as aneurysmal bone cysts and chondroblastoma, because they may potentially help the pathologist to distinguish them from giant cell tumors.

Two studies have demonstrated that P63 immunostaining may be a useful tool in the differential diagnosis of giant cell-rich tumors [44,45]. A P63 expression was thus identified in 69 to 100% of giant cell tumor of bone cases studied, whereas it was detected in a smaller proportion of cases of chondroblastoma and aneurysmal bone cyst (20 and 4%, respectively) and was lacking in central giant cell granuloma and giant cell tumor of tendon sheet/pigmented villonodular synovitis.

In giant cell tumor of bone, immunostaining for P63 shows a nuclear expression, predominantly in mononuclear tumor cells (Figure 19.5).

Concerning prognostic factors, in a series of 58 giant-cell tumors, Horvai *et al.* showed that human telomerase reverse transcriptase (h-TERT) expression may predict recurrence in giant-cell tumor insofar as positive immunostaining correlates with shorter recurrence-free survival [46].

VIII. OSTEOFIBRODYSPLASIA AND ADAMANTINOMA

Osteofibrodysplasia (OFD) and amantinoma have several common clinical, immunohistochemical and cytogenetic features, suggesting a relationship between the two entities [47]. Both lesions almost exclusively involve the tibia

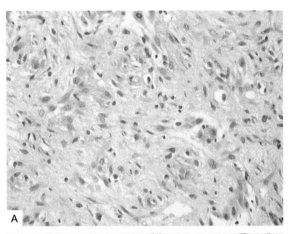

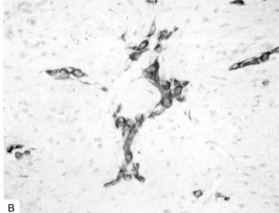

FIGURE 19.6 Differentiated or osteofibrodysplasia-like adamantinoma: small groups of cohesive cells may be detected by careful searching on HE (hematein and eosin) staining (A) or by immunohistochemistry for cytokeratin (B).

and/or the fibula and exhibit epithelial differentiation, following different patterns. The epithelial component in adamantinoma may vary in histologic appearance, providing basaloid, spindle cell, tubular and squamous variants, frequently associated with osteofibrodysplasia-like areas. A differentiated or OFD-like form of adamantinoma has also been described, in which small groups of epithelial cells are only detected by careful searching or immunohistochemistry for keratins (Figure 19.6A, B). In OFD, the differentiation consists of the presence of single cytokeratin-positive cells in about 90% of the lesions (Figure 19.7). Both entities have a common cytokeratin expression profile (CK19+, CK8–, CK18–), common expression of certain oncoproteins (such as c-jun and c-fos) and bone matrix proteins (such fibronectin and osteonectin) and common cytogenetic abnormalities (trisomies 7, 8 and 12) [48]. Moreover, a few cases of OFD-like adamantinoma evolving into a classic variant of adamantinoma have been reported. Although a common histogenesis for OFD and adamantinomas seems likely on the basis of all of these findings, two theories remain, differing from each other by the place occupied by OFD-like adamantinoma in the lesional spectrum. The first

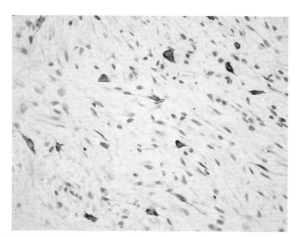

FIGURE 19.7 Immunostaining for cytokeratin in a case of osteofibrodysplasia showing single sparse positive cells.

considers OFD-like adamantinoma as a regressive form of adamantinoma in which the fibro-osseous component took over the epithelial component. The second consists of a multi-stage histogenesis in which OFD adamantinoma represents an intermediate stage between OFD and classic adamantinoma. Further studies are required to elucidate this.

IX. 'PSEUDO NEOPLASTIC PROCESS'

A. Aneurysmal Bone Cyst

An aneurysmal cyst is a lesion composed histologically of cavernous spaces filled with blood and delimited by fibrous walls containing spindle cells of fibroblastic-type histiocytes and osteoclast-like giant cells. An aneurysmal bone cyst may be a primitive, isolated lesion, known as a primary aneurysmal bone cyst, or may be 'secondary', associated with another coexisting lesion, such as giant cell tumor, chondroblastoma, osteoblatoma, etc. A solid variant of a primary aneurysmal bone cyst, composed of a proliferation of spindle cells intermixed with giant cells and histiocytes but lacking cavernous cavities, has been described. Rare cases of primitive aneurysmal cysts of soft tissues have been also reported.

Cytogenetic and molecular findings have opened up new perspectives in the understanding and characterization of aneurysmal bone cysts. Several studies have reported translocations involving chromosome 17 in aneurysmal bone cysts. Recurrent t(16; 17), t(1; 17), (3; 17), (9; 17) and (17; 17) translocations, at the origin of a fusion gene involving oncogene USP6, located in 17p13, and genes CDH11,TRAP150, ZNF9, Osteomodulin and COL1A1, respectively, have been described [49]. These different genes play the role of promoters inducing the activation and overexpression of USP6. These new findings support the neoplastic nature of aneurysmal cysts, regarded since its initial description as a reactive process. Oliveira *et al.* reported

USP6 and/or CDH11 rearrangements in 69% of the 52 cases of primary aneurysmal cysts they studied, whatever the variants (conventional, solid or primary developed in soft tissues), but not in any of the 17 cases of secondary aneurysmal cysts explored. The demonstration of a genetic link between the different variants of primitive aneurysmal cyst leads to the concept of the primary aneurysmal cyst as a particular neoplastic entity, from which secondary aneurysmal cysts are excluded. The latter probably represents a non-specific morphological pattern, mimicking the features of a true aneurysmal bone cyst [50]. USP6 rearrangements have been identified in two patients with myositis ossificans [51]. The value of this genetic tool in diagnostic routine remains to be evaluated.

B. Bizarre Parosteal Osteochondromatous Proliferation (Nora's Lesion) and Subungueal Exostosis

Bizarre parosteal osteochondromatous proliferations (Nora's lesion) and subungueal exostosis are regarded as reactive processes composed of bone and cartilage and involving the small bones of the hands and feet.

Recurrent t(1; 17) and t(X; 6) translocations have been reported in Nora's lesion and subungueal exostosis, respectively, raising questions regarding the reactive nature of these entities [52,53].

1. FIBROUS DYSPLASIA

Fibrous dysplasia is composed of fibrous stroma containing regular small spindle cells and of trabeculae of immature bone appearing as irregular networks and round islands.

Major progress has now been made in the understanding of the histogenesis of fibrous dysplasia. The molecular basis of fibrous dysplasia consists of activating mutations of the Gsα protein, inducing abnormalities in the proliferation and differentiation of osteoblastic precursors by means of increased levels of cAMP [54]. It has also been shown that the small spindle cells in the fibrous stroma of fibrous dysplasia lesions do not in fact belong to the fibroblastic lineage but have the phenotype of preosteoblastic cells. These cells therefore express bone matrix protein such as osteonectin and osteocalcin. They also have been shown to express transcription factors involved in osteoblastic differentiation such as CBFA1 (Runx2) and MSX2. Increased interleukin-6 production has also been observed among the molecular changes in fibrous dysplasia [55].

The potential value of these different markers in the differential diagnosis of histologically atypical fibroosseous bone lesions should be explored. Toyosawa *et al.* [56] reported that osteocalcin immunoreactivity was strong throughout calcified regions of fibrous dysplasia but weak in ossifying fibroma suggesting that this marker could be used for differential diagnosis.

X. CONCLUSION

Cytogenetics and molecular biology have, and will continue to have, a significant impact on the understanding of the histogenesis and probably the classification of bone tumors. These approaches should make it possible to define new diagnostic criteria, new prognostic markers and new therapeutic targets over the next few years and to provide better characterization of tumor response to specific chemotherapy.

Such new markers should be adopted by pathologists and ideally be evaluated by easily performed and reproducible *in situ* techniques such as immunohistochemistry. Nevertheless, their diagnostic and/or prognostic value should first be compared to the current reference markers when they exist. The Tissue MicroArray (TMA) technique, allowing simultaneous study of the expression of a marker on a great number of tumors, constitutes a preferred approach for the validation of candidate markers.

References

1. J.X. O'Connell, S.S. Nanthakumar & G.P. Nielsen, et al., Osteoid osteoma: the uniquely innervated bone tumor, Mod Pathol 1 (1998) 175–180.

2. D.R. Lucas, K.K. Unni & R.A. McLeod, et al., Osteoblastoma: clinicopathologic study of 306 cases, Hum Pathol 25 (1994) 117–134.

3. J. Szymanska, N. Mandahl & F. Mertens, et al., Ring chromosomes in parosteal osteosarcoma contain sequences from 12q13-15: a combined cytogenetic and comparative genomic hybridization study, Genes Chromosomes Cancer 16 (1996) 31–34.

4. J.S. Wunder, K. Eppert & S.R. Burrow, et al., Co-amplification and overexpression of CDK4, SAS and MDM2 occurs frequently in human parosteal osteosarcomas, Oncogene 18 (2000) 783–788.

5. H.R. Park, W.W. Jung & F. Bertoni, et al., Molecular analysis of p53, MDM2 and H-ras genes in low-grade central osteosarcoma, Pathol Res Pract 200 (2004) 439–445.

6. K.D. Bunting & R.G. Hawley, Integrative molecular and developmental biology of adult stem cells, Biol Cell 95 (2003) 563–578.

7. M.B. Mintz, R. Sowers & K.M. Brown, et al., An expression signature classifies chemotherapy-resistant pediatric osteosarcoma, Cancer Res 65 (2005) 1748–1754.

8. K. Scotlandi, M.C. Manara & C.M. Hattinger, et al., Prognostic and therapeutic relevance of HER2 expression in osteosarcoma and Ewing's sarcoma, Eur J Cancer 41 (2005) 1349–1361.

9. K. Okada, T. Hasegawa & R. Yokoyama, et al., Prognostic relevance of rosette-like features in osteosarcoma, J Clin Pathol 56 (2003) 831–834.

10. C. Khanna, J. Khan, P. Nguyen & J. Prehn, et al., Metastasis-associated differences in gene expression in a murine model of osteosarcoma, Cancer Res 61 (2001) 3750–3759.

11. C. Khanna, X. Wan & S. Bose, et al., The membrane-cytoskeleton linker ezrin is necessary for osteosarcoma metastasis, Nat Med 10 (2004) 182–186.

12. M.S. Kim, W.S. Song & W.H. Cho, et al., Ezrin expression predicts survival in stage IIB osteosarcomas, Clin Orthop Relat Res 459 (2007) 229–236.

13. S. Salas, C. Bartoli & J.L. Deville, et al., Ezrin and alpha-smooth muscle actin are immunohistochemical prognostic markers in conventional osteosarcomas, Virchows Arch 451 (2007) 999–1007.

14. M. Forest & G. de Pinieux, Chondroblastoma and its differential diagnosis, Ann Pathol 21 (2001) 468–478.

15. C. Povysil, R. Tomanova & Z. Matejovsky, Muscle-specific actin expression in chondroblastomas, Hum Pathol 28 (1997) 316–320.

16. D.J. Papachristou, M.A. Goodman & K. Cieply, et al., Comparison of allelic losses in chondroblastoma and primary chondrosarcoma of bone and correlation with fluorescence *in situ* hybridization analysis, Hum Pathol 37 (2006) 890–898.

17. S. Soder, A.M. Oliveira & C.Y. Inwards, et al., Type II collagen, but not aggrecan expression, distinguishes clear cell chondrosarcoma and chondroblastoma, Pathology 38 (2006) 35–38.

18. S. Salas, G. De Pinieux & A. Gomez-Brouchet, et al., Ezrin immunohistochemical expression in cartalaginous tumours: a useful tool for differential diagnosis between chondroblastic osteosarcoma and chondrosarcoma, Virchows Arch 454 (2008) 81–87.

19. S. Romeo, B. Eyden & F.A. Prins, et al., TGF-beta1 drives partial myofibroblastic differentiation in chondromyxoid fibroma of bone, J Pathol 208 (2006) 26–34.

20. J.M. Mirra, R. Gold & J. Downs, et al., A new histologic approach to the differentiation of enchondroma and chondrosarcoma of the bones. A clinicopathologic analysis of 51 cases, Clin Orthop 201 (1985) 214–237.

21. J.V. Bovee, AM. Cleton-Jansen & A.H. Taminiau, et al., Emerging pathways in the development of chondrosarcoma of bone and implications for targeted treatment, Lancet Oncol 6 (2005) 599–607.

22. K.M. Sutton, M. Wright & G. Fondren, et al., Cyclooxygenase-2 expression in chondrosarcoma, Oncology 66 (2004) 275–280.

23. M.L. Ranty, C. Michot & F. Le Pessot, et al., PAS inclusions, immunoreactive tenascin and proliferative activity in low-grade chondrosarcomas, Pathol Res Pract 199 (2003) 29–34.

24. H.M. van Beerendonk, L.B. Rozeman & A.H. Taminiau, et al., Molecular analysis of the INK4A/INK4A-ARF gene locus in conventional (central) chondrosarcomas and enchondromas: indication of an important gene for tumour progression, J Pathol 202 (2004) 359–366.

25. D.J. Papachristou, G.I. Papachristou & O.A. Papaefthimiou, et al., The MAPK-AP-1/-Runx2 signaling axes are implicated in chondrosarcoma pathobiology either independently or via up-regulation of VEGF, Histopathology 47 (2005) 565–574.

26. N. Mandahl, P. Gustafson & F. Mertens, et al., Cytogenetic aberrations and their prognostic impact in chondrosarcoma, Genes Chromosomes Cancer 33 (2002) 188–200.

27. L.B. Rozeman, K. Szuhai & Y.M. Schrage, et al., Array-comparative genomic hybridization of central chondrosarcoma: identification of ribosomal protein S6 and cyclin-dependent kinase 4 as candidate target genes for genomic aberrations, Cancer 107 (2006) 380–388.

28. L. Hameetman, P. Kok & P.H. Eilers, et al., The use of Bcl-2 and PTHLH immunohistochemistry in the diagnosis of

peripheral chondrosarcoma in a clinicopathological setting, Virchows Arch 446 (2005) 430–437.

29. L. Hameetman, G. David & A. Yavas, et al., Decreased EXT expression and intracellular accumulation of heparan sulphate proteoglycan in osteochondromas and peripheral chondrosarcomas, J Pathol 211 (2007) 399–409.

30. A.A. Sandberg, Decreased EXT expression and intracellular accumulation of heparan sulphate proteoglycan in osteochondromas and peripheral chondrosarcomas, Curr Opin Oncol 16 (2004) 342–409.

31. B.M. Wehrli, W. Huang & B. De Crombrugghe, et al., Sox9, a master regulator of chondrogenesis, distinguishes mesenchymal chondrosarcoma from other small blue round cell tumors, Hum Pathol 34 (2003) 263–269.

32. E.I. Hauben, G. Jundt & A.M. Cleton-Jansen, et al., Desmoplastic fibroma of bone: an immunohistochemical study including beta-catenin expression and mutational analysis for beta-catenin, Hum Pathol 36 (2005) 1025–1030.

33. F. Bertoni, P. Calderoni & P. Bacchini, et al., Benign fibrous histiocytoma of bone, J Bone Joint Surg Am 68 (1986) 1225–1230.

34. M. Tarkkanen, M.L. Larramendy & T. Bohling, et al., Malignant fibrous histiocytoma of bone: analysis of genomic imbalances by comparative genomic hybridisation and C-MYC expression by immunohistochemistry, Eur J Cancer 42 (2006) 1172–1180.

35. A.L. Folpe, J.R. Goldblum & B.P. Rubin, et al., Morphologic and immunophenotypic diversity in Ewing's family tumors: a study of 66 genetically confirmed cases, Am J Surg Pathol 29 (2005) 1025–1033.

36. F. Tirode, K. Laud-Duval & A. Prieur, et al., Mesenchymal stem cell features of Ewings' tumors, Cancer Cell 11 (2007) 421–429.

37. T. Yamaguchi, S. Suzuki & H. Ishiiwa, et al., Intraosseous benign notochordal cell tumours: overlooked precursors of classic chordomas?, Histopathology 44 (2004) 597–602.

38. C. Gavril, C. Bouvier & A. Liprandi, et al., Pathology of myxoid bone tumors of the skull base, Ann Pathol 22 (2002) 259–266.

39. T. Naka, Y. Oda, Y. Iwamoto & N. Shinohara, et al., Immunohistochemical analysis of E-cadherin, alpha-catenin, beta-catenin, gamma-catenin, and neural cell adhesion molecule (NCAM) in chordoma, J Clin Pathol 54 (2001) 945–950.

40. S. Vujovic, S. Henderson & N. Presneau, et al., Brachyury, a crucial regulator of notochordal development, is a novel biomarker for chordomas, J Pathol 209 (2006) 157–165.

41. P. O'Donnell, R. Tirabosco & S. Vujovic, et al., Diagnosing an extra-axial chordoma of the proximal tibia with the help of brachyury, a molecule required for notochordal differentiation, Skeletal Radiol 36 (2007) 59–65.

42. A. Murata, T. Fujita & N. Kawahara, et al., Osteoblast lineage properties in giant cell tumors of bone, J Orthop Sci 10 (2005) 581–588.

43. L. Huang, X.Y. Teng & Y.Y. Cheng, et al., Expression of preosteoblast markers and Cbfa-1 and Osterix gene transcripts in stromal tumour cells of giant cell tumour of bone, Bone 34 (2004) 393–401.

44. C.H. Lee, I. Espinosa & K.C. Jensen, et al., Gene expression profiling identifies p63 as a diagnostic marker for giant cell tumor of the bone, Mod Pathol 21 (2008) 531–539.

45. B.C. Dickson, S.Q. Li & J.S. Wunder, et al., Giant cell tumor of bone express P63, Modern Pathol 21 (2008) 369–375.

46. A.E. Horvai, M.J. Kramer & J.J. Garcia, et al., Distribution and prognostic significance of human telomerase reverse transcriptase (hTERT) expression in giant-cell tumor of bone, Modern Pathol 21 (2008) 423–430.

47. L.B. Kahn, Adamantinoma, osteofibrous dysplasia and differentiated adamantinoma, Skeletal Radiol 32 (2003) 245–258.

48. M. Maki & N. Athanasou, Osteofibrous dysplasia and adamantinoma: correlation of proto-oncogene product and matrix protein expression, Hum Pathol 35 (2004) 69–74.

49. A.M. Oliveira, A.R. Perez-Atayde & P. Dal Cin, et al., Aneurysmal bone cyst variant translocations upregulate USP6 transcription by promoter swapping with the ZNF9, COL1A1, TRAP150, and OMD genes, Oncogene 24 (2005) 3419–3426.

50. A.M. Oliveira, A.R. Perez-Atayde & C.Y. Inwards, et al., USP6 and CDH11 oncogenes identify the neoplastic cell in primary aneurysmal bone cysts and are absent in so-called secondary aneurysmal bone cysts, Am J Pathol 165 (2004) 1773–1780.

51. W.R. Sukov, M.F. Franco & M. Erickson-Johnson, et al., Frequency of USP6 rearrangements in myositis ossificans, brown tumor, and cherubism: molecular cytogenetic evidence that a subset of 'myositis ossificans-like lesions' are the early phases in the formation of soft-tissue aneurysmal bone cyst, Skeletal Radiol 37 (2008) 321–327.

52. M. Nilsson, H.A. Domanski & F. Mertens, et al., Molecular cytogenetic characterization of recurrent translocation breakpoints in bizarre parosteal osteochondromatous proliferation (Nora's lesion), Hum Pathol 35 (2004) 1063–1069.

53. C.T. Storlazzi, A. Wozniak & I. Panagopoulos, et al., Rearrangement of the COL12A1 and COL4A5 genes in subungual exostosis: molecular cytogenetic delineation of the tumor-specific translocation t(X;6)(q13-14;q22), Int J Cancer 118 (2006) 1972–1976.

54. M. Riminucci, B. Liu & A. Corsi, et al., The histopathology of fibrous dysplasia of bone in patients with activating mutations of the Gs alpha gene: site-specific patterns and recurrent histological hallmarks, J Pathol 187 (1999) 249–258.

55. P.J. Marie, Cellular and molecular basis of fibrous dysplasia, Histol Histopathol 16 (2001) 981–988.

56. S. Toyosawa, M. Yuki & M. Kishino, et al., Ossifying fibroma vs fibrous dysplasia of the jaw: molecular and immunological characterization, Mod Pathol 20 (2007) 389–396.

CHAPTER **20**

Ewing's Sarcoma Family of Tumors

JOSEPH D. KHOURY[1]

[1]*Department of Pathology, Nevada Cancer Institute and Quest Diagnostics, Las Vegas, Nevada, USA.*

Contents

I. INTRODUCTION

The terms 'Ewing's sarcoma', 'peripheral primitive neuro-ectodermal tumor (PNET)', and 'malignant small cell tumor of the thoracopulmonary region' [1] (Askin tumor) are currently regarded as manifestations of a single neoplastic entity with underlying common phenotypic and molecular features. These tumors are now grouped under the general eponym Ewing's sarcoma family of tumors (ESFT) and are characterized by non-random translocations involving the *EWS* gene and one of several members of the ETS family of transcription factors [2].

The Ewing's sarcoma family of tumors is the second most common malignant neoplasm of bone arising in children and adolescents, with osteosarcoma being the most common. In the United States, the annual incidence rate of ESFT in the general population is three per million [3]. Boys are more commonly affected than girls, and the disease exhibits marked predilection for whites and is particularly rare among black people (Table 20.1). Most patients are between the ages of 5 and 20 years at the time of diagnosis (median, 14 years), and the disease is rare in individuals older than 40 and younger than 5 years [4–6].

There is no evidence that ESFT is associated with any familial predisposition syndrome or environmental factors. Several studies have demonstrated an increased cumulative risk of secondary cancers following therapy for ESFT, with radiation-induced osteosarcoma and therapy-related acute myeloid leukemia being the most frequent [7–10]. Conversely, the occurrence of ESFT as a second neoplasm after therapy for other tumors is rare [11,12].

TABLE 20.1 Incidence of Ewing's sarcoma family of tumors according to the International Classification of Childhood Cancer*

	Incidence rate (per 10^6 persons)	
Patient group	**Ewing's sarcoma**	**PNET**
All races		
Boys	4.0	0.5
Girls	2.8	0.6
White race		
Boys	4.6	0.6
Girls	3.2	0.7
Other races		
Boys	3.1	~
Girls	~	~

*From US Cancer Statistics Working Group. *United States Cancer Statistics: 1999–2001 Incidence and Mortality Web-based Report Version.* Atlanta (GA): Department of Health and Human Services, Centers for Disease Control and Prevention, and National Cancer Institute, 2004.
~Numbers are suppressed due to low incidence. PNET: primitive neuroectodermal tumor.

II. PATHOGENESIS

A. Cell of origin

The cell of origin of ESFT is still unknown. The most widely held view at present is that ESFT is derived from pluripotent neural crest cells that have features of parasympathetic post-ganglionic cholinergic neurons [13–16]. One study using cDNA expression microarrays revealed a high similarity between the pattern of gene expression in ESFT cells and that in endothelial and fetal neural crest-derived cells [17]. In another study, it was demonstrated that *in vitro* expression of EWS-FLI1 or EWS-ERG in bone marrow stromal cells alters their morphology and blocks their differentiation along osteogenic and adipogenic lineages [18].

Bone Cancer
ISBN: 978-0-12-374895-9

B. Molecular features

At present, the hallmark feature of ESFT is the presence of non-random translocations leading to the fusion of the *EWS* gene with one of several members of the ETS family of transcription factors [19] (Table 20.2). The most frequent of these translocations is t(11;22)(q24;q12), which is detected in 90–95% of cases [20,21]. This leads to in-frame fusion of *EWS* at 22q12 to *FLI1* at 11q24 and the formation of EWS-FLI1 on der(22) comprising the 5′ end of *EWS* and the 3′ end of *FLI1* [21] (Figure 20.1). The fusion gene encodes an oncoprotein consisting of the N-terminal domain of EWS and the DNA-binding domain of FLI1 [22].

TABLE 20.2   Recurrent chromosomal translocations in the Ewing's sarcoma family of tumors

Translocation	Fusion gene	Prevalence
t(11;22)(q24;q12)	EWS-FLI1	90%
t(21;22)(q22;q12)	EWS-ERG	10%
t(7;22)(p22;q12)	EWS-ETV1	<1%
t(17;22)(q12;q12)	EWS-E1AF	<1%
t(2;22)(q33;q12)	EWS-FEV	<1%
inv(22)	EWS-ZSG	<1%

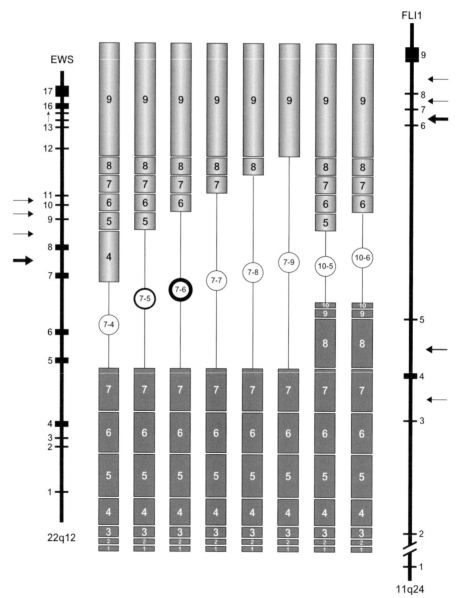

FIGURE 20.1   Schematic depiction of the *EWS* and *FLI1* genes and the most common fusion products resulting from the t(11;22) translocation. Arrows highlight the most common breakpoints. All translocations include exons encoding the N-terminal domain of EWS (exons 1–7) and the DNA-binding domain of FLI1 (exon 9). EWS-FLI1 transcripts are referred to by the exon numbers involved (not drawn to scale).

The second most common non-random translocation is t(21;22)(q22;q12), which is identified in approximately 5–10% of cases and leads to the fusion of *EWS* to *ERG* at 21q22 [23]. Other translocations, which are seen in less than 1% of cases, include t(7;22)(p22;q12), t(17;22)(q12;q12), t(2;22), and inv(22) and lead to fusion of *EWS* with the ETS genes *ETV1, E1AF, FEV,* and *ZSG,* respectively [24–28].

The *EWS* gene spans approximately 40 kb of DNA and is composed of 17 exons [29]. The first seven exons encode the N-terminal region, which is involved in regulating the specificity of the RNA-binding capability of EWS [30]. The RNA-binding capability is localized to the 86 amino acids that comprise the C-terminal region [30]. Three key features indicate that this protein is encoded by a housekeeping gene: EWS is expressed ubiquitously, its expression is stable throughout the cell cycle, and its mRNA has a long half-life [31]. EWS belongs to a subgroup of RNA-binding proteins called the TET family, which also includes TLS/FUS and hTAFII68 [31,32]. Although more remains to be known about the role of native EWS, it is a nuclear protein that appears to be recruited to promoter regions where it associates with other factors to act as a promoter-specific transactivator [33]. It is noteworthy that TET family members are associated with nearly half of sarcomas with characteristic non-random chromosomal translocations, including ESFT, clear cell sarcoma, desmoplastic small round cell tumor, myxoid chondrosarcoma, and myxoid liposarcoma [34]. Interestingly, rare cases of tumors with ESFT-like features harboring FUS-ERG fusion transcripts have recently been reported [35].

The ETS family of transcription factors is defined by a conserved ETS domain that recognizes a core DNA motif of GGAA/T [36]. This family of approximately 30 genes including *FLI1, ERG, ETV1, E1AF, FEV,* and *ZSG* controls a variety of cellular functions in cooperation with other transcription factors and cofactors. Target genes include oncogenes, tumor suppressor genes, and genes related to apoptosis, differentiation, angiogenesis, and invasion [36,37]. Unlike *EWS,* which is ubiquitously expressed, native *FLI1* expression is highly restricted to endothelial and hematopoietic cells [38,39]. FLI1 expression is crucial for hematopoiesis and early vascular development, as demonstrated in knockout mice [40] and zebrafish [41].

The EWS/ETS fusion proteins appear to modulate the expression of target genes in a sequence-specific manner that is determined by the ETS component coming under the control of the potent EWS transactivation component. EWS-FLI1 transforms NIH3T3 mouse fibroblasts when both the EWS and FLI1 functional domains are intact [42]. However, neither FLI1 overexpression nor mutations in its DNA-binding domain are capable of recapitulating the transforming properties of EWS-FLI1, which suggests that the chimeric protein affects target genes that are different from those recognized by FLI1 [22,42,43]. Importantly, when EWS-FLI1 expression is reduced by antisense

oligonucleotides, small interfering RNA (siRNA), or competitive inhibitors, ESFT cell lines die and tumors in nude mice regress [44–48].

III. CLINICAL FEATURES

A. Symptoms

Most patients with ESFT present with localized pain and a visible or palpable mass [49]. Systemic symptoms, especially fever and weight loss, are also common particularly among patients who present with advanced-stage disease. In patients with systemic symptoms, osteomyelitis constitutes an important clinical differential diagnostic consideration. Fractures are identified in up to 15% of patients with ESFT of long bones, most commonly at the time of diagnosis [50].

B. Sites of Disease

In bone, ESFT arise with equal frequency in the appendicular and the axial skeletons, commonly involve the diaphysis, and are more common in flat bones than is osteosarcoma [51]. The femur is the most common long bone involved, followed by the tibia, fibula, and humerus. Bones of the pelvis are the next most common group involved. Nevertheless, ESFT may affect any bone, including the ribs, scapula, spine, clavicle and skull [5,6,52]. Extraosseous ESFT may arise anywhere in the body, including soft tissue, skin, and visceral organs [53–55].

C. Imaging Studies

Imaging studies commonly included in the evaluation of patients with ESFT are plain radiographs of primary and metastatic sites, bone scintigraphy, plain radiographs and computed tomography of the chest, and magnetic resonance imaging (MRI) of the primary site. MRI is the most sensitive imaging modality for delineating the extent of tumor in the medullary cavity and in soft tissue. Imaging features favoring ESFT include diaphyseal location and permeation into soft tissue without frank cortical destruction (Figure 20.2). The major differential diagnostic considerations on diagnostic imaging are usually osteosarcoma and osteomyelitis.

IV. PATHOLOGY

A. Histology

As a group, ESFT exhibits a wide spectrum of cellular morphologic features. Tumors arising in bone (Ewing's sarcoma) are usually composed of uniform small round cells with round nuclei containing fine chromatin and small nucleoli, scant clear or eosinophilic cytoplasm, and indistinct

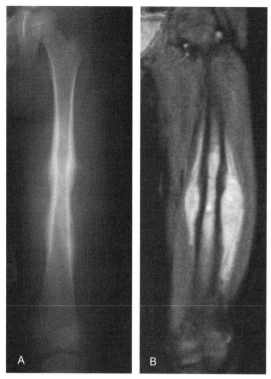

FIGURE 20.2 Ewing's sarcoma family tumor (ESFT) arising in the left femoral diaphysis of a 10-year old girl. (A) Plain radiograph demonstrates a permeative aggressive lytic bone lesion with soft tissue involvement. Codman triangles are present at the proximal aspect of the tumor; (B) post-contrast magnetic resonance imaging (MRI) reveals the extent of bone marrow and soft tissue involvement. The mid-diaphyseal location, the permeative nature of the tumor, and the presence of a soft tissue mass without frank cortical destruction, are all features of ESFT (Courtesy Dr. M. Beth McCarville, St. Jude Children's Research Hospital, Memphis, Tennessee).

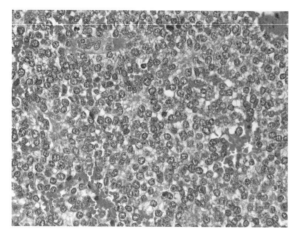

FIGURE 20.3 Microscopic features of the Ewing's sarcoma family of tumors (ESFT). This case is comprised of uniform, small, undifferentiated cells with scant cytoplasm and vesicular chromatin.

cytoplasmic membranes (Figure 20.3) True rosette structures may be identified occasionally [56]. Mitotic figures and necrosis are variable in frequency. A small subset of tumors is composed of relatively larger cells with irregular nuclear contours and prominent nucleoli [57].

Intracytoplasmic glycogen within neoplastic cells may be demonstrated using PAS staining and diastase digestion. While of historical value, this technique lacks specificity and is not recommended currently for the diagnostic workup for ESFT. Primitive intercellular junctions, indicating epithelial differentiation, and dense core granules, indicating neural differentiation, may be identified by electron microscopy [58].

B. Immunohistochemistry

Most ESFT express CD99 which is a cell membrane protein encoded by the *MIC2* gene located in the pseudoautosomal region at the end of the short arms of the X and Y chromosomes [59–64]. CD99 is a 32-kDa cell surface antigen with broad cellular expression whose function remains incompletely understood but believed to be involved in T-cell regulation [65–68].

While expressed by most ESFT, CD99 expression is not specific for ESFT and may be detected in lymphoblastic lymphoma, embryonal rhabdomyosarcoma, and other soft tissue sarcomas [59,64,69,70]. Nevertheless, in the absence of conclusive molecular data, strong diffuse CD99 immunostaining constitutes a useful marker for ESFT in tumors lacking features suggestive of other round cell malignancies. CD99 is most useful as part of a panel of immunostains that also includes myogenin-D1, TdT, and NB84 synaptophysin, which are helpful in ruling out the major differential diagnostic considerations rhabdomyosarcoma, lymphoblastic lymphoma, and neuroblastoma, respectively (Table 20.3) Distinction between ESFT and small cell osteosarcoma rests on the absence of CD99 expression and identification of osteoid deposition in the latter and on identification of ESFT-specific translocations.

C. Molecular Diagnostics

Translocations   involving the EWS gene are detected in the vast majority of ESFT, most commonly using reverse transcriptase polymerase chain reaction (RT-PCR) and fluorescence *in situ* hybridization (FISH).

1. RT-PCR

Up to 18 types of in-frame *EWS-FLI1* chimeric transcripts are possible and, of note, all contain the transactivating amino-terminal domain of EWS (exons 1 to 7) and the ETS-type DNA-binding domain of FLI1 (exon 9) [71]. The portion of the chimeric protein between these two domains is variable in size and composition, reflecting genomic breaks in one of four *EWS* introns and one of six *FLI1* introns [29,71]. The two main fusion types, fusion of *EWS* exon 7

TABLE 20.3   Immunohistochemistry panel frequently employed when working up Ewing's sarcoma family of tumors (ESFT)

	ESFT	ALL	Neuroblastoma	Rhabdomyosarcoma
CD99	+	+/−	+/−	+/−
TdT	−	+	−	−
Synaptophysin	−/+	−	+	−
NB84	−	−	+	−
Myogenin	−	−	−	+
MyoD1	−	−	−	+

ESFT: Ewing's sarcoma family of tumors; ALL: acute lymphoblastic leukemia/lymphoma.

to *FLI1* exon 6 (so-called type 1) and fusion of *EWS* exon 7 to *FLI1* exon 5 (so-called type 2), account for about 85% of *EWS-FLI1* fusions [72,73]. All other *EWS-FLI1* fusion types are designated by the exons involved, by convention.

EWS exon 7 forward and *FLI1* exon 9 reverse primers should amplify all forms of *EWS-FLI1*, with potential amplification products of variable sizes. However, using this approach may result in false negative results in tumors harboring large fusions such as types 9-4 or 10-5, especially if sample RNA is partially degraded. An alternative approach entails using initially an *FLI1* exon 6 reverse primer in combination with an *EWS* exon 7 forward primer. Such a primer pair will yield small RT-PCR products in more than 85% of cases with *EWS-FLI1*. To ensure detection of a minority of possible false-negative cases, a second-line reaction in which the *EWS* exon 7 forward primer is paired with an *FLI1* exon 9 reverse primer and an *ERG* reverse primer is performed.

Approximately 5% of ESFT harbor a complex or cryptic t(21;22)(q22;q12) that rearranges *EWS* with another ETS family gene, *ERG* [23,74]. With an exon structure highly analogous to *FLI1*, several translocation variants of *EWS-ERG* have been noted [71,74,75]. It is noteworthy that enough molecular homology exists between *FLI1*, *ERG*, and *FEV* to allow the design of consensus reverse primers that could detect all the corresponding translocations using one assay.

The use of PCR methods for detection of t(11;22) in formalin-fixed, paraffin-embedded tissue is currently feasible, provided the tissue has not been subjected to acid decalcification [76–80].

2. FLUORESCENCE *IN SITU* HYBRIDIZATION

At present, FISH is regarded as the technique of choice in confirming the presence of EWS/ETS translocations. The reasons include technical ease, low cost, high sensitivity and specificity when analyzing tumor samples, ability to use minimal frozen tissue, non-decalcified paraffin-embedded tissue, or adequately prepared cytology material. In retrospective studies, both the sensitivity and specificity of FISH were found to be superior to those of RT-PCR [81, 82]. One of the major limitations of FISH is its inability to delineate the type of EWS-FLI1 translocation.

A variety of FISH assays have been described for the detection of non-random translocations in ESFT [83–86]. Two testing strategies using the FISH technique have evolved over the past decade: the break apart and the fusion strategies.

Using the break apart strategy, FISH is performed using a dual-color cocktail of DNA probes flanking the EWS breakpoint region on chromosome 22 to detect breaks at the EWS locus [83]. This EWSR1 dual color break apart set is currently available commercially (Vysis Inc., Downers Grove, IL, USA). It combines a 500 kb Spectrum Orange-labeled probe on the centromeric side of the 7 kb EWSR1 breakpoint region between exons 7 and 10 of the EWS gene with an 1100 kb Spectrum Green-labeled probe localizing just telomeric to this breakpoint region. If a translocation involving the EWS gene is present, the signals (usually red and green pseudocolors) would be spatially apart within nuclei of the tumor cells (Figure 20.4). While this approach is capable of detecting any translocation involving EWS,

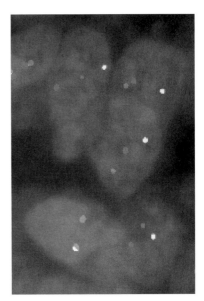

FIGURE 20.4   Fluorescence *in situ* hybridization using a cocktail of probes specific for the *EWS* gene at 22q12 (red) and the *FLI1* gene at 11q24 (green). Juxtaposition of the red and green pseudocolors (occasionally manifesting as a yellow signal) indicates the presence of the EWS-FLI1 translocation.

it is not specific for ESFT by virtue of its inherent inability to demonstrate the nature of the translocation partner.

V. THERAPY AND CLINICAL OUTCOME

A. Therapy

Treatment of ESFT consists of two major components: systemic chemotherapy and local control. These two components are carried out in three phases: (1) induction chemotherapy, the goal of which is to achieve rapid initial cytoreduction and facilitate local control; (2) local control using surgery, radiation therapy, or both, usually after 10 to 12 weeks of induction chemotherapy; and (3) continuation therapy, which consists of chemotherapeutic regimens similar to those used for induction [87].

B. Outcome and Prognostic Factors

Survival estimates for patients with metastatic ESFT at diagnosis are significantly lower than those for patients who present with localized disease [5,87]. Furthermore, pelvic ESFT is commonly insidious, and patients tend to present later in the disease course with advanced-stage disease. In one study, 25% of patients with primary pelvic ESFT had metastasis at diagnosis compared to 16% for patients with tumors arising at other sites [5]. In another study, 32% of patients with pelvic ESFT had metastatic disease at the time of diagnosis [52]. The most common sites of metastasis are the lungs, bone, and bone marrow. Metastasis to other sites is less common, except in late stages of the disease. Furthermore, patients with metastasis restricted to lungs appear to have a better clinical outcome in comparison to patients with metastasis restricted to skeletal sites or patients with both skeletal and lung metastasis [88].

Detection of submicroscopic disease in the bone marrow by RT-PCR has been associated with metastatic disease, and it appears to denote a more adverse clinical outcome among patients with apparently localized disease [89–92]. Although some data demonstrate no correlation between the detection of fusion-positive cells in peripheral blood and tumor size, primary site, metastasis, or survival, other data suggest that the presence of fusion transcript-positive cells in peripheral blood is associated with and may be predictive of disease progression [89, 92].

Two studies have indicated that patients with localized tumors harboring the EWS-FLI1 type 1 fusion transcript may have a more favorable clinical outcome than do patients with other EWS-FLI1 fusion types [93,94]. The underlying cause for such a difference has been postulated to result from the type 1 fusion transcript encoding a less active chimeric transcription factor [93]. There is no evidence, however, that EWS-FLI1 and EWS-ERG are associated with different clinical characteristics [95].

Chromosomal abnormalities in ESFT can also include both numerical and structural findings. The most common are gains of chromosomes 8, 12, 20, and 1q, losses of 16q and 19q, and the translocation der(16)t(1;16)(q12;q11.2) [96–101]. The presence and frequency of secondary chromosomal changes may be associated with worse clinical outcome [100,102,103]. In one study, deletions at the short arm of chromosome 1 were associated with an unfavorable outcome in patients with localized disease [103]. In another study, multivariate analysis revealed that the loss of 16q was an independent prognostic factor [100].

References

1. F.B. Askin, J. Rosai & R.K. Sibley, et al., Cancer 43 (1979) 2438–2451.
2. U. Ushigome, R. Machinami & P.H. Sorensen, in: C.D.M. Fletcher, K.K. Unni & F. Mertens (Eds.), World Health Organization Classification of Tumours. Pathology and Genetics of Tumours of Soft Tissue and Bone, IARC Press, Lyon, 2002, pp. 298–300.
3. L.A.G.E.M. Ries, C.L. Kosary & B.F. Hankey, et al., SEER Cancer Statistics Review, 1975–2001, National Cancer Institute, Bethesda, MD, 2004.
4. R.M. Wilkins, D.J. Pritchard, E.O. Burgert Jr. & K.K. Unni, Cancer 58 (1986) 2551–2555.
5. S.J. Cotterill, S. Ahrens & M. Paulussen, et al., J Clin Oncol 18 (2000) 3108–3114.
6. K. Fizazi, N. Dohollou & J.Y. Blay, et al., J Clin Oncol 16 (1998) 3736–3743.
7. L.B. Travis, R.E. Curtis, B.F. Hankey & J.F. Fraumeni Jr., Med Pediatr Oncol 22 (1994) 296–297.
8. M. Gasparini, F. Lombardi & E. Ballerini, et al., Med Pediatr Oncol 23 (1994) 406–412.
9. J.F. Kuttesch Jr., L.H. Wexler & R.B. Marcus, et al., J Clin Oncol 14 (1996) 2818–2825.
10. J. Dunst, S. Ahrens & M. Paulussen, et al., Int J Radiat Oncol Biol Phys 42 (1998) 379–384.
11. S.L. Spunt, C. Rodriguez-Gahindo & C.E. Fuller, et al., Cancer 107(1) (2006) 201–206.
12. R. Fisher, S.C. Kaste & D.M. Parham, et al., J Pediatr Hematol Oncol 17 (1995) 76–80.
13. F. van Valen, W. Winkelmann & H. Jurgens, J Cancer Res Clin Oncol 118 (1992) 529–536.
14. S. O'Regan, M.F. Diebler & F.M. Meunier, et al., J Neurochem 64 (1995) 69–76.
15. M. Lipinski, K. Braham & I. Philip, et al., Cancer Res 47 (1987) 183–187.
16. M. Lipinski, K. Braham & I. Philip, et al., J Cell Biochem 31 (1986) 289–296.
17. M.S. Staege, C. Hutter & I. Neumann, et al., Cancer Res 64 (2004) 8213–8221.
18. E.C. Torchia, S. Jaishankar & S.J. Baker, Cancer Res 63 (2003) 3464–3468.
19. O. Delattre, J. Zucman & T. Melot, et al., N Engl J Med 331 (1994) 294–299.
20. C. Turc-Carel, I. Philip & M.P. Berger, et al., C R Seances Acad Sci III 296 (1983) 1101–1103.

21. O. Delattre, J. Zucman & B. Plougastel, et al., Nature 359 (1992) 162–165.

22. W.A. May, M.L. Gishizky & S.L. Lessnick, et al., Proc Natl Acad Sci USA A 90 (1993) 5752–5756.

23. P.H. Sorensen, S.L. Lessnick & D. Lopez-Terrada, et al., Nat Genet 6 (1994) 146–151.

24. I.S. Jeon, J.N. Davis & B.S. Braun, et al., Oncogene 10 (1995) 1229–1234.

25. Y. Kaneko, K. Yoshida & M. Handa, et al., Genes Chromosomes Cancer 15 (1996) 115–121.

26. F. Urano, A. Umezawa & W. Hong, et al., Biochem Biophys Res Commun 219 (1996) 608–612.

27. M. Peter, J. Couturier & H. Pacquement, et al., Oncogene 14 (1997) 1159–1164.

28. T. Mastrangelo, P. Modena & S. Tornielli, et al., Oncogene 19 (2000) 3799–3804.

29. B. Plougastel, J. Zucman & M. Peter, et al., Genomics 18 (1993) 609–615.

30. T. Ohno, M. Ouchida & L. Lee, et al., Oncogene 9 (1994) 3087–3097.

31. P. Aman, I. Panagopoulos & C. Lassen, et al., Genomics 37 (1996) 1–8.

32. A. Bertolotti, Y. Lutz & D.J. Heard, et al., Embo J 15 (1996) 5022–5031.

33. K.L. Rossow & R. Janknecht, Cancer Res 61 (2001) 2690–2695.

34. L.J. Helman & P. Meltzer, Nat Rev Cancer 3 (2003) 685–694.

35. D.C. Shing, D.J. McMullan & P. Roberts, et al., Cancer Res 63 (2003) 4568–4576.

36. V.I. Sementchenko & D.K. Watson, Oncogene 19 (2000) 6533–6548.

37. A.D. Sharrocks, Nat Rev Mol Cell Biol 2 (2001) 827–837.

38. A.L. Folpe, E.M. Chand & J.R. Goldblum, et al., Am J Surg Pathol 25 (2001) 1061–1066.

39. A.H. Truong & Y. Ben-David, Oncogene 19 (2000) 6482–6489.

40. A. Hart, F. Melet & P. Grossfeld, et al., Immunity 13 (2000) 167–177.

41. L.A. Brown, A.R. Rodaway & T.F. Schilling, et al., Mech Dev 90 (2000) 237–252.

42. W.A. May, S.L. Lessnick & B.S. Braun, et al., Mol Cell Biol 13 (1993) 7393–7398.

43. S. Jaishankar, J. Zhang & M.F. Roussel, et al., Oncogene 18 (1999) 5592–5597.

44. A. Prieur, F. Tirode & P. Cohen, et al., Mol Cell Biol 24 (2004) 7275–7283.

45. M. Ouchida, T. Ohno & Y. Fujimura, et al., Oncogene 11 (1995) 1049–1054.

46. K. Tanaka, T. Iwakuma & K. Harimaya, et al., J Clin Invest 99 (1997) 239–247.

47. A. Maksimenko, G. Lambert & J.R. Bertrand, et al., Ann NY Acad Sci 1002 (2003) 72–77.

48. G. Lambert, J.R. Bertrand & E. Fattal, et al., Biochem Biophys Res Commun 279 (2000) 401–406.

49. B. Widhe & T. Widhe, J Bone Joint Surg Am 82 (2000) 667–674.

50. L.M. Wagner, M.D. Neel & A.S. Pappo, et al., J Pediatr Hematol Oncol 23 (2001) 568–571.

51. D.M. Parkin, C.A. Stiller & J. Nectoux, Int J Cancer 53 (1993) 371–376.

52. C. Hoffmann, S. Ahrens & J. Dunst, et al., Cancer 85 (1999) 869–877.

53. M.J. O'Sullivan, E.J. Perlman & J. Furman, et al., Hum Pathol 32 (2001) 1109–1115.

54. S.L. Hasegawa, J.M. Davison & A. Rutten, et al., Am J Surg Pathol 22 (1998) 310–318.

55. R.E. Jimenez, A.L. Folpe & R.L. Lapham, et al., Am J Surg Pathol 26 (2002) 320–327.

56. R. Jaffe, M. Santamaria & E.J. Yunis, et al., Am J Surg Pathol 8 (1984) 885–898.

57. A.G. Nascimento, K.K. Unii & D.J. Pritchard, et al., Am J Surg Pathol 4 (1980) 29–36.

58. C.H. Suh, N.G. Ordonez & J. Hicks, et al., Ultrastruct Pathol 26 (2002) 67–76.

59. E.J. Fellinger, P. Garin-Chesa & T.J. Triche, et al., Am J Pathol 139 (1991) 317–325.

60. I.M. Ambros, P.F. Ambros & S. Strehl, et al., Cancer 67 (1991) 1886–1893.

61. G.S. Banting, B. Pym & S.M. Darling, et al., Mol Immunol 26 (1989) 181–188.

62. S.M. Darling, P.J. Goodfellow & B. Pym, et al., Cold Spring Harb Symp Quant Biol 51 Pt 1 (1986) 205–212.

63. H. Kovar, M. Dworzak & S. Strehl, et al., Oncogene 5 (1990) 1067–1070.

64. E.J. Perlman, P.S. Dickman & F.B. Askin, et al., Hum Pathol 25 (1994) 304–307.

65. C. Gelin, F. Aubrit & A. Phalipon, et al., Embo J 8 (1989) 3253–3259.

66. M. Waclavicek, O. Majdic & T. Stulnig, et al., J Immunol 161 (1998) 4671–4678.

67. D. Wingett, K. Forcier & C.P. Nielson, Cell Immunol 193 (1999) 17–23.

68. G. Bernard, J.P. Breittmayer & M. de Matteis, et al., J Immunol 158 (1997) 2543–2550.

69. E.J. Fellinger, P. Garin-Chesa & D.B. Glasser, et al., Am J Surg Pathol 16 (1992) 746–755.

70. K. Scotlandi, M. Serra & M.C. Manara, et al., Hum Pathol 27 (1996) 408–416.

71. J. Zucman, T. Melot & C. Desmaze, et al., Embo J 12 (1993) 4481–4487.

72. A. Zoubek, C. Pfleiderer & M. Salzer-Kuntschik, et al., Br J Cancer 70 (1994) 908–913.

73. A. Zoubek, B. Dockhorn-Dworniczak & O. Delattre, et al., J Clin Oncol 14 (1996) 1245–1251.

74. M. Giovannini, J.A. Biegel & M. Serra, et al., J Clin Invest 94 (1994) 489–496.

75. K. Ida, S. Kobayashi & T. Taki, et al., Int J Cancer 63 (1995) 500–504.

76. V. Adams, M.A. Hany & M. Schmid, et al., Diagn Mol Pathol 5 (1996) 107–113.

77. M.K. Fritsch, J.A. Bridge & A.E. Schuster, et al., Pediatr Dev Pathol 6 (2003) 43–53.

78. M. Hisaoka, S. Tsuji & Y. Morimitsu, et al., Apmis 107 (1999) 577–584.

79. T.B. Lewis, C.M. Coffin & P.S. Bernard, Mod Pathol 20 (2007) 397–404.

80. S. Stegmaier, I. Leuschner & E. Aakcha-Rudel, et al., Klin Padiatr 216 (2004) 315–322.

81. R.S. Bridge, V. Rajaram & L.P. Dehner, et al., Mod Pathol 19 (2006) 1–8.

82. X. Qian, L. Jin & B.M. Shearer, et al., Diagn Mol Pathol 14 (2005) 23–28.

83. C.E. Fuller, J. Dalton & J.J. Jenkins, et al., Mod Pathol 17 (2004) 329a.

84. S. Kumar, S. Pack & D. Kumar, et al., Hum Pathol 30 (1999) 324–330.

85. K. Nagao, H. Ito & H. Yoshida, et al., J Pathol 181 (1997) 62–66.

86. C. Taylor, K. Patel & T. Jones, et al., Br J Cancer 67 (1993) 128–133.

87. C. Rodriguez-Galindo, Expert Opin Pharmacother 5 (2004) 1257–1270.

88. M. Paulussen, S. Ahrens & S. Burdach, et al., Ann Oncol 9 (1998) 275–281.

89. C. Fagnou, J. Michon & M. Peter, et al., J Clin Oncol 16 (1998) 1707–1711.

90. A. Zoubek, R. Ladenstein & R. Windhager, et al., Int J Cancer 79 (1998) 56–60.

91. D.C. West, H.E. Grier & M.M. Swallow, et al., J Clin Oncol 15 (1997) 583–588.

92. G. Schleiermacher, M. Peter & O. Oberlin, et al., J Clin Oncol 21 (2003) 85–91.

93. P.P. Lin, R.I. Brody & A.C. Hamelin, et al., Cancer Res 59 (1999) 1428–1432.

94. E. de Alava, A. Kawai & J.H. Healey, et al., J Clin Oncol 16 (1998) 1248–1255.

95. J.P. Ginsberg, E. de Alava & M. Ladanyi, et al., J Clin Oncol 17 (1999) 1809–1814.

96. G. Armengol, M. Tarkkanen & M. Virolainen, et al., Br J Cancer 75 (1997) 1403–1409.

97. F. Mugneret, S. Lizard & A. Aurias, et al., Cancer Genet Cytogenet 32 (1988) 239–245.

98. D. Maurici, A. Perez-Atayde & H.E. Grier, et al., Cancer Genet Cytogenet 100 (1998) 106–110.

99. M. Tarkkanen, S. Kiuru-Kuhlefelt & C. Blomqvist, et al., Cancer Genet Cytogenet 114 (1999) 35–41.

100. T. Ozaki, M. Paulussen & C. Poremba, et al., Genes Chromosomes Cancer 32 (2001) 164–171.

101. S. Brisset, G. Schleiermacher & M. Peter, et al., Cancer Genet Cytogenet 130 (2001) 57–61.

102. M. Zielenska, Z.M. Zhang & K. Ng, et al., Cancer 91 (2001) 2156–2164.

103. C.M. Hattinger, S. Rumpler & S. Strehl, et al., Genes Chromosomes Cancer 24 (1999) 243–254.

CHAPTER 21

The Histopathology of Skeletal Metastases

PING TANG[1] AND DAVID G. HICKS[1]

[1]*Department of Pathology and Laboratory Medicine, University of Rochester Medical Center, Rochester, NY, USA.*

Contents

I. INTRODUCTION

Bone is one of the most common sites for metastasis in patients with solid tumors arising from breast, prostate, lung, thyroid and kidney, with over 400,000 individuals affected in the United States annually [1]. Approximately 70% of patients with advanced prostate or breast cancer, and up to 40% of patients with other advanced solid tumors, will develop bone metastases over the course of their disease. In addition, more than 50% of advanced prostate cancer cases and 20% of advanced breast cancer cases will have metastatic disease clinically confined to the skeleton [2]. The development of bone metastasis from a solid tumor is a devastating complication and usually means that their diseases have reached the point of being incurable. The clinical manifestation of bone metastases is associated with considerable morbidity including intractable bone pain, decreased mobility, and pathologic bone loss associated with fractures, spinal compression and sequelae related to hypercalcemia [3]. Given the prevalence of these malignant diseases, bone metastasis constitutes a major clinical problem with significant implications for health care resources.

There have been great advancements in the treatment and prevention of metastatic diseases of the bone in recent years. The bisphosphonates, a group of compounds that ultimately cause apoptosis of osteoclasts, have been shown to reduce skeletal morbidity by 30–50% in multiple myeloma as well as in a wide range of solid tumors. They have been increasingly used to prevent skeletal complications and relieve bone pain [4–6]. Other agents such as cathepsin K inhibitors and matrix metalloproteinase inhibitors have also been proposed as therapeutic agents [7,8].

II. PATTERNS OF BONE INVOLVEMENT BY SKELETAL METASTASIS

Bone seems to be the preferred site of metastasis for a subset of solid tumors, which may be at least partly related to its unique anatomic vascular system—sinusoidal systems of red marrow that are lined by endothelium with large intercellular gaps and 'Batson's vertebral venous plexus' that lack venous valves [9]. Also, bone is a dynamic tissue with a unique microenvironment that undergoes continuous turnover to help maintain skeletal integrity and structural support for the body as well as providing a source of ions to support mineral homeostasis. The maintenance of skeletal mass in the face of these conflicting demands requires the coordinated activity of the two principal cell types responsible for bone resorption and formation: the osteoclast and the osteoblast [10]. The physiologic balance of ongoing bone remodeling cycles that occur throughout the skeleton are both temporally and spatially coupled, involving a regulatory mechanism that closely links the activity of these two important cell types. Therefore, complex regulatory interactions must exist between metastatic tumor cells and the host bone that interrupts this balance, facilitating the establishment and progression of the tumor within the bone microenvironment. Indeed, current evidence suggests that, in order for metastatic tumor cells to establish and grow within skeletal tissue, they must be able to interfere with normal bone cell function, tipping the balance in favor of osteoclast activation and bone resorption [11–13].

Skeletal involvement by metastatic disease can be classified as either osteolytic or osteoblastic, based on radiographic findings. This classification, while useful clinically, in fact represents two extremes of a continuum in which dysregulation of the processes of normal bone remodeling has occurred [14]. While metastatic deposits within the skeleton originating from different primary sites can show varying degrees of lytic and blastic reaction within the affected bone, virtually all tumors cause osteolysis. On one end of this spectrum, tumors such as myeloma and metastases from lung, kidney and thyroid are usually purely lytic in nature. Metastatic breast cancer to the bone, on the other hand, can be purely lytic or mixed lytic and blastic [15]. Purely blastic lesions are far less common and are usually seen in metastatic carcinomas from the prostate [16].

The mechanisms for bone metastasis are complex, involving many steps which include angiogenesis, invasion, and proliferation in the bone microenvironment. Tumor cells in the bone microenvironment produce a large number of cytokines disrupting osteoclastic and/or osteoblastic activities, causing an imbalance of the processes of bone formation and resorption. This imbalance in turn may facilitate the proliferation of metastatic foci in bone [17,18]. The activation of osteoclastic bone resorption will release numerous growth factors into the local bone environment, which can stimulate metastatic tumor cell deposits in a paracrine fashion, promoting tumor progression [17]. Studies have also indicated the potential prognostic clinical significance of finding disseminated tumor cells within the bone marrow of cancer patients [19]. The primary tumors that affect the bone most frequently are cancers of the breast, prostate, lungs, thyroid and kidneys [20]. The affinity for skeletal dissemination displayed by this select group of primary tumors suggests that these diseases share common biological characteristics that allow malignant cells from them to establish and grow in the bone microenvironment [21].

III. SPECIFIC PRIMARY TUMORS WITH A PREDILECTION FOR SKELETAL METASTASIS

More than 80% of bone metastases are from carcinomas of the breast, prostate, lung, kidney, and thyroid. The most common sites of involvement are the spine, femur, and skull. Among patients whose malignant disease presents with bone metastases from a tumor of unknown origin, the most likely primary sites are lung, kidney, pancreas, gastrointestinal tract, liver, thyroid, and melanoma. Pain is the most common symptom, present in two-thirds of patients with a radiologically detectable lesion. Pathological fracture is a major complication, and is more frequently associated with lytic skeletal lesions.

A. Breast (Figure 21.1A–F)

Breast carcinoma is the most common source of bone metastasis. At least 80% of patients who develop metastatic breast cancer will, at some point during their disease, develop bone metastasis [22]. Bone represents the first site of metastasis in more than 50% of patients who fail systemically [23]. The average age of a patient with breast cancer metastasis is 50, and the average interval from treatment of

the primary tumor to bone metastasis is about 30 months. However, it is not unusual to see metastasis 10 years or occasionally 20 years after initial treatment. The most common sites for metastatic breast cancer to bone are spine, pelvis, ribs, skull, femur, humerus, and scapula. Metastatic bone lesions from breast are 65% lytic, 25% mixed with lytic and blastic, and 10% blastic. Grossly, the lesions are usually firm grayish tissue, and microscopically the malignant glands showing varying degrees of differentiation (Figure 21.1A–C) are usually associated with fibrosis and thickened reactive bone formation. Despite the variable radiographic patterns that can be seen with breast cancer metastases to the bone, one of the histopathologic hallmarks is the activation of osteoclastic bone resorption in proximity to foci of metastatic tumor deposits. Immunohistochemical stains for mammaglobulin, estrogen receptor (Figure 21.1D) and GCDFP-15 (Figure 21.1F) may be helpful and could be used if there is a doubt as to the origin of the metastatic tumor.

The most common clinic opathological factors associated with bone metastasis include lower histological grade, estrogen receptor (ER) positivity, and lymph node staging [15,24,25]. It has also been suggested that factors such as S-phase fraction <5% [25], expression of parathyroid hormone-related peptide [26], bone sialoprotein [27], calcium-sensing receptor [28], lack of squamoid differentiation and involucrin expression [29], strand growth pattern and presence of fibrotic foci in invasive ductal carcinoma [30] are also associated with bone metastasis. In addition, Smid *et al.* [31] have identified a 69-gene panel that is relevant to bone metastasis, and many of the genes seem to be involved in the fibroblast growth factor receptor signaling pathway. We reported that ER+/PR-phenotype and AR positivity are also strongly associated with bone metastasis [32]. A review by Sleeman and Cremers [33] summarized current understanding of the importance of tumor initiating cells and the microenvironment they create in tumor metastasis.

B. Prostate (Figure 21.2A and B)

Although relatively few prostate cancer patients will manifest bone involvement at their initial diagnosis, approximately 90% of hematogenous metastasis in the course of prostate cancers occurs in bone, making skeletal complications the leading cause of morbidity and mortality in these patients [34–36]. By the time of death from their disease, skeletal involvement by metastatic tumor may be seen in 85–100% of patients [37]. The median time between the diagnosis of a clinically evident metastasis in bones and death is approximately 3–5 years [38]. Radiologically, foci of bony metastasis from prostate cancer are frequently osteoblastic (75%), with 10% lytic and 15% mixed. Most patients will have an elevated serum acid phosphatase. Histologically, most metastatic foci show small closely packed glands and cells with a pale cytoplasm, surrounded

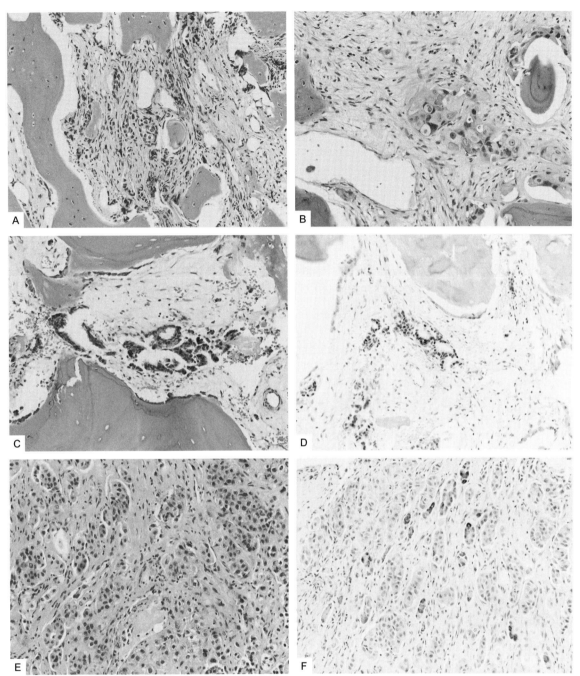

FIGURE 21.1 Metastatic breast cancer to bone, (A) hematoxylin and eosin stained section of metastatic breast cancer to bone (200 × original magnification). Nests of moderately differentiated tumor cells are seen replacing the marrow space with a characteristic fibrous response seen in the surrounding stroma; (B) hematoxylin and eosin stained section of another case of metastatic breast cancer to bone (200 × original magnification). This case shows a higher grade tumor with pleomorphic nuclei and a similar fibrous stromal response; (C) hematoxylin and eosin stained section of another case of metastatic breast cancer to bone (200 × original magnification). This low grade tumor shows evidence of estrogen receptor expression by immunohistochemistry (D) which is not specific for breast cancer; however, this degree of reactivity supports the origin from a breast primary for this metastatic tumor; (E) hematoxylin and eosin stained section of another case of metastatic breast cancer to bone (200 × original magnification). This moderately differentiated tumor shows a similar fibrous reaction and evidence of gross cystic disease fluid protein expression by immunohistochemistry (F). The expression of gross cystic disease fluid protein by metastatic tumor can be used as evidence for origin from a breast primary.

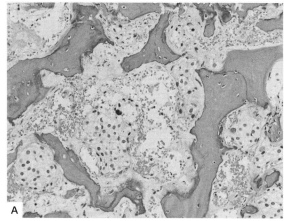

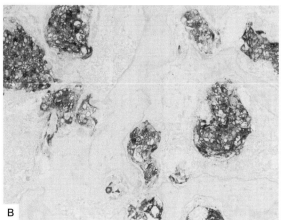

FIGURE 21.2   Metastatic prostate cancer to bone. (A) Hematoxylin and eosin stained section of metastatic prostate cancer to bone (200 × original magnification). Note the nests of tumor cells within a hypervascular marrow space. The tumor cells demonstrate oval uniform nuclei and abundant pink cytoplasm. There is abundant woven new bone formation associated with host trabeculae which would give rise to an osteoblastic radiographic appearance for this lesion; (B) immunohistochemical stain for prostate-specific antigen (200 × original magnification) from the same case. Tumor cells within the marrow space show strong cytoplasmic reactivity for prostate-specific antigen, confirming their origin from a carcinoma of the prostate.

by fibrous or fibroosseous tissue with new bone formation. Usually, the neoplastic glands are well differentiated with nuclei that are round, small, and eccentrically placed (Figure 21.2A). Immunohistochemical stains for prostate-specific acid phosphatase could be used if there is a doubt as to the origin of the metastatic tumor (Figure 21.2B).

Studies of prostate metastases suggested that these lesions can be osteolytic or osteoblastic with osteoblastic lesions largely composed of undermineralized woven bone [39–41]. Junior *et al.* [42] reported that loss of expression of E-cadherin and beta-catenin is related to bone metastasis in prostate cancer. Liao *et al.* [43] also showed that PTHrP (parathyroid hormone-related protein) facilitates prostate cancer-induced osteoblastic lesions. One study showed that

the presence of disseminated tumor cells in the bone marrow of prostate cancer patients before neoadjuvant hormone therapy and subsequent surgery is an independent prognostic factor correlating with a poor prognosis [44]. Dai *et al.* [45] showed that one of the mechanisms of prostate cancer induced bone metastasis is the promotion of osteoblast differentiation through the canonical and non-canonical Wnt signaling pathway by stimulating both bone morphogenetic protein dependent and independent osteoblast differentiation.

C. Lung (Figure 21.3A–C)

About 15% of lung cancers metastasize to bone, with 80% being lytic, 15% mixed, and 5% blastic. Unlike other tumors, lung carcinomas are among the most frequent tumors to metastasize to hands or feet (acral metastasis). Although most lung cancer metastases are lytic, osteoblastic metastases are much more frequently associated with adenocarcinoma (Figure 21.3A) and small cell carcinoma [46]. Hiraoka *et al.* [47] showed that tumor associated macrophages/monocytes are associated with promoting bone metastasis. Patients with lung cancer can demonstrate bone metastases as the first presentation of their malignant disease. Such cases are usually poorly differentiated carcinomas (Figure 21.3B). Immunohistochemical staining for TTF-1 (Figure 21.3C) could be used to help confirm the origin of the tumor as a lung primary in the appropriate clinical context.

D. Kidney (Figure 21.4A and B)

Among the approximately 51,000 patients diagnosed with renal cell carcinoma (RCC) annually, 30% will present as metastatic disease, and another 30% will develop local or systematic recurrence after a potentially curative nephrectomy [48]. Bone metastases represent the second most common site of recurrence in renal cell carcinoma, accounting for 16–27% of all recurrent sites [49,50]. Renal cell carcinoma and thyroid carcinoma are the most common tumors presenting as a solitary bone metastasis. Bone metastases in RCC are usually symptomatic, discovered either as a result of local pain or abnormal alkaline phosphatase levels [51]. More than 90% of the cases are pure to predominantly lytic causing the destruction of cortical bone which can predispose to pathologic fractures. Grossly these lesions are highly vascular, and the tumor cells typically demonstrate a clear cell appearance in nesting, alveolar, or tubular patterns (Figure 21.4A). Renal cell carcinoma to the bone is frequently osteolytic and is typically characterized by extensive activation of osteoclastic bone resorption, which can be seen at the interface between the host bone and the adjacent tumor cells (Figure 21.4B).

Metastatic sarcomatoid RCC to bone, due to its spindle cell proliferation and rarely intense stimulation of reactive host woven bone and osteoid, can be mistaken for fibrosarcoma or osteosarcoma. The treatment of bone metastasis in RCC is usually palliative. Shvarts *et al.* [52] showed that

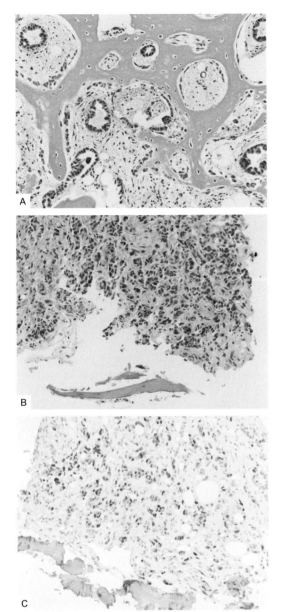

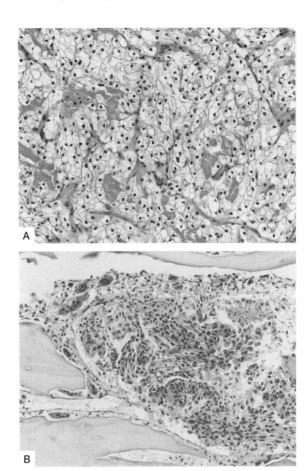

FIGURE 21.3 Metastatic lung cancer to bone. (A) Hematoxylin and eosin stained section of metastatic adenocarcinoma of the lung to bone (200 × original magnification). Note the nests of tumor cells within the marrow space with glandular acinar formation consistent with an adenocarcinoma. Although metastatic lung cancer is frequently osteolytic, this case demonstrates extensive woven new bone formation which would give rise to an osteoblastic radiographic appearance; (B) hematoxylin and eosin stained section of another case of metastatic lung cancer to bone (200 × original magnification). This case demonstrates a poorly differentiated carcinoma on needle core biopsy with few morphologic clues as to the tissue of origin for the tumor. Correlation with clinical and radiographic information for the patient would be necessary if these bone metastases were the initial presentation for this patient's malignancy. An immunohistochemical stain for thyroid transcription factor-1 for this case (C) shows strong nuclear staining within tumor cells supporting the diagnosis of a metastatic carcinoma from either a thyroid or a lung primary. The clinical context can help to establish the correct diagnosis for the patient.

FIGURE 21.4 Metastatic renal cell cancer to bone. (A) Hematoxylin and Eosin stained section of metastatic renal cell carcinoma to bone (200 × original magnification). This lytic lesion has extensively replaced the medullary cavity with destruction of surrounding cancellous bone. The tumors cells demonstrate a nested pattern of growth with abundant clear cytoplasm, which is characteristic for carcinomas arising from the kidney. Note the prominent sinusoidal vascular pattern surrounding individual nests of tumor cells. The prominent vasculature associated with renal metastases can result in excessive bleeding during surgical intervention; (B) hematoxylin and eosin stained section of another case of metastatic renal to bone (200 × original magnification). The tumor cells within the marrow space from this case show granular pink cytoplasm. Renal cell carcinoma to the bone is typically osteolytic which is characterized by extensive activation of osteoclastic bone resorption (which can be seen at the interface between the host bone and the adjacent tumor cells).

the Eastern Cooperative Oncology Group Performance Status is also a good predictor for bone metastasis in RCC, with a poor score having higher risk of bone metastasis.

E. Thyroid (Figure 21.5A and B)

About 8% of thyroid carcinoma has clinical metastasis to bone, and its radiologic features are similar to what is seen clinically from renal cell carcinoma. The sites include spine, pelvis, ribs, etc. Grossly, these lesions are hemorrhagic, like

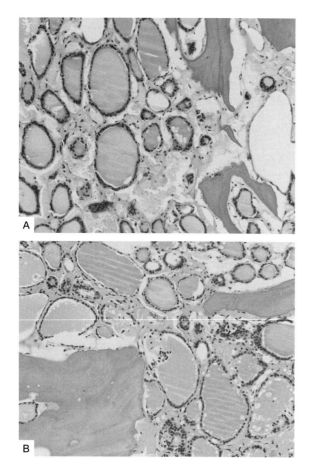

FIGURE 21.5 Metastatic thyroid cancer to bone. (A and B) hematoxylin and eosin stained section of metastatic thyroid cancer to bone (200 × original magnification). The marrow space is extensively replaced with well-differentiated tumor cells showing follicular formation with colloid production. Colloid production by metastatic carcinoma to the bone is virtually pathognomonic for thyroid cancer. The adjacent host bone demonstrates irregular scalloped surfaces (Howship's lacunae) consistent with evidence of extensive prior osteoclastic bone resorption.

the typical lesions associated with metastatic RCC. Histologically, thyroid carcinomas with skeletal dissemination frequently demonstrate well differentiated follicular formations (Figure 21.5A and B), or follicular variant histology of papillary carcinoma as well as papillary formation. They often are associated with colloid production (Figure 21.5A and B), which is pathognomonic for the diagnosis.

IV. OTHER PRIMARY TUMORS

Other tumors that can metastasize to bone include melanoma, neuroblastoma, hepatocellular carcinoma, carcinoid tumor, paraganglioma, as well as a number of additional solid tumors, although the incidence of such metastases is less common. Five percent of melanoma patients will have clinically evident skeletal metastasis. Subungual melanoma is characterized by massive destruction of a distal digit. Diagnostic clues include multiple lesions, mixed spindle and round cells with large nucleoli, minimal collagen production and minimal melanin pigment. The most frequent sites for neuroblastoma metastasis are the skull and long bones. Most carcinoid tumors are indolent low-grade lesions that can occasionally metastasize to bone. Histologically these tumors demonstrate typical neuroendocrine features including a nest or cord-like arrangement of tumor cells with fine chromatin and distinct nuclear membranes. Immunohistochemical stains for neuroendocrine markers such as chromogranin and synaptophysin may be helpful in establishing a diagnosis of metastatic carcinoid tumor. Carcinoid tumors associated with serotonin production produce extensive fibrosis and blastic lesions similar to those from prostate cancer.

V. METASTATIC CARCINOMA OF UNKNOWN PRIMARY SITE

Patients with an undiagnosed malignancy can present with bone metastases as the first manifestation of their disease [53]. The clinical evaluation of such patients begins with a careful medical history, physical examination, laboratory and imaging studies and an analysis of a diagnostic tissue biopsy. A biopsy of such lesions usually reveals an adenocarcinoma or a poorly differentiated carcinoma [54]. Routine morphology can at times be helpful in suggesting the origin of the metastatic tumor. Breast cancer is often associated with glandular formation and a prominent fibrous reaction, tumors from the GI tract with mucin production, tumors from the kidney with clear cell changes and tumors from the thyroid with follicular formation and colloid production. A number of immunohistochemical markers can also be helpful in suggesting the primary site and include cytokeratin 7 and 20, prostate-specific antigen, gross cystic disease fluid protein and thyroid transcription factor 1. However, in some cases the primary site may be indeterminate even after extensive clinical, laboratory, imaging and pathologic evaluation. An extensive immunohistochemical evaluation of biopsy material may be inconclusive and should not be considered a substitute for the careful clinical evaluation of the patient.

VI. CONCLUSION

The bone is the most common site of metastases for tumors from breast, prostate, lung, kidney and thyroid. An accurate diagnosis is dependent upon the combination of clinical, radiological, and pathological clues. With the development of more effective treatment, prophylactic strategies and preventive agents for bone metastases, the need for pathologists to diagnose and predict the likelihood of bone metastasis is more urgent than ever. The discovery of tumor profiles and new biomarkers that could help to accurately predict which patients are at high risk for skeletal metastases would be an important step toward developing effective prophylactic strategies to prevent this dreaded complication for patients diagnosed with a variety of common solid tumors.

References

1. R.T. Greenlee, M.B. Hill-Harmon & T. Murray, et al., Cancer Statistics, 2001, CA Cancer J Clin 51 (2001) 15–36.

2. J.E. Brown, R.J. Cook & P. Major, et al., Bone turnover markers as predictors of skeletal complications in prostate cancer, lung cancer, and other solid tumors, J Natl Cancer Inst 97 (2005) 59–69.

3. M.L. Cher, D.A. Towler & S. Rafii, et al., Cancer interaction with the bone microenvironment. A workshop of the National Institutes of Health Tumor Microenvironment Study Section, Am J Pathol 168 (2006) 1405–1412.

4. H.T. Hatoum, S.J. Lin & M.R. Smith, et al., Zoledronic acid and skeletal complications in patients with solid tumors and bone metastases, Cancer 113 (2008) 1438–1445.

5. T.A. Guise, Antitumor effects of bisphosphonates: promising preclinical evidence, Cancer Treat Rev 34 (Suppl 1) (2008) S19–S24.

6. R.E. Coleman, T.A. Guise & A. Lipton, et al., Advancing treatment for metastatic bone cancer: consensus recommendations from the second Cambridge Conference, Clin Cancer Res 14 (2008) 6387–6395.

7. C. Le Gall, E. Bonnelye & O. Clezardin, Cathepsin K inhibitors as treatment of bone metastasis, Curr Opin Support Palliat Care 2 (2008) 218–222.

8. R.D. Bonfil, R. Fridman & S. Mobashery, et al., Are matrix metalloproteinases relevant therapeutic targets for prostate cancer bone metastasis?, Curr Oncol 15 (2008) 188–192.

9. O.V. Batson, The function of the vertebral veins and their role in the spread of metastases, Ann Surg 112 (1940) 138–149.

10. L. Masi & M.L. Brandi, Physiopathological basis of bone turnover, Q J Nucl Med 45 (2001) 2–6.

11. R.E. Coleman, Metastic bone disease: clinical features, pathophysiology and treatment strategies, Cancer Treat Rev 27 (2001) 165–176.

12. T. Taube, I. Elomaa & C. Blomqvist, et al., Histomorphometric evidence for osteoclast-mediated bone resorption in metastatic breast cancer, Bone 15 (1994) 161–166.

13. D. Goltzman, Osteolysis and cancer, J Clin Invest 107 (2001) 1219–1220.

14. G.D. Roodman, Mechanisms of bone metastasis, N Engl J Med 350 (2004) 1655–1664.

15. J.J. James, A.J. Evans & S.E. Pinder, et al., Bone metastases from breast carcinoma: histopathological-radiological correlations and prognostic features, Br J Cancer 89 (2003) 660–665.

16. M. Koutsilieris, Osteoblastic metastasis in advanced prostate cancer, Anticancer Res 13 (1993) 443–449.

17. T.A. Guise, K.S. Mohammad & G. Clines, et al., Basic mechanisms responsible for osteolytic and osteoblastic bone metastases, Clin Cancer Res 12 (2006) 6213s–6216s.

18. J.T. Buijs & G. van der Pluijm, Osteotropic cancers: from primary tumor to bone, Cancer Lett 273 (2008) 177–193.

19. S. Riethdorf, H. Wikman & K. Pantel, Review: biological relevance of disseminated tumor cells in cancer patients, Int J Cancer 123 (2008) 1991–2006.

20. B.A. Berrettoni & J.R. Carter, Mechanisms of cancer metastasis to bone [Review], J Bone Joint Surg Am 68 (1986) 308–312.

21. T.A. Guise, Molecular mechanisms of osteolytic bone metastases, Cancer 88 (2000) 2892–2898.

22. M. Tubiana-Hulin, Incidence, prevalence and distribution of bone metastases, Bone 12 (Suppl 1) (1991) S9–S10.

23. R.E. Coleman & R.D. Rubens, The clininical course of bone metastases from breast cancer, Br J Cancer 55 (1987) 61–66.

24. M. Colleoni, A. O'Neill & A. Goldhirsch, et al., Identifying breast cancer patients at high risk for bone metastases, J Clin Oncol 18 (2000) 3925–3935.

25. E.F. Solomayer, I.J. Diel & G.C. Meyberg, et al., Metastatic breast cancer: clinical course, prognosis and therapy related to the first site of metastasis, Breast Cancer Res Treat 59 (2000) 271–278.

26. Z. Bouizar, F. Spyratos & S. Deytieux, et al., Polymerase chain reaction analysis of parathyroid hormone-related protein gene expression in breast cancer patients and occurrence of bone metastases, Cancer Res 53 (1993) 5076–5078.

27. I.J. Diel, E.F. Solomayer & M.J. Seibel, et al., Serum bone sialoprotein in patients with primary breast cancer is a prognostic marker for subsequent bone metastasis, Clin Cancer Res 5 (1999) 3914–3919.

28. R. Mihai, J. Stevens & C. McKinney, et al., Expression of the calcium receptor in human breast cancer—a potential new marker predicting the risk of bone metastases, Eur J Surg Oncol 32 (2006) 511–515.

29. H. Tsuda, C. Sakamaki & T. Fukutomi, et al., Squamoid features and expression of involucrin in primary breast carcinoma associated with high histological grade, tumour cell necrosis and recurrence sites, Br J Cancer 75 (1997) 1519–1524.

30. T. Koyama, T. Hasebe & H. Tsuda, et al., Histological factors associated with initial bone metastasis of invasive ductal carcinoma of the breast, Jpn J Cancer Res 90 (1999) 294–300.

31. M. Smid, Y. Wang & J.G. Klijn, et al., Genes associated with breast cancer metastatic to bone, J Clin Oncol 24 (2006) 2261–2267.

32. B. Wei, J. Wang & P. Bourne, et al., Bone metastasis is strongly associated with estrogen receptor-positive/progesterone receptor negative breast carcinomas, Hum Pathol 39 (2008) 1809–1815.

33. J.P. Sleeman & N. Cremers, New concepts in breast cancer metastasis: tumor initiating cells and the microenvironment, Clin Exp Metastasis 24 (2007) 707–715.

34. L. Bubendorf, A. Schopfer & U. Wagner, et al., Metastatic patterns of prostate cancer: an autopsy study of 1,589 patients, Hum Pathol 31 (2000) 578–583.

35. B.I. Carlin & G.L. Andriole, The natural history, skeletal complications, and management of bone metastases in patients with prostate carcinoma, Cancer 88 (2000) 2989–2994.

36. M.P. Roudier, L.D. True & C.S. Higano, et al., Phenotypic heterogeneity of end-stage prostate carcinoma metastatic to bone, Hum Pathol 34 (2003) 646–653.

37. W.J. Whitmore, Natural history and staging of prostate cancer, Urol Clin North Am 11 (1984) 205–220.

38. C.R. Pound, A.W. Partin & M.A. Eisenberger, et al., Natural history of progression after PSA elevation following radical prostatectomy, JAMA 281 (1999) 1591–1597.

39. R.C. Percival, G.H. Urwin & S. Harris, et al., Biochemical and histological evidence that carcinoma of the prostate is associated with increased bone resorption, Eur J Surg Oncol 13 (1987) 41–49.

40. E.T. Keller & J. Brown, Prostate cancer bone metastases promote both osteolytic and osteoblastic activity, J Cell Biochem 91 (2004) 718–729.

41. M.P. Roudier, C. Morrissey & L.D. True, et al., Histopathological assessment of prostate cancer bone osteoblastic metastases, J Urol 180 (2008) 1154–1160.

42. J.P. Junior, M. Srougi, P.M. Borra, et al., E-cadherin and beta-catenin loss of expression related to bone metastasis in prostate cancer. Appl Immunohistochem Mol Morphol Aug 5 (2008) (Epub ahead of print).

43. J. Liao, X. Li & A. Koh, et al., Tumor expressed PTHrP facilitates prostate cancer-induced osteoblastic lesions, Int J Cancer 123 (2008) 2267–2278.

44. J. Kollermann, S. Weikert & M. Schostak, et al., Prognostic significance of disseminated tumor cells in the bone marrow of prostate cancer patients treated with neoadjuvant hormone treatment, J Clin Oncol 26 (2008) 4928–4933.

45. J. Dai, C.L. Hall & J. Escara-Wilke, et al., Prostate cancer induces bone metastasis through Wnt-induced bone morphogenetic protein-dependent and independent mechanisms, Cancer Res 68 (2008) 5785–5794.

46. F.M. Muggia & H.H. Hansen, Osteoblastic metastases in small-cell (oat-cell) carcinoma of the lung, Cancer 30 (1972) 801–805.

47. K. Hiraoka, M. Zenmyo & K. Watari, et al., Inhibition of bone and muscle metastases of lung cancer cells by a decrease in the number of monocytes/macrophages, Cancer Sci 99 (2008) 1595–1602.

48. A. Jemal, R. Siegel & E. Ward, et al., Cancer Statistics, 2007, CA Cancer J Clin 57 (2007) 43–66.

49. B. Ljungberg, F.I. Alamdari & T. Rasmuson, et al., Follow-up guidelines for non-metastatic renal cell carcinoma based on the occurrence of metastases after radical nephrectomy, BJU Int 84 (1999) 405–411.

50. K.S. Hafez, A.C. Novick & S.C. Campbell, Patterns of tumor recurrence and guidelines for followup after nephron sparing surgery for sporadic renal cell carcinoma, J Urol 157 (1997) 2067–2070.

51. N.K. Janzen, H.L. Kim & R.A. Figlin, et al., Surveillance after radical or partial nephrectomy for localized renal cell carcinoma and management of recurrent disease, Urol Clin North Am 30 (2003) 843–852.

52. O. Shvarts, J.S. Lam & H.L. Kim, et al., Eastern Cooperative Oncology Group performance status predicts bone metastasis in patients presenting with renal cell carcinoma: implication for preoperative bone scans, J Urol 172 (2004) 867–870.

53. B.T. Rougraff, J.S. Kneisl & M.A. Simon, Skeletal metastases of unknown origin. A prospective study of a diagnostic strategy, J Bone Joint Surg Am 75 (1993) 1276–1281.

54. M.S. Didolkar, N. Fanous, E.G. Elias & R.H. Moore, Metastatic carcinomas from occult primary tumore. A study of 254 patients, Ann Surg 186 (1977) 625–630.

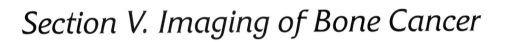

Section V. Imaging of Bone Cancer

CHAPTER **22**

Interventional Radiologic Techniques and their Contribution to the Management of Bone Tumors

ROBERT G. JONES[1], ERIC J. HEFFERNAN[1], FAISAL RASHID[1] AND PETER L. MUNK[1]

[1]Vancouver General Hospital, Department of Radiology, Vancouver, BC V5Z 1M9, Canada.

Contents

I. INTRODUCTION

Until as recently as 25 to 30 years ago the principal role of radiology in the work-up and management of bone tumors was almost exclusively diagnostic. Since then a wide variety of new techniques have been developed which allow the interventional radiologist to contribute in new and exciting ways to the management of the patient with bone tumors. These facilitate not only diagnosis but actual treatment of the lesions, often replacing or supplementing other methods.

This review will be divided into three principal sections. The first of these will be on imaging guided bone biopsy. In many institutions virtually all biopsies are done under imaging guidance either fluoroscopic, CT (computed tomography) and less frequently MRI (Magnetic Resonance Imaging).

The second section is on therapeutic embolization. This has become a very important adjunct in facilitating the performance of at times complex and difficult surgery by minimizing the frequently profuse bleeding that would otherwise occur. Embolization is also invaluable in palliating patients with lesions that are unresponsive to other conventional techniques such as chemotherapy, radiation therapy or surgery, either alone or in combination.

The last segment is on vertebroplasty and osteoplasty, a very exciting development which particularly in the last 10 years has provided an entirely new avenue for providing high quality palliation of patients with difficult to treat

destructive lesions of the spine and pelvis. Radiofrequency ablation can be used in conjunction with cement injection to provide pain relief as well as structural support of the treated bone.

II. IMAGE-GUIDED BONE BIOPSY

The first reported core biopsy of bone was performed by Ellis in 1947 [1]. The first image-guided bone biopsies were carried out with the help of radiographs only; real-time, fluoroscopy-guided bone biopsy was subsequently introduced in the 1960s [2]. Since then, with the accumulation of experience by radiologists, the improvement in biopsy needles and techniques and the development of CT and MRI, image-guided bone biopsy has replaced open surgical biopsy as the method of choice for definitive evaluation of bone lesions [3,4].

Image-guided percutaneous bone biopsy has a number of advantages over the traditional, open technique: it is performed as an outpatient procedure under local anaesthesia, it is relatively straightforward in experienced hands, and it is safe and cost-effective, with a low complication rate [5].

The indications for percutaneous bone biopsy are:

- Lesion of unknown aetiology
- Suspected metastatic lesion in patient with known primary malignancy elsewhere
- Lesion suggestive of infection but specific organism required in order to guide treatment
- Symptomatic vertebral compression fracture when unclear if aetiology is osteoporotic or neoplastic
- Assessment of effectiveness of chemo- or radio-therapy
- Cytogenetic evaluation of multiple myeloma

In the literature, the most commonly reported indication for biopsy is metastatic bone disease [6]; however, this varies from institution to institution: in our own center, a tertiary referral unit, primary bone lesions are more commonly referred for biopsy than metastases. The current widespread use of CT, MRI and positron emission tomography (PET) has led to a huge increase in the number of ambiguous bone lesions identified during the staging of tumors elsewhere, or as incidental findings on imaging for other indications; as a result, the demand for bone biopsy is steadily rising [7,8].

Contraindications to biopsy include a bleeding diathesis, inaccessible sites such as C1 and the odontoid process of C2, bone that is surrounded by infected soft tissue or where the planned access route would traverse infected skin or soft tissue, and an uncooperative patient [5]. An additional relative contraindication is a suspected hypervascular metastasis (such as renal cell carcinoma) in the spine; hemorrhage from such lesions following biopsy may lead to spinal cord compression and an open biopsy may be preferable [2].

Prior to the procedure, any available imaging should be reviewed by the radiologist who will perform the biopsy [6]. Additional imaging may be indicated: for example, where multiple lesions are suspected, a radionuclide bone scan may identify a lesion, which is easier and safer to biopsy [9]. The planning of a bone biopsy should be a multidisciplinary process [10]. Most importantly, if a primary bone neoplasm is suspected, biopsy should only be considered following consultation with the surgeon who will be resecting the lesion [11], as a poorly planned biopsy may have devastating consequences [12]. The biopsy needle path must be in the same location as the surgeon's planned incision for resection, so that the biopsy track is removed with the tumor. This is because of the small but well-documented risk of tumor seeding [13]. If the needle traverses an uninvolved anatomical compartment or joint, a more radical resection or even amputation may become necessary. In one large series of sarcoma patients who underwent biopsy preoperatively, the optimum treatment plan was adversely affected in 18% of cases due to poor biopsy technique, leading to unnecessary amputation in 5% [14].

Percutaneous bone biopsy may be performed under ultrasound, fluoroscopy, CT, MRI or CT-fluoroscopy guidance. While ultrasound has the advantage of being fast, inexpensive, and free of ionizing radiation, it is of limited use in the biopsy of bone lesions unless there is complete cortical destruction with extension of a lytic tumor into the soft tissues [2,15]. Like ultrasound, fluoroscopic guidance allows real-time imaging of the biopsy needle as it is advanced into the lesion. However, it is difficult to assess the depth of the needle as it is advanced unless biplane fluoroscopy is used, and it does not allow visualization of soft tissue abnormalities, therefore its use is generally limited to superficial, easily visible lesions (Figure 22.1) or biopsy of spinal tumors when performed as a component of a vertebroplasty procedure. MRI-guided biopsy is not yet widely available. However, the available literature suggests that it is a safe and accurate alternative [16–18]. Its main

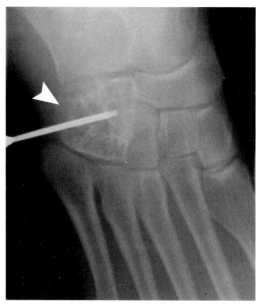

FIGURE 22.1 Fluoroscopy-guided biopsy of a lytic lesion filling the right cuboid (arrowhead) in a 25-year-old male. Biopsy revealed epithelioid hemangioma.

advantages over CT-guided biopsy are the absence of any ionizing radiation, the ability to see lesions that are not visible on other imaging modalities (e.g., edematous marrow lesions), and better contrast resolution even without intravenous contrast medium [17]. A considerable disadvantage is its cost, as MRI-compatible needles and instruments remain relatively expensive; in addition, the materials used in the biopsy needles (such as nickel alloy and carbon fiber) are softer and blunter than the stainless steel equipment that is standard when using other imaging modalities, making sampling of sclerotic lesions a difficult task [18]. CT-fluoroscopy is not yet widely available. This modality combines the real-time capabilities of fluoroscopy with the contrast-resolution and depth information provided by CT, but is associated with a high radiation dose both to the patient and radiologist.

Currently, CT guidance remains the technique of choice for percutaneous bone biopsy [4]. Almost every part of the skeleton can be reached [9], it retains superior spatial resolution to MRI [18], it is relatively cheap [5], and biopsies typically take less than one hour to perform. It is also a reliable and accurate procedure [14].

Depending upon the location and size of the lesion, fine-needle aspiration (FNA) or core biopsy may be performed. FNA can be carried out using a spinal or a Chiba needle. There is a variety of commercially-available core biopsy needles for use in bone lesions (e.g., Cook Bone Biopsy Needle, Cook Australia, Queensland, Australia (Figure 22.2A. In addition, when a lytic bone lesion is encountered, a soft-tissue core biopsy gun (e.g., Tru-Cut spring-loaded biopsy gun, Baxter Healthcare Corp., Deerfield, Illinois, USA) may be useful. When a lytic lesion

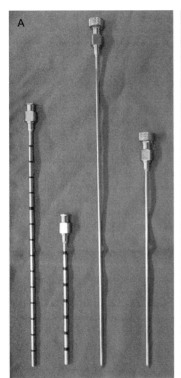
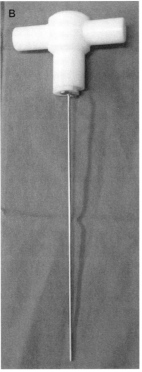
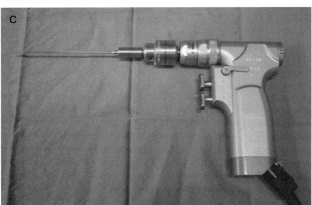

FIGURE 22.2 (A) Cook bone biopsy set. On the left, disposable 15.0 cm and 7.5 cm 12G guide cannulae. On the right, disposable 19.5 cm and 12.0 cm 14G bone biopsy needles. (B) Reusable sterile handle attached to a 14G bone biopsy needle. (C) Sterile hand-held drill, with disposable 14G bone biopsy needle attached. The device allows two different drill speeds and permits both clockwise and anti-clockwise drilling.

is surrounded by intact cortex, a combined approach can be performed, using a 14G bone biopsy needle to make a window through the cortex through which an 18G Tru-Cut needle can be inserted co-axially for sampling of the soft-tissue component [5,11]. Penetration of intact cortex or of sclerotic bone lesions can be difficult, but is facilitated by the use of a sterile, reusable handle for the biopsy needle (Figure 22.2B), or a sterile hand-held drill (Figure 22.2C).

In the authors' practice, we generally obtain an MRI prior to biopsy. In addition to facilitating staging of the tumor, this may also identify tumor heterogeneity and necrosis, and

guide planning of the biopsy in order to maximize the diagnostic yield. Informed consent is obtained from the patient, including an explanation of the small risks of hemorrhage, infection, tumor seeding and fracture; the potential need for a repeat percutaneous or open biopsy is also discussed. The biopsy is planned with the surgeon who will be performing resection if it turns out to be a primary lesion, ensuring that uninvolved compartments are not traversed while also checking that the proposed path is free of major vessels, nerves and pleura; the surgeon chooses his preferred incision site and marks the patient's skin accordingly. In the authors' experience, conscious sedation is usually required, particularly when deep or painful lesions are being biopsied. The patient is positioned appropriately on the CT table and a metallic object (such as a straightened paper clip) is taped to the skin over the surgeon's mark (Figure 22.3A). A preliminary CT is performed using 5 mm slices, the distance from the skin marker to the bone lesion is measured, and the angle at which the needle will have to be introduced is estimated. The skin and subcutaneous tissues are infiltrated with 1% lidocaine, initially with a short 25G needle then with a 22G spinal needle; the latter is advanced as far as the periosteum, and a small number of CT slices are performed at this site to check the position and angle of the needle (Figure 22.3B). The needle is repositioned if necessary, and the periosteum is infiltrated with local anesthetic. This minimizes the discomfort the patient will feel during penetration of the cortex, and reduces the chance of patient motion during the procedure. A longitudinal incision is made in the skin; while this need only be 3 or 4 mm in length to allow the needle to be inserted, we routinely make the incision larger than this so that the scar from the biopsy is unambiguous when the surgeon returns at a later date for definitive resection. A 11G co-axial needle guide is inserted along the same path as the spinal needle and position is rechecked with CT (Figure 22.3C). Through this, the 14G bone biopsy needle is introduced and either manually pushed through the cortex or, more commonly, drilled into the lesion (Figure 22.3D). Multiple (at least three) cores are obtained; different regions of the tumor can be sampled without repositioning the needle, simply by making slight changes to the angle of the outer needle guide. When dealing with a predominantly lytic lesion, Tru-Cut biopsies are obtained once any overlying cortex has been penetrated with the 14G needle.

The procedure is similar whether extremity or spinal lesions are being biopsied. Several approaches have been described for biopsy of vertebral tumors [2,5,19]. In the lower cervical spine and the thoracic spine, a posterolateral or transpedicular approach can be used (Figure 22.4). In the lumbar spine, a lateral approach is also feasible. For upper cervical spine lesions, transoral or transpharyngeal access is necessary.

CT-guided bone biopsy is an extremely safe procedure, with reported complication rates ranging from 0 to 7.4%

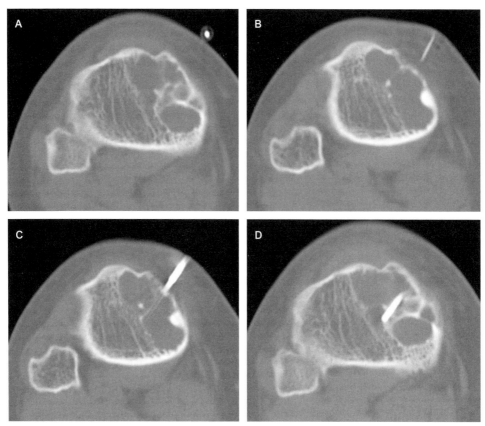

FIGURE 22.3   CT-guided bone biopsy technique. Twenty-three-year-old male with a lytic lesion in his proximal tibia. (A) An 18G needle, in its sheath, has been taped onto the patient's skin where it was marked by the referring surgeon. (B) Local anesthetic has been infiltrated, and the needle position and angulation are checked with CT. (C) Minor correction to the trajectory has been made, the periosteum infiltrated with local anesthetic, the skin incised and a 12G guide cannula inserted as far as the cortex. (D) The 14G bone biopsy needle has been drilled through the cortex into the lesion. Biopsy revealed giant cell tumor of bone.

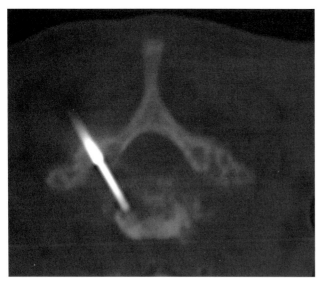

FIGURE 22.4   Transpedicular approach for CT-guided biopsy of a destructive lesion in the 5th cervical vertebra in a 47-year-old male. Biopsy revealed metastatic pancreatic adenocarcinoma.

[3]; complications requiring treatment are more frequent following spine biopsy [20]. The most commonly encountered complications are outlined in Table 22.1 [21]. Apparent neurologic injury following biopsy is most commonly related to the infiltration of local anesthetic, and can be expected to resolve within 3 to 4 hours. Actual injury to nerves, nerve roots or the spinal cord is relatively uncommon but is more likely to be encountered when biopsying spinal lesions. Thoracic spine biopsy is the most prone to complications, such as pneumothorax, cerebrospinal fluid leak from a thecal sac laceration, and paraplegia [2]. Fracture is an uncommon but well-documented risk following bone biopsy, particularly in weight-bearing bones like the femur (Figure 22.5), and should be discussed with the patient when obtaining consent. The exact incidence of tumor seeding is not known but appears to be very rare [22].

The diagnostic accuracy of CT-guided bone biopsy, which can be defined as the proportion of cases in which the biopsy diagnosis is in concordance with the final pathological diagnosis, has been reported to vary from 74 to 96%

TABLE 22.1 Complications of percutaneous bone biopsy

Major	Minor
Hemorrhage requiring transfusion	Wound infection
Osteomyelitis	Hematoma
Neurologic injury (transient or permanent)	Pain
Pneumothorax	
Cerebrospinal fluid leak	
Fracture	
Tumor seeding	

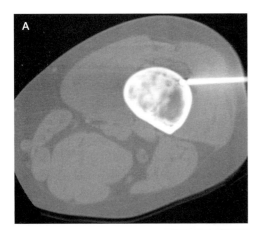

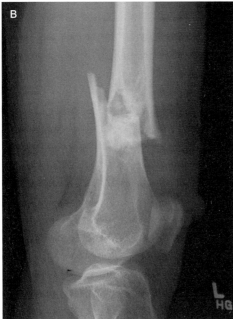

FIGURE 22.5 (A) CT-guided biopsy of a mixed sclerotic/lytic lesion in the distal diaphysis of the left femur in a 19-year-old female. Biopsy revealed liposclerosing myxofibrous tumor. (B) Two weeks later the patient returned with a fracture through the biopsy site.

[3,5,11,23]. Similar accuracy has been reported with MRI-guided bone biopsy [17]. The most commonly reported reason for an inaccurate image-guided biopsy is failure to obtain enough tissue for analysis [11]. Other reasons include sampling of necrotic areas within a tumor or sampling of the lower-grade component of a heterogenous tumor [5,10]. To avoid this, biopsies should be obtained from several different areas within a lesion, if possible. If pre-procedure imaging reveals a mixed lytic/sclerotic tumor, biopsies should be preferentially obtained from the lytic component as this has a higher diagnostic yield [9,10]. In addition, CT or MRI may reveal areas of probable necrosis, which should be avoided. Nonetheless, when imaging-guided percutaneous biopsy has been performed by an experienced team but is non-diagnostic, repeat percutaneous biopsy is of limited use and may place the patient under undue psychological stress, therefore a low threshold for proceeding to open biopsy is recommended [5,10].

In summary, image-guided percutaneous biopsy, generally performed using CT, is a safe, cost-effective and accurate method of diagnosis of bone lesions when performed in the setting of a multidisciplinary musculoskeletal tumor practice.

III. THERAPEUTIC EMBOLIZATION

Embolization is the intentional fluoroscopic guided, transcatheter occlusion of blood vessels. Early attempts at applying this principle pre-date the discovery of x-rays. As far back as 1831, physicians placed large needles into aneurysms in an attempt to induce thrombosis [24]. This early work was limited by technology and the lack of a 'true endovascular' approach and technique. Most of the pioneering work on modern techniques of catheter directed embolization was carried out by neuroradiologists with a landmark achievement in 1960 by Lussenhop and Spence who successfully occluded a cerebral arteriovenous malformation under radiographic and catheter guidance [25]. Technical advancements (for example, microcatheter systems) have increased the potential for safe and effective treatment of life threatening hemorrhage with an endovascular approach [26–28]. In addition to managing acute hemorrhage, the application of this endovascular therapy can be extended to nearly every organ system with a vascular abnormality or tumor.

The earliest report of embolization of hypervascular bone tumors was described by Feldman *et al.* in 1975 [29]. In this case, hypervascular renal metastases were treated. Hypervascular metastatic disease is the commonest bone abnormality to be managed using embolization, particularly with a renal cell or thyroid primary. Embolization is utilized predominantly where reducing blood supply has a therapeutic or adjuvant affect.

A. Metastatic Bone Lesions

It is estimated that 30–40% of patients with renal cell or thyroid carcinoma have bone metastasis [30,31]. Up to 75% of these lesions are hypervascular, mimicking the primary tumor. Bone metastasis is treated if they become symptomatic. The vascularity of these tumors can cause a multitude of problems including blood loss during surgery and intractable pain. Up to 7 liters of blood loss may occur during surgical excision or fracture fixation [32]. Pain generally occurs as a result of compression of local structures such as nerves and organs (e.g., bladder). Bone pain can be secondary to pathological fracture of a weakened bone or periosteal infiltration, as this has a rich nerve supply.

The role and indication for trans-arterial embolization in the management of hypervascular metastasis is:

1. Control of bleeding: both to control pain and as an adjuvant to surgical excision where excessive intra-operative blood loss can lead to considerable mortality and morbidity. Ideally, surgery should be performed immediately after embolization [33] or at least within 3 days [34].
2. Inhibition of tumor growth, particularly after radiotherapy has had limited effect. Renal bone metastasis are relatively radiotherapy resistant and re-growth of tumor following this form of treatment is common [35].
3. Relief of pain caused by mass effect. Embolization can provide up to 6 months of pain relief in renal cell bone metastasis [36].

B. Technique

Prior to embolization basic principles of angiography should be first applied. These include ensuring the patient is prehydrated and that renal function is adequate as iodinated contrast volumes can be high in this procedure, possibly causing decline in renal function. Pain control and conscious sedation is of utmost important as embolization can often lead to a transient increase in pain, especially in the immediate post procedural period. This is due to a transient expansion of the mass secondary to tissue necrosis and inflammation. Narcotic analgesia is often required.

Following standard arterial access, focus should be turned to the anatomical area of interest with careful arterial mapping, including selective angiography of the entire region as hypervascular metastasis can recruit supply from surrounding vascular territories [37] (Figure 22.6A–C).

Vertebral metastases often share vascular supply with spinal arteries and, therefore, pre-embolization arteriography is important to avoid non-target (or unintentional) embolization. A similar scenario exists in the pelvis where the blood supply to the sciatic nerve can be affected during embolization. The target vessel in this instance is the inferior gluteal artery which supplies the sciatic nerve. If selective and super-selective catheterization cannot be achieved using conventional catheters, then microcatheter systems should be utilized to achieve a safe result. The catheter

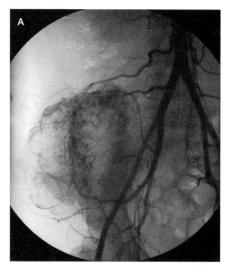
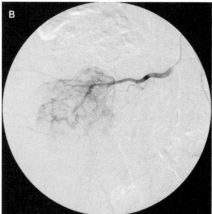
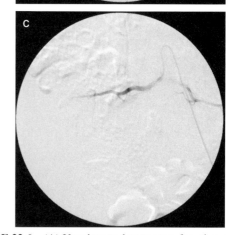

FIGURE 22.6   (A) Unsubtracted aortogram focusing on the arterial supply to the right hemi-pelvis in a 25-year-old female with known metastatic rhabdomyosarcoma to the right iliac bone. The angiogram demonstrates a large hypervascular tumor with multiple, hypertrophied feeding arteries from a variety of territories including lumbar arteries and branches of the internal iliac artery; (B) selective Digital Subtraction Angiography (DSA) of a lumbar artery found to be contributing supply to the tumor. A Mickelson catheter was used; (C) post-embolization DSA of the selected lumbar artery from (B) demonstrating lack of tumor hypervascularity and a satisfactory angiographic result. In this artery 355–500 micron diameter PVA particles were used as embolization material. Embolization was carried out for symptomatic control.

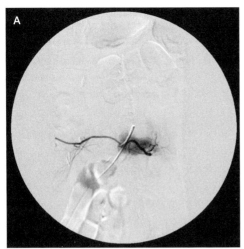
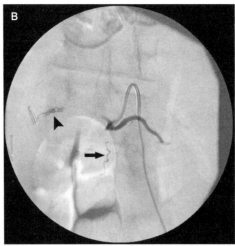

FIGURE 22.7 (A) Selective Digital Subtraction Angiogram (DSA) using a Mickelson catheter of a common L4 lumbar artery trunk supplying both left and right lumbar arteries at this level. The patient was a 50-year-old male with known renal cell carcinoma metastases to lumbar vertebra. Note an intense arterial blush within the hypervascular metastatic deposit; (B) post-embolization unsubtracted angiogram demonstrating a satisfactory angiographic result. Embolization coils were placed in a deep muscular arterial branch (arrow head) and a median sacral branch (arrow) to prevent non-target embolization and redirect higher concentration of PVA particles towards the malignant target which is now devascularized (compare to (A)).

should be positioned as close to the target as possible before embolization (see Figure 22.7A).

In Figure 22.7, a selective angiogram of the left 7th thoracic (T7) body artery is shown. This patient had multiple level thoracic and lumbar vertebral body metastasis. In mapping out the adjacent vertebral body arteries, the artery of Adamkewicz was identified originating at the T7 level. This vertebral body itself was unaffected. An understanding of the spinal cord blood supply is particularly important before attempting embolization procedures involving vertebral bodies. The blood supply to the human spinal cord is provided by a single anterior spinal artery, which supplies most of the cord and a pair of posterior spinal arteries. Six to eight radicular arteries arise from the posterior wall of the aorta and anastomose with the anterior spinal artery at several levels. The most caudad artery is the major anterior radicular artery of Adamkewicz and may be found anywhere from the level of T7 to L4 (Figure 22.8). This artery may supply the lower two thirds of the spinal cord [38].

A wide variety of embolization materials are available and can be safely used in this setting. These include thrombogenic embolization coils, polyvinyl alcohol (PVA) particles, gelatine sponge (gelfoam) and tissue adhesives. Coils and PVA particles are the commonest agents used. When considering PVA particles (which are available in a variety of sizes from 250 microns diameter to 1200 microns), particles smaller than 355 microns tend to cause excessive tissue necrosis and these should be avoided. The particles are suspended in iodinated contrast and injected through the safely positioned catheter under fluoroscopic control. In the setting of palliative embolization care should be taken not to over-embolize and subsequently render the target and

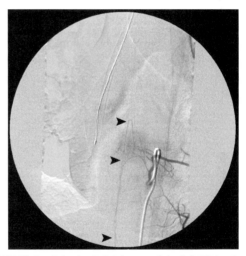

FIGURE 22.8 Selective DSA image of the left T7 lumbar artery using a Mickelson-type catheter demonstrating the major anterior radicular artery of Adamkewicz (arrow heads).

remaining normal tissue avascular. The injection of particles should generally cease when reflux past the catheter tip occurs or when flow has considerably diminished in the target vessel. This observation develops with operator experience.

Embolization using coils tends to occlude the target vessel and although a satisfactory angiographic result may be obtained, distal recruitment from collaterals is a common observation. If surgery is immediately imminent, the use of coils is more acceptable as recruitment takes some time. If palliation is the main objective, better results are achieved using particulate embolic material. Coiling can be used to occlude non-target vessels distal to the target. The principle here is that particles can then be more focally directed towards the target, minimizing the risk of distal embolization. The tissues beyond this then recruit collateral circulation and are preserved (see Figure 22.7B).

Ethanol can be used and is an excellent vascular occlusive agent due to its low viscosity and non-adhesive nature. It is also inexpensive and readily available. One of the drawbacks of using ethanol is intense pain caused due to its sclerotic properties and general anesthesia is often required for its anticipated use.

Post-procedural completion angiography should always be carried out within the surrounding arterial territory to identify any collaterals that may have developed or become more significant and apparent since embolization. This phenomenon can occur within minutes.

C. Complications and Post-embolization Scenarios

One of the most frequently encountered complications is that of the post-embolization syndrome. This occurs to some degree in every patient. It may last up to seven days. It is characterized by a low-grade fever, pain and nausea caused by the release of toxins from ischemic tissue. This can be managed with analgesia, antiemetic and anti-inflammatory medication.

Non-target embolization of the spinal arteries and inferior gluteal arteries can lead to significant morbidity due to ischemia of the spinal cord and sciatic nerve [39]. Embolization of the inferior gluteal artery can usually be tolerated if embolization of this vessel is absolutely necessary but spinal arterial embolization should never be carried out.

Skin ulceration and necrosis can occur if the tumor is close to the skin [40].

Remineralization has been observed but any significant degree of new bone formation following embolization is extremely unlikely to occur [41].

D. Embolization of Non-metastatic Bone Lesions

The utilization of embolization in the management of primary bone tumors is less well established than that of metastatic disease. Osteosarcoma is the most common primary malignant bone tumor in children and adolescents. Limb salvage surgery is becoming a more accepted replacement for amputation in the treatment of this aggressive primary bone tumor [42,43]. Pre-operative chemotherapy and/or embolization has improved the prognosis and made limb salvage surgery possible in many cases. This is largely due to pre-operative reduction or stabilization of tumor size and limiting peri-operative blood loss [44]. Trans-arterial chemoembolization (TACE) has also been applied and may be

beneficial as an adjuvant therapy in the management of osteosarcoma [45]. This procedure is well described in the treatment of hepatocellular carcinoma of the liver [46]. This involves the delivery of a chemotherapy agent directly into the arterial supply of a tumor in combination with an embolic agent. The principle is that the tumor receives a direct, calibrated dose of chemotherapy which has an increased contact time in the target tissue due to diminished blood flow caused by the embolic component of the compound. Indications for TACE in the treatment of osteosarcoma are: malignant bone tumor prior to limb salvage surgery; hypervascular bone tumor, or unresectable bone tumor due to a complicated anatomic position; osseous metastasis in the advanced stage [45]. The catheter principles used in the treatment of metastatic tumors described earlier apply in this setting.

Primary pelvic bone tumors are usually asymptomatic until they grow to a considerable size and at this stage are, in the majority of circumstances, inoperable. Normal limb function is usually preserved. Radiotherapy has limited effect; however, embolization may be of considerable benefit in symptom control.

Other rarer bone tumors have also been successfully treated by embolization, these include giant cell tumors (GCT) and vertebral hemangiomas.

GCTs of bone are generally considered benign entities. They can behave in an aggressive manner and even metastasize [47]. In some cases, uncontrolled growth can even be fatal, as a result of either local effect or metastatic spread. Sacral GCTs can grow to large sizes before they become symptomatic and can be difficult to manage. The sacrum is the commonest place in the axial skeleton for GCTs to occur and recurrence rates here are higher than any other area of the human skeleton [48,49].

Effective treatment of these tumors is important in the first instance due to their recurrent nature. The accepted treatment of sacral GCTs is subject of debate given the variable results and associated morbidity and mortality experienced with surgical resection and primary radiotherapy [50]. Serial arterial embolization may serve useful in treatment as most patients demonstrate an immediate objective and subjective response to embolization and this modality should be included in the armamentarium of treatments for patients with this disease [51].

Vertebral hemangiomas are relatively common, benign hypervascular tumors affecting the vertebral column and they contribute to 2–3% of all spinal tumors [52]. These lesions are largely asymptomatic and are often picked up incidentally. They can occasionally enlarge and cause pain or even spinal cord compression leading to neurological deficit. Treatments are traditionally radiotherapy or decompressive surgery with or without post-operative radiotherapy [53]. Embolization can be carried out in this setting as a pre-operative measure to limit intraoperative blood loss (which itself allows a more aggressive surgical approach), or it can be used as a pain controlling measure [53].

Technically, the procedure is identical to that used in the treatment of vertebral metastatic lesions.

IV. VERTEBROPLASTY AND OSTEOPLASTY

Vertebroplasty was initially described in the 1980s when percutaneous injection of methylmethacrylate cement was utilized as an alternative to surgery and arterial embolization in the treatment of spinal hemangiomas [54]. In contrast to spine surgery, which carries significant morbidity, is time consuming and expensive, vertebroplasty is minimally invasive, of inherently low morbidity and relatively inexpensive. These advantages have been reflected in continued reports appearing in the literature advocating the procedure in the treatment of refractory vertebral compression fractures [55–57].

Osteoporotic compression fractures are the most common indication for vertebroplasty in North America [58–62]. This is also the indication for which vertebroplasty has been most successful.

Osteoporosis is extremely common in the Western world. Despite advances in investigation and management [63–70] there remains an enormous burden on health care spending. It is estimated that the annual cost of inpatient treatment of osteoporosis in the USA is approximately 750 million dollars with approximately 700,000 osteoporotic compression fractures occurring each year [68]. In two thirds of these patients, pain resolution is either spontaneous or achieved with only medical therapies within 6 weeks. Vertebroplasty has gained utility in the treatment of the non-responsive osteoporotic compression fractures. In these patients, who are often elderly and deconditioned, the goal is to maximize quality of life by reducing pain, increasing mobility and reducing analgesic requirements. The ultimate aim is to reduce osteoporotic fracture associated mortality, which may increase 23–34% in untreated fractures. Ideally, increased use of vertebroplasty would be reflected in reduced spending on the treatment of osteoporotic compression fractures.

Pathologic vertebral compression fractures (those resulting from the fracture of a bone weakened by a pathologic process, often malignancy) are the second largest indication for vertebroplasty. Growth in the use of vertebroplasty in this setting partially reflects the limitations of traditional therapeutic options. Radiotherapy, the accepted gold standard in the treatment of bone malignancy, fails in 10–50% of patients as evidenced by there being no response, or an insufficient response despite the maximum safe dose having been reached. Chemotherapy, which is occasionally used in combination, is systemically toxic. Both have a delayed onset of action, typically between 12 and 20 weeks. Analgesic agents such as non-steroidal inflammatory drugs and opiates have well-documented side effect profiles and are subject to tolerance.

The remaining indications for vertebroplasty include trauma-induced fractures including burst fractures [69], Paget's disease [70], osteogenesis imperfecta [71,72] and aneurysmal bone cysts.

Although various figures have been published, dramatic or very significant improvement in pain has been consistently reported in approximately 75% and 85% of patients treated for pathologic and osteoporotic compression fractures, respectively. The onset of pain relief is rapid, typically within hours to 1 week almost always following a degree of local discomfort related to the procedure.

The natural history in most patients undergoing vertebroplasty is of an acute vertebral compression fracture (VCF) complicated by pain persisting beyond 4 to 6 weeks despite conservative measures and medical therapy (the non-responsive subacute VCF). As mentioned, this group comprises approximately one third of patients who have vertebral fractures [73,74]. In selected instances treatment in the initial 4 weeks (the acute phase) [75] is performed. This, however, may lead to a higher risk of complications such as cement leakage [76,77]. Pre-procedural cross-sectional imaging, either computed tomography (CT) or magnetic resonance imaging (MRI) is essential for procedural planning. This includes a decision as to which vertebral segments will be treated, the size of the needle that will be used, the expected needle approach and whether radiofrequency (RF) ablation or cavity creation will be used in conjunction. MRI may be preferable. It both better images all components of the neural axis and is more sensitive in detecting confounding pathologies (such as disc herniations). MRI utilizing a short tau inversion recovery (STIR) sequence is also highly sensitive in the detection of marrow edema [78,79], which correlates with pain and therefore the sites that should be targeted for treatment.

Several contraindications of vertebroplasty exist. Coagulopathy, specifically an INR of greater than 1.2, is an absolute contraindication due to the risk of uncontrolled bleeding. Unstable vertebral body fractures, particularly those involving the posterior vertebral body wall with a retro-pulsed fragment causing greater than 40% reduction in the anteroposterior dimension of the canal, preclude vertebroplasty due to both the risk of direct mechanical cord or cauda equina injury by displacement of retro-pulsed fragments and of potential thermal neural injury by extravasated methylmethacrylate. Local or systemic infection must be eradicated prior to the procedure due to the risk of vertebral osteomyelitis and discitis by direct inoculation. Vertebral body collapse with greater than 90% loss of vertebral body height effectively excludes patients from treatment as appropriate intravertebral needle placement is not possible. Neurological symptoms provide another contraindication as their presence often heralds preexisting canal compromise, which could be exacerbated.

Informed consent is obtained from all patients, which includes a general discussion of risks associated with

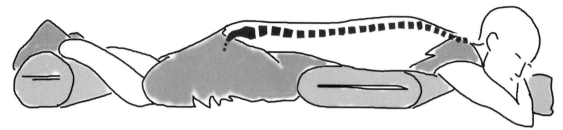

FIGURE 22.9   Standard patient position in vertebroplasty. Padding placed under the patient is used to straighten the spine.

vertebroplasty as well as a discussion of risks specific to the region being treated. For example, in consenting for treatment of a thoracic vertebra, the potential for anterior cement extravasation resulting in thermal injury to the structures within the visceral space is mentioned. Anesthetic support is invaluable. At our institution, the choice of local anesthetic, conscious sedation or general anesthetic is left to the anesthesiologist.

In conventional vertebroplasty, the patient is placed prone with padding beneath the thorax and ankles in order to maximize comfort and straighten the vertebral column as much a possible (Figure 22.9). Some time is taken with patient positioning. The PA projection over the vertebrae to be treated is magnified and obliqued such that the ideal needle trajectory through the pedicle is visualized en face. Similarly, the lateral projection is adjusted such that a true lateral projection is acquired with clear visualization of the vertebral bodies, end plates and overlap of any visualized ribs. A biplane fluoroscopic unit or a C-arm with an isocenter function is required. This enables rapid switching between the posteroanterior (PA) and lateral projections to assess cement distribution during the injection.

The puncture site is localized with a skin marker such as a Kelly's forcep, which is then used to guide the local anesthetic needle. Local anesthetic agent is used to create a subcutaneous bleb over the puncture site and then infiltrate the subcutaneous tissues, muscle and the pain sensitive periosteum (Figure 22.10). The local anesthetic needle is used as a guide to the trajectory required for the vertebroplasty needle. The vertebroplasty needle is held with forceps and passed through a skin nick formed by a scalpel until it engages the periosteum. Its position can be altered using fluoroscopic guidance. A range of needle sizes can be used. Small caliber (15G) needles are typically chosen when accessing small pedicles such as in the upper thoracic spine and in the treatment of severely crushed vertebrae (vertebrae plana's). Large (8G) needles are used in the cavity creation techniques (kyphoplasty and Skyphoplasty). A transpedicular approach is generally preferred in which the upper outer quadrant of the pedicle is punctured and a medial needle trajectory is taken through the pedicle and vertebral body with the aim being a final needle position in the anterior third of the lower portion of the vertebra in the midline (Figure 22.11). This maximizes the chance of

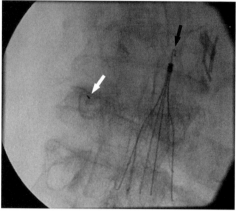

FIGURE 22.10   Oblique posteroanterior projection demonstrating a severe compression fracture of L4. A 22 gauge spinal needle (white arrow) is placed at the periosteum of the left pedicle, which is visualized en face with the patient prone. Note the IVC filter (black arrow).

optimal vertebral cement opacification, which ideally encompasses most of the superoinferior dimension of the vertebral body with cement crossing the midline. In thoracic vertebrae, which are smaller than lumbar vertebrae with correspondingly smaller pedicles, a costotransverse puncture is occasionally used. Other described approaches include anterolateral and posterolateral punctures. More novel access routes including transoral puncture of C2 and transdiscal access have been reported [80,81]. Planned bipedicular punctures may be mandated by unique anatomic features of the vertebrae being treated; for example, a heavily compressed vertebrae with near complete loss of vertebral body height centrally preventing needle placement in the midline.

Bone cement is mixed once satisfactory needle tip position has been achieved. Osteofirm radio-opaque bone cement can be used. This cement is backfilled into 1 ml syringes and is initially of a fluid consistency. Within minutes, the cement reaches a toothpaste-like consistency [82] at which time it is cautiously injected under continuous biplane fluoroscopic guidance utilizing both planes (Figure 22.12). Should a region of cement extravasation be suspected, the injection is ceased briefly to allow the cement to polymerize and harden. Often the needle will be rotated causing the bevel to turn in an attempt to redirect the

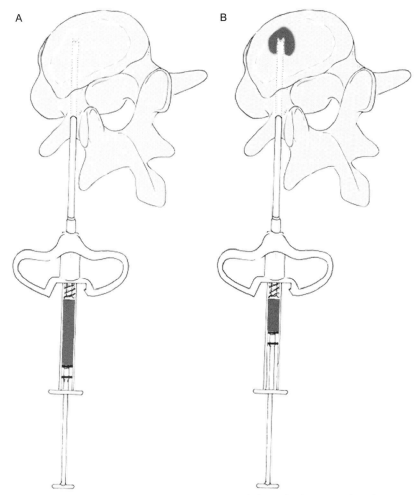

FIGURE 22.11 Schematic showing transpendicular vertebroplasty. (A) Schematic demonstrating the expected needle trajectory in a transpedicular puncture during percutaneous vertebroplasty; (B) schematic demonstrating cement injection.

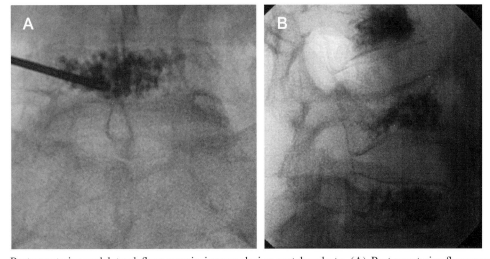

FIGURE 22.12 Posteroanterior and lateral fluoroscopic images during vertebroplasty. (A) Posteroanterior fluoroscopic image during vertebroplasty via a left transpedicular puncture with the needle *in situ* demonstrating an ideal cement distribution; (B) lateral fluoroscopic image during vertebroplasty in the same patient as (A).

injection. In selected cases the needle may be withdrawn slightly under fluoroscopic guidance and further injection made to maximize vertebral body filling. The methylmethacrylate has a limited useful working time, hardening as it polymerizes to a level inhibiting further injection. If opacification is suboptimal a contralateral puncture may be required to complete the procedure. Once complete the needles are rotated to fracture the cement column and local dressings are applied. In our institution intraprocedural images are stored in orthogonal planes using a last image hold function.

Immediate post-procedural multi-detector CT scanning is advised, to assist the cement distribution, potential height restoration and any change in kyphotic angle (Figure 22.13).

Neurological observations and wound site assessment are performed during a 4-hour period of observed bed rest before discharge. We usually recommend that the patient returns to normal activities as tolerated the following day with caution.

A number of complications with vertebroplasty have been documented. The published frequency of complications is 1.3% for osteoporosis, 2.5% for hemangioma and 10% in the treatment of metastatic disease [83]. Complications are almost always self-limited. In general there is a slightly higher risk of cement extravasation and periprocedural hemorrhage in the treatment of pathologic crush fractures. Cement extravasation is the most frequent complication occurring in up to 72.5% of malignant and 65% of osteoporotic compression fractures treated [84]. In almost all cases this is self-limited extravasation into either the vertebral venous plexus or directly into the Para spinal soft tissues. More worrisome examples of extravasation are rare. These include pulmonary cement embolization, thermal neural injury resulting from foraminal or epidural

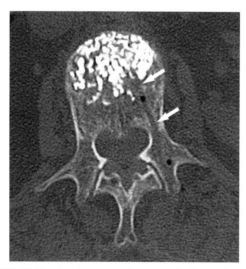

FIGURE 22.13 Axial computed tomography image demonstrating the ideal intravertebral cement distribution post vertebroplasty with cement crossing the midline and no extravasation. The transpedicular needle tract is clearly visible (arrow).

extravasation [85–90] and pedicle fractures during needle placement resulting in dural and neural injuries. In addition, rib and sternal fractures may complicate vigorous patient positioning. Up to 30% of patients will experience a transient exacerbation of pain usually lasting hours.

The mechanism of action of vertebroplasty is not fully understood. It is hypothesized that reduced motion between fracture fragments and microtrabecular stabilization reduces activity in pain sensitive periosteal nerves. In addition, direct chemical and thermal cauterization of these pain sensitive nerve fibers is thought to make a contribution. It has also been suggested that it is in preventing further compression that vertebroplasty has some of its effect.

Various reports have described incidences of new fractures post-treatment within adjacent vertebrae shortly after treatment. It has been suggested that with pain reduction, increased load is placed upon an abnormal (often osteoporotic) spine, which, when combined with the increased tendency for elderly patients to fall, has been felt likely to contribute to incidences of post-treatment fractures in adjacent levels.

Kyphoplasty, also known as 'balloon assisted vertebroplasty', is another method of percutaneous spinal augmentation. Patient workup, anesthesia, positioning and access are as for conventional vertebroplasty. Unlike vertebroplasty, a larger (8–10G) cannula is used to gain access and a degree of pre-insertion, monitoring and preparation of the device is required. A bone biopsy drill is passed through the access cannula to create a channel for an inflatable bone tamp. This is placed and inflated to create an intravertebral cavity. It can be deflated and repositioned to extend the created cavity as required by the configuration of the lesion being treated.

SKyphoplasty is the latest method of percutaneous vertebral method of augmentation. As with kyphoplasty, it is a cavity creation technique. It utilizes a device known as the SKy Bone Expander (disc orthopedic technology/Disc-O-Tech Monroe Township, New Jersey), which comprises a stiff plastic tube, which is deployed through an 8-gauge cannula introduced in a similar fashion to vertebroplasty. It is subsequently deployed into a popcorn-like crenulated configuration to create an intravertebral cavity. Unlike kyphoplasty, the device can only be used once. Theoretic risks of cavity creation devices such as height restoration, kyphotic angle correction, reduced cement extravasation and more predictable cement flow have not definitively been proven.

The basic technique of vertebroplasty has been adapted to treating lesions in the pelvis, with most experience in the sacrum and acetabulum. The indication is almost exclusively malignancy, the exception being the treatment of sacral insufficiency fractures. Pelvic procedures tend to be more complex, often employing combined cement injection, RF ablation and cavity creation. Early results with these combined techniques are promising and suggest that they provide additional benefit when used in combination rather than singly.

Radiofrequency ablation has long been used in the treatment of osteoid osteomas, a benign but painful lesion of the skeleton. Investigators have begun to treat painful bone tumors, especially metastases, with good success particularly when the tumor—normal bone interface—is ablated. The injection of bone cement following RF ablation helps provide additional structural support. The exact role for each of these techniques alone or in combination will be an active area of clinical research in the coming years.

References

1. F. Ellis, Needle biopsy in the clinical diagnosis of tumors, Br J Surg 34 (1974) 240–261.
2. J. Tehranzadeh, C. Tao & C.A. Browing, Percutaneous needle biopsy of the spine, Acta Radiol 48 (2007) 860–868.
3. M.A. Hau, J.I. Kim & S. Kattapuram, et al., Accuracy of CT-guided biopsies in 359 patients with musculoskeletal lesions, Skeletal Radiol 31 (2002) 349–353.
4. J. Issakov, G. Flusser & Y. Kollender, et al., Computed tomography-guided core needle biopsy for bone and soft tissue tumors, Isr Med Assoc J 5 (2003) 28–30.
5. A. Puri, V.U. Shingade & M.G. Agarwal, et al., CT-guided percutaneous core needle biopsy in deep seated musculoskeletal lesions: a prospective study of 128 cases, Skeletal Radiol 35 (2006) 138–143.
6. B. Ghelman, Biopsies of the musculoskeletal system, Radiol Clin North Am 36 (1998) 576–580.
7. KH. Ahlstrom & K.G.O. Astrom, CT-guided bone biopsy performed by means of a coaxial biopsy system with an eccentric drill, Radiology 188 (1993) 549–552.
8. J.S. Jelinek, M.J. Kransdorf & R. Gray, et al., Percutaneous transpedicular biopsy of vertebral body lesions, Spine 21 (1996) 2035–2040.
9. W. Berning, J. Freyschmidt & H. Ostertag, Percutaneous bone biopsy, techniques and indications, Eur Radiol 6 (1996) 875–881.
10. E.F. McCarthy, CT-guided needle biopsies of bone and soft tissue tumors: a pathologist's perspective, Skeletal Radiol 36 (2007) 181–182.
11. M.P. Logan, D.G. Connell & J.X. O'Connell, et al., Image-guided percutaneous biopsy of musculoskeletal tumors: an algorithm for selection of specific biopsy techniques, AJR Am J Roentgenol 166 (1996) 137–141.
12. M.W. Anderson, H.T. Temple & R.G. Dussault, et al., Compartmental anatomy: relevance to staging and biopsy of musculoskeletal tumors, AJR Am J Roentgenol 173 (1999) 1663–1671.
13. L. Yao, S.D. Nelson & L.L. Seeger, et al., Primary musculoskeletal neoplasms: effectiveness of core-needle biopsy, Radiology 212 (1999) 682–686.
14. H.J. Mankin, T.A. Lange & S.S. Spanier, The hazards of biopsy in patients with malignant primary bone and soft-tissue tumors, J Bone Joint Surg Am 64A (1982) 1121–1127.
15. M. Kang, S. Gupta & N. Khandelwal, et al., CT-guided fine-needle aspiration biopsy of spinal lesions, Acta Radiol 40 (1999) 474–478.
16. A. Saifuddin, B.S. Mann & S. Mahroof, et al., Dedifferentiated chondrosarcoma: use of MRI to guide needle biopsy, Clin Radiol 59 (2004) 268–272.
17. R. Blanco-Seqeuiros, R. Klemola & R. Ojala, et al., MRI-guided trephine biopsy and fine-needle aspiration in the diagnosis of bone lesions in low-field (0.23 T) MRI system using optical instrument tracking, Eur Radiol 12 (2002) 830–835.
18. J. Alanen, L. Keski-Nisula & R. Blanco-Seqeuiros, et al., Cost-comparison analysis of low-field (0.23 T) MRI- and CT-guided bone biopsies, Eur Radiol 14 (2004) 123–128.
19. J. Garces & G. Hidalgo, Lateral access for CT-guided percutaneous biopsy of the lumbar spine, AJR Am J Roentgenol 174 (2000) 425–426.
20. D. Yaffe, G. Greenberg & J. Leitner, et al., CT-guided percutaneous biopsy of thoracic and lumbar spine: a new coaxial technique, AJNR Am J Neuroradiol 24 (2003) 2111–2113.
21. O. Buckley, W. Benfayed & T. Geoghegan, et al., CT-guided bone biopsy: initial experience with a commercially available hand held Black and Decker drill, Eur J Radiol 61 (2007) 176–180.
22. K. Iemsawatdikul, C.A. Gooding & E.L. Twomey, et al., Seeding of osteosarcoma in the biopsy tract of a patient with multifocal osteosarcoma, Pediatr Radiol 35 (2005) 717–721.
23. S.G. Leffler & F.X. Chew, CT-guided percutaneous biopsy of sclerotic bone lesions: diagnostic yield and accuracy, AJR Am J Roentgenol 172 (1999) 1389–1392.
24. A. Velpeau, Memoire sur la piqure ou l'acupuncture des arteres dans le traitement des aneurismes, Gaz Med Paris 2 (1831) 1–4.
25. A.J. Luessenhop & W.T. Spence, Artificial embolization of cerebral arteries. Report of use in a case of arteriovenous malformation, JAMA 172 (1960) 1153–1155.
26. S.K. Seppanen & M.J. Leppanen, et al., Microcatheter embolisation of hemorrhages, Cardiovasc Intervent Radiol 20 (3) (1997) 174–179.
27. G.P. Teitelbaum & R.A. Reed, et al., Microcatheter embolisation of non-neurologic traumatic vascular lesions, J Vasc Interv Radiol 4 (1) (1993) 149–154.
28. A.A. Nicholson, Vascular radiology in trauma, Cardiovasc Intervent Radiol 27 (2004) 105–120.
29. F. Feldman, W.J. Casarella & H.M. Dick, et al., Selective intra-arterial embolization of bone tumors. A useful adjunct in the management of selected lesions, AJR 123 (1975) 130–139.
30. J. Weber, Palliative embolization in bone metastasis of hypernephroma using oily contrast-labelled gel, Ann Radiol 25 (1982) 460–462.
31. D.M. Rowe, G.J. Becker & F.E. Rabe, et al., Osseous metastasis from renal cell carcinoma: embolization and surgery for restoration of function, Radiology 150 (1984) 673–676.
32. T.A. Bowers, J.A. Murray & C. Charnsangavej, et al., Bone metastasis from renal carcinoma, J Bone Joint Surg 64A (1982) 749–754.
33. F.E. Gellard, N. Sadato & Y. Numaguchi, et al., Vascular metastatic lesions of the spine: preoperative embolization, Radiology 176 (1990) 683–686.
34. M. Reuter, M. Heller & U. Heise, et al., Transcatheter embolization of tumors of the musculo-skeletal system, Fortschr Rontgenstr 156 (1992) 182–188.
35. R. Nickolisen & B. Fallon, Locally recurrent hypernephroma treated by radiation therapy and embolization, Cancer 56 (1985) 1049–1051.
36. G.V. O'Reilly, J. Kleefield & L.A. Klein, et al., Embolization of solitary spinal metastases from renal cell carcinoma:alternative

therapy for spinal cord or nerve root compression, Surg Neurol 31 (1989) 268–271.

37. P.L. Munk, M.J. Lee & D.C. Morris, et al., Embolisation of renal cell carcinoma bone metastasis, Journal of the Hong Kong College of Radiology 2 (4) (1999) 327–335.

38. T.H. Suh, Vascular system of the human spinal cord, Arch Neurol Psychia 41 (1939) 559–677.

39. A.P. Hemingway & D.J. Allison, Complications of embolization: analysis of 410 procedures, Radiology 669 (1988).

40. J. Varma, R.P. Huben & Z. Wajsman, et al., Therapeutic embolization of pelvic metastasis of renal cell carcinoma, Urology 131 (1984) 647–649.

41. C.S. Soo, S. Wallace & V.P. Chuang, et al., Lumbar artery embolization in cancer patients, Radiology 145 (1982) 655–659.

42. A. Basile, T. Rand & F. Lomoschitz, et al., Trisacryl gelatin microscheres versus polyvinyl alcohol particles in the progressive embolization of bone neoplasms, Cardiovasc Intervent Radiol 27 (2004) 495–502.

43. P. Picci, L. Sangiorgi & L. Bahamonde, et al., Risk factors for local recurrences after limb-salvage surgery for high grade osteosarcoma of the extremities, Ann Oncol 8 (1997) 899–903.

44. T.E. Gellad, N. Sadato & Y. Numaguchi, et al., Vascular metastatic lesions of the spine: preoperative embolization, Radiology 176 (1990) 683–686.

45. Chu Jian-Ping, Chen Wei & Li Jia-ping, et al., Clinicopathologic features and results of transcatheter arterial chemoembolization for osteosarcoma, Cardiovasc Intervent Radiol 30 (2007) 201–206.

46. R. Yamada, T. Kishi & T. Sonomura, et al., Transcatheter arterial embolization in unresectable hepatocellular carcinoma, Cardiovasc Intervent Radiol 13 (1990) 135–139.

47. K.M. Yip, P.C. Leung & S.M. Kumta, Giant cell tumor of bone, Clin Orthop 323 (1996) 60–64.

48. R.E. Turcotte, F.H. Sim & K.K. Unni, Giant cell tumor of the sacrum, Clin Orthop 291 (1993) 215–221.

49. M. Campanacci, N. Baldini & S. Boriani, et al., Giant cell tumor of bone, J Bone Joint Surg Am 69 (1987) 106–114.

50. H.S. Hosalkar, K.J. Jones & J.J. King, et al., Serial arterial embolization for large sacral giant-cell tumors. Mid to long-term results, Spine 10 (2007) 1107–1115.

51. P.P. Lin, V.B. Guzel & M.F. Moura, et al., Long-term follow-up of patients with giant cell tumor of the sacrum treated with selective arterial embolization, Cancer 95 (6) (2002) 1317–1325.

52. M.W. Fox & B.M. Onofrio, The natural history and management of asymptomatic vertebral hemangiomas, J Neurosurg 78 (1993) 36–45.

53. F.L. Acosta, C.F. Dowd & C. Chin, et al., Current treatment strategies and outcomes in the management of symptomatic vertebral hemangiomas, Neurosurgery 58 (2) (2006) 287–294.

54. P. Galibert, H. Deramond & P. Rosat, et al., Preliminary note on the treatment vertebral angioma by percutaneous acrylic vertebroplasty, Neurochirurgie 33 (1987) 166–168.

55. L. Ramos, A. de Las Heras & S. Sanchez, et al., Medium-term results of percutaneous vertebroplasty in multiple myeloma, Eur J Haematol 77 (2006) 7–13.

56. M.K. Heran, G.M. Legiehn & P.L. Munk, Current concepts and techniques in percutaneous vertebroplasty, Orthop Clin North Am 37 (2006) 409–434.

57. P. Kammerlen, P. Thiesse & H. Bouvard, et al., Percutaneous vertebroplasty in the treatment of metastases. Technique and results, J Radiol 70 (10) (1989) 557–562.

58. J.M. Lane, C.E. Johnson & S.N. Khan, et al., Minimally invasive options for the treatment of osteoporotic vertebral compression fractures, Orthop Clin North Am 33 (2) (2002) 431–438.

59. T.A. Predey, L.E. Sewall & S.J. Smith, Percutaneous vertebroplasty: new treatment for vertebral compression fractures, Am Fam Physician 66 (4) (2002) 611–615.

60. S. Larsson, Treatment of osteoporotic fractures, Scand J Surg 91 (2) (2002) 140–146.

61. H. Deramond & J.M. Mathis, Vertebroplasty in osteoporosis, Semin Musculoskeletal Radiol 6 (3) (2002) 263–268.

62. F.M. Phillips, B.A. Pfeifer & I.H. Lieberman, et al., Minimally invasive treatments of osteoporotic vertebral compression fractures: vertebroplasty and kyphoplasty, Instr Course Lect 52 (2003) 559–567.

63. A. Papaioanou, N.B. Watts & D.L. Kendler, et al., Diagnosis and management of vertebral fractures in elderly adults, Am J Med 113 (3) (2002) 220–228.

64. S. Bajaj & K.G. Saag, Osteoporosis: evaluation and treatment, Curr Womens Health Rep 3 (5) (2003) 418–424.

65. D.H. Kim, J.S. Silber & T.J. Albert, Osteoporotic vertebral compression fractures, Instr Course Lect 52 (2003) 541–550.

66. S.D. Glassman & G.M. Alegre, Adult spinal deformity in the osteoporotic spine: options and pitfalls, Instr Course Lect 52 (2003) 579–588.

67. S.S. Wu, E. Lachmann & W. Nagler, Current medical, rehabilitation and surgical management of vertebral compression fractures, J Womens Health (Larchmt) 12 (1) (2003) 17–26.

68. B.L. Riggs & L.J. Melton, The worldwide problem of osteoporosis: insights afforded by epidemiology, Bone 17 (S) (1995) 505–511.

69. J.F. Chen & S.T. Lee, Percutaneous vertebroplasty for treatment of thoracolumbar spine bursting fracture, Surg Neurol 62 (6) (2004) 494–500 (discussion 500).

70. M.A. Kremer, A. Fruin & T.C., Larson, III, et al., Vertebroplasty in focal Paget disease of the spine. Case Report, J Neurosurg 99 (1 Suppl) (2003) 110–113.

71. Pm. Rami, J.K. McGraw & E.V. Heatwole, et al., Percutaneous vertebroplasty in the treatment of vertebral body compression fracture secondary to osteogenesis imperfecta, Skeletal Radiol 31 (3) (2002) 162–165.

72. G. Kasó, C. Varjú & T. Dóczi, Multiple vertebral fractures in osteogenesis imperfecta treated by vertebroplasty, J Neurosurg (Spine 1) 2 (2004) 237.

73. K.J. Murphy & D.D. Lin, Vertebroplasty: a simple solution to a difficult problem, J Clin Densitom 4 (3) (2001) 189–197.

74. S.L. Silvermann, The clinical consequences of vertebral compression fracture, Bone 13 (1992) S27–S531.

75. Th. Diamond, T. Hartwell & W. Clarke, et al., Percutaneous vertebroplasty for acute vertebral body fracture and deformity in multiple myeloma: a short report, Br J Haematol 124 (4) (2004) 485–487.

76. S.W. Yu, P.C. Lee & C.H. Ma, et al., Vertebroplasty for the treatment of osteoporotic spinal compression fracture: comparison of remedial action at different stages of injury, J Trauma 56 (3) (2004) 629–632.

77. M.M. Teng, H. Cheng & D.M. Ho, et al., Intraspinal leakage of bone cement after vertebroplasty: a report of 3 cases, AJNR Am J Neuroradiol 27 (1) (2006) 224–229.

78. H.M. Do, Magnetic resonance imaging in the evaluation of patients for percutaneous vertebroplasty, Top Mag Reson Imaging 11 (4) (2000) 235–244.

79. N. Tanigawa, A. Komemushi & S. Kariya, et al., percutaneous vertebroplasty: relationship between vertebral body bone marrow edema pattern on MR images and initial clinical response, Radiology 239 (2006) 195–200.

80. J.B. Martin, P. Gailloud & P.Y. Dietrich, et al., Direct transoral approach to C2 for percutaneous vertebroplasty, Cardiovasc Intervent Radiol 25 (6) (2002) 517–519.

81. A. Mehdizade, M. Payer & T. Somon, et al., Percutaneous vertebroplasty through a transdiscal access route after lumbar transpedicular instrumentation, Spine J 4 (4) (2004) 475–479.

82. M.E. Jensen, A.J. Evans & J.M. Mathis, et al., Percutaneous polymethylmethacrylate vertebroplasty in the treatment of osteoporotic vertebral body compression fractures: technical aspects, AJNR Am J Neuroradiol 18 (10) (1997) 1897–1904.

83. J. Chiras, C. Depriester & A. Weill, et al., Percutaneous vertebral surgery: techniques and indications, J Neuroradiol 24 (1997) 45–59.

84. J.D. Laredo & B. Hamze, Complications of percutaneous vertebroplasty and their prevention, Semin Ultrasound CT MR 26 (2) (2005) 65–80.

85. J. Ratliff, T. Nguyen & J. Heiss, Root and spinal cord compression from methylmethacrylate vertebroplasty, Spine 261 (13) (2001) E300–E302.

86. N.M. Lopes & V.K. Lopes, Paraplegia complicating percutaneous vertebroplasty for osteoporotic compression fracture. A case report, Arq Neuropsiquiatr 62 (3B) (2004) 879–881.

87. P. Kammerlen, P. Thiesse & H. Bouvard, et al., Percutaneous vertebroplasty in the treatment of metastases. Technique and results, J Radiol 70 (10) (1989) 557–562.

88. A. Cotton, N. Boutry & B. Cortet, et al., Percutaneous vertebroplasty: state of the art, Radiographics 18 (2) (1998) 311–320 (discussion 320–323).

89. B.J. Lee, S.R. Lee & T.Y. Yoo, Paraplegia as a complication of percutaneous vertebroplasty with polymethylmethacrylate: a case report, Spine 27 (19) (2002) E419–E422.

90. S. Shapiro, T. Abel & S. Purvines, Surgical removal of epidural and intradural polymethylmethacrylate extravasation complicating percutaneous vertebroplasty for a osteoporotic lumbar compression fracture. Case report, J Neurosurg 98 (1 Suppl) (2003) 90–92.

CHAPTER **23**

Imaging of Bone Metastases

NIEROSHAN RAJARUBENDRA[1] AND NATHAN LAWRENTSCHUK[1]

[1]*University of Melbourne, Department of Surgery, Urology Unit, Austin Hospital, Heidelberg, Melbourne, Australia.*

Contents

TABLE 23.2   Radiological features of bony lesions [6]

Commonly lytic	Commonly blastic	Commonly mixed
Kidney	Bladder, with prostate	Lung
Thyroid	Bronchial carcinoid	Ovary
Adrenal		Testis
Uterus		Cervix

I. INTRODUCTION

Bone provides an ideal environment for metastases of cancer. For cancers such as breast, lung and prostate, the incidence of bony metastatic spread is as high as 70% [1]. Other malignancies that metastasize to bone are kidney, thyroid, bladder and colon (refer to Table 23.1). The complications attributed to bone metastases can be debilitating. They can result in severe pain, pathological fractures, spinal cord compression, hypercalcemia and nerve compression syndromes.

The presence of bony metastases is a survival predictor. For example, the five-year survival for patients with bony spread of breast cancer is 20% [3]. In the United States there are more than 350,000 people who die with bone metastases [4].

Bone is a preferred site for spread as blood flow is high in areas of red marrow. Adhesive molecules produced by tumor cells bind to marrow stromal cells and bone matrix. Furthermore, there is a large reservoir for immobilized growth factors [1]. It is difficult to determine the tendency of tumors to spread to bone because patients who succumb to cancer early from an aggressively growing malignancy do not have enough time for metastases to develop.

Bone metastases are classified as either being osteoblastic (bone forming) or osteolytic (bone destructive) (refer to Table 23.2). However, the majority of cancers have a combination of the two. At the extreme end of the spectrum, multiple myeloma is lytic, while prostate cancer is predominately osteoblastic [5].

Prevention of complications of bony metastases by early detection can reduce morbidity to patients as well as the cost to the community. It will allow the implementation of treatment strategies such as surgical fixation, radiotherapy or bisphosphonate therapy. As part of the assessment and surveillance of malignancies, radiological imaging modalities are vital in the diagnosis of bony spread.

TABLE 23.1   Frequency of metastatic spread to bone [2]

Order of frequency	Whole population
1	Breast
2	Prostate
3	Bronchus
4	Colon
5	Stomach
6	Bladder
7	Uterus
8	Rectum
9	Thyroid
10	Kidney
11	Ovary

II. IMAGING MODALITIES

There are several methods used in analyzing and assessing bone metastases. The most common forms include the following.

A. Plain Radiography

An x-ray beam is projected through a patient and is absorbed in varying degrees by the different structures within the body. Only a small percentage of the beam strikes the detector plate forming the image.

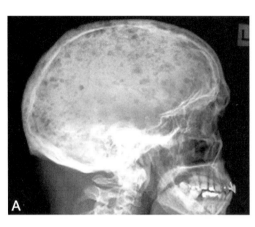
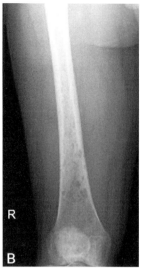

FIGURE 23.1 A 48-year-old male diagnosed with multiple myeloma. (A) Skull showing multiple lesions—'pepper pot' skull appearance; (B) distal right femur with multiple lytic lesions.

The final result of bone destruction and repair is seen with plain radiography. Usually lysis or sclerosis predominates and will characterize that particular bone metastasis. Lytic lesions are commonly found in breast, lung, thyroid, kidney and myeloma. These lesions have a thinning of trabeculae and ill-defined margins that represent regions of destroyed trabeculae between the central destruction and the radiological normal bone (Figure 23.1).

Prostate cancer predominantly has sclerotic lesions. However, it can also be found in breast and carcinoid tumors. Radiologically they appear as nodular, rounded and fairly well-circumscribed sclerotic areas due to the thickened coarse trabeculae (Figure 23.2).

Plain radiographs visualize bone structure and as a result 30 to 75% of normal bone mineral content must be lost before they become apparent. Therefore, it may take several months before they can be detected using this modality. It is less sensitive, ranging from 44 to 50% (level II-III evidence) than bone scintigraphy [7].

B. Computed Tomography

CT operates by rotating a continuous fan beam of radiation through a patient and measuring the transmission at thousands of points. The data obtained is calculated by a computer, which determines the exact exposure of radiation at a given location. The information produced is presented as segmental slices or as reconstructed three-dimensional images. Conventional scanners, called spiral or helical scanners, work by rotating the x-ray tube around the patient while the table which they are on is moving.

New scanners such as the multidetector CT, which has multiple rows of detectors, can obtain up to 16 slices at once. This allows for results to be obtained faster and at high spatial resolution [8] (Figure 23.3).

As a cautionary note, it is acknowledged that the amount of radiation exposure is high with the use of CT. In the 1990s, the Royal College of Radiologists in the UK compared CT with conventional x-ray. It was determined that a

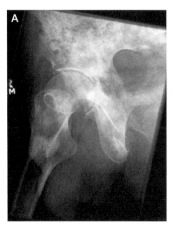
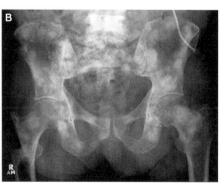

FIGURE 23.2 An 82-year-old male was diagnosed with metastatic prostate cancer. (A and B), Plain radiographs of the right hip and pelvis show multiple sclerotic lesions.

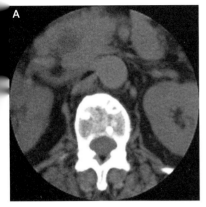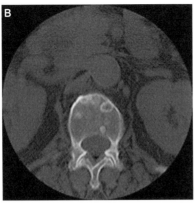

FIGURE 23.3 Conventional CT imaging of spinal column with the presence of bony metastases is seen in A. Bony windows in B show greater detail in the bone structure and the lesions are seen with more definition in comparison to the conventional window.

CT of the abdomen was equivalent to the radiation exposure equivalent to 500 chest x-rays [9]. It is recommended that patient selection and benefits of the use of CT compared to unnecessary radiation exposure should be assessed before ordering this investigation.

However, the benefit of the images produced by a CT scanner of bony metastases is in the detail. It is able to show both osteolytic and osteoblastic lesions as well as soft tissue extension. CT visualizes bone structure, tumors in bone marrow and can detect potentially small bone marrow metastases early. The sensitivity of CT has been reported ranging from 71 to 100% (level II-III evidence) [7].

Despite having the ability to show spinal metastases well with the use of bony windows, the entire vertebral column cannot be scanned due to the limitations with the CT table movement. As a result it is employed to assess suspicious lesions questioned by other imaging modalities.

C. Bone Scintigraphy

Images are produced by administration of a radionucleotide, usually ^{99m}Tc-methylene diphosphonate (^{99m}Tc-MDP) and the distribution of radioactivity is recorded by a gamma camera. The radionucleotide is absorbed onto the calcium of hydroxyapatite in the bone, which is influenced by increased local blood flow and osteoblastic activity (Figure 23.4).

Bone scintigraphy has a high sensitivity of 95% in detecting metastatic bone disease but poor specificity [10]. Degenerative changes, infections and fractures can produce a false positive (Figure 23.5). As a result, further imaging is required to make the diagnosis. Initially a plain radiograph is taken; however, if the results appear to be normal but the suspicion of metastasis persists, further imaging in the form of CT or MRI is warranted.

False-positive results are a known drawback of bone scintigraphy but false-negative results have been reported (Figures 23.5 and 23.6). In purely osteolytic metastases that are aggressively developing, when bone turnover is labile

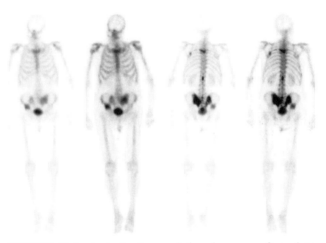

FIGURE 23.4 A staging bone scintigraphy was performed on a 77-year-old male with prostate cancer. Metastases are seen in the left 6th rib posteriorly, the right 5th and 6th ribs laterally, T6, spinous process of L2, sacrum and both ilia adjacent to sacroiliac joints and in the right superior acetabulum.

or the site is avascular (cold spot), it may fail to diagnose these lesions.

D. Positron Emission Tomography

Malignant tumors exhibit increased glucolysis due to upregulation of intracellular hexokinase activity [11]. The most commonly used radiopharmaceutical in PET is 2-deoxy-2-[^{18}F]-fluoro-D-glucose (FDG), which behaves as a glucose analog. It is able to provide qualitative and quantitative metabolic information allowing assessment of a lesion as being benign or malignant.

It is useful in the follow-up of patients after chemotherapy or surgical resection as the function capacity of the tumor is measured. Scarring or fibrosis does not affect its results. It is a whole-body technique and therefore detects disease in regions not routinely included in anatomical studies (Figure 23.7). Inadequacies have been addressed with its fusion with CT; see later.

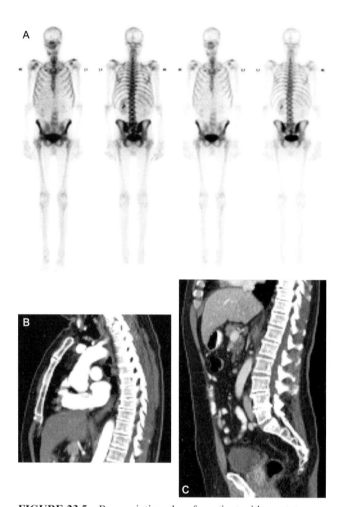

FIGURE 23.5   Bone scintigraphy of a patient with prostate cancer showed increased uptake in the lumbosacral spine and sternum (A). However, CT evaluation of these sites, images B and C, proved that there was no evidence of metastatic lesions but there was evidence of degenerative changes.

PET visualizes tumor metabolism and early tumor formation in marrow. Sensitivity for detecting bone metastases ranges from 62 to 100% and specificity from 96 to 100% (level II-III evidence) [7].

In the future, whole-body PET can be used to stage for not only bony metastases but also nodal and visceral disease.

E. Magnetic Resonance Imaging

MRI has the advantage of not using ionizing radiation and being non-invasive. It uses radiofrequency radiation in the presence of a carefully controlled magnetic field in order to produce high quality cross-sectional images of the body in any plane (Figure 23.8).

The difference in the magnetic signal intensity between the tumor tissue and normal bone marrow allows for the detection of bone metastases. With MRI, the metastatic tumor is visualized directly whereas plain radiography and bone scintigraphy visualize indirect changes. Like CT, it is more useful in assessing suspicious lesions found by other modalities.

MRI is the only imaging modality that allows direct visualization of the bone marrow. As a result, it can detect an intramedullary lesion before any cortex destruction and before any osteoblastic reaction is detected on a bone scan [12]. It is the often the technique of choice for cord compression.

It is able to produce wide sagittal views allowing for the entire spine to be imaged. As a result MRI is able to provide more information on the spine for patients with spinal symptoms in comparison to bone scintigraphy.

MRI like CT can visualize bone marrow and detect early tumors in marrow before structural changes in cortical bone are seen.

The images of bone marrow produced by MRI have better resolution than that by CT. On T1 imaging, bone marrow

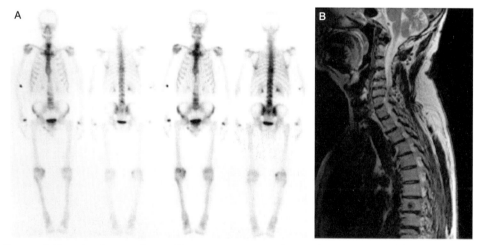

FIGURE 23.6   Bone scintigraphy in a patient with prostate cancer shows the presence of bone metastases in L4 vertebra (A). However, further imaging with MRI shows the presence of other bony lesions in T8 as seen in image B and also in T3, L1 and L2.

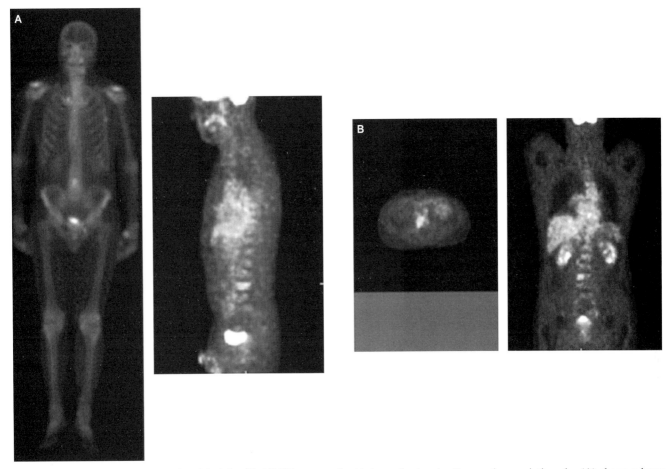

FIGURE 23.7 A 61-year-old male with right sided RCC presented with lower back pain. Reverse bone scintigraphy (A) shows a bony lesion at the L4 level. The group of images in B were performed with PET, which shows increased activity at the L4 level. Note increased activity is seen in the upper pole of the right kidney, depicting the RCC.

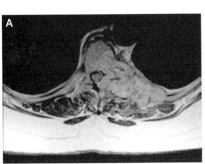

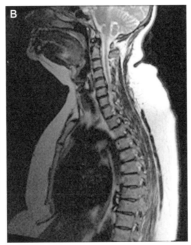

FIGURE 23.8 Metastatic RCC in a 59-year-old female. A metastatic lesion is seen in T8 and T9 extending into the left pedicle and left 9th rib. One third of the spinal canal is encroached upon by the malignancy.

produces a high intensity signal and metastases have a low signal as they replace the fat in the marrow. However, MRI is unable to depict destruction of bone structure as well as plain radiography and CT because cortical bone does not produce a signal.

F. PET/CT

The combination of a PET camera and a CT scanner allows for the amalgamation of functional and anatomical studies. It permits rapid and accurate anatomical localization of abnormal uptake.

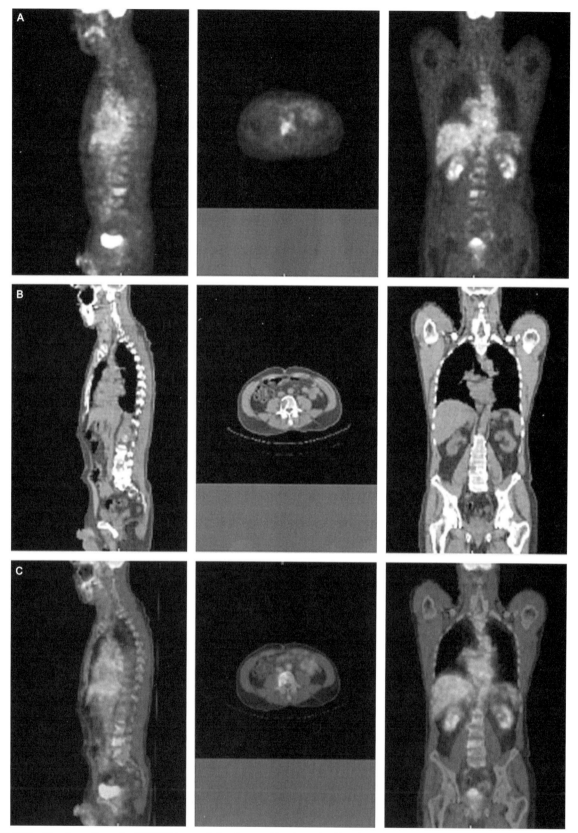

FIGURE 23.9   The formation of a PET/CT image is by the combination of a PET image with a CT scan. Image A shows the PET of the patient seen above with metastatic RCC. The CT image in B is able to show the anatomical location of the lesion in L4. The final product, image C, shows the PET/CT depicting the L4 lesion. It shows the metabolic activity as well as the anatomical location of the lesion.

A study by Nakamoto *et al.* indicated that CT only showed morphological changes in half of the patients who were identified as having bone metastases using PET [13]. However, in combination with PET, it was able to show precise locations of bone metastases allowing for targeted treatment (Figure 23.9).

The use of CT images enables for attenuation correction of PET emission data. It not only reduces scanning time by 40% but also produces noiseless attenuation-correction factors compared to the standard PET transmission measurements [14].

A study comparing PET and PET/CT indicated that the sensitivity of detecting bone metastases was 88 and 100%, respectively (*P* < 0.05) and specificity was 56 and 88%, respectively (not statistically significant) [15]. PET/CT has been shown to have a greater ability in differentiating between benign and malignant bony lesions.

III. MALIGNANCY

A. Breast Cancer

Bone metastases are very common in metastatic breast cancer. It has been reported that 30 to 85% of patients with metastatic breast cancer have bony lesions during their time course [16–18]. Morphology of breast cancer bone metastases can vary from osteoblastic to osteolytic to mixed. Breast cancer favors spread to the vertebra and pelvis and then to ribs, skull and femur as it is the location of red bone marrow [19,20].

Bone scintigraphy is the most common imaging modality used to assess for metastatic spread of breast cancer to bone. For breast cancer the published data have varied in terms of sensitivity and specificity. It has been reported in the range of 62 to 100% in sensitivity and 72 to 100% in specificity (level II-III evidence) [7] (Figure 23.10).

Plain radiography is useful in evaluating abnormal lesions on bone scintigraphy or symptomatic sites and should not be used as a screening tool due to its low sensitivity.

CT is much more useful in assessing bone lesions after treatment, as it is not affected by the 'flare phenomenon'.

The use of MRI in assessing for breast cancer bone metastases is as a supportive method to delineate if a lesion is metastatic which was initially investigated by other imaging modalities. Due to its high costs, it is not chosen as a screening tool.

In breast cancer the use of PET has high sensitivity of 67 to 100% in detecting occult primary breast lesions and in detecting bony metastases 84 to 100% (level II-III evidence) [7]. PET is more sensitive in detecting osteolytic metastases but less sensitive in detecting osteoblastic lesions [21]. The use of bone scintigraphy is advocated as a whole-body screening

modality for detecting bone metastases of breast cancer than PET due to cost and availability.

BOX 23.1

For screening, bone scintigraphy is the first choice and then plain radiography, CT and MRI are used to ascertain metastatic lesions if suspicious lesions are identified.

For focal symptoms, a plain radiograph should be used before CT and MRI to establish the anatomical changes.

CT is preferred for axial bone metastases.

MRI should be utilized for suspected lesions affecting the bone marrow or spinal cord compression.

PET and PET/CT can be used as a first line investigation in the future provided that its costs and availability have been addressed.

B. Prostate

Bone is the commonest site for the spread of prostate cancer, where it accounts for up to 80% of all metastases [22].

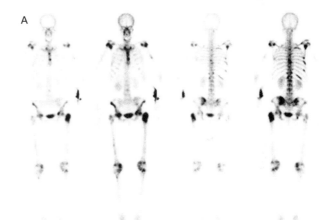

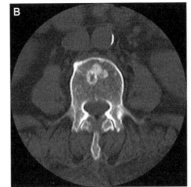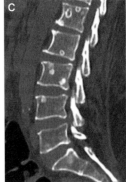

FIGURE 23.10 A 66-year-old female diagnosed with metastatic breast cancer. Image A shows widespread disease. Mixed lytic and sclerotic lesions measuring up to 1 cm in the lumbar vertebrae are seen on CT using bony windows (B and C).

Prostate cancer cells most commonly metastasize via the haematogenous route to well-vascularized areas of the skeleton, particularly the red bone marrow of the axial skeleton. These cells invade Batson's plexus, which is a low-pressure, high-volume communication venous network between the pelvis and vertebral veins. As a result the vertebral column is the first site for prostate cancer spread [22].

Early metastases can be missed because bone scintigraphy looks for osteoblastic reaction rather than tumor proliferation. Its sensitivity is impaired when assessing for microscopic or marrow-infiltrate-only disease or osteolytic lesions (which are uncommon in prostate cancer) [23].

According to the European Association of Urology guidelines, published in 2007 for the detection of bone metastases from prostate cancer, bone scintigraphy was recommended as the first line modality. An elevated Prostate Specific Antigen, PSA > 20 μg/L, increases the probability of detecting prostate cancer bone metastases (grade B recommendation) [24]. Other factors that increase the detection of bone metastases are when the patient has a locally advanced disease or with a Gleason score 8 or greater [25]. However, to overcome the deficiency with reduced specificity, other imaging modalities such as a plain radiograph, CT or MRI are needed to confirm the diagnosis as suspect lesions (Figure 23.11).

Bone scintigraphy can distinguish the site of metastases in relation to axial or appendicular distribution in the skeleton. This ability has been shown to assist with gauging prognosis. Axial metastases have a better prognosis than appendicular metastases [26].

When compared to bone scintigraphy, PET has been reported as not being as efficient in detecting bone metastases [27,28]. However, it could have a role in detecting local recurrence and distant spread after treatment failure [28,29]. Over time PET will improve and may challenge bone scintigraphy, but further studies are needed and data currently still strongly favor bone scintigraphy as the first line imaging modality.

Another radiotracer utilized for bone metastases, ^{18}F-fluoride-PET, has been shown to be more sensitive than bone scintigraphy. However, the data to support this is limited and further research is needed to establish this practice [15].

Groves *et al.* investigated the use of multidetector CT for the identification of bony metastases. They concluded that CT could not be validated to replace bone scintigraphy [30]. CT should be used as a complimentary investigative tool for assessing suspicious regions determined by bone scintigraphy or plain radiography. The combination of PET and CT as mentioned earlier is able to localize metastatic disease as well as be used to follow up treated patients. PET/CT has been put forward as being used as a first-line measure in re-staging prostate cancer after radical prostatectomy. However, it is still recommended that further data are needed before implementation of this technique as best practice [31].

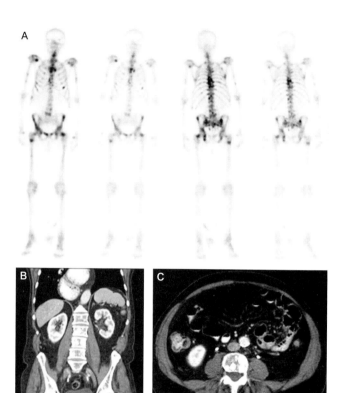

FIGURE 23.11 A patient diagnosed with hormone refractory prostate cancer shown here to have widespread osseous metastatic disease involving the axial and appendicular skeleton (A). Images B and C show multiple sclerotic lesions in the lumbar spine.

The use of MRI as a first-line imaging modality has been considered as not being feasible due to the limited availability, costs, and supportive data [32]. However, there have been studies indicating MRI as being much more sensitive and specific in detecting prostate cancer bone metastases in the spinal column than bone scintigraphy in high grade prostate cancer [33,34]. It is able to detect early stage bone metastases, before osteoblastic reactions appear visible on bone scintigraphy or plain radiography.

BOX 23.2

Bone scintigraphy should be used as first-line modality for screening for metastatic bone disease in prostate cancer.

Plain radiography, CT and MRI are important in distinguishing metastatic lesions questioned by bone scintigraphy.

PET and PET/CT are better for assessing bone metastases after treatment—however, further evidence is needed to support this methodology.

C. Lung

Lung cancer is the leading cause of deaths in the United States with the estimated deaths for 2007 being 160,390 [4]. It is categorized into two broad classifications, small cell carcinoma which accounts for 20%, and non-small cell carcinoma (NSCLC) for the remaining 80% [35]. The commonest sites of metastatic spread are the liver, adrenal gland, brain, bone, kidney, and abdominal lymph nodes [36]. The commonest site of bone metastases is in the axial skeleton. The majority of metastases from squamous cell carcinoma are osteolytic whereas adenocarcinoma and bronchial carcinoid tumors produce blastic lesions (Figure 23.12).

Accurate staging of lung cancer is paramount before therapeutic measures can be implemented. Radiological examination for the detection of metastatic spread is guided after clinical history, physical examination and blood indices (alkaline phosphatase, hematocrit, gamma-glutamyl-transpeptidase and aspartate aminotransferase) have been explored. If this work-up does not elicit any signs of metastatic spread, the negative predictive value has been shown to be greater than 95% and routine radiological evaluation of extrathoracic spread is not warranted [37].

For patients with NSCLC, the incidence of bone metastasis at the time of diagnosis is 10% [38]. Most of these patients have localized symptoms or laboratory markers indicating the possibility of bony spread. Plain radiograph, bone scintigraphy and MRI should be used to make the diagnosis (Figure 23.13).

In 2003, the American College of Chest Physicians published guidelines for the staging of NSCLC [39]. They recommend for localized symptoms, bone scintigraphy and plain radiography as the appropriate study to evaluate for bone metastases (grade A evidence). Patients with stage I or II lung cancer and who have normal clinical evaluation, do not require any extrathoracic imaging (grade A evidence) (Table 23.3). However, patients with stage IIIA and IIIB disease, bone scintigraphy should be used to screen for bone metastases, irrespective of clinical assessment (grade C evidence).

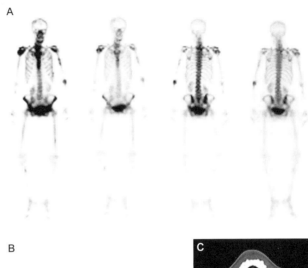

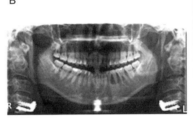

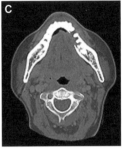

FIGURE 23.12 A 57-year-old female with NSCLC noted to have increased tracer uptake in multiple regions on bone scintigraphy (A). Tracer uptake is seen in left mandible, right humeral head, sternum, spinal column and right sacroiliac joint. An OPG and CT (B and C, respectively) show a lytic lesion in the mandible highlighting the presence of mixed lesions occurring in lung cancer.

As a modality, whole-body PET can detect both intra- and extrathoracic metastatic spread with the one examination. Van Tinteren *et al.* have shown that for patients who were considered to have operable NSCLC, the addition of PET as part of the initial screening process was able to detect metastatic disease in 20% of these patients and prevent unnecessary thoracotomy [41]. FDG PET has also been shown to

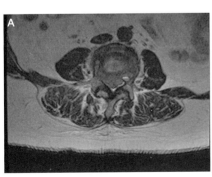

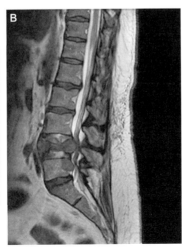

FIGURE 23.13 A 58-year-old female with NSCLC presented with right foot drop and sensation and power loss in L4-5 region. MRI shows a pathological fracture of L4 resulting in narrowing of the spinal canal by 75% (A and B). Also there is metastatic deposit seen on L5.

TABLE 23.3   Staging of NSCLC using TNM classification [40]

Stage	TNM
0	Carcinoma *in situ*
IA	T1N0M0
IB	T2N0M0
IIA	T1N1M0
IIB	T2N1M0
	T3N0M0
	T3N1M0
IIIA	T3N1M0
	T1-3N2M0
IIIB	Any T4
	Any N3
IV	Any M1

T = tumor, N = lymph node, M = distant metastases.

be more accurate than bone scintigraphy in NSCLC. It was more specific and had a higher positive predictive value than bone scintigraphy [42]. The accuracy of PET could eventually replace the use of bone scintigraphy but the lack of availability and costs detract from its universal use.

BOX 23.3

Where there are clinical and laboratory indicators suggesting possible bone metastases, plain radiography, bone scintigraphy and MRI can be employed to detect disease.

Patients with stage IIIA and IIIB lung cancer should have bone scintigraphy as part of work-up.

PET has shown to have great potential as a future staging modality for detecting intra- and extrathoracic metastases.

D. Renal

Renal cell carcinoma (RCC) accounts for 90% of all primary renal tumors [43]. In the United States the prevalence of new cases of renal tumors is over 50,000 [4]. On initial diagnosis of RCC, distant metastases have been found in 30 to 60% of patients and these lesions are predominantly osteolytic [44].

According to guidelines released by the European Association of Urology in 2007 for the staging of RCC, the use of bone scintigraphy for detection of bone spread should only be utilized in high-risk patients, e.g. raised alkaline phosphatase or bone pain (grade A recommendation) [45]. As a result, bone scintigraphy should not be employed as a screening modality in RCC. As discussed earlier, further imaging is required to confirm diagnosis of suspect lesions questioned by bone scintigraphy (Figure 23.14).

It has been reported that the sensitivity of FDG-PET in the detection of metastases in RCC is as high as 63 to 100% [46–50]. In cases where conventional studies have been inconclusive, PET has been able to assist with attaining a diagnosis. However, other studies have shown the sensitivity in screening for bone lesions in RCC to be less than conventional imaging [47]. With conflicting reports on sensitivity, it is difficult to justify its use in routine assessment of metastatic RCC.

However, for re-staging of RCC, FDG-PET has been reported to have sensitivities ranging between 87 and 100% [46]. Large trials are needed prior to implementing it as a follow-up tool.

BOX 23.4

Bone scintigraphy is recommended where symptoms or laboratory markers indicate a high possibility of bony spread. Further evaluation of suspect lesions can be assessed with plain radiography, CT and MRI where indicated.

PET possesses the possibility of becoming an imaging modality for screening and re-staging in the future. Further evidence is still required.

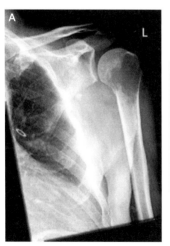
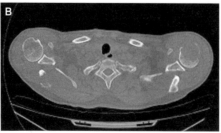

FIGURE 23.14 A 55-year-old male with renal cell carcinoma presented with left shoulder pain. A lytic lesion is seen in the proximal humerus with over 50% loss of cortex (A and B). The risk of developing a fracture was high and subsequently surgical fixation was conducted to prevent morbidity.

E. Thyroid

Papillary and follicular carcinoma account for 90% of all thyroid carcinoma and they are referred to as differentiated thyroid cancer (DTC); the remainder are anaplastic and medullary carcinoma, lymphoma and sarcoma [51]. Bone is the second commonest site of metastases of thyroid cancer after lung. Metastases to bone have been reported as ranging from 7 to 23% [52,53].

The majority of metastases to bone are lytic in nature. [131]I whole-body scan is used in the assessment for recurrence post-treatment; however, it has poor sensitivity in detecting bone metastases [54–57]. The more commonly used imaging modality for detecting metastatic spread to bone is plain radiography and bone scintigraphy. Plain radiography is used for localized symptoms whereas bone scintigraphy is employed for looking at the entire skeleton. Again, further imaging such as CT and MRI are used to clarify suspicious sites (Figure 23.15).

The use of FDG PET in thyroid cancer is gaining further support. A report by Ito *et al.* showed that FDG PET had a sensitivity of 87.4% and specificity of 99.6% compared with bone scintigraphy, which had a sensitivity of 78% and specificity of 91.4% [58]. FDG PET was also shown to have low false positive results in detection of bone metastases of DTC. Another study by Phan *et al.* concluded from their study that bone scintigraphy was more valuable in detecting bone metastases from DTC than FDG PET [59]. Despite conflicting evidence regarding the use of PET, it has shown great potential for superseding bone scintigraphy. The advent of PET/CT has been shown to improves diagnostic value in restaging DTC and also provides accurate information regarding subsequent treatment [60].

BOX 23.5

Bone scintigraphy or plain radiography should be used to assess for metastatic bony spread in symptomatic patients. Further imaging with CT and MRI should be employed to delineate suspect lesions.

PET and PET/CT have shown for potential use in the restaging process.

F. Bladder

The majority of bladder cancers are transitional cell carcinoma (TCC) (>90%) followed by squamous cell (5 to 10%), mixed transitional and squamous (<5%) and adenocarcinoma (2 to 3%) [61,62]. One third of the patients with TCC

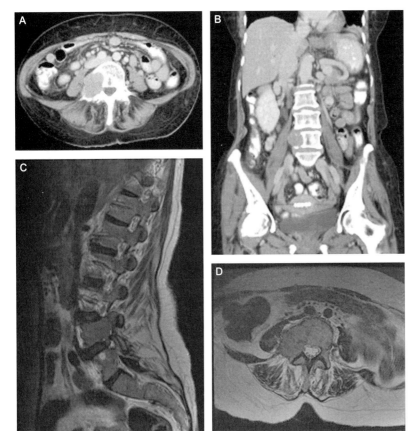

FIGURE 23.15 A 62-year-old female was diagnosed with thyroid cancer and presented with a four-day history of lower back pain. CT imaging showed multiple lesions in the spinal column in particular a large metastasis is seen in the right side of the L4 vertebrae (A and B). MRI at the same level illustrates no evidence of cauda equina compression (C and D).

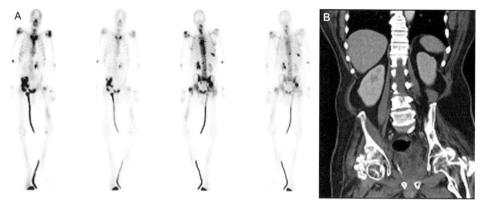

FIGURE 23.16   Image A shows radiotracer uptake in the posterior aspect of the right 9th rib and right ilium in a 62-year-old male with TCC of the bladder (indwelling catheter *in situ*). The destructive lesion located in the wing of the right ilium is visualized in the CT as shown in image B.

will have muscle invasive or metastatic disease and 30% of superficial TCC will progress to an invasive tumor [63].

Transitional cell carcinoma preferentially spreads via the lymphatic system as opposed to the hematogenous route, due to a large lymphatic network draining the bladder. However, there can be hematogenous spread to bone, lung, liver, and directly to the retroperitoneum [64]. Bone metastases are usually lytic but can occasionally be osteoblastic. Autopsy reports have shown a 25% incidence in bone metastases in patients who succumbed to bladder cancer [65,66].

The imaging modality for assessing bone metastases for patients with TCC is bone scintigraphy (Figure 23.16). The 2006 European Association of Urology guidelines for muscle invasive bladder carcinoma advocate the use of bone scintigraphy only for patients with symptoms of bone involvement [63]. This has been supported by other reports indicating that there is no role for routine screening for bone metastases [61,67–70].

The use of PET in bladder cancer is still being evaluated. It has been shown to be useful in staging lymph nodes and assessment of local recurrence [71]. Further studies with 11C-methionine-PET have also been used in the staging process and its advantage over conventional PET is that it is not excreted renally so that it does not obscure the bladder and the surrounding region.

BOX 23.6

For symptoms indicating possible bony spread of bladder cancer, bone scintigraphy should be employed.

There is no evidence indicating the use of PET to assess for bony lesions in bladder cancer.

IV. CONCLUSION

The detection of bone metastases in a patient with cancer will alter the treatment plan. It allows for appropriate measures to be taken to prevent complications and improve quality of life. Apart from a pathological diagnosis, radiological diagnosis is the most common approach to locating metastatic spread. The utilization of imaging modalities depends on many factors such as accuracy, timing, cost-effectiveness and availability.

Table 23.4 shows a summary of the recommended imaging techniques for specific malignancies.

With evolving technology, detection rates are improving, and early and appropriate measures can be instituted to

---

TABLE 23.4   Imaging recommendations

Malignancy	Symptoms	Screening	Follow-up	Future role
Breast	PR	BS	BS	PET
Prostate	PR, BS	BS	BS, PET	PET
Lung	PR, BS, MRI	BS (stage IIIA & IIIB)	PET	PET
Renal	BS	–	If symptomatic	PET
Thyroid	PR, BS	–	PET	PET
Bladder	BS	–	If symptomatic	–

PR, Plain radiography; BS, Bone scintigraphy; PET, Positron emission tomography; MRI, Magnetic resonance imaging.

obtain better patient outcomes. The use of PET and PET/CT has shown promising results and will have a greater role in the future for determining metastatic spread.

References

1. G.D. Roodman, Mechanisms of bone metastasis. [See comment.], N Engl J Med 350 (16) (2004) 1655–1664.
2. H.L. Abrams, R. Spiro & N. Goldstein, Metastases in carcinoma; analysis of 1000 autopsied cases, Cancer 3 (1) (1950) 74–85.
3. R. Coleman, Metastatic bone disease: clinical features, pathophysiology and treatment strategies, Cancer Treat Review 27 (2001) 165–176.
4. A. Jemal, R. Siegel & E. Ward, et al., Cancer Statistics, 2007, CA Cancer J Clin 57 (1) (2007) 43–66.
5. G.R. Mundy, Metastasis to bone: causes, consequences and therapeutic opportunities, Nature Reviews Cancer 2 (2002) 584–593.
6. D.I. Rosenthal, 1997 Radiologic diagnosis of bone metastases. Cancer 80 (8 Suppl), 1595–1607.
7. T. Hamaoka, J.E. Madewell & D.A. Podoloff, et al., Bone imaging in metastatic breast cancer. [See comment.], J Clin Oncol 22 (14) (2004) 2942–2953.
8. W.D. Foley, Renal MDCT, Eur J Radiol 45 (Suppl 1) (2003) S73–S78.
9. Radiologists RCo, Making the Best Use of a Department of Clinical Radiology, 4th edn., Royal College of Radiology, London, 1998.
10. M.L. Brown, Bone scintigraphy in benign and malignant tumors, Radiol Clin North Am 31 (4) (1993) 731–738.
11. T.A. Smith, FDG uptake, tumor characteristics and response to therapy: a review, Nucl Med Commun 19 (2) (1998) 97–105.
12. D. Vanel, J. Bittoun & A. Tardivon, MRI of bone metastases, Eur Radiol 8 (8) (1998) 1345–1351.
13. Y. Nakamoto, C. Cohade & M. Tatsumi, et al., CT appearance of bone metastases detected with FDG PET as part of the same PET/CT examination, Radiology 237 (2) (2005) 627–634.
14. T.M. Blodgett, C.C. Meltzer & D.W. Townsend, PET/CT: form and function, Radiology 242 (2) (2007) 360–385.
15. E. Even-Sapir, U. Metser & G. Flusser, et al., Assessment of malignant skeletal disease: initial experience with 18F-fluoride PET/CT and comparison between 18F-fluoride PET and 18F-fluoride PET/CT, J Nucl Med 45 (2) (2004) 272–278.
16. R.E. Coleman & R.D. Rubens, The clinical course of bone metastases from breast cancer, Br J Cancer 55 (1) (1987) 61–66.
17. G.N. Hortobagyi, Bone metastases in breast cancer patients, Semin Oncol 18 (4 Suppl 5) (1991) 11–15.
18. E.F. Solomayer, I.J. Diel & G.C. Meyberg, et al., Metastatic breast cancer: clinical course, prognosis and therapy related to the first site of metastasis, Breast Cancer Res Treat 59 (3) (2000) 271–278.
19. M. Tubiana-Hulin, Incidence, prevalence and distribution of bone metastases, Bone 12 (Suppl 1) (1991) S9–S10.
20. D.J. Perez, T.J. Powles & J. Milan, et al., Detection of breast carcinoma metastases in bone: relative merits of X-rays and skeletal scintigraphy, Lancet 2 (8350) (1983) 613–616.
21. G.J. Cook & I. Fogelman, The role of positron emission tomography in the management of bone metastases, Cancer 88 (12 Suppl) (2000) 2927–2933.
22. R. Thurairaja, J. McFarlane & Z. Traill, et al., State-of-the-art approaches to detecting early bone metastasis in prostate cancer, BJU Int 94 (3) (2004) 268–2671.
23. N. Lawrentschuk, I.D. Davis & D.M. Bolton, et al., Diagnostic and therapeutic use of radioisotopes for bony disease in prostate cancer: current practice, Int J Urol 14 (2) (2007) 89–95.
24. A. Heidenreich, G. Aus, C. Abbou, et al. Guidelines on Prostate Cancer: European Association of Urology (2007).
25. S. Abuzallouf, I. Dayes & H. Lukka, Baseline staging of newly diagnosed prostate cancer: a summary of the literature, J Urol 171 (6 Pt 1) (2004) 2122–2127.
26. J. Rigaud, R. Tiguert & L. Le Normand, et al., Prognostic value of bone scan in patients with metastatic prostate cancer treated initially with androgen deprivation therapy, J Urol 168 (4 Pt 1) (2002) 1423–1426.
27. O. Akin & H. Hricak, Imaging of prostate cancer, Radiol Clin North Am 45 (1) (2007) 207–222.
28. H. Schoder & S.M. Larson, Positron emission tomography for prostate, bladder, and renal cancer, Semin Nucl Med 34 (4) (2004) 274–292.
29. C. Hofer, H. Kubler & R. Hartung, et al., Diagnosis and monitoring of urological tumors using positron emission tomography, Eur Urol 40 (5) (2001) 481–487.
30. A.M. Groves, C.J. Beadsmoore & H.K. Cheow, et al., Can 16-detector multislice CT exclude skeletal lesions during tumor staging? Implications for the cancer patient, Eur Radiol 16 (5) (2006) 1066–1073.
31. M. Picchio, C. Messa & C. Landoni, et al., Value of [11C]choline-positron emission tomography for re-staging prostate cancer: a comparison with [18F]fluorodeoxyglucose-positron emission tomography, J Urol 169 (4) (2003) 1337–1340.
32. H. Schirrmeister, A. Guhlmann & J. Kotzerke, et al., Early detection and accurate description of extent of metastatic bone disease in breast cancer with fluoride ion and positron emission tomography, J Clin Oncol 17 (8) (1999) 2381–2389.
33. E., Gosfield 3rd., A. Alavi & B. Kneeland, Comparison of radionuclide bone scans and magnetic resonance imaging in detecting spinal metastases. [See comment.], J Nucl Med 34 (12) (1993) 2191–2198.
34. F.E. Lecouvet, D. Geukens & A. Stainier, et al., Magnetic resonance imaging of the axial skeleton for detecting bone metastases in patients with high-risk prostate cancer: diagnostic and cost-effectiveness and comparison with current detection strategies, J Clin Oncol 25 (22) (2007) 3281–3287.
35. S. Sachs & J.J. Fiore, An overview of lung cancer, Respir Care Clin N Am 9 (1) (2003) 1–25.
36. R.F. Munden, S.S. Swisher & C.W. Stevens, et al., Imaging of the patient with non-small cell lung cancer, Radiology 237 (3) (2005) 803–818.
37. G.A. Silvestri, B. Littenberg & G.L. Colice, The clinical evaluation for detecting metastatic lung cancer. A meta-analysis, Am J Respir Crit Care Med 152 (1) (1995) 225–230.
38. J.J. Erasmus, M.T. Truong & R.F. Munden, CT, MR, and PET imaging in staging of non-small-cell lung cancer, Semin Roentgenol 40 (2) (2005) 126–142.

39. G.A. Silvestri L.T. Tanoue & American College of Chest Physicians, et al., The noninvasive staging of non-small cell lung cancer: the guidelines, Chest 123 (1 Suppl) (2003) 147S–156S.

40. J.G. Ravenel, Lung cancer staging, Semin Roentgenol 39 (3) (2004) 373–385.

41. H. van Tinteren, O.S. Hoekstra & E.F. Smit, et al., Effectiveness of positron emission tomography in the preoperative assessment of patients with suspected non-small-cell lung cancer: the PLUS multicentre randomised trial. [See comment.], Lancet 359 (9315) (2002) 1388–1393.

42. T. Bury, A. Barreto & F. Daenen, et al., Fluorine-18 deoxyglucose positron emission tomography for the detection of bone metastases in patients with non-small cell lung cancer, Eur J Nucl Med 25 (9) (1998) 1244–1247.

43. V. Lindner, H. Lang & D. Jacqmin, Pathology and genetics in renal cell cancer. EUA Update Series, Renal Cell Cancer (2003) 197–208.

44. S. Mani, M.B. Todd & K. Katz, et al., Prognostic factors for survival in patients with metastatic renal cancer treated with biological response modifiers, J Urol 154 (1) (1995) 35–40.

45. B. Ljungberg, D. Hanbury, M. Kuczyk, et al. Guidelines on Renal Cell Carcinoma: European Association of Urology (2007).

46. S. Ramdave, G.W. Thomas & S.U. Berlangieri, et al., Clinical role of F−18 fluorodeoxyglucose positron emission tomography for detection and management of renal cell carcinoma, J Urol 166 (3) (2001) 825–830.

47. D.E. Kang & R.L., White, Jr., et al., Clinical use of fluorodeoxyglucose F 18 positron emission tomography for detection of renal cell carcinoma, J Urol 171 (5) (2004) 1806–1809.

48. N. Aide, O. Cappele & P. Bottet, et al., Efficiency of [(18)F]FDG PET in characterising renal cancer and detecting distant metastases: a comparison with CT. [See comment.], Eur J Nucl Med Mol Imaging 30 (9) (2003) 1236–1245.

49. N.S. Majhail, J.-L. Urbain & J.M. Albani, et al., F-18 fluorodeoxyglucose positron emission tomography in the evaluation of distant metastases from renal cell carcinoma, J Clin Oncol 21 (21) (2003) 3995–4000.

50. A. Safaei, R. Figlin & C.K. Hoh, et al., The usefulness of F-18 deoxyglucose whole-body positron emission tomography (PET) for re-staging of renal cell cancer. [See comment.], Clin Nephrol 57 (1) (2002) 56–62.

51. M. Haq & C. Harmer, Thyroid cancer: an overview, Nucl Med Commun 25 (9) (2004) 861–867.

52. M. Shoup, A. Stojadinovic & A. Nissan, et al. Prognostic indicators of outcomes in patients with distant metastases from differentiated thyroid carcinoma, J Am Coll Surg 197 (2) (2003) 191–197.

53. F. Pacini, M. Schlumberger H. Dralle, et al. European consensus for the management of patients with differentiated thyroid carcinoma of the follicular epithelium. [Erratum appears in Eur J Endocrinol 155 (2), 385.] Eur 154 (6) (2006) 787–803.

54. M. Iwata, K. Kasagi & T. Misaki, et al., Comparison of whole-body 18F-FDG PET, 99mTc-MIBI SPET, and post-therapeutic 131I-Na scintigraphy in the detection of metastatic thyroid cancer, Eur J Nucl Med Mol Imaging 31 (4) (2004) 491–498.

55. F. Grunwald, T. Kalicke & U. Feine, et al., Fluorine-18 fluorodeoxyglucose positron emission tomography in thyroid cancer: results of a multicentre study, Eur J Nucl Med 26 (1999) 1547–1552.

56. M. Dietlein, K. Scheidhauer & E. Voth, et al., Fluorine-18 fluorodeoxyglucose positron emission tomography and iodine-131 whole-body scintigraphy in the follow-up of differentiated thyroid cancer, Eur J Nucl Med 24 (11) (1997) 1342–1348.

57. J.A. Wexler & J. Sharretts, Thyroid and bone, Endocrinol Metab Clin North Am 36 (3) (2007) 673–705.

58. S. Ito, K. Kato & M. Ikeda, et al., Comparison of 18F-FDG PET and bone scintigraphy in detection of bone metastases of thyroid cancer, J Nucl Med 48 (6) (2007) 889–995.

59. H.T.T. Phan, P.L. Jager & J.T.M. Plukker, et al., Detection of bone metastases in thyroid cancer patients: bone scintigraphy or 18F-FDG PET?, Nucl Med Commun 28 (8) (2007) 597–602.

60. M. Zoller, S. Kohlfuerst & I. Igerc, et al., Combined PET/CT in the follow-up of differentiated thyroid carcinoma: what is the impact of each modality?, Eur J Nucl Med Mol Imaging 34 (4) (2007) 487–495.

61. W. Oosterlinck, B. Lobel & G. Jakse, et al., Guidelines on bladder cancer, Eur Urol 41 (2) (2002) 105–112.

62. F. Mostofi, Histological Typing of Urinary Bladder Tumours, Springer-Verlag, 1999 pp. 3–27.

63. G. Jakse, F. Algaba, S. Fossa, et al. Guidelines on Bladder Cancer – Muscle-invasive and metastatic: European Association of Urology (2006).

64. M.A. Saksena, D.M. Dahl & M.G. Harisinghani, New imaging modalities in bladder cancer, World J Urol 24 (5) (2006) 473–480.

65. R.J. Babaian, D.E. Johnson & L. Llamas, et al., Metastases from transitional cell carcinoma of urinary bladder, Urology 16 (2) (1980) 142–144.

66. K. Kishi, T. Hirota & K. Matsumoto, et al., Carcinoma of the bladder: a clinical and pathological analysis of 87 autopsy cases, J Urol 125 (1) (1981) 36–39.

67. P. Davey, M.V. Merrick & W. Duncan, et al., Bladder cancer: the value of routine bone scintigraphy, Clin Radiol 36 (1) (1985) 77–79.

68. M. Braendengen, M. Winderen & S.D. Fossa, Clinical significance of routine pre-cystectomy bone scans in patients with muscle-invasive bladder cancer, Br J Urol 77 (1) (1996) 36–40.

69. G.L. Berger, R.W. Sadlowski & J.R. Sharpe, et al., Lack of value of routine preoperative bone and liver scans in cystectomy candidates, J Urol 125 (5) (1981) 637–639.

70. A. Lindner & J.B. deKernion, Cost-effective analysis of pre-cystectomy radioisotope scans, J Urol 128 (6) (1982) 1181–1182.

71. C.S. Ng, Radiologic diagnosis and staging of renal and bladder cancer, Semin Roentgenol 41 (2) (2006) 121–138.

CHAPTER **24**

Diagnosis of Skeletal Metastases in Malignant Extraskeletal Cancers

HOLGER SCHIRRMEISTER[1] AND COSKUN ARSLANDEMIR[2]

[1]*Department of Nuclear Medicine, Westküstenklinikum Heide, Germany.*
[2]*Department of Nuclear Medicine, University Hospital, Kiel, Germany.*

Contents

I. INTRODUCTION

The incidences of metastatic bone disease are particularly high in those carcinomas which are most common in the Western world. In post-mortem studies, the incidence of breast cancer amounts to 73%, up to 68% in prostate cancer, and 35% in lung cancer [1].

Up until now, the ability to be able to change a patient's prognosis for the better via more sensitive detection of metastases and, therefore, earlier therapy has not materialized. This leaves a palliative situation for most patients with bone metastases.

It is therefore necessary to exclude metastatic bone disease before starting a potentially curative therapy.

An exact localization and description of the extent of metastatic bone disease is required for patients with known skeletal metastases in order to reassess the efficiency of a follow-up systemic therapy and further assess the risk of fracture. Apart from bone scintigraphy with technetium labeled polyphosphonates, other diagnostic methods such as magnetic resonance imaging (MRI) as a whole-body technique, positron emission tomography with fluor-18 sodium fluoride (F-18 NaF) or F-18 fluordesoxyglucose (F-18 FDG), as well as a combination of PET and CT, are clinically important. Current literature regarding these diagnostic techniques and some aspects regarding the interpretation of these data are presented in the following pages.

II. DEFINITION AND ORIGIN

The term 'metastasis' basically describes a migration of tumor cells via the blood or lymphstream into other primarily unaffected areas of the body. Thus the term 'bone metastasis' describes the appearance of secondary tumors in the skeletal system after groups of tumor cells enabled to leave the primary tumor have reached the skeletal system. Damage of the skeleton occurs when those cells affect the continuous remodeling of the bone, thereby leading to an increased sclerosis or bone resorption. Typically a combination of increased bone resorption and formation is observed. In this connection, radiographs or computed tomography (CT) show which one of these processes prevails. When bone resorption is dominant metastases appear osteolytic. In the case of predominating bone formation they appear sclerotic (osteoblastic metastases). New bone is formed predominantly in osteoblastic metastases by the production of new matrix on the surface of existing trabeculae. And the production of new bone within the marrow cavity between existing trabeculae by means of membranous ossification. The radiologically noticeable increment of density and the scintigraphic accumulation reflect these processes.

By contrast, a reactive bone sclerosis is an attempt to repair the damage caused by tumor cells. Owing to this reaction, osteolytic metastases often appear as areas of increased activity at the bone scintigraphy.

Bone Cancer
ISBN: 978-0-12-374895-9

Currently the RANK/RANKL system has attached great importance to the onset of osteolyses. Receptor activator of nuclear factor-κ-B (RANKL) is considered to be the determining factor in the genesis of osteolyses. RANKL is expressed by osteoblasts, stroma cells and some tumor cells and exists both bound to membranes and in soluble form. It is part of the tumor necrosis factor (TNF) super family. The interaction of RANKL with its receptor RANK (receptor activator of nuclear factor-κ-B) induces the development and further differentiation of pre-stages of osteoclasts to mature osteoclasts and the activation of mature osteoclasts. It also causes a delayed initiation of apoptosis and thereby longer survival of osteoclasts. The protein osteoprotegerin (OPG) is also secreted by osteoblasts. OPG is considered to be an antagonist to RANKL. It is a soluble receptor which binds RANKL and neutralizes its biological effects. A balanced RANKL/OPG ratio is indispensable for the equilibrium of bone formation and resorption. Disturbances in this balance were also described in other bone affecting diseases like multiple myeloma and postmenopausal or gluco-corticoid-induced osteoporosis.

Along with metabolic changes via the RANK/RANKL/OPG system, tumor cells can exert an activating influence on osteoblasts via the synthesis of parathormone (PTH) or PTH-related peptide (PTHrP) and other mediators, as well. Additionally, a direct destruction of the bone by carcinoma cells was discussed [2].

At the time of the primary diagnosis of solid cancers, tumor cells are already found in 30% of all patients in bone marrow aspirates. However, in the follow-up of the disease, lesions suspicious of metastases only appear in a small number of patients in medical imaging or autopsy. These days it is well known that single cells, and even smaller groups of tumor cells up to a diameter of 2–3 mm, can subsist by diffusion. Beyond this size an additional vessel supply is needed. Due to this, metastases smaller than 2–3 mm are often defined as micro-metastases. Yet, until now, there is no exact scientific definition of the point of time when potentially reversible micro-metastases change into irreversible bone metastases.

III. SKELETAL METASTASES ARE NOT A UNIFORM TUMOR ENTITY

It is customary to subsume the topic of skeletal metastases to gain some clarity. Similarities in the onset and description are usually accentuated to form the impression of a relatively uniform tumor entity.

However, bone metastases often vary in their genetic equipment to a great extent. For this reason they often possess different abilities to emerge new metastases, to influence the osseous metabolism, and have variable prognostic impacts. Independent from the primary tumor bone, metastases can

have similar appearances radiologically and scintigraphically. Yet in some cases their distribution, their localization or their morphological appearance can indicate the origin. Dependent on blood supply of the primary tumor, metastases reach the skeleton in different ways through the vascular system. This implies that the expected infestation pattern is dependent on the localization, as well as the blood supply, of the primary tumor. The most common infestation is the vertebral column. For the most part, early metastases are located in the vertebrae near the corticalis in the ingress areas of the vessels.

Early metastases in the pelvis and the lumbar region are relatively typical in prostate cancer. The metastatic disease spreads cranially via a paravertebral vascular network, called 'Batson's plexus' which brings forward the venous spreading of the metastases. At this tumor entity osteoblastic metastases, in particular, are often observed. Predominantly osteolytic metastases occur typically in thyroid cancer, lung cancer, renal cell cancer and cancers of the gastrointestinal tract. Metastases in the fingers, especially the distal phalanx (acrometastases) are extremely rare, but arise most probably from a cancer of the lung, kidneys or breast.

Metastases of a thyroid cancer are more commonly located in 'flat' bones as the scapula, pelvis, skull, ribs or the sternum. In contrast to other solid cancers, 50% of the affected patients have only one or two metastases at the time of initial diagnosis. After resection of these metastases and a subsequent radio-iodine-therapy and radiotherapy, 70% of patients can be cured despite distant metastases.

IV. THE SIGNIFICANCE OF DIAGNOSTIC TESTS AND STUDIES COMPARING DIFFERENT METHODS

A major issue of medical diagnostics is that the accuracy of a method is closely linked to the prevalence of a disease. The sensitivity and specificity are test parameters that are often used to evaluate the quality of a test. However, for medical determinations it is important to know the probability of a positively tested patient actually being sick and a negatively tested patient being in good health. The post test probability (positive predictive value, PPV) describes the percentage of patients who are actually sick when tested positive. This connection can be derived from Bayes' theorem [3]. It allows for calculations with limited probabilities, especially the reversal of conclusions. For clinical practice this means that physicians who rarely request skeletal diagnostics may get false negative findings; whereas those who request skeletal surveys too often may get false positive results. For the significance of clinical studies dealing with the comparison of imaging methods, this applies equally. For example, when only patients who have bone metastases on plain radiographs are included in a study, the pre-test probability for the existence of these metastases in this collective is 100%, even before conducting additional tests due to the low sensitivity of radiographs. In an MRI, CT scan or bone scintigraphy carried out later additionally discovered areas suspicious of metastases will nearly always be true positive because of the high pre-test probability for having further metastases.

V. MEANING OF THE GOLD STANDARD

In the assessment of a diagnostic test it is essential to consider that the diagnostic statement can never be absolutely 'reliable' but only 'probable'. The physician can only make more or less well-founded assumptions. It would be wrong to 'trust' a diagnostic method to provide 'objective', 'absolute' findings, which unfortunately is often postulated in medical practice or in the conclusions of studies comparing diagnostic methods. A lot of information – like a clinical follow-up regarding former medical treatment, results of other examinations and the stage of the tumor – is used to reach a correct diagnosis. Findings are assessed in prospective studies that are generally blinded in order to depict the calculative accuracy of a single diagnostic method. Compared to daily clinical practice this is a rather theoretical situation. The validity of such results is not assured unless an objective test standard, independent of competing diagnostic methods, exists. As there is no way to affirm or discard a diagnosis with absolute certainty, a 'gold standard' needs to be defined in diagnostic studies.

In the evaluation of a primary tumor the histological finding is often defined as the gold standard. It is considered quite reliable, but can nevertheless reveal false results due to sampling errors or an interim carried out therapy.

Contrary to the relatively safe histological gold standard, it is almost impossible to define a reliable gold standard for secondary tumors. It is especially difficult for bone metastases because, owing to their high number and inaccessibility, a histological confirmation of metastases is often impossible. Therefore, other imaging modalities or a combination of methods are commonly used for definition of the gold standard. Due to an improvement in quality and availability in diagnostic methods over previous decades and the development of new methods, the general opinion on the accuracy of diagnostic methods has changed drastically.

To give a simple example regarding the valuation of bone scintigraphy: since the 1960s we have known that metastatic bone disease can be diagnosed by using bone scintigraphy months before metastases appear on X-rays. Typically in the first studies patients with known skeletal metastases were examined, which could be detected at the bone scintigraphy as expected. As no other method with a higher sensitivity than the bone scintigraphy existed, it was considered 100% sensitive. It can be derived from Bayes' theorem that,

because of the pre-test probability of 100% (only patients with known bone metastases were recruited), the specificity was also considered to be almost 100%. With the introduction into daily routine and application in routine aftercare the pre-test probability changed to a value of lower than 10%. As no other method for medical imaging than the less sensitive radiologic diagnostics was available, the specificity was considered to be only 50% in later studies, even though image quality had improved meanwhile. This shows that the sensitivity and specificity of diagnostic methods are not fixed parameters, and that results of studies can be influenced or even predetermined by the selection of the collective or the definition of the gold standard.

VI. EXPERIENCE

Statistical parameters like sensitivity and specificity are important criteria to describe the reliability of a diagnostic method. But applicability in clinical practice is limited by the experience of the diagnostician and the technical equipment available. For example, students reached a value of 97% for sensitivity in the assessment of bone scintigraphies, while specificity was only at 57% [4]. With experienced diagnosticians the use of additional information raised the specificity up to 95% with a sensitivity of 95%. By evaluating bone scintigraphies without additional information they only reached 74% for specificity. Similar phenomena are also revealed in scientific literature. In monocentric studies, institutions with many years of experience generally report a much higher accuracy in the evaluation of a method than in multicentric studies under the same conditions.

VII. X-RAY AND COMPUTED TOMOGRAPHY

Planar radiographs and computed tomography are not used to screen for skeletal metastases. The detection of bone metastases is not possible with conventional X-ray technology unless at least 30 to 50% of bone mineral is destroyed [5]. In known metastases, especially suspicious lesions, it is nevertheless indispensable to assess the risk of a fracture. There are no specific characteristics of x-ray examinations that exclusively apply to bone metastases. The type of bone destruction can be geographic, moth-eaten or permeative. The edges can be sharp or blurred. Periostal reactions and expansion into surrounding soft tissue parts can be present or absent. The differentiation between osteolytic, osteoblastic or mixed metastases is made according to x-ray or CT criteria.

Especially in patients with skeletal metastases of an unknown primary tumor, knowledge about differences of the infestation pattern and presentation on the x-ray image can be very helpful. For lung cancer, a relatively characteristic type of destruction is reported, the 'cookie-bite' or 'cookie-cutter' which affects the corticalis. This type of metastatic bone disease presumably emerges by hematogenic distribution of tumor cells via cortical vessel anastomoses which arise from the periosteum. Along with lung cancer, even renal cell cancer, bladder cancer, and the malignant melanoma, can cause these cortical metastases. Bullous, very expansively growing 'blow-out' metastases were described in renal cell cancer and thyroid cancer.

VIII. BONE SCINTIGRAPHY

As mentioned above, since the early 1960s bone scintigraphy was considered the diagnostic method with the highest sensitivity for the aftercare of cancer due to its higher sensitivity compared to planar x-ray technology [6,7].

As it shows a higher sensitivity and a better spatial resolution, the scintigraphy with Tc-99m polyphosphonate replaced the scintigraphy with F-18 sodium fluoride [7,8]. Along with the currently used Tc-99m polyphosphonate a number of other radiotracers were tested for skeletal imaging. Of these, F-18 sodium fluoride (F-18 NaF)—already introduced into practice by Blau *et al.* [6]—proved to be superior to substances of the calcium family (Sr-85, Ba-131, Ca-45) as a standard tracer.

Bone scintigraphy is generally considered to be very reliable for predominantly osteoblastic metastases. However, disseminated bone metastases were even described on MRI in patients with prostate cancer but normal bone scintigraphy [9]. In contrast to a relatively high sensitivity for osteoblastic metastases, a markedly lower sensitivity was postulated in osteolytic metastases [4].

Single Photon Emission Computed Tomography (SPECT) is often only used as a supplementary in indeterminate lesions seen with the planar bone scintigraphy. One reason for this is the noticeable duration of time needed for the examination.

In a retrospective study by Kosuda *et al.* [10] a comparable sensitivity as with MRI was achieved in a routine use of SPECT of the vertebral column for the detection of bone metastases. In another prospective study [11] the accuracy of bone scintigraphy, based on a lesion-by-lesion analysis of patients with predominantly osteoblastic or osteolytic metastases, was examined. A group of patients with prostate cancer was scrutinized for the evaluation of the sensitivity of bone scintigraphy in detecting osteoblastic metastases. In a second group, patients with thyroid cancer or lung cancer were included to evaluate the sensitivity of bone scintigraphy in osteolytic metastases. Contrary to the generally stated hypothesis of a lower sensitivity of bone scintigraphy for osteolytic metastases, there was no statistically significant difference in the sensitivity for both groups. However, for detecting lesions, the anatomical localization gains in higher importance. With bone scintigraphy a sensitivity of 80 to 90% was achieved for the thorax, the skull and the extremities; whereas the sensitivity for the pelvis and vertebral column ranged between 20.5 and 43.2%. Therefore, the sensitivity of bone scintigraphy for detection of skeletal lesions with less superposition by other anatomical parts was considerably higher than for subjacent bone. This superposition is of no importance in tomographic techniques. Consequently, in a published prospective study [12,13] of 103 patients with initial diagnoses of lung cancer, the sensitivity of bone scintigraphy could be raised considerably by using a supplementary SPECT of the vertebral column (Figures 24.1–24.3).

With an area under the ROC curve of 0.875 a significantly higher accuracy was achieved by the combination of SPECT and planar bone scintigraphy than without SPECT. In this case, the accuracy decreased to 0.771. Owing to the increase of the accuracy, nine patients who would have been diagnosed as false negative on a single use of planar bone scintigraphy were diagnosed with metastatic bone disease. Because of this, the therapeutic regimen changed for at least eight of the 103 patients examined. As in this study, two SPECT acquisitions per patients were needed, the time of examination increased up to 150 minutes. Consequently, a lower image quality had to be taken into account owing to motion artifacts.

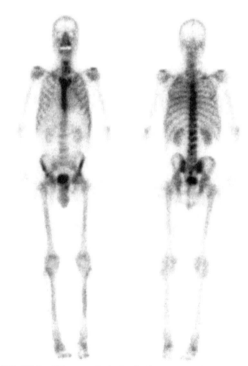

FIGURE 24.1 Planar whole-body bone scan in a patient with non-small cell lung cancer (pT2 N0). The patient was restaged because of increased CEA levels after surgery. The bone scan shows physiologically increased tracer uptake in the sternum after sternotomy (previous bypass surgery). There is inhomogeneous indeterminate tracer uptake in the spine but no typical bone metastasis.

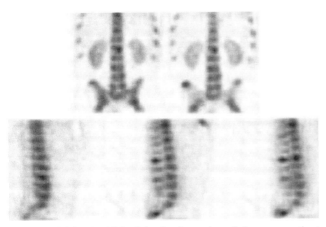

FIGURE 24.2 SPECT of the lumbar spine of the same patient as presented in Figure 24.1. Multiple hot spots are typical for disseminated metastatic bone disease.

IX. POSITRON EMISSION TOMOGRAPHY WITH F-18 SODIUM FLUORIDE

Gamma cameras used for conventional whole-body bone scintigraphy are commonly single-crystal cameras. The photomultipliers directly connected to the scintillation crystal and the photocathode are connected to each other via a network of electrical resistances.

Through analysis of differences in voltage in the network of resistances, the localization where a photon hits the crystal is calculated (Anger principle). The resolution of a conventional gamma camera is, among other things, dependent on the collimator. A drawback of the collimator is that only less than 1 per mill of all photons can penetrate it. Thereby the sensitivity of the system is reduced. In contrast to a conventional gamma camera, PET scanners are multi-crystal cameras. Detection of radioactivity results from coincidental stimulation of two opposite crystals in the ring system. This principle of measuring coincidences has the advantage that a collimator is not needed. As a result, a PET scanner delivers a higher number of impulses and a higher spatial resolution compared to conventional gamma camera systems. Because PET is a tomographic method, small structures are shown without superposition and are detected with a higher sensitivity than with planar imaging methods. Compared to SPECT, the duration of F-18 sodium fluoride PET is only 70–80 min so that the risk of movement artifacts is reduced compared to SPECT imaging. As well as technical advantages there is a further advantage because of the better pharmacokinetics of F-18 sodium fluoride compared to the Tc-99m labeled polyphosponates which are used for bone scintigraphy. F-18 sodium fluoride was considered an ideal tracer due to its favorable half-life time of 110 min, the possibility of oral application [14] and the excellent bone-to-soft tissue ratio [15–17]. The 'first-pass' extraction of a fluoride ion is almost 100% [18]. Comparatively, the 'first-pass' extraction out of the blood in the bone for the Tc-99m polyphosphonate complexes is only 64% [18].

The maximum absorption for fluoride is reached after 60 min with 60–70% of the administered activity [19]. The maximum osseous activity for the commonly used Tc-99m Polyphosphonate is at 30–40% and is reached 2 to 4 hours after the injection. Both radiotracers are excreted through the kidneys. The elimination is much faster for F-18 sodium fluoride (bloodpool after 1 hour: 1.6% [20], retention in soft tissue: 10–15% [15–17]. Because of this, the contrast between bone and soft tissue and the bone-to-lesion ratio are significantly higher for F-18 sodium fluoride than for Tc-99m polyphosphonate [15–17]. With F-18 PET, it is possible to depict very small structures, like the atlantoaxial and atlantodental joint, the foramina transversalia and the spinous processes of the cervical vertebrae.

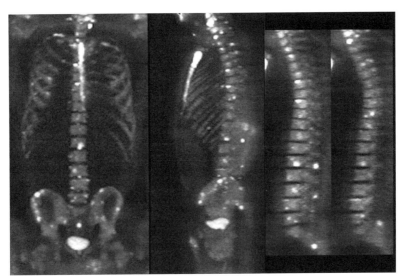

FIGURE 24.3 F-18 sodium fluoride PET of the same patient as presented in Figures 24.1 and 24.2. Multiple small osteosclerotic metastases present as focal lesions with intensively increased tracer uptake.

In section findings, osteoarthrithis of the vertebral column could be proven in 90% of men above 50 years of age and 90% of all women above 60 years of age [21]. According to this 80–90% of all lesions not suspicious of metastases that were detected with F-18 PET were caused by intervertebral arthritis. These lesions showed an accumulation pattern [22] that is known from conventional radiographs [23,24] and can therefore be easily discerned from metastases (Figure 24.4).

For bone metastases two different accumulation patterns are observed. Osteolytic metastases often present as cold lesions surrounded by a small rim of increased activity.

Benign tumors that could be mistaken for metastases are rarely located in the spinal column [25,26] (Figure 24.5). According to this, focal lesions that have no contact to surfaces of joints and do not show the typical accumulation pattern of fractures of the ribs or endplates, are suspicious of metastasis. Because initial metastases are often located at the vascular entry points, a peripheral accumulation cannot be qualified as benign in any case.

Bone metastases were diagnosed using ^{18}F-PET with two-fold higher sensitivity of conventional skeletal scintigraphy in a prospective study [11]. The previous opinion, that conventional skeletal scintigraphy shows a lower sensitivity for osteolytic than for osteoblastic metastases [4], was not confirmed in this study. Furthermore, it is often postulated that tumor cells cause replacing and oedema at an early stage in bone marrow. They affect the osseous metabolism only after advanced expansion of the metastasis [27–30]. Because of this, bone metastases should be detected with MRI or bone marrow scintigraphy at an earlier stage than with bone scintigraphy. Because the enrichment of fluoride principally represents the regional mineralization of the bone, this theory does not hold in view of the high number of very small metastases of the vertebral column, which are reliably detected using MRI and concordant with ^{18}F-PET (Figure 24.6).

In a highly selected series [31] of patients with breast cancer and a high risk of metastatic bone disease the therapy regimen was changed in 4 of 34 [11.7%] patients. In

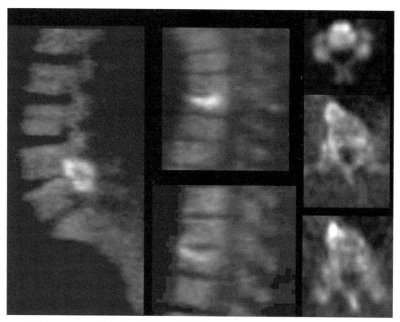

FIGURE 24.4   Typical accumulation pattern of benign lesions with F-18 sodium fluoride PET.

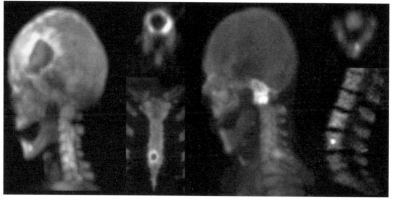

FIGURE 24.5   F-18 sodium fluoride PET—osteolytic (left) and osteosclerotic (right) metastases.

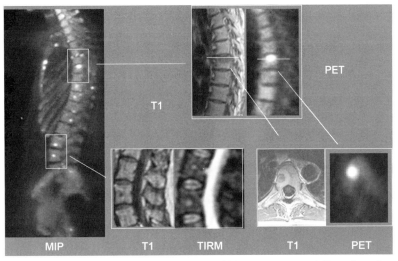

FIGURE 24.6 F-18 sodium fluoride PET and MRI of a female patient with breast cancer and disseminated metastatic bone disease.

that study the number of skeletal metastases was also significantly underestimated using planar bone scintigraphy in comparison to F-18 PET in 11 of 17 (64.7%) patients.

In another study [32] whole with body PET using the glucose analogue 18F-FDG, metastases of the lungs and liver were detected with the same sensitivity as with the standard imaging methods (sonography of the liver, chest x-ray, bone scintigraphy).

In this collective only two out of 89 patients had osseous metastases. These were correctly detected with both bone scintigraphy and FDG-PET. Therefore, the conclusion that bone scintigraphy should be replaced by F-18 PET for the primary staging of breast cancer is not realistic. In breast cancer F-18 PET might be helpful in a patient's unclear increase of tumor markers but negative for standard imaging procedures or for verification of suspicious lesions detected in MRI but negative bone scans.

In another study 103 patients with the initial diagnosis of a lung cancer were examined [12]. The high accuracy of F-18 PET was confirmed in this study. Because metastases were diagnosed with F-18 PET, the therapeutic approach changed for 10 out of the 103 patients (9.7%) who had false negative planar bone scintigraphy. For four of these patients a planned surgery was canceled and radiotherapy was canceled for the other six patients, which implied a reduction of costs overall, despite the higher costs for pre-therapeutic diagnostics.

X. POSITRON EMISSION TOMOGRAPHY WITH FLUORINE-18 DESOXYGLUCOSE

The glucose analog FDG is currently the most commonly used radiotracer in oncology for PET imaging. This surrogate marker for glucose metabolism enters the cell via the glucose transporter membrane proteins glut-1 and glut-5.

FDG is then phosphorylated by the enzyme hexokinase. In contrast to glucose, FDG-6-phospate is not a substrate of glucose-6-phophate isomerase and is therefore trapped within the tumor cell. Although the exact mechanism of FDG uptake in bone metastases is not yet known, it is assumed that FDG is taken directly into the tumor tissue of skeletal metastases and not into reactive bone as F-18 sodium fluoride. Unlike evaluation of the primary tumor and its lymph nodes, there are only a few reports that address the accuracy of FDG-PET in detecting skeletal metastases. From the malignant tumors that are typically associated with skeletal metastases, some cancers such as well-differentiated thyroid or prostate cancer show either no or only slightly increased glucose metabolism. This means that sensitivity for the detection of metastases of these tumors using FDG is limited. In one study by Yeh *et al.* [33] on a small collective of 13 patients with bone metastases of a prostate cancer, only 18% of metastases pre-known from skeletal scintigraphy were detected on FDG-PET. In another study, Shreve *et al.* [34] reported a sensitivity of 65% for the proof of skeletal metastases of the prostate cancer. And a higher sensitivity of 77% was reported for a collective of 17 patients with progressive prostate cancer (Figure 24.7).

Additionally, a study by Cook *et al.* [35] suggests that there are differences in the glucose metabolism of osteoblastic and osteolytic metastases. He and his coworkers evaluated a series of 23 women with metastatic bone disease from breast cancer FDG uptake in osteosclerotic and osteolytic bone metastases by calculation of standardized uptake values. In this series uptake was approximately 7-fold higher in osteolytic metastases than in osteosclerotic metastases (Figures 24.8 and 24.9). Compared to bone scintigraphy, FDG detected more metastases in the entire patient group. Bone scintigraphy, however, was more sensitive in a subgroup of patients with predominantly osteoblastic disease.

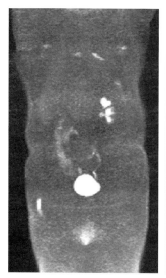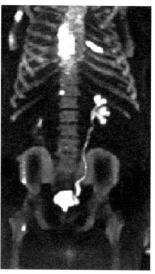

FIGURE 24.7 PET with F-18 FDG and F-18 sodium fluoride (maximum intensity projection images, MIP) of a patient with prostate cancer. The ostesclerotic bone metastases (right scapula, sternum, ribs, T12, right femur) show no or very slight FDG uptake but are easy to identify with F-18 sodium fluoride (NaF). The left ureter is obstructed in the vicinity of the prostate.

In a further study, Ohta and coworkers [36] compared the accuracy of conventional bone scans and FDG-PET in detecting bone metastases in 51 female patients with breast cancer. The sensitivity of both PET and bone scintigraphy was 58%. The specificity was higher at 98% for FDG-PET than for bone scintigraphy with 80%. A higher specificity of FDG-PET in comparison to bone scintigraphy with identical sensitivity for both methods was also reported by Yang *et al.* [37] in a series of 48 patients with breast cancer. A comparable accuracy of bone scintigraphy and FDG-PET was also described by Kao *et al.* [38] in 24 patients with breast cancer.

In contrast to the low incidence of bone metasases at initial staging of breast cancer there is a significantly higher incidence at initial diagnosis of lung cancer. Unlike metastases from cancer of the prostate or thyroid, the metastases from lung cancer typically present with elevated glucose consumption. Therefore, meaningful studies dealing with initial staging of malignant tumors can be planned in patients with an initial diagnosis of lung cancer. In a study by Marom *et al.* [39] an FDG-PET was carried out in 100 patients with non-small cell lung cancer. Bone scintigraphy was carried out for 90 patients. In this study 12 patients had bone metastases. The FDG-PET was correctly positive in 11 (90%) and the bone scintigraphy in only six (50%) patients. In another study by Bury *et al.* [40], 110 patients with non-small cell lung cancer were examined with FDG-PET as well as with conventional bone scintigraphy. Forty-three of these patients had bone metastases. Metastatic bone disease was proven in only 21 patients. With FDG-PET as well as with bone scintigraphy, 19 of 21 patients were true positive. However, the FDG-PET, in contrast to bone scintigraphy, produced a higher rate of true negative patients. In a study by Gayed *et al.* [41] a mixed collective of 85 patients with lung cancer was examined. In this study, 80 patients had non-small cell cancer, four patients had small cell lung cancer and one patient had bronchioloalveolar cancer. FDG-PET correctly diagnosed eight patients with bone metastases, while bone scintigraphy correctly diagnosed 10 patients. When comparing correctly diagnosed lesions in this study, 16 false positive findings were reported for FDG-PET and 27 for bone scintigraphy.

A significant limitation of the above-named studies is that planar bone scintigraphy was compared with PET, which is a tomographic imaging method. In general, tomographic imaging methods are more sensitive at detecting small lesions than planar imaging is. The general validity of this statement is affirmed by the comparison of planar x-ray technology and computer tomography for detecting lung

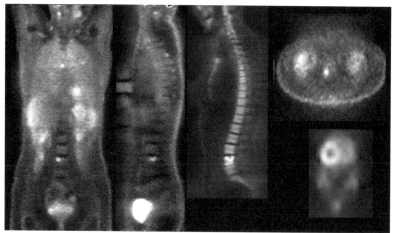

FIGURE 24.8 A single osteolytic metastasis in a patient with breast cancer is presented as a hot spot on FDG-PET and as a cold lesion surrounded by a rim of increased activity on F-18 sodium fluoride PET.

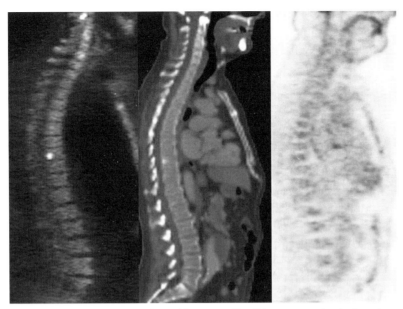

FIGURE 24.9   A small osteosclerotic metastasis in a patient with non-small cell lung cancer (sagittal sections, right: F-18 sodium fluoride PET, middle: computed tomography, left: FDG PET). Note that there is no increased glucose metabolism visible on the FDG PET.

metastases. Even though both imaging techniques are based on the same principle of differences in the absorption of x-rays in different types of tissue, small metastases in the lungs are detectable with a higher sensitivity using CT than with planar x-ray images, because the images are free of superposition by other anatomical structures. The same applies for the detection of metastases of the vertebral column using SPECT, MRI, F-18 PET or CT, which might be missed with planar bone scintigraphy (Figure 24.10).

Accordingly, Kosuda *et al.* [10] found an identical sensitivity for the detection of metastases in the vertebral column when comparing bone SPECT and MRI. The sensitivity of

SPECT was even higher in the transverse and spinous processes. In that study, both technologies proved to be much more sensitive than planar bone scintigraphy.

XI. MAGNETIC RESONANCE IMAGING

MRI enables early detection of pathological changes in the bone marrow. Bone metastases present as focal lesions with high signal intensity on T2 images and low signal intensity on T1 images. Commonly, metastases present with gadolinium uptake. The Short Tau Inversion Recovery Sequence

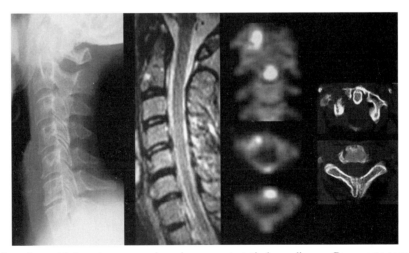

FIGURE 24.10   A female patient with breast cancer and pre-known metastatic bone disease. Bone metastases were seen on a previous planar bone scan in the thoracic spine, pelvis and femora. After an accident the patient complained of neck stiffness. A radiograph does not show suspicious lesions (left). On MRI (middle-left) there is a lesion suspicious for metastasis at the ventral edge of C2. This lesion, however, does not explain the patient's symptoms. On F-18 sodium fluoride PET (middle-right) the metastasis in C2 was confirmed and a second metastasis which appears osteolytic on CT (right) was detected in C1.

(STIR) is very useful for the proof of bone metastases, because it detects edema or blood with a high sensitivity. The edema caused by metastases is shown as hyperintense for these sequences, while the fatty bone marrow shows no signal or is shown as hypointense. Morphologically metastases in the bone marrow appear initially as round lesions with sharp edges. In the further course an edema around these lesions is often observed. For metastases in a vertebral body this can result in a pathological change of the signal for the entire vertebral body. As the inorganic part of the osseous matrix contains only a few protones, the bone itself is not shown on MRI tomography. This means that the exact size of the metastasis and the assessment of the risk of a fracture can be evaluated more accurately when using conventional x-ray technology or computed tomography. In several studies it was reported that significantly more metastases in the spine can be detected using MRI than with planar bone scans. Nevertheless, for a long time MRI was considered to be unsuitable for whole-body screening because of the long duration of examination and its limited availability. New sequences now enable whole-body imaging in 45 minutes. In a mixed collective of 18 patients with breast cancer Steinborn *et al.* [42] compared the sensitivity of MRI and bone scintigraphy. In this study, 91% of the metastases were correctly diagnosed with MRI and 85% with planar bone scintigraphy. Leyer *et al.* [43] compared the accuracy of both methods in 52 patients with small cell lung cancer and 33 patients with breast cancer. Of these 25, five had bone metastases. In this study, MRI and bone scintigraphy showed concordant results in the patients with breast cancer. However, in the subgroup of patients with small cell lung cancer, MRI showed pathological lesions significantly more often than bone scintigraphy. In 19 patients with prostate cancer Friedman *et al.* [44] found concordant results with MRI and bone scintigraphy in 14 cases. Interestingly, bone scintigraphy was false negative in one case and MRI in two cases. Tausig *et al.* [45] also compared bone scintigraphy to MRI in 20 patients with breast cancer. Five patients already had known bone metastases. With MRI as well as with conventional planar bone scans the skeletal status was interpreted true negative in nine patients and true positive in 11 patients. Nevertheless, for the comparison of both methods on a lesion-by-lesion analysis MRI was more sensitive. It is interesting to see that when using MRI, a higher number of metastases was detected in the proximal extremities, the pelvis and the vertebral column. Conversely, more metastases were detected in the skull, the sternum and especially in the ribs when using bone scintigraphy.

Because of its high sensitivity, no adequate gold standard for non-invasive confirmation of lesions interpreted as metastases detected with MRI but negative with other imaging methods exists. Therefore, the specificity of this method cannot be sufficiently assessed. In a large prospective trial [13] 157 patients with the initial diagnosis of lung cancer were screened for bone metastases with F-18 PET, MRI as well as with conventional bone scintigraphy with and without SPECT. MRI was defined as part of the gold standard in this study. If there was a discrepancy between MRI and the other methods then, instead of assuming a higher accuracy, the possibility of false positive MRT findings was considered. The discrepant findings were clarified by using a combination of FDG-PET, CT, the clinical course over 1–5 years and, if possible, by autopsy. This procedure was required for 12 patients. Only in one of these patients was MRI true positive. Metastatic bone disease was excluded in the autopsy of another patient. For 10 further patients, medical imaging was without suspicious findings over the next 1–5 years which did not affirm the assumption of metastases because of the low life expectancy following the initial diagnosis of skeletal metastases.

XII. CONCLUSIONS AND PERSPECTIVES

Because of the above-named different characteristics of bone metastases in reference to the distribution pattern and their influence on bone metabolism, it is evident that no existing imaging method is generally better than another for the detection of bone metastases.

For the detection of metastases with FDG and PET a sufficiently high glucose metabolism is needed; this is not given in the case of prostate cancer or the iodine accumulating thyroid cancer. With MRI, an earlier diagnosis of metastases confined to the vertebral bodies, in the pelvis and the proximal extremities should be possible. Nevertheless, metastases in the skull, the vertebral pedicles and the distal extremities might be missed and the specificity has not yet been sufficiently assessed. Additionally, at the time of writing, there were no representative prospective publications for the primary staging of cancer of the breast, prostate, lung, kidney or thyroid, so that a diagnostic advantage in comparison to conventional bone scintigraphy was not shown.

Sensitivity of bone scintigraphy is limited for the detection of metastases in the vertebral bodies because of the superposition of anatomical structures. In contrast, there is a markedly higher sensitivity for the detection of metastases in the peripheral skeletal regions such as in the skull or the extremities. The result of comparative studies was therefore often predetermined, since they compared planar bone scanning with tomographic imaging methods such as PET, CT or MRI for the sensitivity in detecting metastases in the vertebral bodies. Furthermore, the significance of studies that included various different tumor entities was more dependent on the choice of the collective, the examined skeletal regions, and the definition of the gold standard than on the actual accuracy of the tested methods.

These limitations mean that the transferability of these studies to the daily clinical practice is limited. Therefore, conventional bone scintigraphy can still be regarded as the standard method for the screening for skeletal metastases. Due to its limited sensitivity in detecting vertebral lesions, additional tomographic imaging methods like SPECT, MRI, PET or CT should be used in the case of unclear lesions or in patients with a high risk of metastatic bone disease.

References

1. R.D. Rubens & I. Fogelman, Bone Metastases, Springer-Verlag, London (1991).

2. F.W. Orr, O.H. Sanchez & P. Kostenuik, et al., Tumor interactions in skeletal metastasis, Clin Orthop 312 (1995) 19–33.

3. R.S. Ledley & L.B. Luisted, Reasoning foundations of medical diagnosis, symbolic logic, probability, and value theory aid our understanding of how physicians reason, Science 130 (1959) 9–21.

4. D.L. Munz, Ist die Skelettszintigraphie zum Metastasenscreening noch erforderlich?, Nuklearmedizin 32 (1994) 5–10.

5. A.S. Bachman & E.E. Sproul, Correlation of radiographic and autopsy findings in suspected metastases in the spine, Bull NY Acad Med 44 (1940) 169–175.

6. M. Blau, 18F-Fluoride for bone imaging, Semin Nucl Med 2 (1972) 131–133.

7. E.R. Silberstein, E.L. Saenger & A.J. Tofe, et al., Imaging of bone metastases with ^{99m}Tc-Sn-HEDP (diphosphonate), ^{18}F and skeletal radiography, Radiology 107 (1973) 551–555.

8. D.A. Weber, J.W. Keyes & S. Landmann, et al., Comparison of Tc-polyphosphate and F18 for bone imaging, Am J Roentgen Rad Ther Nucl Med 121 (1974) 184–190.

9. S. Venz, N. Hosten & R. Friedrichs, et al., Osteoplastische Knochenmetastasen beim Prostatakarzinom: Magnetresonanztomographie und Knochenmarkszintigraphie, Fortschr Röntgenstr 161 (1994) 64–69.

10. S. Kosuda, K. Tatsumi & H. Yokoyama, et al., Does bone SPECT actually have lower sensitivity for detecting vertebral metastases than MRI?, J Nucl Med 37 (1996) 975–978.

11. H. Schirrmeister, A.C. Guhlmann & K. Elsner, et al., Sensitivity in detecting osseous lesions depends on anatomical localization: planar bone scintigraphy vs 18F-PET, J Nucl Med 40 (1999) 1623–1629.

12. H. Schirrmeister, G. Glatting & J. Hetzel, et al., Prospective evaluation of the clinical value of planar bone scans, SPECT and 18F-labeled NaF PET in newly diagnosed lung cancer, J Nucl Med 42 (2001) 1800–1804.

13. M. Hetzel, C. Arslandemir & J. Hetzel, et al., F-18 NaF PET in lung cancer – Accuracy, cost-effectiveness and impact on patient management, J Bone Miner Res 18 (2003) 2206–2214.

14. A.E. Jones, N. Ghaed & G.L. Dunson, et al., Clinical evaluation of orally administered fluorine-18 for bone scanning, Radiology 107 (1973) 129–131.

15. H. Creutzig, A. Creutzig & K.G. Gerdts, et al., Vergleichende Untersuchungen mit osteotropen Radiopharmaka. I. Tierexperimentelle Untersuchungen zur Anreicherung von ^{18}F, ^{85}Sr und ^{99m}Tc-EHDP, Fortschr Röntgenstr 123 (1975) 137–143.

16. H. Creutzig, Vergleichende Untersuchungen mit osteotropen Radiopharmaka. II. Plasmaclearance von ^{18}F und ^{99m}Tc-EHDP, Fortschr Röntgenstr 123 (1975) 313–318.

17. H. Creutzig, A. Creutzig & K.G. Gerdts, et al., Vergleichende Untersuchungen mit osteotropen Radiopharmaka. I. Tierexperimentelle Untersuchungen zur Anreicherung von ^{18}F, ^{85}Sr und ^{99m}Tc-EHDP, Fortschr Röntgenstr 123 (1975) 137–143.

18. R. Wootton & C. Dore, The single-passage extraction of ^{18}F in rabbit bone, Clin Physiol Meas 7 (1986) 333–343.

19. N.D. Charkes, P.T. Makler & C. Philips, Studies of skeletal tracer kinetics. I. Digital computer solution of a five-compartment model of ^{18}F fluoride kinetics in humans, J Nucl Med 19 (1978) 1301–1309.

20. G.T. Krishnamurthy, R.J. Huebotter & M. Tubis, et al., Pharmakokinetics of current skeletal-seeking radiopharmaceuticals, Am J Roentgen Rad Ther Nucl Med 126 (1976) 293–301.

21. W.E. Goldhahn, G. Goldhahn & I. Mohsenipur, et al., Degenerative Erkrankungen der Halswirbelsäule, Hippokrates-Verlag, Stuttgard, 1994.

22. H. Schirrmeister, J. Kotzerke & M. Rentschler, et al., Die Positronenemissionstomographie des Skelettsystems mit 18FNa: Häufigkeit, Befundmuster und Verteilung benigner Veränderungen, Fortschr Röntgenstr 169 (1998) 309–314.

23. W. Dihlmann, Röntgendiagnostische Basisinformation: Vertebralosteophyten, Akt Rheumatol 2 (1977) 139–142.

24. W. Dihlmann, Gelenke, Wirbelverbindungen. 3. Aufl., Thieme, New York: Stuttgart (1987).

25. R. Erlemann, A. Roessner & P.E. Peters, et al., Tumoröse Raumforderungen der Wirbelsäule, Fortschr. Röntgenstr 146 (1987) 403–409.

26. R. Erlemann, M. Reiser & A. Roessner, et al., Primäre Knochentumoren und tumorähnliche Läsionen in der Wirbelsäule, Fortschr Röntgenstr 147 (1987) 131–137.

27. J.A. Frank, A. Ling & N.J. Patronas, et al., Detection of malignant bone tumors: MR imaging vs scintigraphy, Amer J Roentgenol 155 (1990) 1043–1048.

28. S.N. Reske, J.H. Karstens & W.M. Glöckner, et al., Nachweis des Knochenmarksbefalls beim Mammakarzinom und bei malignen Lymphomen durch Immunszintigraphie des hämatopoetischen Knochenmarks, Fortschr Röntgenstr 152 (1990) 60–66.

29. Z. Traill, M.A. Richards & N.R. Moore, Magnetic resonance imaging of metastatic bone disease, Clin Orthop 312 (1995) 76–88.

30. K. Pantel, J. Izbicki & B. Passlick, et al., Frequency and prognostic significance of isolated tumor cells in bone marrow of patients with non-small-cell lung cancer without overt metastases, Lancet 347 (1996) 649–653.

31. H. Schirrmeister, A.C. Guhlmann & J. Kotzerke, et al., Early detection and accurate description of extent of metastatic bone disease in breast cancer with 18F-fluoride ion and positron emission tomography, J Clin Oncol 17 (1999) 2381–2389.

32. H. Schirrmeister, T. Kühn & A.C. Guhlmann, et al., [F-18] 2-deoxy-2-fluoro D-glucose PET in preoperative staging of breast cancer—comparison with the standard staging procedures, Eur J Nucl Med 28 (2001) 351–358.

33. S.D. Yeh, M. Imbriaco & S.M. Larson, et al., Detection of bony metastases of androgen-independent prostate cancer by FDG-PET, Nucl Med Biol 23 (1996) 693–697.

34. P.D. Shreve, H.B. Grossman & M.D. Gross, et al., Metastatic prostate cancer: initial findings of PET with 2-deoxy-2-[F-18] fluoro-D-glucose, Radiology 199 (1996) 751–756.

35. G.J. Cook, S. Houston & R. Rubens, et al., Detection of bone metastases in breast cancer by 18FDG PET: differing metabolic activity in osteoblastic and osteolytic lesions, J Clin Oncol 16 (1998) 3375–3379.

36. M. Ohta, Y. Tokuda & Y. Suzuki, et al., Whole body PET for the evaluation of bony metastases in patients with breast cancer: comparison with 99mTc-MDP bone scintigraphy, Nucl Med Commun 22 (2001) 875–879.

37. S.N. Yang, J.A. Liang & F.J. Lin, et al., Comparing whole body (18)F-2-deoxyglucose positron emission tomography and technetium-99m methylene diphosphonate bone scan to detect bone metastases in patients with breast cancer, J Cancer Res Clin Oncol 128 (2002) 325–328.

38. C.H. Kao, J.F. Hsieh & S.C. Tsai, et al., Comparison and discrepancy of 18F-deoxyglucose-positron emission tomography and Tc-99m MDP bone scan to detect bone metastases, Anticancer Res 20 (2000) 2189–2192.

39. E.M. Marom, H.P. McAdams & J.J. Erasmus, et al., Staging non-small cell lung cancer with whole-body PET, Radiology 212 (2002) 803–809.

40. T. Bury, A. Barreto & F. Daenen, et al., Fluorine-18 deoxyglucose positron emission tomography for detection of bone metastases in patients with non-small cell lung cancer, Eur J Nucl Med 25 (1998) 1244–1247.

41. I. Gayed, T. Vu & M. Johnson, et al., Comparison of bone and [18]2-deoxy-2-[18F]fluoro-D-glucose positron emission tomography in the evaluation of bony metastases in lung cancer, Mol Imaging Biol 5 (2003) 26–31.

42. M.M. Steinborn, A.F. Heuck & R. Tiling, et al., Whole-body bone marrow MRI in patients with metastatic disease to the skeletal system, J Comput Assist Tomogr 23 (1999) 123–129.

43. G. Layer, A. Steudel & F. Grünwald, et al., Magnetic resonance imaging to detect bone marrow metastases in the initial staging of small cell lung carcinoma and breast carcinoma, Cancer 85 (1999) 1004–1009.

44. G.M. Freedman, W.G. Negendank & G.R. Hudes, et al., Preliminary results of a bone marrow magnetic resonance imaging protocol for patients with high risk prostate cancer, Urology 54 (1999) 118–123.

45. A. Tausig, N. Manthey & F. Berger, et al., Vorzüge und Limitationen der Ganzkörper-MRT mit Turbo-STIR Sequenzen im Vergleich zur planaren Skelettszintigraphie, Nuklearmedizin 39 (2000) 174–179.

Section VI. Pain Control in Bone Cancer

CHAPTER **25**

Pain Control with Palliative Radiotherapy in Bone Metastases

ALYSA FAIRCHILD[1], AMANDA HIRD[2] AND EDWARD CHOW[2]

[1]*Department of Radiation Oncology, University of Alberta, Cross Cancer Institute, Edmonton, Alberta, Canada.*
[2]*Rapid Response Radiotherapy Program, Odette Cancer Centre, Sunnybrook Health Sciences Centre, Toronto, Ontario, Canada.*

Contents

I. INTRODUCTION

Palliation of bone metastases (BM) comprises a significant proportion of the workload in the specialty of radiation oncology. About 50% of cancer patients will receive palliative radiotherapy (RT) during the course of their disease [1]. Seventy percent of BM occur in the axial skeleton (spine, pelvis, ribs and skull) and 10% in the appendicular skeleton, usually the proximal ends of long bones [2].

Symptoms secondary to BM are common, with up to 75% of patients experiencing pain. Moreover, hypercalcemia, fractures and spinal cord compression can occur [3]. These adverse outcomes are referred to as skeletal-related events or SREs; nerve root compression, impaired mobility, myelosuppression and the need for palliative RT or surgery are also frequent complications.

Radiation therapy is frequently employed with palliative intent in order to minimize tumor-related symptoms. Radiotherapy delivery can be broadly classified as via an

external beam ('teletherapy') or via radioactive sources implanted or inserted into a body surface, tissue or cavity near to the tumor, or into the tumor itself ('brachytherapy'). External beam radiation therapy (EBRT) utilizes high-energy gamma rays produced by a linear accelerator, or x-rays given off by a radioactive cobalt source housed within the head of a treatment machine. This chapter will be focusing primarily on EBRT, delivered as either local fields or wide fields.

II. PRINCIPLES OF PALLIATIVE RADIATION THERAPY

RT exposes both cancerous and non-cancerous cells in the treatment field to ionizing radiation, which penetrates individual cells and induces damage through direct and indirect effects. Direct DNA damage includes base deletions, single and double strand breaks. Indirect damage occurs when radiation ionizes water molecules, producing free radicals, which in turn damage DNA. Repair of DNA damage is possible both in normal cells and cancer cells, but cancer cells have less capacity to do so, creating a therapeutic ratio that can be exploited. 'Fractionation', or dividing the total dose of radiation into a number of smaller doses ('fractions') delivered over time, allows normal tissues to repair damage that cancer cells cannot [4,5]. Typically, patients are treated once per day, Monday through Friday, a schedule which has evolved empirically to balance normal tissue repair with tumor cell kill, although there are clinical scenarios where more than one treatment is given per day, or is administered on weekends. Radiation dose is measured in Gray (Gy); 1 Gy is one joule of absorbed energy per kilogram. One centigray (cGy) is equivalent to 0.01 Gy (or 1 rad in the old system of measurement).

Tumors do not usually have to be completely eradicated in order to relieve symptoms [4], and therefore doses lower than that required for total lesion ablation are used in palliative situations. The use of a lower total dose than that required for cure, but which still achieves symptom control, has several advantages: the risk of acute side effects is minimized, which increases patient quality of life (QoL) and acceptance of treatment; RT can be delivered over fewer fractions, which decreases transportation and hospital admission requirements; it is more convenient for the patient; patient discomfort with positioning is decreased; resources are freed for others; and 'opportunity cost' is decreased. Kirkbride has described the latter as the cost associated with lost opportunities for patients to spend their remaining days as they choose [4]. Although the possibility of long-term side effects should be considered, this is usually less of an issue in patients with limited lifespan [4,5].

III. MECHANISM OF ACTION IN RELIEF OF PAINFUL BONE METASTASES

The exact mechanism of action of EBRT in relieving pain secondary to metastatic bone lesions is still uncertain; however, tumor cell kill may indeed be an important contributor, especially in pain due to periosteal or nerve root compression. Rapid responses and poor correlation of symptom relief with tumor regression suggest that an effect on host mechanisms of pain could also be important. RT may damage radiosensitive host cells (i.e., osteoclasts and macrophages), and in turn inhibit both bone breakdown and the chemical mediators of pain, such as PGE2. Disturbance of neuronal transmission by RT may destroy or exhaust resources for neurotransmission of the pain signal [6]. Effects on blood vessels have been postulated but are yet to be elucidated.

IV. PAIN MONITORING

Cancer pain is a complex and multidimensional construct, and unfortunately is very common [7]. Frequency, severity and impact of symptoms, including pain, vary tremendously in patients with incurable cancer and can affect the patient's sense of well-being and physical and social functioning. Part of the difficulty in assessing pain, and pain relief, is the subjectivity involved.

Clinical assessment of bony metastatic pain can be achieved through one of three methods: verbal rating scales, numerical rating scales, and visual analog scales. Although verbal rating scales (i.e., none, mild, moderate, or severe) are the easiest to use, the sensitivity of such scales is questionable. Eleven point (0–10) numerical rating scales are particularly advantageous in the cancer research setting since such scales enable the detection of meaningful change in pain scores [8].

The Brief Pain Inventory (BPI) is a commonly employed measure of pain intensity and functional interference in cancer-related research [8]. Developed by Cleeland and Ryan [9], this validated patient-based assessment tool evaluates pain on three dimensions: worst pain, average pain, and current pain. In addition, seven indicators of function interference are explored: general activity, normal work, walking ability, mood, sleep, relationships with others, and enjoyment of life [9]. Both components of the BPI utilize an 11-point scale with '0' representing an absence of pain/absence of functional interference, and '10' representing the worst pain imaginable/complete functional interference. Analgesic consumption over the preceding 24-hour period is recorded. Utilizing this pain assessment tool in the palliative cancer population has revealed varying levels of correspondence of the three dimensions of pain (mild, moderate, or severe) with functional interference [8]. Multiple studies have shown the intensity of the worst pain rating correlates most substantially to functional interference [8–14]. As such, a patient's worst pain score should be used in the assessment of overall RT response [8].

Attempts have been made to validate developed pain measurement instruments in an effort to improve the clinical management and research of cancer pain. Furthermore, the absence of universally accepted endpoints for the evaluation of partial response, complete response, and pain progression has prevented a thorough appraisal of the overall efficacy of palliative radiotherapy. Response rate is a function of endpoint [15], and thus different conclusions can be reached based solely on the methods of data interpretation employed. Specifically, the absence of widely accepted endpoints has contributed to the barriers surrounding the establishment of optimal dose fractionation in the palliative care setting [15].

In 2002, the Bone Metastases Consensus Working Party introduced the International Consensus Endpoints for the evaluation of palliative response to radiotherapy [15]. According to the authors' recommendations, evaluation of pain response should occur at 1, 2, and 3 months following completion of RT. Complete response was defined as a pain score of zero at the radiated site with no simultaneous increase in analgesic consumption employing daily oral morphine equivalents. Partial response was defined as one of the following:

- decrease in pain score of 2 or more, on a 0–10 scale, without analgesic increase;
- analgesic reduction of 25% or more from baseline without an increase in pain.

Pain progression was defined as an increase in pain score of 2 or more points above the reported baseline pain score at the radiated site with a stable analgesic regimen, or an increase in daily analgesic consumption (oral morphine equivalent) of 25% or more compared with baseline with a stable pain score, or an increase in pain of 1 or more [15].

V. LOCAL FIELD RADIATION THERAPY: CLINICAL TRIALS

A growing body of empirical evidence describes results of randomized controlled trials (RCTs) of different dose fractionation schedules for uncomplicated BM [16]. While there is no specific, accepted definition of 'uncomplicated', it is generally taken to mean the absence of associated complications such as impending or established fracture.

There have been approximately 25 RCTs published, the vast majority of which have shown that single fraction (SF) palliative RT provides equivalent pain relief for uncomplicated BM as multiple fractions (MF). This topic has been controversial for more than two decades, with analysis of one of the first randomized studies performed twice, each coming to different conclusions [17,18]. Publications from the 1980s contributed to initial controversy, as most had one or more serious design flaws [15]. Not until the late 1990s did more consistent and conclusive data begin to emerge from several, large, multicenter, phase III randomized trials, supported by the results of three meta-analyses [16,19–24].

In general, no differences have been found to date in the proportion of patients achieving complete or partial pain relief from RT regardless of dose employed [19,20,23,24]. No differences in quality of life, time to first improvement in pain, time to complete pain relief, or time to pain progression have been found in studies examining these endpoints [19,20,24]. Narcotic use at three months was not found to be statistically different in the one trial which reported it [23].

The data on pathological fracture are less consistent. In two publications, for example, patients receiving SF RT had higher fracture rates [17,24]. However, in two others, incidence was higher in the MF arms [19,21] (Table 25.1).

In several trials, there have been no significant differences in the incidence of nausea, vomiting, spinal cord compression or pathological fracture [19,20]. However, in two trials, fewer patients on the single fraction arm experienced toxicity [23,24]. Grade two to four acute toxicity, for example, was experienced by 10% in the SF arm compared to 17% in the multifraction arm ($p = 0.002$) [24] (Table 25.2).

The two meta-analyses published in 2003 each showed no significant difference in complete and overall pain relief between single and multiple fraction EBRT for bone metastases [21,22]. Results were remarkably similar, with the Wu paper reporting a complete response rate (absence of pain) of 33% and 32% after single and multiple fraction RT, respectively, compared to 34% and 32% for Sze. Wu's overall response rates were 62 and 59%, compared to 60 and 59% for Sze, for single and multiple fraction RT, respectively. When restricted to evaluable patients, overall response rates became 73% for each arm [22]. Most patients experienced pain relief in the first 2 to 4 weeks after radiotherapy of any duration [22]. Side effects consisting generally of nausea and vomiting were similar in severity for both treatment arms.

An updated meta-analysis reviewed 16 randomized trials which compared SF and multifraction schedules [16]. Studies included were published in full or in abstract form, and totaled 2513 randomizations to SF arms and 2487 to MF arms, respectively. The overall response rate to SF RT was 58%, and complete response rate was 23%, which was not significantly different from the 59 and 24% experienced by patients randomized to MF RT, confirming the conclusions of the 2003 systematic reviews. Generally, no differences in acute toxicity, pathological fracture or spinal cord compression incidence were found. It was determined that 3.2% of patients fractured after SF versus 2.8% after MF ($p = 0.75$).

To date, controversy over the optimal dose fractionation has almost entirely ignored patient choice. Three studies

TABLE 25.1   Incidence of pathologic fracture, from selected randomized controlled trials and meta-analyses

Trial	Dose	Fracture rate	Dose	Fracture rate	*P* value
RTOG 7402[*], 1982	Low	5%	High	8%	No *p* value
RTOG 7402[†], 1982	20 Gy/5	4%	40.5 Gy/15	18%	$p = 0.02$
BPTWP, 1999	8 Gy/1	2%	20 Gy/5 or 30 Gy/10	0.5%	NS
Dutch, 1999	8 Gy/1	4%	24 Gy/6	2%	$p < 0.05$
RTOG, 2005	8 Gy/1	5%	30 Gy/10	4%	No *p* value
TROG 9605, 2005	8 Gy/1	4%	20 Gy/5	4%	NS
Scandinavian[††], 2006	8 Gy/1	4%	30 Gy/10	11%	No *p* value
Sze, 2003§	Single fraction	3%	Multiple fraction	2%	$p = 0.03$
Wu, 2003§[ρ]	Single fraction	Not pooled	Multiple fraction	Not pooled	N/a
Chow, 2007§	Single fraction	3%	Multiple fraction	3%	NS

[*]Multiple metastases cohort, [†]solitary metastasis cohort, [††]not referable to treatment site only and proportions calculated based on absolute number reported, § meta-analysis, [ρ]not pooled due to trial heterogeneity. Abbreviations: n/a—not assessable; NS—not significant.

TABLE 25.2   Incidence of toxicity, from selected randomized controlled trials and meta-analyses

Trial	Dose	Toxicity	Dose	Toxicity	*P* value
RTOG 7402, 1982	Lower	Not reported	Higher	Not reported	N/a
BPTWP, 1999	8 Gy/1	30%	20 Gy/5 or 30 Gy/10	32%	NS
Dutch, 1999	8 Gy/1	Not reported	24 Gy/6	Not reported	NS
RTOG, 2005	8 Gy/1	Grade 2–4—10%	30 Gy/10	Grade 2–4—17%	*p* = 0.002
TROG 9605, 2005	8 Gy/1	Grade 3—2%	20 Gy/5	Grade 3—2%	No *p* value
Scandinavian, 2006	8 Gy/1	'Fewer'* Patients	30 Gy/10	More patients	No *p* value No *p* value
Sze, 2003[†]	Single fraction	'Similar in severity'	Multiple fraction	'Similar in severity'	No *p* value
Wu, 2003[†],[††]	Single fraction	Not pooled	Multiple fraction	Not pooled	N/a
Chow, 2007[†]	Single fraction	'Generally similar'	Multiple fraction	'Generally similar'	N/a

*Absolute numbers not stated, [†] meta-analysis, [††] not pooled due to trial heterogeneity. Abbreviations: n/a—not assessable; NS—not significant.

have investigated patients' preferences of RT schedules [25–27]. In one study, 21 Australian patients with BM who had received RT between 6 weeks and 2 years prior participated in structured interviews where they were asked to indicate the relative priority attributed to different aspects of treatment [25]. Participants generally considered medical appointments to be physically demanding, and rated sustained pain relief and reduced risk of future complications as their highest priorities. Convenience was acknowledged, but factors such as traveling distance and brevity of treatment were considered of secondary importance to overall QoL and treatment efficacy. Most patients favored SF RT, assuming equivalent outcomes.

Patients in Singapore and Canada were studied using the same patient-preference instrument, which presented differences and similarities between SF and MF radiotherapy [26,27]. In the Singapore study, 85% of patients would choose extended courses of RT (24 Gy/6 fractions) compared to a single treatment due to lower retreatment rates and decreased fracture risk; choice did not seem to depend on age, performance status, primary cancer site, cost, or pain score [26].

Seventy-six percent of Canadian patients would choose a single 8 Gy, as opposed to 1 week of RT, due to greater convenience [27]. Preference for the MF treatment regimen was largely the result of the perceived decreased likelihood of pathologic fracture. Older and retired patients were more likely to select SF. Differences in the above three studies may be explained in part by cultural differences and potentially by differences in the decision aid instrument [28].

Despite the overwhelming amount of randomized evidence and obvious advantages for patients, there has been a reluctance to adopt SF schedules as global standard practice to date. An article reviewed surveys published between 1988 and 2006 on prescription patterns for RT for bone metastases [28]. American respondents indicated an overwhelming preference for the 30 Gy/10 schedule, and 90–100% of radiation oncologists preferred multiple to single fractions. Approximately 85% of Canadian Radiation Oncologists preferred multiple fractions, most often as 20 Gy/5 over 1 week. Multiple fractions were again commonly used in the UK, Western Europe, Australia and New Zealand, and India; however, oncologists in these countries would consider SF schedules in up to 42% of cases [28].

Nonetheless, first indications of a shift in prescription patterns have begun to appear. In the UK, a practice audit performed in 2003 revealed the most common palliative RT schedule to be delivery of a single fraction [29]. In Sweden, a 2001 national audit reported that 'the principle of irradiation of skeletal metastases with a single or few fractions has been widely adopted in clinical practice' since 1992 [30]. After the Dutch trial was published in 1999, 'almost all Dutch institutions either changed or [were] planning to change their protocols to SF for palliation of bone metastases' [31]. A Scandinavian trial was terminated early due to slow recruitment, blamed on physician reluctance to randomize between single and multiple fractions [24].

VI. WIDE FIELD RADIATION THERAPY: CLINICAL TRIALS

Patients with bone metastases can have multiple sites of disease causing diffuse symptoms. Wide field (also known as 'hemi-body irradiation' or HBI) differs from localized EBRT mainly in the volume of tissue and BM included in a single treatment portal. HBI is usually delivered either to the upper half (base of skull to iliac crest) or to the lower half (iliac crest to ankles) of the body, to a total dose of 6 Gy and 8 Gy, respectively [32].

Single fraction HBI has been shown in retrospective and prospective phase I and II studies to provide pain relief in 70–80% of patients [33–36]. Since pain relief is apparent within 24–48 hours [36,37], it is suggested that cells of the inflammatory response pathway may be the initial target, as tumor cell kill is unlikely to be accomplished so quickly.

Fractionated HBI was investigated in a randomized phase II study involving 29 patients, comparing a single dose with MF (25–30 Gy in 9–10 fractions) [38]. Pain relief was achieved in over 94% of patients. At 1 year, 70% in the fractionated and 15% in the single fraction group had pain control, and repeat radiation was required in 71% of the single and 13% of the fractionated group. Fractionation is thought to allow delivery of a higher overall dose with less toxicity [39].

Poulter *et al.* reported results of a randomized trial of 499 patients comparing local radiation alone versus local RT and single fraction HBI. A lower incidence of new bone metastases (50% vs 68%) and fewer patients requiring further local RT at 1 year after HBI (60% vs 76%) were reported [40].

In a randomized trial of 156 patients, Salazar *et al.* investigated the choice of dose-fractionation schedules for HBI [32]. Among the three trial arms (15 Gy/5 over 1 week, 8 Gy/2 fractions in 1 day, 12 Gy/4 over 2 days), the 15 Gy/5 arm not only provided equivalent pain relief, but also a longer survival duration compared with the other schedules. The 2- and 5-day regimens gave similar results (except for prostate patients where the 2-day arm was inferior), with pain relief seen in 91% of patients by day 3. The 1-day regimen resulted in inferior pain relief and poorer QoL [32].

VII. SIDE EFFECTS OF RADIATION THERAPY

A. Local Field RT

Due to the nature of palliative radiotherapy and the existing level of discomfort within the treatment population, it is imperative to minimize adverse side effects. Treating the tumor while limiting dose to surrounding normal tissue can accomplish this [4]. As local EBRT is a focused treatment modality, benefits and potential side effects are site-specific; the only exception to this is fatigue, the etiology of which is unknown [5].

Treatment-related side effects are classified in terms of when they present relative to RT. Acute side effects arise within 90 days of RT, while late toxicities occur following this cut-off point. Acute side effects are self-limited, lasting days to weeks, and their severity cannot generally be predicted *a priori*. Most acute side effects do not peak until after treatment completion [4]. Late side effects are

generally infrequent due to patients' limited remaining life expectancies.

Skin reactions are usually minimal during RT for bone metastases, are limited to the radiation field, and treated similarly to sunburns [5]. Patients receiving treatment to large volumes encompassing the pelvis, epigastrium or thoracolumbar spine may experience nausea and/or emesis [41]. Prophylactic anti-emetics should be prescribed orally 30–60 minutes prior to RT, and continued on an as-needed basis between fractions. Hematologic side effects are usually mild and transient, but bone marrow suppression may occur if the treatment portals are large, the total dose is moderate to high, and a significant proportion of marrow is included, especially in heavily pretreated patients [42]. Mucositis and esophagitis causing difficult, painful swallowing occur after treatment to the head and neck or thorax, and are treated with dietary modifications, oral rinses, antifungals, analgesics and cytoprotective agents [5,42]. If large amounts of small intestine are included in the fields, radiation enteritis may occur, manifested by cramping; frequent, loose stools; and occasionally bleeding [42]. Treating the pelvis may also result in short-lived diarrhea, the risk of which is diminished in view of the large doses of opioids patients are commonly taking [41]. Bone weakened by disease will not be strengthened immediately by EBRT. Fractures after RT have been reported in up to 18% of patients [17] (Table 25.1).

B. Wide Field RT

After wide-field or HBI radiation therapy, toxicities include minor bone marrow suppression and acute gastrointestinal side effects such as nausea, vomiting and diarrhea. Patients should be premedicated with intravenous fluids, anti-emetics and corticosteroids, and provided with analgesics for pain flare [37,43,44]. Sequential treatment of both upper and lower body requires a 4–6 week gap for interval recovery of myelosuppression. Pulmonary toxicity is limited provided that the lung dose is no more than 6 Gy [45].

C. Pain Flare

After a course of RT to a treatment field that includes bony metastases, pain flare, a self-limited worsening of symptoms within a week of commencing treatment, can be problematic [46]. Definitions of pain flare in the literature vary, for example, in terms of whether they take into account concomitant changes in analgesic usage. In order to distinguish pain flare from disease progression, pain scores and analgesic intake usually must return to baseline after the transient increase [47]. Estimates of incidence of pain flare vary from 10 to 44% following EBRT, and in one trial duration was a median of 3 days [48–50]. The proportion of patients experiencing pain flare is reported to be higher after large, single fractions than after completing multiple, smaller fractions [50].

Pain flare usually occurs in the first few days following RT. In a palliative population, the potential for treatment-induced pain crisis is concerning. Patients can be instructed to take extra breakthrough analgesic doses should they experience increased pain; however, preventive measures are always preferred. Dexamethasone, a well-known adjuvant analgesic and anti-inflammatory, is a good choice as a prophylactic agent because of a long half-life (36–54 hours) that corresponds to the time frame following RT in which pain flare incidence is greatest [48–50].

The first study reporting a potential role for dexamethasone in the prophylaxis of pain flare after single fraction RT has been published [47]. One dose (8 mg by mouth) was administered 1 hour prior to 8 Gy/1 for painful bone metastases. Patients completed the Brief Pain Inventory at baseline and daily for 10 days. Pain flare was defined as a 2-point increase in worst pain on an 11-point numerical rating scale with no decrease in analgesic, or a 25% increase in analgesic intake without a decrease in worst pain score. In the 33 patients entered, median total oral morphine equivalent at baseline was 18 mg per day, and baseline mean worst pain was 7.8/10. No significant toxicity was observed secondary to the medication. Twenty-four percent (8/33) experienced pain flare, starting anywhere from day 3 to day 7 after RT, and lasting from 1 to 6 days. The incidence of flare in the first 2 days after dexamethasone was 3%. A multicenter phase II Canadian trial investigating the effectiveness of Dexamethasone in prevention of pain flare is ongoing, with a phase III trial planned.

VIII. COMPLICATIONS OF BONE METASTASES

A. Pathologic Fracture

Pathologic fractures may be the first sign of metastatic disease to bone. A review of 1800 patients reported an 8% incidence of pathologic fracture, of which >50% were due to breast cancer [51]. Annual fracture rates of 20% may be seen in hormone resistant prostate cancer [52]. Other malignancies such as kidney, lung and thyroid carcinoma each account for 5–10% of fractures [51]. Approximately 1% of bone metastases fracture. Ten percent of all BM, usually located in the femur, require some form surgical intervention. The femoral neck is responsible for 50% of proximal femoral fractures, the subtrochanteric region for 30%, and the intertrochanteric region 15% [53].

B. Impending Fracture and Risk Prediction

An impending fracture is defined as a bony metastasis that, if not addressed, has a significant likelihood of fracture

under normal physiological stresses. Although some physicians believe that all patients with proximally located femoral metastases should undergo preventive surgery, this would result in a large number of unnecessary surgical procedures [54]. Therefore, many studies, mostly in the context of femoral fractures, have attempted to predict fracture risk based on clinical and/or radiologic findings [3,53–69]. Incidence of long bone fractures has been found to be related to many patient and tumor factors (Table 25.3). For example, functional pain is caused by a bone which is mechanically weak, and can no longer support the normal stresses of daily activities; this is the most strongly positive predictor of fracture in some series [53].

However, many of these retrospective studies were based on two-dimensional imaging and surgical data only. Additionally, most investigators did not specifically state how they measured such parameters as circumferential cortical involvement. In the reporting of fracture post-radiotherapy in the dose-finding RCTs, risk was almost never assessed pretreatment, making definitive conclusions from these data difficult.

Perhaps the best known scoring system, that of Mirels, is a useful guide for non-orthopedists for directing referrals [65]. Based on 78 cases, he devised a system grading the site, pain pattern, lesion size, and radiographic appearance (Table 25.4). Each factor was given a score of 0 to 3. For total scores of ≤7, the risk of fracture is <5%; for these cases non-invasive management is appropriate. For scores of 9 or greater, fracture can almost be said to be inevitable, and fixation should be performed. Lesions scoring 8 are intermediate, with a risk of fracture of 15%, and should be assessed on a case-by-case basis. However, Damron has suggested that this classification has a high false negative rate, with a specificity of only 35% [70].

In the randomized Dutch Bone Metastasis Study on the palliative effect of a single fraction of 8 Gy versus 24 Gy/6, database analysis revealed 14 fractures in 102 patients with femoral metastases [54]. (Patients with lesions suspected to be at high risk of fracturing at baseline were ineligible for study entry.) Twenty-three percent (10/44) had received SF and 7% (4/58) had received MF. In general, SF patients had a higher chance of experiencing a pathological fracture than MF patients, with a median time to fracture of 7 weeks (SF) versus 20 weeks (MF). Results suggest that MF postponed fracturing longer than SF. Patients who remained free from fracturing were not retreated more often; therefore, higher total dose of RT was not a valid explanation for the absence of expected fractures. On pretreatment radiographs, the amount of axial cortical involvement was the only predictive parameter for fracturing. The authors recommended treating femoral metastases with an axial cortical involvement length of >30 mm with prophylactic surgery due to a 25% fracture incidence. Although more fractures occurred after a single dose of 8 Gy, they could not prove the treatment schedule to be predictive [54].

TABLE 25.3 Indications for surgery in impending fractures of the femur

References	Indication for surgical intervention
[53,55–57,59,65,66,68,69]	Increasing pain during or after radiotherapy, especially with weight-bearing
[53,55–57,69]	Lesion size >25 mm
[62]	Lesion size >20 mm
[53,55–57,59,62,65–67]	Osteolytic appearance on radiographs
[55,57,59]	Transverse cortical destruction
[55,59,63]	Axial cortical destruction (present)
[54,64]	Axial cortical destruction >30 mm*
[68]	Axial cortical destruction >38 mm
[54,55,59,62]	Circumferential cortical destruction (present)
[53,56,58,61,64,66,69]	Circumferential cortical destruction (>50%)
[65]	Circumferential cortical destruction (>66%)
[59]	Cortical lesion of any size secondary to lung carcinoma
[3]	Lesser trochanter avulsion fracture
[60,62,65]	Any proximal lesion
[60]	Diffusely mottled lesion
[62]	Increased body weight and activity
[64]	Ratio of width of metastasis/width bone >0.6
[68]	Ratio of width of metastasis/width bone >0.9
[53]	General health adequate to tolerate surgery and remaining bone adequate to support the surgical construct
[53]	Life expectancy ≥1 month (weight-bearing bone)
[53]	Life expectancy ≤3 months (non-weight-bearing bone)

*Except lesions in femoral neck where axial cortical destruction >13 mm is considered significant.

TABLE 25.4 Mirel's criteria for risk prediction of fracture

Variable	Score 1	2	3
Site	Upper limb	Lower limb	Peritrochanter
Pain	Mild	Moderate	Functional
Lesion	Blastic	Mixed	Lytic
Size	<1/3	1/3–2/3	>2/3

From: Mirels, H. (1989) *Clin Orthop Relat Res 249*, 256.

C. Impending or Established Pathologic Fractures Treated with Radiotherapy Alone

Although there are multiple benefits to prophylactic fixation followed by post-operative radiotherapy (PORT) (see below), a proportion of patients will not be candidates for an operative procedure, or will refuse surgical intervention. Often a minimum life expectancy (6–12 weeks) is required, in order that the patient survives a sufficient time to justify the morbidity and mortality risk. Patients also must have a reasonable performance status, manageable comorbidities, and adequate remaining bone to support any implanted hardware [53].

Otherwise, patients may receive RT alone. Although it can provide pain relief and tumor control, it does not restore bone stability, and remineralization will take weeks to months [41]. Patients should be warned of the increased risk of fracture in the peri-radiation period due to an induced hyperemic response at the periphery of the tumor that weakens the adjacent bone in the short term. As such, it is routine to introduce measures to reduce anatomic forces across the lesion during this time, such as crutches, a sling or a walker.

Although there is no consensus on appropriate dose fractionation, most authors recommend a multifraction course of EBRT in a patient with an impending or established fracture [54]. One retrospective series analyzed 27 pathologic fractures in various sites treated with doses of 40–50 Gy over 4–5 weeks. Healing with remineralization was seen in 33%, with pain relief in 67% [71]. In practice, 20–40 Gy for established pathologic fracture is generally given over 1–3 weeks. In the specific case of an apparently solitary, histologically-confirmed metastasis, especially after a long disease-free interval, some clinicians may wish to give higher dose under the assumption that this will provide long term control (e.g., 40–50 Gy).

D. Post-Operative Radiotherapy (PORT)

An implant will fail from repetitive loading unless the bone heals. Since cancerous bone heals slower than normal bone, adjunctive modalities, such as RT, are often required to promote healing, presuming that the site has not yet been radiated. Additional supportive care such as physiotherapy and comfort measures to assist with analgesia and prevent contractures should always be considered.

Traditionally, PORT is used to suppress tumor growth and prevent destabilization of the prosthesis by maintaining the structural integrity of the bone in which the implant is fixed [72]. Post-operative treatment is thought to decrease pain, minimize the risk of disease progression, minimize implant failure, and reduce the risk of refracture [73]. In a review of 64 orthopedic procedures performed on 60 patients, Townsend *et al.* reported normal use of extremity (with or without pain) in 53% of patients receiving PORT versus 11.5% after surgery alone. Repeated orthopedic procedures were more frequent in the group that received surgery alone. Interestingly, the actuarial median survival for the surgery-alone group was 3.3 months, compared with 12.4 months for the PORT group. However, this study needs to be interpreted with caution due to its retrospective nature and possible selection biases.

Concrete evidence regarding the optimal dose in the post-operative setting does not exist. Nonetheless, most radiation oncologists use a multifraction schedule, similar to that of patients receiving RT alone for impending fracture, such as 20–40 Gy over 1–4 weeks [1,42,73]. The portal usually encompasses the entire implant with a margin, and in many cases this will involve treating the entire bone. Following intramedullary nailing, the entire length of bone is thought to be at risk of seeding. Thus, the whole surgical field and all implanted hardware should be included in the radiation field. Treatment is generally started within 2 to 4 weeks of surgery, after the wound has healed. Patients should be assessed 4 weeks after RT and if there has been no improvement in pain control, especially if mechanical or functional pain still exists, they should be referred to an appropriate orthopedic specialist [53].

Some authors have suggested that, in patients whose prognosis may be only a few weeks or months, pain relief may be a more reasonable goal than rehabilitation and mobilization [72]. In this situation, consideration could be given to single dose RT, with the understanding that supporting evidence is non-existent [1]. In extremely debilitated patients, EBRT may not be indicated at all. Prospective trials are urgently needed to clarify this issue, and to give some guidance on the issues of technique and dose fractionation schedule.

E. Neuropathic Pain

Neuropathic pain is defined as pain initiated or caused by a primary lesion or other dysfunction in the nervous system [74]. Neuropathic pain associated with bone metastases can be difficult to treat effectively, as it is generally considered to be not as predictively responsive to standard analgesics [75]. Characteristic symptoms include spontaneous pain in a dermatomal distribution, altered sensation (hypoesthesia or hyperesthesia) and allodynia (pain evoked by a non-noxious stimulus) [76,77]. Neuropathic pain is often described by patients as burning or electric shock-like [41]. The primary approaches to treating tumor-related neurologic injury are control of the underlying disease, and use of concomitant symptomatic measures.

There is some evidence to suggest that radiation oncologists are more reluctant to use single fractions of RT when neuropathic pain is present [46,78]. Possible reasons for this include the belief that tumor shrinkage is required to relieve mechanical pressure on nerves, concern about occult spinal cord or cauda equina compression, or the general exclusion of patients with neuropathic pain in trials examining efficacy of single fraction EBRT [46].

Roos *et al.* compared a single 8 Gy versus 20 Gy/5 for 245 per protocol patients with bone metastases causing neuropathic pain in the only RCT of its kind [46]. Both schedules were highly effective: pain relief was seen in 53–61% of patients, with 26–27% experiencing complete response. Time to treatment failure was higher in the fractionated arm (3.7 vs 2.4 months), but, like the response rates, the difference did not reach statistical significance. Rates of spinal cord compression, pathological fracture and retreatment with RT in relation to the index site were not significantly different (Tables 25.1, 25.2 and 25.5). The authors concluded that a single dose was not as effective as MF for the treatment of neuropathic pain, but was also not significantly worse. It was recommended that 20 Gy/5 fractions be used as the standard schedule. In situations in which the patient has an unfavorable prognosis or poor performance status, or the cost and/or inconvenience of multiple treatments is a factor, SF should be considered.

Pollicino *et al.* performed a cost-effectiveness reanalysis of the TROG 9605 trial data. The authors determined that larger retreatment costs were associated with the SF arm; however, these were offset by savings in medication and hospital admission costs, as well as by the lower cost of initial RT [79]. For more on cost-effectiveness, see below.

IX. RE-IRRADIATION

External beam RT has many benefits: generally mild toxicity, few patient-related contraindications, fewer stringent functional status and expected lifespan requirements than surgery, and non-invasiveness. Nevertheless, drawbacks include the sometimes lengthy planning process and dosage

TABLE 25.5 Incidence of re-irradiation, from selected randomized controlled trials and meta-analyses

Trial	Dose	Re-irradiation rate	Dose	Re-irradiation rate	P value
RTOG 7402, 1982	Lower	Not reported	Higher	Not reported	N/a
BPTWP, 1999	8 Gy/1	23%	20 Gy/5 or 30 Gy/10	10%	$p < 0.001$
Dutch, 1999	8 Gy/1	25%	24 Gy/6	7%	p = Sig (no value)
RTOG, 2005	8 Gy/1	18%	30 Gy/10	9%	$p < 0.001$
TROG 9605, 2005	8 Gy/1	29%	20 Gy/5	24%	$p = 0.41$
Scandinavian, 2006[*]	8 Gy/1	16%	30 Gy/10	4%	No p value
Sze, 2003[†]	Single fraction	22%	Multiple fraction	7%	$p < 0.0001$
Wu, 2003[†,††]	Single fraction	Not pooled	Multiple fraction	Not pooled	N/a
Chow, 2007[†]	Single fraction	20%	Multiple fraction	8%	$p < 0.0001$

[*]Proportions calculated based on absolute number reported in paper, [†]meta-analysis, [††]not pooled because of trial heterogeneity. Abbreviations: n/a—not assessable; sig—significant.

limits to normal tissues. Since there is a maximal amount of RT that can be delivered to normal tissue before irreversible damage results, patients can face a situation in which no further RT can be delivered to a painful site.

Certain subsets of patients with metastatic disease have longer life expectancies than in the past, in large part due to advances in systemic therapy. More and more patients therefore outlive the duration of benefit provided by their initial palliative RT, requiring consideration of re-irradiation of previously treated sites at a later date. Re-irradiation can be offered in clinical situations in which other modalities, such as surgery or chemotherapy, are either ineffective or not indicated [80].

Painful bony metastases are so prone to causing difficulty with pain that a significant body of literature has emerged concerning repeat irradiation to the same site over time. There are three scenarios where re-irradiation may be considered, and it is unclear whether response to retreatment is similar for each:

• The patient experiences no pain relief or pain progression after initial RT;
• The patient experiences partial response after initial RT, but hopes to achieve a greater response with further treatment;
• The patient experiences partial or complete response after initial RT, but subsequently has a recurrence of pain.

When assessing retreatment rates after RT, it is important to be aware that one reason why more patients receive repeat treatment after a single dose of radiation therapy is because of the comparatively low total dose of RT they have received [81]. Many radiation oncologists are reluctant to prescribe a second course of treatment after a patient has had in excess of 30 Gy, particularly if the spinal cord or another sensitive normal tissue is in the treatment volume [42,81]. Consideration of retreatment should be delayed until 4 to 6 weeks after initial RT to allow response to the

first course to be adequately assessed and to allow any pain flare to resolve [41]. Unfortunately, patients who could potentially benefit from further treatment may be lost to follow-up or may not be referred back to the cancer center after this time interval.

The clinical indications, optimal dose and fractionation, and techniques for retreatment are controversial and vary among physicians. The response to re-irradiation is variable and no consistent policy is recommended or followed. Individual oncologists may find decision-making difficult because of the multiple 'one-off' situations which make general guidelines impossible [82]. Many radiation oncologists are reluctant to re-irradiate because of a lack of precise quantitative data on the time course, magnitude and tissue specificity of long-term occult radiation injury recovery [83].

Re-irradiation in the RCTs for BM was delivered at the discretion of the treating physicians who were not blinded to initial RT received. Additionally, there were no guidelines explaining when, why and what dose of radiation should be prescribed for the second course. Retreatment rates after 8 Gy/1 varied from 18 to 25%, and after multifraction RT varied from 7 to 9% [19,20,23,24]. Only two out of the three published meta-analyses have pooled this outcome, with Sze finding a significantly higher retreatment rate across studies with SF (22 vs 7%, $p < 0.0001$) [21]. This was echoed by Chow *et al.*, who reported 20% (SF) versus 8% (MF) retreatment rates ($p < 0.0001$) [16] (see Table 25.5).

In the most robust data reported to date, the Dutch Bone Metastases Study Group re-analyzed their data to specifically report the efficacy of re-irradiation [54]. Of patients not responding to initial radiation, 66% who initially received 8 Gy/1 responded to retreatment, compared to 33% of patients who initially received a multifraction course. Retreatment in patients after pain progression was successful in 70% of those who received SF initially, as compared with 57% of those who received more than one fraction. Overall, re-irradiation was effective in 63% of all such treated patients.

It is therefore worth considering re-irradiation of sites of metastatic bone pain after initial RT, particularly where this follows an initial period of response. There is also evidence that a proportion of initial non-responders will respond. The preferred dose schedule, however, is unknown. To date, no prospective randomized study has been completed.

However, a large, prospective, randomized intergroup study employing common re-irradiation schedules has been launched [84]. Patients with painful BM who have received prior palliative RT will be included. The initial dose to extremities or ribs can be 6 Gy/1, 8 Gy/1, 18 Gy/4, 20 Gy/5, 24 Gy/6 or 30 Gy/10. The initial dose to metastases in the spine and pelvis can be 6 Gy/1, 8 Gy/1, 18 Gy/4 or 20 Gy/5. Patients are randomized to either 8 Gy/1 or 20 Gy in five or eight daily fractions; 20 Gy/8 is delivered if the initial RT course was multifraction and included the spine or whole pelvis. The primary endpoint is pain relief after re-irradiation. Secondary objectives pertain to side effects and QoL.

X. COST-EFFECTIVENESS

Nowhere is the urgent need to consider economic factors in day-to-day practice more pressing than in the field of radiation oncology, where a combination of better screening, early diagnosis, improved survival due to systemic therapies, and innovative technology for treatment delivery mean a higher cost of delivering RT than ever before.

Several economic analyses have compared different schedules of RT, or RT with another treatment modality. A cost-utility analysis was conducted prospectively within the Dutch randomized trial comparing a single 8 Gy to 24 Gy/6 dose, which reported equivalent symptom palliation in 1999. When considering the estimated quality-adjusted life years, including the effect of retreatment, single fraction RT provided an additional 1.7 quality-adjusted weeks and saved USD$1753 compared to multiple fractions [85].

Through the use of a Markov model, Konski estimated that SF RT was more cost-effective for painful BM than either multifraction RT, chemotherapy (mitoxantrone and prednisone) or analgesics (oxycontin with senokot bowel routine) [86]. Chemotherapy had the highest expected mean total cost. MF RT had only slightly more quality-adjusted life months than SF but cost USD$1300 more. The improved cost-effectiveness of RT in comparison to narcotic analgesics and bisphosphonates has also been reported by other investigators [41].

Most studies indicate that RT provides good value for the money when compared with other palliative treatments. From a resource perspective, SF or short course RT should always be considered when treating pain arising from uncomplicated BM.

XI. OTHER TREATMENT MODALITIES AND THEIR INTEGRATION WITH RADIATION THERAPY

With advances in minimally invasive surgery, innovative radiopharmaceuticals, and newer generation bisphosphonates and systemic therapy, new combinations of modalities are being explored for additive or synergistic effects to improve clinical outcomes in the treatment of bone metastases.

A. Radiotherapy and Minimally Invasive Surgical Techniques

The need for multidisciplinary, cooperative assessment is nowhere more imperative from a patient QoL perspective than in the area of balancing the need for surgical intervention for advanced cancer with its potential side effects.

Percutaneous vertebroplasty (PVP) and kyphoplasty are minimally invasive surgical techniques that are alternatives to open surgery for restoring stability to BM in the spine, pelvis and elsewhere [77]. These are potential treatment options for patients who are not suitable for invasive spinal surgery due to medical comorbidities, multilevel disease or profound neurologic deficits [87]. Both involve percutaneous needle placement into the vertebral body under IV sedation. Injection of radio-opaque polymethylmethacrylate (PMMA; bone cement) takes place under radiologic guidance via a parapedicular or transpedicular approach. The difference between the two procedures is whether or not a balloon is used prior to create or enlarge a cavity for the PMMA; this is the case in kyphoplasty, but not in PVP.

Typically, pain relief is early and significant. Weill showed in 37 patients undergoing vertebroplasty that 73% had pain relief immediately and at six months, but cement extrusion occurred in three cases [88]. Complication rates are around 10% in metastatic disease [89]. Furthermore, PVP in particular has been used to salvage patients experiencing progression of pain after external beam radiotherapy [90].

B. Radiotherapy and Radiopharmaceuticals

Bone-seeking radiopharmaceuticals, or radionuclides, have several mechanisms of action: direct substitution for stable analogs in the hydroxyapatite mineral, or formation of insoluble salts with bone [91]. Radiopharmaceutical uptake is greater where new reactive bone is being formed, such as in areas of osteoblastic metastases. These agents, though administered systemically, have localized effects, as the mean range of the radiation particles is 0.2–3.0 mm. Therefore, surrounding normal tissue is relatively spared, which is an advantage in terms of retreatment, and in simultaneously alleviating pain from several sites of painful BM.

There seem to be no differences between agents in terms of pain relief, and each works equally well in different cancer types, without evidence of dose response [91,92].

Randomized studies of strontium (89Sr) and samarium (153Sm-EDTMP) indicate improved pain control and decreased analgesic consumption. Response usually takes 2–3 weeks after administration. Response rates are 55–95%, with complete relief in 5–20%, and mean duration of pain relief is 3–6 months. In terms of side effects, flare reaction occurs in approximately 10% of patients. Anecdotally, patients who experience flare may be more likely to respond. The degree of myelosuppression in a particular patient cannot be reliably estimated, but is usually grade 2 or less, self-limited, and recovers in 8–12 weeks. However, eligibility criteria are quite strict, and radionuclides cannot be used in the presence of impending or established pathologic fracture, spinal cord or nerve root compression [93]. Clinical use may be more limited than evidence would suggest due to cost and availability.

Improved outcomes have been demonstrated by some studies when radionuclides have been combined with RT. The multicenter Trans-Canada study found that 40% of strontium patients were pain-free at 3 months, compared with 23% of placebo patients [94]. Seventeen percent of patients receiving adjuvant 89Sr discontinued analgesics as compared to 2%. At 3 months, 59% of strontium patients were free of new painful metastases versus 34% of the placebo arm ($p < 0.05$), with an increased median time to further local RT of 35 weeks versus 20 weeks. QoL, pain relief and improvement in physical activity were also statistically significantly superior in the 89Sr arm with acceptable hematologic toxicity and overall management cost savings. A Norwegian randomized trial, however, reported no advantage in pain relief with the addition of 89Sr to local RT [95]. Canadian practice guidelines do not currently recommend 89Sr as a routine adjuvant to local RT because of conflicting trial results [92].

Quilty and colleagues compared radionuclides to local EBRT, and also to hemi-body irradiation [44]. A total of 284 patients with metastatic prostate cancer and painful bone metastases were randomized to either local field RT, HBI or 89Sr. HBI resulted in pain relief in 64%, compared to 66% in the 89Sr group and 61% in the local RT group. Fewer patients reported new painful metastatic sites after 89Sr treatment than after HBI or local field RT alone.

C. Local RT, HBI and Radionuclides: A Comparison

The pain relief achieved with HBI and radionuclides is comparable; however, the onset of pain relief is faster with HBI [32]. Administration of a systemic radionuclide has the advantage of targeting all bony lesions simultaneously and is given on an outpatient basis as a single injection. HBI affects both osseous and extra-osseous tumors, whereas 89Sr only affects bone metastases which have adequate radioisotope uptake. Both are associated with transient myelosuppression, but with HBI, acute GI toxicity is worse,

with added concerns of late toxicity to visceral structures. Radionuclides are recommended for blastic cancers, in patients with painful BM on both sides of the diaphragm, not adequately controlled with conventional analgesics, and in whom the multiple fields of local EBRT or HBI may cause unacceptable toxicity. HBI is an effective treatment option for patients with diffuse lytic disease, who are not candidates for radionuclides.

D. Systemic Therapy

Systemic therapy can be targeted against the tumor itself (for example, traditional chemotherapy), or directed toward blocking the effect of tumor products on host cells (for example, bisphosphonates' action on osteoclasts; see below).

In certain settings, systemic therapy has been shown to improve pain, quality of life and to prolong survival in patients with BM, such as hormone-refractory prostate cancer [96]. Chemotherapy could also be considered in patients with bone lesions due to chemosensitive tumors such as multiple myeloma, lymphoma or germ cell tumors. However, response is nearly always partial, with a median duration of 9–12 months. In more resistant solid tumors, such as melanoma, benefits of systemic therapy are limited. Additionally, chemotherapy can be hazardous for patients with extensive bone marrow disease, especially if heavily pretreated. Whether combining RT and chemotherapy concurrently improves symptom relief is unknown, and has not yet been investigated in patients with BM. Patients with hormonally responsive cancers usually gain some relief of symptoms, with a median response of 15–24 months.

E. Radiotherapy and Bisphosphonates

Bisphosphonates are analogs of pyrophosphate that bind avidly to exposed bone mineral. During bone resorption, they are internalized by the osteoclast and subsequently cause cell death, preventing further osteolysis. Bisphosphonates have now become established as a valuable adjunctive approach to other systemic treatments, becoming the standard of care for breast cancer and multiple myeloma. Benefits have also been demonstrated in prostate cancer and other solid tumors [97]. A meta-analysis of 33 studies that included patients with bone lesions from many different tumor types found significantly reduced odds ratios for fracture (0.65, 95%CI 0.55–0.78); need for RT (0.67, 95%CI 0.57–0.79); and hypercalcemia (0.54, 95%CI 0.36–0.71) [98]. Other benefits include improvement in quality of life and delay in second and subsequent complications [99–101]. The role of bisphosphonates in combination with EBRT has also been investigated.

The first report to explore differences in clinical and radiologic responses to concurrent RT and ibandronate by different types of metastases (lytic, sclerotic, and mixed) has been published [102]. Patients received 30–40 Gy concurrent with the first dose of intravenous ibandronate, which was repeated monthly to a maximum of ten injections. Fifty two out of 70 patients enrolled were evaluable at 3 months, of which 22 patients had bone lesions classified as lytic, 16 mixed and 14 sclerotic. All groups experienced significant reduction in pain and opioid requirements, and significant improvement in performance status and quality of life at each follow-up visit (3, 6 and 10 months) compared to baseline. At 3 months, pain responses were: 41% complete response and 59% partial response (lytic), 75% complete and 25% partial (mixed), and 79% complete and 21% partial (sclerotic metastases group). Bone density was significantly increased in all groups at all time points compared to baseline, except for the sclerotic group at 3 months [102]. This approach clearly shows promise, but further studies are needed in this area to define the optimal duration of use.

XII. PERSPECTIVES AND CONCLUSIONS

With an increasing number of treatment modalities effective for relief of pain secondary to bone metastases, the multidisciplinary approach to patient assessment has never been more important to derive a management plan best suited for the individual. Clinical experience and published literature support the continuing role of external beam radiation as a well-tolerated modality able to relieve pain and treat complications of BM. Wide-field RT, HBI and radionuclides all have benefits for diffuse disease beyond that of localized RT, but have greater potential morbidity. There is an urgent need for large, well-designed prospective clinical trials in many areas of palliative radiation, such as complicated BM settings of impending pathologic fracture and re-irradiation. Additional study of radiopharmaceuticals as adjuvants to RT would also serve to further elucidate the optimal treatment for these patients. From a common sense perspective, the shortest possible palliative radiotherapy treatment schedule which maximizes functional outcome is preferable.

References

1. D. Hoegler, Radiotherapy for palliation of symptoms in incurable cancer, Curr Prob Cancer 21 (1997) 129–183.
2. W.D. Hage, Incidence, location, and diagnostic evaluation of metastatic bone disease, Orthop Clin N Am 31 (2000) 515–528.
3. BASO: British Association of Surgical Oncology, The management of metastatic bone disease in the United Kingdom, Eur J Surg Onc 25 (1999) 3–23.
4. P. Kirkbride & R. Barton, Palliative radiation therapy, J Pall Med 2 (1999) 87–97.
5. R. Samant & A.C. Gooi, Radiotherapy basics for family physicians, Can Fam Physician 51 (2005) 1496–1501.
6. E.H. Rutten, B.J. Crul & P.P. van der Toorn, et al., Pain characteristics help to predict the analgesic efficacy of radiotherapy for the treatment of cancer pain, Pain 69 (1997) 131–135.
7. K.M. Foley, Supportive care and quality of life, in: V.T. DeVita, S. Hellman & S.A. Rosenberg (Eds.) Cancer: Principles and Practice of Oncology, 6th Edn., Philadelphia, PA, Lippincott Williams & Wilkins, 1993, pp. 2977–3011.
8. K. Harris, K. Li & C. Flynn, et al., Worst, average or current pain in the Brief Pain Inventory: which should be used to calculate the response to palliative radiotherapy in patients with bone metastases? Clin Oncol 19 (2007) 523–527.
9. C.S. Cleeland & K.M. Ryan, Pain assessment: global use of the Brief Pain Inventory, Ann Acad Med Singapore 23 (1994) 129–138.
10. R.L. Daut, C.S. Cleeland & R.C. Flanery, Development of the Wisconsin Brief Pain Questionnaire to assess pain in cancer and other diseases, Pain 17 (1983) 197–210.
11. L.P. Ger, S.T. Ho & W.Z. Sun, et al., Validation of the Brief Pain Inventory in a Taiwanese population, J Pain Symp Manage 18 (1999) 316–322.
12. K. Li, K. Fung & E. Sinclair, et al., Correlation of pain score with functional interference in the Brief Pain Inventory, Curr Oncol 12 (2005) 37–43.
13. S.C. McMillan, M. Tittle & S. Hagan, et al., Management of pain and pain-related symptoms in hospitalized veterans with cancer, Cancer Nurs 23 (2000) 327–336.
14. R.C. Serlin, T.R. Mendoza & Y. Nakamura, et al., When is cancer pain mild, moderate, or severe? Grading pain severity by its interference with function, Pain 61 (1995) 277–284.
15. E. Chow, J. Wu & P. Hoskin, et al., International consensus on palliative radiotherapy endpoints for future clinical trials in bone metastases, Radiother Oncol 64 (2002) 275–280.
16. E. Chow, K. Harris & G. Fan, et al., Palliative radiotherapy trials for bone metastases: a systematic review, J Clin Oncol 25 (2007) 1423–1436.
17. D. Tong, L. Gillick & F. Hendrickson, The palliation of symptomatic osseous metastases: final results of the Study by the Radiation Therapy Oncology Group, Cancer 50 (1982) 893–899.
18. P. Blitzer, Reanalysis of the RTOG study of the palliation of symptomatic osseous metastasis, Cancer 55 (1985) 1468–1472.
19. E. Steenland, J.W. Leer & H. van Houwelingen, et al., The effect of a single fraction compared to multiple fractions on painful bone metastases: a global analysis of the Dutch Bone Metastasis Study, Radiother Oncol 52 (1999) 101–109.
20. Bone Pain Trial Working Party, 8 Gy single fraction radiotherapy for the treatment of metastatic skeletal pain: randomised comparison with a multifraction schedule over 12 months of patient follow-up, Radiother Oncol 52 (1999) 111–121.
21. W.M. Sze, M.D. Shelley & I. Held, et al., Palliation of metastatic bone pain: single fraction versus multifraction radiotherapy—a systematic review of randomised trials, Clin Oncol 15 (2003) 345–352.
22. J.S. Wu, R. Wong & M. Johnston, et al., Cancer Care Ontario Practice Guidelines Initiative Supportive Care Group. Meta-analysis of dose-fractionation radiotherapy trials for the palliation of painful bone metastases, Int J Radiat Oncol Biol Phys 55 (2003) 594–605.

23. W.F. Hartsell, C.B. Scott & D.W. Bruner, et al., Randomized trial of short- versus long-course radiotherapy for palliation of painful bone metastases, J Natl Cancer Inst 97 (2005) 798–804.
24. S. Kaasa, E. Brenne & J.A. Lund, et al., Prospective randomised multicenter trial on single fraction radiotherapy (8 Gy × 1) versus multiple fractions (3 Gy × 10) in the treatment of painful bone metastases, Radiother Oncol 79 (2006) 278–284.
25. M.B. Barton, R. Dawson & S. Jacob, et al., Palliative radiotherapy of bone metastases: an evaluation of outcome measures, J Eval Clin Pract 7 (2001) 47–64.
26. T.P. Shakespeare, J.J. Lu & M.F. Back, et al., Patient preference for radiotherapy fractionation schedule in the palliation of painful bone metastases, J Clin Oncol 21 (2003) 2156–2162.
27. E. Szumacher, H. Llewellyn-Thomas & E. Franssen, et al., Treatment of bone metastases with palliative radiotherapy: patients' treatment preferences, Int J Radiat Oncol Biol Phys 61 (2005) 1473–1481.
28. N.M. Bradley, J. Husted & M.S. Sey, et al., Review of patterns of practice and patients' preferences in the treatment of bone metastases with palliative radiotherapy, Support Care Cancer 15 (2007) 373–385.
29. M.V. Williams, N.D. James & E.T. Summers, et al., National survey of radiotherapy fractionation practice in 2003, Clin Onc 18 (2006) 3–14.
30. T.R. Moller, B. Brorsson & J. Ceberg, et al., A prospective survey of radiotherapy practice 2001 in Sweden, Acta Oncol 42 (2003) 387–410.
31. Y. Van der Linden & J. Leer, Impact of randomized trial-outcome in the treatment of painful bone metastases; patterns of practice among radiation oncologists. A matter of believers vs. non-believers?, Radiother Oncol 56 (2000) 279–281.
32. O.M. Salazar, T. Sandhu & N.W. da Motta, et al., Fractionated half-body irradiation (HBI) for the rapid palliation of widespread, symptomatic, metastatic bone disease: a randomized Phase III trial of the International Atomic Energy Agency (IAEA), Int J Radiat Oncol Biol Phys 50 (2001) 765–775.
33. P.F. Fitzpatrick & WD. Rider, Half-body radiotherapy of advanced cancer, Int J J Can Assoc Radiol 27 (1976) 75–79.
34. P.J. Hoskin, H.T. Ford & C.L. Harmer, Hemibody irradiation (HBI) for metastatic bone pain in two histologically distinct groups of patients, Clin Onc 1 (1989) 67–69.
35. D.A. Kuban, T. Delbridge & A.M. el-Mahdi, et al., Half-body irradiation for treatment of widely metastatic adenocarcinoma of the prostate, J Urol 141 (1989) 572–574.
36. O.M. Salazar, P. Rubin & F.R. Hendrickson, et al., Single-dose half-body irradiation for palliation of multiple bone metastases from solid tumors. Final Radiation Therapy Oncology Group report, Cancer 58 (1986) 29–36.
37. D.P. Dearnaley, R.J. Bayly & R.P. A'Hern, et al., Palliation of bone metastases in prostate cancer. Hemibody irradiation or strontium-89? Clin Onc 4 (1992) 101–107.
38. M.J. Zelefsky, H.I. Scher & J.D. Forman, et al., Palliative hemiskeletal irradiation for widespread metastatic prostate cancer: a comparison of single dose and fractionated regimens, Int J Radiat Oncol Biol Phys 17 (1989) 1281–1285.
39. O.M. Salazar & C.W. Scarantino, Theoretical and practical uses of elective systemic (half-body) irradiation after 20 years of experimental designs, Int J Radiat Oncol Biol Phys 39 (1997) 907–913.
40. C.A. Poulter, D. Cosmatos & P. Rubin, et al., A report of RTOG 8206: a phase III study of whether the addition of single dose hemibody irradiation to standard fractionated local field irradiation is more effective than local field irradiation alone in the treatment of symptomatic osseous metastases, Int J Radiat Oncol Biol Phys 23 (1992) 207–214.
41. J.P. Agarawal, T. Swangsilpa & Y. van der Linden, et al., The role of external beam radiotherapy in the management of bone metastases, Clin Onc 18 (2006) 747–760.
42. D.A. Frassica, General principles of external beam radiation therapy for skeletal metastases, Clin Orth Rel Res 415S (2003) S158–S164.
43. T.J. Priestman, J.T. Roberts & H. Lucraft, et al., Results of a randomized, double-blind comparative study of ondansetron and metoclopramide in the prevention of nausea and vomiting following high-dose upper abdominal irradiation, Clin Onc 2 (1990) 71–75.
44. P.M. Quilty, D. Kirk & J.J. Bolger, et al., A comparison of the palliative effects of strontium-89 and external beam radiotherapy in metastatic prostate cancer, Radiother Oncol 31 (1994) 33–40.
45. J. Van Dyk, T.J. Keane & S. Kan, et al., Radiation pneumonitis following large single dose irradiation: a re-evaluation based on absolute dose to lung, Int J Radiat Oncol Biol Phys 7 (1981) 461–467.
46. D.E. Roos, S.L. Turner & P.C. O'Brien, et al., Randomized trial of 8 Gy in 1 versus 20 Gy in 5 fractions of radiotherapy for neuropathic pain due to bone metastases (Trans-Tasman Radiation Oncology Group, TROG 96.05), Radiother Oncol 75 (2005) 54–63.
47. E. Chow, A. Loblaw & K. Harris, et al., Dexamethasone for the prophylaxis of radiation-induced pain flare after palliative radiotherapy for bone metastases: a pilot study, Support Care Cancer 15 (2007) 643–647.
48. P. Kirkbride & J. Aslanidis, Single fraction radiation therapy for bone metastases—a pilot study using a dose of 12 Gy, Clin Invest Med 19 (1996) S87 (Abstr 581).
49. P. Foro, M. Algara & A. Reig, Randomized prospective trial comparing three schedules of palliative radiotherapy [in Spanish], Preliminary results. Oncologia 21 (1998) 55–60.
50. D.A. Loblaw, J.S. Wu & P. Kirkbride, et al., Pain flare in patients with bone metastases after palliative radiotherapy—a nested randomized control trial, Support Care Cancer 15 (2007) 451–455.
51. N.L. Higinbotham & R.C. Marcove, The management of pathological fractures, J Trauma 5 (1965) 792–798.
52. R.E. Coleman, Clinical features of metastatic bone disease and risk of skeletal morbidity, Clin Cancer Res 12 (20 Suppl) (2006) 6243–6249.
53. J.H. Healey & H.K. Brown, Complications of bone metastases: surgical management, Cancer 88 (2000) 2940–2951.
54. Y.M. van der Linden, H.M. Kroon & S.P. Dijkstra, et al., Simple radiographic parameter predicts fracturing in metastatic femoral bone lesions: results from a randomised trial, Radiother Oncol 69 (2003) 21–31.

55. W.E. Snell & R.K. Beals, Femoral metastases and fractures from breast cancer, Surg Gynecol Obstet 119 (1964) 22–24.

56. F.F. Parrish & J.A. Murray, Surgical treatment for secondary neoplastic fractures. A retrospective study of ninety-six patients, J Bone Joint Surg Am 52 (1970) 665–686.

57. R.K. Beals, G.D. Lawton & W.H. Snell, Prophylactic internal fixation of the femur in metastatic breast cancer, Cancer 28 (1971) 1350–1354.

58. M. Fidler, Prophylactic internal fixation of secondary neoplastic deposits in long bones, Br Med J 1 (1973) 341–343.

59. R.E. Zickel & W.H. Mouradian, Intramedullary fixation of pathological fractures and lesions of the subtrochanteric region of the femur, J Bone Joint Surg Am 58 (1976) 1061–1066.

60. D.S. Cheng, C.B. Seitz & H.J. Eyre, Nonoperative management of femoral, humeral, and acetabular metastases in patients with breast carcinoma, Cancer 45 (1980) 1533–1537.

61. M. Fidler, Incidence of fracture through metastases in long bones, Acta Orthop Scand 52 (1981) 623–627.

62. F. Miller & R. Whitehill, Carcinoma of the breast metastatic to the skeleton, Clin Orthop 184 (1984) 121–127.

63. J.S. Keene, D.S. Sellinger & A.A. McBeath, et al., Metastatic breast cancer in the femur. A search for the lesion at risk of fracture, Clin Orthop Relat Res 203 (1986) 282–288.

64. H. Mencke, S. Schulze & E. Larsen, Metastasis size in pathologic femoral fractures, Acta Orthop Scand 59 (1988) 151–154.

65. H. Mirels, Metastatic disease in long bones, a proposed scoring system for diagnosing impending pathologic fractures. Clin Orthop Relat Res 249 (1989) 256–264.

66. Y. Yazawa, F.J. Frassica & E.Y. Chao, et al., Metastatic bone disease. A study of the surgical treatment of 166 pathologic humeral and femoral fractures, Clin Orthop Relat Res 251 (1990) 213–219.

67. R.W. Bunting, M. Boublik & F.T. Blevins, et al., Functional outcome of pathologic fracture secondary to malignant disease in a rehabilitation hospital, Cancer 69 (1992) 98–102.

68. P. Dijkstra, M. Oudkerk & T. Wiggers, Prediction of pathological subtrochanteric fractures due to metastatic lesions, Arch Orthop Trauma Surg 116 (1997) 221–224.

69. KD. Harrington, Orthopedic surgical management of skeletal complications of malignancy, Cancer 80 (8 Suppl) (1997) 1614–1627.

70. T.A. Damron, H. Morgan & D. Prakash, et al., Critical evaluation of Mirels' rating system for impending pathologic fractures, Clin Orthop Relat Res 415 (Suppl) (2003) S201–S207.

71 K. Rieden, B. Kober & U. Mende, Radiotherapy of pathological fractures and skeletal lesions in danger of fractures, Strahlenther Onkol 162 (1986) 742–749.

72. P.J. Hoskin, Radiotherapy in the management of bone pain, Clin Orth Rel Res 312 (1995) 105–119.

73. P.W. Townsend, H.G. Rosenthal & S.R. Smalley, et al., Impact of postoperative radiation therapy and other perioperative factors on outcome after orthopedic stabilization of impending or pathologic fractures due to metastatic disease, J Clin Oncol 12 (1994) 2345–2350.

74. H. Merskey & N. Bogduk, Classification of Chronic Pain, IASP Press, Seattle, 1994.

75. S. Grond, L. Radbruch & T. Meuser, et al., Assessment and treatment of neuropathic cancer pain following WHO guidelines, Pain 79 (1999) 15–20.

76. R. Kanner, Diagnosis and management of neuropathic pain in patients with cancer, Cancer Invest 19 (2001) 324–333.

77. D.R. Fourney, D.F. Schomer & R. Nader, et al., Percutaneous vertebroplasty and kyphoplasty for painful vertebral body fractures in cancer patients, J Neurosurg 98 (1 Suppl) (2003) 21–30.

78. A.M. Crellin, A. Marks & E.J. Maher, Why don't British radiotherapists give single fractions of radiotherapy for bone metastases?, Clin Onc 1 (1989) 63–66.

79. C.A. Pollicino, S.L. Turner & D.E. Roos, et al., Costing the components of pain management: analysis of Trans-Tasman Radiation Oncology Group trial (TROG 96.05): one versus five fractions for neuropathic bone pain, Radiother Oncol 76 (2005) 264–269.

80. D.E Morris, Clinical experience with retreatment for palliation, Sem Rad Onc 10 (2000) 210–221.

81. S.T. Lutz, E.L. Chow & W.F. Hartsell, et al., A review of hypofractionated palliative radiotherapy, Cancer 109 (2007) 1462–1470.

82. B. Jones & P.R. Blake, Retreatment of cancer after radical radiotherapy, Br J Rad 72 (1999) 1037–1039.

83. C. Nieder, L. Milas & K.K. Ang, Tissue tolerance to reirradiation, Sem Rad Onc 10 (2000) 200–209.

84. E. Chow, P.J. Hoskin & J. Wu, et al., A phase III international randomised trial comparing single with multiple fractions for re-irradiation of painful bone metastases: National Cancer Institute of Canada Clinical Trials Group (NCIC CTG) SC 20, Clin Onc 18 (2006) 125–128.

85. W.B. van den Hout, Y.M. van der Linden & E. Steenland, et al., Single- versus multiple-fraction radiotherapy in patients with painful bone metastases: cost-utility analysis based on a randomized trial, J Natl Cancer Inst 95 (2003) 222–229.

86. A. Konski, Radiotherapy is a cost-effective palliative treatment for patients with bone metastasis from prostate cancer, Int J Radiat Oncol Biol Phys 60 (2004) 1373–1378.

87. L. Alvarez, A. Perez-Higueras & D. Quinones, et al., Vertebroplasty in the treatment of vertebral tumors: postprocedural outcome and quality of life, Eur Spine J 12 (2003) 356–360.

88. A. Weill, J. Chiras & J.M. Simon, et al., Spinal metastases: indications for and results of percutaneous injection of acrylic surgical cement, Radiology 199 (1996) 241–247.

89. J. Chiras, C. Depriester & A. Weill, et al., Percutaneous vertebral surgery. Techniques and indications, J Neuroradiol 24 (1997) 45–59.

90. E. Chow, L. Holden & C. Danjoux, et al., Successful salvage using percutaneous vertebroplasty in cancer patients with painful spinal metastases or osteoporotic compression fractures, Radiother Onc 70 (2004) 265–267.

91. E.B. Silberstein, Teletherapy and radiopharmaceutical therapy of painful bone metastases, Sem Nucl Med 35 (2005) 152–158.

92. G. Bauman, M. Charette & R. Reid, et al., Radiopharmaceuticals for the palliation of painful bone metastasis-a systemic review, Radiother Oncol 75 (2005) 258–270.

93. N.A. Iscoe, E. Bruera & R.C. Choo, Prostate cancer: 10. Palliative care, CMAJ 160 (1999) 365–371.

94. A. Porter, A. McEwan & J. Powe, Results of a randomized phase-III trial to evaluate the efficacy of strontium-89 adjuvant to local field external beam irradiation in the management of endocrine resistant metastatic prostate cancer, Int J Radiat Oncol Biol Phys 25 (1993) 805–813.

95. S. Smeland, B. Erikstein & M. Aas, et al., Role of strontium-89 as adjuvant to palliative external beam radiotherapy is questionable: results of a double-blind randomized study, Int J Radiat Oncol Biol Phys 56 (2003) 1397–1404.

96. I.F. Tannock, R. de Wit & W.R. Berry, et al., Docetaxel plus prednisone or mitoxantrone plus prednisone for advanced prostate cancer, New Engl J Med 351 (2004) 1502–1512.

97. R.E. Coleman, Bisphosphonates: clinical experience, Oncologist 7 (Suppl 4) (2004) 14–27.

98. J.F. Ross, Y. Saunders & P.M. Edmonds, Systematic review of role of bisphosphonates on skeletal morbidity in metastatic cancer, British Med J 327 (2003) 469.

99. J.J. Body, I.J. Diel & M.R. Lichinitser, et al., Intravenous ibandronate reduces the incidence of skeletal complications in patients with breast cancer and bone metastases, Ann Oncol 14 (2003) 1399–1405.

100. F. Saad, D.M. Gleason & R. Murray, et al., Long-term efficacy of zoledronic acid for the prevention of skeletal complications in patients with metastatic hormone-refractory prostate cancer, J Natl Cancer Inst 96 (2004) 879–882.

101. L.S. Rosen, D. Gordon & N.S. Tchekmedyian, et al., Long-term efficacy and safety of zoledronic acid in the treatment of skeletal metastases in patients with nonsmall cell lung carcinoma and other solid tumors: a randomized, Phase III, double-blind, placebo-controlled trial, Cancer 100 (2004) 2613–2621.

102. V. Vassiliou, C. Kalogeropoulou & E. Giannopoulou, et al., A novel study investigating the therapeutic outcome of patients with lytic, mixed and sclerotic bone metastases treated with combined radiotherapy and ibandronate, Clin Exp Metastasis 24 (2007) 169–178.

CHAPTER **26**

Mechanisms and Management of Bone Cancer Pain

MA'ANN C. SABINO[1] AND DENIS R. CLOHISY[2]

[1] Division of Oral and Maxillofacial Surgery, School of Dentistry, University of Minnesota, Minneapolis, MN.
[2] Department of Orthopedic Surgery and Cancer Center, School of Medicine, University of Minnesota, Minneapolis, MN, USA.

Contents

I. INTRODUCTION

A. Epidemiology of Bone Cancer Pain

Pain is the most common presenting symptom in patients with skeletal metastases and is directly proportional to its impact on the cancer patient's quality of life [1,2]. Two main types of cancer pain exist: ongoing pain and incident or breakthrough pain. Ongoing pain is typically described as a dull and aching pain that is constant in nature and progresses in accordance with the disease process. Incident or breakthrough pain is most commonly associated with bone metastases and is characterized by sharp pains that are intermittent in nature and exacerbated by both volitional and non-volitional movements. The latter type of pain is difficult to treat due to its intermittence and intensity [3,4] and can be found in as high as 80% of patients with advanced disease [5].

B. Mechanisms of Bone Cancer Pain

1. ANIMAL MODELS OF CANCER PAIN

Rodent and canine models of osteolytic and osteoblastic bone cancer pain have been described in the literature in the past decade. Each model differs in the route of inoculation of tumor cells [6–8], type of tumor cells [9,10], immuno-competency of the host [10], and species of host [11,12]. Despite these differences, a wealth of information has been gleaned on the pathophysiologic mechanisms which drive bone cancer pain. Bone cancer pain is a multi-factorial process which arises from different cells within the cancerous bone and whose signals extend towards the central nervous system for sensory processing.

2. PERIPHERAL MECHANISMS OF CANCER PAIN

Pain generally occurs during tissue ischemia and/or damage and is a result of release of neurotransmitters, cytokines and factors from damaged cells, adjacent blood vessels and nerve terminals. Pain is transduced at the level of the primary afferent nerve fiber which innervates peripheral tissues including bone. Recently, we have shown that bone is densely innervated by both sensory and sympathetic nerve fibers within bone marrow, mineralized bone and periosteum (Figure 26.1; see Plate 12) [13]. Sensory and sympathetic neurons are present within all three anatomic locations and are influenced by fractures, ischemia or the presence of tumor cells and may play a unique but coordinated role in the generation of bone cancer pain.

The majority of metastatic skeletal malignancies are destructive in nature and produce regions of osteolysis (bone destruction). This primarily occurs via activation, recruitment and proliferation of osteoclasts and is characterized by an increased number and size of osteoclasts found in tumor-bearing sites [14–18]. The activation and proliferation of osteoclasts is mediated by the interaction between receptor activator for nuclear factor κB (RANK) expressed on osteoclasts and precursors with RANK ligand (RANKL) expressed on osteoblasts and stromal cells. An increased expression of both RANK and RANKL has been found in tumor-bearing sites [19,20]. Selective destruction of osteoclasts utilizing the soluble decoy receptor for RANKL, osteoprotegerin (OPG) results in inhibition of cancer-induced osteolysis, cancer pain behaviors and neurochemical markers of peripheral and central sensitization [19–23]. Osteoclasts have now been shown to play a pivotal role in the development and progression of bone cancer pain.

Tumor-derived cytokines, growth factors and peptides have been shown to activate primary afferent nerve fibers that innervate bone. Prostaglandins, interleukins, protons, bradykinin, chemokines, tumor-necrosis alpha and endothelins are all examples of chemical mediators released from

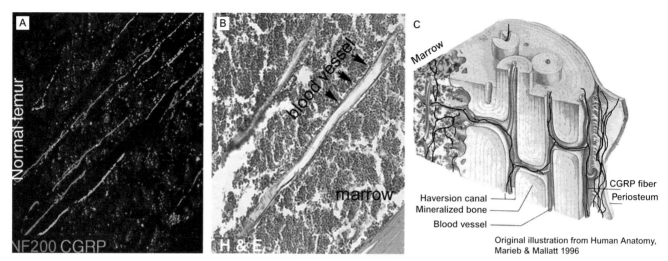

FIGURE 26.1   Innervation of bone. Histophotomicrographs of (A) confocal and (B) histologic serial images of normal bone. Note the extensive myelinated (red, NF200) and unmyelinated (green, CGRP) nerve fibers within bone marrow which appear to course along blood vessels (arrowheads, B). (C) Schematic diagram demonstrating the innervation within periosteum, mineralized bone and bone marrow. All three tissues may be sensitized during the various stages of bone cancer pain.

tumor cells and have been shown to sensitize nerve terminals [24–29] resulting in cancer pain. Each mediator has a specialized cognate channel or receptor to which it binds resulting in conversion from a chemical to electrical signal (Figure 26.2). In the bone cancer pain state, chemical mediators are released then bind to their respective receptor or channel, and pain transduction occurs and resolves over time. *Peripheral sensitization* occurs where the peripheral nerve becomes sensitized due to constant stimulation and activation. This may be in the form of decreased excitation thresholds, upregulation of receptors and/or channels in both nerve terminals and sensory neurons, or recruitment of previously silent pain receptors or nociceptors and have been shown to occur in bone cancer pain models [8,30–33].

Destruction or direct damage to peripheral nerves innervating bone has been postulated as another mechanism by which bone cancer exists. This neuropathic pain condition is supported by clinical findings of resistance to traditional opioid therapy known to be ineffective in managing neuropathic pain. Animal models of bone cancer pain have also shown damaged peripheral nerve terminals within cancerous bone and increased expression of neurochemical markers of injury in sensory neurons that innervate bone. Gabapentin (Neurontin®), a common drug used to manage neuropathic pain, was efficacious in reducing neuropathic pain behaviors but did not affect tumor-induced bone destruction or tumor proliferation [34].

3. CENTRAL SENSITIZATION

Central sensitization refers to the heightened reactivity of central nervous system neurons in the face of sustained peripheral neural input. While this may occur within the thalamus and cortex, research has been primarily focused on the dorsal horn of the spinal cord. Electrophysiologic and anatomic studies have demonstrated a change in the activity and responsiveness of dorsal horn neurons in response to persistent painful stimulation.

Persistent stimulation of unmyelinated C fibers results in the increased activity and responsiveness of spinal neurons which receive input from the stimulated unmyelinated C fiber. This increased responsiveness is of short (10 sec) duration and is known as *wind-up*. Sensitization can also occur when persistent stimulation results in phenotypic changes in neurons that do not receive, but are adjacent to, neurons that receive the persistent painful stimulation. Typically these neurons receive input from A-beta fibers that normally do not transmit painful stimuli. However, once sensitized, these neurons are capable of transmitting both non-painful and painful information. Central sensitization is mediated in part by glutamate, substance P, prostaglandins and growth factors. These receptors/ion channels are known as N-methyl-D-aspartate (NMDA), neurokinin-1 (NK-1), EP and tyrosine kinase B (trkB), respectively. Upregulation of transient receptor potential (TRPV1) and sodium channels have also been reported in central sensitization. Allodynia is a condition where normally non-noxious stimulation is painful and a condition which can result from central sensitization [6,15].

4. REORGANIZATION OF PERIPHERAL AND CENTRAL NERVOUS SYSTEM IN RESPONSE TO CANCER PAIN

There are several examples of nociceptor peripheral sensitization in experimental cancer models [6,11,21,24,29,33]. In normal mice, the neurotransmitter substance P is synthesized by nociceptors and released in the spinal cord when noxious—but not non-noxious—mechanical stress is

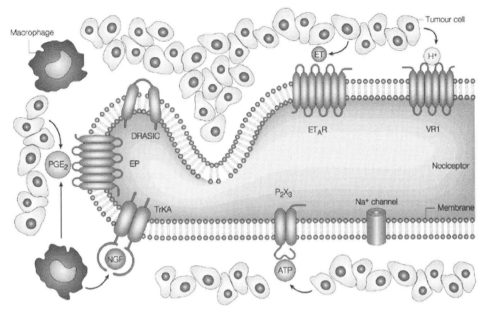

Nature Reviews | Cancer

FIGURE 26.2 Interaction between chemical mediators and receptors. Schematic diagram of a peripheral pain fiber expressing receptors and ion channels. Interaction between neurotransmitters and chemical mediators and their cognate receptor results in pain transduction and signaling (Reprinted with permission, Mantyh, P.W. *et al., Nature Cancer Rev,* 2002). (H+-protons; ET-endothelin; VR1-vanilloid receptor-1; ETAR-endothelin A receptor; DRASIC-dorsal root acid sensing ion channel; EP-prostaglandin E receptor; PGE2-prostaglandin E2; TrkA-high affinity nerve growth factor tyrosine kinase receptor A; NGF-nerve growth factor; ATP-adenosine triphosphate; P2×3-purinergic ion-gated receptor; Na+-sodium).

applied to the femur. In mice with bone cancer, what would normally be a non-painful level of mechanical stress can induce the release of substance P from primary afferent fibers that terminate in the spinal cord. Substance P, in turn, binds to and activates the neurokinin-1 receptor that is expressed by a subset of spinal cord neurons [6].

Similar to phenotypic alterations and sensitization of peripheral nerves, studies involving a murine model of bone cancer pain also showed extensive neurochemical reorganization in the spinal cord segments that receive input from primary afferent neurons that innervate the tumor-bearing bone [6]. This includes an astrocyte hypertrophy, which may be

accompanied by a decreased expression of glutamate reuptake transporters resulting in increased extracellular levels of the excitatory neurotransmitter glutamate leading to excitotoxicity within the central nervous system. This and other spinal cord changes could be attenuated by blocking the tumor-induced tissue destruction and pain [21,22,29,32,35]. These findings indicate that cancer pain induces, and is at least partially maintained by, a state of central sensitization, in which neurochemical changes in the spinal cord and forebrain promote an increased transmission of nociceptive information, so that normally non-noxious input is amplified and perceived as a noxious stimulus (Figure 26.3; see Plate 13).

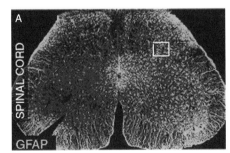
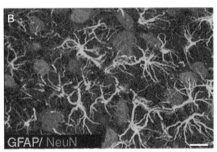

FIGURE 26.3 Neurochemical changes in the spinal cord and dorsal root ganglia (DRG) in bone cancer pain. (A) Confocal imaging of glial fibrillary acidic protein (GFAP) expressed by astrocytes in a spinal cord of a tumor-bearing mouse. Note increased expression only on side ipsilateral to tumorous limb. (B) High power magnification of spinal cord showing hypertrophy of astrocytes (green) without changes in neuronal numbers (red, stained with neuronal marker, NeuN).

The constant barrage of neurochemicals that are implicated in pain transmission results in changes in the activity and phenotype of nerve fibers and neurons within the peripheral and central nervous system. These changes result in a chronic and debilitating condition that is recalcitrant to many conventional modes of acute pain therapy. The chronic bone cancer pain patient has a 'pain portrait' that is distinct from the acute pain patient and its management reflects this difference.

C. Therapeutic Strategies: Past, Present and Future

Pain research has significantly improved our understanding of acute and chronic pain mechanisms. By highlighting key molecular mechanisms involved in pain transmission, new drugs are currently being investigated as potential novel and selective therapies. Currently available medications such as the opioids are certainly fraught with side effect profiles that may limit their clinical efficacy and patient quality of life. Research is now focused on specific receptor or channel targets within the nervous system that limits systemic complications.

1. Therapeutic Targets: Ion Channels
The transient receptor potential (TRPV1) family of channels is located on unmyelinated C fibers and spinal nociceptive neurons that mediate pain transmission. TRPV1 channels can be activated by noxious heat, capsaicin and acid. Mice that lack the channel are unable to develop chronic pain states and when antagonists to TRPV1 are administered orally or into the intrathecal space, chronic pain is markedly reduced [27,36]. Interestingly, intrathecal admistration of resiniferatoxin, a potent capsaicin analog, in a canine bone cancer model resulted in reductions in pain behaviors and selective destruction of small, but not medium or large-diameter sensory neurons [12]. Long-term efficacy or safety has not been established in animal models but TRPV1 is only expressed on nociceptive peripheral terminals and spinal neurons therefore its selective blockade may limit its side effect profile.

2. Therapeutic Targets: Growth Factors
Growth factors are important in the differentiation, maturation and plasticity of cells within the nervous system. Key growth factors that have been implicated in pain include nerve growth factor (NGF), glial-derived growth factor (GDNF), and brain-derived growth factor (BDNF) (for review, see [37]). Receptors for such growth factors are expressed on C fibers and Aδ fibers which terminate within the spinal cord. In animal models of chronic pain, NGF levels are elevated in damaged peripheral tissues. Neutralizing antibodies against NGF are effective, at least in animal models, in reducing and in some cases preventing chronic pain. Interestingly, administration of NGF has also been

shown to reduce neuropathic pain. Phase III clinical trials are currently under way assessing the efficacy of recombinant NGF to treat diabetic neuropathy. BDNF has been implicated in the modulation of central sensitization as its expression is increased in nociceptive neurons in models of peripheral neuropathy. BNDF sensitizes C fiber activity resulting in hyperalgesia and allodynia. Inhibition of BNDF and its cognate receptor, trkB results in decreased C fiber firing and a reduction in pain behaviors. Finally, GDNF is important in the survival of sensory neurons and supporting cells. Neuropathic pain behaviors commonly observed in animal models of chronic pain are prevented or reversed following GDNF administration. The timing of administration determined whether treatment was protective or therapeutic in nature.

3. Therapeutic Targets: Cytokines
Endothelin antagonists are another type of pharmacological agent that may show significant promise in the management of cancer pain [28,38,39]. Endothelins are a family of vasoactive peptides that are expressed by several tumors, especially prostate cancer, with levels that appear to correlate with pain severity [40]. Endothelins could contribute to cancer pain by directly sensitizing or exciting nociceptors, as a subset of small unmyelinated primary afferent neurons express endothelin A receptors [41]. Direct application of endothelin to peripheral nerves induces activation of primary afferent fibers and an induction of pain behaviors [42] while selective blockade of endothelin A receptors blocked bone cancer pain-related behaviors and spinal changes indicative of peripheral and central sensitization [28]. Like prostaglandins, endothelins that are produced by cancer cells are also thought be involved in regulating angiogenesis [43] and tumor growth [44]. These findings indicate that endothelin antagonists may be useful not only in inhibiting cancer pain but in reducing tumor growth and metastasis.

4. Therapeutic Targets: Osteoclast
Experiments in a murine model of bone cancer pain reported that osteoclasts play an essential role in cancer-induced bone loss and that osteoclasts contribute to the etiology of bone cancer pain [21,22,29,45]. Osteoprotegerin (OPG) is a soluble target that holds significant promise for alleviating bone cancer pain [20,46]. OPG is a secreted soluble receptor that is a member of the tumor necrosis factor receptor (TNFR) family [47]. This decoy receptor prevents the activation and proliferation of osteoclasts by binding to and sequestering osteoprotegerin ligand (OPGL; also known as receptor for activator of NFκB ligand, RANKL) [47]. While OPG has been shown to decrease pain behaviors in an animal model of bone cancer [21,22], it is still being developed for use in cancer patients. OPG has been shown to increase bone mineral density and bone volume and inhibit bone resorption in women with osteoporosis [48]

BOX 26.1

Pain definitions, *Classification of Chronic Pain,* 2nd Edn, IASP Task Force on Taxonomy (Merskey, H. and Bogduk, N. eds), Seattle: IASP Press, © 1994, pp. 209–214.

Allodynia	Pain evoked with stimulus that normally does not provoke pain
Analgesia	Absence of pain in response to stimulation that would normally be painful
Arthralgia	Pain within a joint
Causalgia	A syndrome of sustained burning pain, allodynia, and hyperpathia after a traumatic nerve lesion, often combined with vasomotor and sudomotor dysfunction and later trophic changes
Central Pain	Pain initiated or caused by a primary lesion or dysfunction in the central nervous system
Dysesthesia	An unpleasant abnormal sensation, whether spontaneous or evoked
Hyperesthesia	Increased sensitivity to stimulation
Hypoesthesia	Diminished sensitivity to stimulation
Hyperalgesia	An increased response to a stimulus that is normally painful
Hypoalgesia	Diminished sensitivity to noxious stimulation
Hyperpathia	A painful syndrome, characterized by increased reaction to a stimulus, heightened with repetition. Hyperpathia may occur with hyperesthesia, hyperalgesia, or dysesthesia
Neuralgia	Pain in distribution of nerve or nerves
Neuropathic Pain	Pain initiated or caused by a primary lesion or dysfunction in the nervous system
Neuropathy	A disturbance of function or pathological change in a nerve: in one nerve, mononeuropathy; in several nerves, mononeuropathy multiplex; if diffuse and bilateral, polyneuropathy
Paresthesia	An abnormal sensation, whether spontaneous or evoked

and has anti-resorptive effects comparable to pamidronate when administered as a single dose to patients with bony malignancies [49]. Phase II clinical trials of Denusomab (AMG-162, Amgen), a human monoclonal antibody against RANKL in postmenopausal osteoporotic women, show significant promise although its analgesic efficacy for managing bone cancer pain remains unanswered [50].

Bisphosphonates are pyrophosphate analog that are commonly used to manage osteolytic and osteoblastic processes such as primary bone tumors (i.e., multiple myeloma), metastatic bone cancers, humoral hypercalcemia of malignancy, and moderate to severe osteoporosis and osteopenia. Nitrogen-containing bisphosphonates are available in both intravenous (zoledronic acid/Zometa®, Novartis Pharmaceuticals; pamidronate/Aredia®, Novartis Pharmaceuticals) and oral forms (alendronate/Fosamax®, Merck and Co.; ibandronate/ Boniva®, Roche Baboratories; risedronate/Actonel®, Procter and Gamble) with differing potencies. Bisphosphonates act by disrupting the activity of osteoclasts, one of the principle bone cells responsible for bone metabolism [51].

Administration of bisphosphonates have a clear and positive impact on skeletal health and quality of life in people who suffer from destructive bone diseases and have also been reported to reduce pain in patients with osteoclast-induced skeletal metastases [52,53]. The long-term beneficial effects of bisphosphonate treatment on reductions in bone pain and skeletal related events (e.g., spinal compression, fractures) and an improvement in overall quality of life are clearly obvious from clinical trials in multiple myeloma, breast cancer [54,55] and prostate cancer [56] patients. Because of the potentially beneficial and skeletal protective effects of bisphosphonates, recommendations may evolve to include prophylactic treatment of prostate cancer patients without evidence of skeletal metastases with bisphosphonates [56].

References

1. R.E. Coleman, Clinical features of metastatic bone disease and risk of skeletal morbidity, Clin Cancer Res 12 (20) (2006) 6243s–6249s.
2. N. Coyle, et al., Character of terminal illness in the advanced cancer patient: pain and other symptoms during the last four weeks of life, J Pain Symptom Manage 5 (2) (1990) 83–93.
3. S. Mercadante, Malignant bone pain: pathophysiology and treatment, Pain 69 (1–2) (1997) 1–18.
4. C. Ripamonti & F. Fulfaro, Malignant bone pain: pathophysiology and treatments, Current Review of Pain 4 (3) (2000) 187–196.
5. S. Mercadante, et al., Episodic (breakthrough) pain: consensus conference of an expert working group of the European Association for Palliative Care, Cancer 94 (3) (2002) 832–839.
6. M.J. Schwei, et al., Neurochemical and cellular reorganization of the spinal cord in a murine model of bone cancer pain, J Neurosci 19 (24) (1999) 10886–10897.
7. R.-X. Zhang, et al., Spinal glial activation in a new rat model of bone cancer pain produced by prostate cancer cell inoculation of the tibia, Pain 118 (1–2) (2005) 125–136.
8. D.M. Cain, et al., Functional interactions between tumor and peripheral nerve: changes in excitability and morphology of

primary afferent fibers in a murine model of cancer pain, J Neurosci 21 (23) (2001) 9367–9376.

9. K.G.B.A. Halvorson, et al., Similarities and differences in tumor growth, skeletal remodeling and pain in an osteolytic and osteoblastic model of bone cancer, Clin J Pain 22 (7) (2006) 587–600.

10. M.A. Sabino, et al., Different tumors in bone each give rise to a distinct pattern of skeletal destruction, bone cancer-related pain behaviors and neurochemical changes in the central nervous system, Int J Cancer 104 (5) (2003) 550–558.

11. K. Walker, et al., Disease modifying and anti-nociceptive effects of the bisphosphonate, zoledronic acid in a model of bone cancer pain, Pain 100 (3) (2002) 219–229.

12. D.C. Brown, et al., Physiologic and antinociceptive effects of intrathecal resiniferatoxin in a canine bone cancer model, Anesthesiology 103 (5) (2005) 1052–1059.

13. D.B. Mach, et al., Origins of skeletal pain: sensory and sympathetic innervation of the mouse femur, Neuroscience 113 (1) (2002) 155–166.

14. T. Taube, et al., Histomorphometric evidence for osteoclast-mediated bone resorption in metastatic breast cancer, Bone 15 (2) (1994) 161–166.

15. D.R. Clohisy, S.L. Perkins & M.L. Ramnaraine, Review of cellular mechanisms of tumor osteolysis, Clin Orthop Relat R (373) (2000) 104–114.

16. D.R. Clohisy & M.L. Ramnaraine, Osteoclasts are required for bone tumors to grow and destroy bone, J Orthopaed Res 16 (6) (1998) 660–666.

17. D.R. Clohisy, et al., Human breast cancer induces osteoclast activation and increases the number of osteoclasts at sites of tumor osteolysis, J Orthopaed Res 14 (3) (1996) 396–402.

18. D.R. Clohisy, et al., Localized, tumor-associated osteolysis involves the recruitment and activation of osteoclasts, J Orthopaed Res 14 (1) (1996) 2–6.

19. D.R. Clohisy, et al., Osteoprotegerin inhibits tumor-induced osteoclastogenesis and bone tumor growth in osteopetrotic mice, J Orthopaed Res 18 (6) (2000) 967–976.

20. D.R. Clohisy, et al., Bone cancer pain and the role of RANKL/OPG, J Musculoskelet Neuronal Interacts 4 (3) (2004) 293–300.

21. N.M. Luger, et al., Osteoprotegerin diminishes advanced bone cancer pain, Cancer Res 61 (10) (2001) 4038–4047.

22. P. Honore, et al., Osteoprotegerin blocks bone cancer-induced skeletal destruction, skeletal pain and pain-related neurochemical reorganization of the spinal cord. [See comment] [erratum appears in Nat Med 2000 Jul;6(7):838], Nat Med 6 (5) (2000) 521–528.

23. M. Roudier, S. Bain & W. Dougall, Effects of the RANKL inhibitor, osteoprotegerin, on the pain and histopathology of bone cancer in rats, Clin Exp Metastasis 23 (3) (2006) 167–175.

24. P.W. Wacnik, et al., Functional interactions between tumor and peripheral nerve: morphology, algogen identification, and behavioral characterization of a new murine model of cancer pain, J Neurosci 21 (23) (2001) 9355–9366.

25. P.W. Wacnik, et al., Nociceptive characteristics of tumor necrosis factor-[alpha] in naive and tumor-bearing mice, Neuroscience 132 (2) (2005) 479–491.

26. I.A. Khasabova, et al., Chemical interactions between fibrosarcoma cancer cells and sensory neurons contribute to cancer pain, J Neurosci 27 (38) (2007) 10289–10298.

27. J.R. Ghilardi, et al., Selective blockade of the capsaicin receptor TRPV1 attenuates bone cancer pain, J Neurosci 25 (12) (2005) 3126–3131.

28. C.M. Peters, et al., Endothelin and the tumorigenic component of bone cancer pain, Neuroscience 126 (4) (2004) 1043–1052.

29. M.A. Sabino, et al., Simultaneous reduction in cancer pain, bone destruction, and tumor growth by selective inhibition of cyclooxygenase-2, Cancer Res 62 (24) (2002) 7343–7349.

30. S.P. Hunt & P.W. Mantyh, The molecular dynamics of pain control, Nature Reviews Neuroscience 2 (2) (2001) 83–91.

31. L.S. Gilchrist, et al., Re-organization of P2 × 3 receptor localization on epidermal nerve fibers in a murine model of cancer pain, Brain Res 1044 (2) (2005) 197–205.

32. K.G. Halvorson, et al., A blocking antibody to nerve growth factor attenuates skeletal pain induced by prostate tumor cells growing in bone, Cancer Res 65 (20) (2005) 9426–9435.

33. P. Honore, et al., Cellular and neurochemical remodeling of the spinal cord in bone cancer pain, Prog Brain Res 129 (2000) 389–397.

34. C.M. Peters, et al., Tumor-induced injury of primary afferent sensory nerve fibers in bone cancer pain, Exp Neurol 193 (1) (2005) 85–100.

35. M.A. Sevcik, et al., Anti-NGF therapy profoundly reduces bone cancer pain and the accompanying increase in markers of peripheral and central sensitization, Pain 115 (1–2) (2005) 128–141.

36. M. Cui, et al., TRPV1 receptors in the CNS play a key role in broad-spectrum analgesia of TRPV1 antagonists, J Neurosci 26 (37) (2006) 9385–9393.

37. D.W. Sah, M.H. Ossipov & F. Porreca, Neurotrophic factors as novel therapeutics for neuropathic pain, Nat Rev Drug Discov 2 (6) (2003) 460–472.

38. M.A. Carducci, et al., Atrasentan, an endothelin-receptor antagonist for refractory adenocarcinomas: safety and pharmacokinetics, J Clin Oncol 20 (8) (2002) 2171–2180.

39. M.A. Carducci & A. Jimeno, Targeting bone metastasis in prostate cancer with endothelin receptor antagonists, Clin Cancer Res 12 (2006) 6296s–6300s.

40. J.B. Nelson, et al., Endothelin-1 production and decreased endothelin B receptor expression in advanced prostate cancer, Cancer Res 56 (4) (1996) 663–668.

41. J.D. Pomonis, et al., Expression and localization of endothelin receptors: implications for the involvement of peripheral glia in nociception, J Neurosci 21 (3) (2001) 999–1006.

42. G. Davar, Endothelin-1 and metastatic cancer pain, Pain Medicine 2 (1) (2001) 24–27.

43. K. Dawas, et al., Angiogenesis in cancer: the role of endothelin-1, Ann Roy Coll Surg 81 (5) (1999) 306–310.

44. E.H. Asham, M. Loizidou & I. Taylor, Endothelin-1 and tumour development, Eur J Surg Oncol 24 (1) (1998) 57–60.

45. M. Goblirsch, et al., Radiation treatment decreases bone cancer pain, osteolysis and tumor size, Radiat Res 161 (2) (2004) 228–234.

46. P.W. Mantyh, et al., Molecular mechanisms of cancer pain, Nat Rev Cancer 2 (3) (2002) 201–209.

47. W.S. Simonet, et al., Osteoprotegerin—a novel secreted protein involved in the regulation of bone density, Cell 89 (2) (1997) 309–319.

48. P.J. Bekker, et al., The effect of a single dose of osteoprotegerin in postmenopausal women, J Bone Miner Res 16 (2) (2001) 348–360.

49. J.J. Body, et al., A phase I study of AMGN-0007, a recombinant osteoprotegerin construct, in patients with multiple myeloma or breast carcinoma related bone metastases, Cancer 97 (3 Suppl) (2003) 887–892.

50. M.R. McClung, et al., Denosumab in postmenopausal women with low bone, Mineral Density (2006) 821–831.

51. J. Green, Bisphosphonates: preclinical review, Oncologist 9 (Suppl 4) (2004) 3–13.

52. A. Lipton, E. Small, F. Saad & D. Gleason, et al., The new bisphosphonate, Zometa (zoledronic acid), decreases skeletal complications in both osteolytic and osteoblastic lesions: a comparison to pamidronate, Cancer Invest 20 (Suppl 2) (2002) 45–54.

53. J.R. Berenson, et al., Zoledronic acid reduces skeletal-related events in patients with osteolytic metastases, Cancer 91 (7) (2001) 1191–1200.

54. G. Carteni, et al., Efficacy and safety of zoledronic acid in patients with breast cancer metastatic to bone: a multicenter clinical trial, Oncologist 11 (7) (2006) 841–848.

55. A. Lipton, et al., The new bisphosphonate, Zometa (zoledronic acid), decreases skeletal complications in both osteolytic and osteoblastic lesions: a comparison to pamidronate, Cancer Invest 20 (Suppl 2) (2002) 45–54.

56. F. Saad, J. McKiernan & J. Eastham, Rationale for zoledronic acid therapy in men with hormone-sensitive prostate cancer with or without bone metastasis, Urol Oncol 24 (1) (2006) 4–12.

CHAPTER **27**

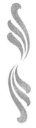

Malignant Skeletal Pain: Mechanisms and Potential Therapeutic Opportunities

MONICA HERRERA[1], JUAN MIGUEL JIMENEZ-ANDRADE[1], MARINA VARDANYAN[1]
AND PATRICK W. MANTYH[1]

[1]*Department of Pharmacology, University of Arizona, Tucson, AZ 85724, USA.*

Contents

I. INTRODUCTION

With more than 10 million people being diagnosed with cancer annually, by 2020 it is estimated that 20 million new cases will be diagnosed each year [1,2]. In 2005, cancer caused 7.6 million deaths worldwide [3]. In the United States, cancer is a major health problem, being the second leading cause of death. Currently, 25% of US deaths are cancer related [4].

Cancer-associated pain can be present at any time during the course of the disease, but the frequency and intensity of cancer pain tends to increase with advancing stages of cancer. In patients with advanced cancer, 62 to 86% experience significant pain that is described as 'moderate to severe' in approximately 40–50% and as 'very severe' in 25–30% [5]. Bone cancer pain is the most common pain in patients with advanced cancer as two thirds of patients with metastatic bone disease experience severe pain [6,7]. Most common tumors including breast, prostate, thyroid, kidney and lung have a remarkable affinity to metastasize to bone [7].

Currently, the factors that drive bone cancer pain are poorly understood; however, several recently introduced models of bone cancer pain are not only providing insight into the mechanisms that drive bone cancer pain but are guiding the development of novel mechanism-based therapies to treat the pain and skeletal remodeling that accompany metastatic bone cancer. As analgesics can also influence disease progression, findings from these studies may lead to therapies that have the potential to improve the quality of life and survival of patients with skeletal malignancies.

II. THE CHALLENGE OF BONE CANCER PAIN

Although bone is not a vital organ, most common tumors have a strong predilection for bone metastasis. Tumor metastases to the skeleton are major contributors to morbidity and mortality in metastatic cancer. Tumor growth in bone results in pain, hypercalcemia, anemia, increased susceptibility to infection, skeletal fractures, compression of the spinal cord, spinal instability and decreased mobility; all of which compromise the patient's survival and quality of life [7,8]. Once tumor cells have metastasized to the skeleton, tumor-induced bone pain is usually described as dull in character, constant in presentation, and gradually increasing in intensity with time [9]. As bone remodeling progresses, severe spontaneous pain frequently occurs [10] and given that the onset of this pain is both acute and unpredictable, this component of bone cancer pain can be particularly debilitating to the patient's functional status [10,11]. Breakthrough pain, which is an intermittent episode of extreme pain, can occur spontaneously or more commonly is induced by movement of, or weight bearing on, the tumor-bearing bone(s) [12].

Currently, the treatment of pain from bone metastases involves the use of multiple complementary approaches, including radiotherapy, surgery, chemotherapy, bisphosphonates, calcitonin, and analgesics [6,10]. However, bone cancer pain is one of the most difficult of all persistent pains to fully control [10], as the metastases are generally not limited to a single site and the analgesics most commonly used to treat bone cancer pain, NSAIDS [10] and opioids [10,13–15], are limited by significant adverse side effects [16,17].

The onset of clinically apparent bone metastases marks a crucial moment in the natural history of cancer, sharply decreasing expected survival (on average, 12 months for prostate cancer patients after the diagnosis of bone metastasis) [18]. However, the length of survival continues to increase for cancer patients [4], so to maintain the patient's quality of life and functional status, it is essential that new therapies be developed that can be administered over several years to control bone pain without the side effects commonly encountered with the currently available analgesics.

In the last decade, the first animal models of bone cancer pain were developed. These models, in terms of tumor growth, bone remodeling and bone pain, appear to mirror several aspects of human bone cancer pain [19–23]. Information engendered from these models has begun to provide insight into the mechanisms that generate and maintain bone cancer pain. Nevertheless, what remains still unclear is how the primarily osteolytic animal models (which are the models that have been the most utilized to date) compare with common osteoblastic tumors that avidly metastasize to bone in regards to bone remodeling and tumor-induced bone pain. In this chapter we examine the similarities and differences between a primarily osteolytic sarcoma tumor versus a primarily osteoblastic prostate tumor in terms of bone destruction, bone formation, tumor growth, macrophage infiltration, osteoclast and osteoblast number and type and severity of bone cancer-related pain. Additionally, we discuss the remodeling of the sensory innervation of bone in osteolytic and osteoblastic bone cancer models.

III. PAIN TRANSMISSION

Primary afferent sensory neurons are the gateway by which sensory information from peripheral tissues is transmitted to the spinal cord and brain. These sensory neurons innervate every organ of the body with exception of the brain. The cell bodies of sensory fibers that innervate the head and body are housed in the trigeminal and dorsal root ganglia, respectively, and can be divided into three major categories, large diameter myelinated A fibers, small diameter unmyelinated C-fibers and finely myelinated A fibers (Fig. 27.1).

Large diameter myelinated A beta fibers originating in skin, joints and muscles normally conduct non-noxious stimuli including fine touch, vibration and proprioception. In contrast, most small diameter sensory fibers are specialized sensory neurons known as nociceptors. Nociceptors have the remarkable ability to detect a wide range of stimulus modalities including those of physical and chemical nature by expressing an extremely diverse repertoire of receptors and transduction molecules that can sense forms of noxious stimuli including thermal, mechanical and chemical albeit with varying degrees of sensitivity (Fig. 27.1). These unmyelinated C fibers and finely myelinated A sensory neurons are involved in generating the chronic pain that accompanies many cancers. Following tissue injury induced by the tumor or tumor associated cells, many nociceptors alter their pattern of neurotransmitter, receptor, growth factor expression and response properties. All these neurochemical changes in part underly the development of peripheral sensitization so that normally non-noxious sensory stimulation is now perceived as noxious stimuli resulting in a chronic pain state.

This chapter will focus on involvement of sensory neurons in the generation and maintenance of tumor-induced pain. However, it should be stressed that following cancer-induced injury to sensory neurons, areas of the spinal cord and CNS involved in the processing of somatosensory information also undergo a variety of neurochemical and cellular changes known as central sensitization (see Fig. 27.2; Plate 14) that facilitate the transmission and conscious appreciation of both noxious and non-noxious sensory information. Thus, during the development of cancer, there is probably a slow, but progressive neurochemical and cellular remodeling of both the peripheral and central nervous system that inhibits, facilitates or otherwise alters the transmission of somatosensory information from the damaged peripheral sensory fibers to the cerebral cortex that results in an altered and unwanted perception of both noxious and non-noxious sensory information.

IV. TUMOR GROWTH, SKELETAL REMODELING AND PAIN INDUCED BY PRIMARILY OSTEOLYTIC OR OSTEOBLASTIC TUMORS

When primarily osteolytic 2472 murine osteosarcoma tumor cells are injected and confined to the intramedullary space of the femur, these tumor cells grow in a highly reproducible fashion as they proliferate, replacing the hemopoetic cells in the bone marrow [20–22]. Eventually, the entire marrow space is homogeneously filled with tumor cells and tumor-associated inflammatory/immune cells. In contrast, following injection and confinement of the primarily osteoblastic ACE-1 prostate cells into the mouse femur, the tumor cells are present in small clonal colonies throughout the marrow space of the femur and these small colonies

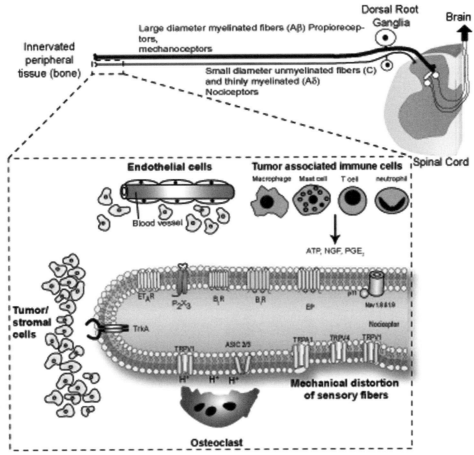

FIGURE 27.1   Primary afferent sensory nerve fibers involved in generating the bone cancer pain. Primary afferent neurons innervating the body have their cell bodies in the dorsal root ganglia (DRG) and transmit sensory information from the periphery to the spinal cord and brain. Myelinated A fibers (Aβ) containing large diameter cell bodies, which project centrally to the dorsal column nuclei and deep spinal cord, are involved in detecting non-noxious sensations including light touch, vibration, and proprioception. Unmyelinated C fibers and thinly myelinated Aδ fibers contain small diameter cell bodies which project centrally to the superficial spinal cord. These fibers are involved in detecting multiple noxious stimuli (chemical, thermal, and mechanical). Box: Nociceptors use several different types of receptors to detect and transmit signals about noxious stimuli that are produced by cancer cells (yellow), tumor associated immune cells (orange) or other aspects of the tumor microenvironment. There are multiple factors that may contribute to the pain associated with cancer. The transient receptor potential vanilloid receptor-1 (TRPV1) and acid sensing ion channels (ASICs) detect extracellular protons produced by tumor induced tissue damage or abnormal osteoclast mediated bone resorption. Several mechanosensitive ion channels may be involved in detecting high threshold mechanical stimuli that occurs when distal aspects of sensory nerve fiber are distended from mechanical pressure due to the growing tumor or as a result of destabilization or fracture of bone. Tumor cells and associated inflammatory (immune) cells produce a variety of chemical mediators including prostaglandins (PGE$_2$), nerve growth factor (NGF), endothelins, bradykinin, and extracellular ATP. Several of these proinflammatory mediators have receptors on peripheral terminals and can directly activate or sensitize nociceptors.

of osteoblastic tumor cells are separated from each other by extensive matrices of newly formed woven bone (Fig. 27.2; see Plate 14).

In regards to bone remodeling, injection of osteosarcoma cells to the femur induces predominant bone destruction along the entire bone. In sharp contrast, prostate tumor cells induce significant formation of new woven bone at the proximal and distal head of the femur as well as the diaphysis of the bone (Fig. 27.2; see Plate 14). The marked bone formation induced by prostate cancer cells is also accompanied by bone destruction giving the tumor-bearing femur a unique scalloped appearance when assessed by μCT or with

traditional histological methodology. The pathological features are similar in appearance to that observed in human patients with prostate tumor metastases [24].

The concurrent bone destruction and formation in the prostate cancer model is quite distinct from that observed in tumors such as sarcoma [21,25] or breast [26], where the tumor is primarily osteolytic as bone destruction predominates [21,25]. This mixed bone remodeling in the prostate tumor-bearing femurs is characterized by an increase in: (a) the number of osteoclasts throughout the intramedullary space which drive osteolytic bone remodeling; and (b) the number of macrophages scattered throughout the tumor and

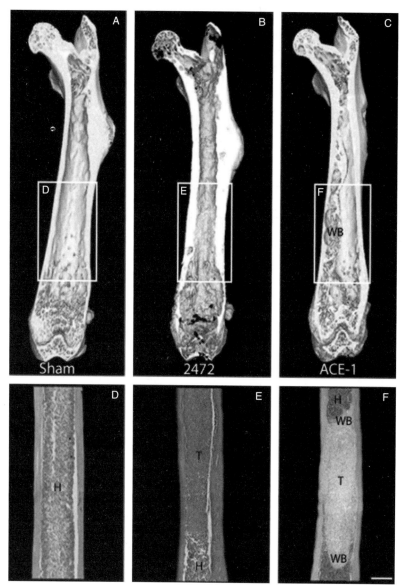

FIGURE 27.2   Bone remodeling and tumor growth in the 2472 sarcoma and ACE-1 prostate carcinoma-injected femurs have different characteristics depending on the osteolytic or osteoblastic component of the tumor cells as assessed by μCT imaging and hematoxilin and eosin (H&E) staining. Sham-injected femurs present relative absence of bone formation or bone destruction (A, D). The 2472 sarcoma-injected femurs display a primarily osteolytic appearance visible as regions absent of trabecular bone at the proximal and distal heads (B) as well as replacement of normal hematopoietic cells by tumor cells (E). The ACE-1 prostate carcinoma-injected femurs mainly present an osteoblastic appearance which is characterized by pathologic bone formation in the intramedullary space (C) surrounding pockets of tumor cells which generate diaphyseal bridging structures (F). A–F: Scale bar, 0.5 mm. T, tumor; H, normal hematopoietic cells; WB, ACE-1-induced woven bone formation.

remaining hematopoietic spaces in the bone. In the sarcoma bone cancer pain model there is an upregulation in the number of osteoclasts and macrophages (2-fold greater increase in macrophages than the prostate cancer line). However, it is the increase in the number of osteoblasts found throughout the tumor-bearing intramedullary space that ultimately separates the prostate tumor from the primarily osteolytic bone tumors in which few osteoblasts are observed and little or no bone formation occurs.

In these developed models, baseline spontaneous and evoked pain behaviors were assessed in the hind limb following tumor cell injection into the intramedullary space of the femur. Ongoing and movement evoked pain related behaviors increased in severity with time. These pain behaviors correlate with the progressive tumor-induced bone destruction or bone formation. This appears to mimic the condition in patients with primary or metastatic bone cancer.

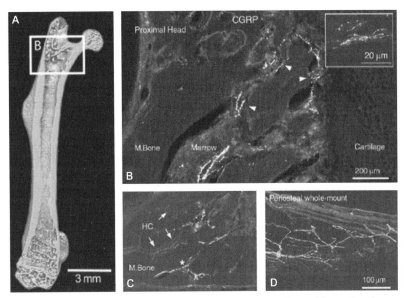

FIGURE 27.3   Sensory innervation of the mouse bone. A μCT 3D image of a mouse femur illustrating the areas used for analysis of bone innervation (A). Confocal photomicrograph showing CGRP in the mouse femur (B). Low power photomicrograph of the proximal head of the mouse femur where the CGRP-positive (+) fibers are bright white and are present in the marrow and surround the trabeculae (white arrowhead). The inset in the top right of (B) shows the average diameter of individual fibers in a bundle of CGRP fibers found in the marrow. High power photomicrographs of CGRP expressing fiber in the marrow (C) and periosteum (D). Note that the CGRP+ nerve fibers are in close proximity to blood vessels within the Haversian canal system, while in the periosteum CGRP+ nerve fibers form a dense net-like meshwork. Reprinted with permission, Mach, et al., *Neuroscience*, 2000.

V. NEUROPATHIC COMPONENT OF BONE CANCER PAIN

Numerous studies have demonstrated that the periosteum is densely innervated by both sensory and sympathetic fibers [27–29] and that it receives the greatest density of nerve fibers per area as compared to mineralized bone and bone marrow [30]. Using a combination of minimal decalcification techniques and antigen amplification techniques it has also been demonstrated that the bone marrow, mineralized bone and periosteum all receive a significant innervation by both sensory and sympathetic nerve fibers (Fig. 27.3) [31–33]. Since sensory and sympathetic neurons are present within the bone marrow, mineralized bone and periosteum and all aspects of the bone are ultimately impacted by fractures, ischemia or the presence of tumor cells, sensory fibers in any of these compartments may play a role in the generation and maintenance of bone cancer pain.

In examining the changes in the sensory innervation of bone induced by the primarily osteolytic sarcoma cells, sensory fibers were observed at and within the leading edge of the tumor. Additionally, these sensory nerve fibers displayed a discontinuous and fragmented appearance, suggesting that following initial activation by the osteolytic tumor cells, the distal processes of the sensory fibers were ultimately injured by the invading tumor cells. In contrast, in examining the sensory innervation of bone following injection of the primarily osteoblastic prostate cancer cells, data suggest that there is simultaneous injury and sprouting of sensory fibers in the bone.

In the sarcoma-injected animals, there was expression of activating transcription factor-3 (ATF-3) in the nucleus of sensory neurons that innervate the femur (Fig. 27.4; see Plate 15). ATF-3 is a member of the ATF/CREB family of transcription factors, which is not expressed at detectable levels in normal sensory neurons or in sensory neurons following peripheral inflammation, but is strongly expressed in sensory neurons following injury to peripheral nerves in neuropathic pain models [34]. It is likely that the expression of ATF-3 in sensory neurons of tumor-bearing animals is a result of peripheral nerve destruction within the tumor-bearing femur [35].

This tumor-induced injury of sensory nerve fibers in the sarcoma model was also accompanied by an increase in ongoing and movement-evoked pain behaviors, an upregulation of galanin by sensory neurons that innervate the tumor-bearing femur, upregulation of glial fibrillary acidic protein (GFAP) (Fig. 27.5; see Plate 16) and hypertrophy of satellite cells surrounding sensory neuron cell bodies within the ipsilateral dorsal root ganglia (DRG), and macrophage infiltration of the DRG ipsilateral to the tumor-bearing femur [25,36,37]. Similar neurochemical changes have been described following peripheral nerve injury and in other non-cancerous neuropathic pain states [38]. Chronic treatment with gabapentin in the sarcoma model also did not influence tumor growth, tumor-induced bone destruction or the tumor-induced neurochemical reorganization that occurs in sensory neurons or the spinal cord, but did attenuate both ongoing and movement-evoked bone cancer-related pain

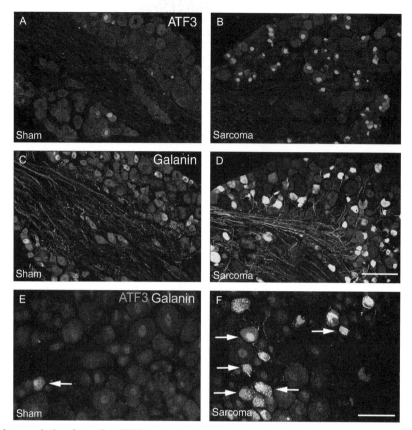

FIGURE 27.4   Activated transcription factor-3 (ATF-3) and galanin are upregulated in primary sensory neurons that innervate the tumor-bearing femur 14 days following injection of osteolytic sarcoma cells into intramedullary space of the femur. Neurons in the sham-vehicle L2 dorsal root ganglia express low levels of both activating transcription factor-3 (A) or the neuropeptide galanin (C), whereas 14 days following injection and confinement of sarcoma cells to the marrow space there is a marked upregulation of both ATF-3 (B) and galanin (D) in sensory neurons in the L2 dorsal root ganglia ipsilateral to the tumor-bearing bone. Many sensory neurons which show an upregulation of galanin in response to tumor-induced injury of sensory fibers in the bone also show an upregulation of ATF-3 in their nucleus (compare E vs F, arrows). These data suggest tumor cells invading the bone injure the sensory nerve fibers that normally innervate the tumor-bearing bone. Scale bar = 200 μm (A–D), Scale bar = 100 μm (E, F). Reprinted with permission, Peters, et al., *Experimental Neurology*, 2005.

behaviors [25]. These results suggest that even when the tumor is confined within the bone, a component of bone cancer pain is due to tumor-induced injury to primary afferent nerve fibers that normally innervate the tumor-bearing bone.

VI. SKELETAL REMODELING AND ACIDOSIS IN BONE CANCER PAIN

Experiments in a murine model of bone cancer pain have reported that osteoclasts play an essential role in cancer-induced bone loss and that osteoclasts contribute to the etiology of bone cancer pain [21,39]. Osteoclasts are terminally differentiated, multinucleated, monocyte lineage cells that resorb bone by maintaining an extracellular microenvironment of acidic pH (4.0–5.0) at the osteoclast-mineralized bone interface [40]. Tumor-induced release of protons and acidosis may be particularly important in the generation of bone cancer pain. Both osteolytic (bone destroying) and osteoblastic (bone forming) cancers are characterized by osteoclast proliferation and hypertrophy [41].

Bisphosphonates, a class of anti-resorptive compounds which induce osteoclast apoptosis, have also been reported to reduce pain in patients with osteoclast-induced skeletal metastases [42–44]. In a study of the bisphosphonate alendronate in the sarcoma model, a reduction in the number of osteoclasts and osteoclast activity was noted, as evidenced by the reduction in tumor-induced bone resorption and a reduction in the number of osteoclasts displaying the clear zone at the basal bone resorbing surface that is characteristic of highly active osteoclasts [45]. In this model, alendronate also attenuates ongoing and movement-evoked bone cancer pain, and the neurochemical reorganization of the peripheral and central nervous system while at the same time promoting both tumor growth and tumor necrosis. The present results suggest that in bone cancer, alendronate can simultaneously modulate pain, bone destruction, tumor growth and tumor necrosis.

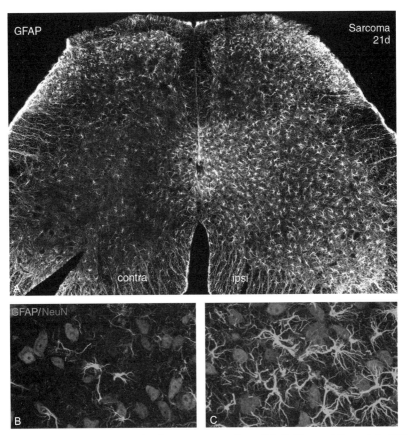

FIGURE 27.5　Confocal images showing the increase in the astrocyte marker glial fibrillary acidic protein (GFAP) in a mouse with bone cancer pain in the right femur. Coronal sections of the L4 spinal cord 21 days following injection of osteolytic sarcoma cells into the intramedullary space of the femur. In (A) the GFAP is bright orange and in (B, C) GFAP is green and the NeuN staining (which labels neurons) is in red. A low power image (A) shows that the upregulation of GFAP is almost exclusively ipsilateral to the femur with the intraosseous tumor. Higher magnification of GFAP contralateral (B) and ipsilateral (C) to the femur with cancer shows that on the ipsilateral side, there is marked hypertrophy of astrocytes characterized by an increase in both the size of the astrocyte cell bodies and the extent of the arborization of their distal processes. Additionally, this increase in GFAP (green) is observed without a detectable loss of neurons, as NeuN (red) labeling remains unchanged. These images, from 60 μm thick tissue, are projected from 6 optical sections acquired at 4 μm intervals with a 20× lens, scale bar = 200 μm (A), and from 12 optical sections acquired at 0.8 μm intervals with a 60× lens, scale bar = 30 μm (B, C). Reprinted with permission, Schwei, et al., *Journal of Neuroscience*, 1999.

Osteoprotegerin (OPG) is a secreted soluble receptor that is a member of the tumor necrosis factor receptor (TNFR) family [46,47]. This decoy receptor prevents the activation and proliferation of osteoclasts by binding to and sequestering OPG ligand (OPGL; also known as receptor for activator of NFκB ligand, RANKL) [48–51]. OPG has been shown to decrease pain behaviors in the sarcoma model of bone cancer [39]. These results suggest that a substantial part of the actions of OPG seems to result from inhibition of tumor-induced bone destruction via a reduction in osteoclast function. This reduction of osteoclast function in turn inhibits the neurochemical changes in the spinal cord that are thought to be involved in the generation and maintenance of cancer pain which demonstrates that excessive tumor-induced bone destruction is involved in the generation of bone cancer pain.

The finding that sensory neurons can be directly excited by protons or acid originating from cells like osteoclasts in bone has generated intense clinical interest in pain research [52,53]. Studies have shown that subsets of sensory neurons express different acid-sensing ion channels [54,55]. The two major classes of acid sensing ion channels expressed by nociceptors are TRPV1 [56,57] and the acid-sensing ion channel-3 (ASIC-3) [52,54,58]. Both of these channels are sensitized and excited by a decrease in pH. Tumor stroma [59] and areas of ischemic necrosis [60] such as that observed in the 2472 or ACE-1 prostate bone cancer model typically exhibit lower extracellular pH than surrounding normal tissues. As inflammatory cells invade tumor stroma, they release protons that generate local acidosis. The large amount of apoptosis that occurs in the tumor environment may also contribute to the acidotic environment.

It has been shown that TRPV1 is present on a subset of sensory neuron fibers and on those that innervate the mouse femur (Fig. 27.1). TRPV1 antagonist or disruption of the TRPV1 gene results in a significant attenuation of both ongoing and movement-evoked nocifensive behaviors in a model of bone cancer pain [37]. In addition, previous studies have also shown in the 2472 model that administration of a TRPV1 antagonist retains its efficacy at early, middle and late stages of tumor growth [37]. The ability of a TRPV1 antagonist to maintain its analgesic potency with disease progression is probably influenced by the fact that sensory nerve fibers innervating the tumor-bearing mouse femur maintain and upregulate the expression of TRPV1 even as tumor growth and tumor-induced bone destruction progresses [61]. All together these results suggest that the TRPV1 channel plays a role in the integration of nociceptive signaling in a severe pain state.

VII. TUMOR-DERIVED PRODUCTS IN GENERATION OF BONE CANCER PAIN

The tumor stroma is made up of many different cell types apart from cancer cells, including immune cells such as macrophages, neutrophils and T-lymphocytes. They secrete a variety of factors that have been shown to sensitize or directly excite primary afferent neurons, such as prostaglandins [62,63], tumor necrosis factor alpha [64–67], endothelins [68,69], interleukin-1 and -6 [64,70,71], epidermal growth factor [72], transforming growth factor-beta [73,74], and platelet-derived growth factor [75–78]. Receptors for many of these factors are expressed by primary afferent neurons.

A. Prostaglandins

Cancer cells and tumor-associated macrophages have both been shown to express high levels of cyclooxygenase (COX) isoenzymes, leading to high levels of prostaglandins [79–83]. Prostaglandins are lipid-derived eicosanoids that are synthesized from arachidonic acid by COX isoenzymes COX-1 and COX-2. Prostaglandins have been shown to be involved in the sensitization and/or direct excitation of nociceptors by binding to several prostanoid receptors expressed by nociceptors [84] (Fig. 27.1).

Studies have shown in the sarcoma model of bone cancer pain that chronic inhibition of COX-2 activity with selective COX-2 inhibitors resulted in significant attenuation of bone cancer pain behaviors as well as many of the neurochemical changes suggestive of both peripheral and central sensitization [21]. In addition, prostaglandins have been shown to be involved in tumor growth, cell survival, and angiogenesis [85–91]. Therefore, as well as having the ability to block cancer pain, COX-2 inhibitors are also capable of retarding tumor growth within bone [21]. Chronic administration of a selective COX-2 inhibitor significantly reduced tumor burden in sarcoma-bearing bones which may, in turn, reduce factors released by tumor cells

capable of exciting primary afferent fibers [68]. Acute or chronic administration of a selective COX-2 inhibitor significantly attenuated both ongoing and movement-evoked pain. Whereas acute administration of a COX-2 inhibitor presumably reduces prostaglandins capable of activating sensory or spinal cord neurons, chronic inhibition of COX-2 also appears to simultaneously reduce osteoclastogenesis, bone resorption, and tumor burden. Together, suppression of prostaglandin synthesis and release at multiple sites by selective inhibition of COX-2 may synergistically improve the survival and quality of life of patients with bone cancer pain.

B. Endothelins

Endothelins (endothelin-1, -2 and -3) are a family of vasoactive peptides that are expressed at high levels by several types of tumors, including those that arise from the prostate [69]. Clinical studies have shown a correlation between the severity of the pain and plasma levels of endothelins in prostate cancer patients [92]. Endothelins could contribute to cancer pain by directly sensitizing or exciting nociceptors, as a subset of small unmyelinated primary afferent neurons express endothelin A receptors [93] (Fig. 27.1). Furthermore, direct application of endothelin to peripheral nerves induces activation of primary afferent fibers and an induction of pain-related behaviors [94]. Like prostaglandins, endothelins that are produced by cancer cells are also thought be involved in regulating angiogenesis [95] and tumor growth [96,97].

In the sarcoma model, acute or chronic administration of the endothelin A receptor (ET_AR) selective antagonist ABT-627 significantly attenuated ongoing and movement-evoked bone cancer pain. Chronic administration of ABT-627 also reduced several neurochemical indices of peripheral and central sensitization without influencing tumor growth or bone destruction [98]. As tumor expression and release of ET-1 has been shown to be regulated by the local environment, location-specific expression and release of ET-1 by tumor cells may provide insight into the mechanisms that underlie the heterogeneity of bone cancer pain that is frequently observed in humans with multiple skeletal metastases.

C. Kinins

Previous studies have shown that bradykinin and related kinins are released in response to tissue injury and these kinins play a significant role in driving the acute and chronic inflammatory pain [99]. The action of bradykinin is mediated by two receptors termed B_1 and B_2. Whereas the B_2 receptor is constitutively expressed at high levels by sensory neurons, the B_1 receptor is normally expressed at low but detectable levels by sensory neurons and these B_1 receptors are significantly upregulated following peripheral inflammation and/or tissue injury [100]. Tumor metastases to the skeleton induce significant bone remodeling with accompanying tissue injury, which presumably induces the release of bradykinin. It has been demonstrated that both bone cancer-induced ongoing and movement-evoked nocifensive behaviors were reduced following the pharmacologic blockade of the B$_1$ receptor [101].

D. Nerve Growth Factor

One important concept that has emerged over the past decade is that, in addition to nerve growth factor (NGF) being able to directly activate sensory neurons that express the trkA receptor, NGF modulates expression and function of a wide variety of molecules and proteins expressed by sensory neurons that express the trkA or p75 receptor. Some of these molecules and proteins include: neurotransmitters (substance P and CGRP), receptors (bradykinin R), channels (P2 $\times$ 3, TRPV-1, ASIC-3 and sodium channels), transcription factors (ATF-3), and structural molecules (neurofilaments and the sodium channel anchoring molecule p11) [102,103] (Fig. 27.1). Additionally, NGF has been shown to modulate the trafficking and insertion of sodium channels such as Nav 1.8 [104] and TRPV1 [105] in the sensory neurons as well as modulating the expression profile of supporting cells in the dorsal root ganglia (DRG) and peripheral nerve, such as non-myelinating Schwann cells and macrophages [106,107]. Therefore, anti-NGF antibody therapy may be particularly effective in blocking bone cancer pain as NGF appears to be integrally involved in the upregulation, sensitization and disinhibition of multiple neurotransmitters, ion channels and receptors in the primary afferent nerve and DRG fibers that synergistically increase nociceptive signals originating from the tumor-bearing bone.

In two studies where the same analgesic therapy was used in the primarily osteolytic 2472 sarcoma and the primarily osteoblastic ACE-1 prostate bone cancer model, it was demonstrated that administration of an anti-NGF antibody was not only highly efficacious in reducing both early and late stage bone cancer pain-related behaviors but that this reduction in pain-related behaviors was greater than that achieved with acute administration of 10 or 30 mg/kg of morphine sulfate [19,36]. In light of these findings, the mechanisms that contribute to the efficacy of anti-NGF in blocking sarcoma or prostate tumor-induced bone pain remain a critical matter that requires further investigation.

VIII. CONCLUSIONS

For the first time, animal models of cancer pain are now available and effectively mirror the clinical picture observed in humans with bone cancer pain. Information generated from these models has begun to provide insight into the mechanisms that generate and maintain bone cancer pain

and helped target potential mechanism-based therapies to treat this chronic pain state. It is noteworthy that in these models analgesics such as a bisphosphonate, osteoprotegerin and a cyclooxygenase-2 inhibitor appear to influence disease progression in the tumor-bearing bone. Together these and other studies using models of bone cancer suggest that it may be possible to develop novel mechanism-based therapies that not only reduce tumor-induced bone pain but may provide added benefit in synergistically reducing disease progression. Successful development and clinical use of these therapies has the potential not only to positively impact survival, but also to improve the cancer patient's quality of life.

Acknowledgements

This work was supported by National Institutes of Health grants NS23970, NS048021 and a Merit Review from the Veterans Administration.

References

1. B. Stewart, P. Kleihues, World Cancer Report Lyon: IARC Press, 2003.
2. F. Brennan, D.B. Carr & M. Cousins, Pain management: a fundamental human right, Anesth Analg 105 (2007) 205–221.
3. WHO. Cancer Control, in: Vol. http://www.who.int.cancer, 2006.
4. A. Jemal, R. Siegel & E. Ward, et al., Cancer statistics, CA Cancer J Clin 58 (2008) 71–96.
5. M. van den Beuken-van Everdingen, J. de Rijke & A. Kessels, et al., Prevalence of pain in patients with cancer: a systematic review of the past 40 years, Ann Oncol 18 (9) (2007) 1437–1449.
6. S. Mercadante & F. Fulfaro, Management of painful bone metastases, Curr Opin Oncol 19 (2007) 308–314.
7. R.E. Coleman, Clinical features of metastatic bone disease and risk of skeletal morbidity, Clin Cancer Res 12 (2006) 6243s–6249s.
8. R.E. Coleman, Risks and benefits of bisphosphonates, Br J Cancer 98 (2008) 1736–1740.
9. S.M. Dy, S.M. Asch & A. Naeim, et al., Evidence-based standards for cancer pain management, J Clin Oncol 26 (2008) 3879–3885.
10. S. Mercadante, Malignant bone pain: pathophysiology and treatment, Pain 69 (1997) 1–18.
11. R.E. Coleman, Skeletal complications of malignancy, Cancer 80 (1997) 1588–1594.
12. S. Mercadante, P. Villari & P. Ferrera, et al., Optimization of opioid therapy for preventing incident pain associated with bone metastases, J Pain Symptom Manage 28 (2004) 505–510.
13. N. Cherny, New strategies in opioid therapy for cancer pain, J Oncol Manag 9 (2000) 8–15.
14. C.M. Reid, R. Gooberman-Hill & G.W. Hanks, Opioid analgesics for cancer pain: symptom control for the living or comfort for the dying? A qualitative study to investigate the factors influencing the decision to accept morphine for pain caused by cancer, Ann Oncol 19 (2008) 44–48.

15. D. Lussier, A.G. Huskey & R.K. Portenoy, Adjuvant analgesics in cancer pain management, Oncologist 9 (2004) 571–591.

16. M. Weber & C. Huber, Documentation of severe pain, opioid doses, and opioid-related side effects in outpatients with cancer: a retrospective study, J Pain Symptom Manage 17 (1999) 49–54.

17. J.D. Harris, Management of expected and unexpected opioid-related side effects, Clin J Pain 24 (Suppl 10) (2008) S8–S13.

18. J.A. Storey & F.M. Torti, Bone metastases in prostate cancer: a targeted approach, Curr Opin Oncol 19 (2007) 254–258.

19. K.G. Halvorson, K. Kubota & M.A. Sevcik, et al., A blocking antibody to nerve growth factor attenuates skeletal pain induced by prostate tumor cells growing in bone, Cancer Res 65 (2005) 9426–9435.

20. P. Honore, S.D. Rogers & M.J. Schwei, et al., Murine models of inflammatory, neuropathic and cancer pain each generates a unique set of neurochemical changes in the spinal cord and sensory neurons, Neuroscience 98 (2000) 585–598.

21. M.A. Sabino, J.R. Ghilardi & J.L. Jongen, et al., Simultaneous reduction in cancer pain, bone destruction, and tumor growth by selective inhibition of cyclooxygenase-2, Cancer Res 62 (2002) 7343–7349.

22. M.J. Schwei, P. Honore & S.D. Rogers, et al., Neurochemical and cellular reorganization of the spinal cord in a murine model of bone cancer pain, J Neurosci 19 (1999) 10886–10897.

23. T.A. Guise, K.S. Mohammad & G. Clines, et al., Basic mechanisms responsible for osteolytic and osteoblastic bone metastases, Clin Cancer Res 12 (2006) 6213s–6216s.

24. J.J. Body, Metastatic bone disease: clinical and therapeutic aspects, Bone 13 (1992) S57–S62.

25. C.M. Peters, J.R. Ghilardi & C.P. Keyser, et al., Tumor-induced injury of primary afferent sensory nerve fibe 18(9): 1437–1449rs in bone cancer pain, Exp Neurol 193 (2005) 85–100.

26. B.F. Boyce, T. Yoneda & T.A. Guise, Factors regulating the growth of metastatic cancer in bone, Endocrine-Related Cancer 6 (1999) 333–347.

27. S.E. Asmus, S. Parsons & S.C. Landis, Developmental changes in the transmitter properties of sympathetic neurons that innervate the periosteum, J Neurosci 20 (2000) 1495–1504.

28. C.D. Martin, J.M. Jimenez-Andrade & J.R. Ghilardi, et al., Organization of a unique net-like meshwork of CGRP+ sensory fibers in the mouse periosteum: implications for the generation and maintenance of bone fracture pain, Neurosci Lett 427 (2007) 148–152.

29. K. Irie, F. Hara-Irie & H. Ozawa, et al., Calcitonin gene-related peptide (CGRP)-containing nerve fibers in bone tissue and their involvement in bone remodeling, Microsc Res Tech 58 (2002) 85–90.

30. D.B. Mach, S.D. Rogers & M.C. Sabino, et al., Origins of skeletal pain: sensory and sympathetic innervation of the mouse femur, Neuroscience 113 (2002) 155–166.

31. A. Bjurholm, A. Kreicbergs & E. Brodin, et al., Substance P- and CGRP-immunoreactive nerves in bone, Peptides 9 (1988) 165–171.

32. A. Bjurholm, A. Kreicbergs & L. Terenius, et al., Neuropeptide Y-, tyrosine hydroxylase- and vasoactive intestinal polypeptide-immunoreactive nerves in bone and surrounding tissues, J Auton Nerv Syst 25 (1988) 119–125.

33. Z. Tabarowski, K. Gibson-Berry & S.Y. Felten, Noradrenergic and peptidergic innervation of the mouse femur bone marrow, Acta Histochem 98 (1996) 453–457.

34. H. Tsujino, E. Kondo & T. Fukuoka, et al., Activating transcription factor 3 (ATF3) induction by axotomy in sensory and motoneurons: a novel neuronal marker of nerve injury, Mol Cell Neurosci 15 (2000) 170–182.

35. P. Honore, N. Luger & M. Sabino, et al., Osteoprotegerin blocks bone cancer-induced skeletal destruction, skeletal pain and pain-related neurochemcial reorganization of the spinal cord, Nat Med 6 (2000) 521–528.

36. M.A. Sevcik, J.R. Ghilardi & C.M. Peters, et al., Anti-NGF therapy profoundly reduces bone cancer pain and the accompanying increase in markers of peripheral and central sensitization, Pain 115 (2005) 128–141.

37. J.R. Ghilardi, H. Rohrich & T.H. Lindsay, et al., Selective blockade of the capsaicin receptor TRPV1 attenuates bone cancer pain, J Neurosci 25 (2005) 3126–3131.

38. K. Obata, H. Yamanaka & T. Fukuoka, et al., Contribution of injured and uninjured dorsal root ganglion neurons to pain behavior and the changes in gene expression following chronic constriction injury of the sciatic nerve in rats, Pain 101 (2003) 65–77.

39. N.M. Luger, P. Honore & M.A. Sabino, et al., Osteoprotegerin diminishes advanced bone cancer pain, Cancer Research 61 (2001) 4038–4047.

40. J.M. Delaisse & G. Vaes, Mechanism of mineral solubilizationand matrix degradation in osteoclastic bone resorption, in: B.R. Rifkin & C.V. Gays (Eds.) Biology and Physiology of the Osteoclast, CRC, Ann Arbor, 1992, pp. 289–314.

41. D.R. Clohisy, S.L. Perkins & M.L. Ramnaraine, Review of cellular mechanisms of tumor osteolysis, Clin Orthop Rel Res 373 (2000) 104–114.

42. J.R. Berenson, L.S. Rosen & A. Howell, et al., Zoledronic acid reduces skeletal-related events in patients with osteolytic metastases, Cancer 91 (2001) 1191–1200.

43. P.P. Major, A. Lipton, J. Berenson & G. Hortobagyi, Oral bisphosphonates: a review of clinical use in patients with bone metastases, Cancer 88 (2000) 6–14.

44. L. Costa, A. Lipton & R.E. Coleman, Role of bisphosphonates for the management of skeletal complications and bone pain from skeletal metastases, Support Cancer Ther 3 (2006) 143–153.

45. A. Horton, S. Nesbitt, J. Bennett & G. Stenbeck, Integrins and other cell surface attachment molecules of bone cells, in: J.P. Bilezikian, L.G. Raisz & G.A. Rodans (Eds.) Principles of Bone Biology, Academic Press, San Diego, 2002, pp. 265–286.

46. H. Min, S. Morony & I. Sarosi, et al., Osteoprotegerin reverses osteoporosis by inhibiting endosteal osteoclasts and prevents vascular calcification by blocking a process resembling osteoclastogenesis, J Exp Med 192 (2000) 463–474.

47. N.A. Hamdy, Denosumab: RANKL inhibition in the management of bone loss, Drugs Today (Barc) 44 (2008) 7–21.

48. D.M. Anderson, E. Maraskovsky & W.L. Billingsley, et al., A homologue of the Tnf receptor and its ligand enhance T-cell growth and dendritic-cell function, Nature 390 (1997) 175–179.

49. G.A. Rodan & T.J. Martin, Therapeutic approaches to bone diseases, Science 289 (2000) 1508–1514.

50. W.S. Simonet, D.L. Lacey & C.R. Dunstan, et al., Osteoprotegerin—a novel secreted protein involved in the regulation of bone density, Cell 89 (1997) 309–319.

51. M.S. Ominsky, X. Li & F.J. Asuncion, et al., RANKL inhibition with osteoprotegerin increases bone strength by improving cortical and trabecular bone architecture in ovariectomized rats, J Bone Miner Res 23 (2008) 672–682.

52. S. Sutherland, S. Cook & E.W. McCleskey, Chemical mediators of pain due to tissue damage and ischemia, Progress in Brain Research 129 (2000) 21–38.

53. C.J. Woolf, Pain: moving from symptom control toward mechanism-specific pharmacologic management, Annals of Internal Medicine 140 (2004) 441–451.

54. T.H. Olson, M.S. Riedl & L. Vulchanova, et al., An acid sensing ion channel (ASIC) localizes to small primary afferent neurons in rats, Neuroreport 9 (1998) 1109–1113.

55. D. Julius & A.I. Basbaum, Molecular mechanisms of nociception [Review], Nature 413 (2001) 203–210.

56. M.J. Caterina, M.A. Schumacher & M. Tominaga, et al., The capsaicin receptor: a heat-activated ion channel in the pain pathway, Nature 389 (1997) 816–824.

57. M. Tominaga, M.J. Caterina & A.B. Malmberg, et al., The cloned capsaicin receptor integrates multiple pain-producing stimuli, Neuron 21 (1998) 531–543.

58. F. Bassilana, G. Champigny & R. Waldmann, et al., The acid-sensitive ionic channel subunit ASIC and the mammalian degenerin MDEG form a heteromultimeric H+-gated Na+ channel with novel properties, J Biol Chem 272 (1997) 28819–28822.

59. R.A. Gatenby, E.T. Gawlinski & A.F. Gmitro, et al., Acid-mediated tumor invasion: a multidisciplinary study, Cancer Res 66 (2006) 5216–5223.

60. H.P. Deigner & R. Kinscherf, Modulating apoptosis: current applications and prospects for future drug development, Curr Med Chem 6 (1999) 399–414.

61. Y. Niiyama, T. Kawamata & J. Yamamoto, et al., Bone cancer increases transient receptor potential vanilloid subfamily 1 expression within distinct subpopulations of dorsal root ganglion neurons, Neuroscience 148 (2) (2007) 560–572.

62. C.S. Galasko, Diagnosis of skeletal metastases and assessment of response to treatment, Clinical Orthopaedics and Related Research 312 (1995) 64–75.

63. O.S. Nielsen, A.J. Munro & I.F. Tannock, Bone metastases: pathophysiology and management policy, J Clin Oncol 9 (1991) 509–524.

64. J.A. DeLeo & R.P. Yezierski, The role of neuroinflammation and neuroimmune activation in persistent pain, Pain 90 (2001) 1–6.

65. L.R. Watkins & S.F. Maier, Implications of immune-to-brain communication for sickness and pain, Proceedings of the National Academy of Sciences of the United States of America 96 (1999) 7710–7713.

66. R.B. Nadler, A.E. Koch & E.A. Calhoun, et al., IL-1beta and TNF-alpha in prostatic secretions are indicators in the evaluation of men with chronic prostatitis, J Urology 164 (2000) 214–218.

67. M. Khatami, 'Yin and yang' in inflammation: duality in innate immune cell function and tumorigenesis, Expert Opin Biol Ther 8 (2008) 1461–1472.

68. G. Davar, Endothelin-1 and metastatic cancer pain, Pain Medicine 2 (2001) 24–27.

69. J.B. Nelson & M.A. Carducci, The role of endothelin-1 and endothelin receptor antagonists in prostate cancer, BJU International 85 (2000) 45–48.

70. A. Opree & M. Kress, Involvement of the proinflammatory cytokines tumor necrosis factor-alpha, IL-1 beta, and IL-6 but not IL-8 in the development of heat hyperalgesia: effects on heat-evoked calcitonin gene-related peptide release from rat skin, J Neurosci 20 (2000) 6289–6293.

71. L.R. Watkins, L.E. Goehler & J. Relton, et al., Mechanisms of tumor necrosis factor-alpha (Tnf-alpha) hyperalgesia, Brain Res 692 (1995) 244–250.

72. B.W. Purow, T.K. Sundaresan & M.J. Burdick, et al., Notch-1 regulates transcription of the epidermal growth factor receptor through p53, Carcinogenesis 29 (2008) 918–925.

73. R.T. Poon, S.T. Fan & J. Wong, Clinical implications of circulating angiogenic factors in cancer patients, J Clin Oncol 19 (2001) 1207–1225.

74. C. Roman, D. Saha & R. Beauchamp, TGF-beta and colorectal carcinogenesis, Microsc Res Techniq 52 (2001) 450–457.

75. R. Radinsky, Growth factors and their receptors in metastasis, Seminars in Cancer Biology 2 (1991) 169–177.

76. F. Kuhnert, B.Y. Tam & B. Sennino, et al., Soluble receptor-mediated selective inhibition of VEGFR and PDGFRbeta signaling during physiologic and tumor angiogenesis, Proc Natl Acad Sci USA 105 (2008) 10185–10190.

77. M. Ono, Molecular links between tumor angiogenesis and inflammation: inflammatory stimuli of macrophages and cancer cells as targets for therapeutic strategy, Cancer Sci 99 (2008) 1501–1506.

78. S.Y. Lin, J. Yang & A.D. Everett, et al., The isolation of novel mesenchymal stromal cell chemotactic factors from the conditioned medium of tumor cells, Exp Cell Res 314 (17) (2008) 3107–3117.

79. S.B. Shappell, S. Manning & W.E. Boeglin, et al., Alterations in lipoxygenase and cyclooxygenase-2 catalytic activity and mRNA expression in prostate carcinoma, Neoplasia 3 (2001) 287–303.

80. N. Kundu, Q.Y. Yang & R. Dorsey, et al., Increased cyclooxygenase-2 (cox-2) expression and activity in a murine model of metastatic breast cancer, Int J Cancer 93 (2001) 681–686.

81. R. Ohno, K. Yoshinaga & T. Fujita, et al., Depth of invasion parallels increased cyclooxygenase-2 levels in patients with gastric carcinoma, Cancer 91 (2001) 1876–1881.

82. D. Wang & R.N. Dubois, Pro-inflammatory prostaglandins and progression of colorectal cancer, Cancer Lett 267 (2008) 197–203.

83. M. Farooqui, Y. Li & T. Rogers, et al., COX-2 inhibitor celecoxib prevents chronic morphine-induced promotion of

angiogenesis, tumour growth, metastasis and mortality, without compromising analgesia, Br J Cancer 97 (2007) 1523–1531.

84. H. Baba, T. Kohno, K.A. Moore & C.J. Woolf, Direct activation of rat spinal dorsal horn neurons by prostaglandin E2, J Neurosci 21 (2001) 1750–1756.

85. M. Sonoshita, K. Takaku & N. Sasaki, et al., Acceleration of intestinal polyposis through prostaglandin receptor EP2 in Apc(Delta 716) knockout mice, Nature Medicine 7 (2001) 1048–1051.

86. C.S. Williams, M. Tsujii & J. Reese, et al., Host cyclooxygenase-2 modulates carcinoma growth, J Clin Invest 105 (2000) 1589–1594.

87. J.L. Masferrer, K.M. Leahy & A.T. Koki, et al., Antiangiogenic and antitumor activities of cyclooxygenase-2 inhibitors, Cancer Res 60 (2000) 1306–1311.

88. R.E. Harris, G.A. Alshafie & H. Abou-Issa, et al., Chemoprevention of breast cancer in rats by celecoxib, a cyclooxygenase 2 inhibitor, Cancer Res 60 (2000) 2101–2103.

89. B.S. Reddy, Y. Hirose & R. Lubet, et al., Chemoprevention of colon cancer by specific cyclooxygenase-2 inhibitor, celecoxib, administered during different stages of carcinogenesis, Cancer Res 60 (2000) 293–297.

90. G. Lal, C. Ash & K. Hay, et al., Suppression of intestinal polyps in Msh2-deficient and non-Msh2-deficient multiple intestinal neoplasia mice by a specific cyclooxygenase-2 inhibitor and by a dual cyclooxygenase-12 inhibitor, Cancer Res 61 (2001) 6131–6136.

91. S. Yaqub, K. Henjum & M. Mahic, et al., Regulatory T cells in colorectal cancer patients suppress anti-tumor immune activity in a COX-2 dependent manner, Cancer Immunol Immunother 57 (2008) 813–821.

92. M. Smollich & P. Wulfing, Targeting the endothelin system: novel therapeutic options in gynecological, urological and breast cancers, Expert Rev Anticancer Ther 8 (2008) 1481–1493.

93. J.D. Pomonis, S.D. Rogers & C.M. Peters, et al., Expression and localization of endothelin receptors: implication for the involvement of peripheral glia in nociception, J Neurosci 21 (2001) 999–1006.

94. H. Yuyama, A. Koakutsu & N. Fujiyasu, et al., Effects of selective endothelin ET(A) receptor antagonists on endothelin-1-induced potentiation of cancer pain, Eur J Pharmacol 492 (2004) 177–182.

95. L. Boldrini, S. Pistolesi & S. Gisfredi, et al., Expression of endothelin 1 and its angiogenic role in meningiomas, Virchows Arch 449 (2006) 546–553.

96. E.H. Asham, M. Loizidou & I. Taylor, Endothelin-1 and tumour development, Eur J Surg Oncol 24 (1998) 57–60.

97. E. Herrmann, M. Bogemann & S. Bierer, et al., The endothelin axis in urologic tumors: mechanisms of tumor biology and therapeutic implications, Expert Rev Anticancer Ther 6 (2006) 73–81.

98. C.M. Peters, T.H. Lindsay & J.D. Pomonis, et al., Endothelin and the tumorigenic component of bone cancer pain, Neuroscience 126 (2004) 1043–1052.

99. R. Couture, M. Harrisson & R.M. Vianna, et al., Kinin receptors in pain and inflammation, Eur J Pharmacol 429 (2001) 161–176.

100. A. Fox, G. Wotherspoon & K. McNair, et al., Regulation and function of spinal and peripheral neuronal B1 bradykinin receptors in inflammatory mechanical hyperalgesia, Pain 104 (2003) 683–691.

101. M.A. Sevcik, J.R. Ghilardi & K.G. Halvorson, et al., Analgesic efficacy of bradykinin B1 antagonists in a murine bone cancer pain model, J Pain 6 (2005) 771–775.

102. F.F. Hefti, A. Rosenthal & P.A. Walicke, et al., Novel class of pain drugs based on antagonism of NGF, Trends Pharmacol Sci 27 (2006) 85–91.

103. S. Pezet & S.B. McMahon, Neurotrophins: mediators and modulators of pain, Annu Rev Neurosci 29 (2006) 507–538.

104. H.J. Gould 3rd, T.N. Gould & J.D. England, et al., A possible role for nerve growth factor in the augmentation of sodium channels in models of chronic pain, Brain Res 854 (2000) 19–29.

105. R.R. Ji, T.A. Samad & S.X. Jin, et al., p38 MAPK activation by NGF in primary sensory neurons after inflammation increases TRPV1 levels and maintains heat hyperalgesia, Neuron 36 (2002) 57–68.

106. A. Brown, M.J. Ricci & L.C. Weaver, NGF message and protein distribution in the injured rat spinal cord, Exp Neurol 188 (2004) 115–127.

107. Z.L. Chen, W.M. Yu & S. Strickland, Peripheral regeneration, Annu Rev Neurosci 30 (2007) 209–233.

Section VII. New Therapeutic Advances in Primary Bone Cancers and Bone Metastases

CHAPTER **28**

Animal Models of Malignant Primary Bone Tumors and Novel Therapeutic Approaches

JULIE ROUSSEAU[1,2], FRANÇOIS LAMOUREUX[1,2], GAËLLE PICARDA[1,2], FRANÇOIS GOUIN[1,2,3], VALÉRIE TRICHET[1,2] AND FRANÇOISE RÉDINI[1,2]

[1]Université de Nantes, Nantes Atlantique Universités, Laboratoire de Physiopathologie de la Résorption Osseuse et Thérapie des Tumeurs Osseuses Primitives, EA3822, Nantes, F-44035, France.
[2]INSERM, U957, Nantes, F-44035, France.
[3]CHU de Nantes, Nantes, F-44000 France.

Contents

I. INTRODUCTION

A. Pathophysiology, Available Therapeutic Approaches

Primary tumors of bone include benign and malignant tumors, the term 'Benign Bone Tumors' covering a wide variety of disorders such as isolated and transmissible pathologies, malformations, endocrine and metabolic abnormalities, reactional lesions, real tumor development of varying evolution ranging from spontaneous regression to benign metastatic spread (e.g., exostoses, synovial chondromatosis, fibrous or osteofibrous dysplasia, aneurismal cyst, giant cell tumors, chondromyxoide fibroma). Benign tumors induce bone fragility, and some of them may degenerate into malignant tumors (chondroma—chondrosarcoma). Malignant primary bone tumors, mainly represented by osteosarcoma, Ewing's sarcoma and chondrosarcoma, have the ability to spread out of the tumors, leading to metastasis dissemination, the main cause of patient deaths. In all cases, these aggressive tumors induce functional problems that may become vital when pulmonary metastase development occurs, representing 25–50% of patients with osteosarcoma and Ewing's sarcoma with initially non-metastatic disease. The management of malignant primary tumors necessitates multidisciplinary approaches including surgeons, pathologists, oncologists and radiologists.

With an estimated incidence of 2 cases per million persons per year, osteosarcoma is the most common malignant primary bone tumor excluding hematopoietic intraosseous tumors. Osteosarcomas generally affects the young, with 60% of cases occurring before the age of 25 and a peak of incidence at 18. An additional smaller peak after age 50 corresponds to osteosarcoma arising in patients with Paget's disease of bone, fibrous dysplasia or an irradiated site [1].

The conventional osteosarcoma type arising in the intramedullary cavity of bone represents 75% of all osteosarcomas [2]. These tumors frequently penetrate and destroy the cortex of the bone and extend into the surrounding tissues. The unifying histologic feature present in all types and subtypes of osteosarcomas is the presence of osteoid produced by the neoplastic cells [3]. Surgical removal of the primary tumor is followed by distal recurrence in 80–90% of cases, implying that the majority of patients with osteosarcoma have microscopic metastatic spread at the time of diagnosis. A preference for pulmonary metastases compared with other metastatic sites is a distinct feature of osteosarcoma, and 5-year survival rates after the detection of lung metastasis are less than 30%. Thus, the prognosis of patients is highly dependent on the presence or absence of lung metastasis and on the effectiveness of treatment against it. This dismal outlook prompted interest in the use of adjuvant chemotherapy associated with surgical resection of the tumor. Over time, single-agent trials led to the development of multi-agent chemotherapies, and marked improvements have been seen over the past three decades, with current survival rates for non-metastatic disease reaching 75% overall survival at 5 years. Current treatment for non-metastatic disease includes the use of doxorubicin, cisplatin, and methotrexate with aggressive surgery. Ifosfamide and etoposide have also been shown to be active agents and are generally used for high-risk (metastatic) or recurrent disease that occurs in approximately 30–40% of patients who have non-metastatic disease at diagnosis. Salvage therapy for these patients is poor, with only 25% surviving at 5 years [4]. As these survival rates have not improved for at least two decades, there is an urgent need for new therapeutic strategies, adjuvant to surgery and chemotherapy.

The clinical data reveal the need to develop animal models of osteosarcoma and set up new therapeutic strategies against primary tumor and pulmonary metastases—the main causes of patient deaths. Although numerous osteosarcoma cell lines have been established and characterized *in vitro*, there is a scarcity of reliable and reproducible *in vivo* animal models that mimic all aspects of the human conditions at the temporal, physiological and histopathological levels. Therefore, the accurate testing of new therapeutic strategies is rendered difficult. Satisfactory experimental models for preclinical studies in cancerology must answer several criteria: reproducibility of the method used for inducing tumors, and clinical, pathological and kinetic similarity with the corresponding human osteosarcoma.

II. CURRENT ANIMAL MODELS

Several animal models of osteosarcoma have been developed and described in the literature, induced by: (i) irradiation in rats; (ii) inoculation of virus or osteosarcoma cells infected by M-MSV; (iii) transplantation of tumor fragment; (iv) injection of tumor cells at different localizations, including into the tail vein to study their metastasis abilities. In all of these models, the authors distinguished two phenomena: the development of primary bone tumor (with osteolytic or bone-formation characteristics) or the ability to induce metastasis dissemination to the lungs.

A. Radiation-induced Osteosarcomas

Described by several groups, radiation-induced osteosarcomas occur in rats 4–8 months after irradiation (60 Co gamma rays) [5]. Witzel and colleagues described a radiation-induced osteosarcoma transplanted in nude rats that showed a high similarity to human osteosarcoma [6]. In other experiments, a colloidal suspension of radioactive cerium was inoculated to the hind legs of rats, inducing the development of bone and soft-tissue tumors at the site of inoculation [7,8]. All bone tumors were osteogenic sarcoma and pulmonary metastases were frequent (53.8%). However, in these radiation-induced models, the doubling time of the tumor is very low, with the development of detectable osteosarcoma in several months, up to 600 days in Klein's study [8]. If the similarities between these bone-tissue sarcomas induced by radioactive element and their counterparts in humans are striking, these models are difficult to use in experimental therapeutic assays as their manipulation is heavy and the development is long to achieve.

B. Inoculation of Virus or M-MSV Infected Osteosarcoma Cells

Osteosarcomas were induced by the intratibial inoculation of New Zealand black rats with Moloney sarcoma virus (MSV) [9]. Radiographic evidence of osteosarcoma was first demonstrated at 10 to 15 days post-inoculation. Rats had a 93% metastasis rate involving either sublumbar nodes, lungs or both. The high tumor incidence after a short latent period and the morphologic and biochemical similarities between the MSV-induced murine osteosarcoma and the osteosarcoma in humans make this tumor a valuable model for the evaluation of new therapeutic regimens. Another model can be induced in anti-lymphocyte serum treated hamsters by the injection of TE-85 human osteosarcoma cells infected with M-MSV virus [10]. Tumors were palpable 10 to 14 days after the cells were injected and grew progressively until the animals died. All animals have pulmonary metastases. The osteosarcoma adjacent to the femur and scapula contained collagen, osteoid and calcified bone when observed by light and electron microscopy, indicating that the TE-85-M-MSV cell-hamster system is an attractive model for the study of osteosarcomas of human cell origin.

C. Tumor Transplantation in Syngenic Rats or Not

The group of Mii and colleagues established a spontaneously derived transplantable osteosarcoma in syngenic F344 rats, the success rate becoming 100% within five passage generations [11–13]. A highly lung metastatic variant has been derived that could be used to compare the different genes expressed between highly and low metastatic rat osteosarcomas [13]. Another group developed a transplantable model of osteosarcoma in Sprague-Dawley rats that was initially radio-induced as described above [7,8,14]. Whatever the graft localization (intra- or para-osseous), the normal bone is rapidly invaded, partly lysed and remodeled. The tumor is made of a hard pathological bone tissue, highly calcified if the receiver of the graft is older than 1 month. The histological structure is comparable to that of human osteosarcoma composed of differentiated osteoblasts that produce an abundant osteoid framework more or less calcified. These transplantable rat models induce an osteogenic sarcoma together with pulmonary metastases thus presenting high similarities with the human osteosarcoma. The only disadvantage of these experimental osteosarcomas lies in the poor reproducibility of the model due to the high heterogeneity in cell composition, with a variable proportion of tumoral and necrotic tissue. Therefore, the use of osteosarcoma cell lines gives better reproducible models.

D. Injection of Transformed or Tumor Cells

These may have different localizations: adjacent to the femur or the scapula [10], subcutaneously between the scapula [15], intracerebrally [16], femoral or tibial intra-medullary [9,17–19], or into the tail vein of nude mice to study the metastatic ability of these cells [20]. For example, when inoculated subcutaneously between the scapula, canine osteosarcoma cells have the ability to produce tumors in nude mice, typical of canine and human osteosarcoma with a similar pathological and biological behavior [15]. However, in the hamster this model, together with that developed by Singh and colleagues, had a subcutaneous implantation that is not relevant with the intra-osseous development of the primary osteosarcoma in humans [10]. K7M2 and K12 mouse osteosarcoma cell lines, originally derived from spontaneous BALB/c mouse osteosarcoma, have been successfully used as metastatic models of osteosarcoma with difference in their aggressive phenotype when injected intravenously [21]. The biological behaviors of K7M2 and K12 implanted orthotopically were considerably distinct: K7M2 tumors were characterized by higher tumor take rates, shorter and more consistent time to tumor detection, and more rapid tumor growth as compared to K12. Therefore, as the human condition often manifests with different degrees of aggression, this model using both cell lines is useful; it allows for the study of the various mechanisms associated with metastasis and the possibility of testing novel therapeutic interventions. UMR 106 is a rat osteosarcoma cell line that was developed from a ^{32}P-induced tumor [22]. Intramedullary injections of transformed or tumor cells have been previously described to establish osteosarcoma that induced either osteolysis [18] or bone formation [19], but with manipulated cells [10].

One of the former experimental models contributes to the detailed understanding of the cellular mechanisms of tumor osteolysis that could be used to examine therapeutic modalities aimed at inhibiting tumor osteolysis [18]. However, this model does not present high similarities with osteogenic sarcomas that appear in humans. The other model consists of the inoculation of rat osteosarcoma cells (UMR 106) into the tibia of athymic mice [19]. This model leads to the development of osteosarcoma which shows radiographic changes, including osteolysis and new bone formation. Lung metastases developed spontaneously. The latter model effectively induces osteogenic sarcoma but involves manipulated cells or viruses that could change biological behaviors of the cells or environmental conditions of the hosts for therapeutical studies [9,10]. The OSRGa cell line isolated from a rat transplantable model of osteosarcoma was passaged many times in culture and characterized both for its *in vitro* phenotype and for its tumor development ability *in vivo* [23]. When injected into the medullar cavity of rat femur, these cells induce the local development of an osteogenic sarcoma associated with pulmonary metastasis dissemination providing a reproducible model for preclinical studies.

However, kinetic, clinical and pathological similarities with the corresponding human tumor are essential criteria that must be followed for the setting up of satisfactory experimental models for preclinical studies.

E. *In vivo* Model of Human Osteosarcoma

Although several human osteosarcoma cell lines have been studied in depth *in vitro*, there is still the need for an *in vivo* model of human osteosarcoma that can be used to more accurately study the key genetic aberrations contributing to tumor invasion and metastasis, and also to develop specific agents. Therefore, there was a dramatic trend during the most recent decades towards using an immunocompromised or immunodeficient host to study the *in vivo* behavior of allotransplanted or xenotransplanted human tumor cells. Among human osteosarcoma cell lines used to develop *in vivo* models, three of the most described will be discussed. The human U2OS was originated from a biopsy of a moderately differentiated osteosarcoma obtained from the tibia of a 15-year-old Caucasian girl. Although this cell line has been extensively characterized *in vitro* [24,25], only one study by Manara and colleagues reported its tumorigenic ability *in vivo* [26]. Tumor cells were injected subcutaneously inducing tumor development in 63% of mice or via the tail vein, with 100% mice developing pulmonary lesions at 8 weeks. SaOS-2 was derived by Fogh and colleagues in 1973 from a primary osteosarcoma in an 11-year old Caucasian girl [27]. Development of tumors *in vivo* has been described after subcutaneous injection of cells into nude mice [28]. Jia and colleagues then established an SaOS-2 metastasis model that was derived from lung metastases of nude mice [29]. Sub-clones of these lung metastases (SaOS-LM) were established after cells were isolated and re-injected. Another human cell line, HOS (originally M.T., then TE-85) was originally derived from the distal femur of a 13-year-old Caucasian girl [30]. HOS cells have been studied extensively *in vitro*, particularly for the detection of possible causative viral agents. However, despite several attempts, consistent *in vivo* growth of HOS after subcutaneous and orthotopic inoculation have all been unsuccessful. Tumorigenic potential, however, could only be achieved after HOS was further genetically altered and, as a result, many *in vivo* models have been established using cell line derivatives. Successful *in vivo* growth of HOS in mice has been achieved using the viral agents Kirsten murine sarcomavirus (Ki-MSV) and Moloney sarcoma virus (M-MSV RD-114) and the chemical agent N-methyl-N′-nitro-N-nitroguanidine (MNNG). The KRIB model developed using the HOS cells transformed with the oncogene v-Ki-ras had the propensity to form pulmonary metastases in nude mice when injected as a single i.v. bolus. Intratibial inoculation of tumor cells resulted in tumor formations in 100% of mice at 4 weeks that were similar both radiologically and histologically to the primary human condition. Moreover, spontaneous pulmonary metastases also developed at 4 weeks in all mice that were inoculated. This model was the first successful orthotopic xenotransplantation osteosarcoma model that had the ability to form pulmonary metastases. Although this model has been further studied by other investigators, its main limitation is that it is essentially a transformed osteosarcoma cell line, and thus is not a true representation of the human condition. Nakano and colleagues established a useful and convenient animal model to provide valuable information for metastasis ability of human osteosarcoma [20]. In this model, sublines with high- and low-metastatic potential to lungs were established from the parental Hu09 osteosarcoma cell line, and injected into the tail vein of nude mice. However, this model is only valuable for the study of pulmonary metastasis dissemination and not for primary tumor development.

All of these models show advantages and disadvantages that should be taken into account when establishing pre-clinical protocols.

III. NEW THERAPEUTIC APPROACHES

Despite chemotherapy and surgical resection, 30–40% of patients with localized osteosarcoma and 80% with diagnosed metastases usually relapse within the first 3 years. New directions for bone tumor treatment are given by rapid advances in molecular medicine and research into the basic tumor biology and its microenvironment.

A. Immune-based Therapies

Several attempts have been made to utilize immuno-stimulatory therapies, such as granulocyte-macrophage colony-stimulating factor (GM-CSF) and liposomal muramyl tripeptide phoshatidylethanolamine (MTP-PE) to treat and prevent lung metastases. Other strategies including IFN, IL-2, IL-12 and cellular immune-based therapies are also presented.

GM-CSF has been shown to have many antitumor effects in multiple tumor models mediated by augmentation of antibody-dependent cellular toxicity [31], functioning as an adjuvant for the generation of immune responses to tumor vaccines and enhancement of Natural Killer (NK) functions. Because pulmonary relapses are a significant cause of morbidity and mortality in patients with osteosarcoma, pulmonary deliveries of GM-CSF have been tested and with minimal toxicity have shown stabilization and even a reduction in the pulmonary metastases in some cases [32,33].

MTP-PE is a synthetic lipophilic analog of muramyl dipeptide, a component of the cell wall of mycobacterium that is able to stimulate monocytes and macrophages. This effect is further enhanced by encapsulation in liposomes that preferentially deliver the dipeptide to pulmonary macrophages. Laboratory and animal studies demonstrating

promising results have led to human trials. These trials have shown a prolongation of relapse-free survival in patients with recurrent osteosarcoma [34]. MTP-PE was also evaluated in patients with non-metastatic osteosarcoma in a randomized phase III trial of combination chemotherapy comparing chemotherapy with and without ifosfamide and with or without MTP-PE [35]. The results suggest a potential interaction between MTP-PE and ifosfamide, as both may upregulate the Fas/Fas ligand pathway, thereby inducing tumor cell apoptosis.

Interferons (IFNs) have a variety of biological effects in innate and adaptive immune response and have also shown moderate antitumor effects when given therapeutically [36]. Despite reports of osteosarcoma growth inhibition and enhanced chemosensitivity *in vitro* [37], clinical trials of IFN in osteosarcoma are sparse and conflicting [38–41]. Although the role of IFN in the treatment of osteosarcoma is unclear, it may be beneficial in minimal residual diseases; for example, at the end of standard chemotherapy.

Cellular immune-based therapies were used in two approaches. A first approach indicated that Tumor Infiltrating Lymphocytes (TILs) therapy could be a very efficient strategy for the treatment of osteosarcoma [42]. Human TILs were isolated and characterized (phenotype, lytic activity) from patients with bone-associated tumors. While TILs with a main CD4+ profile were easily extracted from most of the tumor samples, only TILs extracted from osteosarcoma were cytotoxic against allogenic tumor cells. In all cases, TIL lytic activity was significantly higher compared to autologous peripheral blood leukocytes.

A second approach reveals that active immunotherapy of osteosarcoma is also promising. Indeed, we have demonstrated that a CD4-subset of rat spleen dendritic cells (DC) incubated one night in the presence of rat osteosarcoma OSRGa cells before being injected as a vaccination protocol to rats bearing osteosarcoma induces tumor growth inhibition and survival rate augmentation, as compared to DC incubated with human lymphoma cells. These results suggest that active immunotherapy in this model involves the recognition of tumor antigens specifically expressed by rat osteosarcoma cells and their presentation by dendritic cells [43]. Moreover in one study, bone marrow dendritic cells showed efficacy towards lung metastases from murine osteosarcoma [44].

B. Gene Therapies and Conventional Tumor Targets

Conventional targets of tumor gene therapy have been tested in various osteosarcoma models. They concern three main strategies: (1) mutation compensation of tumor-suppressor genes; (2) induction of suicide genes; and (3) activation of immune response.

1. TUMOR-SUPPRESSOR GENE THERAPY

One goal of gene therapy is to replace mutated or deleted tumor-suppressor genes with their wild-type forms to gain anti-tumor effects. As the tumor-suppressor genes *pRb* and *p53* are mutated in most human osteosarcomas [45–47], the majority of preclinical studies have targeted these genes. In an early study, the re-established wild-type pRb had resulted in growth inhibition of at least one osteosarcoma cell line (SaOS-2) [48]. Nevertheless, the pRb replacement effects have been shown to be variable and incomplete in a large panel of human tumor cell lines, including osteosarcoma derivatives [49]. Furthermore, pRb was shown to interfere with the growth of normal cells [50] and with p53 dependent and independent apoptosis [51,52]. The usage of pRb gene therapy needs more guarantees, but it deserves further investigation [53].

By using different non-viral vectors, p53 gene transfer induced an inhibition of human osteosarcoma progression in mice. Densmore and colleagues reported a successful aerosol administration of p53 gene combined with polyethylenimine (PEI) to treat osteosarcoma lung metastases which were induced in nude mice after SaOS cell line injection [54]. In another study, the p53 gene was associated with a cationic liposome supplemented with transferrin, and this complex was sequentially injected in tumors which were induced by HOSM-1 human osteosarcoma cell line inoculation in nude mice. Beside control groups, the group that received p53/liposome/transferrin complexes showed a significant reduction of tumor growth [55]. Moreover, such an approach could provide beneficial effects when used in combination with chemotherapeutic agents, such as doxorubicin and cisplatin. Indeed the viral-mediated wild-type p53 expression was able to sensitize osteosarcoma cell lines to apoptotic death [56,57]. Despite these encouraging results, significant improvements are needed to bypass the resistance towards p53 treatment [58], as 30% of osteosarcomas overexpress MDM2 which links and inhibits p53 [59].

Although clinical trials using p53 gene replacement were successful for the treatment of head and neck cancers [60], to date they have failed for other cancers [61]. Such p53-based gene therapy has not yet been recommended to patients with osteosarcomas, partly because it is conduced by an adenovirus vector whose high-affinity receptor (CAR) is weakly expressed on primary human bone tumors. Retargeting adenovirus towards human epidermal growth factor receptor may represent a more efficient option, as demonstrated by Witlox and colleagues [62].

2. SUICIDE GENE THERAPY

Using this strategy, tumor cell death would result from the delivery of a gene encoding a specific enzyme which converts a non-toxic prodrug into a substance toxic for cell metabolism. Three prodrug-converting enzymes have been tested in the context of osteosarcomas: the Herpes Simplex Virus—Thymidine Kinase (HSV-TK), the cytosine deaminase (CD), and the carbocylesterase-2 (CE-2).

Osteosarcoma primary cultures and cell lines were variably killed (in a range of 0 to 60%) by ganciclovir (GCV) addition following adenovirus-mediated HSV-TK gene transfer [62]. In the same study, the authors observed improvements by using epidermal growth factor receptor redirected adenovirus, reaching 40 to 80% cell deaths for either osteosarcoma primary cells or established cell lines [62]. *In vivo*, the efficiency of HSV-TK plus GCV therapy had been demonstrated earlier by Charissoux and colleagues [63]. Packaging cells modified *ex vivo* by retroviral vector encoding HSV-TK have been inoculated into osteosarcoma grafts on rat hind limb. The following GCV addition reduced the tumor mass and prevented lung metastase development. Dong and colleagues demonstrated that cell transfected by the HSV-TK gene followed by GCV delivery allowed tumor eradication within immunocompetent mouse models [64]. In order to drive the HSV-TK gene expression specifically in osteoblast-like cells, the promoter of osteocalcin (OC) was chosen in a first attempt and a highly effective inhibition of osteosarcoma growth was observed both *in vitro* and *in vivo* [65]. In addition, such Ad-OC-TK/acyclovir treatment was able to sensitize both rat and human osteosarcomas to methotrexate [66]. The OC promoter was also used to restrict the viral replication and subsequent lysis to osteocalcin expressing tumors, by cloning it upstream from the adenovirus gene encoding the E1a protein [67]. This virus-mediated suicide therapy resulted in lung metastasis reduction in osteosarcoma animal models. Results of a first clinical trial using HSV-TK gene transfer plus ganciclovir treatment demonstrated that this combination was feasible and well tolerated. A phase III clinical trial using this suicide gene strategy was conducted for glioblastoma but the published results reported no significant improvement for HSV-TK/GCV treated patients compared with control group [68]. The failure of such treatment could be due either to the presumed poor rate of delivery to tumor cells or the resistance mechanisms to enzyme-activated drug [69].

The cytosine deaminase (CD) and the carboxylesterase (CE) convert respectively, the 5-fluorocytosine (5FC) and the agent CPT-11 into active drugs. A bacterial CD fusion gene demonstrated a direct and bystander killing effect *in vitro* for sarcoma cells, but was inefficient *in vivo* [70]. By contrast, a yeast CD fusion gene was effective in decreasing bone sarcoma growth in mice treated with 5FC with a diminution of bone destruction [70]. Given this osteolysis inhibition, osteoclasts were tested for 5FC treatment sensitivity. Transgenic mice overexpressing the CD gene under an osteoclast-specific promoter (TRAP (tartrate-resistant acid phosphatase)) were of particular interest as the 5FC treatment allowed high reduction to complete killing of bone tumors. Importantly, osteoclasts isolated from CD transgenic mice were resistant to the 5FC treatment *in vivo*, suggesting that they have directed bystander killing of bone tumor cells without being affected by the active drug [71]. Finally, osteoclasts were designed as cell candidate for CD gene delivery.

In order to explore the CE gene therapeutic potential, various osteosarcoma cell lines and primary cultures were modified with adenovirus units encoding a secreted form of carboxylesterase (Ad-sCE2). These modifications resulted in sensitization to CPT-11 up to 2800-fold for cell lines and 70-fold for primary cultures. Moreover, the injections of Ad-sCE2 plus CPT-11 within osteosarcoma xenografts allowed a significant reduction of tumor volume in comparison with animals treated with Ad-sCE2 or CPT-11 alone [72].

Despite the satisfactory preclinical results, the efficacy of the three suicide genes reviewed above showed no beneficial effect yet for patients with osteosarcoma.

3. IMMUNO-POTENTIATION GENE THERAPY

Although several interleukins have been identified as good candidates for enhancement of tumor cell recognition and elimination by the immune system, their systemic administration is not always possible because of consecutive toxic effects. Beside this problem, the interleukin gene therapy could provide survival advantages.

Among these cytokines, interleukin-12 (IL-12) is of particular interest. Indeed, it promotes the production of interferon (IFN)-gamma by natural killer cells and T-lymphocytes and inhibits angiogenesis, but provokes undesirable side effects when injected in blood. The UMR 108 osteosarcoma cells transfected with plasmid encoding IL-12 were used to develop osteosarcomas in rats [73]. Then the local IL-12 secretion led to intratumoral IFN-gamma induction. The IL-12 gene delivered in combination with polyethylenimine (PEI) by aerosol in a model of osteosarcoma lung metastases in mice induced a significant nodule reduction [74]. Using the same mouse model of lung metastases, the combination of PEI:IL-12 with ifosfamide was studied. Both ifosfamide and PEI:IL-12 alone significantly inhibited lung metastases when compared to control groups. However, the most significant anti-tumor effect was observed in mice receiving the combined treatment [75]. Kleinerman's laboratory studied IL-12 gene therapy in the primary bone tumor model of Ewing's sarcoma developed on nude mice. Significant tumor growth inhibition was observed with a single injection of adenovirus encoding murine IL-12 in each tumor [76]. Moreover, the IL-12 local secretion inhibited the growth of an untreated tumor that was developed in the controlateral limb. In nude mice depleted in T-lymphocytes, the IL-12-activated tumor elimination could imply the NK cell activation, but also an upregulation of death receptors on tumor cells as shown for Fas expression in human osteosarcoma [77].

Concerning the use of another interleukin, IL-2, the proof-of-principle has been demonstrated in the control of osteosarcoma in a phase II clinical trial [78]. In this study,

IL-2 was administrated as a recombinant protein and the consecutive NK activation correlated with clinical outcome. The delivery of IL-3 and IL-2 by gene transfer using adenovirus was tested in the context of osteosarcoma animal models. In the ROS-1 rat model, the rat IL-3 expression was driven by either a strong (Ad-CMV-rIL-3) or a weak (Ad-MLP-rIL-3) promoter and the IL-3 adenovirus units were injected only once using three distinct protocols: limb perfusion, intra-tumoral injection, or intravenous administration [79]. The tumor growth inhibition was efficient only with the single perfusion of Ad-CMV-rIL-3. In a murine osteosarcoma model, the single intra-tumoral injection of adenovirus units encoding IL-2 suppressed primary tumor growth, eradicated disseminated micro-metastases and avoided side effects, but only in the case of the optimal doses [80]. In conclusion, cytokine gene therapy is feasible, but difficulties reside in the gene transfer control to get the more efficient dose of produced molecule.

C. Therapies Targeting Tumor Bone Micro-environment

Given advances in basic bone tumor biology, the bone environment is evidenced as the soil favoring progression of bone metastases and primary bone tumors [81]. A vicious cycle arises from the tumoral and stromal cell secretions that activate the osteoclastic bone resorption which, in turn, delivers growth factors stocked from the bone matrix to the tumor cells and osteoblasts. Bone resorption can be targeted by bisphosphonate treatment that are used to reduce the skeletal disorders associated with bone metastases secondary to prostate or breast carcinomas [82,83]. Our group demonstrated that the bisphosphonate zoledronic acid was also effective in reducing morbidity in osteosarcoma models [14,84]. These results provided the rationale for the French clinical trial 'OS2006' designed to test the impact of zoledronic acid in association with chemotherapy and surgery in children and adult patients with osteosarcomas. Despite the possibility that zoledronic acid effects could result from inhibition of both osteoclast and osteosarcoma cell activities as demonstrated *in vitro* [85,86], osteolysis is considered as a pertinent target for improving the primary bone tumor treatments.

Two gene therapies could be proposed to inhibit osteoclastogenesis: the overexpression of anti-bone resorption molecules such as Osteoprotegerin (OPG) or Receptor Activator of NF-kB (RANK)-Fc, or the inhibition of pro-bone resorption molecules such as RANK Ligand (RANKL) (Figure 28.1).

1. OVEREXPRESSION OF DECOY/SOLUBLE RECEPTORS FOR RANKL BY GENE TRANSFER

The OPG acts as a decoy receptor for RANKL preventing it from binding to its receptor RANK expressed on osteoclast

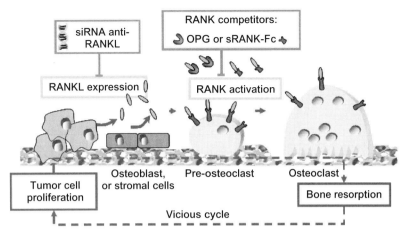

FIGURE 28.1 Anti-RANKL therapeutic strategies to inhibit bone tumor development. The biological problematic of tumor development in bone site relies on the existence of a vicious cycle between tumor cell proliferation and bone resorption. As Receptor Activator of NF-κB Ligand (RANKL) plays a pivotal role in the regulation of bone resorption mechanisms, inhibition of its expression by siRNA anti-RANKL or its activity (RANK activation) by using soluble or competitor receptors (sRANK-Fc or osteoprotegerin (OPG)) may represent a promising challenge in primary bone tumor therapy.

precursors or mature osteoclasts. Thereby, OPG over-expression is expected to inhibit osteoclast formation, function and survival. Supporting this therapeutic hypothesis, injections of recombinant OPG were effective in inhibiting osteolysis and skeletal tumor burden in different murine models of myeloma, bone metastases secondary to breast and prostate carcinomas [87–89]. Advanced bone cancer pain was diminished by OPG administration to mice with sarcoma-induced bone destruction [90]. As OPG is also able to bind TNF-Related Apoptosis Inducing Ligand (TRAIL), a truncated form of OPG must be used in therapeutic approaches of osteolysis from tumor origin. Indeed, OPG was described as a survival factor for numerous tumor cells, by its ability to inhibit TRAIL activity [91].

Our group studied OPG effects in osteosarcoma by using two gene-transfer strategies: adenovirus and synthetic vectors, demonstrating that injections of adenovirus encoding OPG were effective in protecting from bone remodeling and slowing down the tumor progression [92]. A plasmid encoding OPG was associated with the amphiphilic polymer Lutrol® and administrated intramuscularly in mice bearing POS-1 osteosarcomas. This non-viral OPG gene delivery was effective in preventing the formation of osteolytic lesions associated with osteosarcoma development [92]. Interestingly, OPG gene delivered by Lutrol® in the mouse model of osteosarcoma was not able to prevent the development of pulmonary metastasis alone, suggesting that bone environment is necessary for OPG therapeutic efficacy. Moreover, as no direct binding of OPG on osteosarcoma cells could be evidenced *in vitro*, it can be suggested that OPG acts indirectly on osteoblastic tumor cell growth through inhibition of bone resorption (Figure 28.1). In contrast, OPG was shown to act directly on signal transduction of osteoclasts, indicating that it is more than a

decoy receptor for RANKL, but can also act as a cytokine on osteoclast functions [93]. In conclusion, the OPG therapeutic effects demonstrated in two murine osteosarcoma models are very likely mediated by the inhibition of RANKL, as demonstrated by Jones and colleagues using a mouse model of bone metastases secondary to melanoma [94]. Indeed, they observed the neutralization of RANKL by recombinant OPG administration which resulted in complete protection from paralysis and a marked reduction in tumor burden in bones, but not in other organs. Another study by Heath and colleagues also evidenced the potential therapeutic role of osteolysis inhibition by using an OPG-like peptidomimetic in a model of myeloma [95].

Besides the decoy receptor OPG, the soluble form of RANKL receptor (sRANK) has proved effective in several preclinical models of osteolytic bone tumors, such as myeloma, bone metastases or malignant hypercalcemia [96–98]. It is therefore a good candidate for therapeutic application in primary bone tumors.

2. RANKL DOWN-EXPRESSION BY RNA

INTERFERENCE

RANKL is enhanced in the bone tumor environment where it stimulates osteoclast differentiation and activation. Therefore, the RANKL expression has to be reduced to inhibit osteoclastogenesis activation. Regarding the positive therapeutic effect of RANKL inhibition by OPG [94], it would be worth blocking the RANKL secretion in the context of primary osteolytic bone tumor.

The antisense oligonucleotide strategy was used early in the 1990s to downregulate the expression of a targeted protein by specific sequence recognition of its encoding RNA. The proto-oncogene cyclin G1, which regulates cell cycle control, is frequently overexpressed in human osteosarcoma cells. It has been thus targeted by long anti-sense RNA molecules that were transcribed from retrovirus. In the MG-63 human osteosarcoma cell line, the cyclin G1 anti-sense RNA which were 3421 base long induced cell division arrest [99]. Even more interesting, the retroviruses producing these cyclin G1 anti-sense RNAs were injected into HOS-derived human osteosarcomas developed in nude mice and were able to inhibit tumor growth [100]. However, the observed effects using long anti-sense RNA may have resulted from side effects rather than from a specific decrease of cyclin G1 expression. Indeed, the understanding of RNA interference mechanisms has since revealed that long double-stranded RNA molecules induce a general arrest of translation leading to cell death, especially in mammalian cells [101]. In contrast, small interfering RNA molecules (siRNA) have been demonstrated to evade from the interferon response leading to translations arrest and yet to be still effective mediators of sequence-specific degradation of complementary mRNA [102]. The siRNA are 21 base pair long, with two nucleotides overhanging at the 3' ends and a core sequence of 19 nucleotides whose one strand is the perfect complementary sequence of 19 nucleotides of the targeted mRNA. The siRNA molecules are synthetic or result from cell enzyme-modified short hairpin RNA (shRNA) molecules that could be transcribed from DNA vector sequences. Before acting as RNA interference mediators, the siRNA or the shRNA-expressing vectors must be transported into the cells where the targeted protein is translated.

In the context of osteosarcoma, the RANKL secretion could be targeted by such siRNA or shRNA molecules directed against RANKL mRNA. The first challenge of such therapeutic strategy would be to transport the siRNA/shRNA molecules into cells that produce RANKL (i.e., neoplasic and

non-neoplasic osteoblastic cells). Indeed, RANKL molecules were detected by immuno-histochemistry within the bone tumor, suggesting that the osteoblastic tumor cells produce RANKL *in vivo*, in response to micro-environmental factors [92]. A challenge to get therapeutic success with siRNA will be the improvement of delivery protocols (quantity, frequency and way of injection) to osteoblastic tumor cells.

D. Bioluminescence as a New Tool to Follow Tumor Responses to Therapeutic Protocols

By cloning the firefly luciferase gene into a lentiviral vector, it is possible to produce viral units which are highly efficient in stably transferring the transgene luciferase into various tumor cell types, including osteosarcoma cells (Figure 28.2; see Plate 17). Two murine osteosarcoma cell lines overexpressing luciferase, POS-luc and OSRGa-luc have been developed in our laboratory for osteosarcoma imaging (Figure 28.2; see Plate 17). These cells are used to induce osteosarcoma in rodents, then to follow and quantify the progression of the tumor in response to therapeutic protocols. This methodology has already proved its interest in other bone tumor experimental models, such as bone metastases [103]. This technology could also be applied to plasmid constructions combining the expression of therapeutic gene and luciferase, to follow the targeting of tumor cells by luciferase-modified therapeutic genes. Concerning the siRNA strategy, Derek and colleagues showed how the live-animal bioluminescent imaging is useful for following the siRNA effect against the luciferase protein whose enzymatic activity is detectable *in vivo* [104]. The development of murine models expressing the luciferase is first needed to further develop a therapeutic approach of primary bone tumors based on siRNA strategy.

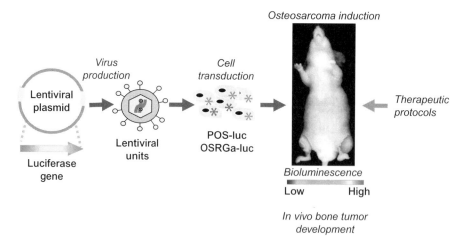

FIGURE. 28.2 *In vivo* bioluminescence imaging to follow and quantify the progression or regression of bone tumor in response to therapeutic protocols. By cloning the firefly luciferase gene into a lentiviral plasmid, it is possible to produce lentiviral units which are highly efficient in stably transferring the transgene luciferase into various tumor cell types, including murine POS and rat OSRGa osteosarcoma cells. These cells are then injected into mice/rats to develop the corresponding osteosarcoma model. The measurement of *in vivo* bioluminescence further allows us to quantify tumor progression, regression or recurrence, together with pulmonary metastases dissemination in response to the applied therapeutic protocol.

IV. CONCLUSION AND PERSPECTIVES

A comprehensive multidisciplinary approach has transformed osteosarcoma from a disease with a modest long-term survival to one in which at least two thirds of patients will be cured. Surgery remains a vital modality for treating primary tumors, whereas adjuvant chemotherapy plays an essential role in the control of subclinical metastatic disease. Some groups of patients who remain at a high risk of eventual relapse may benefit from future investigations into innovative approaches such as immune-based therapies or gene transfer, novel agents such as biological response modifiers, anti-angiogenesis factors or growth receptor modulation. Data emphasize the relevance of targeting tumor microenvironment in the case of bone tumors. The importance of the local host tissue microenvironment that actively participates in the propensity of certain cancers to metastasize to bone has been studied, confirming the 'seed and soil' hypothesis proposed by Paget [105]. Among the homeostatic factors that promote tumor-cell growth in the bone, RANKL is a good candidate influencing the local bone resorption process that is necessary for tumor development in bone sites [106]. The combined use of emerging technologies such as RNA interference and *in vivo* bio-imaging will create opportunities for evaluating the potency of the RANKL downregulation strategy for osteosarcoma therapy in preclinical studies.

References

1. M.S. Linet, L.A. Ries & M.A. Smith, et al., Cancer surveillance series: recent trends in childhood cancer incidence and mortality in the United States, J Natl Cancer Inst 91 (1999) 1051–1058.
2. F. Mertens, N. Mandahl & C. Orndal, et al., Cytogenetic findings in 33 osteosarcomas, Int J Cancer 55 (1993) 44–50.
3. M. Link, M. Gebhardt & P. Meyers, Osteosarcoma, in: P. Pizzo & D. Poplack (Eds.) Principles and Practice of Pediatric Oncology, Lippincott Williams & Wilkins, Philadelphia, 2002, pp. 1051–1089.
4. W.G. Ward, K. Mikaelian & F. Dorey, et al., Pulmonary metastases of stage IIB extremity osteosarcoma and subsequent pulmonary metastases, J Clin Oncol 12 (1994) 1849–1858.
5. P.T. Tinkey, T.M. Lembo & G.R. Evans, et al., Postirradiation sarcomas in Sprague-Dawley rats, Radiat Res 149 (1998) 401–404.
6. J.G. Witzel, A. Prescher & H. Weisser, Experimental animal model for the evaluation of chemotherapeutical effects on osteosarcoma, Chemotherapy 38 (1992) 251–260.
7. J.P. Thiéry, B. Perdereau & R. Gongora, et al., Un modèle experimental d'ostéosarcome chez le rat. II L'ostéosarcome greffable du rat, Sem Hôp Paris 58 (1982) 1686–1689.
8. B. Klein, S. Pals & R. Masse, et al., Studies of bone and soft-tissue tumours induced in rats with radioactive cerium chloride, Int J Cancer 20 (1977) 112–119.
9. H.M. Olson & C.C. Capen, Virus-induced animal model of osteosarcoma in the rat: morphologic and biochemical studies, Am J Pathol 86 (1977) 437–458.
10. I. Singh, J.M. Hatheway & K.Y. Tsang, et al., An animal model for human osteosarcoma, Surgery 81 (1977) 168–175.
11. Y. Mii, M. Tsutsumi & K. Shiraiwa, et al., Transplantable osteosarcomas with high lung metastatic potential in Fischer 344 rats, Jpn J Cancer Res 79 (1988) 589–592.
12. T. Morishita, Y. Miyauchi & Y. Mii, et al., Delay in administration of CDDP until completion of AGM-1470 treatment enhances antimetastatic and antitumor effects, Clin Exp Metastasis 17 (1999) 15–18.
13. T. Fukuda, A. Kido & K. Kajino, et al., Cloning of differentially expressed genes in highly and low metastatic rat osteosarcomas by a modified cDNA-AFLP method, Biochem Biophys Res Commun 261 (1999) 35–40.
14. D. Heymann, B. Ory & F. Blanchard, et al., Enhanced tumor regression and tissue repair when zoledronic acid is combined with ifosfamide in rat osteosarcoma, Bone 37 (2005) 74–86.
15. A.M. Shoieb, K.A. Hahn & M.A. Barnhill, an in vivo/in vitro experimental model system for the study of human osteosarcoma: canine osteosarcoma cells (COS31) which retain osteoblastic and metastatic properties in nude mice, In Vivo 12 (1998) 463–472.
16. W. Cosolo & N. Christophidis, Blood-brain barrier disruption and methotrexate in the treatment of a readily transplantable intracerebral osteogenic sarcoma of rats, Cancer Res 47 (1987) 6225–6228.
17. I. Kjonniksen, M. Winderen & O. Bruland, et al., Validity and usefulness of human tumor models established by intratibial cell inoculation in nude rats, Cancer Res 54 (1994) 1715–1719.
18. D.R. Clohisy, C.M. Ogilvie & R.J. Carpenter, et al., Localized, tumor-associated osteolysis involves the recruitment and activation of osteoclasts, J Orthop Res 14 (1996) 2–6.
19. J.L. Fisher, P.S. Mackie & M.L. Howard, et al., The expression of the urokinase plasminogen activator system in metastatic murine osteosarcoma: an *in vivo* mouse model, Clin Cancer Res 7 (2001) 1654–1660.
20. T. Nakano, M. Tani & Y. Ishibashi, et al., Biological properties and gene expression associated with metastatic potential of human osteosarcoma, Clin Exp Metastasis 20 (2003) 665–674.
21. C. Khanna, J. Prehn & C. Yeung, et al., An orthotopic model of murine osteosarcoma with clonally related variants differing in pulmonary metastatic potential, Clin Exp Metastasis 18 (2000) 261–271.
22. T.J. Martin, P.M. Ingleton & J.C. Underwood, et al., Parathyroid hormone-responsive adenylate cyclase in induced transplantable osteogenic rat sarcoma, Nature 260 (1976) 436–438.
23. B. Cherrier, F. Gouin & M.F. Heymann, et al., A new experimental rat model of osteosarcoma established by intrafemoral tumor cell inoculation, useful for biology and therapy investigations, Tumour Biol 26 (2005) 121–130.
24. M. Lind, E.F. Eriksen & C. Bunger, Bone morphogenetic protein-2 but not bone morphogenetic protein-4 and -6 stimulates chemotactic migration of human osteoblasts, human marrow osteoblasts, and U2-OS cells, Bone 18 (1996) 53–57.
25. Y. Sun, Y. Sun & L. Wenger, et al., p53 down-regulates human matrix metalloproteinase-1 (Collagenase-1) gene expression, J Biol Chem 274 (1999) 11535–11540.

26. M.C. Manara, N. Baldini & M. Serra, et al., Reversal of malignant phenotype in human osteosarcoma cells transduced with the alkaline phosphatase gene, Bone 26 (2000) 215–[220].

27. J. Fogh, J.M. Fogh & T. Orfeo, One hundred and twenty-seven cultured human tumor cell lines producing tumors in nude mice, J Natl Cancer Inst 59 (1977) 221–226.

28. Y. Zhou, S. Mohan & T.A. Linkhart, et al., Retinoic acid regulates insulin-like growth factor-binding protein expression in human osteoblast cells, Endocrinology 137 (1996) 975–983.

29. S.F. Jia, L.L. Worth & E.S. Kleinerman, A nude mouse model of human osteosarcoma lung metastases for evaluating new therapeutic strategies, Clin Exp Metastasis 17 (1999) 501–506.

30. R.M. McAllister, M.B. Gardner & C. Bradt, et al., Cultivation *in vitro* of cells from a human osteosarcoma, Cancer 27 (1971) 397–402.

31. G. Masucci, P. Wersall & P. Ragnhammar, et al., Granulocyte-monocyte-colony-stimulating factor augments the cytotoxic capacity of lymphocytes and monocytes in antibody-dependent cellular cytotoxicity, Cancer Immunol Immunother 29 (1989) 288–292.

32. P.M. Anderson, S.N. Markovic & J.A. Sloan, et al., Aerosol granulocyte macrophage-colony stimulating factor: a low toxicity, lung-specific biological therapy in patients with lung metastases, Clin Cancer Res 5 (1999) 2316–2323.

33. R.D. Rao, P.M. Anderson & C.A. Arndt, et al., Aerosolized granulocyte macrophage colony-stimulating factor (GM-CSF) therapy in metastatic cancer, Am J Clin Oncol 26 (2003) 493–498.

34. E.S. Kleinerman, J.B. Gano & D.A. Johnston, et al., Efficacy of liposomal muramyl tripeptide (CGP 19835A) in the treatment of relapsed osteosarcoma, Am J Clin Oncol 18 (1995) 93–99.

35. P.A. Meyers, C.L. Schwartz & M. Krailo, et al., Osteosarcoma: a randomized, prospective trial of the addition of ifosfamide and/or muramyl tripeptide to cisplatin, doxorubicin, and high-dose methotrexate, J Clin Oncol 23 (2005) 2004–2011.

36. M. Decatris, S. Santhanam & K. O'Byrne, Potential of interferon-alpha in solid tumours: part 1, BioDrugs 16 (2002) 261–281.

37. S.F. Jia, T. An & L. Worth, et al., Interferon-alpha enhances the sensitivity of human osteosarcoma cells to etoposide, J Interferon Cytokine Res 19 (1999) 617–624.

38. H. Strander, H.C. Bauer & O. Brosjo, et al., Long-term adjuvant interferon treatment of human osteosarcoma. A pilot study, Acta Oncol 34 (1995) 877–880.

39. U. Nilsonne, L.A. Brostrom & T. Aparisi, Local tumour resection in interferon treated osteosarcoma patients, Ann Chir Gynaecol 84 (1995) 63–70.

40. K. Winkler, G. Beron & R. Kotz, et al., Neoadjuvant chemotherapy for osteogenic sarcoma: results of a Cooperative German/Austrian study, J Clin Oncol 2 (1984) 617–624.

41. J.H. Edmonson, H.J. Long & S. Frytak, et al., Phase II study of recombinant alfa-2a interferon in patients with advanced bone sarcomas, Cancer Treat Rep 71 (1987) 747–748.

42. S. Theoleyre, K. Mori & B. Cherrier, et al., Phenotypic and functional analysis of lymphocytes infiltrating osteolytic tumors: use as a possible therapeutic approach of osteosarcoma, BMC Cancer 5 (2005) 123–127.

43. C. Chauvin, J.-M. Philippeau & F.-X. Hubert, et al., Killer dendritic cells link innate and adaptive immunity against established osteosarcoma in rats, Cancer Res 68 (2008) 9433–9440.

44. S. Joyama, N. Naka & Y. Tsukamoto, et al., Dendritic cell immunotherapy is effective for lung metastasis from murine osteosarcoma, Clin Orthop Relat Res 453 (2006) 318–327.

45. C.W. Miller, A. Aslo & A. Won, et al., Alterations of the p53, Rb and MDM2 genes in osteosarcoma, J Cancer Res Clin Oncol 122 (1996) 559–565.

46. H. Masuda, C. Miller & H.P. Koeffler, et al., Rearrangement of the p53 gene in human osteogenic sarcomas, Proc Natl Acad Sci USA 84 (1987) 7716–7719.

47. B.D. Ragland, W.C. Bell & R.R. Lopez, et al., Cytogenetics and molecular biology of osteosarcoma, Lab Invest 82 (2002) 365–373.

48. H.J. Huang, J.K. Yee & J.Y. Shew, et al., Suppression of the neoplastic phenotype by replacement of the RB gene in human cancer cells, Science 242 (1988) 1563–1566.

49. M.M. Muncaster, B.L. Cohen & R.A. Phillips, et al., Failure of RB1 to reverse the malignant phenotype of human tumor cell lines, Cancer Res 52 (1992) 654–661.

50. Y.K. Fung, A. T'Ang & A.L. Murphree, et al., The Rb gene suppresses the growth of normal cells, Oncogene 8 (1993) 2659–2672.

51. Y. Haupt, S. Rowan & M. Oren, p53-Mediated apoptosis in HeLa cells can be overcome by excess pRB, Oncogene 10 (1995) 1563–1571.

52. D.A. Haas-Kogan, S.C. Kogan & D. Levi, et al., Inhibition of apoptosis by the retinoblastoma gene product, Embo J 14 (1995) 461–472.

53. D. Goodrich, The retinoblastoma tumor-suppressor gene, the exception that proves the rule, Oncogene 25 (2006) 5233–5243.

54. C.L. Densmore, E.S. Kleinerman & A. Gautam, et al., Growth suppression of established human osteosarcoma lung metastases in mice by aerosol gene therapy with PEI-p53 complexes, Cancer Gene Ther 8 (2001) 619–627.

55. M. Nakase, M. Inui & K. Okumura, et al., p53 Gene therapy of human osteosarcoma using a transferrin-modified cationic liposome, Mol Cancer Ther 4 (2005) 625–631.

56. S.U. Song & F.M. Boyce, Combination treatment for osteosarcoma with baculoviral vector mediated gene therapy (p53) and chemotherapy (adriamycin), Exp Mol Med 33 (2001) 46–53.

57. H. Ganjavi, M. Gee & A. Narendran, et al., Adenovirus-mediated p53 gene therapy in pediatric soft-tissue sarcoma cell lines: sensitization to cisplatin and doxorubicin, Cancer Gene Ther 12 (2005) 397–406.

58. O.J. Hellwinkel, J. Muller & A. Pollmann, et al., Osteosarcoma cell lines display variable individual reactions on wildtype p53 and Rb tumour-suppressor transgenes, J Gene Med 7 (2005) 407–419.

59. J.D. Oliner, K.W. Kinzler & P.S. Meltzer, et al., Amplification of a gene encoding a p53–associated protein in human sarcomas, Nature 358 (1992) 80–83.

60. Z. Peng, Current status of gendicine in China: recombinant human Ad-p53 agent for treatment of cancers, Hum Gene Ther 16 (2005) 1016–1027.

61. A.G. Zeimet & C. Marth, Why did p53 gene therapy fail in ovarian cancer?, Lancet Oncol 4 (2003) 415–422.

62. M. Witlox, V.W. Van Beusechem & J. Grill, et al., Epidermal growth factor receptor targeting enhances adenoviral vector based suicide gene therapy of osteosarcoma, J Gene Med 4 (2002) 510–516.

63. J.L. Charissoux, L. Grossin & M.J. Leboutet, et al., Treatment of experimental osteosarcoma tumors in rat by herpes simplex thymidine kinase gene transfer and ganciclovir, Anticancer Res 19 (1999) 77–80.

64. D. Dong, L. Dubeau & J. Bading, et al., Spontaneous and controllable activation of suicide gene expression driven by the stress-inducible grp78 promoter resulting in eradication of sizable human tumors, Hum Gene Ther 15 (2004) 553–561.

65. S.C. Ko, J. Cheon & C. Kao, et al., Osteocalcin promoter-based toxic gene therapy for the treatment of osteosarcoma in experimental models, Cancer Res 56 (1996) 4614–4619.

66. J. Cheon, S.C. Ko & T.A. Gardner, et al., Chemogene therapy: osteocalcin promoter-based suicide gene therapy in combination with methotrexate in a murine osteosarcoma model, Cancer Gene Ther 4 (1997) 359–365.

67. R. Benjamin, L. Helman & P. Meyers, et al., A phase I/II dose escalation and activity study of intravenous injections of OCaP1 for subjects with refractory osteosarcoma metastatic to lung, Hum Gene Ther 12 (2001) 1591–1593.

68. N.G. Rainov, A phase III clinical evaluation of herpes simplex virus type 1 thymidine kinase and ganciclovir gene therapy as an adjuvant to surgical resection and radiation in adults with previously untreated glioblastoma multiforme, Hum Gene Ther 11 (2000) 2389–2401.

69. U. Fischer, S. Steffens & S. Frank, et al., Mechanisms of thymidine kinase/ganciclovir and cytosine deaminase/5-fluorocytosine suicide gene therapy-induced cell death in glioma cells, Oncogene 24 (2005) 1231–1243.

70. M. Ramnaraine, W. Pan & M. Goblirsch, et al., Direct and bystander killing of sarcomas by novel cytosine deaminase fusion gene, Cancer Res 63 (2003) 6847–6854.

71. M.L. Ramnaraine, W.E. Mathews & J.M. Donohue, et al., Osteoclasts direct bystander killing of bone cancer, Cancer Res 66 (2006) 10929–10935.

72. D. Oosterhoff, M.A. Witlox & V.W. van Beusechem, et al., Gene-directed enzyme prodrug therapy for osteosarcoma: sensitization to CPT-11 *in vitro* and *in vivo* by adenoviral delivery of a gene encoding secreted carboxylesterase-2, Mol Cancer Ther 2 (2003) 765–771.

73. C. Liebau, C. Roesel & S. Schmidt, et al., Immunotherapy by gene transfer with plasmids encoding IL-12/IL-18 is superior to IL-23/IL-18 gene transfer in a rat osteosarcoma model, Anticancer Res 24 (2004) 2861–2867.

74. S.F. Jia, L.L. Worth & C.L. Densmore, et al., Aerosol gene therapy with PEI: IL-12 eradicates osteosarcoma lung metastases, Clin Cancer Res 9 (2003) 3462–3468.

75. X. Duan, S.F. Jia & N. Koshkina, et al., Intranasal interleukin-12 gene therapy enhanced the activity of ifosfamide against osteosarcoma lung metastases, Cancer 106 (2006) 1382–1388.

76. S.F. Jia, X. Duan & L.L. Worth, et al., Intratumor murine interleukin-12 gene therapy suppressed the growth of local and distant Ewing's sarcoma, Cancer Gene Ther 13 (2006) 948–957.

77. E.A. Lafleur, S.F. Jia & L.L. Worth, et al., Interleukin (IL)-12 and IL-12 gene transfer up-regulate Fas expression in human osteosarcoma and breast cancer cells, Cancer Res 61 (2001) 4066–4071.

78. R. Luksch, D. Perotti & G. Cefalo, et al., Immunomodulation in a treatment program including pre- and post-operative interleukin-2 and chemotherapy for childhood osteosarcoma, Tumori 89 (2003) 263–268.

79. J.H. de Wilt, A. Bout & A.M. Eggermont, et al., Adenovirus-mediated interleukin 3 beta gene transfer by isolated limb perfusion inhibits growth of limb sarcoma in rats, Hum Gene Ther 12 (2001) 489–502.

80. S. Nagano, K. Yuge & M. Fukunaga, et al., Gene therapy eradicating distant disseminated micro-metastases by optimal cytokine expression in the primary lesion only: novel concepts for successful cytokine gene therapy, Int J Oncol 24 (2004) 549–558.

81. T.A. Guise, K.S. Mohammad & G. Clines, et al., Basic mechanisms responsible for osteolytic and osteoblastic bone metastases, Clin Cancer Res 12 (2006) 6213s–6216s.

82. F. Saad, D.M. Gleason & R. Murray, et al., A randomized, placebo-controlled trial of zoledronic acid in patients with hormone-refractory metastatic prostate carcinoma, J Natl Cancer Inst 94 (2002) 1458–1468.

83. A. Lipton, R.L. Theriault & G.N. Hortobagyi, et al., Pamidronate prevents skeletal complications and is effective palliative treatment in women with breast carcinoma and osteolytic bone metastases: long-term follow-up of two randomized, placebo-controlled trials, Cancer 88 (2000) 1082–1090.

84. B. Ory, M.F. Heymann & A. Kamijo, et al., Zoledronic acid suppresses lung metastases and prolongs overall survival of osteosarcoma-bearing mice, Cancer 104 (2005) 2522–2529.

85. A. Evdokiou, A. Labrinidis & S. Bouralexis, et al., Induction of cell death of human osteogenic sarcoma cells by zoledronic acid resembles anoikis, Bone 33 (2003) 216–228.

86. D. Heymann, B. Ory & F. Gouin, et al., Bisphosphonates: new therapeutic agents for the treatment of bone tumors, Trends Mol Med 10 (2004) 337–343.

87. P.I. Croucher, C.M. Shipman & J. Lippitt, et al., Osteoprotegerin inhibits the development of osteolytic bone disease in multiple myeloma, Blood 98 (2001) 3534–3540.

88. S. Morony, C. Capparelli & I. Sarosi, et al., Osteoprotegerin inhibits osteolysis and decreases skeletal tumor burden in syngeneic and nude mouse models of experimental bone metastasis, Cancer Res 61 (2001) 4432–4436.

89. H. Yonou, N. Kanomata & M. Goya, et al., Osteoprotegerin/osteoclastogenesis inhibitory factor decreases human prostate cancer burden in human adult bone implanted into non-obese diabetic/severe combined immunodeficient mice, Cancer Res 63 (2003) 2096–2102.

90. N.M. Luger, P. Honore & M.A. Sabino, et al., Osteoprotegerin diminishes advanced bone cancer pain, Cancer Res 61 (2001) 4038–4047.

91. I. Holen & C.M. Shipman, Role of osteoprotegerin (OPG) in cancer, Clin Sci (Lond) 110 (2006) 279–291.

92. F. Lamoureux, P. Richard & Y. Wittrant, et al., Therapeutic relevance of osteoprotegerin gene therapy in osteosarcoma: blockade of the vicious cycle between tumor cell proliferation and bone resorption, Cancer Res 67 (2007) 7308–7318.

93. S. Theoleyre, Y. Wittrant & S. Couillaud, et al., Cellular activity and signaling induced by osteoprotegerin in osteoclasts: involvement of receptor activator of nuclear factor kappaB ligand and MAPK, Biochim Biophys Acta 1644 (2004) 1–7.

94. D.H. Jones, T. Nakashima & O.H. Sanchez, et al., Regulation of cancer cell migration and bone metastasis by RANKL, Nature 440 (2006) 692–696.

95. D.J. Heath, K. Vanderkerken & X. Cheng, et al., An osteoprotegerin-like peptidomimetic inhibits osteoclastic bone resorption and osteolytic bone disease in myeloma, Cancer Res 67 (2007) 202–208.

96. B.O. Oyajobi, D.M. Anderson & K. Traianedes, et al., Therapeutic efficacy of a soluble receptor activator of nuclear factor kappaB-IgG Fc fusion protein in suppressing bone resorption and hypercalcemia in a model of humoral hypercalcemia of malignancy, Cancer Res 61 (2001) 2572–2578.

97. R.N. Pearse, E.M. Sordillo & S. Yaccoby, et al., Multiple myeloma disrupts the TRANCE/osteoprotegerin cytokine axis to trigger bone destruction and promote tumor progression, Proc Natl Acad Sci USA 98 (2001) 11581–11586.

98. J. Zhang, J. Dai & Z. Yao, et al., Soluble receptor activator of nuclear factor kappaB Fc diminishes prostate cancer progression in bone, Cancer Res 63 (2003) 7883–7890.

99. M. Skotzko, L. Wu & W.F. Anderson, et al., Retroviral vector-mediated gene transfer of antisense cyclin G1 (CYCG1) inhibits proliferation of human osteogenic sarcoma cells, Cancer Res 55 (1995) 5493–5498.

100. D.S. Chen, N.L. Zhu & G. Hung, et al., Retroviral vector-mediated transfer of an antisense cyclin G1 construct inhibits osteosarcoma tumor growth in nude mice, Hum Gene Ther 8 (1997) 1667–1674.

101. G.R. Stark, I.M. Kerr & B.R. Williams, et al., How cells respond to interferons, Annu Rev Biochem 67 (1998) 227–264.

102. S.M. Elbashir, J. Harborth & W. Lendeckel, et al., Duplexes of 21-nucleotide RNAs mediate RNA interference in cultured mammalian cells, Nature 411 (2001) 494–498.

103. G. van der Pluijm, I. Que & B. Sijmons, et al., Interference with the microenvironmental support impairs the *de novo* formation of bone metastases *in vivo*, Cancer Res 65 (2005) 7682–7690.

104. D.W. Bartlett & M.E. Davis, Insights into the kinetics of siRNA-mediated gene silencing from live-cell and live-animal bioluminescent imaging, Nucleic Acids Res 34 (2006) 322–333.

105. S. Paget, The distribution of secondary growths in cancer of the breast, Lancet 1 (1889) 571–572.

106. J.M. Chirgwin, K.S. Mohammad & T.A. Guise, Tumor-bone cellular interactions in skeletal metastases, J Musculoskelet Neuronal Interact 4 (2004) 308–318.

CHAPTER **29**

In vivo Models Used in Studies of Bone Metastases

INGUNN HOLEN[1] AND MICHELLE A. LAWSON[2]

[1]*Academic Unit of Clinical Oncology, School of Medicine and Biomedical Sciences, University of Sheffield, Sheffield S10 2RX, UK.*
[2]*Academic Unit of Bone Biology, School of Medicine and Biomedical Sciences, University of Sheffield, Sheffield S10 2RX, UK.*

Contents

I. INTRODUCTION

In human disease, bone metastasis formation is a slow process often developing years after the initial tumor has been diagnosed and treated. The presence of bone metastases is commonly only detected when patients present with late stage and therefore symptomatic disease, at a point when the tumors are fairly big and extensive bone lesions have developed. In addition, bone is an inaccessible site that is not routinely biopsied or otherwise sampled. Studies using human material are further complicated by the fact that this group of patients may have undergone extensive therapeutic interventions during the treatment of their primary tumor, which may also affect the subsequent development of bone metastases. As a result, our understanding of the precise biological mechanisms responsible for bone metastases formation is incomplete, hampering the development of successful treatment and prevention strategies. In order to address this problem, researchers have turned increasingly to the use of animal models, although these generally represent only particular stages of human disease rather than the gradual transition from benign disease through hyperplasia and subsequent aggressive and advanced metastatic disease. Bone metastases represent a particular challenge, as these are often preceded or accompanied by visceral metastasis that have profound effects on morbidity and survival [1].

The majority of *in vivo* studies of bone metastases use rodents, mainly mice, as these are widely available, have a short life span, and a relatively large number of animals can be easily investigated. Only a few specialist facilities have the capacity to carry out research using larger animals (primarily dogs), and as a result only a limited amount of work is carried out using such models. However, rodents do not naturally develop bone metastases, suggesting that they do not provide the optimal setting to study this aspect of human cancer, and key molecules and mechanisms that drive human disease may potentially be missed in murine model systems. Despite their clear limitations, *in vivo* models of bone metastases have provided valuable insights into the molecules and pathways that may play a role in the development of human disease, as well as the effects of a range of therapies.

II. MODELS USED IN STUDIES OF BREAST CANCER BONE METASTASES

Patients with advanced breast cancer are at high risk of developing bone metastases, associated with a high degree of morbidity and mortality. As covered elsewhere in this volume, the bone lesions arise as a result of complex molecular interactions and involve a range of cell types, including tumor cells, osteoblasts, osteoclasts, immune cells and cells of the vasculature [2]. The net outcome is excessive bone resorption leading to generation of lytic lesions. In order to increase our understanding of the processes underlying the development of breast cancer bone metastases, a number of different models have been described [3–5]. The main focus has been on generation of models that display the characteristic lytic lesions associated with breast cancer-induced bone disease, and examples of these will be described in the following sections.

A. Xenograft Models

The majority of *in vivo* studies of bone metastases have used xenograft models, where human tumor cells are implanted in immunocompromised animals, most often mice [6], although corresponding models using rats are also available [7]. The human tumor cells are now routinely engineered to express either green fluorescent protein (GFP) or luciferase, allowing non-invasive *in vivo* monitoring of tumor development. Depending on the cell line used, the age and strain of the animal as well as the route of implantation, tumors will develop in bone within 3–5 weeks, providing the opportunity to study both the biological aspects of bone metastases as well as the effects of therapeutics [8–10].

1. INTRACARDIAC INJECTION

By injecting human breast cancer cells into the left ventricle of the heart of immunocompromised mice, the cells will bypass the pulmonary vasculature resulting in widespread metastasis formation in several sites including bone within 4–5 weeks [11]. This method requires a high degree of technical skill, but does provide a model of early growth and development of breast cancer bone metastases. However, it does not represent the initial steps in the disease process, where tumor cells leave a primary site (breast), enter the circulation and subsequently re-colonize a distant site (bone). Intracardiac injection of breast cancer cells has been used to investigate the role of tumor cell derived factors in accelerated bone turnover, as well as the ability of bone-derived molecules to support tumor cell growth. The effects of therapeutic agents like anti-resorptives on bone metastases and the associated bone disease have also been studied using this type of model.

Mechanisms of Bone Metastasis Formation The intracardiac injection model was used by Phadke and colleagues to perform a detailed and informative study of the kinetics of breast cancer cell trafficking in bone [12]. Following injections of 1.5×10^6 GFP-expressing MDA-MB-435 cells into the left ventricle of female athymic mice (4–6 weeks of age), animals were sacrificed at different time points ranging from very early (1, 2, 4, 8 hour post injection), intermediate (days 1, 2, 3) and after longer periods (2, 4 and 6 weeks). Bones were isolated and extensive histological and histomorphometric analysis of the femurs carried out combined with fluorescence microscopy, FACS analysis and real time PCR for detection of tumor cells. This allowed charting the precise localization of breast cancer cells during progression of bone metastases, from the initial colonization to advanced bone disease. The study showed that 1 hour following injection, tumor cells can be detected in the highly vascularized methaphysis of the femur, but that these then gradually cleared over the next 72 hours. One week after injection small tumor cell foci (around 10 cells) were detected in bone, mainly located to the distal methaphysis. During the next 2–3 weeks, a few of these develop

into larger tumors that eventually are associated with loss of the majority of the trabecular bone and replacing the bone marrow in the medullary canal. In addition to generating information on early tumor growth in bone, this study also provided new knowledge relating to the effects of increasing numbers of tumor cells on osteoblasts and osteoclasts, and how this relates to the extent of bone destruction. The analysis revealed that tumor growth was associated with an increase in the number of apoptotic osteoblasts, resulting in a substantial decrease in osteoblast number. Surprisingly, there was also a decrease in the number of osteoclasts of up to 60% compared to control 4 weeks after tumor cell injection. By determining the osteoblast:osteoclast ratio at different time points the authors found that this was reduced from around 40:1 to 4:1 by 4 weeks, indicating that bone turnover would be shifted towards increased resorption. These data show that an early event following the arrival of breast cancer cells in bone is a rapid depletion of bone forming cells mediated by an as yet unknown mechanism, probably preventing repair of tumor-induced lytic lesions. The implications for human disease are that an effort should be made to develop therapeutic strategies to protect the osteoblast from the detrimental effects of tumor cells, for use in combination with anti-resorptive agents.

The Effects of Therapies Models based on intracardiac injection of breast cancer cells have also been used to study effects of therapeutics on cancer-induced bone disease. Changes in the normal ratio of receptor activator of NF-kappaB ligand (RANKL) and its soluble decoy receptor osteoprotegerin (OPG) may lead to increased osteolysis in human bone metastases. Canon and colleagues investigated how administration of recombinant osteoprotegerin (Fc-OPG) influenced bone disease and survival of mice with bone metastases following intracardiac injection of 1×10^5 luciferase expressing MDA-MB-231Luc cells [13]. Bioluminescence imaging revealed that OPG-Fc inhibited growth of MDA-MB-231 tumor cells in bony sites *in vivo* when given both as a preventative (day 0) and as a therapeutic agent for established bone metastases (day 7). OPG-Fc inhibited tumor-induced osteoclastogenesis and osteolysis in a dose-dependent fashion, 3 mg/kg OPG-Fc causing complete inhibition of osteoclast formation, accompanied by reduced tumor burden and increased levels of tumor cell apoptosis. These results support that RANKL is an important regulator of bone metastases and therefore an attractive therapeutic target. This study was the first to show that survival of mice with established bone metastases could be improved by treatment with OPG-Fc, and demonstrated the importance of tumor cell-stromal interactions for the development and progression of cancer-induced bone disease.

By genetic manipulation of the cancer cells prior to intracardiac injection, the role of particular molecules in bone metastases formation can be elucidated. This has been done by the group of Teti, who transfected MDA-MB-231 cells to overexpress the proto-oncogene c-Src, to investigate how this affected the ability of the cells to metastasize [14]. Female BALB/c-nu/nu mice injected with 1×10^5 MDA-231 cells stably transfected with wild-type c-Src (MDA-231-SrcWT) had increased metastatic disease compared to control. Injection of cells transfected with a c-Src kinase-dead dominant-negative construct (MDA-231-SrcDN) resulted in reduced levels of metastases, accompanied by reduced IL-6 and IL-1b expression by osteoblasts. The authors conclude that c-Src may be a suitable therapeutic target in breast cancer, as disruption of c-Src activity affects the metastatic process both in bone and in soft tissue.

B. Intravenous Injection

In view of the technical challenges associated with intracardiac injection of tumor cells, several groups have developed particular breast cancer cell lines that have the ability to home to bone following intravenous injection. These have been generated by isolation of cells from bone metastases (originally introduced by intracardiac injection), expanding the cells in culture and re-inoculating them into the left ventricle. Following a number of passages through bone [5–6] clones that home specifically to bone following intravenous injection have been isolated and characterized.

1. MECHANISMS OF BONE METASTASIS FORMATION

Using this approach, the group of Clezardin developed the BO2 model, generating a bone-homing strain of MDA-MB-231 breast cancer cells [15]. This was used to investigate whether therapeutic targeting of tumor alphavbeta3 integrin prevents bone metastasis formation [16]. Alphavbeta3-overexpressing or mock-transfected BO2 breast cancer cells were injected i.v. in immunocompromised mice, and the levels of bone metastasis and osteolytic lesions compared. Both tumor burden and extent of bone disease were found to be increased in animals injected with alphavbeta3-overexpressing cells. The ability of this model to reveal the molecules involved in very early stages of bone metastases formation is supported by the fact that direct intratibial inoculation of alphavbeta3-overexpressing cells did not increase skeletal tumor burden or bone destruction, compared to that caused by mock transfected tumor cells. Subsequent studies using an inhibitor of alphavbeta3 (PSK1404) showed significant inhibition of bone marrow colonization by alphavbeta3-expressing tumor cells *in vivo*, supporting that this integrin may be a potential therapeutic target for the prevention of skeletal metastases.

The BO2 model was used by Peyruchaud *et al.* to determine the potential role of platelet-derived lysophosphatidic acid (LPA) in the progression of breast cancer bone metastases [17]. MDA-BO2 cells overexpressing the LPA$_1$ receptor promoted bone metastasis formation in mice by increasing skeletal breast tumor growth and the extent of lytic bone lesions. BO2 cells did not produce LPA, but were found to induce the release of LPA from activated platelets, resulting in secretion of IL-6 and IL-8 leading to cytokine-induced osteoclast-mediated bone destruction. When animals bearing LPA1-overexpressing BO2 tumors were treated with the platelet antagonist Integrilin, progression of bone metastases was strongly inhibited. This study illustrates the important role of the microenvironment in the development of bone metastases, and was the first to show that platelet-derived factors may drive parts of the metastatic process in breast cancer.

2. THE EFFECTS OF THERAPIES

The effects of therapeutic agents used to treat cancer-induced bone disease have also been investigated using the BO2 model. Daubine and colleagues compared the anti-tumor effects of clinical dosing regimens of the two bisphosphonates zoledronic acid (98–100µg/kg) and clodronate (530µg/kg/day) [18]. Treatment administered prior to injection of tumor cells (preventive protocols) was compared to treatment starting once lytic bone lesions had developed (treatment protocols). Bone destruction was measured by radiography, x-ray absorptiometry or tomography, and histomorphometry. The BO2 cells used expressed both GFP and luciferase, and skeletal tumor burden was assessed by histomorphometry and luciferase activity. Mice treated with a daily preventive regimen of clodronate, or with a daily or weekly preventive regimen of zoledronic acid, showed a decreased tumor burden compared to that in mice treated with vehicle, whereas a single preventive dose of zoledronic acid had no effect. The authors concluded that daily or repeated intermittent therapy with clinical doses of bisphosphonates inhibits skeletal tumor growth in this mouse model.

Successful eradication of tumor cells in bone may require the combination of therapeutic agents that target the tumor cells with agents that modify the bone microenvironment. The effects of the chemotherapeutic agent doxorubicin combined with a single administration of the potent anti-resorptive agent zoledronic acid on tumor growth in bone has been reported using the BO2 model [19]. In this study, treatment commenced once lytic bone lesions were evident, when mice with equal tumor burden were divided into the following treatment groups: placebo, 2 mg/kg doxorubicin weekly, 100 µg/kg zoledronic acid (once), doxorubicin and zoledronic acid simultaneously, or doxorubicin followed 24 hours later by zoledronic acid. The study showed that a single administration of zoledronic acid did prevent the progression of lytic bone lesions, whether given alone or in combination with doxorubicin. In contrast, tumor volume was only significantly reduced in the animals receiving the sequential administration of doxorubicin followed 24 hours later by zoledronic acid. No effects of any of the treatments were found when extra-osseous tumor growth was assessed, suggesting that the doses of the therapeutic agents sufficient to affect tumor growth directly are only available within the bone marrow cavity. The data generated in this study suggest that breast cancer patients may benefit from the use of combined therapies even in the advanced setting.

3. Intra-osseous Implantation

Bone metastases can also be generated by implantation of human breast cancer cells directly into bone of immuno-compromised mice, most commonly following intratibial injection (example described in Gordon and colleagues). These models are generally used to investigate late stage disease, as a large number of tumor cells are introduced directly into bone, bypassing the early steps of homing and colonization [20]. In this method, holes are drilled in the tibia of anesthetized animals, and the bone marrow flushed out and replaced by a suspension of GFP-expressing tumor cells. This technique will inevitably cause some damage to the bone near the injection site, which may compli-cate analysis of the subsequent tumor-induced changes of bone structure. In the first few days following injection the majority of the tumor cells will die, as determined by the loss of detectable GFP, but sufficient numbers survive to generate bone tumors within 3–4 weeks. These are gener-ally restricted to trabecular areas, and develop rapidly once established. It is assumed that the tumor cells will prefer-ably colonize areas associated with active bone resorption, although the importance of the putative stem cell niche in initial tumor cell growth has now become a novel area of interest [21]. One hypothesis is that only tumor cells with stem cell characteristics that reach specific stem cell niches in bone (possibly the hemapoetic stem cell niche) are able to develop into new tumors. This may explain why less than 0.1% of tumor cells that are injected directly into bone sub-sequently establish colonies. Intratibial injection of breast cancer cells has been used in a number of studies both of molecular pathways involved in tumor cell-bone cell inter-actions, and of effects of therapeutics of bone metastases.

Mechanisms of Bone Metastasis Formation Fisher and colleagues used intratibial implantation of MCF-7 cells overexpressing PTHrP and osteoprotegerin (OPG) in athymic nude mice to examine the effect of local tumor production of OPG on the ability of breast cancer cells to establish and grow in bone [22]. The study showed that there was increased tumor growth and osteolysis in mice receiving MCF-7 cells overexpressing PTHrP and OPG, compared to that seen in mice receiving the paren-tal MCF-7 cells. In marked contrast, administration of recombinant Fc-OPG reduced tumor growth and limited osteolysis even in mice inoculated with OPG overexpress-ing cells. The data suggest that there may be a difference between the biological actions of tumor cell-derived OPG, compared to therapeutically administered recombinant constructs like Fc-OPG.

The effects of high versus low bone turnover on bone metastases formation has been studied following intrati-bial implantation of 5×10^4 MDA-MB-231 Tx-SA cells in nude mice maintained on a normal (0.6%) or a low (0.1%) calcium diet that were treated with either recombinant osteoprotegerin OPG (1 mg/kg/d s.c.) or vehicle [23]. OPG treatment increased serum PTH levels but caused substan-tial inhibition of bone resorption. In mice receiving low Ca alone, lytic lesion area, tumor area, and cancer cell prolifer-ation increased by 43, 24, and 24%, respectively, compared with mice receiving normal Ca ($p < 0.01$). In the low Ca group, OPG treatment reduced total tumor area in bone as well as prevented the appearance of lytic lesions, decreased cancer cell proliferation, and increased cancer cell apop-tosis. The authors conclude that increased bone turnover due to dietary calcium deficiency promotes tumor growth in bone, independent of the action of PTH, suggesting that breast cancer patients may benefit from treatments to nor-malize calcium both in the adjuvant and advanced setting.

The Effects of Therapies Intratibial tumor cell injec-tion has been used to investigate the effects of therapies on breast cancer-induced bone disease; in particular in relation to reducing the number and severity of lytic bone lesions. Zheng and colleagues investigated the potential anti-tumor effects of OPG and the anti-resorptive agent ibandro-nate (IBN), alone and in combination, on intratibial tumor growth [24]. Tumors could be detected 10 days following implantation of MDA-MB-231 cells, and mice were then treated with vehicle, OPG (1 mg/kg/day), IBN (160 microg/kg/day) or IBN and OPG at the same doses (IBN + OPG) for a week, and the effects on lytic lesions, tumor cell growth, apoptosis and proliferation were measured by radiography, immunohistochemistry and histomorphom-etry. The development of lytic lesions was inhibited by all treatments compared to vehicle controls, accompanied by a reduction in tumor area. OPG and IBN alone, and in com-bination, each produced a similar increase in cancer cell apoptosis (OPG 330%, IBN 342%, IBN and OPG 347%, $p < 0.01$ vs vehicle) and a decrease in cancer cell prolifera-tion (OPG 59%, IBN 62%, IBN and OPG 58%, $p < 0.05$ vs vehicle). The authors conclude that there is no additional benefit by combining OPG and IBN compared to using the single agents, and that both agents seem mainly to affect tumor volume indirectly by preventing the development of tumor-induced bone disease.

C. Syngeneic Models

Whereas the xenograft models described above represent several of the stages of tumor development in bone, they do not include the initial steps of bone metastasis forma-tion. Syngeneic models (e.g., 4T1) have therefore been developed, where implantation of murine tumor cells into the mammary fat pad of female, immunocompe-tent, Balb/c mice results in subsequent tumor spread and development of bone and visceral metastasis (lung, liver, kidney) within 3–4 weeks. 4T1 is a mammary carcinoma originally derived from a spontaneously arising mammary tumor in BALB/cfC3H mice [25]. This model includes the growth of the initial mammary tumor in an anatomically correct site, followed by metastatic spread to a range of distant organs, thereby mimicking human breast cancer. By using immunocompetent animals the model has the advantage that it can be used to study the role of the immune system, both in tumor progression in bone as well as in response to anti-cancer therapy. However, syngeneic models do have some important limitations. The murine tumor cells differ from human breast cancer cells in the genetic makeup and potentially in their growth characteristics and responses to anti-cancer agents. In addition, the primary mammary tumors grow quickly once established, leaving a limited window of opportunity for studies of the metastases before animals must be sacrificed for welfare reasons. Alternatively, the primary tumor may be removed, but this complicates the model and requires surgical skills. The 4T1 model has been used to study effects of therapies on early stages of tumor spread to bone, and detection of tumor growth has been aided by stable transfection of the cells with a luciferase reporter gene (4T1/Luc).

1. MECHANISMS OF BONE METASTASIS FORMATION

A version of the model using luciferase expressing 4T1-12B cells has been developed by Tao and colleagues for studies of the role of innate and acquired immunity in metastasis formation [26]. They found that following implantation of the original 4T1-12B cell line only 2/6 animals developed bone metastases, and these were evident throughout the skeleton including skull, sternum and ribs as well as long bones. The animals also displayed brain, intestine and kidney metastasis. In contrast, implantation of a different version of the line (4T1-1V) caused skeletal metastases in 6/7 animals. This study is highlighting the differential ability of closely related cells to spread to the bone microenvironment, and illustrates some of the problems associated with studying bone metastases in a model where visceral metastasis are also prevalent.

Rose and colleagues have used the 4T1 model to identify novel genes involved in bone metastases formation [27]. By *in vivo* selection, several populations of 4T1 cells with increased capacity to form bone metastasis were identified, displaying increased capacity for invasion and migration. Subsequent comparative gene expression analysis revealed a subset of genes that were associated with the increased bone metastatic potential. Overexpression of one of the factors identified, osteoactivin, was shown to increase bone metastatic capability and subsequent osteolysis of weak bone metastatic cells. The authors suggest that osteoactivin is a protein that is capable of promoting breast cancer metastasis to bone.

2. THE EFFECTS OF THERAPIES

Hiraga and colleagues used the 4T1 model to examine the effects of the anti-resorptive agent zoledronic acid (ZOL) on metastasis formation [28]. Following orthotopic implantation of 1×10^6 4T1/luc cells in the mammary fat pad in 6-week-old female BALB/c mice, metastases were detected in multiple organs including bone, lung, and liver. The mice received single or four i.v. injections of ZOL (0.5 or 5 μg/mouse), and metastasis formation evaluated. In this study, only treatment with the highest dose of ZOL (5 μg) was found to cause a marked reduction in bone, lung and liver metastases, resulting in prolonged overall survival of the tumor-bearing mice. Detailed analysis of the metastasis revealed that ZOL treatment induced increased levels of tumor cell apoptosis in the bone metastases, but not in the visceral metastases. These results support the theory that, in addition to causing tumor cell death in bone, zoledronic acid affects breast cancer metastasis to visceral organs, potentially by inhibiting migration and invasion of breast cancer cells.

The role of vacuolar ATPase (V-ATPase) in cancer-induced bone disease has been investigated by administration of the V-ATPase inhibitor FR202126 (3.2 mg/kg orally, daily for 29 days) following injection [29] of 1×10^6 4T1 into the mammary fat pad in 6-week-old immunocompetent BALB/c mice. Bone mineral density (BMD) of the proximal tibia was measured using peripheral quantitative computed tomography, and the number of osteoclasts determined following histomorphometric analysis. Administration of the V-ATPase inhibitor caused a reduction in the levels of osteolysis reflected by decreased numbers of osteoclasts, compared to vehicle treated animals. The authors suggest that the V-ATPase inhibitor might be a useful anti-resorptive agent, potentially able to alleviate bone pain associated with metastatic bone disease caused by stimulation of acid-sensitive receptors.

D. Human-to-Human Models

In an effort to capture the species-specific organ tropism involved in homing of breast cancer cells to bone, 'human-to-human' models have been developed, using subcutaneous implantation of pieces of human bone in immunocompromised animals. Human breast cancer cells are subsequently injected, either i.v., in the mammary fat pad or directly into the marrow cavity of the human bone. Alternatively, tumor cells and bone fragments are implanted together. One obvious advantage of these models is that they provide the tumor cells with access to the appropriate human bone microenvironment, as opposed to the murine xenograft systems described above. Indeed this may be a requirement for some human cancer cells to grow in bone. However, the bone fragments used have frequently either been fetal or from patients undergoing hip replacements, and not from breast cancer patients with bone metastases. In order to generate consistent bone metastasis the cancer cells must be introduced directly into the bone, whereas tumors implanted in the mammary fat pad generate low frequency of bone colonization. These results are in agreement with the observation that not all breast cancer cells home to bone even when the right microenvironment is available. A complication of this model is that there may be problems with a graft versus graft immune response, as the human bone and the human tumor cells are of different origin. Despite these limitations, human-to-human models are likely to become increasingly important as we seek to understand the pivotal role of the bone microenvironment in the development of bone metastases.

1. Mechanisms of Bone Metastasis Formation

The Rosenblatt group has developed a model to investigate the breast cancer colonization of human bone [30]. In their initial experiments, fragments of human adult bone were implanted in the flanks of female NOD/SCID mice, and the implants harvested and characterized at different time points post implantation. The fragments were viable for up to 12 weeks and contained osteoblasts, osteoclasts and a range of stromal cells including endothelial cells. The bone was well vascularized with both mouse and human-derived vessels contributing, and by week 12 there was evidence of new bone formation associated with the fragments. High levels of human IgG were detectable in the blood of the animals, indicating human B cells originating from the bone fragments which were present and functional for prolonged periods of time following implantation. The ability of tumor cells to home to the human bone was determined using a range of different breast cancer cell lines, cells were injected i.v. and i.p. 4 weeks following implantation of the bone fragments. These included MDA-MB-231, MCF7, MCF10A cells and a range of SUM lines derived from primary or metastatic breast cancer samples (SUM 159, SUM 149, SUM 225, SUM 229, SUM 190, SUM 1315). Histological examination of the lungs and bone fragments 8 weeks later showed that only one cell line had generated bone metastases (SUM 1315). Subsequent experiments found that orthotopically implanted (mammary fat pad) SUM 1315 cells colonized bone fragments in 4/20 animals, and that these also displayed lung metastases [31]. Importantly, the mice did not have any evidence of bone disease, supporting the species-specific bone tropism of this cell line. Perhaps surprisingly, this study also showed that the MDA-MB-231 cell line commonly used in xenograft bone metastases models was unable to colonize human bone implanted in mice, indicating that these cells do not have a true bone metastatic potential.

The importance of the presence of a human bone microenvironment for human breast cancer cells to metastasize has been investigated by Yang and colleagues, using co-transplantation of GFP-MDA-MB-231 breast cancer cells with human bone fragments (isolated from patients undergoing hip replacements) into NOD/SCID mice [32]. Bone fragments of approximately 1 cm^3 implanted into both flanks of 10-week-old mice were shown to be viable for at least 20 weeks. 5×10^6 GFP-expressing MDA-MB-231 cells were either mixed with morcellized human bone prior to implantation (co-transplantation protocol), or alternatively cells were injected i.v. after implantation of bone fragments (bone-homing protocol). MDA-MB-231 cells were shown to only form lung metastasis following i.v. injection in the absence of human bone implants; whereas tumor growth was detected in the human bone implants in 3/3 animals at 4 weeks. Metastasis from the co-implantation site to the opposite non-tumor bearing human bone fragments were detected in two thrids of animals, whereas no bone metastases were detected in the mouse skeleton. The study also addressed whether cells from human breast cancer bone metastasis specimens would generate new bone metastasis when access was provided to human bone microenvironment. In 4/10 animals, tumor growth was detected at 20 weeks in the tumor-free bone implanted in the opposite flank, showing that the tumor cells had preferentially migrated from the original human bone site to a second distant site providing a favorable bone microenvironment. This pioneering study shows that tumor cells do preferentially colonize sites where the specific local conditions support their expansion, and that the human bone microenvironment is key in the metastatic process. The authors suggest that this model can be further developed as an *in vivo* testing system to identify breast tumors with the capacity to metastasize to bone. However, the importance of the nature and origin of the recipient bone fragment for the metastatic process remains to be established.

III. *IN VIVO* MODELS OF PROSTATE CANCER BONE METASTASES

As in the case for breast cancer, bone metastasis is also a common clinical feature of advanced prostate cancer, associated with accelerated levels of bone turnover and considerable morbidity for the patients. Prostate cancer bone metastases are generally described as osteosclerotic, involving excess bone formation, but there is also a substantial increase in the osteoclastic bone resorption providing a lytic component to the metastatic process. Compared to breast cancer, there are fewer cell lines and *in vivo* model systems available for studies of bone metastases in prostate cancer, and none of these accurately represent the osteoblastic/osteosclerotic phenotype that characterizes human disease [33,34]. Although mixed lesions have been described, the models are mainly restricted to mimicking the osteolytic component of the disease, illustrating our limited understanding of the dysregulation of bone formation caused by prostate cancer cells [35].

A. Xenograft Models

1. INTRACARDIAC INJECTION

As described above for breast cancer, injection of prostate cancer cells via the intracardiac route will lead to tumor cell colonization of distant organs including bone. The majority of published studies report that the tumors that subsequently develop in bone are predominantly associated with the appearance of lytic bone lesions.

Mechanisms of Bone Metastasis Formation The role of active bone turnover for the formation of prostate cancer bone metastasis was investigated by Schneider and colleagues, following intra-cardiac injection of 2×10^5 luciferase-expressing PC-3Luc prostate cancer cells in male athymic mice that had undergone 1 week treatment with PTH to accelerate bone turnover [36]. Groups of young (4-weeks-old) and adult (15-weeks-old) male mice received either PTH (80 µg/kg) or saline daily for 7 days prior to and 7 days after intracardiac inoculation of PC-3Luc cells, and subsequent tumor growth was assessed by bioluminescence imaging weekly for 5 weeks. In young animals, there was no difference in tumor incidence between the saline and PTH treated groups, with tumors associated with lytic bone

lesions appearing in the hind limbs and craniofacial regions. In contrast, there was a marked increase in tumor burden in PTH treated adult mice compared to control, as assessed by intensity of the bioluminescece signals. Only PTH treated animals had evidence of bone metastasis in the hind limbs. Labeling of newly formed bone by injection of calcein prior to sacrifice showed that there was a significant increase in the percentage of calcein uptake at trabecular bone surfaces in PTH treated mice compared to animals treated with saline. This study was the first to clearly show that there are increased levels of bone formation *in vivo* associated with tumors generated by implantation of the predominantly lytic PC3 cell line, and concludes that elevated levels of bone turnover induced by PTH does facilitate the formation of prostate cancer bone metastasis in adult mice. This study supports the theory that increased bone turnover as a consequence of androgen ablation used in the treatment of prostate cancer may increase the risk of subsequent tumor progression in skeletal sites (Table 29.1).

The Effects of Therapies Prior to the introduction of novel therapeutic agents for advanced prostate cancer, testing in *in vivo* model systems is an essential part of the proof of concept required to initiate clinical trials. The effect of

TABLE 29.1 A summary of the current main animal models used in studies of breast cancer-induced bone disease

Model type	Cells administered	Route of administration	No of cells injected	Duration	Disease characteristics and features of models
Xenograft	MDA-MB-231(Luc) MDA-MB-435	Intracardiac	1×10^5–1.5×10^6 1×10^5	3–5 weeks	Bone is the main site of colonization for low frequency lung and liver metastases. Osteolytic bone lesions.
Immuno-deficient animals	MDA-MB-231 MCF7	Intratibial	1–2×10^5	2–4 weeks	Extensive osteolytic disease.
	BO2	Intravenous	1×10^5	2–6 weeks	Cells home specifically to bone, lytic bone disease evident round day 18.
Syngeneic 4T1 Immuno-competent	4T1 Mouse Mammary carcinoma cells	Orthotopic Mammary fat pad	1×10^6	3–4 weeks	Multifocal disease with metastases in lung, liver, kidney, and bone.
Human-to-human models	Human breast cancer cell lines	Intravenous		Tumour cells injected 3–4 weeks following implantation of human adult bone	Cells primarily home to human bone, generating osteolytic disease. No metastases detected in mouse skeleton.
	Primary human breast cancer cells			Sacrifice 8 weeks later	

the EGF-R inhibitor Gefitinib (Iressa; ZD1839) on prostate cancer bone metastasis formation has been reported by Angellucci and colleagues, comparing the parental PC3 prostate cancer cell line and a highly metastatic subline (PCb2) [37]. Following intracardiac injection of 1×10^5 tumor cells into 4-week-old nude mice 150 mg/kg Gefitinib or vehicle (three cycles of 5 days of treatment followed by 2 days of no drug). Tumor burden in bone was assessed at 5 weeks, and 12/16 animals receiving PC3 cells had confirmed bone metastases at this point compared to 16/18 when PCb2 was used. Gefitinib treatment resulted in a decrease in the number of bone metastases by 47% in the PC3 group and by 81% in the PCb2 group, accompanied by a significant reduction in the extent of the associated lytic bone lesions. The data suggest that the PC3 sublines varied in the role of EGF in driving bone metastasis formation, with the more highly metastatic PC2b cells displaying higher sensitivity to Gefitinib. The authors conclude that Gefitinib may be a potential agent in the treatment of advanced prostate cancer with a risk of tumor spread to bone.

2. Intratibial Implantation

Mechanisms of Metastasis As prostate cancer xenografts do not cause bone metastasis following orthotopic implantation in prostate, the ability of different human prostate cancer cell lines to form bone lesions has been determined following direct intratibial implantation in SCID mice. Whereas this does not capture the early stages of bone metastasis formation, interactions between prostate cancer cells and bone cells can be studied in this setting. Using this approach, the group of Corey *et al.* performed detailed characterization of the bone lesions generated by LNCaP, PC-3, LuCaP 35, and LuCaP 23.1 cells [38]. Intratibial injection of $1–2 \times 10^5$ cells in 4-week-old male SCID mice was followed by extensive immunohistochemistry and bone histomorphometry to characterize tumor growth and the associated bone lesions at different time points ranging from 4 to 27 weeks depending on the cell line implanted. Although there was a considerable difference between their growth rate following implantation, all of the tested cell lines were found to have the capacity to form tumors following direct implantation in bone, with LUCaP 23.1 cells generating an osteoblastic response that was evident at the early stages of metastasis development. LNCaP caused mixed bone lesions, whereas LuCaP 35 and PC-3 generated osteolytic responses. Subsequent studies showed that prostate cancer cell growth in bone was associated with tumor expression of a range of molecules involved in regulation of bone turnover, including RANKL, ET-1, PTHrP and OPG, indicating that the nature of the bone lesions is dependent on the levels of tumor-derived factors affecting osteoblast and osteoclast activity. An important characteristic of LuCaP 23.1-generated metastases was that these were able to grow independently of castration, mimicking human advanced hormone-refractory prostate cancer.

Whereas early studies of bone metastasis focused on end stage disease, improved methodology (including *in vivo* imaging techniques) has enabled researchers to investigate early steps in the process involving a low number of tumor cells. Using a xenograft model of early growth of prostate cancer in bone, Cross and colleagues have investigated the role of increased bone remodeling on the ability of tumor cells to form bone metastasis [39]. GFP expressing androgen-independent PC3 cells were injected intratibially in castrated and non-castrated 6–8-week-old MF1 athymic mice, and animals sacrificed 6–9 days following the appearance of GFP-expressing tumors. The presence of tumor and extent of cancer-induced bone disease was determined by micro-CT analysis and histology/immunohistochemistry, and the effects of castration on tumor frequency in bone evaluated. In this study, castration did not affect tumor frequency and volume, or time to initial appearance, despite inducing a significant decrease in trabecular bone volume indicative of increased bone turnover. The presence of PC3 cells had profound effects on bone remodeling, resulting in the suppression of a number of osteoblasts which, coupled with increased numbers of activated osteoclasts, may outweigh the effects of castration-induced bone changes in these experiments. The study illustrates some of the key challenges encountered in studies of complex biological systems like bone metastases, where both physiological and pathological factors contribute to the net outcome.

Effects of Therapies Direct tumor cell implantation in bone is the preferred system for studies of therapeutic agents on established cancer-induced bone disease. Brubaker *et al.* reported a study of the effects of a combination of the antiresorptive agent zoledronic acid (ZOL) and docetaxel (DOC) on LuCaP 23.1, a prostate cancer xenograft that stimulates the osteoblastic reaction following intra-tibial implantation [40]. $1–2 \times 10^5$ LuCap 23.1 cells were injected intratibially in 6–8-week-old male SCID mice which were treated with either saline control, 0.1 mg/kg ZOL 2x pr week s.c., 20 mg/kg DOC i.p. every 2 weeks, or the two drugs in combination. Effects on bone and tumor were evaluated by measurements of bone mineral density and histomorphometrical analysis at week 7. Significant inhibition of tumor growth in bone was observed following treatment with ZOL alone, whereas DOC treatment had no effect compared to saline treated control even though subcutaneous tumor growth was inhibited at this dose of DOC. These results indicate that there is a difference in the responsiveness of tumor cells to therapeutic agents depending on their organ site, and that eradication of tumor cells in bone may require higher doses of a chemotherapy agent than visceral tumors. The highest degree of inhibition of tumor growth was seen in the animals receiving a combination of ZOL and DOC, targeting both tumor cells and the surrounding bone microenvironment. The authors suggest that this combined strategy may be useful in the treatment of prostate cancer patients with advanced bone disease.

3. Orthotopic Implantation

Prostate cancer differs from breast cancer in that orthotopic xenograft models have been developed, where human prostate cancer cells are implanted into mouse prostate, and subsequent metastatic foci detected in a range of organs including bone. Wang *et al.* initially grafted human prostate cancer tissue in testosterone-supplemented male NOD-SCID mice at the subrenal capsule, and following five serial transplantations, into mouse prostate [41]. Further regrafting into prostate and analysis of the metastatic pattern yielded a particular metastatic subline, PCa1-met which, following orthotopic implantation, generated metastasis in lymph nodes, lung, liver, kidney, spleen and bone at around 8 weeks. Metastatic foci were analyzed in detail and found to be of human origin, with few differences detected between the orthotopic tumor grafts and the resulting metastasis. This study shows that it is possible to generate cell lines that form bone metastasis by using the subrenal capsule graft method, whereas this is not seen following direct implantation of primary human prostate tissue. In contrast to the previously described models, this method may provide a model system that captures the early stages of development of prostate cancer bone metastasis.

B. Syngeneic Models

The best characterized syngeneic model of prostate cancer is the TRAMP (Transgenic Adenocarcinoma Mouse Prostate) model, developed and characterized by Greenberg and colleagues [42]. This transgenic mouse model expresses T antigen by week 8 and at 12 weeks displays a characteristic pathology in the dorsolateral prostate. Metastatic foci can be evident from 12 weeks onwards, mainly in the periaortic lymph nodes and lungs, and less frequently in the kidney, adrenal gland, and bone. Whereas this model represents the different stages of prostate cancer development, originating in the prostate and subsequently spreading to distant sites, its use in studies of bone metastases in particular is confounded by the high prevalence of visceral metastasis. In addition, the relatively low frequency of bone metastasis seen in the TRAMP mice means that a large number of animals is required to generate significant numbers of animals with bone metastases. The model is ideally suited for studies of the role of the immune system and of genetic changes associated with tumor progression in general, whereas investigations of effects of therapies on bone metastasis would be complex.

C. Human-to-human Models

As described previously for breast cancer, availability factors provided by the human bone microenvironment may be of crucial importance for the development of bone metastases, as human cancer cells frequently do not home to the skeleton in rodent xenograft models. Prostate cancer models involving implantation of human bone fragments [43] in mice have, therefore, been used to study subsequent growth of human prostate cancer cells in bone. This technique was used by Nemeth *et al.* to compare the ability of different human prostate cancer cell lines to home to human fetal bone implanted in male CB.17 SCID mice following i.v. injection (tail vein), and also to characterize the bone lesions generated following direct implantation of the tumor cells into the bone fragments. In addition, fragments of human fetal lung and intestine, as well as mouse bones, were implanted in order to determine the tissue and species specificity of tumor cell growth. 1×10^6 PC3, DU145, and LNCaP prostate cancer cells were injected 4 weeks after tissue implantation, and the resulting tumor growth characterized 6 weeks later using histology, immunohistochemistry, and chromosomal analysis. In this study, only PC3 cells formed osteolytic tumors in the implanted bone following i.v. injection (5/19 mice, 26%), whereas no tumors were evident using LNCaP or DU145 cells. No tumors were detected in the human lung or intestine fragments following i.v. injection of any of the cell lines, nor was there any evidence of tumor cell colonization of the mouse skeleton, suggesting that bone metastasis formation (PC3) is both species and tissue specific. In contrast, all cell lines generated large tumors with evidence of stromal involvement following direct injection of 10^4 cells into the bone implants, with PC3 and DU145 tumors displaying an osteolytic phenotype and LNCaP a mixed blastic/lytic phenotype. Small tumors with a minor stromal component could also be seen in fetal lung implants following direct tumor cell injection, whereas no tumors were detected in the implanted mouse bones. This study shows that there may be both a species- and tissue-specific requirement for human prostate cancer cells to grow in bone, suggesting that particular tumor-stromal interactions are essential for the development of bone metastases.

A simplified human-to-human model for prostate cancer bone metastasis has been described by Younou *et al.*, where human adult bone fragments are implanted in 6–8-week-old humanized non-obese diabetic/severe combined immunodeficient (NOD/SCID-hu) mice [44]. Three to 4 weeks after implantation of human tissue, LNCaP (1×10^7) or PC-3 (5×10^6) cells were injected in the tail vein of male NOD/SCID-hu mice, and tumor growth in the implants as well as the mouse skeleton determined 8 weeks later following a detailed histological examination. PC3 cells formed osteolytic tumors in the human bone implants in 65% of the mice, whereas LNCaP cells generated osteoblastic tumors in 35% of the implants. No tumors were found in the implanted lung tissues and only very small, sporadic tumors were detected in the mouse lung or bone, supporting the predominant species and tissue specificity of prostate cancer metastasis reported by Nemeth *et al.* This study lends further support to the theory that co-operation between the human microenvironment and the tumor cells is a requirement for bone metastasis formation, an aspect of disease progression that cannot be studied using syngeneic and xenograft models.

IV. MODELS USED IN THE STUDIES OF BONE DISEASE IN MULTIPLE MYELOMA

Multiple myeloma is a B cell neoplasm caused by the monoclonal expansion and infiltration of malignant antibody-producing plasma cells into the bone marrow (BM) compartment. Typical characteristics of the human disease include the development of osteolytic bone lesions, hypercalcemia, susceptibility to bone fractures, abnormally high levels of monoclonal immunoglobulins (also known as paraprotein or the M-spike), and kidney dysfunction. The onset of myeloma bone disease in humans usually occurs in the axial skeleton (spine, skull and pelvis) and can lead to paralysis due to spinal lesions. There are usually no metastases to the lungs, liver, spleen or kidneys.

In multiple myeloma tumors often have low proliferation rates and the malignant plasma cells are usually diffused throughout the BM [45]. This is unlike other cancers, such as breast and prostate, where tumors are solid at the primary site. Despite this, as in other types of cancer, the formation of blood vessels is an important factor in tumor growth [46,47].

Preclinical animal models of multiple myeloma have been described since the late 1970s. These range from syngeneic mouse models to xenograft models of human myeloma in mice. Derivatives of these animal models, which have enhanced our understanding of myeloma and the limitations that these animal models present, are constantly being developed. In the human multiple myeloma disease there is heterogeneity; therefore, no single animal model can reflect all types of multiple myeloma. Here we will discuss the advantages and disadvantages of established animal models that are available to study multiple myeloma (summarized in Table 29.2).

A. 5TMM Multiple Myeloma Syngeneic Murine Models

The 5TMM series of multiple myeloma was first described by Radl *et al.* [48]. It was observed that ageing immune-competent C57BL/KaLwRij mice spontaneously developed a number of clinical features of human multiple myeloma disease [49,50]. These included spontaneous age-related origin, proliferation of plasma cells in the BM; tumor-related levels of paraprotein (mainly of the IgG isotype); development of osteolytic bone disease; and a decrease in normal immunoglobulin levels. The 5TMM models have subsequently been maintained by the *in vivo* transfer of BM plasma cells from C57BL/KaLwRij tumor-bearing mice to young recipient mice of the same strain.

The reproducibility and easy maintenance of the 5T series makes them a good model for studying multiple myeloma. They have been successfully used in a number of preclinical studies [51–55]. The 5T2MM, 5T33MM and, more recently, the 5TGM1 are the best characterized and described models [56–58].

1. THE 5T2MM SYNGENEIC MODEL OF MULTIPLE MYELOMA

The 5T2MM model develops classical features of the human disease of multiple myeloma moderately over a 12 week period. C57BL/KaLwRij mice aged between 6 and 8 weeks are injected intravenously (i.v.) via the tail vein with 2×10^6 cells. After injection, 5T2MM cells home and grow in the BM. In addition, cells are also present in the spleen, probably due to this organ in the mouse being a site of hematopoiesis [59]. As myeloma disease develops paraprotein can be detected after approximately 8 weeks, shortly afterwards bone lesions occur and usually by 12 weeks post-injection animals are sacrificed (Table 29.3).

Vanderkerken *et al.* [58] have previously described detailed analysis methods for the 5T2MM model. Tumor burden can be assessed by measuring serum paraprotein titers; fluorescent activated cell sorting (FACS) or cytosmear analysis of plasma cells from flushed BM cells [58]; or by histological analysis of plasma cells in the tibiae, femora and vertebrae. Bone disease can be measured by radiography typically by micro-computed tomography (μCT) to acquire 3D images of bone lesions and several other bone parameters [60]. On wax embedded bone histological sections the number of osteoclasts and osteoblasts can be counted after tartrate-resistant acid phosphatase (TRAP) and H&E staining, respectively. Bone formation can be measured using fluorescent dyes, such as calcein and/or tetracycline, which bind to bone.

Tumor Homing, Colonization and Development A number of molecules have been identified that are thought to be involved in the homing and adherence of 5T2MM cells to the bone environment [61,62]. Insulin-like growth factor (IGF) has been reported as a BM stroma-derived chemoattractant for 5T2MM cells [61]. The adhesion molecules LFA-1 (CD11a), H-CAM (CD44), VLA-4 α-chain (CD49d) and VLA-5 α-chain (CD49e) are expressed on 5T2MM cells [62] showing a similar adhesion profile to human myeloma cells [62].

Vanderkerken *et al.* [63] have monitored cell homing and distribution patterns in early disease development using radio-labeled 5T2MM cells. After i.v. via tail vein injection of 2×10^6 Cr^{51}-labeled viable 5T2MM cells mice were sacrificed at 1, 2 and 18 hours. The percentage of the total recovered radioactivity was measured in the BM (ribs, vertebrae and legs), spleen, liver, lungs, heart, intestines, kidney and testis. In addition, immunostaining of isolated 5T2MM cells and PCR analysis was performed.

TABLE 29.2   A summary of the current main animal models used in studies of prostate cancer bone metastases

Model type	Cells administered	Route of administration	No of cells injected	Duration	Disease characteristics and features of models
Xenograft	PC3 PC62	Intracardiac	2×10^5 1×10^5	2–5 weeks	Lytic lesions in hind limbs and craniofacial regions. Elevated bone turnover.
Immuno-deficient animals	LNCaP PC3 LUCaP35 LUCaP23.1	Intratibial	1–2×10^5	Up to 30 weeks Up to 5 weeks Up to 7 weeks Up to 25 weeks	Mixed osteolytic and osteoblastic lesions. Osteolytic lesions. Osteolytic lesions. Osteoblastic lesions.
	PCa1-met	Orthotopic prostate	Tissue implanted	2–5 weeks	Multifocal disease lymph nodes, lung, liver, kidney, spleen, bone.
Syngeneic TRAMP model Immuno-competent	Spontaneous Transgenic Andenocarcinoma of Mouse Prostate	NA	NA	12 weeks onward	Multiorgan disease including lymph nodes, lungs, kidney, adrenal gland, bone.
Human-to-human models	PC3 DU145 LNCaP	Direct injection into implanted human foetal bone fragments	1×10^4 1×10^4 5×10^4	Tumor cells injected 4 weeks following implantation of human fetal bone Sacrifice 6 weeks later	Metastases to human bone osteolytic lestions. Metastases to human bone osteolytic lestions. Osteoblastic and osteolytic lesions.
	LNCaP	Intravenous	1×10^7	Tumor cells injected 3–4 weeks following implantation of human adult bone	Metastases to human bone in 35% of cases—osteoblastic lesions.
	PC3	Adult human bone implanted	5×10^6	Sacrifice 8 weeks later	Metastases to human bone in 65% of cases—osteolytic lesions

Collectively this data showed the presence of 5T2MM cells in the BM, spleen and liver. Interestingly, survival of these cells only occurred in the BM and spleen and not in the liver [62].

The Effects of Therapies The effects of a number of therapeutic agents have been tested in the 5T2MM model [51–53,64,65]. These include bisphosphonates which are currently used clinically to treat myeloma bone disease. Croucher *et al.* [53] treated mice with zoledronic acid (ZOL) (120 μg/kg twice a week) either long term (preventative) or short term (established disease). In the long term treatment group, ZOL was given from the time of tumor cell injection until sacrifice (12 weeks later). In the short-term treatment, ZOL was given from the time of paraprotein detection until sacrifice (4 weeks later). Both treatments

prevented cancer-induced bone disease with a significant reduction in the number of osteoclasts and osteolytic lesions; trabecular bone area was preserved; and BMD was increased. A reduction in tumor burden was also seen in ZOL-treated animals when compared to tumor controls. In addition, a single dose of ZOL was shown to prevent osteolytic bone disease. In a separate experiment, short-term treatment with ZOL significantly reduced angiogenesis and increased animal survival from 35 to 47 days.

2. THE 5T33MM SYNGENEIC MODEL OF MULTIPLE MYELOMA

The 5T33MM model is an aggressive form of myeloma developing over a relatively short period of time (approximately 4 weeks). C57BL/KaLwRij mice aged between

TABLE 29.3   A summary of the current main animal models used in studies of multiple myeloma disease

Model type	Cells administered	No of cells injected	Irradiation	Route of administration	Duration	Disease characteristics and features of models
Syngeneic 5T2MM	Isolated from 5T2MM-tumor-bearing mice	2×10^6	Immune competent	Intravenous	12 weeks	Osteolytic lesion, paraprotein detection. Tumor growth restricted to BM and spleen.
5T33MM	Isolated from 5T33MM-tumor-bearing mice	10^5	Immune competent	Intravenous	5–8 weeks	No osteolytic lesions, tumor growth restricted to BM, spleen and liver.
5TGM1	Isolated from 5TGM1MM-tumor-bearing mice	10^6	Immune competent	Intravenous	4 weeks	Osteolytic lesions, environment independent.
ABL-MYC	N/A	N/A	N/A	N/A	9–19 weeks depending on age	Bone lesions and plasma cell tumors.
Xenograft SCID-xeno **SCID-hu**	Human: Cell lines Cell lines Primary cells	$1–2 \times 10^7$ 1×10^7 $1.5–10 \times 10^6$	300 rads	Sub.cut. i.v Intraosseous	9–11 days 33–46 days 2–19 weeks	Logistics are a problem as it takes 4–8 weeks for bone engraftment.
SCID-rab	Primary cells	$3–10 \times 10^6$		Intraosseous	4–6 weeks	No need for human fetal bones.
NOD/SCID	Cell lines Primary	$1–10 \times 10^6$ $10^6 – 3 \times 10^7$	150–450 rads 150–450 rads	i.v s.c.	2–8 weeks	

6 and 8 weeks are injected i.v. via the tail vein with 0.5×10^6 cells. Growth of the 5T33MM cells has been found to be similar to the 5T2MM cells, except that they are also present in the liver. As with 5T2MM cells, IGF-I [59] and laminin-1 [66] are known to be important chemoattractants. Unlike the 5T2MM model, 5T33MM mice do not develop osteolytic bone lesions. After 4 weeks post injection of 5T33MM cells, mice are sacrificed due to a high tumor burden.

A number of derivatives of 5T33MM model have been developed. These include some where cells can be grown *in vitro* (5T33vt) as well as *in vivo* (5T33vv) [59]. An advantage of using *in vitro* cells is they can be manipulated. For example, the expression of green fluorescent protein (GFP) in 5T33vt cells has allowed them to be traced *in vivo* [67].

Tumor Homing, Colonization and Development 5T33MM cells, like 5T2MM cells, are positive for the adhesion molecules LFA-1, H-CAM, VLA-4 α-chain and VLA-5 α-chain [62]. This may explain why the initial distribution pattern of 5T33MM cells is similar to 5T2MM cells. Direct contact of 5T33MM cells with BM endothelium cells *in vivo* causes an upregulation of IGF-1 receptor and CD44v6 [59]. Interestingly, in the later stages of disease the distribution of 5T33MM cells alters compared to 5T2MM cells [62]. 5T33MM cells are not only found in the BM and spleen but also in the liver where, unlike the 5T2MM cells, they survive and grow. It has been speculated that 5T33MM cells survive in the liver due to their proliferative response to IGF-1 [59].

The Effects of Therapies Therapeutic agents that are thought to prevent tumor growth have been tested in the 5T33MM model. These include an inhibitor of p38α mitogen-activated protein kinase [52], a specific inhibitor of cyclin-dependent kinases (Cdk) and a proteosome inhibitor [68]. Menu *et al.* [68] have monitored the effects of a therapeutic combination of PD 0332991 (a specific inhibitor of Cdk4 and Cdk6) and bortezomib (a proteasome inhibitor). Bortezomib (Velcade) is currently used clinically to treat tumor burden in myeloma patients. After injection of 5T33MM cells, mice were treated with PD 0332991 (150 mg daily by gavage) between 7 and 19 days or in a combination study between 4 and 11 days with bortezomib (0.4 mg/kg, every 3 days by subcutaneous s.c. injection) administered between 12 and 24 days. PD 03332991 treatment led to tumor cell suppression and a significant increase in survival of mice from 25 to 35 days. In addition, PD 03332991 treatment was found to sensitize cells to killing by bortezomib, illustrating a promising cell cycle-based combination therapy.

3. THE 5TGM1 SYNGENEIC MODEL OF MULTIPLE MYELOMA

The 5TGM1MM model, like the 5T33MM model, is an aggressive form of myeloma and develops over approximately 4 weeks [55,57]. C57BL/KaLwRij mice aged between 6 and 8 weeks are injected i.v. via the tail vein with 10^6 cells. However, unlike the 5T33MM and 5T2MM models, they appear to be environment independent and tumor growth is not confined to the bone, spleen and liver (sites of hematopoiesis). They develop osetolytic bone lesions and after approximately 4 weeks mice are sacrificed.

Tumor Homing, Colonization and Development Oyajobi *et al.* [69] have monitored 5TGM1 cell distribution. Cells were fluorescently labeled with eGFP, injected *in vivo* and then visualized in live mice by whole body optical fluorescence microscopy. Tumor cell distribution was mainly seen in the axial skeleton (skull, pelvis, vertebrae, ribs, sternum, scapula and clavicle), although extramedullary tumor sites were also found in the spleen and ovaries.

The Effects of Therapies The effects of ibandronate, an anti-marcophage inflammatory protein-1α monoclonal antibody and bortezomib have all been tested in the 5TGM1 model of myeloma [55,69,70]. Oyajobi *et al.* [69] studied the effects of the proteasome inhibitor bortezomib in the 5TGM1 model. Varying doses of bortezomib (0.1, 0.5, 1 and 3 mg/kg of body weight) were administered 3 times a week from the time of tumor cell injection for 4 weeks. An anti-tumor effect was seen at all doses of bortezomib, with the two highest being most effective, using whole body fluorescent imaging. Toxicity was observed using a 3 mg/kg dose of bortezomib but not when this was reduced to 2 mg/kg.

B. Multiple Myeloma Xenograft Models

These models were developed to study the behavior of human myeloma disease. Human myeloma cell lines were initially found to grow readily in these models. Later they were refined to grow patient primary myeloma cells.

1. SCID-XENOGRAFT MODEL

Originally, severe combined immune deficient (SCID) mice were used to study human multiple myeloma as tumor cells were found not to grow in nude mice which are only deficient in T lymphocytes. SCID mice, which in addition to lacking T cells, also have impaired B cell function. Since the early 1990s, myeloma cell lines have been used in this early model of multiple myeloma using different administration routes [71,72]. Mice inoculated s.c. only develop tumors at the site of administration [72]. In contrast, i.v. administration, following irradiation of mice, results in disseminated tumor growth similar to the human myeloma disease [71]. More recently, nonobese diabetic/ SCID (NOD/LtSz-SCID) mice have been used as they are the most immune-deficient of all the SCID strains [73], making them an ideal model system to monitor the growth of human myeloma cells. In this model, human myeloma cell lines or patient cells are administered by s.c. or i.v. injection.

Pilarski *et al.* [74] have shown that, in irradiated mice following intracardiac injection of peripheral cells from myeloma patients, myeloma disease develops. In addition, intraosseous injections of the same primary cells have shown that tumor cells home to new skeletal sites [74]. Mitsiades *et al.* [75] have engineered RPMI8226 cells expressing GFP, to allow the visualization of the diffused tumor sites. This model has also been shown to be effective administering cells i.v. via the tail vein. Bueno *et al.* [76] have reported the development of a novel NOD/SCID model where cells are delivered directly to femora or tibiae. This model bypasses the need for cells to home to the BM niche but has the limitation that mouse cytokines may not cross-react with human patient cells. In addition, some bone architecture maybe destroyed when cells are injected.

Tumor Homing, Colonization and Development Huang *et al.* [71] injected 2×10^7 ARH-77 cells i.v., following 150 rads of γ-irradiation, into SCID mice (C.B.-17 SCID/SCID). Histological analysis showed tumor cell proliferation in vertebrae, skull, brain and meninges. FACS analysis showed 31% of the BM cells from the vertebrae had a similar profile to the injected human ARH-77 cells (CD38$^+$, PCA-1$^+$, HLAclasses I$^+$ and II$^+$) and PCR analysis confirmed the presence of the human cell line.

The Effects of Therapies Wu *et al.* [77] have targeted the IGF-I receptor (IGF-1R) with an anti-IGF-1R antibody. They used this in combination with agents currently used clinically. NOD/SCID mice were injected i.v. with 10^7 MM.1S cells expressing an eGFP-luciferase fusion protein. Mice were grouped into those treated with anti-IGF-1R (A12) alone (40 mg/kg, by intraperitoneal (i.p.) injection, 3 times a week for 4 weeks); melphalan alone (5 mg/kg, by a single i.p. injection); bortezomib alone (0.5 mg/kg, by i.v. injection twice a week for 3 weeks); A12 plus bortezomib; or A12 plus melphalan. Tumor burden was monitored by bioluminescence whole body imaging. When A12 was used alone there was no significant difference in tumor burden compared to control animals. However, when A12 was used in combination with melphalan a significant reduction was observed. Survival was significantly increased in all single agent groups compared to control mice. In addition, survival was significantly increased in both combination groups compared to all the single agent groups. This suggests that the inclusion of an anti-IGF-1R antibody used with currently licensed agents may lead to a prolonged survival of myeloma patients.

2. SCID-HU MODEL

The SCID-hu model was developed to facilitate the growth of human primary myeloma cells in a human bone microenvironment. Typically fetal human bone chips are transplanted into mice and human patient primary cells or cell lines are injected directly into the xenograft bone [78,79].

Other variations of this model have also been developed. For example, Tassone *et al.* [80] have developed a model using the IL-6-dependent human multiple myeloma cell line, INA-6, transduced with GFP. These INA-6 cells can only engraft in implanted human bone chips and not in mouse bone as IL-6 levels are insufficient. This model allows the evaluation of drugs targeting IL-6-dependent myeloma cells in the human bone marrow environment. In addition, the SCID-rab model was developed because of ethical issues and the limited access to xenograft tissue of human origin in the SCID-hu model. It provides an alternative to using human fetal bone chips. Instead, rabbit bones are implanted s.c. and injected with patient primary myeloma cells in SCID mice [81]. This model has shown successful tumor cell engraftment of both patient unsorted BM samples and BM sorted CD138-positive cells. These model mice have measurable paraprotein levels; osteolytic bone lesions in the implanted rabbit bone; and form new blood vessels of rabbit origin [81].

Tumor Homing, Colonization and Development Human primary myeloma cells or human myeloma cell lines do not need to home to bone as they are injected directly into xenograft implanted bones. Cells are then restricted to the human bone microenvironment site where myeloma growth is frequently accompanied by increased osteoclast activity and blood vessel formation of human cells [79].

The Effects of Therapies Since the SCID-hu model was developed, a number of therapeutic agents have been tested in it [82–86]. Notch signaling has been implicated

in protecting myeloma cells from drug-induced apoptosis [87]. Nefedova *et al.* [88] have blocked notch signaling with a γ-secretase inhibitor (GSI) in an SCID-hu model. Six-week-old female SCID-Beige mice were s.c. injected with human fetal bones. Six weeks after implantation, 5×10^4 RPMI-8226 myeloma cells were injected into each implanted bone. Treatment with GSI alone (5 mg/kg by i.p. injection, daily for 14 days), melphalan alone (1.5 mg/kg by i.p. injection, twice with 4 days between each injection), doxorubicin alone (1.5 mg/kg by i.p. injection, 3 times with 4 days between each injection), or in combination studies started 4 weeks after tumor cell injection. The anti-tumor effects of all agents decreased human paraprotein levels in mice sera. This effect was significantly enhanced in all combination treatment groups, suggesting that the inhibition of notch signaling may sensitize myeloma cells to chemotherapy.

V. CONCLUSIONS

As discussed in this chapter, no ideal single *in vivo* model system for studies of cancer progression to bone exists, representing the long process from primary, organ-confined tumor growth through subsequent steps to advanced metastatic disease. What we do have available is a range of different models which may be used to generate valuable knowledge of the molecular and cellular interactions involved at different steps of the disease process, as well as the effects of therapies. Researchers must give careful consideration as to which model is best suited for their particular study. For instance, the role of the immune system and the human bone microenvironment for bone metastasis progression cannot be determined in xenograft models using immunocompromised animals. The initial homing steps of tumor cells to bone require a model where tumor cells are introduced by i.v. injection, rather than directly implanted into bone. In contrast, the effects of therapeutic agents on cancer-induced bone disease can be investigated in a range of models, including xenografts, as here the focus is mainly on established bone metastases rather than the early colonization steps. As outlined in this chapter, a multitude of factors will influence the results generated using *in vivo* models, including the number/type of tumor cells used, the administration route, recipient animal type/strain/age, etc. Despite their limitations, our current understanding of tumor progression in bone is largely based on data from animal models, and the rapid development of new technologies like *in vivo* imaging is extending the type of information obtained from these [89,90].

Finally, as investigations of bone metastases using human material remain limited, well-designed studies using *in vivo* models are expected to be the main source of new knowledge in relation to this important clinical problem for the foreseeable future.

References

1. K.M. Bussard, C.V. Gay & A.M. Mastro, The bone microenvironment in metastasis; what is special about bone?, Cancer Metastasis Rev 27 (2008) 41–55.
2. V.A. Siclari, T.A. Guise & J.M. Chirgwin, Molecular interactions between breast cancer cells and the bone microenvironment drive skeletal metastases, Cancer Metastasis Rev 25 (2006) 621–633.
3. P.D. Ottewell, R.E. Coleman & I. Holen, From genetic abnormality to metastases: murine models of breast cancer and their use in the development of anticancer therapies, Breast Cancer Res Treat 96 (2006) 101–113.
4. K.U. Wagner, Models of breast cancer: quo vadis, animal modeling? Breast Cancer Res 6 (2004) 31–38.
5. J. Jonkers & P.W. Derksen, Modeling metastatic breast cancer in mice, J Mammary Gland Biol Neoplasia 12 (2007) 191–203.
6. A. Fantozzi & G. Christofori, Mouse models of breast cancer metastasis, Breast Cancer Res 8 (2006) 212.
7. S. Blouin, M.F. Basle & D. Chappard, Rat models of bone metastases, Clin Exp Metastasis 22 (2005) 605–614.
8. S.P. Flanagan, 'Nude', a new hairless gene with pleiotropic effects in the mouse, Genet Res 8 (1966) 295–309.
9. M.J. Bosma & A.M. Carroll, The SCID mouse mutant: definition, characterization, and potential uses, Annu Rev Immunol 9 (1991) 323–350.
10. R.B. Lock, N. Liem & M.L. Farnsworth, et al., The nonobese diabetic/severe combined immunodeficient (NOD/SCID). Mouse model of childhood acute lymphoblastic leukemia reveals intrinsic differences in biological characteristics at diagnosis and relapse, Blood 99 (2002) 4100–4108.
11. T. Yoneda, T. Michigami & B. Yi, et al., Actions of bisphosphonate on bone metastasis in animal models of breast carcinoma, Cancer 15 (2000) 2979–2988.
12. P.A. Phadke, R.R. Mercer & J.F. Harms, et al., Kinetics of metastatic breast cancer cell trafficking in bone, Clin Cancer Res 12 (2006) 1431–1440.
13. J.R. Canon, M. Roudier & R. Bryant, et al., Inhibition of RANKL blocks skeletal tumor progression and improves survival in a mouse model of breast cancer bone metastasis, Clin Exp Metastasis 25 (2008) 119–129.
14. N. Rucci, I. Recchia & A. Angelucci, et al., Inhibition of protein kinase c-Src reduces the incidence of breast cancer metastases and increases survival in mice: implications for therapy, J Pharmacol Exp Ther 318 (2006) 161–172.
15. O. Peyruchaud, B. Winding & I. Pecheur, et al., Early detection of bone metastases in a murine model using fluorescent human breast cancer cells: application to the use of the bisphosphanate zoledronic acid in the treatment of osteolytic lesions, J Bone Miner Res 16 (2001) 2027–2034.
16. Y. Zhao, R. Bachelier & I. Treilleux, et al., Tumor alphav-betaa3 integrin is a therapeutic target for breast cancer bone metastases, Cancer Res 67 (2007) 5821–5830.
17. A. Boucharaba, C.M. Serre & S. Gres, et al., Platelet-derived lysophosphatidic acid supports the progression of osteolytic bone metastases in breast cancer, J Clin Invest 114 (2004) 1714–1725.
18. F. Daubine, C. Le Gall & J. Gasser, et al., Antitumor effects of clinical dosing regimens of bisphosphonates in experimental breast cancer bone metastasis, J Natl Cancer Inst 99 (2007) 322–330.
19. P.D. Ottewell, B. Deux & H. Monkkonen, et al., Differential effect of doxorubicin and zoledronic acid on intraosseous versus extraosseous breast tumor growth in vivo, Clin Cancer Res 14 (2008) 4658–4666.
20. A.H. Gordon, R.J. O'Keefe & E.M. Schwarz, et al., Nuclear factor-kappaB-dependent mechanisms in breast cancer cells regulate tumor burden and osteolysis in bone, Cancer Res 65 (2005) 3209–3217.
21. B. Psaila, R.N. Kaplan & E.R. Port, et al., Priming the 'soil' for breast cancer metastasis: the pre-metastatic niche, Breast Dis 26 (2007) 65–74.
22. J.L. Fisher, R.J. Thomas-Mudge & J. Elliott, et al., Osteoprotegerin overexpression by breast cancer cells enhances orthotopic and osseous tumor growth and contrasts with that delivered therapeutically, Cancer Res 66 (2006) 3620–3628.
23. Y. Zheng, H. Zhou & J.R. Modzelewski, et al., Accelerated bone resorption, due to dietary calcium deficiency, promotes breast cancer tumor growth in bone, Cancer Res 67 (2007) 9542–9548.
24. Y. Zheng, H. Zhou & K. Brennan, et al., Inhibition of bone resorption, rather than direct cytotoxicity, mediates the anti-tumor actions of ibandronate and osteoprotegerin in a murine model of breast cancer bone metastasis, Bone 40 (2007) 471–478.
25. D.L. Dexter, H.M. Kowalski & B.A. Blazar, et al., Heterogeneity of tumor cells from a single mouse mammary tumor, Cancer Res 38 (1978) 3174–3181.
26. K. Tao, M. Fang & J. Alroy, et al., Imagable 4T1 model for the study of late stage breast cancer, BMC Cancer 8 (2008) 228.
27. A.A. Rose, F. Pepin & C. Russo, et al., Osteoactivin promotes breast cancer metastasis to bone, Mol Cancer Res 5 (2007) 1001–1014.
28. T. Hiraga, P.J. Williams & A. Ueda, et al., Zoledronic acid inhibits visceral metastases in the 4T1/luc mouse breast cancer model, Clin Cancer Res 10 (2004) 4559–4567.
29. K. Niikura, Effect of a V-APTase inhibitor, FR202126, in syngeneic mouse model of experimental bone metastasis, Cancer Chemother Pharmacol 60 (2007) 555–562.
30. C. Kuperwasser, S. Dessain & B.E. Bierbaum, et al., A mouse model of human breast cancer metastasis to human bone, Cancer Res 65 (2005) 6130–6138.
31. J. Moreau, K.M. Anderson & J.R. Mauney, et al., Studies of osteotropism on both sides of the breast cancer-bone interaction, Ann NY Acad Sci 1117 (2007) 328–344.
32. W. Yang, P. Lam & R. Kitching, et al., Breast cancer metastasis in a human bone NOD/SCID mouse model, Cancer Biol Ther 6 (2007) 1289–1294.
33. A.S. Singh & W.D. Figg, In vivo models of prostate cancer metastasis to bone, J Urol 174 (2005) 820–826.
34. D.J. Lamb & L. Zhang, Challenges in prostate cancer research: animal models for nutritional studies of chemoprevention and disease progression, J Nutr 135 (2005) 3009S–3015S.
35. C. Morrissey & R.L. Vessella, The role of tumor microenvironment in prostate cancer bone metastasis, J Cell Biochem 101 (2007) 873–886.
36. A. Schneider, L.M. Kalikin & A.C. Mattos, et al., Bone turnover mediates preferential localization of prostate cancer in the skeleton, Endocrinology 146 (2005) 1727–1736.

37. A. Angelucci, G.L. Gravina & N. Rucci, et al., Suppression of EGF-R signaling reduces the incidence of prostate cancer metastasis in nude mice, Endocr Relat Cancer 13 (2006) 197–210.

38. E. Corey, J.E. Quinn & F. Bladou, et al., Establishment and characterization of osseous prostate cancer models: intra-tibial injection of human prostate cancer cells, Prostate 52 (2002) 20–33.

39. N.A. Cross, R. Fowles & K. Reeves, et al., Imaging the effects of castration on bone turnover and hormone-independent prostate cancer colonization of bone, Prostate 68 (2008) 1707–1714.

40. K.D. Brubaker, L.G. Brown & R.L. Vessella, et al., Administration of zoledronic acid enhances the effects of docetaxel on growth of prostate cancer in the bone environment, BMC Cancer 6 (2006) 15.

41. Y. Wang, H. Xue & J.C. Cutz, et al., An orthotopic metastatic prostate cancer model in SCID mice via grafting of a transplantable human prostate tumor line, Lab Invest 85 (2005) 1392–1404.

42. J.R. Gingrich, R.J. Barrios & R.A. Morton, et al., Metastatic prostate cancer in a transgenic mouse, Cancer Res 56 (1996) 4096–4102.

43. J.A. Nemeth, J.F. Harb & U. Barroso Jr, et al., Severe combined immunodeficient-hu model of human prostate cancer metastasis to human bone, Cancer Res 59 (1999) 1987–1993.

44. H. Yonou, T. Yokose & T. Kamijo, et al., Establishment of a novel species- and tissue-specific metastasis model of human prostate cancer in humanized non-obese diabetic/severe combined immunodeficient mice engrafted with human adult lung and bone, Cancer Res 61 (2001) 2177–2182.

45. R.A. Kyle & S.V. Rajkumar, Multiple myeloma, N Engl J Med 351 (2004) 1860–1873.

46. A. Vacca, D. Ribatti & L. Roncali, et al., Bone marrow angiogenesis and progression in multiple myeloma, Br J Haematol 87 (1994) 503–508.

47. A. Vacca, M. Di Loreto & D. Ribatti, et al., Bone marrow of patients with active multiple myeloma: angiogenesis and plasma cell adhesion molecules LFA-1, VLA-4, LAM-1, and CD44, Am J Hematol 50 (1995) 9–14.

48. J. Radl, E.D. De Glopper & H.R. Schuit, et al., Idiopathic paraproteinemia. II. Transplantation of the paraprotein-producing clone from old to young C57BL/KaLwRij mice, J Immunol 122 (1979) 609–613.

49. J. Radl, J.W. Croese & C. Zurcher, et al., Animal model of human disease. Multiple myeloma, Am J Pathol 132 (1988) 593–597.

50. J. Radl, Multiple myeloma and related disorders. Lessons from an animal model, Pathol Biol (Paris) 47 (1999) 109–114.

51. D.J. Heath, K. Vanderkerken & X. Cheng, et al., An osteoprotegerin-like peptidomimetic inhibits osteoclastic bone resorption and osteolytic bone disease in myeloma, Cancer Res 67 (2007) 202–208.

52. K. Vanderkerken, S. Medicherla & L. Coulton, et al., Inhibition of p38alpha mitogen-activated protein kinase prevents the development of osteolytic bone disease, reduces tumor burden, and increases survival in murine models of multiple myeloma, Cancer Res 67 (2007) 4572–4577.

53. P.I. Croucher, R. De Hendrik & M.J. Perry, et al., Zoledronic acid treatment of 5T2MM-bearing mice inhibits the development of myeloma bone disease: evidence for decreased osteolysis, tumor burden and angiogenesis, and increased survival, J Bone Miner Res 18 (2003) 482–492.

54. C.M. Shipman, K. Vanderkerken & M.J. Rogers, et al., The potent bisphosphonate ibandronate does not induce myeloma cell apoptosis in a murine model of established multiple myeloma, Br J Haematol 111 (2000) 283–286.

55. S.L. Dallas, I.R. Garrett & B.O. Oyajobi, et al., Ibandronate reduces osteolytic lesions but not tumor burden in a murine model of myeloma bone disease, Blood 93 (1999) 1697–1706.

56. K. Asosingh, J. Radl & I. Van Riet, et al., The 5TMM series: a useful *in vivo* mouse model of human multiple myeloma, Hematol J 1 (2000) 351–356.

57. I.R. Garrett, S. Dallas & J. Radl, et al., A murine model of human myeloma bone disease, Bone 20 (1997) 515–520.

58. K. Vanderkerken, K. Asosingh & A. Willems, et al., The 5T2MM murine model of multiple myeloma: maintenance and analysis, Methods Mol Med 113 (2005) 191–205.

59. K. Asosingh, U. Gunthert & M.H. Bakkus, et al., *In vivo* induction of insulin-like growth factor-I receptor and CD44v6 confers homing and adhesion to murine multiple myeloma cells, Cancer Res 60 (2000) 3096–3104.

60. D.J. Heath, A.D. Chantry & C.H. Buckle, et al., Inhibiting Dickkopf-1 (Dkk1) removes suppression of bone formation and prevents the development of osteolytic bone disease in multiple myeloma, J Bone Miner Res 24 (2009) 425–436.

61. K. Vanderkerken, K. Asosingh & F. Braet, et al., Insulin-like growth factor-1 acts as a chemoattractant factor for 5T2 multiple myeloma cells, Blood 93 (1999) 235–241.

62. K. Vanderkerken, H. De Raeve & E. Goes, et al., Organ involvement and phenotypic adhesion profile of 5T2 and 5T33 myeloma cells in the C57BL/KaLwRij mouse, Br J Cancer 76 (1997) 451–460.

63. K. Vanderkerken, C. De Greef & K. Asosingh, et al., Selective initial *in vivo* homing pattern of 5T2 multiple myeloma cells in the C57BL/KalwRij mouse, Br J Cancer 82 (2000) 953–959.

64. P.I. Croucher, C.M. Shipman & J. Lippitt, et al., Osteoprotegerin inhibits the development of osteolytic bone disease in multiple myeloma, Blood 98 (2001) 3534–3540.

65. M.A. Lawson, L. Coulton & F.H. Ebetino, et al., Geranylgeranyl transferase type II inhibition prevents myeloma bone disease, Biochem Biophys Res Commun 377 (2008) 453–457.

66. I. Vande Broek, K. Vanderkerken & C. De Greef, et al., Laminin-1-induced migration of multiple myeloma cells involves the high-affinity 67kD laminin receptor, Br J Cancer 85 (2001) 1387–1395.

67. E. Alici, K.V. Konstantinidis & A. Aints, et al., Visualization of 5T33 myeloma cells in the C57BL/KaLwRij mouse: establishment of a new syngeneic murine model of multiple myeloma, Exp Hematol 32 (2004) 1064–1072.

68. E. Menu, J. Garcia & X. Huang, et al., A novel therapeutic combination using PD 0332991 and bortezomib: study in the 5T33MM myeloma model, Cancer Res 68 (2008) 5519–5523.

69. B.O. Oyajobi, S. Munoz & R. Kakonen, et al., Detection of myeloma in skeleton of mice by whole-body optical fluorescence imaging, Mol Cancer Ther 6 (2007) 1701–1708.

70. B.O. Oyajobi, G. Franchin & P.J. Williams, et al., Dual effects of macrophage inflammatory protein-1alpha on osteolysis and

tumor burden in the murine 5TGM1 model of myeloma bone disease, Blood 102 (2003) 311–319.

71. Y.W. Huang, J.A. Richardson & A.W. Tong, et al., Disseminated growth of a human multiple myeloma cell line in mice with severe combined immunodeficiency disease, Cancer Res 53 (1993) 1392–1396.

72. A.W. Tong, Y.W. Huang & B.Q. Zhang, et al., Heterotransplantation of human multiple myeloma cell lines in severe combined immunodeficiency (SCID) mice, Anticancer Res 13 (1993) 593–597.

73. L.D. Shultz, P.A. Schweitzer & S.W. Christianson, et al., Multiple defects in innate and adaptive immunologic function in NOD/LtSz-scid mice, J Immunol 154 (1995) 180–191.

74. L.M. Pilarski, G. Hipperson & K. Seeberger, et al., Myeloma progenitors in the blood of patients with aggressive or minimal disease: engraftment and self-renewal of primary human myeloma in the bone marrow of NOD SCID mice, Blood 95 (2000) 1056–1065.

75. C.S. Mitsiades, N.S. Mitsiades & R.T. Bronson, et al., Fluorescence imaging of multiple myeloma cells in a clinically relevant SCID/NOD *in vivo* model: biologic and clinical implications, Cancer Res 63 (2003) 6689–6696.

76. C. Bueno, L.F. Lopes & M. Greaves, et al., Toward development of a novel NOD/SCID-based *in vivo* strategy to model multiple myeloma pathogenesis, Exp Hematol 35 (2007) 1477–1478.

77. K.D. Wu, L. Zhou & D. Burtrum, et al., Antibody targeting of the insulin-like growth factor I receptor enhances the antitumor response of multiple myeloma to chemotherapy through inhibition of tumor proliferation and angiogenesis, Cancer Immunol Immunother 56 (2007) 343–357.

78. W.T. Bellamy, P. Mendibles & P. Bontje, et al., Development of an orthotopic SCID mouse-human tumor xenograft model displaying the multidrug-resistant phenotype, Cancer Chemother Pharmacol 37 (1996) 305–316.

79. S. Yaccoby, B. Barlogie & J. Epstein, Primary myeloma cells growing in SCID-hu mice: a model for studying the biology and treatment of myeloma and its manifestations, Blood 92 (1998) 2908–2913.

80. P. Tassone, P. Neri & D.R. Carrasco, et al., A clinically relevant SCID-hu *in vivo* model of human multiple myeloma, Blood 106 (2005) 713–716.

81. K. Yata & S. Yaccoby, The SCID-rab model: a novel *in vivo* system for primary human myeloma demonstrating growth of CD138-expressing malignant cells, Leukemia 18 (2004) 1891–1897.

82. T. Hideshima, P. Neri & P. Tassone, et al., MLN120B, a novel IkappaB kinase beta inhibitor, blocks multiple myeloma cell growth *in vitro* and *in vivo*, Clin Cancer Res 12 (2006) 5887–5894.

83. E.M. Sordillo & R.N. Pearse, RANK-Fc: a therapeutic antagonist for RANK-L in myeloma, Cancer 97 (2003) 802–812.

84. S. Yaccoby, C.L. Johnson & S.C. Mahaffey, et al., Antimyeloma efficacy of thalidomide in the SCID-hu model, Blood 100 (2002) 4162–4168.

85. S. Yaccoby, A. Pennisi & X. Li, et al., Atacicept (TACI-Ig). Inhibits growth of TACI(high) primary myeloma cells in SCID-hu mice and in coculture with osteoclasts, Leukemia 22 (2008) 406–413.

86. K. Zhu, E. Gerbino & D.M. Beaupre, et al., Farnesyltransferase inhibitor R115777 (Zarnestra, Tipifarnib) synergizes with paclitaxel to induce apoptosis and mitotic arrest and to inhibit tumor growth of multiple myeloma cells, Blood 105 (2005) 4759–4766.

87. Y. Nefedova, P. Cheng & M. Alsina, et al., Involvement of Notch-1 signaling in bone marrow stroma-mediated de novo drug resistance of myeloma and other malignant lymphoid cell lines, Blood 103 (2004) 3503–3510.

88. Y. Nefedova, D.M. Sullivan & S.C. Bolick, et al., Inhibition of Notch signaling induces apoptosis of myeloma cells and enhances sensitivity to chemotherapy, Blood 111 (2008) 2220–2229.

89. V. Fritz, P. Louis-Plence & F. Apparailly, et al., Micro-CT combined with bioluminescence imaging: a dynamic approach to detect early tumor-bone interaction in a tumor osteolysis murine model, Bone 40 (2007) 1032–1040.

90. N.V. Henriquez, P.G. van Overveld & I. Que, et al., Advances in optical imaging and novel model systems for cancer metastasis research, Clin Exp Metastasis 24 (2007) 699–705.

CHAPTER **30**

Cytokine Gene Therapy in Bone Remodeling

CARL D. RICHARDS[1] AND DAVID SMYTH[1]

[1]*Department of Pathology and Molecular Medicine, MDCL-4020, McMaster University, Hamilton, Ontario, Canada, L8N 3Z5.*

Contents

I. OVERVIEW

The prospect of using gene therapeutic approaches in the treatment of disease has been explored on multiple fronts over the last few years. It is based on the potential to provide long-term expression of key genes that encode functioning proteins to replace defective ones or to elevate levels of factors that control disease processes. There has been an expansion of data available with respect to such approaches; including studies on animal models and a more limited number of clinical trials at present regarding genetic deficiencies, chronic musculo-skeletal defective conditions and cancer therapy. This approach is generally in its infancy for clinical applications, but advances are now utilizing creative ways to improve vector design and methods of gene delivery to local or systemic sites. Much information is still needed to better design meaningful experimentation, and this is evident in chronic conditions of musculo-skeletal remodeling which include considerations such as: (1) determination of the best gene or set of genes to overexpress or modify to repress expression; (2) optimal levels of gene expression; (3) timing of such gene modulation necessary for maximal and long-term beneficial effects; and (4) local versus systemic expression of target genes and associated potential side effects. There are some data in animal models regarding the use of gene transfer for conditions of bone loss or fracture, but less for that on the treatment of bone cancer. There have been excellent reviews written

on the subject of general therapy in osteosarcoma [1] and gene therapy approaches for osteosarcoma [2]. For further exploration on the potential of gene therapy in bone cancer, existing data regarding such approaches in generating bone tissue for the purpose of non-cancer bone disease can be informative, and is the primary subject of this chapter. Although a number of growth factors and cytokines can regulate bone metabolism, most work so far, and thus data reviewed here, includes that on the bone morphogenic protein (BMP) family of polypeptides and on osteoprotegerin (OPG).

II. METHODS OF GENE DELIVERY

Gene therapy using overexpression systems for products that modify bone differentiation and generation have potential in the treatment of fractures and/or assisting with joint implants particularly in osteoporotic patients where failure rates are high. This approach has received considerable attention over the last few years, as proteins with osteogenic potential have been characterized in some detail (also reviewed in Refs. [3,4]). An in-depth understanding of the gross and fine control of bone regeneration is not yet clear; possible uses for therapy will require systems that deliver factors at optimal amounts over optimal time periods in a controllable fashion.

Delivering exogenous genes into cells and tissues requires methods that enable stability of the nucleic acid gene sequences of interest *in vitro* and *in vivo*, passage of the genes through cell membranes and subsequent expression of the 'transduced' genes either from episomal DNA or from the gene incorporated into the host cell genome. Although naked DNA can be taken up by cells, it is rapidly degraded by enzymes. Tightly wound DNA, such as that in plasmids, can be taken up by cells and successfully expressed (at relatively low efficiency), particularly by certain tissues such as striated muscle *in vivo*. Such non-viral gene transfer approaches for expression within/adjacent to bone tissue include implantation of collagen sponges with incorporated plasmid DNA or direct injection of viral vectors [5,6]. The use of viral vector systems has enabled gene transduction to a far greater efficacy than plasmid DNA through efficient mechanisms of cell entry and expression of virally-encoded genes. Ideal vectors for the use of gene transduction would be able to: (1) target cell types appropriate for diseases control; (2) enable sustainable and regulated expression of inserted genes; (3) provide minimal risk of insertional mutagenesis; (4) provide minimal risk of pathological side effects and additionally; (5) enable relatively simple methods to produce vectors in high and concentrated yields.

Detailed comprehensive reviews on methods of gene therapy have been published by Vera and Whiteman [7] and Sinn *et al.* [8]. In addition, Witlox *et al.* [2] have reviewed the potential of a number of vectors used to overexpress certain cell-modifying genes within bone cells. Various systems currently used to modify bone remodeling in an array of animal models include adenovirus, adeno-associated virus (AAV), lentiviruses, *ex vivo* delivery of transduced cells and non-viral methods of gene delivery. The various systems have different characteristics that can result in advantages or challenges for their use, and a brief indication of those identified by others [2,7,8] follows.

Adenovirus (Ad) vectors are a popular choice partly because of the ease with which recombinant vectors can be generated, high levels of transgene expression, and a relatively broad array of cells that can be transduced. Adenoviruses are non-enveloped DNA viruses that do not integrate into host DNA and genes are expressed from episomal DNA. Ad can be found in a number of species, and in humans there are at least 50 serotypes, and current adenovirus vectors are commonly derived from Ad type 5. The wild-type viruses have a high affinity for respiratory epithelial cells and can cause mild pathology in respiratory and gastro-intestinal tracts. They can also infect other organs such as the liver. Ad vectors rendered replication incompetent, have been widely used as a safer and better controlled method for transducing cells, and have provided proof of principle in many systems of the effects of transient gene-of-interest expression. They can orchestrate high levels of expression driven off recombinant inserts that also contain strong promoters, and can infect and thus transduce a variety of cell types.

Ad vectors can induce a potent immune response against infected/transduced cells. Since the infected cells are targeted and cleared by cellular immunity mechanisms, targeted cells produce gene inserts for a relatively short period of time (0–7 days) in immuno-competent animals. Pre-existing immunity to wild-type Ad will also affect efficiency of gene expression. Evolution of Ad vector systems has generated newer variations (second and third generation vectors) containing fewer virus protein genes and thus

a reduced capacity for immune stimulation. However, these newer vectors have reduced capacity, reduced levels of protein expression and reduced ease and quantity of vector preparation.

Adeno-associated virus (AAV) is a non-pathogenic DNA parvovirus that can transduce various cell types and tissues. In comparison to Ad vectors, AAV have a more restricted gene size capacity. Production requires a helper virus and vector production/efficiency is more cumbersome than Ad vector preparation. The best characterized serotype, AAV2, is the most frequently used for vector derivation.

Retroviruses (Rv) are double-stranded RNA viruses that integrate in to host the chromosome, and thus provide 'permanent' transfer of genes to a cell. Rv gene transducing systems (such as those derived from the Moloney murine leukemia virus) use recombinant vectors, which retain the machinery to integrate genes into host the chromosome and are thus useful for long-term expression. However, non-dividing somatic cells are not transduced, and random insertion into the host genome does represent a risk that insertion sites could result in inappropriate expression of native genes. **Lentiviruses** are a subset of RV that can transduce dividing or non-dividing cells. Lentivirus vectors, such as those derived from HIV-1, provide stable transduction and tropism for CD4T cells, macrophages and hematopoietic stem cells. By incorporating other envelope proteins into vectors one can increase the breadth of cells transduced.

Cells implanted after *ex vivo* **gene transduction** to elicit bone-generating capacity is another approach to generating bone healing and remodeling. In these systems, autologous (or syngeneic) cells are harvested, cultured *in vitro* and transduced with viral or non-viral vectors. Cells are then administered back to the subject. The use of autologous stem cell populations is a prospect with good potential for clinical applications. However, identification of appropriate cell populations, their subsequent expansion, efficiency of transduction and manipulation and/or function *in vivo* are current challenges in the field. Transduction of cell populations *ex vivo* with virus vectors enabling expression of genes that can control biological function has been explored in a number of systems.

III. CYTOKINE TRANSGENES AND BONE REMODELING

The control of bone development involves various hormones, transcription factors, signaling systems, cytokines and growth factors. Current knowledge regarding bone biology and the roles of cytokines has been reviewed extensively by others [9–19]. Cytokines and growth factors are polypeptides that interact at cell surface receptors and regulate many aspects of hematopoietic immune and inflammatory cell functions. Pro-inflammatory cytokines

Interleukin-1α and β, as well as tumor necrosis factor (TNF), have been shown to stimulate bone resorption, again in systems dependent on the presence of osteoblasts in cell culture [13,20]. Many more cytokines have been shown to contribute to regulation of bone metabolism (reviewed extensively elsewhere, see Refs. [11,21,22]) including G-CSF and M-CSF, insulin-like growth factor-1 (IGF-1), the IL-6-type (or gp130) family of cytokines, the TGF (transforming growth factor α and β) superfamily which includes the Bone Morphogenic Proteins (BMP), and the ligand/receptor system of membrane associated proteins RANK (receptor associated activator of Nf-κB) and RANK ligand (RANKL, also termed osteoprotegerin ligand or OPGL, TRANCE, and ODF) as well as the soluble inhibitor osteoprotegerin (OPG) in this system (see below).

A. Bone Morphogenic Proteins (BMPs)

The BMP family of cytokines has received attention over the past few years in regards to fracture healing on the basis or activity of recombinant proteins. The BMPs (extensively reviewed elsewhere, see Refs. [16,23]) represent molecules that are secreted and are active in the regulation of responses by various cells including osteoblasts. This area was encouraged by initial experiments that showed significant results in animal systems where recombinant BMPs or adenovirus-encoded BMPs induced ectopic bone formation [5,24]. The approval of direct administration of recombinant BMP-2 and BMP-7 by the FDA regulatory body has facilitated interest in assessing the use of gene therapy for BMPs. Clinical trials using the recombinant proteins have not shown the promise of results in animal studies, although the reasons for this are not yet clear.

In context of the complex nature of the osteogeneic process in bone formation and repair, a number of factors may be involved in the eventual maximization of therapeutic intervention, including half-life of the proteins, site of delivery, and which is the best BMP or other growth factor (or cocktail thereof) to use in the human system. Seehermann, Wozney and colleagues have shown in a number of studies (comprehensively reviewed in Refs. [25,26]) that incorporation of recombinant BMP proteins into treatments at sites of bone defects can be effective in enhancement of bone repair in rabbit [27,28] canine [29] and non-human primate [30,31] models. Thus, recombinant human BMP protein can be incorporated into various matrix scaffolds and subsequent administration is shown to be effective at accelerating healing of bone defects in various systems. The effectiveness of recombinant cytokine is hampered by a short half-life *in vivo* and thus is a significant limitation of single administrations.

Clearly these studies show the potential for the use of recombinant BMPs in enhancing the repair of bone defects. The use of gene therapy techniques to enhance and maintain desired protein (or multiple protein factors) expression

could circumvent some of these problems. It could certainly be helpful as an easier and more rapid way for testing for proof of principle of the usefulness of each protein or combination thereof. Indeed, the use of gene therapeutic methodology to introduce genes in local tissue sites has shown that unpredicted results can be the outcome, which then contributes to our knowledge of potential side effects or unpredicted beneficial effects.

1. Adenovirus Vectors Encoding BMPs

There have been studies that have examined different methods of gene transfer of BMP proteins, and among the first were those using adenovirus vectors. Ad vectors do not result in gene integration into host chromosomes and resulting immune targeting of transduced cells limiting the duration of the expression of the gene of interest. Thus, although this does not result in permanent gene transfer, the transient expression of certain genes may, in fact, be more desirable in certain processes including the remodeling of bone defects.

The use of adenoviral vectors as at least proof of principle has supported the potential of gene therapy for enhancement of bone formation. In 1999, Musgrave *et al.* were able to generate ectopic bone formation in muscle upon administration of an adenovirus vector expressing BMP-2 [5]. In 2000, Baltzer *et al.* [32] found that direct administration of first generation adenovirus encoding BMP-2 could enhance repair in surgically created segmental defects in NZ white rabbits. These studies encouraged the forage into the potential of BMP gene therapy for bone generation. Others have gone on to show that an adenovirus encoding BMP-4 can promote spinal fusion (in a NZ white rabbit model) upon implantation of AdBMP-4 within a collagen sponge onto lumbar lamina [33]. While a number of BMP family members have been identified with similar modes of action, different BMPs may show various capabilities to stimulate bone formation *in vivo*.

A number of other studies have used adenovirus and other vector systems to overexpress BMP family members in animal models; these have provided useful information regarding their potential. Li *et al.* [24] compared the efficacy of BMP-2, BMP-4, BMP-6, BMP-7 and BMP-9 encoded adenoviral vectors in models of rat bone formation *in vivo*. In this study, only Ad vector expressing BMP-9 induced detectable bone formation upon injection into the thigh musculature of immuno-competent rats; although all induced significant bone formation in immuno-deficient (athymic) rats and the vectors induced varying amounts of alkaline phosphatase activity in the C2C12 osteoblast cell line *in vitro*. With a helper-dependent Ad virus vector system designed to reduce immunogenicity of the vector, the same group was able to confirm that BMP-9 gene transfer was effective in ectopic bone induction apparently via normal endochondral formation.

The timing of gene transfer and expression may also be critical. In a rat critical-size femoral defect rat model, Betz *et al.* [34] have shown that direct administration of Ad-BMP-2 to the lesion was most beneficial in healing defects if given 5 or 10 days after the surgery. Whether this is true of other proteins awaits further work, but this does indicate that further study is needed on the best time to administer exogenous agents. Furthermore, combinations of specific products may also be superior. Zhu *et al.* [35] have shown that a combination of BMP-2 and BMP-7 adenovirus vectors were more superior at enhancing stable spine fusion and bone formation in rat models.

Use of recombinant adenovirus as gene transducing vectors for prolonged gene expression is limited by the host immune system. Expression of cytokine gene inserts from first generation Ad vectors (E1/E3 deleted) in a variety of tissue sites in immuno-competent rodent models is 3–7 days. Second generation Ad vectors are designed with more viral genes deleted from the genome, and may decrease the immune reactivity and enhance the longevity of expression. Interestingly, using an assay of ectopic bone formation in rats, Li *et al.* [36] found that direct comparison of first (E1/E3 deleted) and second (E1/E3 and E2b deleted) generation vectors encoding either human or rat BMP-6 showed similar levels of BMP-6 expression *in vitro* and *in vivo*, and a similar ability to induce ectopic bone formation. These results suggest that amounts of BMP-6 and the Ad vector used are not crucial in resulting *in vivo* effects on osteogenic potential in immuno-competent animals, although whether this holds true for other BMPs would require further work.

2. AAV VECTORS ENCODING BMP

Adeno-associated virus recombinant vectors have also shown promise as a platform for bone regeneration, although there has not been as much investigation using AAV-BMP encoded constructs as there has been for adenovirus constructs. Gafni *et al.* [37] have published a duo vector AAV system in order to enable control of transgene expression. Thus, one AAV vector encoding the BMP2 gene downstream of a minimal CMV promoter and a tet-inducible transcriptional factor (rtTA) binding site, and another AAV vector encoding the doxycycline-regulated transactivating transcription a factor (rtTA) can render *in vivo* expression of encoded BMP-1 sensitive to doxycycline treatment in drinking water. Although this study examined ectopic bone formation in rat thigh muscle, the principle of the use of AAV encoded BMP and its control by the tet-on system was nicely demonstrated. Using a different system, Koefoed *et al.* [38] showed that AAV encoding LacZ could be used to coat femoral allografts in a mouse model and result in transgene expression in inflammatory cells and osteoblasts in the callus of the femoral allografts. Using an AAV encoding caAlk-2 (the constitutively active BMP2 receptor), these authors also demonstrated that AAVAlk2-coated allografts resulted in significantly more bone formation [38], supporting the potential use of AAV encoding BMPs in enhancing bone formation and repair.

3. RETRO-VIRAL VECTORS ENCODING BMPS

Some studies have examined retrovirus vectors in expressing BMP proteins in animal models. As noted previously, retroviral vectors require transduction in proliferating cells. Using a MLV-based vector system encoding BMP-4 (fused with the BMP-2 secretory signal to enhance BMP-4 transgene secretion), Rundle *et al.* [39] showed that direct administration of MLV-BMP-4/2 could result in detection of transgene in the callus but not in the surrounding skeletal muscle tissue of a rat femoral fracture model. Furthermore, the fracture callus size was markedly increased, and extensive ossification was evident at 14 and 28 days. At day 70 after administration, the hard callus had been remodeled and substantial healing of the fracture was evident. Although this study suggested that Rv was effective at transducing genes at a fracture site, further study is needed to examine the rate and strength of the fracture healing response. Rundle *et al.* [40] have also shown that direct administration of MLV encoding cyclo-oxygenase 2 (COX-2) can enhance rapidity of healing in the fracture in the same rat model, where bony union of the fracture was evident by 21 days. Conversely, control animals need an additional week for such effects at the fracture site. Interestingly, they also observed less ectopic bone formation that is evident with gene therapy using BMP, which also points to an issue regarding potential side effects of BMP overexpression in general.

In directly comparing a lentivirus construct and an adenovirus construct encoding BMP-2 upon transfecting rat bone marrow cells *ex vivo*, Virk *et al.* [41] showed that lentivirus transduction could maintain prolonged expression *in vitro* and prolonged expression *in vivo* upon a subsequent injection of transduced cells into a rat critical-sized defect model. They also suggested better biomechanical properties of the resulting bone, indicating that prolonged expression of BMP-2 in the lentivirus system was superior to the shorter but higher levels of expression by Ad vector. However, subsequent studies have also shown in a mouse model that, although *in vivo* expression of BMP-2 by lentivirus could be detected for 3 months versus 1 month by Ad vector, there was no detectable difference in the amount of bone formed [42].

Plasmid Vectors The use of viral vectors in gene therapy for human conditions includes a number of unknowns that increases risk. Although low in chance, retroviruses may integrate into chromosomal locations that alter gene expression that generate new pathologies. Adenovirus vectors run the risk of recombination with other replication-competent wild-type adenoviruses of concomitant infections, and efficacy is adversely affected by the immune system in immuno-competent subjects *in vivo*. Thus, although markedly less efficient in gene transduction and of protein expression, transducing cells with plasmid DNA is an alternative approach to circumvent such risks. Implanting scaffolds with recombinant BMP proteins integrated can result in remodeling of bone as noted above. Using a similar approach to administer plasmid encoding BMP-4 protein, Chen *et al.* [43] were able to show in a canine jaw alveolar defect model, that plasmid encoding BMP-4 could increase bone density over controls (scaffold only), similar to bone autografts. In another study, the introduction of liposomes encoding BMP-2 into a model of peri-implant bone defects on pig calvariae [44] resulted in more rapid trabecular bone formation. Furthermore, transducing cells *ex vivo* with plasmid DNA is another approach (see below).

***Ex vivo* Gene Transduction** Transducing autologous cells *ex vivo* and subsequent administration of these cell populations into tissue sites is another potential approach for the elevation of specific genes. Advantages include increased specificity of cells transduced (compared to *in vivo* viral vector administration) and ability to assess parameters of gene transfer efficiency and efficacy of protein expression before administration. Robbins and Evans have clearly shown that this is feasible in the clinical setting for metacarpal joint expression of the interleukin-1 receptor antagonist in phase 1 clinical trials [45]. However, the process is technically challenging in the clinical setting, since time and care are needed in cell preparation and successful gene transduction. Careful characterization of cell populations is also needed for their proportion for *in vivo* administration to ensure efficacy in transgene expression, and purity of preparations then administered back to patients. The use of plasmid DNA for the gene transduction can eliminate concerns about the potential transfer of viral vectors upon re-administration of cell populations.

Systems in rodent models using *ex vivo* gene transfer of BMPs have been informative. Cells used for *ex vivo* transduction have included bone marrow-derived or adipose-derived mesenchymal cells. Rat bone marrow cells transduced with lentivirus or adenovirus expressing BMP-2 could be transferred to recipients (hind limb muscle pouch or radial defect) and express inserted BMP-2 for 3 weeks (Ad vector) or 3 months (lentiviral vector), although similar levels of induced bone formation has been observed [42]. Using human cells derived from adipocytes, Kang *et al.* [46] could transduce the human mesenchymal stem cells with AAV encoding human BMP-7 and subsequently implant the transduced cells in rat hind limb pouch of SCID mice. The system expressed product by day 7 and out to day 56 and formed new ectopic bone.

4. Non-viral *ex vivo* Transduction
Using porcine adipose-derived mesenchymal stem cells, Sheyn *et al.* [47] could transfect with plasmid encoding BMP-6 and then administer to lumbar para-vertebral muscle in immuno-deficient mice and obtain bone formation and spinal fusion. Human mesenchymal cells transduced with hBMP-2 or BMP-9 plasmids by nucleofection could express the BMP proteins for 14 days (after which expression waned) and increase ectopic bone formation in NOD/SCID mice [48]. This supports the feasibility of *ex vivo* transfected autologous cell administration, which may represent a safer means of potential treatment in the human system.

B. Osteoprotegerin Transgene and Bone Remodeling

Since overall bone metabolism is based on the balance of osteoblast and osteoclast numbers and relative activities, targeting the osteoclast is also a potential approach for manipulation of bone metabolism. Osteoclast activity is regulated by a number of cytokines. As noted above, factors including macrophage-colony stimulating factor (M-CSF) [49] and proteins RANK (receptor associated activator of Nf-κB) on osteoclasts and RANKLigand (RANKL or osteoprotegerin ligand (OPGL)) on osteoblasts [18,50–53] are important for osteoclast differentiation. Work has shown that RANK/RANKL is expressed at sites of bone erosion in the collagen-induced arthritis animal model [54]. These ligands and receptors are membrane bound, and are thus facilitated by cell–cell contact.

The natural soluble product osteoprotegerin (OPG) can bind RANKL (also termed OPGLigand) and interfere with RANKL/RANK interaction [18,55–57]. This inhibition has been shown to be efficient in suppressing osteoclast formation *in vitro* and a number of studies have been completed to confirm this function in various systems and in animal models *in vivo*. Mice with targeted mutations in OPG have severe osteoporosis [57] and transgenic mice expressing OPG in the liver showed profound but non-lethal osteopetrosis [55].

The action of OPG *in vivo* in investigative studies, as well as preclinical studies, has shown much promise for the therapy of conditions involving bone loss. A recombinant OPG-Fc fusion protein (OPG fused to the immunoglobulin Fc region for increased half-life), used in a number of pre-clinical studies and in current clinical trials, has shown marked effects of repeated OPG-Fc administration in animal systems. For a potential alternative to the preparation and repeated administration of agents such as OPG, gene transfer has been explored in several systems, with the aim of manipulating the RANK/RANKL interaction.

The use of vectors to express systemic levels of OPG has shown significant effects in animal models of osteoporosis. In 2001, Bolon *et al.* [58] showed that Ad encoding OPG or encoding a fusion of OPG-Fc could be administered to mice and induce systemic OPG levels. However, only the Ad OPG-Fc construct resulted in elevated OPG levels for a sustained period of time (18 months). Furthermore, they showed that in ovarectomized female mice, animals treated with Ad OPG-Fc for 4 weeks had significantly more bone volume and decreased osteoclast numbers in appendicular bones when compared to OVX mice treated with control vector.

A further study examined the use of an AAV vector encoding OPG. It showed significant effects in a model of overectomized (OVX)-induced osteopenia in CDF1 mice [59]. In this study, Kosteniuk *et al.* showed that intravenous (i.v.) administration of AAV-OPG led to increases in serum OPG within 7 days and high levels were maintained for up to 10 weeks. Furthermore, one i.v. administration of AAV-OPG vector provided 6 weeks after OVX (established reduction in bone mineral density (BMP)) could significantly increase BMD over control vector when assessed 10 weeks later as compared to the control (AAV-betaGal) vector [58]. The authors also showed that AAV-OPG administration in C57 Bl/6 mice resulted in sustained OPG elevation of OPG in serum for at least 16 months, similar to the advector expressing OPG-Fc [58]. These studies support the use of systemic administration of vectors for sustained elevation OPG levels that have significant effects on the maintenance of bone integrity. The data utilizing gene transfer for maintained OPGL levels have assisted with the rationale and preclinical studies for taking OPG-Fc further in clinical trials for osteoporosis.

Another indication for the use of controlling bone remodeling is aseptic loosening of orthopedic implants, which reduces the longevity of implants and reconstructed joints. This is thought to occur primarily due to debris-induced osteolysis and osteoclastogenesis, and can be modeled using an implantation of titanium wear-debris into mouse calvariae. Ulrich-Vinther *et al.* [60] have shown that an AAV vector encoding OPG and EGFP (when administered intramuscularly) can increase and maintain elevated serum OPG levels and significantly reduce osteoclast numbers and resorption in the bone wafer assay to a greater extent than parathyroid or AAV-LacZ control treatments. In another study, Goater *et al.* [61] used an *ex vivo* system of transfected fibroblast-like synoviocytes (FLS) with OPG. Cells with stable transfection and expressing OPG were implanted with titanium wear debris and significantly reduced osteoclastogenesis of mouse calvariae at the implantation site, whereas untransfected FLS did not. Collectively, these studies provide support for the use of elevated systemic OPG (maintained using gene transduction methods) to increase the longevity of orthopedic implants. Aseptic joint loosening will be an increasing problem due to a demographic driven need for such joint replacement procedures.

Bone remodeling is a dynamic complex process that ultimately results in the coordinated function and balance of osteoblast and osteoclast activity. Thus, one concern regarding the use of OPG is the potential disruption of such coordination essential for normal remodeling in fracture healing and callus formation. Ulrinch-Vinther *et al.* [62] have begun to address this question by using their AAV vector encoding OPG in a rat model of fracture healing and examining callus formation and characteristics. After 3 weeks of healing, animals treated i.m. with AAV-OPG showed reduced number of osteoclasts within the callus, decreased deposition of new woven bone at the fracture line, but increased bone mineral content. Callus dimensions and structural strength of the bone was not affected, thus in this system OPG affected remodeling but not to the extent that structural strength was compromised. More work in this area should further add to data regarding this issue.

The RANK/RANKL/OPGL cell activation network is not limited to osteoblasts and osteoclasts. Interaction between T cells and antigen presenting cells is also facilitated by RANK/RANKL [51], and this can be modified by OPG. As with other biological agents, effects in multiple systems must be considered for potential generation of side effects. For example, the use of OPG in RA may benefit from effects both on bone remodeling and on mitigation of immune activation, whereas the use of OPG in osteoporosis may evoke immune suppression that is undesirable. In 2007, Stolina *et al.* [63] showed that innate and acquired immune responses appeared to be intact in mice and rats transgenic for OPG. This is encouraging since immune suppression would be a consideration for human systems; however, further validation of such findings is merited.

Clearly, other cytokine growth factors or cell-associated molecules may emerge as effective agents or targets in modification of bone remodeling. For example, members of the IL-6-type (or gp130) cytokines are secreted by immune and non-immune cells and function to modulate differentiation, hematopoietic, immune inflammatory cell networks and osteoblast/osteoclast functions. Several reviews provide extensive information regarding the functions of these molecules [64–68] including those in bone metabolism (reviewed in Refs. [11,13]). Family members such as oncostatin M and IL-11 can induce net bone formation *in vivo* [69–71]. However, precise roles for each IL-6/LIF cytokine family member are not yet clearly defined.

IV. PROSPECTS OF CYTOKINE GENE THERAPY IN BONE CANCER

The potential in treating various types of cancers with gene transfer techniques is an exciting new area of investigation. One major target condition for such approaches is osteosarcoma, a malignant tumor of mesenchymal cell origin that can result in extensive bone remodeling. Osteosarcoma associated pathology can vary, including some tumors with excessive osteoid or woven bone, some with predominantly fibroblastic cell proliferation and/or considerable vascularization. The primary lesion is also characterized by a destruction of bone integrity and increased osteoclast activity, and is also considerably metastatic. The varied pathology may be a result of selective stages of mesenchymal cell differentiation of the primary tumor cells and/or the physiological/immunological response to the cancer cells. This may mean that specific targets for therapy can vary in effectiveness in different models/patients. Other tumors, such as prostate cancer, have a significant metastatic potential in bone. These represent a different array of challenges in understanding how to modify both the tumor growth and the associated bone destruction that occurs. The utilization of gene transducing vectors to modulate bone remodeling has been informative in understanding the potential in dramatically altering biological responses. The use of such methods in modulating bone cancer has been investigated to a limited degree at this point in time. An excellent review by Witlox *et al.* [2] details current aspects of gene transfer approaches for osteosarcoma, including those that utilize compensation of tumor suppressor genes such as p53, suicide genes, immunopotentiation as well as vectors with altered cell/molecular receptors or mechanisms to target specific transcriptional machinery in certain cells.

There is good evidence to suggest that the growth of tumors within bone, either of osteosarcoma or myeloma as the primary tumor or of metastasis of breast and prostate cancer, can be nurtured due to factors within the bone microenvironment (reviewed in Ref. [72]). The activation of osteoblasts and/or osteoclasts results in subsequent remodeling and release of a variety of growth factors that contribute to the vicious cycle of bone remodeling and tumor progression. Interference in the bone remodeling, and particularly osteoclast function, could modulate this process and slow tumor growth. Thus, the manipulation of the OPG/RANKL/RANK triad has been a subject of interest in bone cancers and metastasis (reviewed in Refs. [72–76]).

Studies have shown that systemic OPG administration can modify tumor growth in animal models of cancer metastasis. Zheng *et al.* [77] showed that, in a mouse model of osteosclerotic metastasis using human breast cancer MCF-7 cells implanted into the tibia, OPG treatment markedly inhibited osteoclastic activity and significantly reduced tumor burden [77]. In a mouse model using MDA-231 breast carcinoma cells, which show high levels of RANKL on tumor-bearing bone cells, treatment with OPG-Fc resulted in decreased osteoclastogenesis and tumor growth [78]. Thus, although OPG could potentially protect tumor cells from RANK/RANKL-induced apoptosis, these data support its potential in modifying breast cancer metastasis growth in bony tissues. The prostate cancer cell lines PC3 appears to express RANK and metastasis/growth at

bone sites may also be dependent on RANKL/RANK interactions. Treatment of SCID mice with OPG-Fc resulted in the suppression of PC3 tumor burden [79], although it is not yet clear whether OPG-Fc was acting on host–host or host–tumor (or both) RANK/RANKL interactions.

Such data support further work in using gene therapy methodology to transduce and express systemic levels of OPG. Although the OPG-Fc protein possesses considerable half-life, it is expensive. Safety issues for patient treatment may be more straightforward to address than a gene therapeutic approach. Some studies have investigated the potential of OPG gene therapy. Chanda *et al.* [80] have shown that administration of AAV encoding OPG (but not control AAV) resulted in a significant reduction in bone tumor growth and bone loss upon MDA-MB-435 human breast carcinoma cells given by intracardiac injection in athymic *nu/nu* mice. However, long-term survival was not influenced by the treatment [80], likely because there was no beneficial effect of AAV-OPG-Fc on metastasis to non-osseus tissue sites including liver, lung, spleen and lymph nodes. Using an adenovirus encoding OPG in two rodent models of osteosarcoma, Lamoureux *et al.* [81] could markedly inhibit the formation of osteolystic lesions and tumor incidence in bone tissue as well as increase survival of mice at 28 days. Metastasis to the lungs of animals was not affected, indicating that the effects of OPG gene transfer were dependent on its effects on osteoclast function within the bone. Thus, these data support the vicious cycle hypothesis, while also indicating that such approaches must be augmented with other therapies to enable treatment for metastasis outside of the bone environment.

There is currently little published work examining the potential roles of gene therapy and BMPs in cancer therapy; possibly because the potential of these molecules as therapeutic agents for cancer is not clear. Likewise, the potential of IL-6-type cytokines as therapeutic agents in bone cancer is not yet well studied. Chipoy *et al.* [82] have shown that the IL-6 family member oncostatin M can sensitize osteosarcoma cell lines to staurosporine- or TNF-induced apoptosis. Using a systemic expression of OSM with AdOSM administered i.v. or i.m., Brounais *et al.* [83] have shown that tumor burden can be decreased with co-treatment with midostaurin. These studies support the potential of co-treatment regimes and encourage further work in this area.

V. CONCLUSIONS

The use of gene transduction to explore cytokine over-expression in the control of bone metabolism and remodeling has increased our understanding of certain cytokine biological function *in vivo* as well as being a potential for therapeutic purposes. Experimentation with a number of vector technologies has provided more information on the characteristics and activities of different vectors and their payload genes within the bone environment. This has enabled progress in refining the use of gene transduction for bone disease. The potential for BMPs and OPG prolonged overexpression is still to be explored in greater detail for diseases requiring net bone deposition and repair. Although there have been fewer studies that specifically look at gene transduction of cytokines for treatment of bone cancer, certainly those that examine effects of OPG show promise, and current clinical trials with OPG-Fc protein will help to pave the way for addressing safety in future studies involving long-term OPG therapy. A role of OPG in inhibiting the immune function through its ability to modify APC/T cell interaction is still an issue in treatments where immuno-modulation is contraindicated. Clearly, other molecules may emerge with the potential in modulation of bone metabolism through gene transduction approaches. There are still considerable unknowns in the exploration of the maximization of the effectiveness for gene therapeutic approaches in bone disease.

Acknowledgements

This work was in part supported by the Arthritis Society (Canada) and the Canadian Institute for Health Research.

References

1. K. Mori, F. Redini & F. Gouin, et al., Osteosarcoma: current status of immunotherapy and future trends (Review), Oncol Rep 15 (2006) 693–700.

2. M.A. Witlox, M.L. Lamfers & P.I. Wuisman, et al., Evolving gene therapy approaches for osteosarcoma using viral vectors: review, Bone 40 (2007) 797–812.

3. A.W. Baltzer & J.R. Lieberman, Regional gene therapy to enhance bone repair, Gene Ther 11 (2004) 344–350.

4. N. Kimelman, G. Pelled & G.A. Helm, et al., Review: gene- and stem cell-based therapeutics for bone regeneration and repair, Tissue Eng 13 (2007) 1135–1150.

5. D.S. Musgrave, P.P. Bosch & S. Ghivizzani, et al., Adenovirus-mediated direct gene therapy with bone morphogenetic protein-2 produces bone, Bone 24 (1999) 541–547.

6. M. Egermann, E. Schneider & C.H. Evans, et al., The potential of gene therapy for fracture healing in osteoporosis, Osteoporos Int 16 (Suppl 2) (2005) S120–S128.

7. I.M. Verma & M.D. Weitzman, Gene therapy: twenty-first century medicine, Annu Rev Biochem 74 (2005) 711–738.

8. P.L. Sinn, S.L. Sauter & P.B. McCray Jr, Gene therapy progress and prospects: development of improved lentiviral and retroviral vectors—design, biosafety, and production, Gene Ther 12 (2005) 1089–1098.

9. E. Canalis, T.L. McCarthy & M. Centrella, Growth factors and cytokines in bone cell metabolism, Annu Rev Med 42 (1991) 17–24.

10. E.A. Garcia-Zepeda, M.E. Rothenberg & R.T. Ownbey, et al., Human eotaxin is a specific chemoattractant for eosinophil cells and provides a new mechanism to explain tissue eosinophilia, Nat Med 2 (1996) 449–456.

11. D. Heymann & A.V. Rousselle, p130 Cytokine family and bone cells, Cytokine 12 (2000) 1455–1468.

12. G. Karsenty, The central regulation of bone remodeling, Trends Endocrinol Metab 11 (2000) 437–439.

13. T.S. Kwan, M. Padrines & S. Theoleyre, et al., IL-6, RANKL, TNF-alpha/IL-1: interrelations in bone resorption pathophysiology, Cytokine Growth Factor Rev 15 (2004) 49–60.

14. A.I. Alford & K.D. Hankenson, Matricellular proteins: extracellular modulators of bone development, remodeling, and regeneration, Bone 38 (2006) 749–757.

15. G.K. Chan & G. Duque, Age-related bone loss: old bone, new facts, Gerontology 48 (2002) 62–71.

16. Z.L. Deng, K.A. Sharff & N. Tang, et al., Regulation of osteogenic differentiation during skeletal development, Front Biosci 13 (2008) 2001–2021.

17. J.M. Gimble, S. Zvonic & Z.E. Floyd, et al., Playing with bone and fat, J Cell Biochem 98 (2006) 251–266.

18. S. Theoleyre, Y. Wittrant & S.K. Tat, et al., The molecular triad OPG/RANK/RANKL: involvement in the orchestration of pathophysiological bone remodeling, Cytokine Growth Factor Rev 15 (2004) 457–475.

19. D.J. Hadjidakis & I.I. Androulakis, Bone remodeling, Ann NY Acad Sci 1092 (2006) 385–396.

20. B.M. Thomson, I.I. Mundy & T.J. Chambers, Tumor necrosis factors alpha and beta induce osteoblastic cells to stimulate osteoclastic bone resorption, J Immunol 138 (1987) 775–779.

21. D. Heymann, J. Guicheux & F. Gouin, et al., Cytokines, growth factors and osteoclasts, Cytokine 10 (1998) 155–168.

22. Y. Taguchi, M. Yamamoto & T. Yamate, et al., Interleukin-6-type cytokines stimulate mesenchymal progenitor differentiation toward the osteoblastic lineage, Pro Assoc Am Physicians 110 (1998) 559–574.

23. D.J. Hadjidakis & I.I. Androulakis, Bone remodeling, Ann NY Acad Sci 1092 (2006) 385–396.

24. J.Z. Li, H. Li & T. Sasaki, et al., Osteogenic potential of five different recombinant human bone morphogenetic protein adenoviral vectors in the rat, Gene Ther 10 (2003) 1735–1743.

25. H. Seeherman & J.M. Wozney, Delivery of bone morphogenetic proteins for orthopedic tissue regeneration, Cytokine Growth Factor Rev 16 (2005) 329–345.

26. J.M. Wozney & H.J. Seeherman, Protein-based tissue engineering in bone and cartilage repair, Curr Opin Biotechnol 15 (2004) 392–398.

27. R.H. Li, M.L. Bouxsein & C.A. Blake, et al., rhBMP-2 injected in a calcium phosphate paste (alpha-BSM) accelerates healing in the rabbit ulnar osteotomy model, J Orthop Res 21 (2003) 997–1004.

28. H.J. Seeherman, K. Azari & S. Bidic, et al., rhBMP-2 delivered in a calcium phosphate cement accelerates bridging of critical-sized defects in rabbit radii, J Bone Joint Surg Am 88 (2006) 1553–1565.

29. D.R. Sumner, T.M. Turner & R.M. Urban, et al., Locally delivered rhBMP-2 enhances bone ingrowth and gap healing in a canine model, J Orthop Res 22 (2004) 58–65.

30. H.J. Seeherman, M. Bouxsein & H. Kim, et al., Recombinant human bone morphogenetic protein-2 delivered in an injectable calcium phosphate paste accelerates osteotomy-site healing in a nonhuman primate model, J Bone Joint Surg Am 86–A (2004) 1961–1972.

31. H. Seeherman, R. Li & M. Bouxsein, et al., rhBMP-2/calcium phosphate matrix accelerates osteotomy-site healing in a non-human primate model at multiple treatment times and concentrations, J Bone Joint Surg Am 88 (2006) 144–160.

32. A.W. Baltzer, C. Lattermann & J.D. Whalen, et al., Genetic enhancement of fracture repair: healing of an experimental segmental defect by adenoviral transfer of the BMP-2 gene, Gene Ther 7 (2000) 734–739.

33. J. Zhao, D.Y. Zhao & A.G. Shen, et al., Promoting lumbar spinal fusion by adenovirus-mediated bone morphogenetic protein-4 gene therapy, Chin J Traumatol 10 (2007) 72–76.

34. O.B. Betz, V.M. Betz & A. Nazarian, et al., Delayed administration of adenoviral BMP-2 vector improves the formation of bone in osseous defects, Gene Ther 14 (2007) 1039–1044.

35. W. Zhu, B.A. Rawlins & O. Boachie-Adjei, et al., Combined bone morphogenetic protein-2 and -7 gene transfer enhances osteoblastic differentiation and spine fusion in a rodent model, J Bone Miner Res 19 (2004) 2021–2032.

36. H. Li, J.Z. Li & D.D. Pittman, et al., Comparison of osteogenic potentials of human rat BMP4 and BMP6 gene therapy using [E1-] and [E1-, E2b-] adenoviral vectors, Int J Med Sci 3 (2006) 97–105.

37. Y. Gafni, D.D. Pelled & Y. Zilberman, et al., Gene therapy platform for bone regeneration using an exogenously regulated, AAV-2-based gene expression system, Mol Ther 9 (2004) 587–595.

38. M. Koefoed, H. Ito & K. Gromov, et al., Biological effects of rAAV-caAlk2 coating on structural allograft healing, Mol Ther 12 (2005) 212–218.

39. C.H. Rundle, N. Miyakoshi & Y. Kasukawa, et al., *In vivo* bone formation in fracture repair induced by direct retroviral-based gene therapy with bone morphogenetic protein-4, Bone 32 (2003) 591–601.

40. C.H. Rundle, D.D. Strong & S.T. Chen, et al., Retroviral-based gene therapy with cyclooxygenase-2 promotes the union of bony callus tissues and accelerates fracture healing in the rat, J Gene Med 10 (2008) 229–241.

41. M.S. Virk, A. Conduah & S.H. Park, et al., Influence of short-term adenoviral vector and prolonged lentiviral vector mediated bone morphogenetic protein-2 expression on the quality of bone repair in a rat femoral defect model, Bone 42 (2008) 321–931.

42. B.T. Feeley, A.H. Conduah & O. Sugiyama, et al., *In vivo* molecular imaging of adenoviral versus lentiviral gene therapy in two bone formation models, J Orthop Res 24 (2006) 1709–1721.

43. J.C. Chen, S.R. Winn & X. Gong, et al., rhBMP-4 gene therapy in a juvenile canine alveolar defect model, Plast Reconstr Surg 120 (2007) 1503–1509.

44. J. Park, R. Lutz & E. Felszeghy, et al., The effect on bone regeneration of a liposomal vector to deliver BMP-2 gene to bone grafts in peri-implant bone defects, Biomaterials 28 (2007) 2772–2782.

45. C.H. Evans, P.D. Robbins & S.C. Ghivizzani, et al., Gene transfer to human joints: progress toward a gene therapy of arthritis, Proc Natl Acad Sci USA 102 (2005) 8698–8703.

46. Y. Kang, W.M. Liao & Z.H. Yuan, et al., *In vitro* and *in vivo* induction of bone formation based on adeno-associated virus-mediated BMP-7 gene therapy using human adipose-derived mesenchymal stem cells, Acta Pharmacol Sin 28 (2007) 839–849.

47. D. Sheyn, G. Pelled & Y. Zilberman, et al., Nonvirally engineered porcine adipose tissue-derived stem cells: use in posterior spinal fusion, Stem Cells 4 (2008) 1056–1064.

48. H. Aslan, Y. Zilberman & V. Arbeli, et al., Nucleofection-based ex vivo nonviral gene delivery to human stem cells as a platform for tissue regeneration, Tissue Eng 12 (2006) 877–889.

49. H. Kodama, A. Yamasaki & M. Nose, et al., Congenital osteoclast deficiency in osteopetrotic (op/op) mice is cured by injections of macrophage colony-stimulating factor, J Exp Med 173 (1991) 269–272.

50. D.L. Lacey, E. Timms & H.L. Tan, et al., Osteoprotegerin ligand is a cytokine that regulates osteoclast differentiation and activation, Cell 93 (1998) 165–176.

51. Y.Y. Kong, H. Yoshida & I. Sarosi, et al., OPGL is a key regulator of osteoclastogenesis, lymphocyte development and lymph-node organogenesis, Nature 397 (1999) 315–323.

52. H. Yasuda, N. Shima & N. Nakagawa, et al., Osteoclast differentiation factor is a ligand for osteoprotegerin/osteoclastogenesis-inhibitory factor and is identical to TRANCE/RANKL, Proc Natl Acad Sci USA 95 (1998) 3597–3602.

53. B.R. Wong, R. Josien & Y. Choi, TRANCE is a TNF family member that regulates dendritic cell and osteoclast function, J Leukoc Biol 65 (1999) 715–724.

54. E. Lubberts, M.I. Koenders & B. Oppers-Walgreen, et al., Treatment with a neutralizing anti-murine interleukin-17 antibody after the onset of collagen-induced arthritis reduces joint inflammation, cartilage destruction, and bone erosion, Arthritis Rheum 50 (2004) 650–659.

55. W.S. Simonet, D.L. Lacey & C.R. Dunstan, et al., Osteoprotegerin: a novel secreted protein involved in the regulation of bone density, Cell 89 (1997) 309–319.

56. H. Yasuda, N. Shima & N. Nakagawa, et al., Identity of osteoclastogenesis inhibitory factor (OCIF) and osteoprotegerin (OPG): a mechanism by which OPG/OCIF inhibits osteoclastogenesis *in vitro*, Endocrinology 139 (1998) 1329–1337.

57. A. Mizuno, N. Amizuka & K. Irie, et al., Severe osteoporosis in mice lacking osteoclastogenesis inhibitory factor/osteoprotegerin, Biochem Biophys Res Commun 247 (1998) 610–615.

58. B. Bolon, C. Carter & M. Daris, et al., Adenoviral delivery of osteoprotegerin ameliorates bone resorption in a mouse ovariectomy model of osteoporosis, Mol Ther 3 (2001) 197–205.

59. P.J. Kostenuik, B. Bolon & S. Morony, et al., Gene therapy with human recombinant osteoprotegerin reverses established osteopenia in ovariectomized mice, Bone 34 (2004) 656–664.

60. M. Ulrich-Vinther, E.E. Carmody & J.J. Goater, et al., Recombinant adeno-associated virus-mediated osteoprotegerin gene therapy inhibits wear debris-induced osteolysis, J Bone Joint Surg Am 84–A (2002) 1405–1412.

61. J.J. Goater, R.J. O'Keefe & R.N. Rosier, et al., Efficacy of ex vivo OPG gene therapy in preventing wear debris induced osteolysis, J Orthop Res 20 (2002) 169–173.

62. M. Ulrich-Vinther, E.M. Schwarz & F.S. Pedersen, et al., Gene therapy with human osteoprotegerin decreases callus remodeling with limited effects on biomechanical properties, Bone 37 (2005) 751–758.

63. M. Stolina, D. Dwyer & M.S. Ominsky, et al., Continuous RANKL inhibition in osteoprotegerin transgenic mice and rats suppresses bone resorption without impairing lymphorganogenesis or functional immune responses, J Immunol 179 (2007) 7497–7505.

64. T. Kishimoto, S. Akira & M. Narazaki, et al., Interleukin-6 family of cytokines and gp130, Blood 86 (1995) 1243–1254.

65. D. Kamimura, K. Ishihara & T. Hirano, IL-6 signal transduction and its physiological roles: the signal orchestration model, Rev Physiol Biochem Pharmacol 149 (2003) 1–38.

66. M. Murakami, D. Kamimura & T. Hirano, New IL-6 (gp130) family cytokine members, CLC/NNT1/BSF3 and IL-27, Growth Factors 22 (2004) 75–77.

67. D.J. Hilton, LIF: lots of interesting functions, Trends Biochem Sci 17 (1992) 72–76.

68. A.V. Villarino, E. Huang & C.A. Hunter, Understanding the pro- and anti-inflammatory properties of IL-27, J Immunol 173 (2004) 715–720.

69. N. Malik, H.S. Haugen & B. Modrell, et al., Developmental abnormalities in mice transgenic for bovine oncostatin M, Mol Cell Biol 15 (1995) 2349–2358.

70. A.S. de Hooge, F.A. van de Loo & M.B. Bennink, et al., Growth plate damage, a feature of juvenile idiopathic arthritis, can be induced by adenoviral gene transfer of oncostatin M: a comparative study in gene-deficient mice, Arthritis Rheum 48 (2003) 1750–1761.

71. Y. Takeuchi, S. Watanabe & G. Ishii, et al., Interleukin-11 as a stimulatory factor for bone formation prevents bone loss with advancing age in mice, J Biol Chem 277 (2002) 49011–49018.

72. G.D. Roodman & W.C. Dougall, RANK ligand as a therapeutic target for bone metastases and multiple myeloma, Cancer Treat Rev 34 (2008) 92–101.

73. W.C. Dougall & M. Chaisson, The RANK/RANKL/OPG triad in cancer-induced bone diseases, Cancer Metastasis Rev 25 (2006) 541–549.

74. M. Baud'huin, L. Duplomb & V.C. Ruiz, et al., Key roles of the OPG-RANK-RANKL system in bone oncology, Expert Rev Anticancer Ther 7 (2007) 221–232.

75. M. Baud'huin, F. Lamoureux & L. Duplomb, et al., RANKL, RANK, osteoprotegerin: key partners of osteoimmunology and vascular diseases, Cell Mol Life Sci 64 (2007) 2334–2350.

76. D. Dingli & S.J. Russell, Mouse models and the RANKL/OPG axis in myeloma bone disease, Leukemia 21 (2007) 2090–2093.

77. Y. Zheng, H. Zhou & C. Fong-Yee, et al., Bone resorption increases tumour growth in a mouse model of osteosclerotic breast cancer metastasis, Clin Exp Metastasis 25 (2008) 559–567.

78. J.R. Canon, M. Roudier & R. Bryant, et al., Inhibition of RANKL blocks skeletal tumor progression and improves survival in a mouse model of breast cancer bone metastasis, Clin Exp Metastasis 25 (2008) 119–129.

79. A.P. Armstrong, R.E. Miller & J.C. Jones, et al., RANKL acts directly on RANK-expressing prostate tumor cells and mediates migration and expression of tumor metastasis genes, Prostate 68 (2008) 92–104.

80. D. Chanda, T. Isayeva & S. Kumar, et al., Systemic Osteoprotegerin Gene Therapy Restores Tumor-induced Bone Loss in a Therapeutic Model of Breast Cancer Bone Metastasis, Mol Ther 16 (2008) 871–878.

81. F. Lamoureux, P. Richard & Y. Wittrant, et al., Therapeutic relevance of osteoprotegerin gene therapy in osteosarcoma: blockade of the vicious cycle between tumor cell proliferation and bone resorption, Cancer Res 67 (2007) 7308–7318.

82. C. Chipoy, B. Brounais & V. Trichet, et al., Sensitization of osteosarcoma cells to apoptosis by oncostatin M depends on STAT5 and p53, Oncogene 26 (2007) 6653–6664.

83. B. Brounais, C. Chipoy & K. Mori, et al., Oncostatin M induces bone loss and sensitizes rat osteocarcoma to the antitumour effect of midostaurin *in vivo*, Clin Cancer Res 14 (2008) 5400–5409.

CHAPTER **31**

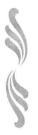

Non-surgical Treatment of Chondrosarcoma: Current Concepts and Future Perspectives

ERIC L. STAALS[1], EMANUELA PALMERINI[2], STEFANO FERRARI[2] AND MARIO MERCURI[1]

[1]Fifth Division of Orthopaedic Surgery, Department of Musculoskeletal Oncology, Istituti Ortopedici Rizzoli, Bologna, Italy.
[2]Chemotherapy Unit, Department of Musculoskeletal Oncology, Istituti Ortopedici Rizzoli, Bologna, Italy.

Contents

I. INTRODUCTION

Chondrosarcoma is a malignant tumor composed of a hyaline cartilage matrix and chondrocytes in lacunae. It is the third most common primary malignant bone tumor, exceeded only by myeloma and osteosarcoma, and accounts for about 10% of all primary malignant bone neoplasms [1–3].

There are several classifications of chondrosarcomas, based on the histologic features, the presence of pre-existing lesions, or the localization of the lesion.

In the classification based on histologic features, conventional chondrosarcoma is the most common type of chondrosarcoma and represents about 90% of all chondrosarcomas. Other histologic variants are dedifferentiated chondrosarcoma, mesenchymal chondrosarcoma and clear cell chondrosarcoma [3].

Chondrosarcoma can arise *de novo* or in pre-existing benign cartilage lesions. When a chondrosarcoma arises *de novo*, it is considered 'primary'. Instead, when a chondrosarcoma arises in a pre-existing osteochondroma or enchondroma, it is called 'secondary'.

According to the site of the lesion, chondrosarcomas are classified as central or peripheral [4]. Central lesions arise within the bone, whereas peripheral lesions occur on the bone surface. The latter are per definition secondary lesions [1].

II. CHONDROSARCOMA SUBTYPES

A. Conventional Chondrosarcoma

Conventional chondrosarcoma is the most common type of chondrosarcoma. It is usually a slow-growing, low-grade cartilaginous lesion. It occurs more frequently in males than in females and usually in adult or elderly patients: more than 60% of the patients are in their fourth through sixth decades of life. When conventional chondrosarcoma involves the long bones, it usually arises in the metaphysis or in the diaphysis. In the pelvis, chondrosarcomas are often located in the periacetabular region. There are three histological grades for conventional chondrosarcoma [1–3]. The incidence for grade 1 is 61%, grade 2 is 36%, and grade 3 is 3% [5].

In cytogenetic studies, conventional chondrosarcoma is characterized by a substantial heterogeneity with respect to karyotypic complexity [6]. The degree of karyotypic complexity [7], as well as aneuploidy [8], has been associated with increased aggressiveness of cartilaginous tumors. Near-diploidy and loss of heterozygosity are typical of low-grade central rather than of peripheral chondrosarcomas [9]. In the oncogenesis and tumor progression of central cartilaginous lesions, important roles are suggested for chromosome 9p21 [6,9,10], the p16 tumor suppressor gene, and p53 alterations [8]. Studies exclusively on peripheral chondrosarcomas are rare. Although the importance of the EXT1 gene in peripheral cartilaginous tumorigenesis has been demonstrated [11], the additional genetic changes that turn an osteochondroma into a peripheral chondrosarcoma are so far unidentified. Nevertheless, advances in the understanding of chondrosarcoma development have suggested that, despite the histological similarities between central and peripheral chondrosarcomas, they differ significantly at a molecular level [12].

The prognosis for patients with conventional chondrosarcoma is closely related to stage of disease, histological grade, size, and surgical margins [1]. The 5-year overall survival rate is 89% for patients with grade 1 lesions, and 57% for the combined group of patients grade 2 and grade 3 lesions [5]. The metastatic rate is close to 0% for grade 1, 10% for grade 2, and 70% for grade 3 lesions [13]. When metastases occur, they generally involve the lungs.

Surgical excision is the main treatment for conventional chondrosarcoma. Although for grades 2 and 3, chondrosarcoma wide surgical margins are mandatory, the best local treatment for grade 1 lesions is controversial and some authors report excellent functional results associated with adequate oncological outcome after curettage and adjuvants for low-grade chondrosarcoma, especially of the long bones [14–17]. Conventional chondrosarcoma has shown to be relatively radiotherapy and chemotherapy resistant [1,2,18]. Therefore, the role of non-surgical treatments for conventional chondrosarcoma is still very limited.

B. Mesenchymal Chondrosarcoma

Mesenchymal chondrosarcoma is a very rare variant of chondrosarcoma. The term 'Mesechymal chondrosarcoma' was introduced in 1959 by Lichtenstein and Bernstein in a series of unusual cartilaginous tumors of bone and soft tissue [19]. Unlike conventional chondrosarcomas, mesenchymal chondrosarcoma tends to affect young adults and about 60% of the patients are in the second and third decade of life [20]. It is characterized by a bimorphic histological pattern in which a relatively well-differentiated cartilage tissue is admixed with a highly undifferentiated small cell component [1,2]. The small cells can appear to be round, oval or spindle-shaped, and this component often resembles a hemangiopericytoma or Ewing's sarcoma. Because of the small cell component, mesenchymal chondrosarcoma always has to be considered as a high-grade (grade 4) malignant tumor.

A chromosome abnormality der(13;21)(q10;q10) was found in two cases [21]. About 60% of tumors demonstrate p53 overexpression; however, no mutation was found [22].

The prognosis is unpredictable; some patients present with disseminated disease and die within a year, others survive for decades. Metastases can occur after 5 years and therefore long-term follow-up is required. The 5-year survival rate has been reported between 42 and 54% [20,23]; the 10-year survival rate between 21 and 28% [23,24].

Due to the rarity of this tumor, a clear treatment strategy in mesenchymal chondrosarcoma has not yet been defined, but these tumors are often managed by a combination of wide surgical excision and chemotherapy. Huvos *et al.* [23] reported results of chemotherapy treatment, in addition to surgery or radiotherapy or both, in 13 patients with mesenchymal chondrosarcoma. They described this combined approach as encouraging, and suggested treating tumors with

a predominant hemangiopericytomatous pattern according to an osteosarcoma protocol, and those with small cells in sheets according to a Ewing's sarcoma protocol. In a review of 111 cases of mesenchymal chondrosarcoma, Nakashima *et al.* did not report any conclusive results on the role of chemotherapy [20]. In another review, using 26 patients from the Rizzoli Institute, Cesari *et al.* [24] showed a statistically significant difference in disease-free survival (DFS) rate for patients treated with chemotherapy (10 years DFS 76% with chemotherapy vs 17% without chemotherapy). Different chemotherapy protocols were used, but all reported regimens contained doxorubicin and ifosfamide. The results were based on a retrospective study with a limited and heterogeneous patient group. The authors recommend the use of chemotherapy in addition to the surgical removal of the tumor, if technically feasible, in cases of mesenchymal chondrosarcoma. Because of the rarity of the tumor, multicenter studies are required to identify the most effective chemotherapy regimen.

C. Dedifferentiated Chondrosarcoma

Dedifferentiated chondrosarcoma is a relatively rare variant, accounting for about 10–15% of chondrosarcomas. This tumor is characterized by a bimorphic histological pattern with areas of low-grade chondrosarcoma juxtaposed to a high-grade spindle cell sarcoma. The high-grade component is usually an osteosarcoma, a malignant fibrous histiocytoma or a fibrosarcoma [1,2]. On this entity, first described by Dahlin and Beabout in 1971 [25], numerous case reports and a few large series have been published [26–34].

Few studies have addressed the genetic abnormalities of dedifferentiated chondrosarcoma, demonstrating concordant genetic aberrations in both the anaplastic and cartilagineous component, indicating a common precursor cell [35–37].

The disease is characterized by an extremely poor prognosis, with the frequent development of distant metastases and consequent death. The 5-year overall survival rate has been reported between 6 and 29% [26–34]. The high-grade spindle cell component is presumably responsible for the poor prognosis of dedifferentiated chondrosarcoma. Given this appalling prognosis, it is not surprising that many attempts have been made to improve the tumor control by adding chemotherapy to the standard surgical treatment. A wide range of drug regimens has been used, the most common being a doxorubicin-based regimen, often in combination with cisplatin, ifosfamide, and/or methotrexate.

However, while for similar aged patients with osteosarcoma and spindle cell sarcoma treated with surgery and chemotherapy the 5-year survival rate is around 50% [38,39], in dedifferentiated chondrosarcoma this rate is less than 30%. Although higher survival rates in dedifferentiated chondrosarcoma have been reported in many papers [32–34], including a relatively high number of patients treated with chemotherapy, no author has ever demonstrated a statistically significant benefit from chemotherapy. Moreover, the studies that assessed tumor necrosis after neoadjuvant chemotherapy reported a poor histological response in almost all cases [29,30,32,34]. The reason why the high-grade spindle cell components in dedifferentiated chondrosarcoma are relatively resistant to chemotherapy remains unclear. However, a common monoclonal origin of both the chondroid and the spindle cell component was demonstrated in genetic studies [35,40], suggesting similar pathways of chemotherapy-resistance between conventional and dedifferentiated chondrosarcoma.

Prospective trials evaluating the role of chemotherapy in dedifferentiated chondrosarcoma are needed. At the present time, the European Musculoskeletal Oncology Society (EMSOS) is performing the EUROBOSS (European over 40 Bone Sarcoma Study), which will include patients with dedifferentiated chondrosarcoma aged between 41 and 64. Patients will undergo chemotherapy using a combination of ifosfamide, adriamycin and cisplatin, with the addition of methotrexate for those with a poor response to neoadjuvant chemotherapy [41].

D. Clear Cell Chondrosarcoma

Clear cell chondrosarcoma is a low grade malignant tumor characterized by tumor cells with clear empty cytoplasms. It was initially described by Unni *et al.* in 1976, and was called 'Clear-cell Variant of Chondrosarcoma' [42]. About two-thirds of the lesions occur in the proximal humerus or proximal femur, and the tumor is usually located in the epiphysis [1–3]. Extra copies of chromosome 20 and loss or rearrangements of 9p were found in a few cases [43].

En bloc excision with clear margins usually results in a cure. However, marginal or intralesional surgery is associated with a very high, more than 80%, recurrence rate and mortality rate between 30 and 50% [42,44]. Although metastases are rare, they may occur even more than 20 years after the initial diagnosis [45]. Dedifferentiation to high grade sarcoma has been reported in three cases [46].

III. TREATMENT

Surgical excision is the main treatment for all chondrosarcoma subtypes. Wide surgical margins are recommended in order to obtain the best chance for local control. Conventional and clear cell chondrosarcoma have shown to be relatively radiotherapy and chemotherapy resistant [1,2,18]. The role of non-surgical treatment of chondrosarcoma is currently very limited. Chemotherapy is used in the clinical practice for the treatment of mesenchymal and dedifferentiated chondrosarcoma, even though there is no statistical evidence of any positive effect on outcome. Radiotherapy has an important role in the treatment of chondrosarcomas located at the skull-base and the cervical

spine, as these lesions are often considered to be inoperable. Both radiotherapy and chemotherapy are occasionally used for metastatic chondrosarcomas, when surgical removal is impossible. Currently, new agents and molecular compounds that could target different pathways of chondrosarcoma development are being investigated and could lead to new treatment strategies in the near future. Hereunder, an overview of the current concepts of non-surgical treatments for chondrosarcoma is presented.

IV. NON-SURGICAL TREATMENT

A. Chemotherapy

Although no prospective trials on chemotherapy efficacy in chondrosarcoma are reported in the literature, conventional chondrosarcomas are generally considered resistant to chemotherapy [1,2,18]. Studies on the underlying mechanisms of chemotherapy resistance in chondrosarcoma are rare. Possible explanations of resistance are the constitutive expression of the multidrug-resistance-1 gene P-glycoprotein [47,48], the large amount of extracellular matrix impending the access of anticancer drugs, and the relatively slow growth of the neoplastic cells [12]. *In vitro*, sensitization of chondrosarcoma cells to doxorubicin treatment was obtained by concomitant wild-type adeno-associated virus type 2 (AAV-2) infection [49]. Anecdotal cases of conventional chondrosarcomas responding to chemotherapy have been reported in the literature [50–52]. Of particular interest is a report by Debruyne *et al.* in 2007 of a partial remission of metastatic chondrosarcoma after trofosfamide, an oral ifosfamide derivate [52].

At present, two non-randomized, open label phase II clinical trials are studying the effect of chemotherapeutic agents on chondrosarcoma: one trial is investigating the effect of pemetrexed, a multitargeted anti-folate that inhibits the formation of precursor purine and pyrimidine nucleotides, in patients with advanced grades 2 and 3 chondrosarcomas [53]. Another trial recruited patients with an unresectable or locally recurrent chondrosarcoma to investigate the response to gemcitabine, followed by docetaxel [54].

B. New Targeted Treatments

New insights in molecular cell biology, cytogenetics, and immunopathology have been reported [12,55]. Better understanding of chondrosarcoma development at a molecular level has resulted in studies of new agents.

1. PROTEIN TYROSINE KINASES INHIBITORS

Protein tyrosine kinases (PTKs) play a fundamental role in the transduction of biochemical signals involved in the regulation of cell proliferation, growth and function [56]. Deregulated activity of these enzymes has been observed in a large number of different diseases. In particular, the chimeric Bcr-Abl fusion protein plays a crucial role in chronic myeloid leukemia (CML) [57], c-KIT receptor in gastrointestinal stromal tumors (GIST) [54], and platelet-derived growth factor receptor-β (PDGFRβ) in dermatofibrosarcoma protuberans [58].

A few studies have evaluated the expression and activation status of platelet-derived growth factor receptor-α (PDGFRα), PDGFRβ, and KIT in conventional chondrosarcomas [59,60]. Co-expression of PDGFRα and PDGFRβ was found, with greater protein expression and higher phosphorylation levels for PDGFRβ. The authors suggest an autocrine/paracrine activation loop of the corresponding receptors since no activating mutations or abnormal genomic profiles were detected. Furthermore, immunohistochemistry expression of tyrosine kinase PDGFRα has been associated with a higher histological grade and shorter survival in conventional chondrosarcoma [60].

Imatinib is a highly selective inhibitor of the protein tyrosine kinase family, registered in 2001 for CML and widely used for GIST. It competitively inhibits the enzyme activity of the protein, by binding to the ATP-binding site. Imatinib is relatively selective for Bcr-Abl but also inhibits other targets mentioned above such as c-KIT and PDGFR [61]. In December 2008, accrual for a prospective phase II study with imatinib in metastatic and locally advanced chondrosarcomas was completed [62].

Dasatinib, a tyrosine kinase inhibitor that was registered for imatinib-resistant GIST, is being investigated in a phase II study on patients with advanced sarcomas, including chondrosarcomas [63].

Perifosine, a mitogen-activated protein kinase (MAPK) inhibitor, modulates the balance between the MAPK and pro-apoptotic stress-activated protein kinase (SAPK/JNK) pathways, thereby inducing apoptosis. Targeting cellular membranes, perifosine modulates membrane permeability, membrane lipid composition, phospholipid metabolism, and mitogenic signal transduction, resulting in cell differentiation and inhibition of cell growth [64]. This orally active alkyl-phosphocholine compound was (at the time of writing) under study in a phase II clinical trial on patients with chondrosarcomas, alveolar soft part sarcomas and extraskeletal myxoid chondrosarcomas [65].

2. MONOCLONAL TRAIL ANTIBODIES
Monoclonal antibodies against TNF-related apoptosis-inducing ligand (TRAIL) death receptors DR4 or DR5 were studied as potential cancer treatments [66]. There are several agonistic humanized or human monoclonal antibodies against DR4 and DR5 that have been tested in Phase I and II trials in patients with advanced cancer. These trials have demonstrated these antibodies to be well tolerated, and to produce prolonged stable disease [67]. Apomab, a monoclonal antibody against the DR5 receptor, was investigated in a phase II study in patients with advanced chondrosarcoma [68]. Preliminary results showed stable disease for 8 out of 14 patients [69].

3. INDIAN HEDGEHOG INHIBITORS
Indian Hedgehog (IHH) signaling plays an important role in growth-plate chondrocyte proliferation [70] and in the development of benign cartilage tumors, such as enchondromas [71] and osteochondromas [11].

In chondrosarcoma cells, the treatment with recombinant hedgehog increased proliferation. At the same time, treatment with hedgehog inhibitors reduced chondrosarcoma tumor proliferation and growth *in vitro* and *in vivo* [72]. In contrast, decreased expression of IHH downstream targets during tumor progression has been identified in peripheral chondrosarcoma [73].

A hedgehog inhibitor, triparanol, has shown to be effective against human chondrosarcomas in a mouse model, but frequent side-effects limited clinical application [72]. Another hedgehog inhibitor, cyclopamine, is a natural product derived from the plant *Veratrum californicum*. This substance was discovered in studies on holoprosencephaly in newborn lambs. It was shown that this agent affects the developing fetus and not the mature sheep ingesting the plant and might be considered for therapeutic use [74]. As newer hedgehog-targeting agents with fewer side-effects are developed, they could be applied in the care of patients with chondrosarcomas and other tumors with active hedgehog signaling [75].

4. PARATHYROID HORMONE-LIKE HORMONE BLOCKADE
Increased activity of parathyroid hormone-like hormone (PTHLH) signaling is active in enchondromas, central and peripheral chondrosarcomas, and increased activity is associated with increased histological grade [76–81]. Therefore, inhibition of PTHLH signaling could be used to decrease the proliferation of chondrosarcomas. Bcl-2 antisense therapy might be useful in this perspective, as Bcl-2 is the downstream effector of PTHLH and is expressed in both peripheral and high-grade central chondrosarcoma [76,77]. Experimental drugs, acting on this pathway have been investigated in clinical trials for melanoma, chronic lymphocytic leukemia, multiple myeloma, and non-small cell lung cancer [82]. A monoclonal murine antibody to PTHLH promoted chondrogenic differentiation and accelerated apoptosis in chondrosarcoma cells, due to downregulation of its downstream target Bcl-2 [83].

5. ANTIANGIOGENESIS THERAPY
The role of angiogenic processes in the development of chondrosarcoma is under investigation. It has been demonstrated that vascularization increases with increasing histological grade of chondrosarcomas [84,85].

In a study carried out in 2006, the expression of the pro-angiogenic molecule vascular endothelial growth factor A (VEGF-A) correlated positively with chondrosarcoma tumor grade [86]. The effect of a combination of an antiangiogenic factor (plasminogen-related protein B) and a marine-derived chemotherapeutic molecule (ecteinascidin-743) has been tested on human chondrosarcoma in a mouse xenograft model. As a single-agent treatment, Ecteinascidin-743 slowed down the tumor growth, with only a modest further repression in combination with plasminogen-related protein B. However, the combination of the two compounds led to a significant increase in tumor necrosis in comparison to the single-drug treatment. Moreover, the co-administration was a highly effective antagonizer of tumor microvessel formation [87]. A phase I clinical study on VEGF-AS, an antisense oligonucleotide that targets VEGF, reported a decline in plasma VEGF levels, and a prolonged stabilization of disease in one patient with chondrosarcoma [88].

Degradation of extracellular matrix and vascular ingrowth are essential in tumor proliferation, growth and metastasis. Matrix metalloproteinases and cathepsins are involved in the destruction of extracellular matrix. Increased activity of matrix metalloproteinases 1, 2, 9, and 13 was associated with high histological grade in chondrosarcoma [8]. Moreover, matrix metalloproteinases 1 antisense *in vitro* decreased invasiveness in chondrosarcoma [89]. Also the overexpression of cathepsin B and L has been associated with increasing histological grade [8], which could suggest a potential role for cathepsin inhibitors in the treatment of chondrosarcoma.

Finally, prostaglandin G/H synthase 2 (COX-2), a mediator of angiogenesis, was shown to be expressed in chondrosarcoma, although no correlation with histological grade was examined [90]. This finding suggests that selective COX-2 inhibitors might be effective in chondrosarcoma.

6. BISPHOSPHONATES

Bisphosphonates are potent inhibitors of osteoclast-mediated bone resorption and widely used in the prevention and treatment of osteoporosis, Paget's disease of bone, bone metastasis, multiple myeloma and other conditions that feature bone fragility. Antitumor activity by several bisphosphonates has been demonstrated in human chondrosarcoma cell lines [91–93].

Zoledronate was tested *in vivo* in a rat chondrosarcoma model and *in vitro* in cells derived from this model, to determine the effect on tumor progression. Zoledronate decreased primary tumor development, tumor progression after intralesional currettage, and increased overall survival. Cell proliferation was inhibited and non-apoptotic cell death was induced [91].

The effect of minodronate, a newly developed third generation nitrogen-containing bisphosphonate, was studied on two chondrosarcoma cell lines. Minodronate inhibited cell viability in both cell lines and induced S-phase arrest and apoptosis in one of them [92].

In a study by Lai *et al.* alendronate showed a dose- and time-dependent inhibitory effect on the invasion and migration of human chondrosarcoma cells. Furthermore, alendronate decreased the activity and mRNA levels of matrix metalloproteinase (MMP)-2 in a concentration-dependent manner [93].

7. HISTONE DEACETYLASE INHIBITORS

Histone acetylation and deacetylation play a key role in the regulation of chondrocytic differentiation. A number of studies have shown that histone deacetylase inhibitors cause a variety of phenotypic changes, such as cell cycle arrest, morphologic reversion of transformed cells, apoptosis, and differentiation [94,95]. One study investigated the antitumor effects of depsipeptide, a histone deacetylase inhibitor, as a differentiating agent on chondrosarcomas. Depsipeptide induced cell cycle arrest, apoptosis, chondrocytic maturation, and it inhibited tumor growth in a xenograft chondrosarcoma murine model [96].

8. HORMONAL THERAPY

Estrogen-mediated signaling is essential in cartilaginous proliferation and differentiation within the growth plate, and is important for the regulation of longitudinal skeletal growth [97]. Aromatase is an enzyme that mediates the last in a series of steps for estrogen synthesis. It was hypothesized that antiestrogen or aromatase inhibitors could potentially have an inhibitory effect on proliferation of chondrosarcomas. The presence of the estrogen receptor and functional aromatase activity were identified in 35 chondrosarcoma samples tested [98]. Growth of chondrosarcoma cells was stimulated by estrogen or androstenedione, and inhibited by an aromatase inhibitor [98].

Another study demonstrated estrogen receptors α and β expression in both benign and malignant cartilage tumors. Both receptors were expressed more frequently in low-grade than in high-grade chondrosarcomas [99].

2-Methoxyestradiol is an endogenous metabolite with estrogen receptor-independent anti-tumor activity. A study on human chondrosarcoma cells demonstrated a time- and dose-dependent cytotoxicity of 2-methoxyestradiol through cell cycle arrest and apoptosis. The same treatment minimally affected primary chondrocytes [100].

C. Radiotherapy

Cartilaginous lesions are considered to be relatively resistant to radiation [2]. The basis of this resistance is not completely understood, although some research has shown that p16(ink4a), one of the major tumor suppressor proteins that regulate the cell cycle, could play a role in radiation resistance in chondrosarcoma cells [101]. Therefore, restoring p16 expression could increase the radiosensitivity of chondrosarcomas. Another possible way of enhancing radiosensitivity in chondrosarcomas is the facilitation of apoptotic pathways by silencing anti-apoptotic genes. Some promising results have been obtained with this method in grade 2 human chondrosarcoma cell lines [102]. The combination of radiotherapy with razoxane, an antiangiogenic topoisomerase II inhibitor, seems to result in a better response than with radiotherapy alone [103].

Irradiation should be considered when surgery would cause major unacceptable morbidity or is technically impossible [104]. Therefore, radiotherapy is usually applied to patients with metastatic or inoperable chondrosarcoma. Chondrosarcomas of the spheno-occipital region and cervical spine are often inoperable. Increasing experience in the radiation treatment of skull-base chondrosarcomas has led to the development of new techniques in this field.

1. STEREOTACTIC RADIOSURGERY
Radiosurgery is the delivery of a single, high dose of radiation to a specific target with surgical precision thanks to stereotactic positioning in a three-dimensional space. Stereotactic radiosurgery (gamma-knife surgery) has been a successful treatment for skull-base [105–107] and spinal [108] chondrosarcomas, especially for those with small sizes, reaching a 5-year local tumor control of 80% [106].

2. PROTON THERAPY
Protons are characterized by low linear energy transfer (LET), but compared with photons and electrons have an improved physical depth dose distribution. Proton radiotherapy has been used for ocular melanoma, chordoma and chondrosarcoma of the skull-base or cervical spine [109]. Compared to conventional radiotherapy, proton radiotherapy seems more effective in skull-base chondrosarcomas [110]. A phase II clinical trial was set up to study the effects of proton beam radiotherapy on skull base chondrosarcomas [111]. A phase I and II clinical trial was set up to investigate if dose intensification of charged particle radiotherapy decreases the local recurrence rate for chordomas and chondrosarcomas of skull base or cervical spine [112].

Promising results were reported after carbon ion radiotherapy in skull base chondrosarcomas [113], with a 4-year local control rate of 90%.

V. CONCLUSIONS

Chondrosarcoma represents a heterogeneous group of malignant cartilage tumors. Surgery is the most important component of treatment. Although convincing evidence of its benefit is lacking, chemotherapy might be useful in the treatment of mesenchymal and dedifferentiated chondrosarcoma.

Radiotherapy plays an important role in the treatment of chondrosarcomas located in the spheno-occipital region and cervical spine. New modern radiation techniques could further improve the outcome for patients with lesions in sites that are surgically difficult to access.

Finally, better understanding of molecular diagnostics and pathogenesis of chondrosarcoma, together with the development of new therapeutic agents, has resulted in numerous studies investigating potentially active treatment approaches to this disease. However, at present, the majority of these new compounds are being tested in preclinical settings, and their future clinical application still needs to be defined.

References

1. K.K. Unni, Dahlin's Bone Tumors: General Aspects and Data on 11,087 Cases, 5th edn., Lippincott-Raven Publishers, Philadelphia (1996) pp. 71–108.
2. M. Campanacci, Bone and Soft Tissue Tumors, 2nd edn., Springer-Verlag, Wien, New York (1999) pp. 283–379.
3. F. Bertoni, P. Bacchini & P.C.W. Hogendoorn, Chondrosarcoma, in: C.D.M. Fletcher, K.K. Unni & F. Mertens (Eds.) World Health Organisation Classification of Tumours. Pathology and Genetics of Tumours of Soft Tissue and Bone, IARC Press, Lyon (2002) pp. 247–251.
4. J. Björnsson, R.A. McLeod & K.K. Unni, et al., Primary chondrosarcoma of long bones and limb girdles, Cancer 83 (10) (1998) 2105–2119.
5. S. Gitelis, F. Bertoni & P. Picci, et al., Chondrosarcoma of bone. The experience at the Istituto Ortopedico Rizzoli, J Bone Joint Surg Am 63 (8) (1981) 1248–1257.
6. A.A. Sandberg, Genetics of chondrosarcoma and related Tumors, Curr Opin Oncol 16 (4) (2004) 342–354.
7. G. Tallini, H. Dorfman & P. Brys, et al., Correlation between clinicopathological features and karyotype in 100 cartilaginous and chordoid tumours. A report from the Chromosomes and Morphology (CHAMP) Collaborative Study Group, J Pathol 196 (2) (2002) 194–203.
8. L.B. Rozeman, P.C. Hogendoorn & J.V. Bovée, Diagnosis and prognosis of chondrosarcoma of bone, Expert Rev Mol Diagn 2 (5) (2002) 461–472.
9. J.V. Bovée, A.M. Cleton-Jansen & N.J. Kuipers-Dijkshoorn, et al., Loss of heterozygosity and DNA ploidy point to a diverging genetic mechanism in the origin of peripheral and central chondrosarcoma, Genes Chromosomes Cancer 26 (3) (1999) 237–246.
10. M.L. Larramendy, M. Tarkkanen & J. Valle, et al., Gains, losses, and amplifications of DNA sequences evaluated by comparative genomic hybridization in chondrosarcomas, Am J Pathol 150 (2) (1997) 685–691.
11. J.V. Bovée, A.M. Cleton-Jansen & W. Wuyts, et al., EXT-mutation analysis and loss of heterozygosity in sporadic and hereditary osteochondromas and secondary chondrosarcomas, Am J Hum Genet 65 (3) (1999) 689–698.
12. J.V. Bovée, A.M. Cleton-Jansen & A.H. Taminiau, et al., Emerging pathways in the development of chondrosarcoma of bone and implications for targeted treatment, Lancet Oncol 6 (8) (2005) 599–607.

13. H.L. Evans, A.G. Ayala & M.M. Romsdahl, Prognostic factors in chondrosarcoma of bone: a clinicopathologic analysis with emphasis on histologic grading, Cancer 40 (2) (1977) 818–831.

14. I.C. Van der Geest, M.H. de Valk & J.W. de Rooy, et al., Oncological and functional results of cryosurgical therapy of enchondromas and chondrosarcomas grade 1, J Surg Oncol 98 (6) (2008) 421–426.

15. T. Leerapun, R.R. Hugate & C.Y. Inwards, et al., Surgical management of conventional grade I chondrosarcoma of long bones, Clin Orthop Relat Res 463 (2007) 166–172.

16. E.R. Ahlmann, L.R. Menendez & A.N. Fedenko, et al., Influence of cryosurgery on treatment outcome of low-grade chondrosarcoma, Clin Orthop Relat Res 451 (2006) 201–207.

17 A. Streitbürger, H. Ahrens, M. Balke, et al. Grade I chondrosarcoma of bone: the Münster experience. J Cancer Res Clin Oncol Oct 15 (2008) [Epub ahead of print].

18. F.Y. Lee, H.J. Mankin & G. Fondren, et al., Chondrosarcoma of bone: an assessment of outcome, J Bone Joint Surg Am 81 (3) (1999) 326–338.

19. L. Lichtenstein & D. Bernstein, Unusual benign and malignant chondroid tumors of bone: a survey of some mesenchymal cartilage tumors and malignant chondroblastic tumors, including a few multicentric ones, as well as many atypical benign chondroblastomas and chondromyxoid fibromas, Cancer 12 (1959) 1142–1157.

20. Y. Nakashima, K.K. Unni & T.C. Shives, et al., Mesenchymal chondrosarcoma of bone and soft tissue. A review of 111 cases, Cancer 57 (12) (1986) 2444–2453.

21. S. Naumann, P.A. Krallman & K.K. Unni, et al., Translocation der(13;21)(q10;q10) in skeletal and extraskeletal mesenchymal chondrosarcoma, Mod Pathol 15 (2002) 572–576.

22. Y.K. Park, H.R. Park & S.G. Chi, et al., Overexpression of p53 and absent genetic mutation in clear cell chondrosarcoma, Int J Oncol 19 (2001) 353–357.

23. A.G. Huvos, G. Rosen & M. Dabska, et al., Mesenchymal chondrosarcoma. A clinicopathologic analysis of 35 patients with emphasis on treatment, Cancer 51 (7) (1983) 1230–1237.

24. M. Cesari, F. Bertoni & P. Bacchini, et al., Mesenchymal chondrosarcoma. An analysis of patients treated at a single institution, Tumori 93 (5) (2007) 423–427.

25. D.C. Dahlin & J.W. Beabout, Dedifferentiation of low-grade chondrosarcomas, Cancer 28 (1971) 461–466.

26. F.J. Frassica, K.K. Unni & J.W. Beabout, et al., Dedifferentiated chondrosarcoma. A report of the clinicopathological features and treatment of seventy-eight cases, J Bone Joint Surg Am 68 (8) (1986) 1197–1205.

27. R. Capanna, F. Bertoni & G. Bettelli, et al., Dedifferentiated chondrosarcoma, J Bone Joint Surg Am 70 (1) (1988) 60–69.

28. M. Mercuri, P. Picci & L. Campanacci, et al., Dedifferentiated chondrosarcoma, Skeletal Radiol 24 (6) (1995) 409–416.

29. A.D. Mitchell, K. Ayoub & D.C. Mangham, et al., Experience in the treatment of dedifferentiated chondrosarcoma, J Bone Joint Surg Br 82 (1) (2000) 55–61.

30. I.D. Dickey, P.S. Rose & B. Fuchs, et al., Dedifferentiated chondrosarcoma: the role of chemotherapy with updated outcomes, J Bone Joint Surg Am 86-A (11) (2004) 2412–2418.

31. J. Bruns, W. Fiedler & M. Werner, et al., Dedifferentiated chondrosarcoma—a fatal disease, J Cancer Res Clin Oncol 131 (6) (2005) 333–339.

32. E.L. Staals, P. Bacchini & F. Bertoni, Dedifferentiated central chondrosarcoma, Cancer 106 (12) (2006) 2682–2691.

33. E.L. Staals, P. Bacchini & M. Mercuri, et al., Dedifferentiated chondrosarcomas arising in preexisting osteochondromas, J Bone Joint Surg Am 89 (5) (2007) 987–993.

34. R.J. Grimer, G. Gosheger & A. Taminiau, et al., Dedifferentiated chondrosarcoma: prognostic factors and outcome from a European group, Eur J Cancer 43 (14) (2007) 2060–2065.

35. J.V. Bovée, A.M. Cleton-Jansen & C. Rosenberg, et al., Molecular genetic characterization of both components of a dedifferentiated chondrosarcoma, with implications for its histogenesis, J Pathol 189 (4) (1999) 454–462.

36. M. Röpke, C. Boltze & H.W. Neumann, et al., Genetic and epigenetic alterations in tumor progression in a dedifferentiated chondrosarcoma, Pathol Res Pract 199 (2003) 437–444.

37. H.J. Grote, R. Schneider-Stock & W. Neumann, et al., Mutation of p53 with loss of heterozygosity in the osteosarcomatous component of a dedifferentiated chondrosarcoma, Virchows Arch 436 (2000) 494–497.

38. V.H. Bramwell, W.P. Steward & M. Nooij, et al., Neoadjuvant chemotherapy with doxorubicin and cisplatin in malignant fibrous histiocytoma of bone: a European Osteosarcoma Intergroup study, J Clin Oncol 17 (1999) 3260–3269.

39. R.J. Grimer, S.R. Cannon & A.M. Taminiau, et al., Osteosarcoma over the age of forty, Eur J Cancer 39 (2003) 157–163.

40. T. Aigner & K.K. Unni, Is dedifferentiated chondrosarcoma a 'de-differentiated' chondrosarcoma?, J Pathol 189 (1999) 445–447.

41. ISG, SSG, COSS (2003). A European treatment protocol for bone sarcoma in patients older than 40 years. Scandinavian Sarcoma Group and Oncologic Center, Lund, Sweden, http://www.ocsyd.se/VP-verksamhet/Hud%20mjukdel%20skelett/Euroboss1.pdf

42. K.K. Unni, D.C. Dahlin & J.W. Beabout, et al., Chondrosarcoma: clear-cell variant. A report of sixteen cases, J Bone Joint Surg Am 58 (1976) 676–683.

43. J. Nishio, J.D. Reith & A. Ogose, et al., Cytogenetic findings in clear cell chondrosarcoma, Cancer Genet Cytogenet 162 (2005) 74–77.

44. J. Bjornsson, K.K. Unni & D.C. Dahlin, et al., Clear cell chondrosarcoma of bone. Observations in 47 cases, Am J Surg Pathol 8 (1984) 223–230.

45. D. Donati, J.Q. Yin & M. Colangeli, et al., Clear cell chondrosarcoma of bone: long time follow-up of 18 cases, Arch Orthop Trauma Surg 128 (2008) 137–142.

46. R.K. Kalil, C.Y. Inwards & K.K. Unni, et al., Dedifferentiated clear cell chondrosarcoma, Am J Surg Pathol 24 (2000) 1079–1086.

47. R.M. Terek, G.K. Schwartz & K. Devaney, et al., Chemotherapy and P-glycoprotein expression in chondrosarcoma, J Orthop Res 16 (5) (1998) 585–590.

48. J.J. Wyman, A.M. Hornstein & P.A. Meitner, et al., Multidrug resistance-1 and p-glycoprotein in human chondrosarcoma cell lines: expression correlates with decreased intracellular doxorubicin and *in vitro* chemoresistance, J Orthop Res 17 (6) (1999) 935–940.

49. M.H. Schwarzbach, S. Eisold & T. Burguete, et al., Sensitization of sarcoma cells to doxorubicin treatment by concomitant wild-type adeno-associated virus type 2 (AAV-2) infection, Int J Oncol 20 (6) (2002) 1211–1218.

50. K.H. Antman, D. Montella & C. Rosenbaum, et al., Phase II trial of ifosfamide with mesna in previously treated metastatic sarcoma, Cancer Treat Rep 69 (5) (1985) 499–504.

51. R.V. La Rocca, K.W. Morgan & K. Paris, et al., Recurrent chondrosarcoma of the cranial base: a durable response to ifosfamide-doxorubicin chemotherapy, J Neuro Oncol 41 (3) (1999) 281–283.

52. P.R. Debruyne, H. Dumez & W. Demey, et al., Recurrent low- to intermediate-grade chondrosarcoma of the thumb with lung metastases: an objective response to trofosfamide, Onkologie 30 (4) (2007) 201–204.

53. Southwest Oncology Group. Pemetrexed disodium in treating patients with recurrent and unresectable or metastatic chondrosarcoma. December 2007. http://clinicaltrials.gov/ct2/show/NCT00107419.

54. Children's Oncology Group (NCI). Gemcitabine and docetaxel in treating patients with recurrent osteosarcoma or Ewing's sarcoma or unresectable or locally recurrent chondrosarcoma. January 2008. http://clinicaltrials.gov/ct2/show/NCT00073983.

55. R.M. Terek, Recent advances in the basic science of chondrosarcoma, Orthop Clin North Am 37 (1) (2006) 9–14.

56. G.D. Demetri, M. von Mehren & C.D. Blanke, et al., Efficacy and safety of imatinib mesylate in advanced gastrointestinal stromal tumors, N Engl J Med 347 (7) (2002) 472–480.

57. H. Kantarjian, C. Sawyers & A. Hochhaus, et al., International STI571 CML Study Group. Hematologic and cytogenetic responses to imatinib mesylate in chronic myelogenous leukemia, N Engl J Med 346 (9) (2002) 645–652.

58. T. Sjöblom, A. Shimizu & K.P. O'Brien, et al., Growth inhibition of dermatofibrosarcoma protuberans tumors by the platelet-derived growth factor receptor antagonist STI571 through induction of apoptosis, Cancer Res 61 (2001) 5778–5783.

59. M.S. Lagonigro, E. Tamborini & T. Negri, et al., PDGFRalpha, PDGFRbeta and KIT expression/activation in conventional chondrosarcoma, J Pathol 208 (5) (2006) 615–623.

60. I. Sulzbacher, P. Birner & K. Trieb, et al., Platelet-derived growth factor-alpha receptor expression supports the growth of conventional chondrosarcoma and is associated with adverse outcome, Am J Surg Pathol 25 (12) (2001) 1520–1527.

61. M.W. Deininger & B.J. Druker, Specific targeted therapy of chronic myelogenous leukemia with imatinib, Pharmacol Rev 55 (3) (2003) 401–423.

62. Italian Sarcoma Group. Studio di fase II sull'utilizzo di imatinib mesilato nel trattamento del tumore Desmoide e del condrosarcoma. February 2008. http://oss-sper-clin.agenziafarmaco.it/.

63. Sarcoma Alliance for Research through Collaboration (SARC). Trial of Dasatinib in Advanced Sarcomas. January 2008. http://clinicaltrials.gov/ct2/show/NCT00464620.

64. B.T. Hennessy, Y. Lu & E. Poradosu, et al., Pharmacodynamic markers of perifosine efficacy, Clin Cancer Res 13 (24) (2007) 7421–7431.

65. Sarcoma Alliance for Research through Collaboration (SARC). A trial of Perifosine in patients with chemoinsensitive sarcomas. January 2008. http://clinicaltrials.gov/ct2/show/NCT00401388.

66. D.J. Buchsbaum, A. Forero-Torres & A.F. LoBuglio, TRAIL-receptor antibodies as a potential cancer treatment, Future Oncol 3 (4) (2007) 405–409.

67. Y. Huang & M.S. Sheikh, TRAIL death receptors and cancer therapeutics, Toxicol Appl Pharmacol 224 (3) (2007) 284–289.

68. Genentech. A study of Apomab in patients with advanced chondrosarcoma. December 2007. http://clinicaltrials.gov/ct2/show/NCT00543712.

69. S. Chawla, G. Demetri, & J. Desai, et al. Initial results of a phase II study of the safety and efficacy of the Apomab DR5 agonist antibody in advanced chondrosarcoma and synovial sarcoma patients. CTOS Annual Meeting 2008, Abstract 35010.

70. B.C. van der Eerden, M. Karperien & E.F. Gevers, et al., Expression of Indian hedgehog, parathyroid hormone-related protein, and their receptors in the postnatal growth plate of the rat: evidence for a locally acting growth restraining feedback loop after birth, J Bone Miner Res 15 (6) (2000) 1045–1055.

71. S. Hopyan, N. Gokgoz & R. Poon, et al., A mutant PTH/PTHrP type I receptor in enchondromatosis, Nat Genet 30 (3) (2002) 306–310.

72. T.D. Tiet, S. Hopyan & P. Nadesan, et al., Constitutive hedgehog signaling in chondrosarcoma up-regulates tumor cell proliferation, Am J Pathol 168 (1) (2006) 321–330.

73. C. Morrison, M. Radmacher & N. Mohammed, et al., MYC amplification and polysomy 8 in chondrosarcoma: array comparative genomic hybridization, fluorescent in situ hybridization, and association with outcome, J Clin Oncol 23 (36) (2005) 9369–9376.

74. J.S. Wunder, T.O. Nielsen & R.G. Maki, et al., Opportunities for improving the therapeutic ratio for patients with sarcoma, Lancet Oncol 8 (6) (2007) 513–524.

75. A.S. Kiselyov, Targeting the hedgehog signaling pathway with small molecules, Anticancer Agents Med Chem 6 (5) (2006) 445–449.

76. L.B. Rozeman, L. Hameetman & A.M. Cleton-Jansen, et al., Absence of IHH and retention of PTHrP signalling in enchondromas and central chondrosarcomas, J Pathol 205 (4) (2005) 476–482.

77. J.V. Bovée, L.J. van den Broek & A.M. Cleton-Jansen, et al., Up-regulation of PTHrP and Bcl-2 expression characterizes the progression of osteochondroma towards peripheral chondrosarcoma and is a late event in central chondrosarcoma, Lab Invest 80 (12) (2000) 1925–1934.

78. M. Amling, M. Pösl & M.W. Hentz, et al., PTHrP and Bcl-2: essential regulatory molecules in chondrocyte differentiation and chondrogenic tumors, Verh Dtsch Ges Pathol 82 (1998) 160–169.

79. T. Kunisada, J.M. Moseley & J.L. Slavin, et al., Co-expression of parathyroid hormone-related protein (PTHrP) and PTH/PTHrP receptor in cartilaginous tumours: a marker for malignancy?, Pathology 34 (2) (2002) 133–137.

80. D.B. Pateder, M.W. Gish & R.J. O'Keefe, et al., Parathyroid hormone-related peptide expression in cartilaginous tumors, Clin Orthop Relat Res 403 (2002) 198–204.

81. L. Hameetman, P. Kok & P.H. Eilers, et al., The use of Bcl-2 and PTHLH immunohistochemistry in the diagnosis of peripheral chondrosarcoma in a clinicopathological setting, Virchows Arch 446 (4) (2005) 430–437.

82. R. Kim, M. Emi & K. Tanabe, et al., Therapeutic potential of antisense Bcl-2 as a chemosensitizer for cancer therapy, Cancer 101 (11) (2004) 2491–2502.

83. T. Miyaji, T. Nakase & E. Onuma, et al., Monoclonal antibody to parathyroid hormone related protein induces differentiation and apoptosis of chondrosarcoma cells, Cancer Lett 199 (2) (2003) 147–155.

84. M.J. Geirnaerdt, P.C. Hogendoorn & J.L. Bloem, et al., Cartilaginous tumors: fast contrast-enhanced MR imaging, Radiology 214 (2) (2000) 539–546.

85. G. Ayala, C. Liu & R. Nicosia, et al., Microvasculature and VEGF expression in cartilaginous tumors, Hum Pathol 31 (3) (2000) 341–346.

86. T. Kalinski, S. Krueger & S. Sel, et al., Differential expression of VEGF-A and angiopoietins in cartilage tumors and regulation by interleukin-1beta, Cancer 106 (9) (2006) 2028–2038.

87. H. Morioka, L. Weissbach & T. Vogel, et al., Antiangiogenesis treatment combined with chemotherapy produces chondrosarcoma necrosis, Clin Cancer Res 9 (3) (2003) 1211–1217.

88. A.M. Levine, A. Tulpule & D.I. Quinn, et al., Phase I study of antisense oligonucleotide against vascular endothelial growth factor: decrease in plasma vascular endothelial growth factor with potential clinical efficacy, J Clin Oncol 24 (11) (2006) 1712–1719.

89. X. Jiang, C.M. Dutton & W. Qi, et al., Inhibition of MMP-1 expression by antisense RNA decreases invasiveness of human chondrosarcoma, J Orthop Res 21 (6) (2003) 1063–1070.

90. K.M. Sutton, M. Wright & G. Fondren, et al., Cyclooxygenase-2 expression in chondrosarcoma, Oncology 66 (4) (2004) 275–280.

91. F. Gouin, B. Ory & F. Rédini, et al., Zoledronic acid slows down rat primary chondrosarcoma development, recurrent tumor progression after intralesional curretage and increases overall survival, Int J Cancer 119 (5) (2006) 980–984.

92. T. Kubo, S. Shimose & T. Matsuo, et al., Inhibitory effects of a new bisphosphonate, minodronate, on proliferation and invasion of a variety of malignant bone tumor cells, J Orthop Res 24 (6) (2008) 1138–1144.

93. T.J. Lai, S.F. Hsu & T.M. Li, et al., Alendronate inhibits cell invasion and MMP-2 secretion in human chondrosarcoma cell line, Acta Pharmacol Sin 28 (8) (2007) 1231–1235.

94. A. Villar-Garea & M. Esteller, Histone deacetylase inhibitors: understanding a new wave of anticancer agents, Int J Cancer 112 (2) (2004) 171–178.

95. R. Sakimura, K. Tanaka & F. Nakatani, et al., Antitumor effects of histone deacetylase inhibitor on Ewing's family tumors, Int J Cancer 116 (5) (2005) 784–792.

96. R. Sakimura, K. Tanaka & S. Yamamoto, et al., The effects of histone deacetylase inhibitors on the induction of differentiation in chondrosarcoma cells, Clin Cancer Res 13 (1) (2007) 275–282.

97. O. Nilsson, R. Marino & F. De Luca, et al., Endocrine regulation of the growth plate, Horm Res 64 (4) (2005) 157–165.

98. A.M. Cleton-Jansen, H.M. van Beerendonk & H.J. Baelde, et al., Estrogen signaling is active in cartilaginous tumors: implications for antiestrogen therapy as treatment option of metastasized or irresectable chondrosarcoma, Clin Cancer Res 11 (22) (2005) 8028–8035.

99. T.J. Grifone, H.M. Haupt & V. Podolski, et al., Immunohistochemical expression of estrogen receptors in chondrosarcomas and enchondromas, Int J Surg Pathol 16 (1) (2008) 31–37.

100. Y.C. Fong, W.H. Yang & S.F. Hsu, et al., 2-Methoxyestradiol induces apoptosis and cell cycle arrest in human chondrosarcoma cells, J Orthop Res 25 (8) (2007) 1106–1114.

101. F. Moussavi-Harami, A. Mollano & J.A. Martin, et al., Intrinsic radiation resistance in human chondrosarcoma cells, Biochem Biophys Res Commun 346 (2) (2006) 379–385.

102. D.W. Kim, S.W. Seo & S.K. Cho, et al., Targeting of cell survival genes using small interfering RNAs (siRNAs) enhances radiosensitivity of Grade II chondrosarcoma cells, J Orthop Res 25 (6) (2007) 820–828.

103. W. Rhomberg, H. Eiter & F. Böhler, et al., Combined radiotherapy and razoxane in the treatment of chondrosarcomas and chordomas, Anticancer Res 26 (3B) (2006) 2407–2411.

104. R. Krochak, A.R. Harwood & B.J. Cummings, et al., Results of radical radiation for chondrosarcoma of bone, Radiother Oncol 1 (2) (1983) 109–115.

105. N. Muthukumar, D. Kondziolka & L.D. Lunsford, et al., Stereotactic radiosurgery for chordoma and chondrosarcoma: further experiences, Int J Radiat Oncol Biol Phys 41 (2) (1998) 387–392.

106. T. Hasegawa, D. Ishii & Y. Kida, et al., Gamma knife surgery for skull base chordomas and chondrosarcomas, J Neurosurg 107 (4) (2007) 752–757.

107. J.J. Martin, A. Niranjan & D. Kondziolka, et al., Radiosurgery for chordomas and chondrosarcomas of the skull base, J Neurosurg 107 (4) (2007) 758–764.

108. G.S. McLoughlin, D.M. Sciubba & J.P. Wolinsky, Chondroma/Chondrosarcoma of the spine, Neurosurg Clin N Am 19 (1) (2008) 57–63.

109. J.J. Mazeron, G. Noel & L. Feuvret, et al., Clinical complementarities between proton and carbon therapies, Radiother Oncol 73 (Suppl 2) (2004) S50–S52.

110. E.B. Hug & J.D. Slater, Proton radiation therapy for chordomas and chondrosarcomas of the skull base, Neurosurg Clin N Am 11 (4) (2000) 627–638.

111. M.D. Anderson, Cancer Center. Proton beam therapy for chondrosarcoma. January 2008. http://clinicaltrials.gov/ct2/show/NCT00496522.

112. Massachusetts General Hospital. Charged particle RT for chordomas and chondrosarcomas of the base of the skull of cervical spine. January 2008. http://clinicaltrials.gov/ct2/show/NCT00592748.

113. D. Schulz-Ertner, A. Nikoghosyan & H. Hof, et al., Carbon ion radiotherapy of skull base chondrosarcomas, Int J Radiat Oncol Biol Phys 67 (1) (2007) 171–177.

CHAPTER **32**

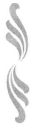

Mechanistic Role of RANKL in Cancer-induced Bone Diseases and Development of a Targeted Therapy to Inhibit this Pathway

WILLIAM C. DOUGALL[1]

[1]*Department of Hematology/Oncology Research, Amgen Washington, Seattle, WA, USA.*

Contents

I. INTRODUCTION

Bone remodeling is a complex process mediated by bone-forming osteoblasts and bone-resorbing osteoclasts. During pathological remodeling resulting from tumor invasion of the skeleton, osteoblastic and osteoclastic activities become unbalanced which leads to a loss of skeletal integrity and clinically-defined skeletal complications of malignancy. Bone metastasis and humoral hypercalcemia of malignancy (HHM) frequently occurs in patients with advanced solid tumors (e.g., breast, prostate, lung, renal, thyroid, colon) and the dysregulated bony response that develops in these patients can include excessive osteoblastic and/or excessive osteolytic activities. Multiple myeloma is a B-cell malignancy in which transformed plasma cells grow within the bone marrow and lead to excessive osteolysis and the suppression of osteoblast activities. Increased osteoclastic activity has been operationally linked to the pathophysiology of these skeletal complications, which include pathologic fracture, hypercalcemia, cytopenias, severe bone pain, and spinal cord compression.

In addition to their role in causing bone lesions which lead to skeletal complications, osteoclasts also contribute to the establishment and progression of skeletal tumors. The observation that breast and prostate cancer will frequently metastasize to the skeleton has suggested that there is a reciprocal interaction (termed a 'seed and soil relationship') between breast or prostate tumor cells and the bone. On the one hand, this interrelationship facilitates the growth of cancer in the skeleton, and, on the other hand, evokes the excessive remodeling and the bony lesions that are so devastating to patients. There is considerable evidence that osteoclastic activity may encourage tumor establishment and growth due to the increased growth factor and calcium release from the bone matrix after bone resorption occurs. This feedback then enhances further production of osteotropic factors such as parathyroid hormone-related peptide (PTHrP), which in turn leads to further bone resorption, creating a 'vicious cycle'.

The RANK, RANKL and OPG proteins are critical for the differentiation, activation, and survival of osteoclasts and therefore control bone resorption, which is integrally part of bone remodeling via the 'coupling' of osteoblast and osteoclast action. Thus, the RANKL signaling pathway has been implicated in the pathological bone resorption evident in diseases such as rheumatoid arthritis, post-menopausal osteoporosis, and the bony lesions which result from malignancies such as MM or solid tumor metastasis to the bone.

Within the bone microenvironment, RANKL protein is produced by bone marrow stromal cells and osteoblasts. It is believed that most tumor-associated osteotropic signals converge on the bone stroma to cause increases in RANKL, which is then responsible for tumor-induced osteoclastogenesis. The corresponding receptor, RANK, is a membrane-bound TNF receptor family member expressed on the surface of osteoclasts and their precursors. OPG, which is also secreted by osteoblasts, limits osteoclastogenesis by functioning as a decoy receptor for RANKL. The level of osteoclast activation is ultimately governed by the ratio of RANKL to OPG proteins and the resulting osteoclastic activity contributes to both physiologic bone resorption (as part of normal bone turnover) and pathologic bone remodeling as observed in bone metastases and myeloma-induced bone disease. This chapter will first summarize the discovery of OPG, RANK and RANKL and then describe the data implicating these proteins in the pathophysiology of skeletal complications of malignancies. Finally, this chapter will summarize the development of a targeted therapy which blocks RANKL (anti-RANKL antibody) and early clinical trial results resulting from this approach.

II. DISCOVERY AND FUNCTIONAL CHARACTERIZATION OF THE RANK/RANKL/OPG PATHWAY

Osteoclasts are hematopoietic cells and are the principal effectors of bone resorption. During normal bone remodeling, a number of cytokines and calciotropic factors including colony stimulating factor-1 [CSF-1], tumor necrosis factor [TNF], interleukin [IL]-1, -6, -11 are secreted by osteoblasts or other cells and have been shown to contribute to osteoclast differentiation or activation. Osteoclastogenesis essentially requires close contact between bone marrow hematopoietic cells and stromal cells [1,2]. Of these pre-defined calciotropic factors, only CSF-1 has been shown to have an essential role in osteoclastogenesis based on the discovery that the op/op mice which lack a functional CSF-1 protein are osteopetrotic [3]. CSF-1 can exist as a soluble or membrane-bound protein [4] and the primary function of CSF-1 in osteoclastogenesis is to provide survival and pro-liferative signals to myeloid osteoclast precursors (reviewed in Ref. [5]). CSF-1 can stimulate the motility and spreading of mature osteoclasts, but fails to provide the necessary signals for osteoclast differentiation. The essential requirement for cell–cell contact between bone marrow and stromal cells [1] suggested that additional factors were necessary for the commitment and differentiation of osteoclasts. Bone marrow stromal or osteoblastic cells were demonstrated to supply both positive and negative signals that would influence

osteoclastogenesis and would regulate the dynamic balance between bone resorption and bone formation [6]. These additional regulatory signals provided by osteoblastic cells were unknown until a series of discoveries revealed the existence of the RANK/RANKL/OPG axis [6–8].

A. Identification of Osteoprotegerin (OPG)

OPG (osteoprotegerin) was identified as a gene/protein member of the tumor necrosis factor receptor (TNFR) superfamily secreted by osteoblastic cells by two independent groups [7,8] (Figure 32.1). Yasuda's group identified an osteoclastogenesis inhibitory factor (OCIF), which would inhibit the *in vitro* formation of osteoclasts from co-cultures of spleen cells and stromal cells [8]. Another group [7] identified the same gene and termed it 'osteoprotegerin' or 'OPG'. This group defined the physiological role of OPG in the regulation of bone mass by observing the increased skeletal radiodensity in transgenic mice that overexpressed OPG, a gene originally identified from a rat intestinal cDNA library. The mice showed significant osteopetrosis as a result of reduced osteoclast numbers [7]. Reciprocally, genetic ablation of OPG resulted in elevated bone resorption and skeletal pathologies reminiscent of osteoporosis [9], confirming the role of OPG as a physiological negative regulator of bone resorption. The OPG protein does not have a transmembrane domain and is synthesized as a monomer and secreted as a disulfide-linked homodimer, distinguishing itself from other TNF receptor superfamily members, which are typically located at the plasma membrane. However, it was clear that the TNFR cysteine-rich repeat motifs of OPG were necessary for the biological action of osteoclast suppression, suggesting that it functioned via binding to a TNF ligand family member.

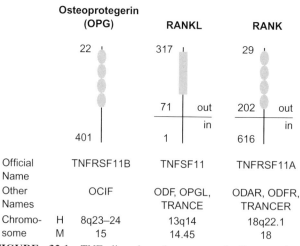

	Osteoprotegerin (OPG)	RANKL	RANK
	22	317	29
		71 out	202 out
		1 in	616 in
	401		
Official Name	TNFRSF11B	TNFSF11	TNFRSF11A
Other Names	OCIF	ODF, OPGL, TRANCE	ODAR, ODFR, TRANCER
Chromosome H	8q23–24	13q14	18q22.1
M	15	14.45	18

FIGURE 32.1 TNF ligand and receptor family members involved in bone mass regulation. Osteoprotegerin (OPG) is a soluble TNF receptor family member. RANKL is a type II TNF ligand family member. RANK is a transmembrane TNF receptor family member. Additional names of each protein and the chromosomal localizations (mouse and human) are also indicated.

B. Receptor Activator of NF-κB Ligand (RANKL)

1. IDENTIFICATION OF RECEPTOR ACTIVATOR OF NF-κB LIGAND (RANKL)

To identify the cognate ligand for OPG, two independent groups [10,11] used a similar expression cloning strategy and identified RANKL, a previously cloned TNF superfamily member [12] as a type II transmembrane protein expressed on the surface of osteoblasts and stromal cells (Figure 32.1). In tissue analyses of adult tissues, RANKL is expressed primarily in bone and peripheral lymph nodes, and also in spleen, thymus, Peyer's patches, intestine, brain, heart, skin, skeletal muscle, kidney, liver, lung, and in mammary tissue of pregnant mice [10,11,13,14]. Cells that express RANKL include cells of the bone microenvironment (e.g., osteoblasts, bone marrow stromal cells) but also activated T cells, B cells, fibroblasts, endothelial cells, chondrocytes, and mammary epithelial cells [11,15–18].

RANKL expression by bone stromal and osteoblast cells is regulated by hormones and other factors that stimulate bone resorption. In the presence of CSF-1, recombinant RANKL can substitute for the stromal cell requirement for osteoclast differentiation [10,11]. A complete absence of osteoclasts, impaired tooth eruption and severe osteopetrosis was observed in the RANKL knockout mice [19], indicating that RANKL, along with CSF-1, are both necessary and sufficient for osteoclastogenesis. Since RANKL has been identified, multiple studies have shown that most calciotropic factors act indirectly, via enhanced production of RANKL by stromal cells, to stimulate osteoclasts (reviewed in Ref. [20]). In a similar fashion, factors released by tumor cells (or the tumor cells themselves) will converge upon the bone stroma to lead to an increase in RANKL and subsequent osteoclastogenesis. These data will be reviewed extensively below (Section IV).

2. MEMBRANE AND SOLUBLE FORMS OF RANKL

RANKL is a type 2 transmembrane protein, and is expressed on the surface of osteoblast precursors in the bone marrow stroma and activated T cells. Early observations have suggested that a cell-to-cell contact between osteoblasts/stromal cells and osteoclast precursors is important for osteoclastogenesis [21]. Indeed, fixed cells expressing the membrane RANKL are capable of inducing osteoclastogenesis [8] suggesting that RANKL is responsible for mediating this cell-to-cell contact-mediated signal. The expression of cell surface RANKL is higher on marrow stromal cells from postmenopausal women compared with premenopausal or postmenopausal women treated with estrogens [16].

In addition to the membrane form of RANKL a soluble form of RANKL has been detected in experimental models of arthritis [19,22] and in other pathological settings such as in serum samples from cancer patients (reviewed below).

The endogenous soluble form can arise from either proteolytic processing or alternative mRNA splicing. Alternative mRNA splicing has been defined for both human and mouse RANKL mRNAs. Ikeda *et al.* [23] identified two shorter versions of the mouse RANKL mRNA including one which would lack the intracellular and transmembrane domain and therefore encode a soluble RANKL protein. Suzuki *et al.* [24] identified three human RANKL mRNA variants which showed similar domain organization as that observed in mice.

Proteolytic processing of RANKL by various metalloproteinases has been demonstrated *in vitro*. The release of soluble RANKL from transfected COS cells were shown to occur through a TACE like protease and could be blocked by MMP inhibitors [25]. Lynch *et al.* [26] showed that MMP-3 and MMP-7 were capable of cleaving RANKL, while MMP-2, MMP-9 and MMP-13 did not. This observation suggests that tumor or osteoclast-derived MMPs may play a role in liberating RANKL from the local site during bone/tumor interactions. The relevance of the MMP-7-dependent cleavage on prostate cancer-induced osteolysis was suggested by decreased bone lesions in the MMP-7 KO mice [26]. However, these authors did not distinguish whether this MMP-7 deficiency altered bone remodeling via altered RANKL cleavage or some other direct effect on osteoclast function. Since most bone destruction mediated by cancer is highly localized to the site of tumor, a membrane form of RANKL may be sufficient for the osteolysis that occurs in skeletal metastasis.

Both soluble and membrane bound forms of RANKL have activity to induce osteoclastogenesis, with some studies indicating that the membrane RANKL has a higher specific activity [27], presumably due to a higher order oligomerization. The *in vivo* activity of a soluble form has been defined by the observation of decreased bone volume and increased osteoclastogenesis in mice treated with a recombinant soluble RANKL form [10]. Additionally, severe osteoporosis in transgenic animals which overexpress a soluble RANKL form [28] has also been documented. A soluble form of RANKL was shown to be secreted or shed from activated T-cells and capable of osteoclast formation *in vitro* [19] and this may explain how both localized bone loss and systemic osteopenia can occur in the adjuvant arthritis model.

C. Identification of Receptor Activator of NF-κB (RANK)

RANKL binds and activates RANK, a member of the TNFR family (Figure 32.1). As in RANKL knockout mice, RANK knockout mice also lack osteoclasts and have osteopetrosis [29,30]. The osteoclast deficiency observed in RANK knockout mice is a cell-autonomous defect of the hematopoietic cells, consistent with the expression of RANK on the surface of myeloid osteoclast precursors [31]. The

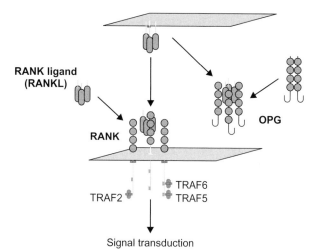

Signal transduction

FIGURE 32.2 The RANKL/RANK/OPG axis:receptor-ligand interactions. RANKL is a type 2 transmembrane protein, and is expressed on the surface of osteoblast precursors in the bone marrow stroma and activated T cells. A soluble form of RANKL has also been described. RANKL binds and activates RANK, a member of the TNFR family. Activation of RANK leads to the recruitment of TRAF adaptor proteins and subsequent signal transduction. OPG acts as a decoy receptor of RANKL by blocking its interaction with RANK.

RANK knockout mice are resistant to the calciotropic effect of factors such as PTHrP, vitamin D3, IL-1 and TNFα [30], proving that these factors require the RANK/RANKL pathway to evoke osteoclastogenesis and calcium mobilization from the skeleton.

The significant osteopetrosis observed in the transgenic mice overexpressing OPG was due to decreases in the number of mature osteoclasts, which resulted in increased bone density [7]. OPG, therefore, acts as a decoy receptor of RANKL by blocking its interaction with RANK and it is ultimately the ratio of RANKL to OPG that determines the degree of osteoclastogenesis and therefore bone resorption. Figure 32.2 depicts the receptor-ligand interactions of this axis.

In addition to the modulation of RANKL and the decoy receptor OPG levels, osteoclastogenesis can be controlled via the upregulation of RANK expression by cytokines such as TNFα and CSF-1 [32–34], which explains, in part, the amplification of osteoclastogenesis by these factors. Moreover, RANK signal transduction can be regulating by the local and systemic signals. For instance, either (IFNβ and IFNγ) can inhibit RANK signaling by lowering cellular levels of key intracellular factors in osteoclastogenesis (e.g., c-fos, TRAF6 and NFATc1) (reviewed in Ref. [35]). While activation of ITAM-containing molecules, DAP12, FcRγ can enhance RANK signal transduction (reviewed in Ref. [36]). The cytokine IL-4 has also been shown to inhibit RANK signaling in osteoclasts through the reversible inactivation of NF-κB, JNK, p38, and ERK pathways [37]. In summary, the interaction of RANKL with RANK is the essential positive signal for osteoclastogenesis that is counterbalanced by the action of OPG.

D. RANKL has a Unique Mechanism of Action in Osteoclastogenesis and Affects Three Distinct Aspects of this Process (Formation, Activation and Survival)

The RANKL system has been identified as an essential mediator of osteoclast formation, function, and survival [5]. RANKL binds RANK on osteoclasts or osteoclast precursors to stimulate or promote differentiation into osteoclasts. This differentiation process includes the transcription of many osteoclast genes (e.g., TRAP, cathepsin K, calcitonin receptor, β3-integrin) as well as the fusion of mononuclear osteoclasts [20]. Importantly, RANKL is essential not only for differentiation, but also for the survival of osteoclasts and the activation of mature osteoclasts, therefore, playing critical roles at multiple stages in the regulation of bone resorption (Figure 32.3). RANK is expressed on mature osteoclasts and RANKL will activate these cells in a dose dependent manner [38] causing the formation of F-actin rings and increasing their ability to resorb bone [39]. *In vivo*, RANKL treatment of mice will lead to an increase in bone resorption and serum calcium within a short time period, indicating that this activity is via pre-existing osteoclasts [10]. Effects on osteoclast apoptosis are observed with either RANKL (increased osteoclast survival *in vitro*) or OPG (increased osteoclast apoptosis). RANKL will enhance osteoclast survival in the presence of CSF-1 [40] while OPG induces apoptosis of osteoclasts in murine bone marrow cultures [41]. Treatment of mice with a single dose of recombinant OPG led to osteoclast apoptosis evident within 18 hours and loss of greater than 90% of osteoclasts within 48 hours, confirming the role of RANKL as a survival factor for differentiated osteoclasts [40].

Bone resorption can be inhibited by preventing the recruitment or activation of osteoclasts or by decreasing their life span. The action of OPG (RANKL inhibition) reduces the terminal differentiation of osteoclasts (thus affecting the pool of mature osteoclasts), as well as the survival and activity of mature osteoclasts [7]. Experiments using OPG-Fc or RANK-Fc as selective pharmacologic inhibitors of RANKL have defined the activity of RANKL on these three distinct steps in osteoclastogenesis: differentiation, activation and survival.

III. CRITICAL INVOLVEMENT OF OSTEOCLASTS IN CANCER-INDUCED BONE DISEASES

A. Role of Osteoclasts in Bone Metastases

The dramatic predilection of some cancers (e.g., breast, prostate, lung) to metastasize to the bone is well established. In 1889 Stephen Paget likened the development of metastases to a tumor 'seed' that is necessary but not

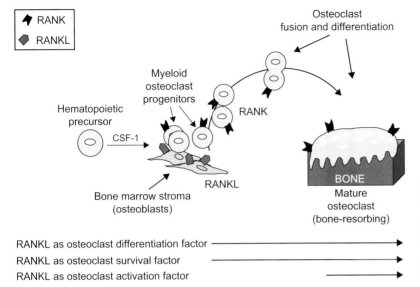

FIGURE 32.3 RANKL is the membrane-bound (and soluble) osteoclast differentiation, survival and activation factor. RANKL is essential not only for differentiation, but also for the survival of osteoclasts and the activation of mature osteoclasts, therefore playing critical roles at multiple stages in the regulation of bone resorption.

sufficient to develop into a plant without 'congenial soil' [42]. A reciprocal relationship between the bone and certain tumors co-opts the skeleton to provide a unique microenvironment ('soil') for the establishment and progression of cancer. As with metastasis to other sites, colonization to the bone requires multiple steps and is a considerably inefficient process. Once a tumor cell escapes the primary site and circulates in the periphery, selective tropism to the bone requires multiple sequential steps including homing to the bone marrow and arrest, adherence and invasion of the bone. The abundant vasculature of the bone ensures a close contact of tumor cells and endothelium. Upon colonization of the bone, tumor growth and neovascularization are initiated, followed by progression of both the tumor and bone lesions. Specific molecular interactions that affect bone tropism have been defined for each of these steps (e.g., chemokine/chemokine receptors, cell adhesion molecules/integrins, matrix metalloproteinases, etc.) and have been the subject of a number of reviews [43,44].

While each of these interactions can enhance bone metastasis, they are neither necessary nor sufficient by themselves. Kang *et al.* [45] used the MDA-231 breast cancer-induced bone metastasis model to define an association between the expression of certain genes and aggressive metastasis to bone. Functional assays demonstrated a causal role for certain genes (e.g., IL-11, CTGF, CXCR4, MMP1) in bone metastasis. However, these studies indicated that a single gene product was not sufficient for bone metastasis but rather that elevated expression of functionally-distinct classes of genes ('tool kits', e.g., homing, invasion, angiogenesis, osteolysis) would cooperate in the different processes, thereby resulting in aggressive bone metastases. The development of bone metastasis therapies based on any of these molecularly-defined targets would thus only have efficacy within the limited patient population which might express the target gene product on tumor cells.

Although these experimental results suggest that there is not a single gene product necessary or sufficient to mediate bone metastasis, one common attribute of tumor cells that metastasize to the bone is the capacity to co-opt the normal regulatory processes of bone remodeling. The hypothesis that increased bone turnover will promote skeletal tumor growth or bone metastasis has been addressed experimentally in several model systems. For instance, Kalikin *et al.* [46] observed significantly faster growth of PC3 prostate tumor burden in the skeletons of young mice than in old mice and hypothesized that the greater rate of bone remodeling in young mice contributed to this observation. Similarly, administration of PTH to mice to induce bone turnover increased the growth rate of PC3 tumor cells in the hind limbs [47]. Androgen ablation will lead to increased osteoclastic activity [48] and accelerated bone turnover resulting from a low calcium diet will enhance the growth of MDA-231 breast cancer cells in the bone and cause greater lytic lesions [49].

The mechanisms by which bone remodeling will enhance tumor metastasis include not only the localized release of growth factors which stimulate tumor growth and survival (discussed in D of this section), but also the elaboration and release of paracrine factors which can support adhesion or stimulate chemotaxis and migration to the skeleton. Overall these studies support the hypothesis that the bone microenvironment undergoing active turnover encourages tumor colonization and/or expansion in bone and would suggest that bone resorption and, by extension, osteoclast action, plays a critical role in this process. These findings suggest that reducing osteoclast activity (e.g., via RANKL inhibition) may then both reduce the growth of established skeletal tumors and prevent the establishment of skeletal tumors in the first place. The pharmacology data using RANKL inhibitors in rodent models of multiple myeloma and bone metastases support this notion and will be addressed in Section V.

B. Role of Osteoclasts in Osteolytic versus Osteoblastic Bone Lesions in Skeletal Metastases

The bone lesions which result from multiple myeloma are almost exclusively osteolytic, due to excessive osteoclast action and suppressed osteoblast function [50]. In the case of bone metastases the classifications of 'osteolytic' and 'osteoblastic' are probably oversimplified and represent two extremes of a continuum of bone lesions in which both osteoclasts and osteoblasts can be involved. Most frequently, bone lesions which occur in breast cancer patients have a more osteolytic radiographic appearance while prostate cancer bone metastases are typically osteosclerotic (as determined by histology) or osteoblastic (according to bone scans).

The concept that osteoclast activation accompanies all bone metastases is supported by the finding that biochemical markers of bone resorption, in particular the N-telopeptide of type I collagen (NTX), are increased in patients with bone metastases, whether they are lytic, blastic, or mixed [51]. A correlation between NTX and clinical outcome (including skeletal related events (SREs) and survival) has been observed in patients with prostate cancer, breast cancer, and other solid tumors (e.g., non-small-cell lung carcinoma, renal carcinoma, small-cell lung carcinoma, thyroid carcinoma) as well as MM [52,53]. Taken together, these findings suggest that the risk of skeletal complications and poor clinical outcome in metastatic bone disease are dependent in part on the capacity to control the level of osteoclast activity and the subsequent osteolysis. Moreover, this relationship appears to hold irrespective of the primary tumor type.

C. Role of Osteoclasts in Skeletal Complications of Malignancies Including Solid Tumor Skeletal Metastasis and Multiple Myeloma

Bone metastases cause considerable morbidity, including pain which requires radiotherapy, reduced mobility, hypercalcemia, spinal cord or nerve root compression and pathologic fracture. One common feature of bone metastases is the increased bone resorption by osteoclasts which leads to osteolysis and the subsequent bone destruction associated with severe skeletal complications and poor clinical outcomes [50,54]. The role of PTHrP in malignant hypercalcemia is well established [55] and is due in part to activated osteoclast-mediated bone resorption caused by increased PTHrP levels. Bone destruction by tumors which cause osteolysis will lead to a loss of bone mass or structure which eventually compromises the stability of a weight-bearing bone [54] leading to fracture or compression of the spinal cord.

Similar mechanical fragility is observed in 'osteodense' prostate cancer bone metastases. In this situation, the bone structure is severely perturbed by pathologically increased bone remodeling which results in heterogeneous, poorly-mineralized [56], woven bone formation [57] and the deterioration of the trabecular structure that provides strength in the normal bone. One hallmark feature of osteolytic and osteoblastic bone metastases is the insufficient mechanical strength due to increased bone turnover as compared to the normal bone [58,59], which can result in pathologic fracture.

The most common source of cancer-related pain is bone metastases [60]. Radiotherapy and opiods are the most common treatments for bone cancer pain [61]; however, the pain symptoms frequently continue to progress as the disease advances. The pathophysiological mechanism of bone pain in patients with bone metastases involves a unique combination of nociceptive and neuropathic pain and cancer-induced bone pain is unusual as compared to inflammatory or neuropathic pain in that it elaborates distinct central changes [60]. Destruction of bone and loss of mechanical stability will lead to microfractures, which can cause pain. The dissolution of the inorganic $CaPO_4$ matrix of the bone by osteoclasts works in part via proton pumps (e.g., ATP6i) which acidify the sealed resorption vacuole. The acidic pH of the bone microenvironment and release of growth factors/cytokines that occur during osteoclast action may activate peripheral neurons [60].

Osteoclast suppression (via RANKL inhibition) has shown a benefit in several models of cancer-induced bone pain. Treatment of mice bearing osteolytic sarcoma cells with OPG not only reduced osteoclast activity and bone destruction [62], but also prevented pain behaviors and pathologic spinal cord changes [63]. In a model of established tumor-induced pain, OPG treatment stabilized pain behavior and improved some of the pathologic spinal cord changes that had already occurred [64]. A role for RANKL as a mediator of pain from malignant breast cancer in bone lesions was observed using a new rat model for bone cancer pain. RANKL inhibition (using OPG-Fc) in the rat mammary tumor (MRMT-1) model reduced mechanical allodynia and prevented central pain sensitization in the spinal cord [65]. These beneficial effects on pain were correlated with the pharmacodynamic effects of RANKL inhibition on osteoclast function including increased BMD, the prevention of tumor-induced bone destruction, reduced osteoclast number and suppression of bone resorption.

Osteoclasts thus play an operative role in the pathophysiology of each type of skeletal complication due to malignancies. Clinical data supports this hypothesis in patients, in which elevated levels of bone turnover markers are associated with an increased risk of skeletal complications, disease progression, and death [52,53,66]. The skeletal morbidities secondary to cancer, particularly the impaired mobility from fractures and the bone pain, significantly reduce the quality of life in these patients. Inhibition of osteoclast function, as measured by decreases in bone resorption, may result in fewer skeletal complications and a more favorable prognosis. A key objective in the management of bone metastases is to minimize skeletal morbidity by 'normalizing' the accelerated rate of bone remodeling which exists in cancer patients. If excessive bone resorption is inhibited, skeletal complications caused by bone metastases may be prevented or delayed.

D. Central Role of RANKL and Osteoclasts in Vicious Cycle

Osteoclastic function will therefore enhance the establishment of skeletal tumor colonization in the bone marrow at early points in metastasis and will also affect skeletal complications as the tumor progresses during later stages. Histological observations of osteolytic bone metastasis reveal a highly reactive microenvironment, with many activated TRAP-positive osteoclasts, evidence of bone and matrix degradation and tumor-induced angiogenesis [67]. Extensive experimental evidence supports the idea that the bone microenvironment provides necessary growth support for the initial establishment of the tumor and progression at later times. This feedback probably occurs via elevated growth factor levels and the increased calcium concentration that exists at sites of active remodeling. The bone contains large amounts of growth factors in latent forms, including transforming growth factor β (TGFβ), fibroblast growth factors (FGF-1 and FGF-2), platelet-derived growth factors (PDGFs), bone morphogenetic proteins (BMPs), and insulin-like growth factors (e.g., IGF-1), which, upon osteoclastic bone resorption, become activated and released into the bone microenvironment. By activating bone resorption

in mouse calvarial organ cultures, Yoneda and colleagues demonstrated elevated levels of IGF-α and TGF-β in the conditioned medium which could support the growth of the MDA-MB-231 breast cancer cells in soft agar [44]. Increased IGF-1 concentration leads to increased cell proliferation, directed migration, and decreased apoptosis of tumor cells [68]. TGFβ will enhance bone metastasis by direct action on the tumor cell as shown by elegant studies using MDA-MB-231 cells transfected with dominant negative forms of the TGFβ receptor in a bone metastasis model [69]. The consequence of locally elevated TGFβ in the bone microenvironment is not the direct increase in tumor growth per se, but rather the elevated production of PTHrP by breast cancer cells locally within the metastatic site [69,70]. Guise *et al.* [71] used neutralizing antibodies to PTHrP to demonstrate the reduced development of MDA-MB-231 bone metastasis, which suggested that tumor-produced PTHrP is causative in the local bone destruction in breast cancer metastatic to bone. Increased PTHrP then contributes to a continuously destructive 'vicious cycle' by enhancing production of RANKL and accelerating bone resorption [72]. The release of calcium from the bone may also stimulate further production of PTHrP from breast cancer [73] or prostate cancer [74] cells, thus exacerbating the osteolytic response.

The release of growth factors and calcium through the resorptive action of osteoclasts may then allow the establishment and progression of the tumor within the skeleton (summarized in Figure 32.4). Taken together,

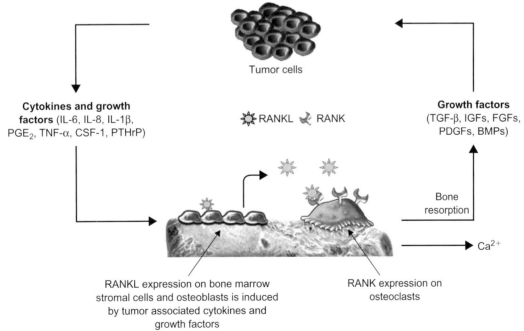

FIGURE 32.4 RANK ligand is an essential mediator in the 'vicious cycle' hypothesis of bone destruction in metastatic cancer. RANKL is necessary for osteoclastogenesis and is generally increased as a result of tumor/bone interactions. The release of growth factors and calcium through the resorptive action of osteoclasts may then allow the establishment and progression of the tumor within the skeleton. The consequence of locally elevated growth factors in the bone microenvironment can include increases in tumor growth and the further release of cytokines and growth factors which would increase RANKL expression.

the evidence suggests that pharmacologic inhibition of bone remodeling will not only reduce the bone lesions, but also may reduce the skeletal tumor burden. A number of the experiments which demonstrate the role of RANKL in both the establishment and progression of skeletal tumor burden will be discussed later in this chapter. RANKL as the key regulator of osteoclastogenesis and bone resorption provides an ideal therapeutic target in this regard.

IV. RANKL AS THE FINAL COMMON MEDIATOR OF TUMOR-INDUCED BONE RESORPTION

Since the discovery of the RANK, RANKL and OPG triad, demonstration of the regulation of RANKL and OPG by various resorptive factors has suggested that the effect of these different factors may converge at the level of RANKL/OPG dysregulation and this signal is the ultimate effector of osteoclast formation, function and survival. Treatment of mice lacking the RANK gene with the major calciotropic factors (IL-1, TNFα, vitamin D3 and PTHrP) failed to elicit osteoclast formation or hypercalcemia [75], confirming that these factors primarily function indirectly, through RANKL, to mediate these effects. Analysis of tumor/bone models have revealed that the tumor cells will employ several mechanisms to dysregulate the RANKL and OPG signal and, therefore, favor osteoclastogenesis. Pharmacologic inhibition of RANKL in animal models of tumor/bone interactions (see below) have also provided evidence that tumor-induced osteoclastogenesis is ultimately dependent upon RANKL.

A. Mechanisms of RANKL and OPG Dysregulation in Cancer

The observations of RANKL and OPG dysregulation in tumors and skeletal metastasis implicate this pathway in the pathophysiology of a wide range of cancer types. The mechanisms responsible for the changes in RANKL and OPG expression include: (1) the induction of RANKL within the tumor stroma and/or bone stroma as a result of tumor-derived factors or cell–cell contact; (2) expression of RANKL by the tumor cell itself; (3) expression of RANKL by activated inflammatory cells within or associated with the tumor; and (4) tumor-associated suppression of OPG production or activity. The preponderance of evidence supports a dominant role for RANKL in tumor-induced osteoclastogenesis. Most, if not all, pre-resorptive factors which operate in the cancer setting will increase RANKL and/or decrease OPG in osteoblasts and stromal cells.

1. THE INDUCTION OF RANKL WITHIN THE STROMA AS A RESULT OF TUMOR-DERIVED FACTORS OR CELL–CELL CONTACT

Tumor associated factors which can influence osteolysis would include IL-1, IL-6, IL-8, IL-11, TNFα, PTHrP, M-CSF, TGF-β and prostaglandins [76]. As in normal bone remodeling, tumor-associated osteoclastogenesis primarily results from the convergence of systemically and locally-produced hormones, cytokines and other factors on the bone microenvironment and causing an increase in local RANKL levels and/or decreases in OPG. In breast cancer and HHM, PTHrP has been identified as one key humoral factor causing osteolysis and subsequent hypercalcemia in a significant fraction of lung and breast cancer patients [55]. Many tumors can release PTHrP into circulation or locally, as in the case of skeletal metastasis. The osteotropic action of PTHrP occurs as a result of activation of the PTH/PTHrP receptor on stromal or osteoblast cells leading to increased expression of RANKL and decreased OPG production [77–79].

Other tumor-associated factors such as IL-1 and TNFα may influence bone metastases through their ability to stimulate bone turnover. IL-1 and TNF have complex effects on osteoclastogenesis. These cytokines are clearly capable of increasing RANKL mRNA within osteoblasts and/or stromal cells, suggesting that these factors increase osteoclastogenesis indirectly, via RANKL. For instance, the inflammatory cytokines IL-1β and TNFα have both been shown to increase RANKL mRNA in osteoblasts [8,80,81] and some tumor cells themselves (e.g., osteosarcoma; [82]).

The ability of IL-6 to alter RANKL levels has been somewhat controversial. In one study, Hofbauer showed that IL-6 was unable to increase RANKL levels from human osteoblast cell lines [81]. However, experiments using mouse calvaria have demonstrated that huIL-6 (in the presence of soluble huIL-6 receptor) can enhance RANKL mRNA and protein production from the calvarial bones [83]. Similar results were observed after treatment of murine bone marrow stromal cells (UAMS-32) with IL-6 plus sIL-6 R [84]. Additionally, other IL-6 like cytokines (e.g., LIF and OSM) also stimulated RANKL production [83,84]. Likewise, IL-11 will increase RANKL in primary mouse osteoblasts [8,77].

In addition, there is some association of elevated levels of C-C chemokines, such as MIP1α, with increased tumor-associated osteolysis. MIP1α levels are elevated in bone marrow samples of 62% of patients with active myeloma [85]. Secretion of MIP1α and MIP1β was detected from a number of MM cell lines and patient samples and these levels correlated with the ability of myeloma cells to enhance osteoclastic bone resorption [86]. Again, each of these factors will induce RANKL on stromal cells which then likely provides the osteoclastogenic signal although there may be species-specific differences in these regulatory pathways.

For instance, there is conflicting data on the effect of MIP-1on RANKL expression with one study demonstrating that MIP-1α stimulates RANKL expression by the mouse stromal cell line ST2 *in vitro* [86]. Other studies [87] using human bone marrow have not observed changes in RANKL after MIP1a treatment.

Other examples of tumor-derived or tumor-induced factors which will contribute to increased osteoclast activation include prostaglandin E2 (PGE2). Elevated levels of PGE2 have also been associated with osteolytic metastases, and are capable of coordinately upregulating RANKL and downregulating OPG levels [11,88]. The alpha chemokine IL-8 will increase RANKL mRNA and protein levels in stromal osteoblast cultures [89].

Co-culture experiments have provided some evidence that tumor cell contact with the stroma lead to increases in RANKL within this latter compartment. For instance, co-culture of MDA-MB-231 cells and the mouse bone marrow stromal cell UAMS-33 caused an increase in stromal RANKL expression [90]. In similar experiments, the addition of MDA-MB-231 cells to bone marrow and osteoblast cultures induce RANKL by osteoblasts, which was dependent upon cell-to-cell contact between tumor and osteoblasts [91]. The expression of RANKL was specifically induced (as determined by RT-PCR) on the mouse stromal cells ST2 or MC3T3-E1 when co-cultured with MDA-231 cells [92] and this co-culture could enhance osteoclastogenesis when bone marrow cells were added. Michigami *et al.* [93] showed that RANKL mRNA levels were increased in co-cultures of NB-19 neuroblastoma cells and bone marrow cells, although it was not clear whether the host or tumor (or both) contributed the RANKL signal. A co-culture of MM cell lines and bone marrow derived endothelial cells led to increased surface RANKL expression on the latter cells [94].

Observations from preclinical animal models and clinical specimens of breast cancer bone metastasis demonstrate local RANKL changes in the bone stroma. For breast cancer, injection of MCF-7 breast cancer cells into rodent bones induced local changes in RANKL that were confined to spindle-shaped stromal cells and osteoblasts residing on the bone surface [72]. Histopathological analysis of the MDA-MB-231 breast cancer bone metastasis model indicated osteoblasts positive for RANKL in close juxtaposition with the TRAP-positive osteoclasts [67]. Ohshiba *et al.* [91] used mRNA analysis to demonstrate a significant increase in local mouse RANKL levels after injection of MDA-231 cells. Similarly, our group has shown local stromal RANKL protein levels increased significantly in the bone in response to the infiltrating MDA-MB-231 breast cancer cells [95]. RANKL was not detected on tumor cells or in serum after MDA-MB-231 innoculation suggesting that RANKL elevations are limited to the local site of bone/tumor interaction.

Analyses of preclinical and clinical samples of prostate tumor skeletal metastasis have shown evidence of RANKL expression in the stromal element. Using different antibodies to detect RANKL by IHC, Roudier *et al.* demonstrated RANKL-positive bone stroma cells in prostate cancer bone metastases while RANKL protein was not detected on tumor cells in this study [96]. The expression of RANKL on tumor cells will be addressed (sub-Section II) below. In our own analysis of the PC3 osteolytic prostate cancer bone metastasis model [97], we demonstrated both local and systemic changes in the RANKL:OPG ratio. For instance, PC3-bearing mice exhibited an increase in RANKL positive stromal cells located at the tumor/bone interface and on stroma found within the tumor mass itself. In the latter preclinical studies, RANKL expression was not detected on the tumor cells themselves.

2. EXPRESSION OF RANKL DIRECTLY BY THE TUMOR CELL ITSELF

While there is clear evidence for RANKL increases in the stroma associated with bone metastases, a number of studies have also indicated that tumor cells can express RANKL in some instances. In the case of multiple myeloma (MM), this expression may correlate with the degree of bone destruction that occurs. High expression of membrane associated RANKL was detected on MM patient samples using flow cytometry [98,99]. In the latter study, the authors correlated the levels of RANKL on MM cells with the bone status of patients. Lai *et al.* [100] showed RANKL not only on MM patient samples, but also on a number of MM tumor cell lines. As described below (sub-Section III), serum samples from MM patients have also shown increases in the ratio of serum RANKL:OPG and this increased ratio was associated with the severity of osteolytic lesions and overall survival [101].

Neuroblastoma can also give rise to osteolytic bone metastasis and in one study, Granchi *et al.* [102] demonstrated that several neuroblastoma cell lines express RANKL mRNA and support osteoclastogenesis *in vitro*. RANKL was also detected in some human squamous carcinoma cell lines derived from patients with humoral hypercalcemia of malignancy [103]. Similarly, adult T-cell leukemia (ATL) patients can often exhibit hypercalcemia and some ATL cells can stimulate osteoclast formation *in vitro*, which correlated with the expression of RANKL by these tumor cells [104]. There has also been a case report of RANKL expression in a patient with follicular lymphoma and bone involvement [105]. Bone sections resected from X patients with primary B-cell lymphoma of the bone have also been shown to express RANKL by IHC [106].

Multiple groups have shown that RANKL is not detectably present (by mRNA analysis) on breast tumor cells either *in vitro* [79] or by mRNA or protein analysis *in vivo* [67,95]. While, at the same time, there is clear evidence of RANKL elevations in breast cancer bone metastasis, particularly in the bone stroma (see above). To date, there are only a few studies that analyze RANKL expression in human breast tumor samples. Analyses of clinical samples using IHC have suggested that RANKL can be expressed by the tumor cell directly in some instances, including examples of primary breast cancer. In a survey of a small series of breast cancers ($n = 40$) by Van Poznak *et al.* [107], RANKL was detected in 55% of invasive cancers (24/40) as well as DCIS (5/11) and LCIS (1/1). The same group used the same antibody for human RANKL detection in a larger study set (395 breast cancer samples with some patient follow-up) and showed expression of RANKL in 14% of cancers [108]. The latter studies suggested a relationship between RANKL expression and a higher histological grade and estrogen receptor negative cancers.

Several studies have demonstrated expression of RANKL on prostate cancer cells *in vitro*. For instance, the C42B, PC3 and LuCap35 cell lines secrete a soluble form of RANKL that can support osteoclastogenesis [109]. Using either mRNA or protein detection methods Armstrong *et al.* [97] did not detect human RANKL in PC3 cells either grown *in vitro* or in a mouse bone metastasis model. Interestingly, one study has demonstrated that treatment of C42B cells with TGF-beta, either *in vitro* or *in vivo*, caused RANKL mRNA levels to increase further [110]. This latter observation suggests that the feedback from the bone (e.g., TGF-beta) will increase further tumor-induced osteolysis via RANKL. Desai *et al.* [111] suggest that overexpression of osteopontin on PC3 cells will cause increases in tumor cell RANKL expression.

Three studies of clinical samples of human prostate cancer using IHC methods to detect RANKL have revealed expression in prostate tumor cells, but not the bone stroma surrounding the tumor [112–114]. These studies are in contrast to a another study cited above which clearly demonstrates RANKL expression by IHC in the bone stroma, but not the prostate tumor cells in bone metastasis [96]. A prostate tumor xenograft study using a human-specific antibody against RANKL has supported the notion that the host/stromal expression of RANKL is the major contributor to tumor-associated osteolysis [115].

It is not clear if the disparate observations of RANKL expression in prostate cancer are due to differences in the specificity of the antibodies used, or the stage of tumor progression in the bone (either pre-clinical models or clinical samples). These *in situ* analyses only represent single 'snapshots' during the natural history of disease *in vivo*, and it is possible that RANKL changes will be specifically observed on skeletal tumor cells early during the establishment or progression of bony metastases. It will be essential for any IHC analysis of RANKL protein expression in tumor samples to demonstrate well-validated controls for the specificity of the reagents used.

The notion that solid tumors of different origin from either breast or prostate would affect the RANKL/OPG axis during bone metastasis is supported by a study by Good *et al.* on 16 cases of bone tumors including primary benign and malignant bone lesions as well as metastatic tumors (renal, lung, and melanoma). The ratio of RANKL to OPG was higher in bone metastases samples (e.g., lung and kidney) and was increased relative to that observed in healthy bone tissue. Good *et al.* [116] demonstrated, using IHC, that RANKL was expressed in 5/8 metastatic bone tumors (including renal and lung cancer); expression was noted in the neoplastic element of these samples. Huang *et al.* [117] analyzed skeletal lesions of breast, lung, prostate and thyroid cancer patients using ISH and IHC and showed greater than 85% of the tissues were RANKL positive, with the tumor cells, osteoblasts and fibroblasts in tissues surrounding the tissue all contributing to the RANKL signal. Grimaud *et al.* [118] used RT-PCR to determine the RANKL and OPG expression in human bone pathologic samples where osteolysis had occurred.

3. EXPRESSION OF RANKL BY ACTIVATED INFLAMMATORY CELLS WITHIN OR ASSOCIATED WITH THE TUMOR

RANKL can be expressed by activated inflammatory cells (e.g., T cells) [19]. Using a co-culture system, Giuliani [119] showed that human MM cell lines stimulated RANKL production and secretion by activated $CD3^+$ cells. Moreover, RANKL mRNA expression was detected from $CD3^+$ T cells purified from MM patients that suffered from greater than 3 osteolytic lesions. Luo *et al.* [120] have reported an increase in RANKL mRNA and protein in prostate tumors in the mouse TRAMP model that occurs coincidentally with the arrival of tumor infiltrating T cells and macrophages.

4. TUMOR-ASSOCIATED REGULATION OF OPG PRODUCTION OR ACTIVITY

While increased local levels of RANKL appear to be a common mechanism by which cancer cells influence increased osteoclastogenesis, tumor metastasis to the bone can also suppress OPG levels, which would also enhance local osteoclast formation. IHC of bone marrow aspirates showed a significantly lower expression of OPG in bone marrow stroma from MM patients [121] and co-culture of MM cells with stromal lines suppressed OPG *in vitro*. In this latter study, IHC and *in situ* hybridization methods clearly demonstrated significantly higher RANKL levels that included stromal elements and activated T cells. In normal marrow, OPG was detected in vessels, stromal cells and megakaryocytes, while in MM marrow lower OPG levels in the latter two tissues were observed. It is believed that MM cells can sequester and degrade OPG through the action of syndecan-1 [122].

There are frequent examples of cancer-associated factors that can not only increase RANKL levels, but will also decrease OPG levels thereby shifting the balance of this axis towards a greater osteoclastogenic signal. For instance,

IL-1 can also decrease OPG expression in osteoblasts [123]. PTHrP will decrease OPG production by stromal cells [77–79]. PGE2, which can be locally increased in bone metastasis, will downregulate stromal OPG [11,88].

EGF-like ligands (e.g., EGF, TGF-α, HB-EGF, amphiregulin/AR) have been shown to stimulate osteoclastogenesis in co-cultures of mouse bone marrow osteoclast precursors and the MC3T3 osteoblast cell line [124]. EGF ligand did not cause detectable changes in RANKL levels; however, OPG expression was decreased. OPG production has been observed in conditioned media of endothelial cells [125]. In human tissue, OPG was apparently absent from normal endothelium, but was observed in endothelial cells associated with malignant tumors. In breast cancer, endothelial OPG expression was associated with a higher tumor grade [125]. The evidence that OPG can be expressed by tumor cells includes mRNA analysis of breast cancer cell lines [79] and the production of OPG protein by cell lines representing prostate cancer (e.g., PC3 and DU145; [126]), colon cancer (e.g., HT-29 and SW-480; [127]) and breast cancer (e.g., MDA-231 and MDA-436; [128]). Patient tumor samples have also shown evidence of OPG expression including 40% of breast tumors in one study [128] and 55% of breast tumors in another study [107].

B. Observations of Serum RANKL and OPG Dysregulation in Cancer Patients

Analysis of clinical bone metastases or preclinical models provides evidence for enhanced RANKL expression and/or altered expression of OPG within the bone stroma, tumor stroma and tumor itself. In solid tumor skeletal metastasis, the bone lesions are highly localized. As described above, increased local RANKL has been detected in the bone stroma proximal to tumor metastasis. While biochemical markers of bone resorption have been shown to be elevated in these patients, there are only a few studies demonstrating alterations in serum levels of RANKL and/or OPG. In a study of patients with newly diagnosed metastasis to the bone with breast cancer ($n = 30$) and non-small cell lung cancer ($n = 14$), significant increases in serum RANKL were detected [129]. While the serum levels of OPG were also increased, the ratio of RANKL:OPG remained higher than in the controls. In the same study, patients with prostate cancer metastatic to the bone ($n = 17$) showed nominal changes in serum RANKL, but significant increases in serum OPG. Interestingly, in a study of a small number of neuroblastoma patients ($n = 54$) serum RANKL levels were increased in patients with advanced neuroblastoma while serum OPG levels were lower in all patients versus controls [130]. However, the ratio of RANKL:OPG did not predict the severity of bone disease observed.

Additional observations of increased serum OPG in patients with bone metastases relative to patients with non-osseous metastases and primary tumors have been made in prostate cancer [112,131,132]. In the study by Eaton [131], higher OPG levels were observed in patients with locally advanced disease compared to those with locally confined disease and also greater in patients with advanced disease who progressed after androgen ablation versus those patients which responded to therapy. The source of the elevated OPG in this setting is not entirely clear and may include osteoblastic and stromal elements (as has been described in Refs [133–135]), endothelium and/or tumor cells themselves (cited in 2 of the section above). Given that prostate cancer patients with bone metastasis have highly elevated bone remodeling (Section III), the increase in OPG may be a compensatory response to excessive skeletal remodeling.

As with solid tumor bone metastasis, MM results in alterations in RANKL and OPG at the site of tumor/bone interaction. As described above, studies using IHC and *in situ* hybridization methods have demonstrated significantly lower expression of OPG and significantly higher RANKL levels (within stromal elements and activated T cells) [121]. However, in MM there is also evidence of a correlation between clinical bony disease and an increased ratio of RANKL: OPG has been observed in the serum of patients. Serum levels of RANKL have been shown to be elevated [101] and the ratio of RANKL:OPG was associated with the severity of bony lesions and was an independent prognostic factor for the disease. The alterations in serum levels of RANKL may be apparent in myeloma also because the disease is hematologic in origin and disseminated systemically. In several independent studies, serum OPG has been shown to be lower in MM patients compared to sex- and age-matched controls and also correlates with bony disease [136,137]. Local changes in RANKL and OPG have been observed in bone marrow biopsies from MM patients as compared with non-MM patients [121] (see above).

Altogether from these observations a few generalizations can be made. For instance, local increases in RANKL at the bone/tumor interface are commonly observed in preclinical models (representing diverse tumor types such as prostate and breast) and in some patient samples of bone metastasis and MM. In MM, local and systemic changes in RANKL and OPG have been documented, which may reflect the marrow dissemination of MM and the observation that RANKL has been shown to be expressed by some myeloma. The correlation in serum RANKL:OPG ratio to the severity of bone lesions may reflect the increased osteoclast activation and/or reflect the greater tumor burden in these patients.

Given the lack of clear evidence for serum RANKL increases, at least for solid tumor bone metastases, it seems likely that most tumor-induced osteoclastogenesis is probably controlled at the local level. As will be described below, pharmacology studies in rodent models using RANKL inhibitors have suggested that RANKL, irrespective of its source (i.e., tumor or stroma), is functionally linked to the tumor-induced osteoclastogenesis. Furthermore as described in Section V below, animal model studies using RANKL inhibitors have also suggested that RANKL control of osteoclasts is important in the pathophysiology of skeletal metastases at both early and late times (e.g., during the establishment and progression, respectively).

V. ANIMAL PHARMACOLOGY DATA WITH RANKL INHIBITORS IN RODENT MODELS OF CANCER-INDUCED BONE DISEASE

Pharmacological inhibition of RANKL in rodent models of bone metastasis and multiple myeloma have been used to define a causal association between RANKL and the skeletal complications of malignancy. Previous sections in this chapter have outlined how osteoclast function plays a fundamental role in the establishment and progression of skeletal metastasis, whether the ultimate lesion is osteolytic, osteoblastic or both. Additionally, osteoclasts are central to bone remodeling and the vicious cycle of tumor/bone interactions, which can lead to stimulation of tumor growth in the skeleton.

Highly specific RANKL inhibitors are unique tools to selectively block osteoclasts *in vivo* and rodent bone tumor models using OPG-Fc or RANK-Fc have provided four key lines of evidence: (1) RANKL is the predominant factor by which tumors (of diverse origins) will induce osteoclastogenesis; (2) RANKL inhibition can reduce both osteolytic and osteoblastic bony lesions; (3) osteoclasts play a critical role not only in the progression of existing skeletal metastases, but also in the establishment of new metastases in the bone; and (4) selective inhibition of osteoclasts via RANKL inhibition can also reduce skeletal tumor burden by attenuating the vicious cycle. The data which supports these four points will be summarized according to the tumor type that has been tested in rodent models, thus the data will be summarized according to the following tumor types: (1) breast cancer; (2) prostate cancer; (3) other solid tumors which metastasize to the bone (e.g., lung, colon, bladder); and (4) multiple myeloma (MM).

A. Role of RANKL in Breast Cancer Bone Metastases

The MDA-MB-231 (MD-231) breast cancer cell line is frequently used to model breast cancer/bone interactions and has been useful to confirm the causative role of RANKL in breast cancer-induced osteolysis. After intracardiac injection of MDA-231 cells, significant increases in osteolytic skeletal lesions and tumor area (as measured either by histology or by *in vivo* imaging) in the bone is observed. Analysis of systemic and local levels of RANKL, OPG and TRAP/TRAP-5b in tumor-bearing animals demonstrated local changes in stromal (murine) RANKL protein

levels which correlated with increased TRAP5b expression and increased osteoclast numbers [95]. Importantly these changes were entirely local, as neither RANKL levels nor TRAP5b were elevated in the serum. These observations underscore the importance and uniqueness of local tumor-bone interactions and confirm previous histopathological analysis of the MDA-231 tumor in the bone which demonstrated RANKL positive osteoblasts in close juxtaposition with the TRAP-positive osteoclasts [67].

To test the effect of RANKL inhibition on pre-existing MDA-231 breast tumors in the bone, OPG-Fc was administered 7 days after intracardiac inoculation of tumor cells. This treatment effectively blocked tumor-induced osteolytic lesions and reduced intra-skeletal tumor burden (as measured by histology and bioluminescent imaging) [95]. Furthermore, RANKL inhibition had a significant impact on survival of animals bearing MDA-231 bone lesions demonstrating the significance and impact of skeletal tumor burden on survival.

Mice treated with OPG-Fc simultaneously with inoculation of the MDA-231 tumor prevented the development of lytic lesions, indicating that RANKL inhibition blocked bone destruction at early stages of tumor establishment [49,95,138]. RANKL inhibition also reduced the MDA-231 tumor burden (by as much as 78%; [95]) within the skeleton. The ability of RANKL inhibition to suppress skeletal tumor localization at early stages in bone metastases may be associated with alterations in the bone microenvironment such that chemotactic, adhesive and growth promoting signals are attenuated.

The reduced skeletal tumor progression after RANKL inhibition was correlated with increased tumor cell apoptosis in two independent studies [49,95] and decreased Ki67 staining as a measure of tumor cell proliferation [49]. Treatment of MDA-231 cells with OPG-Fc had no effect on proliferation *in vitro* [49] or the growth of a subcutaneous MDA-231 tumor [95] suggesting that the effect of RANKL inhibition to reduce tumor burden is likely to be indirect, via inhibition of bone resorption.

Taken together, these data in breast cancer models support a causative role for RANKL in both the establishment of new bone metastases and the progression of pre-existing bone metastases. In addition, osteoclasts probably play a causative role in other paraneoplastic syndromes resulting from breast cancer in the skeleton, in particular hypercalcemia and bone pain (as reviewed in Section III above).

B. Role of RANKL in Prostate Cancer Bone Metastases

As described above (Section III), clinical prostate cancer bony metastases are generally characterized as osteoblastic lesions. However, an osteoclast and osteolytic component of osteoblastic prostate tumors has been revealed by histologic evidence [57] and bone turnover marker data

[51]. Thus, clinical prostate cancer bone metastases probably represents a spectrum of bony lesions from osteolytic to mixed osteolytic/osteoblastic to osteoblastic. A number of xenograft prostate cancer bone metastases models have been developed (reviewed in Ref. [139]) which represent this entire spectrum of bony disease and RANKL inhibition has been tested in multiple animal models which altogether captures this entire spectrum.

The prostate cancer cell line PC3 promotes osteolysis in murine experimental metastases models [140]. Lee *et al.* [141] have demonstrated that the PC3 cells grown in a subcutaneous site can express human mRNAs for RANKL, IL-1 and TNF-α and hypothesized that the production of these factors correlated with the osteolytic phenotype of PC-3 tumors. The expression of IL-1 and TNF-α by PC3 cells within the bone was confirmed by IHC [141]. In another study, Armstrong *et al.* [97] showed that after intracardiac injection of PC3 cells, excessive mouse RANKL levels were detected within the bone stroma (by mRNA and IHC analysis) and an increased ratio of RANKL to OPG was observed at local and systemic levels. The increased RANKL levels within the bone correlated with the increase in osteoclasts associated with tumor and localized osteolysis. These data support a model in which tumor-associated factors converge on the mouse stroma to cause local increases in RANKL, in turn leading to the dramatic increases in osteoclasts.

The causative role for RANKL in the progression of PC3 tumors in the bone was demonstrated using either OPG-Fc [97] or RANK-Fc [142]. In the latter study, mice were treated either early (day 0) or late (4 weeks) with RANK-Fc after intratibial innoculation of PC3 cells. In either setting, RANKL inhibition prevented cortical bone destruction. In the study by Armstrong *et al.* [97], mice with established PC3 lesions were treated with OPG-Fc beginning at day 7 which prevented osteolytic lesions, eliminated tumor-induced osteoclasts and significantly decreased tumor burden as measured by histology. These results have been extended by Miller *et al.* [143]. In these experiments, intracardiac injection of PC3 cells was used to establish skeletal tumors and subsequent treatment with OPG-Fc resulted in a reduction of osteolytic lesions and skeletal tumor burden (as measured by histology and bioluminescent imaging). PC3 tumor cells in bones showed a significantly higher degree of apoptosis after treatment with OPG-Fc. In addition, RANKL inhibition extended the median survival of PC3-tumor bearing mice by 23%. Importantly, OPG-Fc treatment of PC3-tumor bearing animals sensitized the tumor cells to the therapeutic effect of the chemotherapy docetaxel [143]. The effects of RANKL inhibition were likely mediated by blockade of bone resorption as OPG-Fc had no effect on a subcutaneously grown PC3 tumor.

To evaluate the role of RANKL and osteoclasts on the development and progression of a prostate tumor in the bone which gives rise to a mixed osteolytic/osteoblastic lesion, experiments using the C4-2B cell line [144] have been performed. Zhang *et al.* [109] evaluated the effect of OPG-Fc (given at time of tumor inoculation) on the growth of C4-2B cells injected intratibially into SCID mice. RANKL inhibition reduced the tumor-induced osteoclastogenesis to levels similar to that observed in normal bone. In addition, PSA-positive prostate tumor infiltration was reduced as a result of OPG-Fc treatment. RANKL inhibition with OPG-Fc did not affect the growth of a C4-2B subcutaneous tumor suggesting that the effect observed on skeletal tumors was indirect, via inhibition of bone resorption. These data demonstrated that RANKL inhibition blocks the development of C4-2B-derived tumors, which includes both osteolytic and osteoblastic components and suggests that the development of osteoblastic lesions is dependent on osteoclastic activity.

In a study using C4-2 cells, Corey *et al.* [145] overexpressed OPG after direct transfection into these prostate tumor cells in order to determine the effect of OPG expression on tumor growth *in vitro* and *in vivo*. While C4-2 cells overexpressing OPG have similar growth rates to control C4-2 cells *in vitro* and at subcutaneous sites, tumor volume in the bone was significantly reduced. Overexpression of OPG in the prostate cancer cells also resulted in a similar protection against bone lysis as observed with the pharmacologically-delivered OPG-Fc in PC3 or C4-2B-bearing animals [97,109]. The increased bone volume observed after C4-2/OPG cell inoculation was correlated with a decrease in both osteoclast and osteoblast surface area. Interestingly, in 2007, an antibody which specifically blocks the human RANKL was used in a study [115] to demonstrate that the murine (stromal) RANKL is the mediator of the osteolytic lesions in the C4-2 tumor model.

RANKL inhibition has been studied in four separate prostate cancer mouse models which reportedly give rise to 'osteoblastic' bone lesions: LuCaP 23.1 [146], LnCaP [147], LuCAP 35 [148], and LAPC-9 [142]. Inhibition of RANKL using recombinant Fc-OPG in the LuCaP 23.1 model increased bone mineral density at the site of tumor and led to decreased tumor cell growth as measured by histological tumor area within the bone, tumor cell Ki67 staining/proliferative index and serum PSA levels [146]. These results were observed when RANKL inhibition was initiated either at the time of tumor inoculation ('prevention' protocol) or after 4 weeks of tumor establishment ('treatment' protocol). In the LnCaP model studied by Yonou *et al.* [149] prostate tumor cells are injected into human adult bone in NOD/SCID mice, which results in osteoblastic bone metastases. Using this model, RANKL inhibition with recombinant OPG was initiated simultaneously with tumor inoculation and treated for 2 weeks ('early short-term' protocol), then treatment was stopped and tumor and bone were analyzed at 4 weeks. The 'early short-term' protocol with OPG reduced the LnCaP tumor volume in the bone and serum PSA levels, suggesting that RANKL inhibition will suppress the establishment of an osteoblastic prostate tumor. Also, to investigate whether RANKL inhibition would have an effect on the progression of an established tumor, OPG treatment was initiated after 2 weeks of tumor growth and continued until the end of the experiment (at 4 weeks; 'late short-term' protocol). In this latter scenario, RANKL inhibition also led to a smaller skeletal prostate tumor. OPG treatment had no effect on the growth of a subcutaneous LnCaP tumor.

Whang *et al.* [142] demonstrated that RANKL inhibition with RANK-Fc reduced the progression of established osteoblastic LAPC-9 tumors, but did not block the establishment of new tumors (tested by the simultaneous treatment with intratibial injection of tumor cell bolus). The LuCaP 35 prostate xenograft also gives rise to osteoblastic tumors when injected into human bone in SCID mice [148]. As determined by a reduction in serum PSA and histological tumor burden in the bone, treatment of animals with established LuCAP 35 tumors with RANK-Fc reduced tumor burden in the skeleton. Importantly, x-ray and DXA analysis indicated that the increased osteosclerotic response induced by the tumor was also reduced after RANKL inhibition. The reduction in the tumor-induced osteoblastic responses was correlated with a significant decrease in osteoclast numbers and bone volume as well as reduced systemic bone formation markers such as serum osteocalcin, bone-specific alkaline phosphatase and the bone resorption marker N-telopeptide.

In each of these studies, RANKL inhibition was capable of reducing the progression of the prostate tumor in the bone. These observations suggest that osteoclasts and bone resorption promotes the growth of a prostate tumor, even if the resulting bone phenotype is osteoblastic [142,146,148,149]. The mechanism by which RANKL inhibition reduces the progression of prostate tumor in the bone may be similar to that observed with the more lytic breast cancer models described above. That is, a reduction in osteoclast activity and the locally available growth factors and calcium in the bone may result in a slower tumor growth rate. Characterization of the osteoblastic prostate tumor models has provided evidence for increased osteoclast numbers and activity in addition to increased osteoblastic activity. Osteoblasts can also provide growth factors which increase skeletal prostate tumor growth and survival [139] and it is possible that RANKL inhibition will also reduce excessive osteoblast activity by reducing tumor-induced bone remodeling. The study by Zhang *et al.* [148] with the LuCaP 35 cells demonstrated that RANKL inhibition resulted in a normalization of both bone resorption and bone formation markers.

Taken together, the analysis of RANKL inhibition in prostate cancer bone metastases models representing diverse bone lesions (including osteoblastic metastases) provides further support for the notion that inhibition of RANKL and subsequent reduction in osteoclastogenesis may be useful for the treatment of prostate bone metastases. They further suggest that osteoclastic activity may be a requisite element of both osteolytic and osteoblastic lesions.

C. Role of RANKL in Bone Metastases Associated with Other Solid Tumors

Rodent model data suggests that RANKL-dependent osteoclastogenesis operates in humoral hypercalcemia of malignancy (HHM) which is a significant complication of advanced squamous cell, breast, and renal carcinomas. HHM can result from systemic activation of osteoclasts by tumor-derived factors (principally via PTHrP) or local tumor-induced osteoclastogenesis and subsequent osteolysis. While PTHrP may act coordinately with other pro-resorptive factors (e.g., IL-1, TNFα, IL-6) to mediate HHM, *in vitro* data clearly show that PTHrP will disrupt RANKL and OPG regulation to favor greater RANKL and reduced OPG expression [77–79]. Hypercalcemia can result in animals bearing lung or colon cancer cells which express high levels of PTHrP. In the C26 colon carcinoma model, OPG given either at the onset of hypercalcemia or after it had established was capable of reducing tumor-induced bone resorption and normalizing blood ionized calcium [150]. The reversal of established hypercalcemia was extremely rapid and occurred within 24 hours of treatment [151] highlighting the ability of RANKL inhibition to suppress mature osteoclast activity and cause osteoclast apoptosis very rapidly. Treatment of animals bearing a subcutaneous lung squamous cell carcinoma (RWGT2) tumor with RANK-Fc prevented the PTHrP-mediated hypercalcemia and reduced the osteoclastic bone resorption [152]. In an FA-6 model of hypercalcemia, a single injection of OPG was capable of reducing the tumor-induced hypercalcemia [153].

Analysis of OPG-Fc treatment in animals bearing a human lung squamous carcinoma (HARA) which expresses high levels of PTHrP failed to showed a significant decrease in tumor-induced osteoclast numbers or tumor volume [154]. The lack of effects on tumor-induced osteoclastogenesis in this latter study was probably not a true biological phenomenon, as the dose and schedule of OPG-Fc used was suboptimal. In 2007, Miller and colleagues showed that RANKL inhibition effectively decreases both the tumor-induced osteolytic lesions and skeletal tumor burdens in two intracardiac models of lung cancer bone metastases [155]. These data suggest that RANKL will be a common factor induced by solid tumors of diverse origin upon metastasis to the bone. The ability of OPG-Fc or RANK-Fc to control hypercalcemia in parallel with reduced osteolysis in models of HHM suggests that RANKL is a common downstream mediator of this syndrome.

D. Role of RANKL in Multiple Myeloma

The osteolytic bony lesions in MM are a consequence not only of excessive osteoclast activity, but also reduced osteoblastic activity [50]. Mouse models of MM can recapitulate the tumor-induced osteolytic lesions and loss of cancellous bone which is mediated by increased osteoclast formation [156] and have been used to demonstrate a role of

RANKL in MM bone destruction. In the 5T2MM murine MM model, Croucher and colleagues treated animals with Fc-OPG at a point in which tumor was already established and progressing in the bone. This treatment prevented the MM-induced bone loss, lytic lesions and tumor-induced osteoclast formation [157]. In addition, RANKL inhibition was also associated with a 25% reduction in paraprotein, suggesting that osteoclast inhibition resulted in a reduced tumor progression. Further support for the ability of RANKL inhibition to have a therapeutic effect is the observation by Vanderkerken *et al.* [158] that administration of Fc-OPG at time of 5T33MM inoculation resulted in a reduction of both serum paraprotein and MM cells in the bone marrow as well as a significantly improved survival of MM-bearing animals.

The effects of RANKL inhibition on primary human MM tumor growth and osteolytic lesions in human bone implanted in SCID mice have been analyzed in two separate studies. Treatment of Hu/SCID mice bearing primary patient MM tumors with RANK-Fc resulted in a reduction of osteolysis and a decline in tumor burden, as measured by serum paraprotein levels and histology [121,159].

The lack of a therapeutic effect of either RANK-Fc or bisphosphonates on plasma cell leukemias, which no longer require the bone microenvironment to grow, supports the vicious cycle hypothesis [159]. These data suggest that inhibiting RANKL will prevent MM-induced bone lesions and can also result in an indirect anti-myeloma effect. Presumably the tumor is supported by osteoclasts via the 'vicious cycle' of bone destruction that promotes expansion or survival of myeloma that is restricted to the bone marrow. Interestingly, observations have demonstrated that osteoclasts may directly support myeloma cell growth independently of bone resorption [160,161].

E. Role of RANKL and Osteoclasts in Primary Bone Tumors

1. Giant Cell Tumor of Bone

Giant cell tumor of bone (GCTB) is a locally aggressive osteolytic neoplasm characterized histologically by the presence of neoplastic mesenchymal stromal cells surrounded by mononuclear osteoclast precursors and osteoclast-like giant cells that promote bone destruction. There is evidence to suggest that the neoplastic stromal cells are of osteoblastic lineage [162]. Although rarely malignant, severe GCTB is associated with extensive bony lesions, extreme bone pain, and an increased risk of fracture [163]. Immunohistochemistry and mRNA analysis have confirmed the expression of RANKL and RANK in GCTB. The expression of RANKL appears to be confined to the stromal cells [117,162,164–166]. RANKL was highly expressed in GCTB whereas OPG was expressed at very low levels [167]. In a study by Roudier and colleagues using a highly specific antibody to RANKL showed that RANKL protein

is present in the stromal component of all primary GCTB tested ($n = 43$) and was expressed in a significantly higher percentage of recurrent GCTB than primary GCTB [167]. The higher RANKL expression in recurrent GCTB supports the hypothesis that a RANKL-expressing cellular component remained after conservative surgery and drives recurrent tumor growth.

The giant cells are thought to be recruited from normal monocytic precursors by the tumor/stromal cell expression of RANKL within the bone microenvironment [168]. Multinucleated osteoclasts that form giant cells also showed strong RANK expression [169], lending support to the theory that these cells were recruited by RANKL-expressing tumor/stromal cells. The notion that RANKL functions in GCTB-induced osteoclastogenesis and bone resorption has been confirmed by the ability of OPG-Fc to block these processes *in vitro* [164]. RANKL may then play a causative role in this pathologic process and compounds that inhibit RANKL may have potential as therapeutic modalities in primary treatment and recurrent disease.

2. Osteosarcoma

Osteosarcoma is the most common primary malignancy of the skeleton [170]. This is a malignant mesenchymal tumor which causes destructive heterogeneous skeletal lesions with both osteoblastic and osteolytic elements. Treatment typically includes chemotherapy followed by surgical resection of the tumor and post-operative chemotherapy [171]. Similar to breast and prostate cancer bone metastasis, an interaction of the tumor and bone microenvironment may also occur in osteosarcoma. Direct experimental evidence for this hypothesis was provided by Lamoureux *et al.* [172] who showed a role for RANKL in the pathophysiology of osteosarcoma. These authors used gene transfer technology to express the truncated form of OPG in two osteosarcoma cell lines and demonstrated that these engineered lines result in a reduction in the osteolytic lesions, and, importantly, a reduction in tumor incidence and tumor progression.

VI. DO TUMOR-ASSOCIATED FACTORS CIRCUMVENT OR COOPERATE WITH RANKL IN THE PATHOGENESIS OF CANCER-INDUCED OSTEOLYSIS?

In addition to RANKL, several other extracellular factors and hormones have been shown to increase osteoclastogenesis and elevated levels of these factors have been shown, in some circumstances, to be associated with lytic disease in cancer patients [50]. These factors may enhance the lytic bone disease by a number of mechanisms including: (1) increasing stromal RANKL levels and/or decreasing OPG levels resulting in a net increase in the RANKL signal; (2) directly activating mature osteoclasts, or enhancing the survival of osteoclasts, therefore increasing their resorptive capacity; (3) direct effects on osteoclast differentiation; and (4) direct effects on precursor cells to increase the pool of osteoclast precursors.

Elevated levels of IL-1 and TNF-α have been associated with osteolysis in both clinical and preclinical (rodent model) settings. The production of these factors correlated with the osteolytic phenotype of PC-3 tumors [141]. It is well documented (see Section IV on the induction of RANKL) that both IL-1 and TNF will increase RANKL mRNA within osteoblasts and/or stromal cells. However, IL-1 and TNF have pleiotropic actions on osteoclast function and activation and could influence tumor-associated osteolysis beyond alterations in RANKL (or OPG) levels.

For instance, IL-1 has been shown to act directly on osteoclasts and promote multinucleation and enhances the bone resorptive capacity of osteoclasts [173] perhaps by increasing the survival of mature osteoclasts. IL-1 can also influence the differentiation of osteoclasts directly, although this can only occur in the presence of permissive levels of RANKL [174]. TNF-α is capable of directly activating mature osteoclasts that have been generated with RANKL and CSF-1 [175]. Others have demonstrated that TNF can act directly on osteoclast precursors to drive their differentiation [34,176]. TNF can also influence osteoclastogenesis by increasing circulating osteoclast precursors, which require RANKL for ultimate differentiation into resorbing osteoclasts [177].

Importantly, both IL-1 and TNF-α can synergize with exceptionally low (or 'permissive') levels of RANKL to increase osteoclastogenesis [174,178] thereby providing a potential amplification of the osteoclastogenic signal. TNF-α following pre-exposure of purified bone marrow macrophages to RANKL can accelerate this process [178]. Komine *et al.* [34] demonstrated a marked synergy of RANKL and TNF-α in the formation of multinucleated osteoclast like cells. TNF-α can induce RANK expression on osteoclast precursors [33,34] which would provide another mechanism for the amplification of osteoclast differentiation. Later studies indicate that IL-1 is the intermediate between TNFα and RANKL upregulation on stromal cells [174].

There is conflicting data whether MIP1a will increase stromal RANKL levels [86,87]. In one study, MIP1a-induced osteoclastogenesis was not inhibited by RANK-Fc [87] and could synergize with RANKL to cause further osteoclast formation. Multiple groups have demonstrated that TGF-β stimulated osteoclastogenesis was dependent on the presence of M-CSF and RANKL [179–181], while others have argued that TGFβ (with either M-CSF or TNF) will induce osteoclasts independently of RANKL [182,183]. Bendre *et al.* [89] have shown that IL-8 can not only increase RANKL by stromal cells, but can also bind to CXCR1 on osteoclast precursors and promote osteoclast differentiation independently of RANKL. There is also evidence using human peripheral blood mononuclear

cells *in vitro* that OPG-Fc would not block IL-6 and IL-11-induced osteoclastogenesis [184] suggesting that this is a RANKL independent pathway. Lu *et al.* [185] have shown that MCP-1 and IL-8 are produced in the conditioned medium of some prostate cancer cells and that these factors will increase osteoclast formation from human bone marrow mononuclear cells even if a 'neutralizing' antibody to RANKL is included. Whether MCP-1 can truly circumvent RANKL to generate active osteoclasts is confounded by the observations by others [186] that MCP-1 can generate TRAP+ multinuclear cells in the absence of RANKL. However, these 'osteoclast-like' cells are unable to resorb bone unless RANKL is present.

Based on these *in vitro* observations, it seems clear that other tumor associated factors besides RANKL can influence osteolysis via different mechanisms. Pro-osteolytic factors can increase the pool of osteoclast precursors (e.g., TNF-α), increase stromal RANKL levels (e.g., IL-1, IL-6, IL-8, IL-11, MIP1α, PTHrP, TNF-α; reviewed in Section IV), enhance the activity of mature, differentiated osteoclasts (e.g., IL-1, TNF-α) or effect the osteoclast lineage directly, thereby enhancing osteoclast differentiation (TNF-α, IL-6, IL-8, IL-11, MCP-1, MIP1α and TGF-β).

In determining whether any of these tumor-associated factors would mediate osteoclastogenesis independently of RANKL, a number of considerations should be considered and experimentally examined. Firstly, upon examination of knockout animals for these genes there are no reports of an overt bone phenotype indicative of an essential role for IL-1, IL-6, IL-8, IL-11 or TNF-α in osteoclastogenesis. This contrasts significantly to the severe osteopetrosis observed with the RANKL knockout. In fact, studies have shown that RANK, RANKL and M-CSF are the only extracellular factors shown to be essential for osteoclastogenesis *in vivo* [187].

Secondly, there are frequent observations of cooperation between many of these factors and RANKL to promote osteoclastogenesis. Therefore, to exclude any RANKL contribution in any cell culture experiment one would have to ensure that a pharmacologically effective dose of the RANKL inhibitor (e.g., RANK-Fc or OPG-Fc) is maintained throughout the culture conditions. In addition, it is well documented that pre-exposure of osteoclast precursors to RANKL will 'prime' these cells for differentiation by other factors [178], which makes it difficult to definitively eliminate a role for RANKL in osteoclast differentiation *in vitro*.

Finally, there is no evidence using rodent models for the ability of these factors to induce osteoclastogenesis independently of RANKL *in vivo*. In the absence of a RANK/RANKL signal, TNF-α, IL-1, MIP-1α, and PTHrP will not increase serum calcium levels or cause osteoclast formation *in vivo* [30,152]. These genetic approaches suggest that these select tumor associated factors are not individually of circumventing RANKL *in vivo*. In addition, as was reviewed in Section V, multiple proof of concept studies have shown that when tumor-bearing animals are treated with a pharmacologic inhibitor of RANKL at effective doses, there is no evidence of pathways that can circumvent RANKL to form osteoclasts *in vivo*. These data, along with the observation that most cytokines and growth factors associated with tumor cell osteolysis will stimulate stromal cells and osteoblasts to express and secrete RANKL have suggested that RANKL is the key catalyst for osteolytic events in malignant bone conditions.

While other cytokines and factors may influence osteoclastogenesis indirectly (through RANKL) or directly (as described above) in some select circumstances, one clear advantage of a RANKL inhibitor for the treatment and prevention of bone metastases is that this pathway appears to be not only fundamental to osteoclastogenesis, but also generally activated in cancer bone disease irrespective of the origin of the primary tumor.

VII. RANK EXPRESSION ON TUMOR CELLS

Another role for RANK and RANKL in promoting metastasis to bone has been proposed, based on the observation that some tumor cells can express RANK. Wittrant *et al.* [188] detected RANK mRNA on murine POS-1 osteosarcoma cells and demonstrated that RANKL treatment would lead to activation of ERK biochemical signaling and increased BMP-2 induction at the mRNA and protein levels. The authors extended these observations to show that RANK mRNA and protein (using IHC) are expressed on human osteosarcoma cells (Saos-2, MG-63, MNNG/HOS) [189]. Furthermore, RANK protein was also detected in more than 50% of osteosarcoma patient biopsies which represented osteosarcoma isolated from disparate skeletal sites and included both responders and non-responders to chemotherapy.

Holstead-Jones *et al.* showed that certain epithelial (breast and prostate) and melanoma cell lines could express RANK on the surface [190]. Moreover, these authors found that treatment of RANK-expressing breast cancer and melanoma cells with RANKL promote cell migration and this migration was blocked by addition of OPG. RANKL did not apparently alter tumor cell proliferation; however, the positive effects on migration were correlated with RANKL-dependent changes in the cytoskeleton and led the authors to hypothesize that RANKL may act as the 'seed-and-soil' factor that draws certain cancer cells to metastasize to bone. To determine whether the RANKL-induced migration of RANK-expressing cells had a role in bone metastasis *in vivo*, the authors used a clone of B16 melanoma cells that expressed RANK, but did not evoke osteoclast activation. OPG treatment of B16-bearing animals reduced the bone metastasis, but did not have an effect on metastasis to other tissues (e.g., ovaries, adrenal gland, brain), suggesting that RANKL may function as a 'soil' factor which attracts some tumor cells into the bone.

RANK expression has also been observed on prostate cancer cell lines *in vitro* including DU145 [191], PC3 [97,191] and LnCaP [113]. The expression of RANK on these cells has been shown to be biologically active as RANKL treatment of the DU145 cells led to increased biochemical signaling and promoted migration of these cells on plastic [191]. Treatment of PC3 cells with RANKL activated multiple signal transduction pathways [97,191] and increased migration [191] and invasion through a collagen matrix [97]. In the latter study the specificity of the anti-human RANK antibodies was supported by the elimination of antibody reactivity upon suppression of RANK expression with a short-hairpin RNA knockdown construct. Chen *et al.* [113] also demonstrated that RANKL will increase PC3 cell proliferation, although this did not manifest significantly until day 3 in culture. In contrast, in the Chen and Armstrong studies it was also shown that RANKL does not detectably influence prostate tumor cell proliferation or survival of either PC3 or DU145 cells under a variety of conditions. In the case of breast cancer cell lines, RANK expression has been shown on several lines by mRNA analysis [79] and by flow cytometry which demonstrated that some clones of MDA-231 and ZR75-1 expressed RANK, while MCF-7 and T47D cells did not detectably express RANK [192].

The biological relevance of RANK expression on prostate tumor cells has been demonstrated in a publication by Luo *et al.* [120]. Analysis of prostate tumors in the TRAMP transgenic mouse model demonstrated RANK expression on the tumor cells and increases in RANKL expression within the tumor coincidental with increased inflammatory infiltrate. The authors suggest that activated T cells could be a source of RANKL in the tumor. Importantly, RANKL treatment of TRAMP prostate tumors *in vitro* led to the inhibition of maspin, a protein which can suppress prostate cancer metastasis.

To date, there is very little published data describing RANK expression on patient tumor samples representing primary or metastatic disease. The data by Mori *et al.*, which describe RANK expression in greater than 50% of osteosarcoma samples, have already been described above [191]. Bhatia *et al.* [193] described the expression of RANK on 58/58 infiltrating ductal carcinoma and 43/43 breast cancer bony metastases using IHC. In this study there was no documentation of the controls necessary to prove the specificity of the antibody used and it is therefore necessary to confirm their findings of RANK expression on 100% of breast tumors analyzed. Chen *et al.* [113] used a R&D Systems mAb against RANK and revealed that 38% of primary human prostate cancers were RANK positive. To control for antibody specificity, these authors stained tissue with the secondary antibody alone. Until analysis of RANK protein expression on human cancer patient samples is performed using well-validated and specific antibodies, it would seem premature to estimate the significance and relevance of these observations.

Nonetheless, the observations of RANK expression on tumor cells *in vitro* and the implications of the rodent study by Holstead-Jones [190], which showed that RANKL inhibitors could block the metastasis of a RANK-expressing melanoma to the bone, are intriguing and deserve further study. These latter data suggest that inhibition of RANKL will reduce the metastatic behavior of RANK-expressing tumors by directly blocking RANKL effects on the tumor. The extent to which a direct effect of a RANKL inhibitor contributes to the therapeutic efficacy already well documented in rodent pharmacology models (see Section V) or would be a factor in the clinic remains unclear.

VIII. DEVELOPMENT OF TARGETED THERAPIES AGAINST RANKL AND CLINICAL APPLICATIONS IN ONCOLOGY

As described in the previous sections, dysregulation of RANKL and/or OPG was evident in both animal models of MM and bone metastasis and also in the corresponding clinical settings. In the preclinical animal models, the cancer-induced osteoclast hyperactivity was effectively countered by treatment with the RANKL inhibitors RANK-Fc and OPG-Fc. These, and other studies, have provided the proof of concept studies that RANKL is critical for the excessive bone resorption that occurs in cancer-induced bone diseases and provided the rationale for a clinical development program. The development of anti-RANKL therapies in multiple clinical indications has been reviewed [194], so this section will focus on development of therapies for oncology indications. Development of a biological targeted therapy against RANKL first began using recombinant forms of OPG followed by a fully-human monoclonal antibody against RANKL (denosumab).

A small phase I trial evaluated patients with MM (*n* = 28) or breast carcinoma (*n* = 26) who exhibited radiographically confirmed lytic bone lesion after treatment with a genetically engineered human osteoprotegerin-Fc construct (OPG-Fc). The study found that a single s.c. dose of OPG-Fc was able to reduce bone resorption (as assessed by bone turnover markers) similar to that observed after a single dose of intravenous pamidronate treatment (90 mg) [195]. OPG-Fc caused a rapid, sustained dose-dependent decrease in urinary NTX level in this patient population. The reductions in bone turnover after OPG-Fc treatments were approximately 47 and 67% for myeloma and breast cancer patients, respectively (at the 3.0 mg/kg dose). OPG-Fc was well tolerated with no adverse events of concern in this trial.

This study demonstrated that RANKL inhibition therapy was an effective and reversible treatment in cancer patients. However, utility of OPG-Fc in humans may not be feasible in a more chronic setting given the potential risk of developing

neutralizing antibodies against endogenous OPG and the relatively short half-life of OPG-Fc in cancer patients [195]. Although not observed in rodent cancer models, another potential limitation of OPG-Fc is the documented binding of OPG to TNF-related apoptosis-inducing ligand (TRAIL) [196], a survival factor for tumor cells, which may potentially interfere with tumor surveillance mechanisms.

To avoid these limitations, a fully human monoclonal antibody (denosumab) that can bind to and neutralize the activity of human RANKL was developed [197]. Denosumab binding to RANKL prevents the ligand's ability to bind and activate its cognate receptor, RANK. Denosumab inhibits osteoclast function and bone resorption via this mechanism. The osteoclast inhibitory activity of denosumab parallels the properties of native OPG and its engineered variants; however, denosumab is specific for RANKL at high affinity (Kd 3×10^{-12} M) and does not cross-react with other TNF ligand superfamily members (e.g., TNFα, TNFβ, CD40L, or TRAIL) [198]. Because denosumab does not bind murine or rodent RANKL, its activity cannot be studied in rodent models of bone cancer, which necessitated the testing of its anti-resorptive activity in cynomolgus monkeys [199].

Early clinical studies have supported potential application of denosumab in cancer indications including a randomized, active-controlled study to determine the safety and efficacy of denosumab in patients with breast cancer (*n* = 29) or multiple myeloma (*n* = 25) with radiographically evident bone lesions [195]. Changes in uNTX/creatinine from baseline were assessed over 84 days to determine the bone antiresorptive activity of denosumab in humans and to establish the dosage regimen for future studies. Following administration of a single s.c. dose of denosumab, bone turnover decreased within 24 hours in both MM and breast cancer patients. Reductions in uNTX/creatinine were greater than 50% in patients with MM and greater than 75% in patients with breast cancer. Denosumab was generally well tolerated. No related serious adverse events occurred and no patient had detectable anti-denosumab antibodies. The decrease in bone turnover markers was similar in magnitude, but more sustained that the active control (single dose of pamidronate 90 mg i.v.).

The efficacy and safety of denosumab in patients (*n* = 255) with breast cancer-related bone metastases not previously treated with intravenous bisphosphonates (IV BPs) was evaluated. Denosumab was administered s.c. every 4 weeks (30, 120, or 180 mg) or every 12 weeks (60 or 180 mg). The active control was IV BPs (Q4W IV zoledronic acid, pamidronate, or ibandronate), with the majority of this cohort (91%) receiving zoledronic acid. Median percentage reduction in uNTx was 71% for the pooled denosumab treatments, and was similar to the IV BP cohort (79%). A greater proportion of patients achieved a >65% reduction in uNTx in the denosumab pooled arms (74%) than in the IV BP group (63%). The median time to achieve a

>65% reduction in uNTx was shorter for the denosumab pooled arms (13 days) versus 29 days for the IV BP group. Nine percent of denosumab-treated patients experienced one or more on-study SREs, compared to 16% of patients receiving IV BPs. Denosumab appeared to be well tolerated and there were no denosumab-related serious adverse events. This study concluded that subcutaneously administered denosumab may be similar to IV BPs in suppressing bone turnover and reducing SRE risk. These data support further investigation of targeted inhibition of RANKL by denosumab as a potential treatment for bone destruction associated with metastatic cancer.

IX. SUMMARY

This chapter has summarized preclinical data that demonstrated that RANK ligand (RANKL) is essential for osteoclast formation, function, and survival. Furthermore, there is substantial evidence that tumor cell-mediated osteolysis occurs predominantly via induction of RANKL within the bone stroma. The observations that inhibition of RANKL in animal models of bone metastasis blocks tumor-induced osteolysis and prevents the establishment and progression of bony tumors provides the basic rationale for the development of a RANKL inhibitor and application in clinical trials for the treatment and prevention of SREs. Denosumab, a fully human monoclonal antibody with high affinity and specificity for RANKL inhibits osteoclast function and bone resorption by binding and neutralizing RANKL. Currently, large clinical studies are ongoing to provide a more precise estimate of the effect of denosumab treatment on the risk of SREs in cancer patients.

References

1. T. Suda, N. Takahashi & T.J. Martin, Endocr Rev 13 (1992) 66.
2. N. Udagawa, N. Takahashi & T. Akatsu, et al., Proc Natl Acad Sci USA 87 (1990) 7260.
3. H. Yoshida, S. Hayashi & T. Kunisada, et al., Nature 345 (1990) 442.
4. G.Q. Yao, B.H. Sun & E.C. Weir, et al., Calcif Tissue Int 70 (2002) 339.
5. S.L. Teitelbaum & F.P. Ross, Nat Rev Genet 4 (2003) 638.
6. E. Tsuda, M. Goto & S. Mochizuki, et al., Biochem Biophys Res Commun 234 (1997) 137.
7. W.S. Simonet, D.L. Lacey & C.R. Dunstan, et al., Cell 89 (1997) 309.
8. H. Yasuda, N. Shima & N. Nakagawa, et al., Proc Natl Acad Sci USA 95 (1998) 3597.
9. N. Bucay, I. Sarosi & C.R. Dunstan, et al., Genes Dev 12 (1998) 1260.
10. D.L. Lacey, E. Timms & H.L. Tan, et al., Cell 93 (1998) 165.
11. H. Yasuda, N. Shima & N. Nakagawa, et al., Endocrinology 139 (1998) 1329.
12. D.M. Anderson, E. Maraskovsky & W.L. Billingsley, et al., Nature 390 (1997) 175.
13. J.E. Fata, Y.Y. Kong & J. Li, et al., Cell 103 (2000) 41.
14. V. Kartsogiannis, H. Zhou & N.J. Horwood, et al., Bone 25 (1999) 525.
15. P. Collin-Osdoby, L. Rothe & F. Anderson, et al., J Biochem 276 (2001) 20659.
16. G. Eghbali-Fatourechi, S. Khosla & A. Sanyal, et al., J Clin Invest 111 (2003) 1221.
17. L.C. Hofbauer, C. Shui & B.L. Riggs, et al., Biochem Biophys Res Commun 280 (2001) 334.
18. B.R. Wong, R. Josien & S.Y. Lee, et al., J Exp Med 186 (1997) 2075.
19. Y.Y. Kong, H. Yoshida & I. Sarosi, et al., Nature 397 (1999) 315.
20. W.J. Boyle, W.S. Simonet & D.L. Lacey, Nature 423 (2003) 337.
21. N. Takahashi, T. Akatsu & N. Udagawa, et al., Endocrinology 123 (1988) 2600.
22. M. Stolina, S. Adamu & M. Ominsky, et al., J Bone Miner Res 20 (2005) 1756.
23. T. Ikeda, M. Kasai & M. Utsuyama, et al., Endocrinology 142 (2001) 1419.
24. J. Suzuki, T. Ikeda & H. Kuroyama, et al., Biochem Biophys Res Commun 314 (2004) 1021.
25. L. Lum, B.R. Wong & R. Josien, et al., J Biol Chem 274 (1999) 13613.
26. C.C. Lynch, A. Hikosaka & H.B. Acuff, et al., Cancer Cell 7 (2005) 485.
27. T. Nakashima, Y. Kobayashi & S. Yamasaki, et al., Biochem Biophys Res Commun 275 (2000) 768.
28. A. Mizuno, T. Kanno & M. Hoshi, et al., J Bone Miner Metab 20 (2002) 337.
29. W.C. Dougall, M. Glaccum & K. Charrier, et al., Genes Dev 13 (1999) 2412.
30. J. Li, I. Sarosi & X.Q. Yan, et al., Proc Natl Acad Sci USA 97 (2000) 1566.
31. K. Matsuzaki, N. Udagawa & N. Takahashi, et al., Biochem Biophys Res Commun 246 (1998) 199.
32. H. Kitaura, M.S. Sands & K. Aya, et al., J Immunol 173 (2004) 4838.
33. H. Kitaura, P. Zhou & H.J. Kim, et al., J Clin Invest 115 (2005) 3418.
34. M. Komine, A. Kukita & T. Kukita, et al., Bone 28 (2001) 474.
35. M. Asagiri & H. Takayanagi, Bone 40 (2007) 251.
36. T. Wada, T. Nakashima & N. Hiroshi, et al., Trends Mol Med 12 (2006) 17.
37. S. Wei, M.W. Wang & S.L. Teitelbaum, et al., J Biol Chem 277 (2002) 6622.
38. H. Hsu, D.L. Lacey & C.R. Dunstan, et al., Proc Natl Acad Sci USA 96 (1999) 3540.
39. T.L. Burgess, Y. Qian & S. Kaufman, et al., J Cell Biol 145 (1999) 527.
40. D.L. Lacey, H.L. Tan & J. Lu, et al., Am J Pathol 157 (2000) 435.
41. T. Akatsu, T. Murakami & M. Nishikawa, et al., Biochem Biophys Res Commun 250 (1998) 229.
42. S. Paget, Lancet 1 (1889) 571.
43. J.J. Yin, C.B. Pollock & K. Kelly, Cell Res 15 (2005) 57.

44. T. Yoneda & T. Hiraga, Biochem Biophys Res Commun 328 (2005) 679.
45. Y. Kang, P.M. Siegel & W. Shu, et al., Cancer Cell 3 (2003) 537.
46. L.M. Kalikin, A. Schneider & M.A. Thakur, et al., Cancer Biol Ther 2 (2003) 656.
47. A. Schneider, L.M. Kalikin & A.C. Mattos, et al., Endocrinology 146 (2005) 1727.
48. M.R. Smith, F.J. McGovern & A.L. Zietman, et al., N Engl J Med 345 (2001) 948.
49. Y. Zheng, H. Zhou & J.R. Modzelewski, et al., Cancer Res 67 (2007) 9542.
50. G.D. Roodman, N Engl J Med 350 (2004) 1655.
51. L.M. Demers, L. Costa & A. Lipton, Cancer 88 (2000) 2919.
52. J.E. Brown, R.J. Cook & P. Major, et al., J Natl Cancer Inst 97 (2005) 59.
53. R.E. Coleman, P. Major & A. Lipton, et al., J Clin Oncol 23 (2005) 4925.
54. R.E. Coleman, Clin Cancer Res 12 (2006) 6243s.
55. V. Grill, P. Ho & J.J. Body, et al., J Clin Endocrinol Metab 73 (1991) 1309.
56. S.A. Charhon, M.C. Chapuy & E.E. Delvin, et al., Cancer 51 (1983) 918.
57. N.W. Clarke, J. McClure & N.J. George, Br J Urol 68 (1991) 74.
58. J.A. Kanis & E.V. McCloskey, Cancer 80 (1997) 1538.
59. G.H. Urwin, R.C. Percival & S. Harris, et al., Br J Urol 57 (1985) 721.
60. D.R. Clohisy & P.W. Mantyh, J Musculoskelet Neuronal Interact 4 (2004) 293.
61. S. Mercadante, Pain 69 (1997) 1.
62. D.R. Clohisy, M.L. Ramnaraine & S. Scully, et al., J Orthop Res 18 (2000) 967.
63. P. Honore, N.M. Luger & M.A. Sabino, et al., Nat Med 6 (2000) 521.
64. N.M. Luger, P. Honore & M.A. Sabino, et al., Cancer Res 61 (2001) 4038.
65. M.P. Roudier, S.D. Bain & W.C. Dougall, Clin Exp Metastasis 23 (2006) 167.
66. L. Costa, L.M. Demers & A. Gouveia-Oliveira, et al., J Clin Onco 20 (2002) 850.
67. T. Shimamura, N. Amizuka & M. Li, et al., Biomed Res 26 (2005) 159.
68. M.E. Doerr & J.I. Jones, J Biol Chem 271 (1996) 2443.
69. J.J. Yin, K. Selander & J.M. Chirgwin, et al., J Clin Invest 103 (1999) 197.
70. T.A. Guise, Cancer 88 (2000) 2892.
71. T.A. Guise, J.J. Yin & S.D. Taylor, et al., J Clin Invest 98 (1996) 1544.
72. S. Kitazawa & R. Kitazawa, J Pathol 198 (2002) 228.
73. J.L. Sanders, N. Chattopadhyay & O. Kifor, et al., Endocrinology 141 (2000) 4357.
74. J.L. Sanders, N. Chattopadhyay & O. Kifor, et al., Am J Physiol Endocrinol Metab 281 (2001) E1267.
75. J. Li, S. Morony & H. Tan, et al., J Bone Miner Res 16 (2001) S379.
76. M.S. Virk & J.R. Lieberman, Arthritis Res Ther 9 (Suppl 1) (2007) S5.
77. N.J. Horwood, J. Elliott & T.J. Martin, et al., Endocrinology 139 (1998) 4743.
78. S.K. Lee & J.A. Lorenzo, Endocrinology 140 (1999) 3552.
79. R.J. Thomas, T.A. Guise & J.J. Yin, et al., Endocrinology 140 (1999) 4451.
80. N. Giuliani, R. Bataille & C. Mancini, et al., Blood 98 (2001) 3527.
81. L.C. Hofbauer, D.L. Lacey & C.R. Dunstan, et al., Bone 25 (1999) 255.
82. O.N. Vidal, K. Sjogren & B.I. Eriksson, et al., Biochem Biophys Res Commun 248 (1998) 696.
83. P. Palmqvist, E. Persson & H.H. Conaway, et al., J Immunol 169 (2002) 3353.
84. C.A. O'Brien, I. Gubrij & S.C. Lin, et al., J Biol Chem 274 (1999) 19301.
85. S.J. Choi, J.C. Cruz & F. Craig, et al., Blood 96 (2000) 671.
86. M. Abe, K. Hiura & J. Wilde, et al., Blood 100 (2002) 2195.
87. J.H. Han, S.J. Choi & N. Kurihara, et al., Blood 97 (2001) 3349.
88. H. Brandstrom, K.B. Jonsson & C. Ohlsson, et al., Biochem Biophys Res Commun 247 (1998) 338.
89. M.S. Bendre, D.C. Montague & T. Peery, et al., Bone 33 (2003) 28.
90. A.T. Mancino, V.S. Klimberg & M. Yamamoto, et al., J Surg Res 100 (2001) 18.
91. T. Ohshiba, C. Miyaura & M. Inada, et al., Br J Cancer 88 (2003) 1318.
92. H.R. Park, S.K. Min & H.D. Cho, et al., J Korean Med Sci 18 (2003) 541.
93. T. Michigami, M. Ihara-Watanabe & M. Yamazaki, et al., Cancer Res 61 (2001) 1637.
94. T. Okada, S. Akikusa & H. Okuno, et al., Clin Exp Metastasis 20 (2003) 639.
95. Canon, J., Roudier, M., Bryant, R., *et al.,* 2007. In 17th Scientific Meeting of the International Bone and Mineral Society [Abstract 073].
96. M. Roudier, C. Morrissey & L.-Y. Huang, et al., Cancer Treat Rev 32 (Suppl 3) (2006) S13. (abstract 010).
97. A.P. Armstrong, R.E. Miller & J.C. Jones et al., Prostate 68 (2008) 92.
98. A.N. Farrugia, G.J. Atkins & L.B. To, et al., Cancer Res 63 (2003) 5438.
99. U. Heider, C. Langelotz & C. Jakob, et al., Clin Cancer Res 9 (2003) 1436.
100. F.P. Lai, M. Cole-Sinclair & W.J. Cheng, et al., Br J Haematol 126 (2004) 192.
101. E. Terpos, R. Szydlo & J.F. Apperley, et al., Blood 102 (2003) 1064.
102. D. Granchi, I. Amato & L. Battistelli, et al., Int J Cancer 111 (2004) 829.
103. M. Nagai, S. Kyakumoto & N. Sato, Biochem Biophys Res Commun 269 (2000) 532.
104. K. Nosaka, T. Miyamoto & T. Sakai, et al., Blood 99 (2002) 634.
105. V. Barcala, P. Ruybal & H. Garcia Rivello, et al., Eur J Haematol 70 (2003) 417.
106. H. Shibata, M. Abe & K. Hiura, et al., Clin Cancer Res 11 (2005) 6109.

107. C. Van Poznak, S.S. Cross & M. Saggese, et al., J Clin Pathol 59 (2006) 56.

108. S.S. Cross, R. Harrison & S. Balasubramanian, et al., J Clin Pathol 59 (2006) 716–720.

109. J. Zhang, J. Dai & Y. Qi, et al., J Clin Invest 107 (2001) 1235.

110. J. Zhang, Y. Lu & J. Dai, et al., Prostate 59 (2004) 360.

111. B. Desai, M.J. Rogers & M.A. Chellaiah, Mol Cancer 6 (2007) 18.

112. J.M. Brown, E. Corey & Z.D. Lee, et al., Urology 57 (2001) 611.

113. G. Chen, K. Sircar & A. Aprikian, et al., Cancer 107 (2006) 289–298.

114. F.C. Perez-Martinez, V. Alonso & J.L. Sarasa, et al., J Clin Pathol 60 (2006) 290–294.

115. C. Morrissey, P.J. Kostenuik & L.G. Brown, et al., BMC Cancer 148 (2007).

116. C.R. Good, R.J. O'Keefe & J.E. Puzas, et al., J Surg Oncol 79 (2002) 174.

117. L. Huang, Y.Y. Cheng & L.T. Chow, et al., J Clin Pathol 55 (2002) 877.

118. E. Grimaud, L. Soubigou & S. Couillaud, et al., Am J Pathol 163 (2003) 2021.

119. N. Giuliani, S. Colla & R. Sala, et al., Blood 100 (2002) 4615.

120. J.L. Luo, W. Tan & J.M. Ricono, et al., Nature 446 (2007) 690.

121. R.N. Pearse, E.M. Sordillo & S. Yaccoby, et al., Proc Natl Acad Sci USA 98 (2001) 11581.

122. T. Standal, C. Seidel & O. Hjertner, et al., Blood 100 (2002) 3002.

123. T. Murakami, M. Yamamoto & K. Ono, et al., Biochem Biophys Res Commun 252 (1998) 747.

124. J. Zhu, X. Jia & G. Xiao, et al., J Biol Chem 282 (2007) 26656.

125. S.S. Cross, Z. Yang, N.J., Brown, et al., 2005. Int J Cancer.

126. I. Holen, P.I. Croucher & F.C. Hamdy, et al., Cancer Research 62 (2002) 1619.

127. I. Pettersen, W. Bakkelund & B. Smedsrod, et al., Anticancer Res 25 (2005) 3809.

128. I. Holen, S.S. Cross & H.L. Neville-Webbe, et al., Breast Cancer Res Treat 92 (2005) 207.

129. G. Mountzios, M.A. Dimopoulos & A. Bamias, et al., Acta Oncol 46 (2007) 221.

130. D. Granchi, A. Garaventa & I. Amato, et al., Int J Cancer 119 (2006) 146–151.

131. C.L. Eaton, J.M. Wells & I. Holen, et al., Prostate 59 (2004) 304.

132. K. Jung, M. Lein & K. Von Hosslin, et al., Clin Chem 47 (2001) 2061.

133. H.L. Neville-Webbe, N.A. Cross & C.L. Eaton, et al., Breast Cancer Res Treat 86 (2004) 269.

134. R. Nyambo, N. Cross & J. Lippitt, et al., J Bone Miner Res 19 (2004) 1712.

135. H. Yasuda, N. Shima & N. Nakagawa, et al., Bone 25 (1999) 109.

136. A. Lipton, S.M. Ali & K. Leitzel, et al., Clinical Cancer Research 8 (2002) 2306.

137. C. Seidel, O. Hjertner & N. Abildgaard, et al., Blood 98 (2001) 2269.

138. S. Morony, C. Capparelli & I. Sarosi, et al., Cancer Res 61 (2001) 4432.

139. C.J. Logothetis & S.H. Lin, Nat Rev Cancer 5 (2005) 21.

140. E. Corey, J.E. Quinn & F. Bladou, et al., Prostate 52 (2002) 20.

141. Y. Lee, E. Schwarz & M. Davies, et al., J Orthop Res 21 (2003) 62.

142. P.G. Whang, E.M. Schwarz & S.C. Gamradt, et al., J Orthop Res 23 (2005) 1475.

143. R. Miller, M. Roudier & J. Jones, et al., Clin Exp Metastasis 25 (Suppl 1) (2007) 11–68.

144. J. Pfitzenmaier, J.E. Quinn & A.M. Odman, et al., J Bone Miner Res 18 (2003) 1882.

145. E. Corey, L.G. Brown & J.A. Kiefer, et al., Cancer Res 65 (2005) 1710.

146. J.A. Kiefer, R.L. Vessella & J.E. Quinn, et al., Clin Exp Metastasis 21 (2004) 381.

147. H. Yonou, N. Kanomata & M. Goya, et al., Cancer Res 63 (2003) 2096.

148. J. Zhang, J. Dai & Z. Yao, et al., Cancer Res 63 (2003) 7883.

149. H. Yonou, T. Yokose & T. Kamijo, et al., Cancer Res 61 (2001) 2177.

150. C. Capparelli, P.J. Kostenuik & S. Morony, et al., Cancer Res 60 (2000) 783.

151. S. Morony, K. Warmington & S. Adamu, et al., Endocrinology 146 (2005) 3235.

152. B.O. Oyajobi, D.M. Anderson & K. Traianedes, et al., Cancer Res 61 (2001) 2572.

153. T. Akatsu, T. Murakami & K. Ono, et al., Bone 23 (1998) 495.

154. S.H. Tannehill-Gregg, A.L. Levine & M.V. Nadella, et al., Clin Exp Metastasis 23 (2006) 19–31.

155. R. Miller, J. Jones & M. Tometsko, et al., J Bone Miner Res 22 (Suppl 1) (2007) S114. [Abstract S307].

156. P. Croucher, J Musculoskel Neuron Interact 4 (2004) 285.

157. P.I. Croucher, C.M. Shipman & J. Lippitt, et al., Blood 98 (2001) 3534.

158. K. Vanderkerken, E. De Leenheer & C. Shipman, et al., Cancer Res 63 (2003) 287.

159. S. Yaccoby, R.N. Pearse & C.L. Johnson, et al., Br J Haematol 116 (2002) 278.

160. M. Abe, K. Hiura & J. Wilde, et al., Blood 104 (2004) 2484.

161. S. Yaccoby, M.J. Wezeman & A. Henderson, et al., Cancer Res 64 (2004) 2016.

162. T. Morgan, G.J. Atkins & M.K. Trivett, et al., Am J Pathol 167 (2005) 117.

163. M. Szendroi, J Bone Joint Surg Br 86 (2004) 5.

164. G.J. Atkins, S. Bouralexis & D.R. Haynes, et al., Bone 28 (2001) 370.

165. G.J. Atkins, D.R. Haynes & S.E. Graves, et al., J Bone Miner Res 15 (2000) 640.

166. S. Roux, L. Amazit & G. Meduri, et al., Am J Clin Pathol 117 (2002) 210.

167. M.P. Roudier, K.L. Kellar-Graney, L.-Y., Huang, et al. (2007). In: Connective Tissue Oncology Society 13th Annual Meeting.

168. Y.S. Lau, A. Sabokbar & C.L. Gibbons, et al., Hum Pathol 36 (2005) 945.

169. G.J. Atkins, P. Kostakis & C. Vincent, et al., J Bone Miner Res 21 (2006) 1339.

170. M.J. Klein, S. Kenan & M.M. Lewis, Orthop Clin North Am 20 (1989) 327.

171. H. Tsuchiya, Y. Kanazawa & M.E. Abdel-Wanis, et al., J Clin Oncol 20 (2002) 3470.

172. F. Lamoureux, P. Richard & Y. Wittrant, et al., Cancer Res 67 (2007) 7308.

173. E. Jimi, I. Nakamura & L.T. Duong, et al., Exp Cell Res 247 (1999) 84.

174. S. Wei, H. Kitaura & P. Zhou, et al., J Clin Invest 115 (2005) 282.

175. K. Fuller, C. Murphy & B. Kirstein, et al., Endocrinology 143 (2002) 1108.

176. T. Yamashita, Z. Yao & F. Li, et al., J Biol Chem 282 (2007) 18245.

177. Z. Yao, P. Li & Q. Zhang, et al., J Biol Chem 281 (2006) 11846.

178. J. Lam, S. Takeshita & J.E. Barker, et al., J Clin Invest 106 (2000) 1481.

179. K. Fuller, J.M. Lean & K.E. Bayley, et al., J Cell Sci 113 (Pt 13) (2000) 2445.

180. T. Kaneda, T. Nojima & M. Nakagawa, et al., J Immunol 165 (2000) 4254.

181. R.J. Sells Galvin, C.L. Gatlin & J.W. Horn, et al., Biochem Biophys Res Commun 265 (1999) 233.

182. I. Itonaga, A. Sabokbar & S.G. Sun, et al., Bone 34 (2004) 57.

183. N. Kim, Y. Kadono & M. Takami, et al., J Exp Med 202 (2005) 589.

184. O. Kudo, A. Sabokbar & A. Pocock, et al., Bone 32 (2003) 1.

185. Y. Lu, Z. Cai & G. Xiao, et al., Cancer Res 67 (2007) 3646.

186. M.S. Kim, C.J. Day & C.I. Selinger, et al., J Biol Chem 281 (2006) 1274.

187. S.L. Teitelbaum, Am J Pathol 170 (2007) 427.

188. Y. Wittrant, F. Lamoureux & K. Mori, et al., Int J Oncol 28 (2006) 261.

189. K. Mori, B. Le Goff & M. Berreur, et al., J Pathol 211 (2007) 555.

190. D. Holstead Jones, T. Nakashima & O.H. Sanchez, et al., Nature 440 (2006) 692.

191. K. Mori, B. Le Goff & C. Charrier, et al., Bone 40 (2007) 981.

192. M. Tometsko, A. Armstrong & R. Miller, et al., J Bone Miner Res 19 (2004) S25.

193. P. Bhatia, M.M. Sanders & M.F. Hansen, Clin Cancer Res 11 (2005) 162.

194. E.M. Schwarz & C.T. Ritchlin, Arthritis Res Ther 9 (Suppl 1) (2007) S7.

195. J.J. Body, P. Greipp & R.E. Coleman, et al., Cancer 97 (2003) 887.

196. J.G. Emery, P. McDonnell & M.B. Burke, et al., J Biol Chem 273 (1998) 14363.

197. P.J. Bekker, D.L. Holloway & A.S. Rasmussen, et al., J Bone Miner Res 19 (2004) 1059.

198. R. Elliott, P. Kostenuik, C. Chen, et al. (2006). Eur J Cancer Suppl 4, 62 (abstract).

199. J. Atkinson, P. Kostenuik & S. Smith, et al., J Bone Miner Res 18 (2003) S385.

CHAPTER **33**

Chondrosarcoma of Bone: Diagnosis and Therapy

ARNE STREITBUERGER[1], JENDRIK HARDES[1] AND GEORG GOSHEGER[1]

[1]*Department of Orthopaedics, University Hospital of Münster, Germany.*

Contents

I. INTRODUCTION

The chondrosarcoma (CS) is like any other primary malignant bone tumor: a rare entity. Only 1% of all tumors are primary malignant bone tumors. Out of these, the chondrosarcoma is the second most common primary malignant bone tumor in adults. Its incidence is about 3–4/100,000 per year. However, the term 'chondrosarcoma' is not reserved for a single tumor entity, but stands for a heterogeneous group of tumors based on a mesenchymal origin with a malignant cartilage differentiation. Based on the different histomorphogenetic appearances there is a broad variety of clinical courses and therapy. Besides the histological aspect, both the clinical course and the imaging (MRI, CT scan, plain radiographs) are substantial methods for classifying the particular tumor. On the one hand, there are low-grade chondrosarcomas characterized by a relatively benign clinical course with a good overall prognosis. On the other hand, there are highly aggressive chondrosarcomas with overall survival rates of less than 20% after 5 years [1–4]. Because of missing effective adjuvant treatments the therapy of chondrosarcoma is a domain for surgery. However, besides adequate surgery, high rates of metastases and local recurrences are common in high-grade chondrosarcomas [2–4,5]. The overall prognosis in low-grade and intermediate-grade chondrosarcomas is significantly superior to the prognosis of high-grade tumors because of low rates of metastasis even after the development of a local recurrence [2–4,6]. Because of the heterogeneity of cartilage tumors, the therapy, clinical course and prognosis are highly depended on correct diagnosis and staging. Therefore, all chondrosarcomas, even low-grade tumors, should only be treated at a specialized tumor center.

II. CLASSIFICATION

Malignant cartilage tumors are not characterized as a single entity but instead as a heterogeneous group of tumors with a broad spectrum of different histological, radiological and clinical appearances. In the plain radiograph the chondrosarcoma presents normally as an osteolytic lesion with a cortical arrosion and/or destruction. Matrix calcification and extraosseus tumor components are common, but their characteristics depend on the entity and dignity [7]. The commonality of all chondrosarcomas is the histological composition of chondrocyts and chondroid matrix as the tumor basis. However, the histological appearance shows a broad variety. Besides these features, chondrosarcomas can be either primary malignant or secondary malignant. The secondary malignant tumors normally arise out of benign cartilage tumors as enchondroma or osteochondroma and are strongly associated with Ollier's disease or the Maffucci syndrome. The therapy and the prognosis again are associated with the underlying tumor entity and dignity. Additionally, chondrosarcomas are classified either as central or peripheral. The central tumors arise from within the medullary cavity, and the peripheral tumors arise from the bone surface. The primary chondrosarcomas are almost always central, whereas the secondary chondrosarcomas can be either central or peripheral.

Malignant cartilage tumors are classified as follows:

1. Classic chondrosarcoma (grade I–III).
2. Dedifferentiated chondrosarcoma (grade IV).
3. Mesenchymal chondrosarcoma.
4. Clearcell chondrosarcoma.

5. The secondary chondrosarcoma is separated from the primary malignant chondrosarcoma and normally arises from benign cartilage lesions.

A. Classic Chondrosarcomas (Grade I–III)

The classic chondrosarcoma is the most common chondrosarcoma with an estimated annual incidence of 3–4/100,000.

Most of the classic chondrosarcomas are central tumors which arise from within the intramedullary channel of the bones. Subperiosteal and extraosseous chondrosarcoma are rarities. The main tumor site is the pelvic bone, the femur and the shoulder girdle (proximal humerus/scapula) [8–10]. Most of the tumors appear around the sixth decade of life.

The radiological appearance of chondrosarcomas is heterogeneous. They present as ostelytic lesions which represent all grades of the Lodwick classification [11]. Signs of malignancy are a cortical destruction and/or an extraosseous tumor component (Figure 33.1A–C). Further, in the plain radiograph, the scalloping phenomenon is one characteristic sign seen in most of the tumors. However, it is most common in low grade tumors and less often present in the fast-growing high-grade chondrosarcoma. In the CT scan small, amorphous spots of matrix calcification are characteristic for high-grade chondrosarcomas as is a predominance of ostelytic bone destruction [8]. Whereas the low grade chondrosarcoma regularly presents a so-called 'rings and arcs' sign that is based on slow tumor growth and the adaptation of the surrounding bone.

In the MRI scan there is no general pattern for all chondrosarcoma. Again, the appearance depends on the tumor grade. In low-grade chondrosarcomas the imaging presents a more or less homogeneous signal in the T1

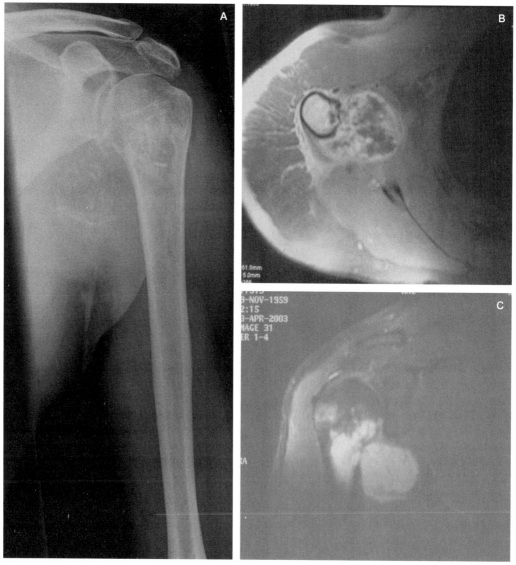

FIGURE 33.1   Grade II chondrosarcoma of the proximal humerus of a 44-year-old patient. The plain radiograph (A) and the MRI scans (B, C) show an osteolytic destruction of the proximal part of the humerus and the extraosseous tumor component.

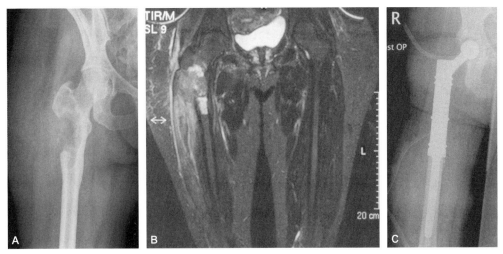

FIGURE 33.2 A 43-year-old patient with a dedifferentiated chondrosarcoma of the proximal part of the right femur. (A) Preoperative plain radiograph with an osteolytic destruction of the lateral cortex and amorphous matrix calcification; (B) MRI STIR sequence showing the bimorphic composition of the tumor; (C) postoperative plain radiograph after wide tumor resection and reconstruction with a (MUTARS®) proximal femur tumour prostheses.

sequences and a signal uptake in T2 that is based on the high percentage of water and the small number of tumor cells in the tumor matrix. Conversely, high-grade chondrosarcomas commonly present larger parts of tumor necrosis, a higher portion of fibrous tissue, a higher cell density and less chondroid matrix and, therefore, are more inhomogeneous [12].

The dignity of chondrosaroma is generally based on histopathological findings. However, in literature several different grading systems have been used over the years. Most of them are based on the cells' morphology, the nucleus size and morphology, the prominence of the nucleoles, the chromatin structure, and the mitotic activity of the tumor chondrocytes. Other criteria are the tumor cell numbers or the rate of necrosis, both of which are associated with the tumor grading. According to these aspects, the tumors are classified into three grades of malignancy in most of the grading systems [13].

B. Dedifferentiated Chondrosarcomas (dd CS)

The dedifferentiated chondrosarcoma is a special form in the group of malignant cartilage tumors. In most of the publications the dedifferentiated CS is classified as a grade IV chondrosarcoma. This tumor is commonly located in the long bones of the extremities and the pelvis. The mean age of the patients range from 65 to 75 years and is therefore slightly older than patients with a classic chondrosarcoma [1,5]. This entity is characterized by its typical bimorphic histological appearance with areas of low-grade chondrosarcomas adjacent to small parts of high-grade sarcoma components. The high-grade component can either be osteosarcoma, malignant fibrous histiozytoma, fibrosarcoma or anaplastic spindle cell sarcoma [14].

In the imaging the dedifferentiated CS is affected mainly by the low-grade component with a scalloping sign and a homogeneous picture in most parts of the tumor. But, in the parts of the high-grade component, there is commonly an aggressive ostelytic tumor growth with cortical destruction, tumor necrosis and frequently an extraosseous component (Figure 33.2A,B). Besides the plain radiograph, the MRI is usually the best method to illustrate the bimorphic composition of the tumor to make the diagnosis (Figure 33.2B).

C. Mesenchymal Chondrosarcomas

The mesenchymal chondrosarcoma is a further rare subentity in the group of malignant cartilage tumors. In contrast to the dedifferentiated and the classic chondrosarcoma this tumor appears mainly in younger patients. The main age at diagnosis is the second and third decade of life. Further, the most common tumor site is the axial skeleton and the extraskeletal soft tissue dissimilar to other chondrosarcomas [15]. From its histological appearance this tumor presents as a tumor with small spindle cell-like tumor cells besides smaller parts of normal cartilage. Especially because of the small cell component, a diagnosis to differentiate it from a Ewing's sarcoma or synovial sarcoma can be difficult. From its dignity the mesenchymal chondrosarcoma has to be classified as a high-grade malignancy on the part of its clinical course and its therapy.

D. Clearcell Chondrosarcomas

This rare type of chondrosarcoma is almost always located at the epiphyseal part of the long bones of the extremities. From its histological appearance it is characterized, like the

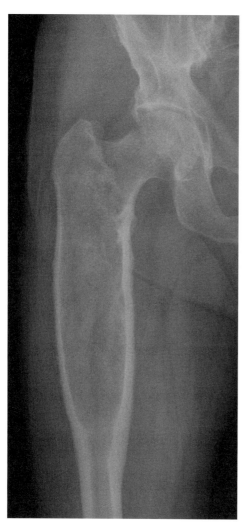

FIGURE 33.3 Plain radiograph of a patient with a clear cell chondrosarcoma of the proximal part of the femur. The image shows an expansive osteolysis with sharp margins and few spots of tumor matrix calcification.

dedifferentiated chondrosarcoma, by its bimorphic composition. These tumors present parts of classic malignant chondrocyts alongside parts of swollen chondocytic cells with a clear cytoplasm that allows the pathologist to separate them easily from other chondrosarcomas [16]. Because of its relatively low proliferation rate, and the slow tumor growth, this tumor appears in the plain radiograph typically as sharp edging ostelytic lesions with a sclerotic border (Figure 33.3).

With regard to its clinical behavior, and the prognosis as the therapy, it must be graduated as an intermediate grade chondrosarcoma [17].

E. Secondary Chondrosarcomas

Secondary chondrosarcomas typically arise from pre-existing benign cartilage lesions like enchondroma or osteochondroma, especially if they are associated with Ollier's disease or the Maffucci syndrome.

Chondrosarcomas arising from osteochondromas are almost solely low-grade chondrosarcomas. Less than 10% seems to be grade II chondrosarcomas as Ahmed presented in his study of 107 patients [18]. The clinical aspect of this secondary malignancy is a new proliferative growth of pre-existing benign lesions after the adolescence and/or newly diagnosed clinical symptoms, such as pain [19]. In these cases, we routinely recommend a further MRI diagnostic with specific cartilage sequences (D3W,FL2D) to judge the cartilage cap of the osteochondroma. A cartilage cap thickness of more than 2 cm and an inhomogeneous appearance of the cartilage cap are strong indications for a malignant transformation and an indication for an open biopsy. The risk of secondary malignancy is about 5–25% in the case of multifocal lesions appearing during the remaining life span of the patient [20,21].

A secondary chondrosarcoma arising from benign enchondroma or in connection with the Maffucci syndrome or Ollier's disease can either be a low-grade or a high-grade chondrosarcoma [22]. The rate of malignant transfer of a benign lesion is about 1% if there is a single lesion and about 10% in the case of multifocal lesions or a syndrome association [23]. In patients with known pre-existing lesions, particularly in combination with a diagnosed syndrome, we attach strong importance on the clinical course. Again, if these patients report on newly occurred pain and clinical symptoms, an advanced diagnosis about the suspicious lesion up to an open biopsy is recommended.

III. DIFFICULTIES IN MAKING THE DIAGNOSIS OF A CHONDROSARCOMA

In patients with cartilage tumors it is important to exclude the benign lesions from the malignant tumors. Normally, benign cartilage tumors do no warrant a biopsy or surgical treatment, in contrast to malignant cartilage tumors. Therefore, the accurate staging of the cartilage tumors with regard to the dignity and the entity is essential for advanced treatment.

The indication for a surgical biopsy is made on the basis of the clinical and radiological appearance of the underlying lesion. However, the histological examination of the specimen is important but is only one component for making the diagnosis. In particular, in low-grade chondrosarcomas the diagnosis can only be made as a consensus of the clinical, radiological and histopathological appearance of the tumor.

A. Biopsy of Chondrosarcomas

Because of the special composition of chondrosarcomas with large parts of myxoid matrix and the broad spectrum of sub-entities, making an accurate biopsy is even more difficult than with other primary malignant bone tumors. For a reliable diagnosis with regard to the dignity and the entity there is a need to get tissue from all parts of the tumor. Especially in the case of dedifferentiated chondrosarcoma with its bimorphic composition, it is essential to detect the small parts of high-grade components for the diagnosis. Therefore, in our clinic we always demand an open biopsy for all chondrosarcomas to be able to get sufficient tissue samples from all parts of the tumor, especially from the heterogeneous parts. A preoperative MRI scan supports the performance of the biopsy by detecting these components (Figure 33.2B). Besides the difficulty in getting a reliable specimen for the histopathological examination, there are further aspects to respect by performing the biopsy. One has to accurately plan the correct biopsy approach in respect of further treatment without unnecessarily contaminating the surrounding soft tissue or adjacent compartments which could lead to serious complications in the definite operation. A true-cut or CT guided needle biopsy cannot be recommended because of the high risk of diagnostic bias due to the small tissue samples that are gained by using this procedure only.

B. Diagnosis of Low-grade Chondrosarcomas

However, even after a sufficient biopsy, there is frequently still the problem of making the diagnosis of a grade I chondrosarcoma. The differentiation of a progressive benign cartilage tumor-like enchondroma from a low-grade chondrosarcoma is still not possible with the histological examination of the biopsy specimen only [19]. But, this important differentiation can only be made as a consensus of the histological appearance, the clinical course and the radiological imaging in most of the tumors.

From our clinical experience, we think that the clinical signs are one of the most important factors for the diagnosis in combination with the plain radiograph and the CT scan. Benign enchondroma are normally detected by chance in the plain radiography in the context of other symptoms caused by, e.g., degenerative joint disease. The low proliferation rate of benign cartilage tumors commonly leads to an adaptation of the tumor surrounding bone to the tumor growth without weakening the bone. Therefore, these tumors are usually asymptomatic. In contrast, in chondrosarcomas, even in grade I tumors, the tumor proliferation rate is much higher, which leads to a pain symptomatic due to tumor affected cortical destruction, bone resorption and consecutive bone weakening. As well as weight-bearing instability pain, most of the patients typically report of a night pain. A pathological fracture of the involved bone is almost always a sign of malignancy except in the case of tumors of the short bones of the hand. In this localization, even in the case of a pathologic fracture, the entity of the cartilage lesion is almost always benign. Chondrosarcomas of the hand are rarities [24]. For all other tumor sides an open biopsy is demanded in case of pathological fracture.

However, decisive for the diagnosis of a grade I chondrosarcoma is the cortical destruction that can be best seen in plain radiographs and CT scans. Therefore, in the case of clinical symptoms we recommend a plain radiograph and a CT scan to classify the lesion. If there is destruction of the cortical bone in combination with clinical symptoms, then an open biopsy has to be done to verify the diagnosis and define further treatment.

IV. THERAPY AND PROGNOSIS

The therapy and prognosis of a chondrosarcoma is strongly associated to the grade of malignancy and the underlying sub-entity.

However, for all types of chondrosarcomas the premise for a curative treatment is surgery. According to Enneking [25], only the wide compartmental tumor resection is able to control the tumor locally and systemically in a curative setting in high- and intermediated-grade tumors. For low-grade chondrosarcomas the intra-lesional or marginal resection can be adequate for some special indications.

A. High-grade Chondrosarcoma

1. SURGERY

The therapy of high-grade chondrosarcomas is a domain for surgery. In a curative setting, the wide compartmental resection is the goal for all high and intermediate-grade chondrosarcomas, irrespective of the tumor site [25]. Besides tumor grading, the type of surgery has been detected as a independent prognostic factor for survival in several studies [2–4]. The limb salvage is possible in most cases; however, this aim is secondary to the oncological outcome. For chondrosarcomas of long bones of the extremities the defect is frequently reconstructed with a tumor endoprostheses while preserving the extremity and its function (Figure 33.2C) [26]. Particularly for tumors of the lower extremities (such as those affecting the knee or hip joint), endoprosthetic reconstruction is the method of choice. This is because of good long-term results that the endoprosthetic device gives regarding the ability of weight-bearing, function, range of motion and stability. The biological reconstruction with allografts or fibula autografts is preserved for tumors of the diaphyseal bone. For tumors of the upper extremity (particularly for proximal humerus and scapula chondrosarcoma affecting the shoulder joint) a biological reconstruction like the Tikoff-Limberg procedure or the clavicula pro humero operation is useful to reconstruct the extremity and its function. The main advantage of these procedures is the fact that these operations can be done even after large soft tissue resections because less soft tissue coverage is needed for the reconstruction compared to a tumor endoprostheses.

Primary amputations are still necessary in about 8–18% [2,26]. Indications for an amputation are preserved for chondrosarcomas in which a wide tumor resection cannot be guaranteed because of a broad soft tissue tumor infiltration and contamination. This could be in the case of infiltration of the neurovascular bundle or in the case of a pathological fracture. In 153 patients, Fiorenza *et al.* reported a primary amputation rate of 18% to achieve adequate margins [2].

For chondrosarcomas of the pelvis, the wide tumor resection is usually possible without sacrificing the extremity. For small tumors, a partial pelvic resection may be sufficient while preserving the pelvic ring and good function of the legs (Figure 33.4). For larger tumors, however, a hemipelvectomy with a hip transposition procedure is frequently needed to achieve wide resection margins (Figure 33.5A,B). An external hemipelvectomy may be necessary in the case of a tumor involved in the neurovascular bundle but remains an exception in the case of a primary tumor resection. However, after the occurrence of local recurrences of pelvic chondrosarcoma an external hemipelvectomy is more frequent [27] to achieve local tumor control.

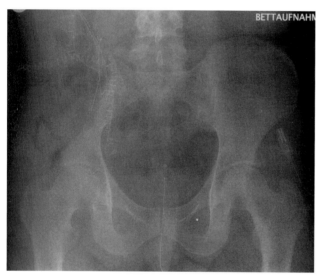

FIGURE 33.4 Postoperative plain radiograph after partial pelvectomy of a grade II chondrosarcoma of the iliac crest preserving the pelvic ring.

2. CHEMOTHERAPY/RADIOTHERAPY

Compared to other primary malignant bone tumors like the osteosarcoma or the Ewing's sarcoma in chondrosarcoma no effective adjuvant therapies have yet been developed. Neither chemotherapy nor radiotherapy showed any positive effect regarding the overall survival in curatively treated patients [1,4,5]. However, most of the patients with grade III and dedifferentiated chondrosarcomas, as patients with mesenchymal chondrosarcomas, are treated with a chemotherapy protocol according to the Euro-BOSS or EURAMOS protocol for osteosarcomas. A published study by the European Musculoskeletal Oncology Society demonstrated that patients with dedifferentiated chondrosarcomas had no benefits from chemotherapy or radiotherapy regarding their overall survival [5]. Early results of patients treated according to the Euro-BOSS and EURAMOS protocol have not been promising with regard to the rate of response to chemotherapy and improvement of survival. However, the chemotherapy regimens have changed over the years, and this earlier study was a multicenter retrospective study, and not homogeneous in the different tumor centers; although several other studies also presented similar results [14,16]. Longer follow-up, similar inclusion criteria and larger study populations are needed for a final conclusion.

Analog results are reported for patients with grade III chondrosarcoma. Larger series did not show significant positive effects of chemotherapy on the overall survival in these patients [3,9,10,28]. Whereas, some patients with a mesenchymal chondrosarcoma a positive effect has been reported with a good response on chemotherapy and significantly improved overall survival in combination with a wide tumor resection [29].

The radiotherapy in the treatment of chondrosarcoma is mainly reserved for palliative indications. However, for some special indications (e.g., tumors of the vertebral bodies or the scull) in which a wide surgical tumor resection is not possible, the heavy weight ion radiation in combination with a photon radiation did show some promising results in small series [30] regarding local tumor control. In patients

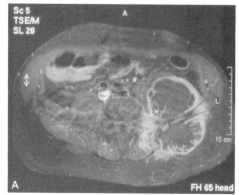
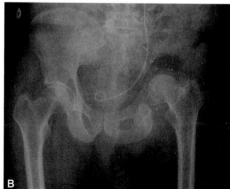

FIGURE 33.5 Grade III chondrosarcoma of a 55-year-old patient of the right iliac crest. (A) T2 sequence of the pelvis with gadolinium enhancement of the tumor. The image shows the huge extraosseous tumor component with infiltration of the surrounding muscles; (B) postoperative plain radiograph after hemipelvectomy and hip transposition procedure.

with inoperable tumors, the radiotherapy is used for temporary local tumor control in a palliative setting. However, a curative treatment is not possible with radiotherapy alone.

Due to the lack of adjuvant therapies, the results regarding local and systemic control despite adequate surgery in high-grade chondrosarcomas are worse than for other primary bone tumors. Patients with grade III and dedifferentiated chondrosarcomas frequently develop distant metastasis in up to 70% and local recurrences in up to 35% [2,3,9,10,26]. Overall survival of patients with grade III chondrosarcomas is less than 60% for 5 years. For patients with dedifferentiated chondrosarcomas, this is even worse, with a median survival rate of about 1.4 years [5,9,10].

B. Therapy Low-grade Chondrosarcoma

The low-grade chondrosarcoma has to be separated from other chondrosarcomas when it comes to its clinical course, therapy and prognosis. For these tumors, surgical resection is the therapy of choice also. However, unlike the high-grade chondrosarcoma, some surgeons prefer intra-lesional resection for special indications because of its low grade malignancy with overall survival rates of more than 90% for 5 and 10 years and rates of metastasis of less than 10% [4]. According to Enneking, for stage IA tumors of the long bones of the extremities an intra-lesional curettage and adjuvant use of cryotherapy and/or PMMA application in the bone cavity without worsening the overall survival, and while preserving a good extremity function, is feasible [27,31,32]. Even the rate of local recurrence decreases only slightly when using conservative surgery. Ahlmann *et al.* reported good results concerning local tumor control in low-grade chondrosarcomas after intralesional tumor curettage and cryotherapy. They observed neither local recurrence nor distant metastasis in 15 treated patients [6]. In most cases, a wide resection of the recurrent tumor is possible without significantly worsening the prognosis and function. This can be done in case a local tumor relapse develops after intralesional resection. Indeed, Enneking recommends a wide resection for tumors of the trunk or the pelvis, as well as for stage II tumors. This is less to improve the overall survival and more to avoid a local recurrence, which is frequently associated with a high complication rate in the case of secondary resection of the relapsed tumor. However, for each patient the risk whether to perform conservative surgery or a wide resection has to be balanced carefully regarding the individual circumstances.

V. PERSPECTIVE OF NEW DIAGNOSTIC AND THERAPEUTIC APPROACHES

New techniques and methods in the staging and new therapeutic approaches in the treatment of chondrosarcomas are under development.

A small selection of possible approaches which may lead to an effective treatment approach in the therapy of chondrosarcoma are presented below.

Degradation and penetration of the extracellular matrix and the basement membrane are important factors in the process of local invasion and metastasis by controlling the ability of the tumor cells to transverse tissue boundaries. Matrix metalloproteinases are one of the depending factors in degradation of extracellular matrix and collagen. TIMP (tissue inhibitors of matrix proteinase) are tissue counterparts of the MMP and are able to inhibit the proteolytic activity of the MMPs. The balance between the activity of the inhibitors and the MMPs determines the proteolytic activity and may be responsible for the invasiveness and the potential of metastasis. Inhibiting the MMP-1 expression in the tumor cells by small inhibitory RNA is a possibility for future chondrosarcoma therapies [33].

As known from other solid tumors, the neovascularization plays an important role in malignant chondrosarcomas regarding tumor growth and metastasis. The tumor grade is positively correlated with the microvascularity of the tumors. Biologically aggressive cartilage tumors have more microvessels than non-aggressive tumors, which correlates with the tumor grade [34]. New anti-angiogenesis agents like the Vascular Endothelial Growth Factor Antisense (VEGF-AS), which is an antisense oligonucleotide that targets VEGF, inhibiting angiogenesis and tumor cell proliferation [35], are being studied *in vitro* and in clinical studies for different tumors and may also be useful in the treatment of chondrosarcoma.

Another approach is, for example, the examination of Indian Hedgehog (IHH) signaling in chondrosarcomas. IHH signaling seems not to be responsible for malignant transformation in cartilage tumors but it likely plays a role in cartilage tumorgenesis by maintaining tumor cells in a less differentiated but proliferative state. Treatment of chondrosarcoma cells with recombinant IHH increased proliferation; whereas IHH signaling inhibitors inhibited tumor proliferation and tumor growth *in vitro* and *in vivo* [36].

Further, biphosphonates are increasingly garnering interest in the treatment of a variety of tumors affecting the bone. Besides their use in patients with metastatic disease from solid tumors like breast or lung cancer, there is increasing evidence of direct antitumor activity of different types of BPs on a broad variety of tumor cells [37]. In *in-vitro* and *in-vivo* studies, antitumor effects have been shown not only for ostesarcoma but also for chondrosarcoma. Clodronat and zoledronat reduced the proliferation rate of chondrosarcoma cells *in vitro* and further zoledronat increased survival in a rat chondrosarcoma model [38,39]. Although clinical studies are not, at the time of writing, published, BP does seem to have a high potential in the therapeutic treatment of chondrosarcoma.

Clearly, preclinical advances on multiple fronts are currently being made. Some of these approaches may lead to the development of novel therapies in the treatment of chondrosarcomas; though, the effectiveness of these newly developed methods in humans has to be proven first. However, surgery still remains the only effective treatment available for most of the patients.

VI. CONCLUSION

Malignant cartilage tumors are characterized by a broad spectrum of different entities. The clinical course and the therapy are strongly associated with the single entity and dignity of the tumor. Therefore, the diagnosis and therapy should remain in the hands of specialized oncologists, radiologists, pathologists and surgeons. Only an interdisciplinary diagnostic and therapeutic approach makes allowances for the variety of these tumors and the difficulties in their treatment. The surgical tumor resection is the only effective curative treatment for all chondrosarcomas, particularly because of missing effective adjuvant chemotherapies. However, to improve the outcome of high-grade chondrosarcomas, new therapeutic approaches have to be developed.

References

1. I.D. Dickey, P.S. Rose & B. Fuchs, et al., Dedifferentiated chondrosarcoma: the role of chemotherapy with updated outcomes, J Bone Joint Surg Am 86-A (11) (2004) 2412–2418.

2. F. Fiorenza, A. Abudu & R.J. Grimer, et al., Risk factors for survival and local control in chondrosarcoma of bone, J Bone Joint Surg Br 84 (1) (2002) 93–99.

3. R.J. Grimer, S.R. Carter & R.M. Tillman, et al., Chondrosarcoma of bone, J Bone Joint Surg Am 82-A (8) (2000) 1203–1204.

4. M. Rizzo, M.A. Ghert & J.M. Harrelson, et al., Chondrosarcoma of bone: analysis of 108 cases and evaluation for predictors of outcome, Clin Orthop Relat Res 391 (2001) 224–233.

5. R.J. Grimer, G. Gosheger & A. Taminiau, et al., Dedifferentiated chondrosarcoma: prognostic factors and outcome from the European group, Eur J Cancer 43 (2007) 2060–2065.

6. E. Ahlmann, L. Memendez & A. Fedenko, et al., Influence of cryosurgery on treatment outcome of low-grade chondorsarcoma, Clin Orthop Relat Res 451 (2006) 201–207.

7. G. Lodwick, Atlas of Tumor Radiology. The Bones and Joints, Year Book Med Publi, Chicago, 1971, pp. 38–39.

8. J. Freyschmidt, H. Ostertag & G. Jundt, Knochentumoren, 2nd edn., Springer-Verlag, Berlin, Heidelberg, New York, 2003.

9. F.Y. Lee, H.J. Mankin & G. Fondren, et al., Chondrosarcoma of bone: an assessment of outcome, J Bone Joint Surg Am 81 (3) (1999) 326–338.

10. M. Soderstrom, T.O. Ekfors & T.O. Bohling, et al., No improvement in the overall survival of 194 patients with chondrosarcoma in Finland in 1971–1990, Acta Orthop Scand 74 (3) (2003) 344–350.

11. R. Erlemann, Benign cartilaginous tumors, Radiology 41 (7) (2001) 548–559.

12. M.J. Geirnaerdt, P.C. Hogendoorn & A.H. Taminiau, et al., Malignant cartilage tumors, Radiology 38 (6) (1998) 502–508.

13. W. Winkelmann, in: C. Wirth & L. Zichner (Eds.), Tumoren und tumorähnliche Erkrankungen, Georg Thieme Verlag KG, Stuttgart, 2005.

14. E. Staals, P. Bacchini & F. Bertoni, Dedifferentiated central chondrosarcoma, Cancer 106 (2006) 2682–2691.

15. Y. Nakashima, K.K. Unni & T.C. Shives, et al., Mesenchymal chondrosarcoma of bone and soft tissue. A review of 111 cases, Cancer 57 (12) (1986) 2444–2453.

16. G. Delling, B. Jobke & S. Burisch, et al., Cartilage tumors. Classification, conditions for biopsy and histologic characteristics, Orthopade 34 (12) (2005) 1267–1281.

17. D. Donati, J.Q. Yin & M. Colangeli, Clear cell chondrosarcoma of bone: long time follow-up of 18 cases, Arch Orthop Trauma Surg 128 (2) (2008) 137–142.

18. A.R. Ahmed, T.S. Tan & K.K. Unni, et al., Secondary chondrosarcoma in osteochondroma: report of 107 patients, Clin Orthop Relat Res 411 (2003) 193–206.

19. K.K. Unni, Cartilaginous lesions of bone, J Orthop Sci 6 (5) (2001) 457–472.

20. P. Canella, F. Gardini & S. Boriani, Exostosis: development, evolution and relationship to malignant degeneration, Ital J Orthop Traumatol 7 (3) (1981) 293–298.

21. M. Altay, K. Bayrakci & Y. Yildiz, et al., Secondary chondrosarcoma in cartilage bone tumors: report of 32 patients, J Orthop Sci 12 (5) (2007) 415–423.

22. J. Liu, P.G. Hudkins & R.G. Swee, et al., Bone sarcomas associated with Ollier's disease, Cancer 59 (7) (1987) 1376–1385.

23. H.S. Schwartz, N.B. Zimmerman & M.A. Simon, et al., The malignant potential of enchondromatosis, J Bone Joint Surg Am 69 (2) (1987) 269–274.

24. S. Patil, M.V. de Silva & R. Reid, Chondrosarcoma of small bones of the hand, J Hand Surg [Br] 28 (6) (2003) 602–608.

25. W.F. Ennking & W. Dunham, A system for the classification of skeletal resections, Chir Organi Mov LXVV (Suppl 1) (1990) 217–240.

26. A. Streitbuerger, J. Hardes & C. Gebert, et al., Cartilage tumors of the bone. Diagnosis and therapy, Orthopade 35 (8) (2006) 871–881 quiz 882.

27. K.L. Weber, M.L. Pring & F.H. Sim, Treatment and outcome of recurrent pelvic chondrosarcoma, Clin Orthop Relat Res 397 (2002) 19–28.

28. J. Bjornsson, R.A. McLeod & K.K. Unni, et al., Primary chondrosarcoma of long bones and limb girdles, Cancer 83 (10) (1998) 2105–2119.

29. M. Cesari, F. Bertoni & P. Bacchini, et al., Mesenchymal chondrosarcoma. An analysis of patients treated at a single institution, Tumori 93 (5) (2007) 423–427.

30. G. Noël, J.L. Habrand & E. Jauffret, et al., Radiation therapy for chordoma and chondrosarcoma of the skull base and the cervical spine. Prognostic factors and patterns of failure, Strahlenther Onkol 179 (4) (2003) 241–248.

31. I.C. van der Geest, M.H. de Valk & J.W. de Rooy, et al., Oncological and functional results of cryosurgical therapy of enchondromas and chondrosarcomas grade 1, J Surg Oncol 98 (6) (2008) 421–426.

32. J. Bickels, Y. Kollender & O. Merinsky, et al., Closed argon-based cryoablation of bone tumors, J Bone Joint Surg [Br] 86-B (2004) 714–718.

33. J. Yuan, C.M. Dutton & S.P. Scully, RNAi mediated MMP-1 silencing inhibits human chondrosarcoma invasion, J Orthop Res 23 (6) (2005) 1467–1474.

34. R.L. McGough, B.I. Asward & R. Terek, Pathologic neovascularization in cartilage tumors, Clin Orthop Relat Res 397 (2002) 76–82.

35. A. Levine, A. Tulpule & D. Quinn, et al., Phase I study of antisense oligonucleotide against vascular endothelial growth factor: decrease in plasma vascular endothelial growth factor with potential clinical efficacy, J Clin Oncol 24 (2006) 1712–1719.

36. T. Tiet, S. Hopyan & P. Nadesan, et al., Constitutive Hedgehog Signaling in Chondrosarcoma Up-Regulates Tumor Cell Proliferation, Am J Pathol 168 (2006) 321–330.

37. D. Santini, U. Vespasiani Gentilucci & B. Vincenzi, et al., The antineoplastic role of bisphosphonates: from basic research to clinical evidence, Annals of Oncology 14 (2003) 1468–1476.

38. F. Gouin, B. Ory & F. Rédine, et al., Zoledronic acid slows down rat primary chondrosarcoma development, recurrent tumor progression after intralesional curretage and increases overall survival, Int J Cancer 119 (5) (2007) 980–984.

39. A. Streitbuerger, J. Hardes, et al. (2006). Zytotoxische Wirkung von Bisphosphonaten auf Chondrosarkom-Zellen 54. Jahrestagung der Vereinigung Süddeutscher Orthopäden e. V.

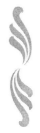

CHAPTER 34

Current Status of Immunotherapy for Osteosarcoma and its Future Trends

KANJI MORI[1], KOSEI ANDO[1], YOSHITAKA MATSUSUE[1] AND DOMINIQUE HEYMANN[2,3,4]

[1]*Department of Orthopaedic Surgery, Shiga University of Medical Science, Tsukinowa-cho, Seta, Otsu, Shiga, 520-2192, Japan.*
[2]*Université de Nantes, Nantes Atlantique Universités, Laboratoire de Physiopathologie de la Résorption Osseuse et Thérapie des Tumeurs Osseuses Primitives, EA3822, Nantes, F-44035, France.*
[3]*INSERM, U957, Nantes, F-44035, France.*
[4]*CHU de Nantes, Nantes, F-44035, France.*

Contents

I. INTRODUCTION

Osteosarcomas, the most frequent primary bone tumor, typically affects children and young adults [1]. Chemotherapy regimens and operating procedures have drastically improved the prognosis of patients with non-metastatic osteosarcoma; however, the prognosis of the patient with recurrence or metastasis is still poor. The overall survival with an aggressive chemotherapy regimen before and after surgery now varies between 50 and 65% [2]. These have led to the exploration of new, more effective and less toxic treatments, such as immunotherapy for curing osteosarcoma.

Immunotherapy is a therapeutic strategy based on the upregulation of the immune response in tumor-bearing hosts. Two immunotherapies can be described: (1) active immunotherapy including pulsed dendritic cells and cytokine treatments that elicit immune response against tumor cells; (2) passive/adoptive immunotherapy consisting in the administration of *ex vivo*-expanded tumor-specific cytotoxic immune cells especially T lymphocytes.

In this chapter, we have summarized accumulating knowledge, strongly underlining the potential interest of these new therapies applicable to osteosarcomas.

II. ACTIVE IMMUNITY

To elicit immunity of tumor-bearing hosts, antigen presenting cells (APCs) such as dendritic cells (DCs)-based therapies, cytokine-based therapies and gene therapies have been demonstrated.

A. Monocyte Lineage

Monocyte lineage constitutes a complex system of professional APCs which can induce primary T and B cell responses.

DCs make up a complex system of professional APCs that have the unique capacity to induce primary T and B cell responses [3]. The main pathway of DC-based immunotherapy is to upregulate lymphocyte activity, such as NK cells and TIL, and the goal will be to optimize the use of DCs (i.e., vaccination) in maintaining T lymphocyte survival and specificity. A number of clinical trials are currently under way studying DCs in a variety of tumors [4]. One clinical phase-I study using DCs against solid tumors in children including osteosarcoma has been reported [5]. In this series, one patient with metastatic fibrosarcoma demonstrated drastic positive response without obvious toxic side effects. Some relevant topics include antigen loading and DCs maturation procedures, frequency and route of DCs administration, efficacy of DCs homing to lymphoid tissues and their durability once there and the role of distinct DCs subsets [3,4].

Monocyte/macrophage-mediated tumor cell killing is a major mechanism of the hosts' defence against primary and/or metastatic neoplasm. Liposome-encapsulated muramyl tripeptide phosphatidylethanolamine (L-MTP-PE) is a peptide that acts as a potent activator of monocytes/

macrophages [6]. Meyers *et al.* reported clear and consistent survival benefits of L-MTP-PE based on the latest follow-up data (6 years EFS, 61% for chemotherapy alone vs 69% with L-MTP-PE; 6 years overall survival improved from 70% with chemotherapy alone to 78% with L-MTP-PE; $p = 0.03$) [7]. Current recommendations are for an initial 12 weeks' dosing bi-weekly followed by weekly dosing for an additional 24 weeks (total 36 weeks) in schedule of L-MTP-PE administration [8]. Since all patients receiving L-MTP-PE on a compassionate basis have had evidence of biologic activity at 2 mg/m^2, pre-medication and use of the fixed 2 mg/m^2 dose is suggested [6].

Whereas the central necrosis pattern is generally seen in conventional chemotherapy treatment, the unique peripheral fibrosis was frequently induced by L-MTP-PE treatment [9,10]. Thus, L-MTP-PE induces peripheral fibrosis of lung metastases indicting an immune mechanism of attack to result in a balanced 'inside-out' plus 'outside-in' attack when used in combination with chemotherapy. Ifosfamide is the most studied and encouraged regimen. A regional delivery route (i.e., aerosol) with Fas/FasL pathway modifying agents should further improve L-MTP-PE efficacy.

B. Cytokines

Most widely used and investigated, cytokines are clearly essential molecules in immunotherapy due to their excellent wide range of abilities. Cytokines represented by interleukins (ILs) play a crucial role in the expression of cellular adhesion molecules (CAMs) and the function of anti-tumor effector cells as the most potent modulators of the immune responses. CAMs play an important role in immune responses including NK cells binding to target [11]. Indeed, melanoma CAM, synonymous MUC18 plays a crucial role in osteosarcoma metastasis [12]. Namely, osteosarcoma cells express this molecule and ABX-MA1, a fully human anti-MUC18 antibody, inhibited the metastasis of human osteosarcoma cells *in vivo* [12].

The most widely studied IL in this field is IL-2 [13]. Luksch *et al.* have reported a clinical trial in osteosarcoma using IL-2 [14], in which 18 children with localized osteosarcoma received four IL-2 courses (9×10^6 IU/ml/day × 4), alternated with pre- and post-operative multiple chemotherapies. The results showed that intensive chemotherapies have no effect on the IL-2-induced immune activation, and suggested a role of the NK cells in the control of osteosarcoma. On the contrary, it has been reported that the clinical use of IL-2 is limited by significant toxic side effects caused by the administration of this cytokine in doses sufficient for cell activation *in vivo* [15]. Therefore, other ILs have been recognized as a candidate for human immunotherapy.

Some studies using IL-12 [16], IL-12 associated with IL-18 [17], IL-18 [18] and IL-17 [19] in osteosarcoma have been already performed. These cytokine-based therapies demonstrated enhanced cytotoxic activity of T cells in osteosarcoma. IL-12 upregulated Fas expression in human osteosarcoma cells [20–23] and ifosfamide induced Fas ligand (FasL) expression in osteosarcoma cells [24]. Thus, a combination therapy of IL-12 with ifosfamide resulted in the upregulation of both Fas and FasL and increased the anti-tumor activity in mice osteosarcoma metastases by an autocrine/paracrine Fas/FasL loop pathway compared with either agent alone [24]. In addition, it has been reported that tumor necrosis factor (TNF)-α and IFN-γ can induce the anti-tumor activity of macrophages [25,26].

C. Gene Therapy

Gene therapy elicits the immune response in tumor-bearing hosts and represents one option of immunotherapy.

In the field of gene therapy for osteosarcoma, several approaches have been envisaged, such as suicide gene therapy [27,28], tumor-suppressor gene therapy [29–32] and cytokine-based gene therapy [18–22]. The most investigated gene transfer vectors is adenoviral vector (Adv) [33]. A single injection of Adv encoding IL-2 gene (Ad IL-2) into a primary tumor lesion elicited anti-tumoral immunity and this immunity has not only suppressed primary tumor growth but also eradicated disseminated micro-metastases in distant organs [34]. Interestingly, in this report, not only minimal side effects but also maximal therapeutic effects were exerted only when injecting the optimal dose (not the highest) of Ad IL-2. Important limitations in this regard are the failure of non-replicating Adv to achieve sufficient tumor-cell transduction and effective solid-tumor penetration. Furthermore, the expression of coxackievirus and adenovirus receptor, which is an important determining factor for adenoviral gene transfer efficiency, in osteosarcoma is controversial [35,36]. Witlox *et al.* demonstrated that targeting a conditionally replicative adenovirus toward integrins Ad5-Δ24RGD [37], providing an alternative viral entry pathway, dramatically enhances its cytotoxicity on osteosarcoma and warrants further exploration of Ad5-Δ24RGD for its utility in osteosarcoma treatment [37].

However, the fetal case report following adenovirus gene transfer [38] sounds a warning against this strategy in humans. As gene transfer vectors other than adenovirus, it has been shown that osteosarcoma cell lines were good targets for lentiviral transduction with favorable gene transfer efficiency [39,40]. After the development of successful safety delivery of therapeutic gene, this strategy demonstrates inestimable potential activities to modulate the prognosis of patients with osteosarcoma.

III. PASSIVE/ADOPTIVE IMMUNITY

Cytotoxic T lymphocytes (CTL) specifically recognizing that tumor cells are the pivot cells of passive/adoptive immunotherapy. Monoclonal, polyclonal and cell lines of

T lymphocytes have been already envisaged to develop such therapeutic strategies.

A. Tumor Antigens

The identification of human cancer antigens restricted to HLA class I has ushered the medical community into the new area of antigen-specific cancer immunotherapy specifically targeting these antigens [3]. Specific immunotherapy utilizing peptides deriving from these antigens are ongoing for the treatment of HLA-A1+ patients suffering from melanoma and resulted in major clinical responses [4,5].

Based on these observations, this therapeutic strategy was extended to other diseases. A number of tumor-associated antigens of several human malignancies have been identified [41,42]. Many of these antigens have been applied to the clinical vaccine trials with successful induction of immune response or tumor regression [43–46]. On the other hand, the reports for tumor antigens of osteosarcoma are limited. Some of the tumor-associated antigens—melanoma-associated antigen (MAGE) [47], squamous cell carcinoma antigen recognized by T cells (SART) 1 [48a,48b], SART3 [49], papillomavirus binding factor (PBF) [50] and clusterin-associated protein 1 (CLUAP1) [51]—were reported to be expressed in osteosarcoma. These findings provided the rationale to develop cellular therapies in osteosarcoma.

Antigenic peptides derived from SART3 and PBF were shown to be recognized by CD8+ CTL from patients with osteosarcoma in MHC class I-restricted manner [49,50]. SART3 was identified from eosophageal cancer cells KE4 [52]. The SART3-derived peptides were able to induce HLA-A2-restricted and tumor-specific CTL in various histological types (squamous cell carcinoma, astrocytoma and adenocarcinoma) [53]. These facts strengthened the potential use of the SART3-derived peptides for specific immunotherapy of HLA-A2+ patients suffering from osteosarcoma. Indeed, SART3-derived peptides induce the production of SART3-specific CTL in an HLA-A24-restricted manner in osteosarcoma [49]. Taken together with the prevalence of HLA-A24 [54], this strategy could be applicable for approximately 60% of HLA-A24+ patients with osteosarcoma. Furthermore, no severe adverse response associated with peptide administration and a significant up-modulation of the cellular immune response against tumor cells in clinical trial using SART3-derived peptides in HLA-A24+ patients with colon cancer [55] encourages further application of this strategy for osteosarcoma.

CLUAP1 is a newly found tumor-associated antigen by the use of serological analysis of recombinant cDNA expression library (SEREX) technique [56]. High expression of CLUAP1 was found not only in osteosarcoma but also in ovarian, colon and lung cancers [51]. These findings suggest that CLUAP1 may play a crucial role in carcinogenesis of multiple types of tumors.

Accumulating evidences revealed that CD4+ T cells also play an important role in anti-tumor immune responses [45,46,57]. However, tumor-associated antigen of osteosarcoma recognized by CT4+ is not determined. Since SEREX antigens were identified by the high-titer immunoglobulin G response of patient sera to the clones from cDNA library, CD4+ T cells were likely to respond to CLUAP1 *in vivo*. The frequency and the degree of the immune response to CLUAP1 in osteosarcoma patients are unclear at present; however, Ishikura *et al.* reported preliminary results that 1 out of 11 sera from osteosarcoma patients but none of the serum from 10 healthy volunteers reacted to CLUAP1 [51]. Further studies are needed to determine whether CLUAP1 is a tumor-associated antigen of osteosarcoma recognized by CT4+, useful as a prognostic/diagnostic marker and/or for a target of immunotherapy of osteosarcoma.

B. Polyclonal Tumor-infiltrating Lymphocytes (TIL)

Polyclonal tumor-infiltrating lymphocytes are a hopeful selected immunotherapeutic weapon which directly induces apoptosis in cancer cells.

An immunohistochemical study has revealed an infiltration of osteosarcomas by T lymphocytes [58]. Phenotypic analyses demonstrated that these TILs were 95% CD3+ and 68% CD8+ [58]. Rivoltini *et al.* have also performed phenotypic analyses of TIL in 37 pediatric tumors including 12 osteosarcomas and revealed their CD8+ predominancy [59]. It is theorized that the infiltrating lymphoid represents a selected population of cells which have preferentially migrated to the tumor secondary to an immune response. These T lymphocytes termed TIL are considered to be more specific in their immunological reactivity to tumor cells than the non-infiltrating lymphocytes [60]. Thus, the identification of tumor-specific lymphocytes has resulted in new therapeutic strategies based on mounting a sustained and effective anti-tumor immune response [60,61]. Théoleyre *et al.* showed that only TIL extracted from osteosarcoma were cytotoxic against allogeneic tumor cells in the analyses of 27 human patients with bone-associated tumors (osteosarcoma, Ewing's sarcoma, giant cell tumor, chondrosarcoma, plasmocytoma and bone metastases) [62]. Furthermore, TIL's lytic activity was significantly higher compared to autologous peripheral blood leukocytes. Moreover, TIL extracted from rat osteosarcoma were very sensitive to the tumor antigens expressed by autologous tumor cells and demonstrated increased proliferation [63]. These findings strongly support the potential capability of TIL therapy for osteosarcoma.

In 1992, Rivoltini *et al.* mentioned that TIL obtained from pediatric patients were difficult to use for immunotherapy at required levels [59]. However, since then, *in vitro* culture methods have shown great advances. Now, one of the most important conditions of T cell immunotherapy is their anergic/tolerant manner against tumor cells [63]. It has been reported that the Fas-mediated apoptosis pathway plays a crucial role in this condition [63,64]. However, these poor immune responses could be normalized on *in vitro* culture [65,66]. Furthermore, immunotherapy in combination with chemotherapeutic agents induces anti-tumor effects in Fas-mediated apoptosis resistant tumors [67–69]. Moreover, interferon (IFN)-γ sensitizes osteosarcoma cells to Fas-induced apoptosis through upregulation of Fas receptor [70]. Combined immunotherapy with IFN-γ and either anti-Fas monoclonal antibody or CTL-bearing Fas ligand (FasL) might be useful. Then, TIL remains a very viable arm of immunotherapy for osteosarcoma as clinical phase-II trials in melanoma [70,71] (Figure 34.1).

Except for tumor immune escape, in osteosarcoma, the Fas/FasL pathway plays a crucial role in chemotherapy-induced apoptosis [69] and metastasis [70,73,74]. Thus, this pathway has been used as a therapeutic target in several strategies [75,76].

Another important factor of T cell therapy is the immunological specificity of T cells for the tumor [63,77]. It is interesting to use *ex vivo*-expanded T cell clones that demonstrate specific lysis of antigen-positive tumor targeting. As shown in a phase-I study in metastatic melanoma, several advantages of the T cell clone strategy were demonstrated without severe toxic side effects [78–80]. Thus, this T cell clone strategy will be able to achieve more effective and less toxic T cell therapy for osteosarcomas.

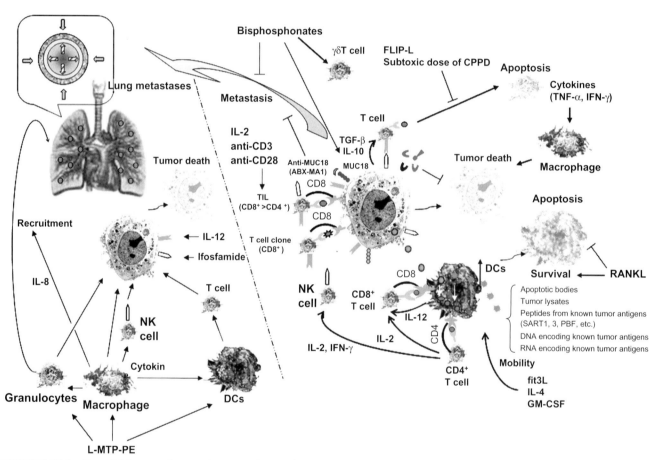

FIGURE 34.1 Potential immunotherapeutic approaches against osteosarcoma cells. T cells, such as TIL and NK cells, directly attack tumor cells in an MHC-restricted manner or not, according to their populations. Administration of DCs induces upregulation of T cells by presenting peptides by an MHC-restricted manner and also directly targets against tumor cells. For priming DCs, several strategies were identified. Cytokines' networks stimulate immune therapeutic cells. Administration of peptides (L-MTP-PE) and cytokines (TNF-α, IFN-γ) stimulate macrophages. Bisphosphonates have potential anti-tumor effects as metastasis inhibitors and modulate immune response as γδT-cells activators. RANKL can not only prolong the survival time of DCs, but also induce T cell growth. OPG acts as a decoy receptor of TRAIL. Left insert: Shadow arrow: central necrosis induced by standard chemotherapy agents, arrow: peripheral fibrosis induced by L-MTP-PE treatment. CAMs: cell adhesion molecules, CDDP: cisplatin, DCs: dendritic cells, fit3L: fit3 ligand, FLIP-L: FLICE inhibitory protein long form, FasL: Fas ligand, GM-CSF: granulocyte macrophage-colony stimulating factor, IFN: interferon, IL: interleukin, L-MTP-PE: liposome-encapsulated muramyl tripeptide phosphatidylethanolamine, RANKL: Receptor Activator of Nuclear Factor-κB ligand, OPG: osteoprotegerin, PBF: papillomavirus binding factor, SART1, 3: squamous cell carcinoma antigen recognized by T cells 1, 3, TCR: T cell receptor, TGF-β: transforming growth factor-β, TIL: tumor-infiltrating lymphocytes, TNF-α: tumor necrosis factor-α, TRAIL: TNF-related apoptosis-inducing ligand. TRAILR: TRAIL receptor.

C. Natural Killer (NK) Cells and T Cell Lines

NK cells have innate anti-tumor functions upon tumor regression [81]. TALL-104 is endowed with MHC non-restricted killer activity against a broad range of tumors across several species, sparing cells from normal tissues [82]. TALL-104 cells were administrated systemically in an adjuvant setting to 23 cases of canine osteosarcoma after surgery and chemotherapy [83]. This therapy achieved favorable median survival times and disease-free intervals compared with canine osteosarcoma treated with standard therapy, and supported the efficacy of adjuvant TALL-104 cell administration. In this series, as severe side effects including TALL-104 cell-induced leukemia were not observed, this strategy is worthwhile to try in humans.

To upregulate NK cell-mediated anti-tumor function, some strategies have been envisaged (cytokines are mentioned above). Kubista *et al.* have reported that hyperthermia increases the susceptibility of osteosarcoma cells to NK-mediated lysis by increased expression of heat shock proteins (hsp) 72 (84). Hsp 72, implicated in tumor immunity [85], is involved in the interaction between T lymphocytes and hsp72+ osteosarcoma cells [86].

IV. SUMMARY AND FUTURE TRENDS

There is no doubt that one of the most significant advances in the field of anti-cancer therapy has been the development of immunotherapy. However, the initial results of human trials were not realized as expected. The reason for this discrepancy has been detailed in a number of issues [63,87], and it is common knowledge that the tumor burden contributes to a significant suppressive environment. Surgery remains the most effective method for debulking tumors and radiation and/or chemotherapy can be used for the removal of remaining and micro-metastatic lesions as well as reducing tumor burden. To achieve desired results, immunotherapies combined with these conventional treatments are recommended.

Incidentally, the number of published data of immunotherapy for bone tumors is very low compared with that of other solid tumors. The reasons for this delay were discussed elsewhere [50,88] and the following reasons were raised: (1) the relatively low immunogenicity of osteosarcoma as only a few examples of spontaneous tumor regression exist [89,90]; (2) the practical difficulty in establishing osteosarcoma cell lines and autologous CTL [91,92]; and (3) the lack of suitable candidate genes for a reverse immunological approach such as a tumor-specific fusion gene [93,94]. However, another hopeful explanation of this delay resides in environmental factors peculiar to bone.

Studies have clarified interesting molecules, receptor activator of nuclear factor-κB ligand (RANKL)/RANK/ osteoprotegerin (OPG), the key regulators of normal and pathological bone metabolism [95–99]. Thus, correlations between the phenotypes of the tumors and changes of RANKL/OPG have been reported [100]. In osteosarcoma, high OPG [101,102] and lack of RANKL at the mRNA level [103] have been reported. To prevent bone destruction due to malignancies, the potential capability of these molecules as therapeutic tools has been proposed [104–107].

Furthermore, direct effects of RANKL/RANK/OPG on the immune response were reported. Specifically, RANKL can dramatically inhibit DCs apoptosis via increased Bcl-x_L expression [108] and induce T cell growth [109]. OPG acts as a weak decoy receptor for TNF-related apoptosis-inducing ligands (TRAIL) [110] and modulates tumor apoptosis [111]. In addition, functional RANK expression on osteosarcoma cells has been reported [112,113]. Targeting RANKL/RANK/OPG should provide a gospel in osteosarcoma treatment.

Bisphosphonates (BPs) can be another therapeutic approach for osteosarcoma [114]. Except for the known function of BPs, the inhibitory effects of BPs on the metastases as well as the potent anti-cancer effect have been suggested [115,116]. Moreover, as BPs can activate γδ-T cells involved in tumor cell surveillance and killing [117], the ability of BPs as γδ-T cell activators is encouraged for further immunotherapy. These results provide the rationale to use these molecules in immunotherapy for osteosarcoma. However, the safety administration of these agents in humans should be addressed carefully.

In conclusion, to date, the limited number of published clinical trials of immunotherapy for osteosarcoma has been reported. However, as mentioned above, there is much evidence that strongly supports the potential capabilities of immunotherapy to eradicate osteosarcoma in combination with conventional treatment. Mainly, osteosarcoma patients die from lung metastasis; its control is very important as well as its primary site. Immunotherapy for osteosarcomas is full of potential capabilities promising hopeful and drastic improvements in the survival rate and quality of life in patients with this tumor.

References

1. A.J. Renard, R.P. Veth & H.W. Schreuder, et al., Osteosarcoma: oncologic and functional results. A single institutional report covering 22 years, J Surg Oncol 72 (1999) 124–129.
2. G. Bacci, A. Briccoli & S. Ferrari, et al., Neoadjuvant chemotherapy for osteosarcoma of the extremity. Long-term results of the Rizzoli's 4th protocol, Eur J Cancer 37 (2001) 2030–2039.
3. J. Banchereau & A.K. Palucka, Dendritic cells as therapeutic vaccines against cancer, Nat Rev Immunol 5 (2005) 296–306.
4. R.M. Steinman & M. Dhodapkar, Active immunization against cancer with dendritic cells: the near future, Int J Cancer 94 (2001) 459–473.

5. J. Geiger, R. Hutchinson & L. Hohenkirk, et al., Treatment of solid tumours in children with tumour-lysate-pulsed dendritic cells, Lancet 356 (2000) 1163–1165.

6. K. Mori, K. Ando & D. Heymann, Liposomal muramyl tripeptide phosphatidyl ethanolamine: a safe and effective agent against osteosarcoma pulmonary metastases, Expert Rev Anticancer Ther 8 (2008) 151–159.

7. P.A. Meyers, C.L. Schwartz & M. Krailo, et al., Osteosarcoma: a randomized, prospective trial of the addition of ifosfamide and/or muramyl tripeptide to cisplatin, doxorubicin, and high-dose methotrexate, J Clin Oncol 23 (2005) 2004–2011.

8. P. Anderson, Liposomal muranyl tripeptide phosphatidyl ethanolamine: ifosfamide-containing chemotherapy in osteosarcoma, Future Oncol 2 (2006) 333–343.

9. E.S. Kleinerman, A.K. Raymond & C.D. Bucana, et al., Unique histological changes in lung metastases of osteosarcoma patients following therapy with liposomal muramyl tripeptide (CGP 19835A lipid), Cancer Immunol Immunother 34 (1992) 211–220.

10. M.A. Gianan & E.S. Kleinerman, Liposomal muramyl tripeptide (CGP 19835A lipid) therapy for resectable melanoma in patients who were at high risk for relapse: an update, Cancer Biother Radiopharm 13 (1998) 363–368.

11. G.K. Koukoulis, C. Patriarca & V.E. Gould, Adhesion molecules and tumor metastasis, Hum Pathol 29 (1998) 889–892.

12. E.C. McGary, A. Heimberger & L. Mills, et al., A fully human antimelanoma cellular adhesion molecule/MUC18 antibody inhibits spontaneous pulmonary metastasis of osteosarcoma cells *in vivo*, Clin Cancer Res 9 (2003) 6560–6566.

13. J.W. Eklund & T.M. Kuzel, A review of recent findings involving interleukin-2-based cancer therapy, Curr Opin Oncol 16 (2004) 542–546.

14. R. Luksch, D. Perotti & G. Cefalo, et al., Immunomodulation in a treatment program including pre- and post-operative interleukin-2 and chemotherapy for childhood osteosarcoma, Tumori 3 (2003) 263–268.

15. S. Nasr, J. McKolanis & R. Pais, et al., A phase I study of interleukin-2 in children with cancer and evaluation of clinical immunologic status during therapy, Cancer 64 (1989) 783–788.

16. E. Mariani, A. Meneghetti & A. Tarozzi, et al., Interleukin-12 induces efficient lysis of natural killer-sensitive and natural killer-resistant human osteosarcoma cells: the synergistic effect of interleukin-2, Scand J Immunol 51 (2000) 618–625.

17. T. Okamoto, N. Yamada & T. Tsujimura, et al., Inhibition by interleukin-18 of the growth of Dunn osteosarcoma cells, J Interferon Cytokine Res 24 (2004) 161–167.

18. L.L. Worth, S.F. Jia & Z. Zhou, et al., Intranasal therapy with an adenoviral vector containing the murine interleukin-12 gene eradicates osteosarcoma lung metastases, Clin Cancer Res 6 (2000) 3713–3718.

19. M.C. Honorati, S. Neri & L. Cattini, et al., IL-17 enhances the susceptibility of U-2 OS osteosarcoma cells to NK cell lysis, Clin Exp Immunol 3 (2003) 344–349.

20. E.A. Lafleur, S.F. Jia & L.L. Worth, et al., Interleukin (IL)-12 and IL-12 gene transfer up-regulate Fas expression in human osteosarcoma and breast cancer cells, Cancer Res 61 (2001) 4066–4071.

21. T. Tamura, T. Nishi & T. Goto, et al., Combination of IL-12 and IL-18 of electrogene therapy synergistically inhibits tumor growth, Anticancer Res 23 (2003) 1173–1179.

22. C. Liebau, C. Roesel & S. Schmidt, et al., Immunotherapy by gene transfer with plasmids encoding IL-12/IL-18 is superior to IL-23/IL-18 gene transfer in a rat osteosarcoma model, Anticancer Res 24 (2004) 2861–2867.

23. X. Duan, Z. Zhou & S.F. Jia, et al., Interleukin-12 enhances the sensitivity of human osteosarcoma cells to 4-hydroperoxycyclophosphamide by a mechanism involving the Fas/Fas-ligand pathway, Clin Cancer Res 10 (2004) 777–783.

24. X. Duan, S.F. Jia & N. Koshkina, et al., Intranasal interleukin-12 gene therapy enhanced the activity of ifosfamide against osteosarcoma lung metastases, Cancer 106 (2006) 1382–1388.

25. G. Brandacher, C. Winkler & K. Schroecksnadel, et al., Antitumoral activity of interferon-gamma involved in impaired immune function in cancer patients, Curr Drug Metab 7 (2006) 599–612.

26. I.D. Kurzman, F. Shi & D.M. Vail, et al., *In vitro* and *in vivo* enhancement of canine pulmonary alveolar macrophage cytotoxic activity against canine osteosarcoma cells, Cancer Biother Radiopharm 14 (1999) 121–128.

27. S.C. Ko, J. Cheon & C. Kao, et al., Osteocalcin promoter-based toxic gene therapy for the treatment of osteosarcoma in experimental models, Cancer Res 56 (1996) 4614–4619.

28. H. Tsuji, S. Kawaguchi & T. Wada, et al., Concurrent induction of T-cell activation and apoptosis of osteosarcoma cells by adenovirus-mediated B7–1/Fas chimeric gene transfer, Cancer Gene Ther 10 (2003) 717–725.

29. H.J. Xu, Y. Zhou & J. Seigne, et al., Enhanced tumor suppressor gene therapy via replication-deficient adenovirus vectors expressing an N-terminal truncated retinoblastoma protein, Cancer Res 56 (1996) 2245–2249.

30. M. Kim, M. Sgagias & X. Deng, et al., Apoptosis induced by adenovirus-mediated p14ARF expression in U2OS osteosarcoma cells is associated with increased Fas expression, Biochem Biophys Res Commun 320 (2004) 138–144.

31. M. Nakase, M. Inui & K. Okumura, et al., p53 gene therapy of human osteosarcoma using a transferrin-modified cationic liposome, Mol Cancer Ther 4 (2005) 625–631.

32. O.J. Hellwinkel, J. Muller & A. Pollmann, et al., Osteosarcoma cell lines display variable individual reactions on wildtype p53 and Rb tumour-suppressor transgenes, J Gene Med 7 (2005) 407–419.

33. M.L. Edelstein, M.R. Abedi & J. Wixon, et al., Gene therapy clinical trials worldwide 1989–2004—an overview, J Gene Med 6 (2003) 597–602.

34. S. Nagano, K. Yuge & M. Fukunaga, et al., Gene therapy eradicating distant disseminated micro-metastases by optimal cytokine expression in the primary lesion only: novel concepts for successful cytokine gene therapy, Int J Oncol 24 (2004) 549–558.

35. W. Gu, A. Ogose & H. Kawashima, et al., High-level expression of the coxsackievirus and adenovirus receptor messenger RNA in osteosarcoma, Ewing's sarcoma, and benign neurogenic tumors among musculoskeletal tumors, Clin Cancer Res 10 (2004) 3831–3838.

36. H.C. Graat, P.I. Wuisman & V.W. van Beusechem, et al., Coxsackievirus and adenovirus receptor expression on

primary osteosarcoma specimens and implications for gene therapy with recombinant adenoviruses, Clin Cancer Res 11 (2005) 2445–2447.

37. A.M. Witlox, V.W. Van Beusechem & B. Molenaar, et al., Conditionally replicative adenovirus with tropism expanded towards integrins inhibits osteosarcoma tumor growth *in vitro* and *in vivo*, Clin Cancer Res 10 (2004) 61–67.

38. S.E. Raper, N. Chirmule & F.S. Lee, et al., Fatal systemic inflammatory response syndrome in a ornithine transcarbamylase deficient patient following adenoviral gene transfer, Mol Genet Metab 80 (2003) 148–158.

39. R. Pellinen, T. Hakkarainen & T. Wahlfors, et al., Cancer cells as targets for lentivirus-mediated gene transfer and gene therapy, Int J Oncol 25 (2004) 1753–1762.

40. A. Ketola, A.M. Maatta & T. Pasanen, et al., Osteosarcoma and chondrosarcoma as targets for virus vectors and herpes simplex virus thymidine kinase/ganciclovir gene therapy, Int J Mol Med 13 (2004) 705–710.

41. P. Van Der Bruggen, Y. Zhang & P. Chaux, et al., Tumor-specific shared antigenic peptides recognized by human T cells, Immunol Rev 188 (2002) 51–64.

42. Y. Kawakami, T. Fujita & C. Kudo, et al., Dendritic cell based personalized immunotherapy based on cancer antigen research, Front Biosci 13 (2008) 1952–1958.

43. S.A. Rosenberg, N.P. Restifo & J.C. Yang, et al., Adoptive cell transfer: a clinical path to effective cancer immunotherapy, Nat Rev Cancer 8 (2008) 299–308.

44. M.E. Dudley & S.A. Rosenberg, Adoptive cell transfer therapy, Semin Oncol 34 (2007) 524–531.

45. H.Y. Wang & R.F. Wang, Regulatory T cells and cancer, Curr Opin Immunol 19 (2007) 217–223.

46. H.Y. Wang & R.F. Wang, Antigen-specific CD4+ regulatory T cells in cancer: implications for immunotherapy, Microbes Infect 7 (2005) 1056–1062.

47. T. Sudo, T. Kuramoto & S. Komiya, et al., Expression of MAGE genes in osteosarcoma, J Orthop Res 15 (1997) 128–132.

48. H. Ishida, S. Komiya, Y. Inoue, et al., Expression of the SART1 tumor-rejection antigen in human osteosarcomas, Int J Oncol 17 (2000) 29–32.

48. E.S. Kleinerman, J.B. Gano & D.A. Johnston, et al., Efficacy of liposomal muramyl tripeptide (CGP 19835A) in the treatment of relapsed osteosarcoma, Am J Clin Oncol 18 (1995) 93–99.

49. N. Tsuda, K. Murayama & H. Ishida, et al., Expression of a newly defined tumor-rejection antigen SART3 in musculoskeletal tumors and induction of HLA class I-restricted cytotoxic T lymphocytes by SART3-derived peptides, J Orthop Res 19 (2001) 346–351.

50. T. Tsukahara, Y. Nabeta & S. Kawaguchi, et al., Identification of human autologous cytotoxic T-lymphocyte-defined osteosarcoma gene that encodes a transcriptional regulator, papillomavirus binding factor, Cancer Res 64 (2004) 5442–5448.

51. H. Ishikura, H. Ikeda & H. Abe, et al., Identification of CLUAP1 as a human osteosarcoma tumor-associated antigen recognized by the humoral immune system, Int J Oncol 30 (2007) 461–467.

52. D. Yang, M. Nakao & S. Shichijo, et al., Identification of a gene coding for a protein possessing shared tumor epitopes capable of inducing HLA-A24-restricted cytotoxic T lymphocytes in cancer patients, Cancer Res 59 (1999) 4056–4063.

53. M. Ito, S. Shichijo & Y. Miyagi, et al., Identification of SART3-derived peptides capable of inducing HLA-A2-restricted and tumor-specific CTLs in cancer patients with different HLA-A2 subtypes, Int J Cancer 88 (2000) 633–639.

54. T. Imanishi, T. Akazawa & A. Kimura, et al., Allele and haplotype frequencies for HLA and complement loci in various ethnic groups, in: K. Tsuji, M. Akizawa & T. Sasazuki (Eds.) HLA, 1991, vol. 1, Oxford Scientific Publications, Oxford, 1992, pp. 1065–1220.

55. Y. Miyagi, N. Imai & T. Sasatomi, et al., Induction of cellular immune responses to tumor cells and peptides in colorectal cancer patients by vaccination with SART3 peptides, Clin Cancer Res 7 (2001) 3950–3962.

56. D. Jäger, Potential target antigens for immunotherapy identified by serological expression cloning (SEREX), Methods Mol Biol 360 (2007) 319–326.

57. C.G. Drake, E. Jaffee & D.M. Pardoll, Mechanisms of immune evasion by tumors, Adv Immunol 90 (2006) 51–81.

58. K. Trieb, T. Lechleitner & S. Lang, et al., Evaluation of HLA-DR expression and T-lymphocyte infiltration in osteosarcoma, Pathol Res Pract 194 (1998) 679–684.

59. L. Rivoltini, F. Arienti & A. Orazi, et al., Phenotypic and functional analysis of lymphocytes infiltrating paediatric tumours, with a characterization of the tumour phenotype, Cancer Immunol Immunother 34 (1992) 241–251.

60. S.A. Rosenberg, P. Spiess & R. Lafreniere, A new approach to the adoptive immunotherapy of cancer with tumor-infiltrating lymphocytes, Science 233 (1986) 1318–1321.

61. P. Aebersold, C. Hyatt & S. Johnson, et al., Lysis of autologous melanoma cells by tumor-infiltrating lymphocytes: association with clinical response, J Natl Cancer Inst 83 (1991) 932–937.

62. S. Théoleyre, K. Mori & B. Cherrier, et al., Phenotypic and functional analysis of lymphocytes infiltrating osteolytic tumors: use as a new therapeutic approach of osteosarcoma, BMC Cancer 5 (2005) 123.

63. W. Zou, Immunosuppressive networks in the tumour environment and their therapeutic relevance, Nat Rev Cancer 5 (2005) 263–274.

64. J. O'Connell, M.W. Bennett & G.C. O'Sullivan, et al., The Fas counter attack: Fas mediated T cell killing by colon cancer cells expressing Fas ligand, J Exp Med 184 (1996) 1075–1082.

65. Y.M. Chen, W.K. Yang & J. Whang-Peng, et al., Restoration of the immunocompetence by IL-2 activation and TCR-CD3 engagement of the *in vivo* energized tumor-specific CTL from lung cancer patients, J Immunother 20 (1997) 354–364.

66. E. Tartour, S. Latour & C. Mathiot, et al., Variable expression of CD3-zeta chain in tumor-infiltrating lymphocytes (TIL) derived from renal-cell carcinoma: relationship with TIL phenotype and function, Int J Cancer 63 (1995) 205–212.

67. P. Frost & B. Bonavida, Circumvention of tumor cell escape following specific immunotherapy, Cancer Biother Radiopharmacol 15 (2000) 141–152.

68. H. . Kinoshita, H. Yoshikawa & K. Shiiki, et al., Cysplatin (CDDP) sensitizes human osteosarcoma cell to Fas/CD95-mediated apoptosis by down-regulating FLIP-L expression, Int J Cancer 88 (2000) 986–991.

69. X. Duan, Z. Zhou & S.F. Jia, et al., Interleukin-12 enhances the sensitivity of human osteosarcoma cells to 4-hydroperoxycyclophosphamide by a mechanism involving the Fas/Fas-ligand pathway, Clin Cancer Res 10 (2004) 777–783.

70. H. Inaba, M. Glibetic & S. Buck, et al., Interferon-gamma sensitizes osteosarcoma cells to fas-induced apoptosis by up-regulating fas receptors and caspase-8, Pediatr Blood Cancer 43 (2004) 729–736.

71. N. Labarriere, M.C. Pandolfino & N. Gervois, et al., Therapeutic efficacy of melanoma-reactive TIL injected in stage III melanoma patients, Cancer Immunol Immunother 51 (2002) 532–538.

72. B. Dreno, J.M. Nguyen & A. Khammari, et al., Randomized trial of adoptive transfer of melanoma tumor-infiltrating lymphocytes as adjuvant therapy for stage III melanoma, Cancer Immunol Immunother 51 (2002) 539–546.

73. L.L. Worth, E.A. Lafleur & S.F. Jia, et al., Fas expression inversely correlates with metastatic potential in osteosarcoma cells, Oncol Rep 9 (2002) 823–827.

74. E.A. Lafleur, N.V. Koshkina & J. Stewart, et al., Increased Fas expression reduces the metastatic potential of human osteosarcoma cells, Clin Cancer Res 10 (2004) 8114–8119.

75. T. Imai, S. Adachi & K. Nishijo, et al., FR901228 induces tumor regression associated with induction of Fas ligand and activation of Fas signaling in human osteosarcoma cells, Oncogene 22 (2003) 9231–9242.

76. K. Watanabe, K. Okamoto & S. Yonehara, Sensitization of osteosarcoma cells to death receptor-mediated apoptosis by HDAC inhibitors through downregulation of cellular FLIP, Cell Death Differ 12 (2005) 10–18.

77. C. Yee, J.A. Thompson & D. Byrd, et al., Adoptive T cell therapy using antigen-specific CD8+ T cell clones for the treatment of patients with metastatic melanoma: *in vivo* persistence, migration, and antitumor effect of transferred T cells, Proc Natl Acad Sci USA 99 (2002) 16168–16173.

78. S.R. Reynolds, E. Celis & A. Sette, et al., HLA-independent heterogeneity of CD8+ T cell responses to MAGE-3, Melan-A/MART-1, gp100, tyrosinase, MC1R, and TRP-2 in vaccine-treated melanoma patients, J Immunol 161 (1998) 6970–6976.

79. B. Thurner, I. Haendle & C. Roder, et al., Vaccination with mage-3A1 peptide-pulsed mature, monocyte-derived dendritic cells expands specific cytotoxic T cells and induces regression of some metastases in advanced stage IV melanoma, J Exp Med 190 (1999) 1669–1678.

80. S.A. Rosenberg, J.C. Yang & D.J. Schwartzentruber, et al., Immunologic and therapeutic evaluation of a systemic peptide vaccine for the treatment of patient with metastatic melanoma, Nat Med 4 (1998) 321–327.

81. J. O'Shea & J.R. Ortaldo, The biology of natural killer cells: insights into molecular basis of function, in: C.E. Lewis & J.O. McGee (Eds.) The Natural Killer Cell, IRL Press, Oxford, 1992, pp. 2–40.

82. A. Cesano & D. Santoli, Two unique human leukemic T-cell lines endowed with stable cytotoxic function and different spectrum of target reactivity. Analysis and modulation of their lytic mechanisms, In vitro Cell Dev Biol 28 (1992) 657–662.

83. S. Visonneau, A. Cesano & K.A. Jeglum, et al., Adjuvant treatment of canine osteosarcoma with the human cytotoxic T-cell line TALL-104, Clin Cancer Res 5 (1999) 1868–1875.

84. B. Kubista, K. Trieb & H. Blahovec, et al., Hyperthermia increases the susceptibility of chondro- and osteosarcoma cells to natural killer cell-mediated lysis, Anticancer Res 22 (2002) 789–792.

85. C. Castelli, L. Rivoltini & F. Rini, et al., Heat shock proteins: biological functions and clinical application as personalized vaccines for human cancer, Cancer Immunol Immunother 53 (2004) 227–233.

86. K. Trieb, S. Lang & R. Kotz, Heat-shock protein 72 in human osteosarcoma: T-lymphocytes reactivity and cytotoxicity, Pediatr Hematol Oncol 17 (2000) 355–364.

87. J.R. Yannelli & J.M. Wroblewski, On the road to a tumor cell vaccine: 20 years of cellular immunotherapy, Vaccine 23 (2004) 97–113.

88. S. Ben-Efraim, Cancer immunotherapy: hopes and pitfalls: a review, Anticancer Res 16 (1996) 3235–3240.

89. Y. Ogihara, K. Takeda & T. Yanagawa, et al., Spontaneous regression of lung metastases from osteosarcoma, Cancer 74 (1994) 2798–2803.

90. J.M. Sabate, J. Llauger & S. Torrubia, et al., Osteosarcoma of the abdominal wall with spontaneous regression of lung metastases, Am J Roentgenol 171 (1998) 691–692.

91. Y. Nabeta, S. Kawaguchi & H. Sahara, et al., Recognition by cellular and humoral autologous immunity in a human osteosarcoma cell line, J Orthop Sci 8 (2003) 554–559.

92. S.F. Slovin, R.D. Lackman & S. Ferrone, et al., Cellular immune response to human sarcomas: cytotoxic T cell clones reactive with autologous sarcomas. I. Development, phenotype, and specificity, J Immunol 137 (1986) 3042–3048.

93. Y. Sato, Y. Nabeta & T. Tsukahara, et al., Detection and induction of CTLs specific for SYT-SSX-derived peptides in HLA-A24(+) patients with synovial sarcoma, J Immunol 169 (2002) 1611–1618.

94. B.S. Worley, L.T. van den Broeke & T.J. Goletz, et al., Antigenicity of fusion proteins from sarcoma-associated chromosomal translocations, Cancer Res 61 (2001) 6868–6875.

95. H. Hsu, D.L. Lacey & C.R. Dunstan, et al., Tumor necrosis factor receptor family member RANK mediates osteoclast differentiation and activation induced by osteoprotegerin ligand, Proc Natl Acad Sci USA 96 (1999) 3540–3545.

96. P. Honore, N.M. Luger & M.A. Sabino, et al., Osteoprotegerin blocks bone cancer-induced skeletal destruction, skeletal pain and pain-related neurochemical reorganization of the spinal cord, Nat Med 6 (2000) 521–528.

97. W.S. Simonet, D.L. Lacey & C.R. Dunstan, et al., Osteoprotegerin: a novel secreted protein involved in the regulation of bone density, Cell 89 (1997) 309–319.

98. E. Tsuda, M. Goto & S. Mochizuki, et al., Isolation of a novel cytokine from human fibroblasts that specifically inhibits osteoclastogenesis, Biochem Biophys Res Commun 234 (1997) 137–142.

99. H. Yasuda, N. Shima & N. Nakagawa, et al., Osteoclast differentiation factor is a ligand for osteoprotegerin/osteoclastogenesis-inhibitory factor and is identical to TRANCE/RANKL, Proc Natl Acad Sci USA 95 (1998) 3597–3602.

100. E. Grimaud, L. Soubigou & S. Couillaud, et al., Receptor activator of nuclear factor kappaB ligand (RANKL)/osteoprotegerin (OPG) ratio is increased in severe osteolysis, Am J Pathol 163 (2003) 2021–2031.

101. L.C. Hofbauer, C.R. Dunstan & T.C. Spelsberg, et al., Osteoprotegerin production by human osteoblast lineage cells is stimulated by vitamin D, bone morphogenetic protein-2, and cytokines, Biochem Biophys Res Commun 250 (1998) 776–781.

102. L.C. Hofbauer, F. Gori & B.L. Riggs, et al., Stimulation of osteoprotegerin ligand and inhibition of osteoprotegerin production by glucocorticoids in human osteoblastic lineage cells: potential paracrine mechanisms of glucocorticoid-induced osteoporosis, Endocrinology 140 (1999) 4382–4389.

103. P. Bhatia, R.J. Leach & G.D. Roodman, Loss of RANKL, a TNF-alpha ligand family member, in sporadic osteosarcoma, J Bone Miner Res 14 (Suppl 1) (1999) F037.

104. Y. Wittrant, S. Theoleyre & C. Chipoy, et al., RANKL/RANK/OPG: new therapeutic targets in bone tumours and associated osteolysis, Biochim Biophys Acta 1704 (2004) 49–57.

105. F. Lamoureux, P. Richard & Y. Wittrant, et al., Therapeutic relevance of osteoprotegerin gene therapy in osteosarcoma: blockade of the vicious cycle between tumor cell proliferation and bone resorption, Cancer Res 67 (2007) 7308–7318.

106. F. Lamoureux, G. Picarda & J. Rousseau, et al., Therapeutic efficacy of soluble receptor activator of nuclear factor-kappa B-Fc delivered by nonviral gene transfer in a mouse model of osteolytic osteosarcoma, Mol Cancer Ther 7 (2008) 3389–3398.

107. B. Brounais, C. Ruiz & J. Rousseau, et al., Novel anti-cancer strategy in bone tumors by targeting molecular and cellular modulators of bone resorption, Recent Patents Anticancer Drug Discov 3 (2008) 178–186.

108. B.R. Wong, R. Josien & S.Y. Lee, et al., TRANCE (tumor necrosis factor (TNF)-related activation-induced cytokine), a new TNF family member predominantly expressed in T cells, is a dendritic cell-specific survival factor, J Exp Med 186 (1997) 2075–2080.

109. D.M. Anderson, E. Maraskovsky & W.L. Billingsley, et al., A homologue of the TNF receptor and its ligand enhance T-cell growth and dendritic-cell function, Nature 390 (1997) 175–179.

110. J.G. Emery, P. McDonnell & M.B. Burke, et al., Osteoprotegerin is a receptor for the cytotoxic ligand TRAIL, J Biol Chem 273 (1998) 14363–14367.

111. R. Nyambo, N. Cross & J. Lippitt, et al., Human bone marrow stromal cells protect prostate cancer cells from TRAIL-induced apoptosis, J Bone Miner Res 19 (2004) 1712–1721.

112. Y. Wittrant, F. Lamoureux & K. Mori, et al., RANKL directly induces bone morphogenetic protein-2 expression in RANK-expressing POS-1 osteosarcoma cells, Int J Oncol 28 (2006) 261–269.

113. K. Mori, B. Le Goff & M. Berreur, et al., Human osteosarcoma cells express functional receptor activator of nuclear factor-kappa B, J Pathol 211 (2007) 555–562.

114. D. Heymann, B. Ory & F. Blanchard, et al., Enhanced tumor regression and tissue repair when zoledronic acid is combined with ifosfamide in rat osteosarcoma, Bone 37 (2005) 74–86.

115. D. Heymann, B. Ory & F. Gouin, et al., Bisphosphonates: new therapeutic agents for the treatment of bone tumors, Trends Mol Med 10 (2004) 337–343.

116. B. Ory, M.F. Heymann & A. Kamijo, et al., Zoledronic acid suppresses lung metastases and prolongs overall survival of osteosarcoma-bearing mice, Cancer 104 (2005) 2522–2529.

117. J.M. Sanders, S. Ghosh & J.M. Chan, et al., Quantitative structure-activity relationships for gammadelta T cell activation by bisphosphonates, J Med Chem 47 (2004) 375–384.

CHAPTER **35**

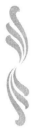

Bisphosphonates, Bone Health and the Clinical Biology of Bone Metastases from Breast Cancer

ALEXANDER H.G. PATERSON

Department of Medicine, Tom Baker Cancer Centre, University of Calgary, Alberta, Canada.

Contents

I. INTRODUCTION

One of the first to observe and document the propensity of cancers of the breast to metastasize to bone was Stephen Paget who reported on the site distribution of metastases in a series of 735 cases of breast cancer, arguing that the frequent association of breast cancer metastases in bone could not be by chance alone. He wrote in the *Lancet* in 1889: 'The evidence seems to be irresistible that in cancer of the breast, the bones suffer in a special way, which cannot be explained by any theory of embolism alone' [1]. Paget also popularized the 'seed and soil' hypothesis. He wrote: 'the best work in pathology of cancer is done by those who... are

studying the nature of the seed... observations of the properties of the soil may also be useful'.

This notion that there might be a local reason for the development of metastases at specific sites beyond a chance colonization following embolism was given a mechanistic twist by Batson [2], who described the connection between the vertebral venous plexus and the bone marrow spaces, hypothesizing a retrograde spread that would allow metastases from a primary prostate cancer to lodge preferentially in the lower vertebrae. Once within the marrow space, metastases have a blood supply for further growth. Mundy has taken the 'seed and soil' idea one step further by adding the concept of a 'vicious cycle', with products from tumor-induced breakdown of bone leading to stimulation and further growth of malignant cells [3,4].

II. INCIDENCE

A. Prevalence and Survival

Coleman and Rubens [5] reported in 1987 that in 587 patients dying of breast cancer, 69% had radiological evidence of bone metastases before death compared to lung and liver metastases (27% each). In this report describing 2240 patients presenting with breast cancer and followed for a median of 5 years, 47% of those relapsing at distant sites relapsed in bone. It is likely that with modern radiological techniques of magnetic resonance imaging this proportion would be found to be higher today.

National Surgical Adjuvant Breast and Bowel Project (NSABP) data also show that bone metastases account for the highest proportion of first sites of distant relapse in breast cancer patients after adjuvant therapy. Nearly half of the patients who developed distant metastases did so in bone either as the sole site of recurrence or simultaneously with other sites of disease. The annual rate of bone metastasis development was higher in node positive patients (approximately 2% per annum) than in node negative (approximately 1% per annum) and higher in ER positive patients than in ER negative [6]. Recurrence rates in bone in current NSABP trials seem to be lower than at the time of the above NSABP report, probably due to a reduced rate of recurrence at all sites (except the central nervous system) because of more effective therapies.

The survival of patients diagnosed with bone metastases also appears to be improving at a rate that cannot be solely explained by diagnostic lead time alone. Over 20 years ago we assessed the median survival of patients diagnosed with bone metastases to be around 16 months. Survival was greater for patients originally presenting with a Stage 1 primary than those presenting with a Stage 2 primary which in turn was greater than for those presenting with a Stage 3 primary [7]. This phenomenon was originally termed 'biological pre-determinism' and described the generally slower growth of metastases from smaller primary tumors with the idea that small tumors were not necessarily small because they were 'early' but because they were growing slowly. The phenomenon is likely to be explained by differing intrinsic genetics of smaller presenting tumors compared to larger ones. In the NSABP series of patients diagnosed in the 1990s the median survival from diagnosis of bone metastases was between 18 and 20 months [6]. During a similar observation period, Coleman and Rubens reported a median survival in the order of 24 months [5].

III. DIAGNOSIS AND TYPES OF BONE METASTASES

The clinical diagnosis of bone metastases can vary from the obvious to the uncertain. Patients who have had a primary breast cancer and who develop bone pain, x-ray evidence of multiple osteolytic, osteosclerotic or mixed lesions on x-ray with typical bone scan changes showing multiple areas of asymmetric uptake, and elevation of bone markers usually require no biopsy or further testing for diagnostic certainty. Much harder to diagnose is the patient who may be asymptomatic but has bone scan findings suspicious of metastases but with no confirmatory x-ray changes. Osteoporosis with vertebral fractures can present this way and indeed the two diagnoses may be concurrent. If bone biopsy is impractical, sometimes serial scanning will clarify the diagnosis. The patient can usually start hormone therapy while the diagnosis is being made. Patients with rarer bone diseases such as Paget's disease of bone or bone histiocytosis usually have x-ray changes which are typical. The patient with a solitary area of increased uptake will require bone biopsy for diagnosis. Some of the hardest cases to diagnose are women with one or two areas of uptake on a bone scan but who are asymptomatic with either no changes or minimal radiological changes. In these instances, biopsy under PET or MRI guidance can be helpful. Sometimes a second malignancy such as bladder, renal, lung or colonic cancer will

metastasise to bone in a patient who has had a primary breast cancer. Likewise, myeloma can occur in women with a previous primary breast cancer.

IV. CLINICAL CONSEQUENCES OF BONE METASTASES

Bone metastases in the absence of fracture can be asymptomatic but often lead to a low to moderate grade aching pain. This pain can fluctuate between sites, sometimes over a few days. In the humerus and femur this is exacerbated by weight bearing and can be a sign of impending fracture. Severe localized back pain can herald a vertebral fracture and spinal cord compression.

Vertebral fracture is particularly common and may occur in the absence of metastases. We have shown that patients presenting with breast cancer have a four to five times higher rate of vertebral fracture on follow-up than an age-matched group of well women [8]. This is most likely related to chemotherapy-induced premature menopause with accelerated bone loss. With the increased use of aromatase inhibitors, this increased fracture rate will continue. The trials of aromatase inhibitors versus tamoxifen show that even without specifically looking for fractures by performing regular thoracic vertebral x-rays, by 5 years 3–4% of patients sustain a fracture on aromatase inhibitors—a figure closely approximating the absolute benefit in disease-free survival at 5 years. The fracture rate appears to stabilize after aromatase inhibitors are stopped [9].

The majority of patients with bone metastases will suffer a fracture or fractures at some point during the trajectory of their illness. Patients who have one fracture are more likely to fracture again. Prior to the routine use of bisphosphonates, hypercalcemia would occur in about 25% of patients. With the widespread use of bisphosphonates, hypercalcemia now occurs more commonly as a terminal event. From time to time, a patient on additive hormone therapy will develop hypercalcemia as a 'flare phenomenon'. Cord compression due to vertebral fracture or a paravertebral mass occurs in 1–3% of patients with bone metastases from breast cancer.

V. RESPONSE IN BONE METASTASES

Assessing response to treatment in patients with bone metastases can be difficult since direct observation of shrinkage of a tumor mass within bone cannot be assessed within two or three months as it can at other sites. PET scanning may turn out to be useful here but studies are few. On rare occasions, lytic bone metastases will heal over and the bone will normalize usually over a period of 12 to 18 months. More frequently, in a responding patient the area of the metastasis will show a rim of sclerosis on x-ray indicating new bone formation. Sclerotic bone metastases may show little change over many years of observation.

Bone scanning can be deceptive for disease monitoring and is best used for diagnosis of sites of disease rather than assessment of response since sites where new bone formation is occurring will display as areas of increased uptake. Even the diagnosis of 'new sites' on a report does not necessarily mean progressive disease since these new sites may have been undetectable on initial scanning but with increased turnover associated with healing become visible on follow-up scanning due to an enhanced tumor: background radionuclide uptake ratio.

Elevations of serum alkaline phosphatase and bone markers such as serum or urine N- or C-telopeptides are suggestive of progression of disease in the presence of increased pain and a scan showing new areas of uptake but in the absence of symptoms can occur with a flare reaction.

Sclerotic bone metastases can be very difficult to assess since extension of sclerotic areas is suggestive of progression but in the absence of new symptoms can be compatible with slow healing and clinically stable disease. In these circumstances it is wise to avoid changing therapy until some additional evidence occurs. The clinical diagnosis of response in bone metastases is an old problem and there has been little change in the associated problems over the last 2 decades [10].

VI. PREDICTING BONE METASTASES

A. Micro-metastases in Bone

The ability to predict which patients are likely to develop bone metastases has received increasing attention with the development of bone active medications which hold the possibility of preventing harmful skeletal events and perhaps even bone metastases.

Studies of bone marrow aspirations in patients presenting with primary breast cancer do suggest poorer prognosis in those patients with detectable cancer cells but there is insufficient evidence to support routine use for prediction of clinical bone metastases [11,12]. While the presence of malignant cells within the marrow at the time of presentation of a breast mass seems to be predictive of a greater likelihood of recurrence, this does not necessarily mean that the first site of recurrence will be within bone. This is similar to the lack of clear correlation of the presence of axillary metastases with relapse in the axilla, although these metastases are predictive of relapse at some site.

B. Bone Markers

Bone markers such as N- or C-telopeptide have not been helpful in predicting bone disease, although they can be helpful in following the course of patients with bone metastases. Bone pain in particular may be correlated with rising levels of N-telopeptide in the serum and urine and dosages of bisphophonates may be adjusted to reduce the bone marker levels and sometimes to relieve bone pain [13].

Osteopontin levels correlate with the progression of bone metastases but they do not rise sufficiently early to use clinically as a predictive marker [14]. Other markers which have been assessed for early diagnosis include bone sialoprotein [15], P1NP [16] and serum alkaline phosphatase levels. Bone sialoprotein may be a candidate marker and confirmatory studies are required. In the case of P1NP, elevation and subsequent drop in levels of this marker of bone turnover (both resorption and formation) may predict in some patients for development of bone metastases and inhibition of these metastases by clodronate but it does not appear to be sufficiently frequently expressed to be used as a routine marker of prediction.

Many studies are ongoing using DNA micro-arrays and genetic profiling looking for a pattern predictive of bone metastases [17]. So far, these are not sufficiently developed to be used in the clinic.

VII. BONE PHYSIOLOGY AND TURNOVER

Bone modeling and remodeling are dynamic processes. Modeling occurs in response to poorly understood physical and chemical forces along lines of stress. Remodeling of damaged bone may result from initial stimulation by osteoblasts derived from bone marrow stromal cells [18]. However, osteocytes, developing from maturing osteoblasts and buried within the bone matrix, send out dendritic appendages to form a network connecting both osteoblasts and osteoclasts. This network may be the primary mechanism of response for detecting micro-fractures and initiating repair and the associated physiology has been reviewed by Pearse [19]. Osteoclasts (derived from hematopoietic precursor cells) are recruited to an area of damaged or worn bone. This effete bone is then broken down by the action of proteases (for example, cathepsin K) secreted by the osteoclast to form a bone resorption bay. These proteases destroy hydroxyapatite crystals and collagen; these are then endocytosed at the basal ruffled border of the osteoclast and transported in vesicles to be released at the apical surface into the extra-cellular milieu and thence into the circulation where they can be measured as breakdown products such as N-telopeptides, C-telopeptides, and others.

A major pathway governing osteoclast/osteoblast functioning and bone turnover is the RANK-L/RANK/osteoprotogerin axis. Differentiation and maturation of osteoclasts derived from macrophage/myeloid cell lines requires stimulation by CSF-1 and RANK-L. This sequence is blocked by osteoprotogerin, a RANK-L decoy receptor produced by immature osteoblasts and stromal cells [20,21]. Modulation of this axis drives osteoclast function.

Osteoblasts then move into the bone resorption bay (Howship's lacuna), and new bone precursor substances, largely consisting of type I collagen, are laid down in layers ('osteoid'), which, over time, become mineralized. Activity can be measured by osteopontin, osteocalcin, osteonectin and bone-specific alkaline phosphatase in the serum. Osteoblast stimulation can occur through many different factors (FGF, PDGF, PTH, BMP and Wnts). The formation of new bone following orderly resorption in the resorption cavities is termed *coupling*. The canonical Wnt signaling pathway and its inhibitors sclerostin, Dkk and Frizzled related protein, are being increasingly recognized as critical to bone health. This topic has been well reviewed by Ott [22].

VIII. PATHOPHYSIOLOGY OF BONE METASTASES IN BREAST CANCER

Cancer cells metastasizing from a primary breast cancer do not all have the capacity for surviving and proliferating in the bone micro-environment. This has been studied by Kang *et al.* [23] who examined the genetic signature of MDA 231 cells serially passaged through immunodeficient mice to produce cells with a tendency to settle and proliferate within bone and bone marrow. They found that gene sets identified by transcriptional profiling included homing (CXCR4), invasion (MMP1), angiogenesis and osteolysis gene sets. It is likely that in human breast cancer, similar genetic signatures will be identified allowing clinicians to select patients for preventive therapies and specific follow-up protocols for diagnosis.

Breast cancer cells within bone release substances such as PTHrP which disrupt the fine balance of RANK-L/OPG secretion by osteoblasts. RANK-L secretion is increased thereby increasing osteoclast function and bone resorption which, in turn, through factors such as IGF-1, TGF-B and calcium stimulates intra-osseous tumor growth. A vicious cycle is established whereby increased tumor growth increases bone breakdown which further increases tumor growth [24]. In addition, bone formation is disrupted and disorganized woven bone is laid down leading to further structural deficiency and increased risk of fracture and other skeletal related events.

IX. TREATMENT OF BONE METASTASES

A. General Principles of Management

Although this chapter focuses on the use of bisphosphonates in the treatment of bone metastases in breast cancer, it is important to recognize that other modalities continue to provide the mainstay of therapy in most patients. Bone pain management includes a thorough history and physical examination, full discussion with the patient about a plan of

action, and attempts to modify the pathological process. These attempts include external beam radiotherapy (still the most effective remedy for alleviation of localized bone pain) and palliative chemotherapy. A good response to chemotherapy includes subjective relief of symptoms, including pain. Hormone therapy can provide a high quality remission in breast cancer patients with bone metastases. Elevation of the pain threshold with the use of non-pharmacological methods as well as analgesics, interruption of pain pathways by local or regional anesthesia or neurolysis, and modification of lifestyle are all helpful, but invariably opioid and other adjuvant analgesic management will be required. Prophylactic surgery and radiation therapy for patients with cortical erosion caused by metastasis in the femur and humerus may prevent the distress of a pathological fracture.

B. Bisphosphonates

Many bisphosphonates have been assessed in the management of malignant bone disease. These include: etidronate, pamidronate, clodronate, residronate, mildronate, neridronate, alendronate, ibandronate, and zoledronate. Pamidronate, ibandronate, zoledronate, and clodronate have been the most extensively studied in neoplastic diseases and are widely available for the treatment of malignant hypercalcemia, prevention of skeletal events in patients with bone metastases, Paget's disease of bone, osteoporosis, and other less common indications. Pamidronate, clodronate, zoledronate, and ibandronate all lead to an effective lowering of serum calcium which is attributable to decreased bone resorption. Pamidronate, an aminobisphosphonate, is not used orally because of dose-related gastrointestinal toxicity. There is evidence that long-term pamidronate administered orally may also induce osteomalacia [25] and this may be the case for most chronically administered bisphosphonates, whether given orally or intravenously. Clodronate is effective when given intravenously for hypercalcemia and bone pain and can be used orally and subcutaneously. Its long-term administration appears not to be associated with a detectable defect in the mineralization of bone [26]. It is important to prescribe supplemental calcium (1–1.5 G/daily) and vitamin D3 (1000 int. units/daily) to all patients receiving long-term bisphosphonate therapy. They should be taken at least 4 hours after or before oral bisphosphonates.

The geminal bisphosphonates are analogs of pyrophosphate characterized by a stable P–C–P bond. They bind with high affinity to hydroxyapatite crystals in bone, and are potent inhibitors of normal and pathological bone resorption [27]. At the cellular level several mechanisms of action seem to operate, the dominant mechanism differing in different compounds, but all appear to have a final common effect of inhibition of osteoclast function. The osteoblast might be the initial target cell for bisphosphonates, exerting an effect on the osteoclast by modulation of stimulating and inhibiting factors, such as the RANK-L/ RANK/osteoprotogerin axis, which control osteoclast function [28].

These agents appear to promote apoptosis in murine osteoclasts both *in vivo* and *in vitro*, the more potent bisphosphonates exhibiting the greatest apoptotic action [29].

In the absence of apoptosis, inhibition of osteoclast function appears to be mediated by osteoblasts. This action does not interfere with the ability of cells of the monocyte–macrophage lineage to produce colonies [30]. Bisphosphonates can also inhibit the proliferation and promote the cell death of macrophages [31,32]. Again, the process is one of apoptosis rather than necrosis and might, in part, explain the pain-relieving properties of bisphosphonates. Shipman *et al.* have described the induction of apoptosis by bisphosphonates in human myeloma cell lines [33].

At the molecular level, bisphosphonates fall into two broad classes: nitrogen containing and non-nitrogen containing. These two groups have different molecular mechanisms of action. Nitrogen-containing bisphosphonates, such as pamidronate, alendronate, and ibandronate, inhibit the mevalonate signaling pathway in osteoclasts while non-nitrogen containing bisphosphonates are incorporated into ATP forming non-hydrolysable analogs [34]. Differences in side-chain moieties account for the variation in potency between the various bisphosphonates, a feature much promoted by the marketing departments of some pharmaceutical companies. There is no level 1 evidence from comparative clinical trials that these differences in potencies translate to major advantages in clinical efficacy.

X. CLINICAL TRIALS AND USE OF BISPHOSPHONATES IN BREAST CANCER

A. Hypercalcemia

As a result of secretion of factors from infiltrating malignant ductal cells acting focally and humorally, osteoclast activity is markedly increased, with a reduction in osteoblast activity, leading to 'uncoupling' of bone resorption and formation [35]. Parathyroid hormone related protein (PTHrP) appears to play a central role in the malignant hypercalcemia of breast cancer [24,36].

We have reviewed the evidence for the treatment of hypercalcemia and have offered some broad guidelines [37]. Randomized trials in hypercalcemic patients are notoriously difficult to carry out due to the poor clinical status of most patients, the questionable ethics of a non-treated control group, the difficulty in obtaining satisfactory consent, and the widely variable response rate which depends on the underlying primary malignancy. For example, the hypercalcemia of myeloma responds more easily to treatment than the hypercalcemia associated with carcinoma of the lung.

Saline rehydration will usually effect a median reduction of 0.25 mM/l but its effect is transient [38]. Rehydration is useful for treating mild degrees of hypercalcemia but usually should be accompanied by bisphosphonate therapy. Symptomatic hypercalcemia, especially with levels of Ca^{2+} greater than 3.0 mM/l, requires vigorous rehydration (N-saline 150–200 ml/hour with KCl 20–40 mEq/l added), and the administration of clodronate 1500 mg in 500 ml physiological saline over 2 hours, or pamidronate 60–90 mg in 250–500 ml physiological saline over 2 hours, or zoledronate 4 mg i.v. over 15 minutes. Pamidronate may give a longer duration of maintenance of normocalcemia than clodronate (28 days median vs 14 days) [39]. Ibandronate at doses of 4–6 mg i.v. and zoledronate at 4 mg i.v. are at least as efficacious as pamidronate and may give a longer duration of normocalcemia [40,41].

Although they are more expensive, it has been suggested that zoledronate or ibandronate may be superior to pamidronate with a higher response rate and longer duration of response, and with the added advantage of a shorter infusion time. These studies are difficult to assess, since results are heavily dependent on the clinical case mix and are of low power, often relying on pooling of trials results (level 2 evidence). Clodronate can be safely and effectively given subcutaneously, normalizing the serum calcium within 5 days in 32 of 43 infusions given in a palliative care unit [42]. Many units use specially prepared baby bottles with balloon bags containing 240 ml of normal saline into which the bisphosphonate can be injected in the pharmacy for outpatient delivery of pamidronate or clodronate. The balloons can be prepared so that delivery rates of around 100 ml/h are achieved.

XI. REDUCTION OF SKELETAL COMPLICATIONS

Early clinical investigations of bisphosphonates were carried out in uncontrolled trials of patients with advanced disease or small non-placebo controlled, open studies [43]. Although these investigators were probably correct in their conclusions, it is difficult to determine the extent to which patient selection and the placebo effect influenced the positive results of the investigations.

One of the first randomized, controlled studies to be published was an open label trial of the aminobisphosphonate, pamidronate, given orally for 2 years at 300 mg daily in patients with bone metastases from breast cancer [44]. The investigators demonstrated a reduction in the skeletal complications of hypercalcemia and vertebral fractures. Radiation treatments for bone pain were also reduced, but there was difficulty in patient compliance due to a high rate of upper gastrointestinal side-effects. In a double-blind, randomized, placebo-controlled trial of oral clodronate, 1600 mg daily for 2 years, we confirmed this beneficial effect on skeletal morbidity in patients with bone metastases from breast cancer [45]. The number of patients suffering from episodes of hypercalcemia was reduced; the number of major vertebral fractures and the vertebral deformity rate were also reduced; and the number of radiation therapy treatments was lower in the clodronate-treated patients. No survival benefit was evident. McCloskey *et al.* reviewed the pre-entry and follow-up vertebral fracture prevalence in 163 of the 173 patients in this trial and found that 46% of the patients had evidence of vertebral fracture at trial entry [46]. The patients deriving the greatest benefit from the oral clodronate were those who had already sustained vertebral fractures and were therefore at greatest risk for sustaining further fractures. This trial enrolled patients with more advanced bone disease and was smaller than later trials of pamidronate and zoledronate.

Pamidronate, which can occasionally induce sclerosis in osteolytic lesions when used as the only therapy [47], has been investigated in several trials. Measurement of response in bone is a difficult process and unless differences in the arms of a trial are large, small but significant differences can be missed. Tumor response in bone and duration of response were assessed in a double-blind, randomized trial, which showed similar response rates in bone but a significantly ($p < 0.02$) increased duration of response for patients receiving pamidronate 45 mg given intravenously every 3 weeks (249 days median time to progression compared to 168 days in controls) [48]. Hortobagyi *et al.* reported a randomized trial of 380 patients with recurrent breast cancer in bone and demonstrated a reduction in the skeletal complications of vertebral fracture, pain, and hypercalcemia with intravenous pamidronate 90 mg given monthly for 2 years [49]. No survival benefit was apparent. A trial of intravenous pamidronate in 372 patients with bone metastases from carcinoma of the breast receiving hormone therapy has shown a similar reduction in skeletal complications [50].

Zoledronate has been assessed in comparison to pamidronate in patients with breast cancer and myeloma. Median time to first event was similar for both agents [51]. Using an Anderson–Gill statistical model (which accounts for the frequency of events subsequent to the first event) it appeared that zoledronate might be the superior agent, although cost considerations come into play here in many countries.

As a result of these trials giving level 1, grade A evidence, we currently recommend the use of either clodronate 1600 mg orally daily (preferably taken one-half hour to 1 hour before breakfast or at least 2 hours away from food) or intravenous pamidronate 90 mg every 4 weeks in patients with radiologically established bone metastases from breast cancer. While the use of bisphosphonates to prevent skeletal complications is an advance, the cost (especially the cost of the high potency agents which are still on patent) to prevent one skeletal complication is high and is at the limits of what some societies would consider worthwhile. The cost of

avoiding one skeletal complication in prostate cancer patients with zoledronate is over US$100,000 [52]. In breast cancer the figure is lower with pamidronate coming in at around US$75,000 per quality adjusted life year. We have performed a comparative cost study suggesting that for many patients, oral clodronate provides a manageable and economic treatment program [53]. Now that pamidronate is off patent in many countries, this provides a reasonably cost-effective intravenous alternative to oral bisphosphonate therapy.

A common clinical question is how long one should continue bisphosphonate therapy. There are no studies to guide the clinician here. It is our practice to continue treatment for as long as the patient has symptoms. There is little evidence that true resistance develops although the common clinical practice of changing bisphosphonates (e.g., from oral clodronate to IV pamidronate or vice versa) on progression of disease has some backing. A study by Clemons suggests that switching to another bisphosphonate augments a fall in markers of resorption [54]. It is likely that tumor burden has increased to a level that bone turnover has further accelerated—increasing the dosage may also produce a reduction in the accelerated turnover.

XII. BONE PAIN

When malignant cells invade inter-trabecular spaces, the malignant cells may form a mass to a size where volume and secreted substances have an impact on pain. But it is too simplistic to explain bone pain on purely mechanistic grounds by suggesting that a bone metastasis causes pain because trabecular fractures occur and bone collapses, leading to compression and distortion of the periosteum, a site known to be innervated by pain fibers. Bone pain can occur in the absence of fracture and this seems to happen commonly. Bone marrow spaces are innervated by nociceptive C-fibers sensitive to changes in pressure, and it is probable that the malignant cells secrete pain-provoking factors such as substance P, bradykinins and other cytokines, which lead to stimulation of C-type fibers within bone. Prostaglandins may also play a role by sensitizing free nerve endings to released vasoactive amines and kinins [55]. The precise interaction between the tumor and bone microenvironment is unknown. Nociceptive nerve fibers staining for substance P have been identified within the trabecular bone of human vertebral bodies [56].

The notion that bisphosphonates might decrease bone pain in some patients with bone metastases arose from clinical observations of patients receiving bisphosphonates for hypercalcemia. Patients experienced not only normalization of serum calcium and relief of the symptoms of hypercalcemia, but also reported relief of pain.

Ernst *et al.* demonstrated, in a double-blind, cross-over trial of intravenous clodronate in patients with bone pain caused by a variety of malignancies, that clodronate had useful analgesic properties [57]. This was confirmed (level 1 evidence) in a larger randomized, double-blind, controlled trial of intravenous clodronate in patients with metastatic bone pain [58]. No dose–response relationship was seen. Improvement in pain and mobility scores had been described in the previously discussed trial of oral pamidronate, although these patients were not selected specifically because of bone pain but because they had osteolytic metastases [44]. However, the modest effect, coupled with its poor oral tolerability as demonstrated by Coleman *et al.* [59] makes oral pamidronate unlikely to be used. Level 1 evidence of pain relief has also been described with intravenous pamidronate in the previously discussed placebo-controlled trial in patients with bone metastases from breast cancer [49].

Ibandronate, a potent nitrogen-containing bisphosphonate, has been shown to reduce skeletal complications of metastatic breast cancer but has also demonstrated significant and lasting pain relief and improved quality of life when given intravenously at a dose of 6 mg repeated monthly in patients with bone metastases from metastatic breast cancer [60]. The drug is also efficacious in reducing the risk of skeletal complications in metastatic breast cancer when used orally and seems to be quite well tolerated at doses of 50 mg daily [61]. Likewise, zoledronic acid has similar effects on bone pain in breast cancer and is modestly effective in patients with prostate cancer [62]. Again it is unclear that one bisphosphonate over another gives superior results.

XIII. SOME PROBLEMS

Bone remodeling is a normal repair mechanism. Basic multicellular units (bone resorption bays) are formed in order to repair areas of effete or damaged bone. Bisphosphonates are potent inhibitors of bone turnover and therefore it is not surprising that the quality of bone formed may differ from normal bone. The more potent bisphosphonates may be particularly problematic in this regard when they are used over a period of several years in the adjuvant setting of women with breast cancer who have normal bone. In experimental animals given high doses of bisphosphonate therapy, an accumulation of microdamage with consequent weakening of bone strength may occur. This has been well discussed by Ott (2005) [63].

Sixty-three cases of osteonecrosis of the maxilla or mandible were reported in patients receiving intravenous pamidronate and zoledronate (55 patients) and oralrisedronate and alendronate (8 patients) [64]. This is a painful, poorly healing or non-healing necrosis of the tooth socket following dental extraction leading to osteonecrosis of the mandible or maxilla. It is a difficult condition to treat, usually requiring excision of bone. The pathological changes seen are similar to those seen with severe radiation necrosis.

Bisphosphonates certainly have the potential for interference with mineralization and healing since their half-life is several years and it is likely that all bisphosphonates might cause this toxicity although it is only occasionally seen with oral clodronate. Increased fractures have been observed in Paget's disease with etidronate [65] and a case report of osteopetrosis in a child on IV pamidronate which also led to increased fractures [66] indicates that these agents must be used with care, using the lowest dose and frequency which is efficacious for the end-point sought. Their routine use for months (and sometimes years) on end with minimum supervision is poor practice.

Renal toxicity can be another problem, especially with IV bisphosphonates. A retrospective analysis of 57 patients with bone metastases from various cancers who were treated with IV bisphosphonates for over 24 months (most switching from IV pamidronate to IV zoledronate given every 3–4 weeks) was conducted to assess long-term renal safety [67]. All patients studied had a normal baseline serum creatinine; 12.2% experienced increased serum creatinine levels, and three patients (5%) suffered osteonecrosis of the jaw. The main message here is that all patients receiving IV bisphosphonates should have a serum creatinine drawn prior to administration as well as an oral examination at each visit. Patients on oral bisphosphonates should have a creatinine drawn and a mouth examination at each 3–6 monthly visit.

XIV. ADJUVANT CLINICAL TRIAL DATA

The antitumor effects of bisphosphonates observed in preclinical studies have not been unequivocally reproduced in the clinical setting to date. Data from clinical trials of adjuvant bisphosphonate therapy suggest that their use in this setting may be beneficial, but these data have been inconsistent across trials. There are three published adjuvant trials of oral clodronate [68–74], and one trial each of pamidronate [75] and zoledronic acid [76].

A. Clodronate

Results obtained from randomized, placebo-controlled clinical trials of adjuvant clodronate suggest that it may increase overall survival for patients with breast cancer. In a single-center trial of 302 women with primary breast cancer, patients received either postoperative treatment with oral clodronate (1600 mg) for 2 years or no treatment [68]. After a 3-year follow-up, patients in the adjuvant clodronate group had a significantly lower incidence of bone metastases than those in the untreated control group ($p = 0.044$). There was a longer overall survival time in the clodronate group ($p < 0.002$).

A 10-year (103 months $\pm$ 12 months) follow-up study of 290 of the original patients found that the significantly longer disease-free survival was not maintained, but that clodronate still improved overall survival ($p = 0.01$); 79.6% of clodronate-treated patients survived compared with 59.3% of patients who received no treatment [73].

Adjuvant oral clodronate was also assessed in a 2-year, randomized, placebo-controlled trial in 1069 women with primary operable breast cancer [71]. Clodronate resulted in a significantly lower incidence of bone metastasis, by 45% during the first 2 years ($p = 0.031$) and by 31% during the 5-year study period ($p = 0.043$) compared with placebo. There was also a significantly longer overall survival time compared with placebo ($p = 0.047$). After a 10.5-year follow-up, oral clodronate was still found to significantly improve overall survival ($p = 0.048$) [72].

In contrast, a third trial did not find a clinical benefit for the use of adjuvant oral clodronate in patients with node positive breast cancer [70]. In a randomized, open label trial of clodronate given for 3 years, the incidence of bone metastases at 5 years was higher in the clodronate-treated patients than in patients in the control arm. Furthermore, both overall and disease-free survival times were significantly shorter in women treated with clodronate compared with those who received placebo. After a 10-year follow-up, no significant difference in survival was seen between patients who received clodronate and those who received placebo, but disease-free survival was still shorter in the clodronate group [74]. The results of this trial are concerning, but they are most likely explained by a randomization bias. Significantly more patients with estrogen receptor (ER)- and progesterone receptor-negative breast cancer were randomized to the clodronate group than the placebo group.

B. Pamidronate

Kokufu and colleagues [75] assessed the effects of pamidronate in a small ($n = 90$), non-randomized study of patients with high-risk breast cancer (four or more positive nodes). With a median follow-up of 5.4 years, patients who received adjuvant pamidronate had a lower incidence of bone metastases ($p = 0.008$) and a higher metastasis-free survival ($p = 0.035$) than controls. These findings require confirmation.

C. Zoledronic Acid

Adjuvant zoledronic acid was studied in a randomized, open-label trial of 40 patients with recurrent solid tumors who did not present with bone metastases at baseline [76]. After 12 months, significantly more patients in the zoledronic acid group were free from bone metastases than patients in the control group (60% vs 10%; $p < 0.0005$). This difference remained significant at 18 months (20% vs 5% for control; $p = 0.0002$).

XV. ONGOING ADJUVANT TRIALS

A number of well-designed, randomized, trials of bisphosphonate therapy for early-stage breast cancer are currently under way. NSABP B-34, assessing oral clodronate versus placebo, may provide further evidence for efficacy in the adjuvant therapy of breast cancer. Because of the low recurrence rates seen in this predominantly Stage 1 trial, results are not expected until late 2009. Trials are also currently evaluating the role of adjuvant IV zoledronic acid, oral clodronate, and oral ibandronate. The S0307 trial is designed to assess the efficacy of bisphosphonates in reducing the incidence of bone metastases. It is a 4-year, joint SWOG/Intergroup/NSABP trial in 6000 women with breast cancer The trial was initiated at the end of 2005 and is due to end in 2015. After 3 years of treatment, patients will be followed up for an additional 3 years. Enrolled patients will randomly receive one of three adjuvant bisphosphonate regimens, in addition to standard systemic therapy [77]. The trial will enroll female patients with histologically confirmed stage I, II, or III non-metastatic breast cancer who are receiving standard adjuvant therapy. Entry criteria are standard, but a new feature in this trial is a requirement for a pretrial dental examination for identification of periodontal disease and exposed bone; this is in an effort to reduce any potential risk factors for osteonecrosis of the jaw or maxilla.

XVI. TREATMENT-INDUCED BONE LOSS

A. Assessing Bone Quality

There is often a mistaken assumption that bone density is the only important consideration in assessing bone quality and a propensity to skeletal events. Bone strength reflects the integration of bone density and bone quality. Bone quality consists of a composite of balanced remodeling adequate mineralization, micro-architecture changes, and accumulation of fatigue damage [78]. Techniques to assess bone quality broadly fall into three categories: radiologic (BMD), biochemical (markers of bone turnover), and histologic (bone biopsies for histomorphometry). Histologic techniques yield the best assessment but are the most invasive and least used routinely, but they are likely to increase in importance in the assessment of new bone active therapies in women with normal bone density. Architecture is of course often disrupted in women with bone metastases but even with sub-clinical disease this may occur with trabecular micro-fractures weakening bone architecture.

Bone turnover is increased in women with breast cancer who have an increased risk of estrogen deficiency due to ovarian failure from systemic chemotherapy quite apart from normal age related menopause [79]. Estrogen exerts a multitude of actions on bone tissues and is integral to bone health. It tends to stimulate TGF-β production, the effect of which may be to decrease osteoblast and stromal cell apoptosis and increase osteoclast apoptosis; it increases the production and secretion of osteoprotogerin, which acts as a decoy receptor for RANK ligand, thereby decreasing osteoclast stimulation. Estrogen not only decreases the production of interleukin (IL)-1 and TNF-α from T cells, but also decreases the production of IL-6 from osteoblasts, all of which substances are stimulators of osteoclast activity. At menopause, therefore, there occurs a general increase in bone turnover, with an increase in bone resorption and formation [80]. The resorption cavities formed tend to be filled in with a slightly lower amount of bone, leading to a net loss of bone over subsequent years, resulting in uncoupling of bone turnover.

Combination chemotherapy is now used in premenopausal women with all stages of breast cancer. One of the effects of these treatments, particularly when the protocol contains alkylating agents or taxanes, is to cause ovarian ablation, leading to premature menopause. This early menopause is associated with a significant increase in bone resorption, which can be detected by bone densitometry and can be substantial, reaching as much as a 7% reduction in the bone density in the first year in some women. This bone density loss can be reduced or prevented by residronate [81], clodronate [82], zoledronate [83], denosumab [84] (a human monoclonal RANK-L inhibitor) and probably most intravenous or oral bisphosphonates. The antiresorptive effect of estrogen appears to be mediated through a direct inhibitor effect on osteoclasts as well as an indirect effect mediated at least in part by the suppression of IL-6, IL-1, TNF, and the augmented TGF-β released by osteoblasts [80].

The skeletal effects of oophorectomy in rats are predictable and consist of an early acceleration of bone turnover and loss of bone, especially cancellous bone. This accelerated bone turnover can be reduced by estrogen or a bisphosphonate. The effect of the estrogen is lost after approximately 90 days from stopping estrogen therapy. In contrast, the bisphosphonate is still effective 180 days after withdrawal [85]. This suggests that intermittent bisphosphonate therapy may be sufficient to prevent or reduce the bone loss associated with treatment-induced premature menopause.

The clinical consequences in bone of the postmenopausal estrogen decrease have been well recognized; in postmenopausal women, there is a tendency to develop fractures in areas of high bone turnover: vertebrae, hip and distal radius. In women who have experienced premature menopause as a result of chemotherapy for breast cancer, there occurs a 4–5-fold increased rate of vertebral fractures compared with an age-matched population of women who do not have breast cancer. In an adjuvant trial of oral clodronate compared with placebo in women with primary carcinoma of the breast, the prevalence of vertebral fracture of

the patients at trial entry was similar to that in a control group of normal women (approximately 5% of the patients had a vertebral fracture at entry to the study, the same as the control population). However, with follow-up, the incidence of new vertebral fractures was 5 times higher in the patients with breast cancer compared with the control group, the incidence in the patients with breast cancer being 2.5% per year compared with 0.5% per year for the control group [8].

In women who receive aromatase inhibitors/inactivators (AIs) as adjuvant therapy for breast cancer, there is an increased risk of fracture. Increased fracture rates (compared to tamoxifen) of between 3–4% at 5 years match the absolute disease-free survival benefit at 5 years of between 3 and 4%. The beneficial effect of AIs on breast cancer recurrence or progression depends on reducing levels of circulating estrogens in the peripheral blood. These agents differ in the magnitude of the effect on serum levels of estradiol, with letrozole generally having the greatest effect. However, this does not necessarily mean it is the most appropriate agent because the beneficial effect on breast cancer cell growth is probably unrelated to the magnitude of the decrease in estrogen levels, and side effects and toxicity of the AI may be greater. There is variation in the effects of AIs in different experimental animals and these effects may also differ in man.

Exemestane has been evaluated in oophorectomized Sprague-Dawley rats. Bone mineral density was 11% higher in the lumbar spine and 7% higher in the femur when exemestane was given to oophorectomized animals compared with control animals that had undergone only an oophorectomy. Furthermore, bending strength and compressive strength improved, trabecular bone volume was higher, and there was a reduction in the oophorectomy-induced increase in serum pyridinoline [86]. In contrast, the AI vorazole leads to an increase in bone resorption markers and a decrease in BMD in an aged male rat model, the effect being reversible with estrogen [87].

In humans, the effect of AIs on bone has been well studied in the Arimidex versus Tamoxifen Alone or in Combination trial (ATAC). In this trial, BMD changes from baseline were significantly different in lumbar spine density for tamoxifen alone compared with anastrozole alone at years 1 and 2. There was an approximately 2.5% loss of BMD at year 1 and a 4% loss at year 2 for anastrozole. Similar changes were observed for hip BMD at years 1 and 2 [88].

Exemestane is associated with a similar incidence of osteoporosis to letrozole when used as adjuvant treatment after tamoxifen in women with primary breast cancer, and any difference may be more apparent than real, as exemestane in the Intergroup Exemestane Study trial [89] is being compared with tamoxifen, a known bone resorption inhibitor, rather than a placebo, as is the case with letrozole in the MA.17 trial 27 [90].

A few studies have been initiated looking at markers of bone resorption in patients receiving AIs. In normal postmenopausal women with low risk breast cancer receiving letrozole 2.5 mgms/per day, there was a 25% increase in the levels of the resorption marker C telopeptide [91]. Lonning *et al.* assessed markers of bone turnover in women with low-risk breast cancers or ductal carcinoma *in situ* receiving exemestane and compared them with women receiving placebo [92]. As expected, estrogen levels decreased in the exemestane group. This resulted in significant increases in markers of bone turnover at 1 and 2 years of follow-up, whereas detectable changes in BMD were minimal over the same period.

Finally, McCloskey has demonstrated in the LEAP study that there is little, if any, difference in markers of bone resorption between the three commonly used AIs [93].

XVII. BONE MINERAL DENSITY AND OSTEOPOROSIS

Indications for the diagnostic use of bone densitometry include the presence of any major risk factors as well as evidence of osteopenia or vertebral deformity on radiography; previous fragility fracture, particularly of the hip, spine, or wrist; and loss of height or kyphosis (with radiographic confirmation of vertebral deformities) [94].

Osteoporosis has been defined as a skeletal disorder characterized by compromised bone strength predisposing a person to an increased risk of fracture. Bone strength reflects the integration of two main features: bone density and bone quality. Bone quality is comprised of a composite of balanced remodeling, adequate mineralization, microarchitecture changes, and accumulation of fatigue damage [95].

Osteoporosis commonly occurs in postmenopausal women in whom trabecular microfractures lead to diminution in the cross-struts of the architecture of bone, leading to a reduction in overall bone strength. Lifetime risks of fracture in a 50-year-old woman are approximately 17.5% for a hip fracture, 15.5% for a vertebral fracture, and 16% for a wrist fracture. In Canadian women ≥50 years of age, the prevalence rates of bone mineral density (BMD) T-scores >-2.5 are 12.1% for the lumbar spine and nearly 8% for the neck of the femur [96]. There are a number of known risk factors for osteoporosis, which have been divided into major and minor categories [97].

Major risk factors include age >65 years, previous vertebral compression fracture, fragility fracture after age 40, systemic glucocorticoids taken for >3 months (this definition might include some chemotherapy regimens that involve high doses of dexamethasone as antinausea medication or antihypersensitivity reactions), malabsorption syndrome, primary hyperparathyroidism, hypogonadism, and menopause occurring at an age ≤45 years. The use of AIs should also be placed within the major risk factor group.

XVIII. RECOMMENDATIONS FROM A MULTIDISCIPLINARY PANEL

For postmenopausal women receiving adjuvant anastrozole or other AIs, a baseline BMD measurement using DEXA is recommended to be repeated every 1–2 years. Regular physical exercise is advised, together with added calcium 1500 mg and vitamin D 1000 U daily. If the T-score reaches a level of >-2.5 or is between -1.5 and -2.5 in the presence of a fragility fracture vertebral compression fracture height loss >2 cm occurs, or there is an annual BMD decrease >3% at the lumbar spine or >5% at the femoral neck, bisphosphonate therapy should be considered [98]. A review panel has further lowered the bar, suggesting that all patients on AIs with a T-score <-2.0 should receive zoledronic acid twice yearly [99].

References

1. S. Paget, The distribution of secondary growths in cancer of the breast, Lancet I (1889) 571–573.
2. O.V. Batson, The function of the vertebral veins and their role in the spread of metastases, Annals of Surgery 112 (1940) 138–149.
3. G.R. Mundy, Mechanisms of bone metastasis, Cancer 80 (Suppl 8) (1997) 1546–1556.
4. G.R. Mundy & T.A. Guise, Pathophysiology of bone metastases, in: R.D. Rubens & G.R. Mundy (Eds.) Cancer and the Skeleton, Martin Dunitz, London, UK, 2000, pp. 43–64.
5. R.E. Coleman & R.D. Rubens, The clinical course of bone metastases from breast cancer, Br J Cancer 55 (1987) 61–66.
6. R. Smith, W. Jiping, J. Bryant, et al., Primary Breast Cancer (PBC) as a risk factor for bone recurrence (BR): NSABP experience. Proceedings of American Society of Clinical Oncology, Vol 18, Abstract 457 (1999).
7. A.H. Paterson, Bone metastases in breast cancer, prostate cancer and myeloma, Bone 8 (Suppl 1) (1987) S17–S22.
8. J.A. Kanis, E.V. McCloskey & T. Powles, et al., A high incidence of vertebral fractures in women with breast cancer, Br J Cancer 79 (1999) 1179–1181.
9. J.F. Forbes, J. Cuzick, A. Buzdar, et al., ATAC: 100 month median follow-up shows continued superior efficacy and no excess fracture risk for anastrozole compared with tamoxifen after treatment completion. Proceedings San Antonio Breast Cancer Symposium December, Abstract 41 (2007).
10. R.C. Coombes, P. Dady & C. Parsons, et al., Assessment of response of bone metastases to systemic treatment in patients with breast cancer, Cancer 52 (4) (1983) 610–614.
11. S. Braun, F.D. Vogl & B. Naume, et al., A pooled analysis of bone marrow micrometastasis in breast cancer, New Engl J of Med 353 (2005) 793–802.
12. L. Harris, H. Fritsche & R. Mennel, et al., American Society of Clinical Oncology 2007 update of recommendations for the use of tumor markers in breast cancer, J Clin Oncol 25 (33) (2007) 5287–5312.
13. J.E. Brown & R.E. Coleman, Assessment of the effects of breast cancer on bone and the response to therapy, Breast 11 (5) (2002) 375–385.

14. V.H. Bramwell, G.S. Doig & A.B. Tuck, et al., Serial plasma osteopontin levels have prognostic value in metastatic breast cancer, Clin Cancer Res 12 (11, Pt 1) (2006) 3337–3343.

15. I.J. Diel, E.F. Solomayer & M.J. Seibel, et al., Serum bone sialoprotein in patients with primary breast cancer is a prognostic marker for subsequent bone metastasis, Clin Cancer Res 5 (12) (1999) 3914–3919.

16. E.V. McCloskey, J. Kanis & A.H. Paterson, et al., Serum P1NP, an index of bone turnover, but not bone mineral density, may be predictive of bone metastases in women with primary operable breast cancer, Breast Cancer Research and Treatment 76 (Suppl 1) (2002) 0. Abstract 565.

17. J. Wang, J. Jarrett & C.C. Huang, et al., Identification of estrogen-responsive genes involved in breast cancer metastases to the bone, Clin Exp Metastasis 24 (6) (2007) 411–422.

18. D.J. Hadjidakis & I. Androulakis, Bone remodeling, Ann NY Acad Sci USA 1092 (2006) 385–396.

19. R.N. Pearse, New strategies for the treatment of metastatic bone disease, Clinical Breast Cancer 8 (Suppl 1) (2008) S35–S45.

20. W.S. Simonet, D.L. Lacey & C.R. Dunstan, et al., Osteoprotogerin: a novel secreted protein involved in the regulation of bone density, Cell 89 (1997) 309–319.

21. D.L. Lacey, E. Timms & H.L. Tan, et al., Osteoprotogerin ligand is a cytokine that regulates osteoclast differentiation and activation, Cell 93 (1998) 165–176.

22. S.M. Ott, Sclerostin and Wnt signaling—the pathway to bone strength (review), J Clin Endocrinol Metab 90 (12) (2005) 6741–6743.

23. Y. Kang, P.M. Siegel & W. Shu, et al., A multigenic program mediating breast cancer metastasis to bone, Cancer Cell 3 (2003) 537–549.

24. G.R. Mundy, Bone resorption and turnover in health and disease, Bone 8 (Suppl 1) (1987) S9–S16.

25. B.B. Adamson, S.J. Gallacher & J. Byars, et al., Mineralization defects with pamidronate therapy for Paget's disease, Lancet 342 (1993) 1459–1460.

26. T. Taube, I. Elomaa & C. Blomqvist, et al., Comparative effects of clodronate and calcitonin in metastatic breast cancer, Eur J Clin Oncol 29 (1993) 1677–1681.

27. H. Fleisch, Bisphosphonates in Bone Disease—From the Laboratory to the Patient, 4th edn., Academic Press, San Diego and London (2000).

28. M. Sahni, H.L. Guenther & H. Fleisch, et al., Bisphosphonates act on rat bone resorption through the mediation of osteoblasts, J Clin Invest 91 (1993) 2004–2011.

29. D.E. Hughes, K.R. Wright & H.L. Uy, et al., Bisphosphonates promote apoptosis in murine osteoclasts in vitro and in vivo, J Bone Mineral Res 10 (1995) 1478–1487.

30. M. Nishikawa, T. Akatsu & Y. Katayama, Bisphosphonates act on osteoblastic cells and inhibit osteoclast formation in mouse marrow cultures, Bone 18 (1996) 9–14.

31. K.S. Selander, J. Monkkonen & E.K. Karhukorpi, et al., Characteristics of clodronate-induced apoptosis in osteoclasts and macrophages, Mol Pharmacol 50 (1996) 1127–1138.

32. M.J. Rogers, K.M. Chilton & F.P. Coxon, et al., Bisphosphonates induce apoptosis in mouse macrophage-like cells in vitro by a nitric oxide independent mechanism, J Bone Mineral Res 11 (1996) 1482–1491.

33. C.M. Shipman, M.J. Rogers & J.F. Apperley, et al., Bisphosphonates induce apoptosis in human myeloma cell lines: a novel anti-tumor activity, Br J Haematol 98 (1997) 665–672.

34. M.J. Rogers, S. Gordon & H.L. Benford, et al., Cellular and molecular mechanisms of action of bisphosphonates, Cancer 88 (S12) (2000) 2961–2978.

35. J.J. Body & P.D. Delmas, Urinary pyridinium cross-links as markers of bone resorption in tumor-associate hypercalcemia, J Clin Endocrinol Metabol 74 (1992) 471–475.

36. V. Grill, P. Ho & J.J. Body, et al., Parathyroid hormone-related protein: elevated levels in both humoral hypercalcemia of malignancy and hypercalcemia complicating metastatic breast cancer, J Clin Endocrinol Metabol 73 (1991) 1309–1315.

37. J.J. Body, R. Bartl & P. Burckhardt, et al., Current use of biphosphonates in oncology. International Bone and Cancer Study Group, J Clin Oncol 16 (1998) 3890–3899.

38. F.R. Singer, P.S. Rich & T.E. Lad for the Hypercalcemia Study Group, et al., Treatment of hypercalcemia of malignancy with intravenous etidronate. A controlled, multicenter study, Arch Int Med 151 (1991) 471–476.

39. O.P. Purohit, C.R. Radstone & C. Anthony, et al., A randomised double-blind comparison of intravenous pamidronate and clodronate in the hypercalcemia of malignancy, Br J Cancer 71 (1995) 1289–1293.

40. S.H. Ralston, D. Thiebaud & Z. Hermann, et al., Dose response study of ibandronate in the treatment of cancer associated hypercalcemia, Br J Cancer 75 (1997) 295–300.

41. P. Major, A. Lortholary & J. Hon, Zoledronic acid is superior to pamidronate in the treatment of hypercalcemia of malignancy: a pooled analysis of two randomized, controlled trials, J Clin Oncol 19 (2001) 558–567.

42. C. Roemer-Becuwe, A. Vigano & F. Romano, et al., Safety of subcutaneous clodronate and efficacy in hypercalcemia of malignancy: a novel route of administration, J Pain Symptom Manage 26 (2003) 843–848.

43. I. Elomaa, C. Blomqvist & L. Porrka, et al., Treatment of skeletal disease in breast cancer: a controlled clinical trial, Bone 8 (Suppl 1) (1987) S53–S56.

44. A.T. van Holten Verzanvoort, O.L. Bijvoet & F.J. Cleton, et al., Reduced morbidity from skeletal metastases in breast cancer patients during long-term bisphosphonates (APD) treatment, Lancet 11 (1987) 983–985.

45. A.H.G. Paterson, T.J. Powles & J.A. Kanis, et al., Double-blind controlled trial of oral clodronate in patients with bone metastases from breast cancer, J Clin Oncol 11 (1993) 59–65.

46. E.V. McCloskey, T.D. Spector & K.S. Eyres, et al., The assessment of vertebral deformity: a method for use in population studies and clinical trials, Osteoporosis Internat 3 (1993) 138–147.

47. R.E. Coleman, P.J. Woll & M. Miles, et al., Treatment of bone metastases from breast cancer with (3-amino-1-hydroxypropylidene)-1, 1-bisphosphonate (APD), Br J Cancer 58 (1988) 621–625.

48. P.F. Conte, J. Latreille & L. Mauriac, et al., Delay in progression of bone metastases in breast cancer patients treated with intravenous pamidronate: results from a multinational randomised controlled trial, J Clin Oncol 14 (1996) 2552–2559.

49. G.N. Hortobagyi, R.L. Theriault & L. Porter, et al., Efficacy of pamidronate in reducing skeletal complications in patients with breast cancer and lytic bone metastases, N Eng J Med 335 (1996) 1785–1791.

50. R.L. Theriault, A. Lipton & G.N. Hortobagy, et al., Pamidronate reduces skeletal morbidity in women with advanced breast cancer and lytic bone lesions: a randomized placebo controlled trial, J Clin Oncol 17 (1999) 846–854.

51. L.S. Rosen, D. Gordon & M. Kaminski, et al., Zoledronic acid versus pamidronate in the treatment of skeletal metastases in patients with breast cancer or osteolytic lesions of multiple myeloma: a phase III, double-blind, comparative trial, Cancer J 7 (2001) 377–387.

52. S.D. Reed, J.I. Radeva & G.A. Glendinning, et al., Cost effectiveness of zoledronic acid for the prevention of skeletal complications in patients with prostate cancer, J Urol 171 (2004) 1537–1542.

53. A.H. Paterson, E.V. McCloskey & J. Redzepovic, et al., Cost-effectiveness of oral clodronate compared with oral ibandronate, intravenous (IV) zoledronate or pamidronate in breast cancer patients, J Int Med Res 36 (3) (2008) 400–413.

54. M. Clemons, G. Dranitsaris & W.S. Ooi, et al., A Phase II trial evaluating the palliative benefit of second-line zoledronic acid in breast cancer patients with either a skeletal related event or progressive bone metastases despite first line bisphosphonate therapy, J Clin Oncol 24 (30) (2006) 4895–4900.

55. S.H. Ferreira, Prostaglandins: peripheral and central analgesia, Adv Pain Res Therapy 5 (1983) 627–634.

56. C. Fras, P. Kravetz & D.R. Mody, et al., Substance P-containing nerves within the human vertebral body: an immunohistochemical study of the basivertebral nerve, Spine J 3 (2003) 63–67.

57. D.S. Ernst, N. MacDonald & A.H.G. Paterson, et al., A double-blind cross-over trial of intravenous clodronate in metastatic bone pain, J Pain Symptom Manage 7 (1992) 4–11.

58. D.S. Ernst, P. Brasher & N.A. Hagen, et al., A randomised, controlled trial of intravenous clodronate in patients with metastatic bone disease and pain, J Pain Symptom Manage 13 (1997) 319–326.

59. R.E. Coleman, S. Houston & O.P. Purohit, et al., A randomized Phase II evaluation of oral pamidronate for advanced bone metastases from breast cancer, Eur J Cancer 34 (1998) 820–824.

60. I.J. Diel, J.J. Body & M.R. Lichinister, et al., Improved quality of life after long-term treatment with the bisphosphonate ibandronate in patients with metastatic bone disease due to breast cancer, Eur J Cancer 40 (2004) 1704–1712.

61. J.J. Body, I.J. Diel & M.R. Lichinitzer, et al., Oral ibandronate reduces the risk of skeletal complications in breast cancer patients with metastatic bone disease: results from two randomized, placebo-controlled Phase 3 studies, Br J Cancer 90 (2004) 1133–1137.

62. K.P. Weinfurt, K.J. Anstrom & L.D. Castel, et al., Effect of zoledronic acid on pain associated with bone metastasis in patients with prostate cancer, Annals of Oncology 17 (6) (2006) 986–989.

63. S.M. Ott, Long-term safety of bisphosphonates, J Clin Endocrinol Metab 90 (3) (2005) 1897–1899.

64. S.L. Ruggiero, B. Mehrotra & T.J. Rosenberg, et al., Osteonecrosis of the jaws associated with the use of bisphosphonates: a review of 63 cases, J Oral Maxillofac Surg 62 (2004) 527–534.

65. K.S. Eyres, P. Marshall & E.V. McCloskey, et al., Spontaneous fractures in a patient treated with low doses of etidronic acid (disodium etidronate), Drug Safety 7 (1992) 162–165.

66. M.P. Whyte, D. Wenkert & K.L. Clements, et al., Bisphosphonate-induced osteopetrosis, N Engl J Med 349 (2003) 457–463.

67. V. Guarneri, S. Donati & M. Nicolini, et al., Renal safety and efficacy of IV bisphosphonates in patients with skeletal metastases treated for up to 10 years, Oncologist 10 (2005) 842–848.

68. I.J. Diel, E.F. Solomayer & S.D. Costa, et al., Reduction in new metastases in breast cancer with adjuvant clodronate treatment, N Engl J Med 339 (1998) 357–363.

69. A. Jaschke, G. Bastert & E.F. Solomayer, et al., Adjuvant clodronate treatment improves the overall survival of primary breast cancer patients with micrometastases to bone marrow—a longtime follow-up, Proc Am Soc Clin Oncol 23 (2004) 9.

70. T. Saarto, C. Blomqvist & P. Virkkunen, et al., Adjuvant clodronate treatment does not reduce the frequency of skeletal metastases in node-positive breast cancer patients: 5-year results of a randomized controlled trial, J Clin Oncol 19 (2001) 10–17.

71. T. Powles, S. Paterson & J.A. Kanis, et al., Randomized, placebo-controlled trial of clodronate in patients with primary operable breast cancer, J Clin Oncol 20 (2002) 3219–3224.

72. T. Powles, A. Paterson & E. McCloskey, et al., Reduction in bone relapse and improved survival with oral clodronate for adjuvant treatment of operable breast cancer, Breast Cancer Res 8 (R13) (2006) 1–7.

73. I.J. Diel, E. Solomayer, C. Gollan, et al., Bisphosphonates in the reduction of metastases in breast cancer—results of the extended follow-up of the first study population, Proc Am Soc Clin Oncol 19 (2000) 82a.

73. A. Jaschke, G. Bastert & E.F. Solomayer, et al., Adjuvant clodronate treatment improves the overall survival of primary breast cancer patients with micrometastases to bone marrow—a longtime follow-up, Proc Am Soc Clin Oncol 23 (2004) 9.

74. T. Saarto, L. Vehmanen & P. Virkkunen, et al., Ten-year follow-up of a randomized controlled trial of adjuvant clodronate treatment in node-positive breast cancer patients, Acta Oncol 43 (2004) 650–656.

75. I. Kokufu, N. Kohno & S. Takao, et al., Adjuvant pamidronate (PMT) therapy for the prevention of bone metastasis in breast cancer (BC) patients (pts) with four or more positive nodes, Proc Am Soc Clin Oncol 23 (2004) 9.

76. K. Mystakidou, E. Katsouda & E. Parpa, et al., Randomized, open label, prospective study on the effect of zoledronic acid on the prevention of bone metastases in patients with recurrent solid tumors that did not present with bone metastases at baseline, Med Oncol 22 (2005) 195–201.

77. J. Gralow & A. Paterson, S0307: a phase III trial of bisphosphonates as adjuvant therapy for primary breast cancer, Bone 38 (Suppl 1) (2006) S74.

78. A.H.G. Paterson, Evaluating bone mass and bone quality in patients with breast cancer. Review, Clinical Breast Cancer 5 (Suppl 2) (2005) S41–S45.

79. B. Winding, H.L. Jorgensen & C. Christiansen, Osteoporosis in patients with a history of breast cancer: causes and diagnosis, in: J.J. Body (Ed.), Tumor Bone Diseases and Osteoporosis in Cancer Patients: Pathophysiology, Diagnosis and Therapy, Marcel Dekker, New York, 2000, pp. 493–514.

80. M. Kassem, Cellular and molecular effects of growth hormone and estrogen on human bone cells, Acta Pathol Microbiol Immunol Scand 71 (suppl) (1997) 1–30.

81. P.D. Delmas, R. Balena & E. Confraveux, The bisphosphonate residronate prevents bone loss in women with artificial menopause due to chemotherapy of breast cancer: a double-blind, placebo-controlled study, J Clin Oncol 15 (1997) 955–962.

82. T.J. Powles, E.V. McCloskey & A.H.G. Paterson, et al., Oral clodronate and reduction in loss of bone mineral density in women with operable primary breast cancer, J Natl Cancer Inst 90 (1998) 704–708.

83. M.F. Gnant, B. Mlineritsch & G. Luschin-Ebengreuth, et al., Zoledronic acid prevents cancer treatment-induced bone loss in premenopausal women receiving adjuvant endocrine therapy for hormone-responsive breast cancer: a report from the Austrian Breast and Colorectal Cancer Study Group, J Clin Oncol 25 (7) (2007) 820–828.

84. G. Ellis, H.G. Bone, R. Chlebowski, et al., A phase 3 study of the effect of denosumab therapy on bone mineral density in women receiving aromatase inhibitors for non-metastatic breast cancer. Proceedings of the San Antonio Breast Cancer Symposium Abstract 47 (2007).

85. T.J. Wronski, L.M. Dann & H. Qi, et al., Skeletal effects of withdrawal of estrogen and diphosphonate treatment in ovariectomised rats, Calcif Tissue Int 53 (1993) 210–216.

86. P.E. Goss, S. Qi & R.G. Josse, et al., The steroidal aromatase inhibitor exemestane prevents bone loss in ovariectomized rats, Bone 34 (2004) 384–392.

87. D. Vanderschueren, S. Boonen & A.G. Ederveen, et al., Skeletal effects of estrogen deficiency as induced by an aromatase inhibitor in an aged male rat model, Bone 27 (2000) 611–617.

88. A. Howell, J. Cuzick & M. Baum, et al., Results of the ATAC trial after completion of 5 years' adjuvant treatment for breast cancer, Lancet 365 (2005) 60–62.

89. R.C. Coombes, E. Hall & L.J. Gibson, et al., A randomised trial of exemestane after two to three years of tamoxifen therapy in postmenopausal women with primary breast cancer, N Engl J Med 350 (2004) 1081–1092.

90. P.E. Goss, J.N. Ingle & S. Martino, et al., A randomised trial of letrozole in post-menopausal women after five years of tamoxifen therapy for early stage breast cancer, N Engl J Med 349 (2003) 1793–1802.

91. C. Harper-Wynne, G. Ross & N. Sacks, et al., Effects of the aromatase inhibitor letrozole on normal breast epithelial cell proliferation and metabolic indices in postmenopausal women: a pilot study for breast cancer prevention, Cancer Epidemiol Biomarkers Prev 11 (2002) 614–621.

92. P.E. Lønning, J. Geisler & L.E. Krag, et al., Effects of exemestane administered for 2 years versus placebo on bone mineral density, bone biomarkers, and plasma lipids in patients with surgically resected early breast cancer, J Clin Oncol 23 (22) (2005) 5126–5137.

93. E.V. McCloskey, R.A. Hannon & G. Lakner, et al., Effects of third generation saromatase inhibitors on bone health and other safety parameters: results of an open, randomised, multi-centre study of letrozole, exemestane and anastrozole in healthy postmenopausal women, Eur J Cancer 43 (2007) 2523–2531.

94. J. Compston, Prevention and treatment of osteoporosis. Clinical guidelines and new evidence, J R Coll Physicians Lond 34 (2000) 518–521.

95. NIH Consensus Development Conference Panel, Osteoporosis prevention, diagnosis, and therapy, JAMA 285 (2001) 785–795.

96. J.D. Adachi, G. Ioannidis & L. Pickard, et al., The association between osteoporotic fractures and health-related quality of life as measured by the Health Utilities Index in the Canadian Multicentre Osteoporosis Study (CaMos), Osteoporos Int 14 (2003) 895–904.

97. J.P. Brown & R.G. Josse, Scientific Advisory Council of the Osteoporosis Society of Canada. 2002 Clinical practice guidelines for the diagnosis and management of osteoporosis in Canada, CMAJ 168 (2003) 675–676.

98. J.R. Mackey & A.A. Joy, Skeletal health in postmenopausal survivors of early breast cancer, Int J Cancer 114 (6) (2005) 1010–1015.

99. P. Hadji, M. Appro & A. Brufsky, et al., Practical guidance for the prevention of aromatase inhibitor-associated bone loss in women with breast cancer. Proceedings of the San Antonio Breast Cancer Symposium Abstract 504 (2007).

CHAPTER **36**

A Multi-targeted Approach to Treating Bone Metastases

ROBERT D. LOBERG[1] AND KENNETH J. PIENTA[1]

Department of Internal Medicine and Urology, University of Michigan Comprehensive Cancer Center, The University of Michigan, Ann Arbor, MI, USA.

Contents

This work was supported by the University of Michigan NIH Cancer Center Core Grant 5P30 CA 46592, PO1 CA093900, University of Michigan NIH SPORE in Prostate Cancer 2P50 CA 69568, and the Prostate Cancer Foundation. Dr. Pienta is an American Cancer Society Clinical Research Professor.

I. INTRODUCTION

Bone metastases are a major cause of morbidity and ultimately mortality for thousands of patients suffering from cancer worldwide each year. It is estimated that there are currently approximately 500,000 cancer patients in the United States and 10 million people worldwide afflicted with bone metastases. In the vast majority of cases, cancer continues to be an incurable disease once it has spread from its primary site to osseous sites [1]. A major focus for treating metastatic cancer has been on designing therapies directed at killing the replicating tumor cells. More attention has been placed on targeting the bone microenvironment as an additional way to achieve therapeutic benefit for patients. This recognition that cancer cells exist within a complex environment requiring the cooperation, or at a minimum, the undermining, of normal functions of multiple normal cell types, has led to a paradigm shift in the treatment of bone metastases. The continued evolution of this treatment paradigm shift requires a further understanding of the vicious cycle in which tumor cells interact with the normal host cells of the bone microenvironment, resulting in normal bone destruction and subsequent morbidity and mortality to the patient.

II. A MODEL FOR SUCCESSFUL CANCER METASTASIS TO BONE

The spread of tumor cells to the bone follows the paradigm established by Stephan Paget in 1889 of seed and soil: the tumor cell (seed) invading the marrow space (fertile soil) to successfully form metastatic lesions [2–4]. We have extended this paradigm and have described metastasis in terms of successful migration from a point of origin to a distant site (Figure 36.1). Cancer cells must successfully leave the primary tumor environment (emigration), travel to a new site (migration), land and establish themselves (immigration), and finally, flourish in their new environment (naturalization) [5]. Each of these steps requires the acquisition of properties or traits that are usually tightly regulated in non-cancerous cells to maintain host homeostasis.

Early in the life of a tumor, cells grow at an uncontrollable rate [6]. As the cancer grows, it must be supplied by new blood vessels or cells start to die from lack of a nutrient supply [7–9]. Hence, hypoxia creates a 'famine' environment for the tumor—analogous to the potato famine in Ireland starting an emigration to new countries [5]. Emigration, however, is only the first step in successful migration. Tumor cells, like migrants, must survive a journey to a distant destination and must find a hospitable place to land, establish themselves, and flourish. To accomplish successful metastasis to the bone marrow, cancer cells hijack several properties exhibited by normal

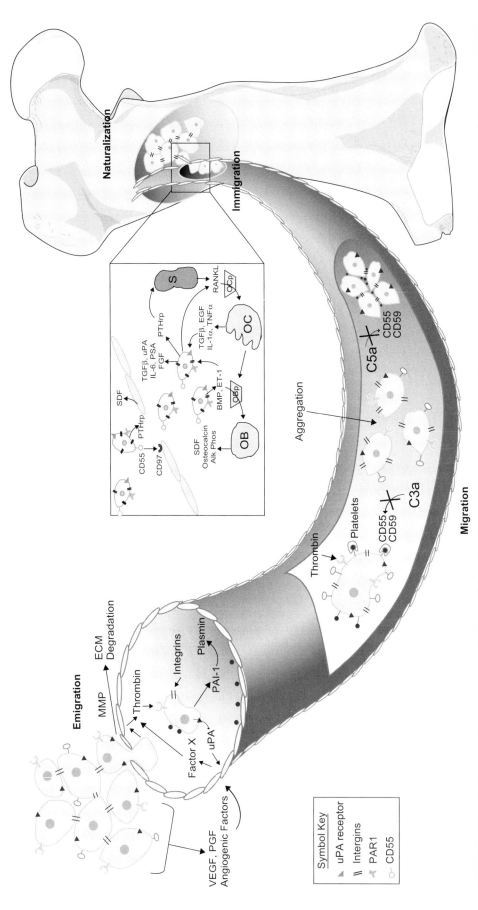

FIGURE 36.1 Mechanisms of cancer metastasis. The initial localized tumor promotes neoangiogenesis by the release of a variety of angiogenic growth factors (e.g. VEGF, PDGF). At the same time, tumor cells secrete matrix metalloproteinases (MMP) that break down the extracellular matrix (ECM) and allow the emigration of tumor cells into the circulation. Several factors are released in response to tumor cell intravasation, including urokinase plasminogen activator (uPA), plasminogen activator inhibitor-1 (PAI-1), and thrombin which promote tumor cell survival and metastasis. The aggregation of tumor cells and platelets during transit (migration) promotes survival and ultimately extravasation at the secondary tumor site. The mechanisms of tumor cell extravasation (immigration) involve docking to the endothelium with subsequent transit into the bone microenvironment. Once established, successful proliferation (naturalization) requires a coordinated, symbiotic relationship between the invading tumor cells and all of the host cells of the bone to create a tumor friendly environment. OBp, osteoblastic progenitor cells; OCp, osteoclastic progenitor cells; OB, osteoblast; OC, osteoclast; S, stromal cell; TFAg, Thomas Friedrich antigen; gal 3, galectin 3 receptor; PTHrp, parathyroid hormone related protein; SDF, stromal derived factor; CD55, decay accelerating factor; CD59, Protectin. Reprinted with permission: K.J. Pienta and R. Loberg. The 'emigration, migration, and immigration' of prostate cancer. *Clinical Prostate Cancer* 4(1) (2005) 24–30.

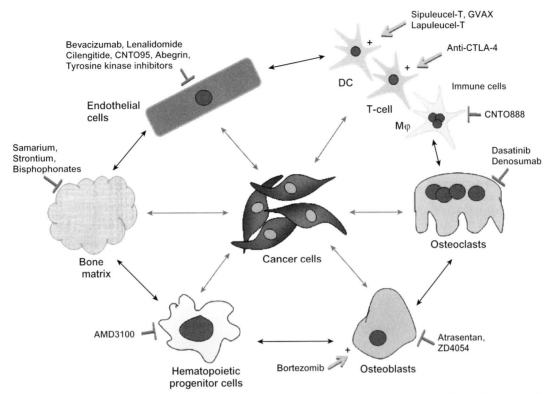

FIGURE 36.2 Tumor cell–bone microenvironment interactions. The relationship between the tumor cell and the surrounding tissue is a complex environment. Tumor cells interact with the bone extracellular matrixstromal cells, osteoblasts, osteoclasts, hematopoietic progenitor cells, endothelial cells, and cells of the immune system to coordinate a sophisticated series of interactions to promote tumor cell survival and proliferation. These interrelationships identify a paradigm shift in understanding cancer growth in bone and lead to the ability to design targeted therapies to interrupt the vicious cycle of the tumor cell with its microenvironment (see text for description of agents). DC, dendritic cells; Mφ, macrophage.

cells that use the circulation and bone marrow as their natural environment. Hypoxia leads to the upregulation of HIF-1α, which activates several cellular programs that mimic those expressed by hematopoietic progenitor cells (HPCs). This includes increased expression of CXC chemokine receptor 4 (CXCR4), the receptor for stromal derived factor-1 (SDF-1, CXCL12). Multiple tumor types, including breast, prostate, and multiple myeloma exhibit osteotropism through mimicry of HPCs which use this receptor to migrate to the bone marrow through chemoattraction to the CXCL12 secreted by osteoblasts [10–12]. Moreover, CXCL12 signaling through CXCR4 triggers an immigrant phenotype by triggering the adhesion of these cells to bone marrow endothelial cells and osteoblasts through activation of CD164 and αvβ3 integrins [13–15]. The high frequency of prostate cancer cell metastasis to bone, which occurs in virtually all patients, may be explained by the fact that these prostate cancer cells also bind to annexin-2, an adhesive-localization molecule used by HPCs [16–18].

Once established in the bone, metastatic cells flourish (naturalize) by utilizing a supporting framework of multiple host cells (Figure 36.2). An understanding of the biologic underpinnings of these interactions has allowed the development of several therapeutic strategies that target the host cells themselves as well as the complex interactions between the cancer cells and the host environment as well as the cross-talk between the different host cells which have been co-opted to support tumor growth (Figure 36.2, Table 36.1).

III. TARGETING OSTEOCLAST FUNCTION

Osteoclasts are active in bone remodeling and offer targets for interruption of the bone destruction associated with metastases. These cells are known to be activated by a variety of growth factors, many of which are secreted by cancer cells (i.e., TGFβ, EGF, IL-1, and IL-6). The activation of osteoclasts leads to the catalysis of the bone matrix and subsequent release of multiple growth factors and cytokines which are capable of stimulating metastatic growth in the bone, thereby creating the vicious cycle of further cancer growth and further bone destruction [19–21].

Bisphosphonates, by binding exposed bone matrix, inhibit osteoclast maturation and function. This poisoning of osteoclast function has been used in multiple

TABLE 36.1 Treating bone metastases: agents and their presumed targets within cells of the bone microenvironment

Cell type	Target	Example agents (Ref)
Osteoblast	Endothelin-1 receptor	Atrasentan, ZD-4054 [35,38]
	Proteosome	Bortezomib [42–44]
Hematopoietic progenitor cells	Stromal derived factor-1	AMD3100 [86–89]
Osteoclast	Pyrophosphate (bone matrix)	Bisphosphonates [22–27], samarium, strontium [45–49]
	RANKL	Denosumab [28–30]
	SRC	Dasatinib [31–33]
Endothelial cell	VEGF	Bevacizumab, VEGF-TRAP thalidomide, lenalidomide [52–57]
	VEGFR	Sunitinib, vatalanib, sorafenib [58–61]
	αvβ3/5 integrin	Cilengitide, Abegrin, CNTO 95 [62–66]
Immunologic activation	Macrophages	CNTO888 [83]
	T cells (CTLA-4)	MDX-010 [70,71]
	Complement (CD55)	105AD7 [72]
	Dendritic cells	sipuleucel-T [67] GVAX [68] Lapuleucel-T [69]

tumor types, including prostate, breast, lung, and multiple myeloma to decrease the morbidity of skeletal metastases [22–24]. For example, zoledronate has been demonstrated to decrease skeletal-related events such as fractures in patients with multiple cancers, including androgen-independent prostate cancer, lung cancer, renal cancer, and multiple myeloma [25–27]. Osteoclast function can also be inhibited through interruption of osteoblast-osteoclast cross-talk via inhibition of the receptor activator of nuclear factor-κB ligand (RANKL)—RANK—osteoprotegerin (OPG) receptor axis. These molecules, by mediating the interaction of osteoblasts with osteoclasts, function as the effector molecules of bone resorption. Inhibition of RANKL leads to osteoclast apoptosis. Denosumab is a fully human mAb directed against RANKL that is being studied in patients with osteoporosis and in patients with metastatic bone lesions [28–30]. Dasatinib is a tyrosine kinase inhibitor that is approved for the treatment of chronic myelogenous leukemia [31]. By targeting the

src pathway, dasatinib acts as an osteoclast inhibitor and therefore has potential to treat cancers that metastasize to bone [31–33].

IV. TARGETING OSTEOBLAST FUNCTION

Osteoblasts play a key role in the bone metastasis microenvironment as several growth factors (e.g., insulin-like growth factor 1, transforming growth factor beta, endothelin-1) produced by osteoblasts and osseous stromal cells act as chemoattractants for cancer cells, as well as promote tumor growth and proliferation [34].

Endothelin-1 (ET-1) is a vasoactive peptide released from the vascular endothelium that serves as a regulator of blood pressure and vascular tone by promoting vasoconstriction [35]. ET-1 is also an important mediator of tumor growth and tumor cell survival in prostate and breast cancers, especially within the bone microenvironment [36–39]. Initial evidence in preclinical models revealed that by using specific receptor antagonists to ET-1 the frequency of bone metastases and the rate of bone formation could be reduced *in vitro* and *in vivo* [35–37]. Several compounds are under investigation as a novel class of chemotherapeutic compounds that target the ETA receptor, including atrasentan, an orally bioavailable compound that has been the subject of several phase III clinical trials in prostate cancer [38–40]. Atrasentan appears to slow the progression of metastatic prostate cancer and interrupting the microenvironment by inhibiting the osteoblast axis appears to have scientific and clinical merit as a potential mode of treatment [35].

Another strategy of clinical importance is to turn on osteoblast function to ameliorate the inappropriate osteolytic activity as seen in diseases such as multiple myeloma [41]. In bone metastases where there is a predominantly lytic component, osteoblast activity is inappropriately repressed [42–44]. The proteosome inhibitor bortezomib has been demonstrated to activate osteoblast activity and is an effective therapy in multiple myeloma, suggesting that this agent may be a useful addition in treating lytic lesions induced by other cancers [41–44].

V. TARGETING BONE MATRIX

Another approach to creating an inhospitable microenvironment for tumor cells utilizes systemic radioisotopes [45,46]. Radioisotopes are effective therapeutic agents for the management and palliation of bone-specific disease due to the high levels of retention by bone metastases (highest in damaged bone, less in normal bone tissue, and no retention outside of bone). The most common radioisotopes are strontium-89 and samarium-135, both beta-emitting radioisotopes [45,46]. The mechanism of radiotherapy-induced palliation is associated with the radioisotopes combining with the calcium component of hydroxyapatite in damaged bone. Radioisotopes have been successfully utilized to palliate pain in patients with bone metastases [47–50]. Adding systemic radioisotopes to chemotherapy regimens for patients with advanced prostate cancer appears to increase response rates and survival [50,51]. Further exploration of how this could be applied to the human disease setting is being investigated in preclinical and clinical settings.

VI. TARGETING ENDOTHELIAL CELL FUNCTION

Cancer metastases, even those in the bone marrow microenvironment, require blood vessels for growth [7]. Multiple strategies are being pursued to block the stimulation of blood vessel proliferation, including the blockade of the interaction of VEGF with its receptors. This can be done by decreasing VEGF production, through antibodies to VEGF (i.e., bevacizumab), antibodies to the VEGF receptors to themselves, or by inhibiting the tyrosine kinase activity of the receptors. The secretion of VEGF by tumor cells as well as many of the supporting cells of the microenvironment can be inhibited by agents such as thalidomide and lenalidomide [52–54]. These agents have demonstrated significant activity in multiple myeloma. The efficacy of directly blocking the growth factor with the anti-VEGF antibody bevacizumab is the subject of a current phase III trial in combination with docetaxel for men with advanced prostate cancer [55–57]. Several small molecule inhibitors of tyrosine kinase activity have demonstrated activity in clinical trials in multiple cancers that metastasize to bone [58–61]. Another strategy targets integrin binding to block the sprouting of new blood vessels into the tumor microenvironment [62–66]. Tumor-related blood vessels sprout into the extracellular matrix through a process that is mediated by the integrins αvβ3 and αvβ5 which bind to a variety of ECM molecules including vitronectin [63]. Integrins αvβ3 and αvβ5 bind molecules containing the amino acid sequence Arg-Gly-Asp (RGD), allowing endothelial cells to attach to the extracellular matrix [63]. EMD 121974 (Cilengitide), a cyclized pentapeptide containing the amino acid sequence Arg-Gly-Asp (RGD), is in clinical trial in patients with advanced prostate cancer [62]. Two different antibodies that block the αvβ3/5 integrins, Vitaxin (Abegrin) and CNTO 95, are also under clinical development in patients with bone metastases [63–66].

VII. ENHANCING IMMUNE RESPONSE

Inhibition of cancer growth through the enhancement of the immune response of the host is also being pursued with a variety of therapies (Table 36.1, Figure 36.2). Several strategies are targeted at stimulating antigen presenting cells to recognize the cancer cells. For prostate cancer patients, Sipuleucel-T (APC8015, Provenge®) is an immunotherapy that exposes autologous dendritic cells to a recombinant fusion protein of prostatic acid phosphatase [67]. GVAX is an immunotherapy that is comprised of two irradiated prostate cancer cell lines which have been genetically modified to secrete granulocyte-macrophage colony-stimulating factor (GM-CSF) [68]. Lapuleucel-T (APC8024) is an autologous active cellular immunotherapy that activates cells with an HER-2-based antigen to treat breast cancer patients [69]. Blockade of the T-cell inhibitory receptor CTL-associated antigen-4 (CTLA-4) augments and prolongs T-cell responses and is under active clinical investigation to elicit antitumor immunity [70]. Blockade of Treg cells through a variety of mechanisms is actively being pursued [71]. An alternative approach within the concept of targeting the immune system is to target the complement system. For example, cancer cells overexpress CD55, a membrane bound complement regulatory protein that is over-expressed in a variety of cancers and protects cells against complement-mediated lysis. Currently, an anti-idiotypic monoclonal antibody, 105AD7, is in clinical trials as a cancer vaccine that mimics the tumor-associated antigen CD55 and has demonstrated the applicability of vaccine-targeted approaches in cancer treatment [72]. These strategies could be used in conjunction with chemotherapy as well as primary therapy early in the disease course.

VIII. TARGETING TUMOR ASSOCIATED MACROPHAGES

Many malignant tumors are associated with a leukocytic infiltrate that consists mainly of macrophages (often called tumor-associated macrophages), which in some instances, comprise up to 70% of the cell tumor mass [73–79]. These cells are an essential cellular component of the innate immune system and are derived from myeloid progenitor cells in the bone marrow compartment. These progenitor cells develop into pro-monocytes and are released into the circulation where they undergo differentiation into monocytes. Monocytes then migrate into tissues where they differentiate into resident tissue macrophages and help to protect these sites from infection and injury (or in the case of cancer monocytes differentiate into TAMs which are capable of promoting tumor growth and metastasis). In addition to this role in innate immunity, further evidence suggests that macrophages also play an important role in the regulation of angiogenesis in both normal and diseased tissues, including malignant tumors [77–79]. When associated with tumors, macrophages demonstrate functional 'polarization' towards one of two phenotypically different subsets of macrophages: T_H1 (also known as M1 macro-phages) or T_H2 (also known as M2 macrophages) [80,81]. The M2 macrophage–tumor associated macrophage population promotes tumor growth and development through stimulation of angiogenesis as well as matrix dissolution. Monocyte chemoattractant protein-1 (MCP-1, CCL2) is an important chemokine that is known to regulate monoctye/macrophage trafficking and has been reported to be present in several solid tumor beds [82–85]. The blockade of tumor associated macrophages induced by CCL-2 is the subject of planned clinical trials with an anti-CCL2 antibody, CNTO888 (Table 36.1) [1,83].

IX. TARGETING HEMATOPOIETIC PROGENITOR CELLS

Hematopoietic progenitor cells (HPCs) are a critical part of the bone microenvironment and the interaction of HPCs with cancer cells is an understudied area. While it may be impractical to target HPC–cancer cell interactions at this time, it is clear that cancer cells that metastasize to bone marrow hijack several properties exhibited by HPCs that traffic through the circulation and bone marrow [1,5]. For example, prostate cancer, breast cancer, and multiple myeloma cells mimic hematopoetic stem/progenitor cells by upregulating the expression of stromal derived factor-1 (SDF-1; also known as CXCL12) receptor CXC chemokine receptor 4 (CXCR4), resulting in chemoattraction to the CXCL12 secreted by the osteoblasts [10–12]. The inhibition of the SDF-1/CXCR4 axis is the target of multiple agents, many of which are already in clinical trials and can serve as a paradigm to further develop this field for the therapy of bone metastasis [14,87–89].

X. CONCLUSION

There is a need for continued therapeutic development based on multi-targeted therapy against the bone microenvironment.

Metastatic cancer in the skeleton is the result of a complex interplay between the cancer cells themselves and the bone microenvironment resulting in a heterogeneous disease that induces a combination of osteolytic and osteoblastic lesions. The pathogenesis of bone metastases includes interactions between the cancer cells and osteoclasts, osteoblasts, endothelial cells, stromal cells, hematopoietic progenitor cells, cells of the immune system, and the bone matrix. A paradigm shift from an initial treatment strategy that primarily targets the tumor cell directly, i.e. traditional chemotherapy, to new therapies that exploit the interactions and contributions of the various cells and elements of surrounding microenvironment to the development of the metastatic lesions is now being explored and already exploited to improve the lives of cancer patients living with skeletal metastases.

References

1. R.D. Loberg, D.A. Bradley & S.A. Tomlins, et al., The lethal phenotype of cancer: the molecular basis of death due to malignancy, CA Cancer J Clin 57 (4) (2007) 225–241.

2. I.J. Fidler, The pathogenesis of cancer metastasis: the 'seed and soil' hypothesis revisited, Nat Rev Cancer 3 (2003) 453–458.

3. S. Paget, The distribution of secondary growths in cancer of the breast, Lancet i (1889) 571–573.

4. J. Ewing. Metastasis, in: *Neoplastics*. 3rd edn. Saunders, Philadelphia (1928), pp. 77–89.

5. K.J. Pienta & R. Loberg, The 'emigration, migration, and immigration' of prostate cancer, Clin Prostate Cancer 4 (1) (2005) 24–30.

6. L.A. Norton, Gompertzian model of human breast cancer growth, Cancer Res 48 (1988) 7067–7071.

7. J. Folkman, Toward an understanding of angiogenesis: search and discovery, Perspect Biol Med 29 (1985) 10–36.

8. J. Carlsson, G.G. Stalnacke & H. Acker, et al., The influence of oxygen on viability and proliferation in cellular spheroids, Int J Radiat Oncol Biol Phys 5 (1979) 2011–2020.

9. L.T. Furcht, Critical factors controlling angiogenesis: cell products, cell matrix, and growth factors, Lab Invest 55 (1986) 505–509.

10. J. Wang, R. Loberg & R.S. Taichman, The pivotal role of CXCL12 (SDF-1)/CXCR4 axis in bone metastasis, Cancer Metastasis Rev 25 (4) (2006) 573–587.

11. A. Kortesidis, A. Zannettino & S. Isenmann, et al., Stromal-derived factor-1 promotes the growth, survival, and development of human bone marrow stromal stem cells, Blood 105 (10) (2005) 3793–3801.

12. Y. Jung, J. Wang & A. Schneider, et al., Regulation of SDF-1 (CXCL12) production by osteoblasts; a possible mechanism for stem cell homing, Bone 38 (4) (2006) 497–508.

13. Y.X. Sun, M. Fang & J. Wang, et al., Expression and activation of alphaVbeta3 integrins by SDF-1/CXCL12 increases the aggressiveness of prostate cancer cells, Prostate 67 (2007) 61–73.

14. Y.X. Sun, A. Schneider & Y. Jung, et al., Skeletal localization and neutralization of the SDF-1(CXCL12)/CXCR4 axis blocks prostate cancer metastasis and growth in osseous sites *in vivo*, J Bone Miner Res 20 (2) (2005) 318–329.

15. A.M. Havens, Y. Jung & Y.X. Sun, et al., The role of sialomucin CD164 (MGC-24v or endolyn) in prostate cancer metastasis, BMC Cancer 6 (2006) 195.

16. Y. Jung, J. Wang & J. Song, et al., Annexin II expressed by osteoblasts and endothelial cells regulates stem cell adhesion, homing and engraftment following transplantation, Blood 25 (2007) 1753–1760.

17. R.A. Sikes, B.E. Nicholson & K.S. Koeneman, et al., Cellular interactions in the tropism of prostate cancer to bone, Int J Cancer 110 (2004) 497–503.

18. L.W. Chung, A. Baseman & V. Assikis, et al., Molecular insights into prostate cancer progression: the missing link of tumor microenvironment, J Urol 173 (2005) 10–20.

19. E.T. Keller, The role of osteoclastic activity in prostate cancer skeletal metastases, Drugs Today (Barc) 38 (2002) 91–102.

20. G.R. Mundy, Metastasis to bone: causes, consequences and therapeutic opportunities, Nat Rev Cancer 2 (2002) 584–593.

21. R.D. Loberg, C.J. Logothetis & E.T. Keller, et al., Pathogenesis and treatment of prostate cancer bone metastasis: targeting the lethal phenotype, J Clin Oncol 23 (2005) 8232–8241.

22. T.C. Ha & H. Li, Meta-analysis of clodronate and breast cancer survival, Br J Cancer 96 (12) (2007) 1796–1801.

23. S. Wu, W.L. Dahut & J.L. Gulley, The use of bisphosphonates in cancer patients, Acta Oncol 46 (5) (2007) 581–591.

24. J.R. Ross, Y. Saunders & P.M. Edmonds, et al., A systematic review of the role of bisphosphonates in metastatic disease, Health Technol Assess 8 (4) (2004) 1–176.

25. A. Veri, M.R. D'Andrea & P. Bonginelli, et al., Clinical usefulness of bisphosphonates in oncology: treatment of bone metastases, antitumoral activity and effect on bone resorption markers, Int J Biol Markers 22 (1) (2007) 24–33.

26. D. Luftner, P. Henschke & K. Possinger, Clinical value of bisphosphonates in cancer therapy, Anticancer Res 27 (4A) (2007) 1759–1768.

27. F. Saad, D.M. Gleason & R. Murray, et al., Long-term efficacy of zoledronic acid for the prevention of skeletal complications in patients with metastatic hormone-refractory prostate cancer, J Natl Cancer Inst 96 (2004) 879–882.

28. E.M. Lewiecki, RANK ligand inhibition with denosumab for the management of osteoporosis, Expert Opin Biol Ther 6 (2006) 1041–1050.

29. E.M. Schwarz & C.T. Ritchlin, Clinical development of anti-RANKL therapy, Arthritis Res Ther 9 (Suppl 1) (2007) S7.

30. J.J. Body, T. Facon & R.E. Coleman, et al., A study of the biological receptor activator of nuclear factor-kappaB ligand inhibitor, denosumab, in patients with multiple myeloma or bone metastases from breast cancer, Clin Cancer Res 12 (4) (2006) 1221–1228.

31. F. Huang, K. Reeves & X. Han, et al., Identification of candidate molecular markers predicting sensitivity in solid tumors to dasatinib: rationale for patient selection, Cancer Res 67 (5) (2007) 2226–2238.

32. Y.M. Chang, H.J. Kung & C.P. Evans, Nonreceptor tyrosine kinases in prostate cancer, Neoplasia 9 (2007) 90–100.

33. S. Nam, D. Kim & J.Q. Cheng, et al., Action of the Src family kinase inhibitor, dasatinib (BMS-354825), on human prostate cancer cells, Cancer Res 65 (2005) 9185–9189.

34. M. Konopleva & M. Andreeff, Targeting the leukemia microenvironment, Curr Drug Targets 8 (6) (2007) 685–701.

35. A. Jimeno & M. Carducci, Targeting bone metastasis in prostate cancer with endothelin receptor antagonists, Clin Cancer Res 12 (2006) 6296s–6300s.

36. A. Bagnato & L. Rosano, Epithelial-mesenchymal transition in ovarian cancer progression: a crucial role for the endothelin axis, Cells Tissues Organs 185 (1–3) (2007) 85–94.

37. M.J. Grimshaw, Endothelins and hypoxia-inducible factor in cancer, Endocr Relat Cancer 14 (2) (2007) 233–244.

38. L. Rosano, V. Di Castro & F. Spinella, et al., ZD4054, a specific antagonist of the endothelin A receptor, inhibits tumor growth and enhances paclitaxel activity in human ovarian carcinoma *in vitro* and *in vivo*, Mol Cancer Ther 6 (7) (2007) 2003–2011.

39. C. Van Sant, G. Wang & M.G. Anderson, et al., Endothelin signaling in osteoblasts: global genome view and implication of the calcineurin/NFAT pathway, Mol Cancer Ther 6 (1) (2007) 253–261.

40. T.A. Guise & K.S. Mohammad, Endothelins in bone cancer metastases, Cancer Treat Res 118 (2004) 197–212.

41. M. Zangari, S. Yaccoby & F. Cavallo, et al., Response to bortezomib and activation of osteoblasts in multiple myeloma, Clin Lymphoma Myeloma 7 (2) (2006) 109–114.

42. E. Terpos, D.J. Heath & A. Rahemtulla, et al., Bortezomib reduces serum dickkopf-1 and receptor activator of nuclear factor-kappaB ligand concentrations and normalises indices of bone remodeling in patients with relapsed multiple myeloma, Br J Haematol 135 (5) (2006) 688–692.

43. R.L. Vessella & E. Corey, Targeting factors involved in bone remodeling as treatment strategies in prostate cancer bone metastasis, Clin Cancer Res 12 (20 Pt 2) (2006) 6285s–6290s.

44. D. Chauhan, T. Hideshima & C. Mitsiades, et al., Proteasome inhibitor therapy in multiple myeloma, Mol Cancer Ther 4 (4) (2005) 686–692.

45. O. Sartor, R.H. Reid & P.J. Hoskins, Quadramet 424Sm 10/11 Study Group, et al., Samarium-153–Lexidronam complex for treatment of painful bone metastases in hormone-refractory prostate cancer, Urology 63 (2004) 940–945.

46. A.T. Porter, A.J. McEwan & J.E. Powe, et al., Results of a randomized phase-III trial to evaluate the efficacy of strontium-89 adjuvant to local field external beam irradiation in the management of endocrine resistant metastatic prostate cancer, Int J Radiat Oncol Biol Phys 25 (1993) 805–813.

47. M.G. Lam, J.M. de Klerk & P.P. van Rijk, et al., Bone seeking radiopharmaceuticals for palliation of pain in cancer patients with osseous metastases, Anticancer Agents Med Chem 7 (4) (2007) 381–397.

48. M. Baczyk, R. Czepczynski & P. Milecki, et al., 89Sr versus 153Sm-EDTMP: comparison of treatment efficacy of painful bone metastases in prostate and breast carcinoma, Nucl Med Commun 28 (4) (2007) 245–250.

49. K. Liepe, R. Runge & J. Kotzerke, Radiopharmaceuticals for the palliation of painful bone metastasis—a systemic review, Radiother Oncol 75 (3) (2005) 258–270.

50. W. Akerley, J. Butera & T. Wehbe, et al., A multiinstitutional, concurrent chemoradiation trial of strontium-89, estramustine, and vinblastine for hormone refractory prostate carcinoma involving bone, Cancer 94 (2002) 1654–1660.

51. S.M. Tu, R.E. Millikan & B. Mengistu, et al., Bone-targeted therapy for advanced androgen-independent carcinoma of the prostate: a randomised phase II trial, Lancet 357 (2001) 336–341.

52. K.V. Rao, Lenalidomide in the treatment of multiple myeloma, Am J Health Syst Pharm 64 (17) (2007) 1799–1807.

53. J. Ghobrial, I.M. Ghobrial & C. Mitsiades, et al., Novel therapeutic avenues in myeloma: changing the treatment paradigm, Oncology (Williston Park) 21 (7) (2007) 785–792.

54. H. Murakami, H. Handa & M. Abe, et al., Low-dose thalidomide plus low-dose dexamethasone therapy in patients with refractory multiple myeloma, Eur J Haematol 79 (3) (2007) 234–239.

55. D.J. Hicklin & L.M. Ellis, Role of the vascular endothelial growth factor pathway in tumor growth and angiogenesis, J Clin Oncol 23 (5) (2005) 1011–1027.

56. J.A. Rumohr & S.S. Chang, Current chemotherapeutic approaches for androgen-independent prostate cancer, Curr Opin Investig Drugs 7 (6) (2006) 529–533.

57. C.J. Ryan, A.M. Lin & E.J. Small, Angiogenesis inhibition plus chemotherapy for metastatic hormone refractory prostate cancer: history and rationale, Urol Oncol 24 (2006) 250–253.

58. K.T. Flaherty, Sorafenib: delivering a targeted drug to the right targets, Expert Rev Anticancer Ther 7 (2007) 617–626.

59. A.J. Pantuck, N. Zomorodian & A.S. Belldegrun, Phase I, open-label, single-center, multiple-dose, dose-escalation clinical study of SUO11248 (sunitinib) in subjects with high-risk prostate cancer who have elected to undergo radical prostatectomy, Curr Urol Rep 8 (2007) 3–4.

60. J. Drevs, U. Zirrgiebel & C.I. Schmidt-Gersbach, et al., Soluble markers for the assessment of biological activity with PTK787/ZK 222584 (PTK/ZK), a vascular endothelial growth factor receptor (VEGFR) tyrosine kinase inhibitor in patients with advanced colorectal cancer from two phase I trials, Ann Oncol 16 (2005) 558–565.

61. S. Baka, A.R. Clamp & G.C. Jayson, A review of the latest clinical compounds to inhibit VEGF in pathological angiogenesis, Expert Opin Ther Targets 10 (2006) 867–876.

62. F.A. Eskens, H. Dumez & R. Hoekstra, et al., Phase I and pharmacokinetic study of continuous twice weekly intravenous administration of Cilengitide (EMD 121974), a novel inhibitor of the integrins alphavbeta3 and alphavbeta5 in patients with advanced solid tumours, Eur J Cancer 39 (2003) 917–926.

63. S.A. Mullamitha, N.C. Ton & G.J. Parker, et al., Phase I evaluation of a fully human anti-alphav integrin monoclonal antibody (CNTO 95) in patients with advanced solid tumors, Clin Cancer Res 13 (7) (2007) 2128–2135.

64. G.C. Tucker, Integrins: molecular targets in cancer therapy, Curr Oncol Rep 8 (2) (2006) 96–103.

65. A. Gramoun, S. Shorey & J.D. Bashutski, et al., Effects of Vitaxin(R), a novel therapeutic in trial for metastatic bone tumors, on osteoclast functions *in vitro*, J Cell Biochem 102 (2007) 341–352.

66. K. Mulgrew, K. Kinneer & X.T. Yao, et al., Direct targeting of alphavbeta3 integrin on tumor cells with a monoclonal antibody, *Abegrin*, Mol Cancer Ther 5 (12) (2006) 3122–3129.

67. R. So-Rosillo & E.J. Small, Sipuleucel-T (APC8015) for prostate cancer, Expert Rev Anticancer Ther 6 (2006) 1163–1167.

68. K.M. Hege, K. Jooss & D. Pardoll, GM-CSF gene-modifed cancer cell immunotherapies: of mice and men, Int Rev Immunol 25 (2006) 321–352.

69. J.W. Park, M.E. Melisko & L.J. Esserman, et al., Treatment with autologous antigen-presenting cells activated with the HER-2 based antigen Lapuleucel-T: results of a phase I study in immunologic and clinical activity in HER-2 overexpressing breast cancer, J Clin Oncol 25 (24) (2007) 3680–3687.

70. E.J. Small, N.S. Tchekmedyian & B.I. Rini, et al., A pilot trial of CTLA-4 blockade with human anti-CTLA-4 in patients with hormone-refractory prostate cancer, Clin Cancer Res 13 (2007) 1810–1815.

71. A. Fulton, F. Miller & A. Weise, et al., Prospects of controlling breast cancer metastasis by immune intervention, Breast Dis 26 (2007) 115–127.

72. K. Pritchard-Jones, I. Spendlove & C. Wilton, et al., Immune responses to the 105AD7 human anti-idiotypic vaccine after

73. J.E. Talmadge, M. Donkor & E. Scholar, Inflammatory cell infiltration of tumors: Jekyll or Hyde, Cancer Metastasis Rev 26 (2007) 373–400.

74. H.J. Knowles & A.L. Harris, Macrophages and the hypoxic tumour microenvironment, Front Biosci 12 (2007) 4298–4314.

75. Y.P. Liao, D. Schaue & W.H. McBride, Modification of the tumor microenvironment to enhance immunity, Front Biosci 12 (2007) 3576–3600.

76. A. Sica & V. Bronte, Altered macrophage differentiation and immune dysfunction in tumor development, J Clin Invest 117 (5) (2007) 1155–1166.

77. A.E. Dirkx, M.G. Oude Egbrink & J. Wagstaff, et al., Monocyte/macrophage infiltration in tumors: modulators of angiogenesis, J Leukoc Biol 80 (6) (2006) 1183–1196.

78. C.E. Lewis & J.W. Pollard, Distinct role of macrophages in different tumor microenvironments, Cancer Res 66 (2) (2006) 605–612.

79. L. Bingle, N.J. Brown & C.E. Lewis, The role of tumour-associated macrophages in tumour progression: implications for new anticancer therapies, J Pathol 196 (3) (2002) 254–265.

80. A. Sica, T. Schioppa & A. Mantovani, et al., Tumour-associated macrophages are a distinct M2 polarised population promoting tumour progression: potential targets of anti-cancer therapy, Eur J Cancer 42 (6) (2006) 717–727.

81. A. Mantovani, T. Schioppa & C. Porta, et al., Role of tumor-associated macrophages in tumor progression and invasion, Cancer Metastasis Rev 25 (3) (2006) 315–322.

82. C. Porta, B. Subhra Kumar & P. Larghi, et al., Tumor promotion by tumor-associated macrophages, Adv Exp Med Biol 604 (2007) 67–86.

83. R.D. Loberg, C. Ying & M. Craig, et al., CCL2 as an important mediator of prostate cancer growth *in vivo* through the regulation of macrophage infiltration, Neoplasia 9 (7) (2007) 556–562.

84. C. Bailey, R. Negus & A. Morris, et al., Chemokine expression is associated with the accumulation of tumour associated macrophages (TAMs) and progression in human colorectal cancer, Clin Exp Metastasis 24 (2) (2007) 121–130.

85. R. Giles & R.D. Loberg, CCL2 (Monocyte Chemoattractant Protein-1) in cancer bone metastases, Cancer Metastasis Rev 25 (4) (2006) 611–619.

86. J. Juarez, L. Bendall & K. Bradstock, Chemokines and their receptors as therapeutic targets: the role of the SDF-1/CXCR4 axis, Curr Pharm Des 10 (11) (2004) 1245–1259.

87. A.F. Cashen, B. Nervi & J. DiPersio, AMD3100: CXCR4 antagonist and rapid stem cell-mobilizing agent, Future Oncol 3 (1) (2007) 19–27.

88. N. Flomenberg, J. DiPersio & G. Calandra, Role of CXCR4 chemokine receptor blockade using AMD3100 for mobilization of autologous hematopoietic progenitor cells, Acta Haematol 114 (4) (2005) 198–205.

89. Y. Alsayed, H. Ngo & J. Runnels, et al., Mechanisms of regulation of CXCR4/SDF-1 (CXCL12)-dependent migration and homing in multiple myeloma, Blood 109 (7) (2007) 2708–2717.

intensive chemotherapy, for osteosarcoma, Br J Cancer 92 (8) (2005) 1358–1365.

CHAPTER **37**

Bone Metastases of Prostatic Cancer: Pathophysiology, Clinical Complications, Actual Treatment and Future Directions

SARA DE DOSSO[1], FERNANDA G. HERRERA[2] AND DOMINIK R. BERTHOLD[3]

[1]*Department of Medical Oncology.*
[2]*Radiation-Oncology, Bellinzona, Switzerland.*
[3]*Centre Pluridisciplinaire d Oncologie, Lausanne, Switzerland.*

Contents

I. MECHANISMS OF BONE METASTASIS

Prostate cancer usually metastasizes to the osseous tissue before other sites, remaining confined to bone in almost 80% of men presenting with advanced disease. Lymph node metastases are detected radiologically in about 20% of patients while lung and liver metastasis is relatively rare. The most commonly accepted mechanism that explains the preference of prostate cancer cells to spread to bone was proposed in 1940 by Batson [1]. By experimenting on animal and human cadavers he demonstrated that spread occurs through a valveless retrograde vertebral venous system that connects the pelvis with the vertebral spine.

Bony metastasis damages the skeleton mechanically, through compression of the vascular system and consequent ischemia, or structurally through a reciprocal cancer-stroma interaction resulting in tumor progression through enhanced paracrine signaling, which will ultimately affect the osteogenesis with consequent bone fragility and density loss [2,3]. The 'seed and soil' theory proposed by Paget in 1889 anticipated the relationship between the tumor and its microenvironment [4,5]. Other physiologic and molecular factors have also been described. As an example, cancer cells produce adhesive molecules that bind them to marrow stromal cells and bone matrix, increasing the production of pro-angiogenic molecules and bone-resorbing factors that

further enhance tumor growth in bone [6]. Blood flow is also high in areas where red marrow resides, explaining the predilection of metastases for those sites [7]. Bone also has a large pool of growth factors (transforming growth factor β, insulin-like growth factors I and II, fibroblast growth factors, platelet-derived growth factors, etc.) which provide a fertile ground in which tumor cells can grow [8,9].

These mechanisms of spread make prostate cancer an interesting experimental model to study the pathogenesis and molecular basis of bone metastatic disease, which may ultimately provide a new insight for novel treatment strategies.

A. Osteolytic Metastases

Osteolytic lesions are usually most frequent in breast, lung, and kidney cancer. Tumor cells secrete factors stimulating, directly or indirectly, the osteoclastic activity. These factors can be local (paracrine) or systemic.

Some well-described paracrine factors are prostaglandin-E (PGE), and a variety of cytokines and growth factors, such as the epidermal growth factor (EGF), tumor necrosis factor (TNF), interleukin-1 (IL-1), and the transforming growth factor (TGF) α and β [10].

In vitro studies of isolated osteoclasts have demonstrated that these factors alone cannot stimulate the growth of active osteoclasts. However, this process may be possible in the presence of osteoblasts. Osteoblasts are key mediators of the osteoclastic activity caused by a mechanism not yet identified but probably related to cell-to-cell contact, and the presence of another, as yet unknown, molecular factors.

Malignant cells can also directly stimulate osteoclastic activity, producing other local paracrine factors such as procathepsin-D and parathyroid hormone-related protein (PTH-rP).

The latter belongs to a family of protein hormones that share the N-terminal end of parathyroid hormone, which is necessary for stimulating osteoclastic bone resorption [11]. In particular, it has been demonstrated that transforming growth factor beta (TGF-3-beta) plays an integral role in promoting the development and progression of osteolytic bone metastases by inducing tumor production of PTHrP and establishing a vicious cycle with the bone microenvironment that has been described in breast cancer cells at the molecular level [12]. Osteolysis can be produced in a systemic manner by stimulating osteoclastic bone resorption: ectopic production of PTH-rP (observed particularly in lung cancer) is involved in the aetiology of systemic hypercalcemia, which is not observed when PTH-rP is secreted in excess in the case of paracrine activity [13].

Human prostate cancer cells line with neuroendocrine differentiation have been found to produce PTH-rP. It has been recognized that osteoclast activation contributes to bone damage in osteoblastic lesions in a similar way to that in osteolytic disease [14].

PTH-rP stimulates osteoblasts and stromal cells production of RANK ligand, which, binding to its receptor RANK-R, promotes their differentiation into mature and active clones [15]. Receptor activator of the nuclear factor-κB ligand (RANKL) is essential for the differentiation, function and survival of osteoclasts, which play a key role in the establishment and propagation of skeletal disease.

Osteolysis and tumor cell accumulation can be interrupted by inhibiting any of these limbs of the vicious cycle. Identification of the molecular mechanisms responsible for osteolytic metastases is crucial in designing effective therapy for this painful complication.

B. Osteoblastic Metastases

Although osteolysis in several types of neoplasms is the most common expression of metastatic bone disease, in prostate cancer osteosclerosis greatly predominates. In contrast to breast and lung cancer, advanced prostate cancer tends to cause osteoblastic lesions in bone, with dense, sclerotic-looking metastases on radiologic imaging. Osteoblast activation can be a consequence of osteoclast activity or directly caused by osteoblast-stimulating factors produced by cancer cells.

Based on the hypothesis that osteoblastic disease is an effect of osteoclast activation, histomorphometric studies and measurement of urinary markers of osteolytic activity have reported an increased bone resorption in biopsies from sites of metastatic osteoblastic disease and elevated levels of biochemical markers of bone resorption. This suggests that in some cases the osteosclerosis process is preceded by osteoclastic bone resorption [16,17]. In prostate cancer cell lines, co-expression of PTH-rP and its receptor has been found, confirming the role of osteoclasts in the development of osteoblastic lesions [18]. Therefore, it has been demonstrated that the formation of osteoblastic disease is not always necessarily preceded by an intense osteoclastic activity and it is, therefore, likely that cancer cells are able to promote both bone lysis and new bone deposition.

Endothelin-1 (ET-1) is produced by prostatic cancer cells and involved in bone lesion development. This protein with a potent vasoconstrictive effect is produced in the normal prostate gland by epithelial cells and found in seminal fluid at the highest concentration. This protein exerts its effects through two receptors, ET-a and ET-b [19]. In cancer cell lines ET-a expression seems to be upregulated. In animal models of prostate cancer ET-1 has been found to induce growth of osteoblasts and to inhibit osteoclast activity driving the osteoblast–osteoclast balance to favor new bone formation [19]. It has also been demonstrated that osteoblastic response to metastatic prostate cancer cells significantly decreases in animals treated with an ET-a antagonist [20].

Further factors that are believed to be responsible for osteoblastic proliferation or differentiation are: insulin-like growth factor (IGF), platelet-derived growth factor (PDGF), vascular endothelial growth factor (VEGF) and bone metastasis related factor (MDA-BF-1). These have all been associated with prostate cancer progression and enhanced osteoblastic disease [21,22].

II. CLINICAL COMPLICATIONS

Bone metastases are the most common cause of morbidity in patients with advanced prostate cancer, significantly affecting their quality of life. Clinical complications consist of intermittent or constant bone pain, malignant spinal cord compression (MSCC), pathologic fracture and bone marrow infiltration. The clinical evaluation typically includes a patient's medical history, physical examination, radiological examinations of plain radiographs, bone scans, computed tomography (CT) or magnetic resonance image (MRI) of suspicious areas, serum calcium and bone-specific alkaline phosphatase (BAP).

A. Bone Pain

Pain is usually the first and most common symptom of a metastatic cancer that has spread to bone. The causes can be different, such as periosteal stretching for the bone invasion due to growing mass, infiltration of nerve roots due to the spread of tumors to surrounding neurological structures, pathological fractures, and the local release of cytokines.

Clinically, bone pain differs from that of joint disorders, because of its characteristic persistence, generally worse during the night. It is usually stabbing, deep, sometimes well localized and fixed, dull, not ameliorating with the change of posture, but exacerbated by movement.

Metastatic bone pain may be poorly localized and in this case it can be particularly difficult to evaluate.

Treatment options include a broad spectrum of possibilities and the selection of therapy may vary depending on different oncological situations (i.e., analgesics, biphosphonates, systemic anti-neoplastic treatment, radiotherapy (RT), and in particular cases, orthopedic stabilization).

1. ROLE OF RADIATION THERAPY IN THE MANAGEMENT OF PAINFUL BONE METASTASIS

Radiotherapy is a well-recognized, effective modality in the palliative treatment of painful bone metastases. About 50–80% of patients experience improvement in their pain, and 20–50% of the treated patients have complete pain relief [23–25].

The optimal dose-fractionation schedule for the treatment of bone metastases is still under debate. It has been suggested that the choice of fractionation is influenced not only by patient-related factors but also by physician education and attitude, treatment toxicity, resource utilization, departmental policy, and economic issues, etc. [26].

Over past decades, significant clinical trial efforts have been devoted to comparing single large-dose radiation (8 Gy to 10 Gy) with multifraction regimens (five to ten fractions) [27–29].

Two large trials were published in 1999 by the Bone Pain Trial Working Party [30], and the Dutch Bone Metastasis Study Group [31]. A third randomized trial was published by the RTOG [25]. Most of these studies included between 20 and 50% patients with prostate cancer, and have shown no statistically significant difference in pain relief between shorter-duration, lower-dose treatments and longer-duration, higher-dose treatments. There were no obvious differences between the various treatment schedules and the incidence of acute or late toxicity in most of the studies, and only one study reported higher rates of acute toxicity among patients receiving 30 Gy in 10 fractions [25].

Metanalysis studies confirm that data, emphasizing that only the re-irradiation rates, pathologic fractures and MSCC were consistently different between the treatment arms (more frequent re-irradiation, pathologic fracture or MSCC in lower dose arms among trials reporting these data) [32–34]. However, a potential physician bias may be responsible for the statistical significant difference in re-irradiation rates (more willingness to give another treatment after a single-dose treatment than after a higher-dose treatment).

In 2000, the Trans-Tasman Radiation Oncology Group undertook a randomized trial comparing the efficacy of a single 8 Gy with 20 Gy in five fractions for neuropathic pain due to bone metastasis, showing the same result [27].

However, there may be subgroups of patients who require fractionated treatments at a higher dose (patients with pathologic fractures, MSCC or at high risk of pathologic fracture or MSCC). Patients with extensive soft-tissue disease arising from bone metastases in which the intent of treatment is not only pain relief but also the reduction of tumor bulk, may also benefit from a higher dose. However, prognostically favorable patients with a relatively long life expectancy did not experience a better response with multifraction radiation, according to the data from the Dutch study. And the evidence supported by the metanalysis did not support the notion of a more durable response with higher dose fractionation.

B. Malignant Spinal Cord Compression

Spinal cord compression is a frequent complication seen in patients with metastatic prostate cancer occurring in 5 to 12% of cases [35]. The spinal cord is compressed by an enlarging extradural mass involving the vertebral body and extending into the spinal canal or by a vertebral dislocation after a pathologic fracture. Less frequently, an intra-spinal metastasis may be responsible for cord compression without involving the bone.

The most common symptoms that may suggest a cord compression are local or radicular back pain, together with neurologic disorders such as motor weakness and sensory loss. Urinary and fecal incontinence or urinary retention may be present when there is compression of the lower tract of the spinal cord. It is a devastating event for both the patient and his or her relatives.

The development of back pain in patients with advanced prostate cancer and radiologic abnormalities at a standard x-ray should preferably be studied with a bone scan followed by MRI to exclude early spinal cord damage. In a study by Bayley *et al.* in patients with metastatic prostate carcinoma, they used a multivariate logistic regression analysis and the extent of disease score and duration of hormonal therapy were predictive of subclinical cord compression ($p = 0.02$ and $p = 0.04$, respectively). Patients with extensive bone scan disease (>20 metastases) had a 32% risk of spinal cord compression before starting hormone therapy, and they were at a 44% risk of compression after 24 months of hormone therapy. The findings of Bayley *et al.* [36] were consistent with those of Talcott *et al.* [37], in that back pain was not predictive of spinal cord compression, and they suggest that patients with high-risk bone scans should be examined further to detect potential MSCC early.

Spinal cord compression represents a medical emergency, necessitating prompt diagnosis and rapid intervention. Corticosteroids, surgery and emergency radiation therapy are all recognized treatments for malignant spinal cord compression and will be further described below.

1. THE ROLE FOR SYSTEMIC CORTICOSTEROIDS

Vecht *et al.* reported the results of a small randomized study that compared high-dose bolus dexamethasone (100 mg) to moderate-dose bolus dexamethasone (10 mg). All patients ($n = 37$) were treated with radiation and maintenance dexamethasone (16 mg/d orally). At 1 week, one (8%) of 13 patients administered moderate-dose dexamethasone and five (25%) of 20 patients administered high-dose dexamethasone showed improved neurologic status, but the difference was not statistically significant [38].

Sorensen and colleagues randomly assigned 57 patients with spinal cord compression treated with radiation to either high-dose maintenance dexamethasone or no corticosteroids (control group). They concluded that high-dose maintenance dexamethasone significantly improves ambulation, but the adverse effects of high-dose maintenance dexamethasone are also greater than with no corticosteroid treatment. Three patients (11%) in the high-dose maintenance dexamethasone group had serious adverse effects, including severe psychoses and gastric ulcers requiring surgery [39].

In conclusion, the current evidence supports the use of moderate doses of dexamethasone in the early phases of therapy. High-dose dexamethasone may be an effective adjunct to RT in improving post-treatment ambulation but carries the risk of serious toxicity. Patients who are ambulatory do not need to be prescribed dexamethasone but should be aware of the symptoms of spinal cord compression.

2. INDICATIONS FOR RT IN THE MANAGEMENT OF MSCC

Several studies support the irradiation of subclinical MSCC as a method of preserving neurologic function. Predictive models may help to define a population of patients at higher risk of developing MSCC, but the optimal screening strategy, population, and intervention have yet to be elucidated [36,37,40]. In a retrospective analysis performed by Huddart *et al.* of 70 patients with prostate cancer and MSCC after RT treatment, 52% had a functional improvement of motor function with 63% of non-ambulant patients becoming ambulant. On multivariate analysis a single level of compression, no previous hormone therapy and a young age (<65 years) predicted for better outcome [41].

Several prognostic scores have been proposed to aid decisions related to a surgical approach according to patient life expectancy, neurologic and performance status as well as predictors of ambulatory function after decompressive surgery [42,43].

A study by Patchell *et al.* has further added evidence to change the management of selected patients with MSCC [44]. They randomly assigned patients with MSCC to either surgery followed by RT 30 Gy in 10 fractions ($n = 50$) or RT alone ($n = 51$). Thirty percent of patients in the entire cohort had metastatic genitourinary cancers. The study was terminated at 50% of accrual (101 patients) when a planned interim analysis met predetermined early stopping rules for the primary outcome. Patients undergoing combined-modality therapy were able to walk further compared with patients

receiving RT alone (median ambulation, 126 vs 35 days, respectively; $p = 0.006$). They also had better pain control, and there was a trend to survival improvement ($p = 0.08$). Furthermore, in the paraparetic group, three (19%) of 16 patients who underwent RT regained ambulation, whereas nine (58%) of 16 patients who received surgery followed by RT recovered the ability to walk ($p < 0.03$).

It is generally accepted that patients who deteriorate neurologically during RT or who recompress after RT should be considered for surgery. Patients who recompress in-field after RT may be considered for re-irradiation, especially if it has been more than 6 weeks since the completion of their last course.

C. Pathologic Fracture

Overall, the pathologic fracture rate from prostate cancer with its predominantly sclerotic nature is relatively low compared to that of other metastatic cancers [45]. However, when bone metastases appear osteoblastic by radiographic imaging, they often show an exuberant osteoclast activity, which is associated with an increased risk of skeletal complications. Men treated with androgen deprivation therapies are at high risk of osteoporosis and therefore at risk of fractures, independently of the presence or absence of bone metastasis [46].

Clinically, anticipatory events of fractures are functional pain, in particular exacerbated with movement. At radiological evaluation the prognostic factors that can preclude a fracture are: the site of metastatic localization in the skeleton (i.e., involving weight-bearing bones, such as proximal femora), the size of the lesions (i.e., greater than two-thirds of the diameter of a long bone), and the extension of bone destruction. Patients presenting bone metastases with such characteristics should be treated with prophylactic procedures in an attempt to prevent possible complications. Axial cortical involvement offers a simple tool for deciding which treatment is appropriate [47].

Surgical fixation is the treatment of choice followed by RT in order to inhibit tumor growth and further bone weakness. Postoperative radiation treatment of pathologic fractures has been demonstrated to be associated with a better recovery of the functional status and a decrease in second procedures [48]. Radiotherapy alone is indicated in patients with poor prognosis disease or who are considered not suitable for surgery [49].

Biphosphonates are used as a prophylactic therapy of pathological fractures in patients with hormone-refractory metastatic prostate cancer, and for reducing the rate of skeletal-related events [45,50].

D. Bone Marrow Infiltration

The replacement of normal bone marrow with cancer cells causes an impaired hematopoiesis, with a low-grade normocytic or occasionally macrocytic anemia and possibly pancytopenia, predisposing patients to infections and hemorrhages. While almost all patients with prostate cancer have some degree of anemia due to hormonal, radiation and chemotherapeutic treatment, thrombocytopenia and leucopenia are usually related to bone marrow infiltration. There are only a few treatment options for this complication, and either treating the metastatic prostate cancer or providing supportive care which includes blood transfusions may improve this hematologic status [51].

III. CURRENT AND EMERGING THERAPEUTIC STRATEGIES IN BONE METASTATIC PROSTATE CANCER

Despite survival rate improvements with the introduction of chemotherapy for treating metastatic prostate cancer, for most patients with refractory disease, bone metastasis remains a significant cause of morbidity. An understanding of prostate cancer cell biology and its mechanisms of interaction with the abnormal tumor microenvironment has led to the development of drugs directed against specific molecular pathways with the aim of improving outcome in this vulnerable group of patients.

Evidence supporting the biological rational for the clinical development of these drugs is strong, and the integration of these agents in the treatment of metastatic disease is discussed here.

While many strategies are directed against bone metastasis, the principal treatment remains the systemic anticancer therapy. Therefore, at the end of this chapter a brief summary about current hormonal and chemotherapeutic treatment is given.

A. Osteoclast Inhibitors

Bisphosphonates are pyrophosphate analogs that inhibit osteoclast-mediated bone resorption, and have been shown to be effective in the treatment of lythic metastatic condition and in patients with hypercalcemia. Biochemical and histopathological studies have shown that metastases from prostate cancer are actually mixed with a significant osteolytic and osteoclastic component. This rapid bone turnover may increase bone fragility and, consequently, the risk of skeletal complications such as fractures, spinal cord compression, and vertebral weaknesses.

Thus, this broad spectrum of mechanisms may be targeted by blocking bone destruction while preserving mineralization. The use of bisphosphonates is a promising treatment strategy for these patients.

The most widely available agent has been zoledronic acid, a nitrogen-containing bisphosphonate. Results of a phase 3 double-blind placebo control trial in patients with hormonal-refractory prostate cancer (HRPC) has shown that the addition of zolendronic acid (4 mg in 15 min intravenous infusion) to conventional treatments significantly reduces pain scores and the probability of skeletal complications [45]. These data led to the approval of zoledronic acid for patients with bone metastasis from prostate cancer. However, the role of this agent in earlier disease settings and its association with androgen deprivation still needs to be elucidated. An ongoing CALGB randomized phase 3 trial is looking at the effectiveness of zolendronic acid in preventing bone-related events in patients who are already receiving androgen deprivation therapy. The study plans to accrue 680 patients, and the primary end point is timed until the first skeletal related event.

Another osteoclast inhibitor, denosumab, a human monoclonal antibody that triggers the nuclear factor kβ receptor activator (RANKL), is a key mediator of osteoclast differentiation and function. It has been shown to reduce bone turnover and resorption in patients with multiple myeloma and metastatic breast cancer [52,53]. A phase 2 randomized study comparing different treatment schedules of subcutaneous denosumab versus zolendronic acid in the treatment of metastatic breast cancers has shown similar effectiveness of both agents in suppressing bone turnover and skeletal events. No serious adverse events related to denosumab were reported, which will probably warrant further development of this drug. An ongoing phase 3 randomized, double-blind, placebo-controlled trial of denosumab investigates the bone metastasis-free survival in men with HRPC.

B. Osteoblast Inhibitors

Patients with prostate cancer develop osteoblastic metastases when tumor cells develop in the bone and stimulate osteoblasts by secreting growth-promoting factors. Endothelin 1 (ET-1) is believed to play a central role in promoting osteoblastic metastasis. Selective blockade of the ET(A) receptor is an established strategy in the development of prostate cancer therapeutics.

Atrasetan (ABT 627), a small molecule that blocks the binding of ET-1 to ET-A, has been shown to interfere in the pathogenesis and progression of osteoblastic lesions [54]. Atrasetan has shown biologic and clinical activity in phase 2 and 3 clinical studies, significantly delaying the time to clinical and PSA progression in men with metastatic prostate cancer compared with placebo-treated patients [55].

A study by Michaelson *et al.* investigated the potential synergistic effect of osteoblast and osteoclast inhibitors. A randomized phase 2 study compared atrasetan alone or in combination with zoledronic acid in men with advanced HRPC. The study failed to demonstrate additive effects from the combined treatment with no significant changes in bone turnover markers [56].

Negative results were also obtained in a phase 3 trial that randomized 809 men with metastatic prostate cancer to receive either atrasetan 10 mg per day or placebo [57].

Atrasetan did not delay disease progression despite evidence of biologic effects on PSA and alkaline phosphatase as markers of disease burden. While there is a biological rational to combine these treatments, an additive effect from these drugs could still not be demonstrated.

The Southwest Oncology Group (SWOG) is currently exploring the combination of docetaxel, prednisone and atrasetan compared to docetaxel and prednisone in HRPC patients.

C. Current Systemic Anticancer Treatment

The relationship between 'testicular factors' and the prostate has been suspected since the eighteenth century and hormonal ablation, achieved through bilateral orchiectomy, was established in 1944. The mechanisms of tumor progression dependent on the androgen receptor have only been elucidated over the last three decades.

Orchiectomy is nowadays rarely offered. Luteinizing hormone-releasing hormone (LHRH)-agonists such as groserelin, leuprolide and triptorelin are easily administered once every 1–4 months achieving similar results compared to surgical castration [58]. Side effects are impotence, modification of the lipid profile and loss of muscle mass [59]. As mentioned, longstanding treatment with an LHRH-agonist increases the risk of osteoporosis and osteoporotic fractures [60]. A slightly increased cardiovascular event rate has also been reported.

Peripheral anti-androgens, agents that block the androgen receptor, are also prescribed to treat advanced prostate cancer. Bicalutamide, given at 150 mg/day has a slightly better toxicity profile in terms of impotence, bone and muscle loss. However, its use is not universally accepted because of lower activity, painful gynecomastia and gastrointestinal side effects [61].

Unfortunately, prostate cancer will ultimately become castration-resistant. While this term is not precise, it usually indicates tumor progression despite hormonal ablation. At that stage further hormonal manipulations are possible but the discussion exceeds the aim of this book.

The standard therapy for men with castration-resistant prostate cancer is currently docetaxel [62,63]. The drug exerts its cytotoxic activity by promoting and stabilizing microtubule assembly of tubulin dimers with blockade of mitotic cell division in the M-phase. The drug is given intravenously every 3 weeks for 30 weeks, depending on efficacy and tolerability. The PSA response rate is around 50% with a survival benefit of 3 months [64]. Toxicity is usually mild to moderate with neutropenia, fatigue, peripheral neuropathy and fluid retention.

Currently, there is no standard treatment for second line therapies [65]. Mitoxantrone, a drug previously used in the treatment of HRPC, has only limited activity [66]. Many trials are ongoing in first and second line therapies and patients should be offered to participate whenever this is possible.

References

1. O.V. Batson, The function of the vertebral veins and their role in the spread of metastases, Ann Surg 112 (1940) 138–149.
2. S.Y. Sung, C.L. Hsieh & A. Law, et al., Coevolution of prostate cancer and bone stroma in three-dimensional coculture: implications for cancer growth and metastasis, Cancer Res 68 (2008) 9996–10003.
3. R. Hill, Y. Song & R.D. Cardiff, et al., Selective evolution of stromal mesenchyme with p53 loss in response to epithelial tumorigenesis, Cell 123 (2005) 1001–1011.
4. S. Paget, The distribution of secondary growths in cancer of the breast. 1889, Cancer Metastasis Rev 8 (1989) 98–101.
5. I.R. Hart & I.J. Fidler, Role of organ selectivity in the determination of metastatic patterns of B16 melanoma, Cancer Res 40 (1980) 2281–2287.
6. G. van der Pluijm, B. Sijmons & H. Vloedgraven, et al., Monitoring metastatic behavior of human tumor cells in mice with species-specific polymerase chain reaction: elevated expression of angiogenesis and bone resorption stimulators by breast cancer in bone metastases, J Bone Miner Res 16 (2001) 1077–1091.
7. D. Kahn, G.J. Weiner & S. Ben-Haim, et al., Positron emission tomographic measurement of bone marrow blood flow to the pelvis and lumbar vertebrae in young normal adults, Blood 83 (1994) 958–963.
8. P.V. Hauschka, A.E. Mavrakos & M.D. Iafrati, et al., Growth factors in bone matrix. Isolation of multiple types by affinity chromatography on heparin-Sepharose, J Biol Chem 261 (1986) 12665–12674.
9. J. Pfeilschifter & G.R. Mundy, Modulation of type beta transforming growth factor activity in bone cultures by osteotropic hormones, Proc Natl Acad Sci USA 84 (1987) 2024–2028.
10. T.A. Guise, K.S. Mohammad & G. Clines, et al., Basic mechanisms responsible for osteolytic and osteoblastic bone metastases, Clin Cancer Res 12 (2008) 6213s–6216s.
11. G.D. Roodman, Mechanisms of bone metastasis, N Engl J Med 350 (2004) 1655–1664.
12. T.A. Guise, Molecular mechanisms of osteolytic bone metastases, Cancer 88 (2000) 2892–2898.
13. S.C. Kukreja, D.H. Shevrin & S.A. Wimbiscus, et al., Antibodies to parathyroid hormone-related protein lower serum calcium in athymic mouse models of malignancy-associated hypercalcemia due to human tumors, J Clin Invest 82 (1988) 1798–1802.
14. M. Iwamura, P.A. Abrahamsson & K.A. Foss, et al., Parathyroid hormone-related protein: a potential autocrine growth regulator in human prostate cancer cell lines, Urology 43 (1994) 675–679.
15. Y. Lu, G. Xiao & D.L. Galson, et al., PTHrP-induced MCP-1 production by human bone marrow endothelial cells and osteoblasts promotes osteoclast differentiation and prostate cancer cell proliferation and invasion *in vitro*, Int J Cancer 121 (2007) 724–733.
16. N.W. Clarke, J. McClure & N.J. George, Morphometric evidence for bone resorption and replacement in prostate cancer, Br J Urol 68 (1991) 74–80.
17. H. Maeda, M. Koizumi & K. Yoshimura, et al., Correlation between bone metabolic markers and bone scan in prostatic cancer, J Urol 157 (1997) 539–543.

18. A.A. Bryden, J.A. Hoyland & A.J. Freemont, et al., Parathyroid hormone related peptide and receptor expression in paired primary prostate cancer and bone metastases, Br J Cancer 86 (2002) 322–325.

19. J. Nelson, A. Bagnato & B. Battistini, et al., The endothelin axis: emerging role in cancer, Nat Rev Cancer 3 (2003) 110–116.

20. J.B. Nelson, S.P. Hedican & D.J. George, et al., Identification of endothelin-1 in the pathophysiology of metastatic adenocarcinoma of the prostate, Nat Med 1 (1995) 944–949.

21. N. Tsuchiya, L. Wang & H. Suzuki, et al., Impact of IGF-I and CYP19 gene polymorphisms on the survival of patients with metastatic prostate cancer, J Clin Oncol 24 (2006) 1982–1989.

22. J. Dai, Y. Kitagawa & J. Zhang, et al., Vascular endothelial growth factor contributes to the prostate cancer-induced osteoblast differentiation mediated by bone morphogenetic protein, Cancer Res 64 (2004) 994–999.

23. T.A. Bates, Review of local radiotherapy in the treatment of bone metastases and cord compression, Int J Radiat Oncol Biol Phys 23 (1992) 217–221.

24. E.J. Maher, The use of palliative radiotherapy in the management of breast cancer, Eur J Cancer 28 (1992) 706–710.

25. W.F. Hartsell, C.B. Scott & D.W. Bruner, et al., Randomized trial of short- versus long-course radiotherapy for palliation of painful bone metastases, J Natl Cancer Inst 97 (2005) 798–804.

26. Y.M. van der Linden & J.W. Leer, Impact of randomized trial-outcome in the treatment of painful bone metastases; patterns of practice among radiation oncologists. A matter of believers vs non-believers? Radiother Oncol 56 (2000) 279–281.

27. D.E. Roos, P.C. O'Brien & J.G. Smith, et al., A role for radiotherapy in neuropathic bone pain: preliminary response rates from a prospective trial (Trans-tasman radiation oncology group, TROG 96.05), Int J Radiat Oncol Biol Phys 46 (2000) 975–981.

28. O.S. Nielsen, S.M. Bentzen & E. Sandberg, et al., Randomized trial of single dose versus fractionated palliative radiotherapy of bone metastases, Radiother Oncol 47 (1998) 233–240.

29. P. Foro Arnalot, A.V. Fontanals & J.C. Galceran, et al., Randomized clinical trial with two palliative radiotherapy regimens in painful bone metastases: 30 Gy in 10 fractions compared with 8 Gy in single fraction, Radiother Oncol 89 (2008) 150–155.

30. Bone Pain Trial Working Party. 8 Gy single fraction radiotherapy for the treatment of metastatic skeletal pain: randomised comparison with a multifraction schedule over 12 months of patient follow-up. Radiother Oncol 52, 111–121.

31. E. Steenland, J.W. Leer & H. van Houwelingen, et al., The effect of a single fraction compared to multiple fractions on painful bone metastases: a global analysis of the Dutch Bone Metastasis Study, Radiother Oncol 52 (1999) 101–109.

32. J.S. Wu, R. Wong & M. Johnston, et al., Meta-analysis of dose-fractionation radiotherapy trials for the palliation of painful bone metastases, Int J Radiat Oncol Biol Phys 55 (2003) 594–605.

33. W.M. Sze, M.D. Shelley & I. Held, et al., Palliation of metastatic bone pain: single fraction versus multifraction radiotherapy—a systematic review of randomised trials, Clin Oncol (R Coll Radiol) 15 (2003) 345–352.

34. E. Chow, K. Harris & G. Fan, et al., Palliative radiotherapy trials for bone metastases: a systematic review, J Clin Oncol 25 (2007) 1423–1436.

35. D.A. Loblaw & N.J. Laperriere, Emergency treatment of malignant extradural spinal cord compression: an evidence-based guideline, J Clin Oncol 16 (1998) 1613–1624.

36. A. Bayley, M. Milosevic & R. Blend, et al., A prospective study of factors predicting clinically occult spinal cord compression in patients with metastatic prostate carcinoma, Cancer 92 (2001) 303–310.

37. J.A. Talcott, P.C. Stomper & F.W. Drislane, et al., Assessing suspected spinal cord compression: a multidisciplinary outcomes analysis of 342 episodes, Support Care Cancer 7 (1999) 31–38.

38. C.J. Vecht, H. Haaxma-Reiche & W.L. van Putten, et al., Initial bolus of conventional versus high-dose dexamethasone in metastatic spinal cord compression, Neurology 39 (1989) 1255–1257.

39. S. Sorensen, S. Helweg-Larsen & H. Mouridsen, et al., Effect of high-dose dexamethasone in carcinomatous metastatic spinal cord compression treated with radiotherapy: a randomised trial, Eur J Cancer 30A (1994) 22–27.

40. D.A. Loblaw, N.J. Laperriere & W.J. Mackillop, A population-based study of malignant spinal cord compression in Ontario, Clin Oncol (R Coll Radiol) 15 (2003) 211–217.

41. R.A. Huddart, B. Rajan & M. Law, et al., Spinal cord compression in prostate cancer: treatment outcome and prognostic factors, Radiother Oncol 44 (1997) 229–236.

42. S. Yilmazlar, S. Dogan & B. Caner, et al., Comparison of prognostic scores and surgical approaches to treat spinal metastatic tumors: A review of 57 cases, J Orthop Surg 3 (2008) 37.

43. K.L. Chaichana, G.F. Woodworth & D.M. Sciubba, et al., Predictors of ambulatory function after decompressive surgery for metastatic epidural spinal cord compression, Neurosurgery 62 (2008) 683–692 (discussion).

44. R.A. Patchell, P.A. Tibbs & W.F. Regine, et al., Direct decompressive surgical resection in the treatment of spinal cord compression caused by metastatic cancer: a randomised trial, Lancet 366 (2005) 643–648.

45. F. Saad, D.M. Gleason & R. Murray, et al., A randomized, placebo-controlled trial of zoledronic acid in patients with hormone-refractory metastatic prostate carcinoma, J Natl Cancer Inst 94 (2002) 1458–1468.

46. F. Saad, J.D. Adachi & J.P. Brown, et al., Cancer treatment-induced bone loss in breast and prostate cancer, J Clin Oncol 26 (2008) 5465–5476.

47. Y.M. Van der Linden, P.D. Dijkstra & H.M. Kroon, et al., Comparative analysis of risk factors for pathological fracture with femoral metastases, J Bone Joint Surg Br 86 (2004) 566–573.

48. P.W. Townsend, H.G. Rosenthal & S.R. Smalley, et al., Impact of postoperative radiation therapy and other perioperative factors on outcome after orthopedic stabilization of impending or pathologic fractures due to metastatic disease, J Clin Oncol 12 (1994) 2345–2350.

49. F. Saad, A. Lipton & R. Cook, et al., Pathologic fractures correlate with reduced survival in patients with malignant bone disease, Cancer 110 (2007) 1860–1867.

50. S.L. Greenspan, J.B. Nelson & D.L. Trump, et al., Skeletal health after continuation, withdrawal, or delay of alendronate in men with prostate cancer undergoing androgen-deprivation therapy, J Clin Oncol 26 (2008) 4426–4434.

51. J.G. Nalesnik, A.G. Mysliwiec & E. Canby-Hagino, Anemia in men with advanced prostate cancer: incidence, etiology, and treatment, Rev Urol 6 (2004) 1–4.

52. J.J. Body, T. Facon & R.E. Coleman, et al., A study of the biological receptor activator of nuclear factor-kappaB ligand inhibitor, denosumab, in patients with multiple myeloma or bone metastases from breast cancer, Clin Cancer Res 12 (2006) 1221–1228.

53. A. Lipton, G.G. Steger & J. Figueroa, et al., Randomized active-controlled phase II study of denosumab efficacy and safety in patients with breast cancer-related bone metastases, J Clin Oncol 25 (2007) 4431–4437.

54. M.A. Carducci & A. Jimeno, Targeting bone metastasis in prostate cancer with endothelin receptor antagonists, Clin Cancer Res 12 (2006) 6296s–6300s.

55. M.A. Carducci, R.J. Padley & J. Breul, et al., Effect of endothelin-A receptor blockade with atrasentan on tumor progression in men with hormone-refractory prostate cancer: a randomized, phase II, placebo-controlled trial, J Clin Oncol 21 (2003) 679–689.

56. M.D. Michaelson, D.S. Kaufman & P. Kantoff, et al., Randomized phase II study of atrasentan alone or in combination with zoledronic acid in men with metastatic prostate cancer, Cancer 107 (2006) 530–535.

57. M.A. Carducci, F. Saad & P.A. Abrahamsson, et al., A phase 3 randomized controlled trial of the efficacy and safety of atrasentan in men with metastatic hormone-refractory prostate cancer, Cancer 110 (2007) 1959–1966.

58. F. Keuppens, L. Denis & P. Smith, et al., Zoladex and fluta-mide versus bilateral orchiectomy. A randomized phase III EORTC 30853 study. The EORTC GU Group, Cancer 66 (1990) 1045–1057.

59. B. Seruga & I.F. Tannock, The changing face of hormonal therapy for prostate cancer, Ann Oncol 19 (Suppl 7) (2008) vii79–vii85.

60. M.R. Smith, R.J. Cook & R. Coleman, et al., Predictors of skeletal complications in men with hormone-refractory metastatic prostate cancer, Urology 70 (2007) 315–319.

61. M.R. Smith, M. Goode & A.L. Zietman, et al., Bicalutamide monotherapy versus leuprolide monotherapy for prostate cancer: effects on bone mineral density and body composition, J Clin Oncol 22 (2004) 2546–2553.

62. I.F. Tannock, R. de Wit & W.R. Berry, et al., Docetaxel plus prednisone or mitoxantrone plus prednisone for advanced prostate cancer, N Engl J Med 351 (2004) 1502–1512.

63. D.P. Petrylak, C.M. Tangen & M.H. Hussain, et al., Docetaxel and estramustine compared with mitoxantrone and prednisone for advanced refractory prostate cancer, N Engl J Med 351 (2004) 1513–1520.

64. D.R. Berthold, G.R. Pond & F. Soban, et al., Docetaxel plus prednisone or mitoxantrone plus prednisone for advanced prostate cancer: updated survival in the TAX 327 study, J Clin Oncol 26 (2008) 242–245.

65. D.R. Berthold, C.N. Sternberg & I.F. Tannock, Management of advanced prostate cancer after first-line chemotherapy, J Clin Oncol 23 (2005) 8247–8252.

66. D.R. Berthold, G.R. Pond & R. de Wit, et al., Survival and PSA response of patients in the TAX 327 study who crossed over to receive docetaxel after mitoxantrone or vice versa, Ann Oncol 19 (2008) 1749–1753.

CHAPTER **38**

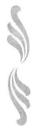

Apoptosis and Drug Resistance in Malignant Bone Tumors

UDO KONTNY[1]

[1]*Division of Pediatric Hematology and Oncology, Center for Pediatrics and Adolescent Medicine, University Medical Center, Freiburg, Germany.*

Contents

I. INTRODUCTION

Apoptosis is a physiological cell death program which occurs in all eukaryotic organisms [1,2]. Its two main purposes for the organism are to allow tissue remodeling, especially during embryogenesis, and to induce cell death in damaged cells in order to prevent genetic instability. Damage of the apoptotic program can lead to tumor formation by shifting the tightly regulated balance between proliferation and apoptosis into the direction of cell growth, and can result in drug resistance, since radiotherapy and most chemotherapeutic agents induce cell death via apoptosis. Knowledge of the apoptotic pathways, therefore, is of utmost importance for the understanding of tumor pathogenesis and of drug resistance.

Apoptosis is an active process in which the caspases, a family of cysteine-proteases are the key mediators [3]. In humans, there are 14 different caspases known. They are synthesized as inactive proenzymes consisting of a prodomain, a large and small subunit. The active caspases are tetramers composed of two large and two small subunits arising from the cleavage of two procaspases. Initiator caspases (such as caspases-8, -9 and -10) receive the apoptotic signal, becoming activated. They then activate themselves by so-called executioner caspases such as caspase-3, -6 and -7. These induce the apoptotic phenotype by the cleavage of enzymes such as the DNA-repair-enzyme PARP, activation of endonucleases and cleavage of structural proteins such as the lamins, which are important for the maintenance of the

nuclear membranes. Activity of the caspases is tightly controlled by proteins from the 'inhibitor of apoptosis family' (IAP), to which the proteins XIAP, c-IAP1, c-IAP2, NAIP, survivin, livin, Ts-IAP, and BRUCE belong [4].

There are two major apoptotic pathways: the intrinsic and extrinsic pathway [1,2]. The intrinsic apoptotic pathway becomes activated when cells are critically damaged. A key event in the intrinsic pathway is the permeabilization of the mitochondrial membrane leading to the release of cytochrome C which binds the cytosolic protein Apaf 1 (apoptosis activating factor 1). Both proteins together bind procaspase-9 and form the apoptosome where procasapase-9 gets cleaved into active caspase-9. In addition, permeabilization of the mitochondria leads to the release of proteins SMAC/DIABLO and HtrA2/Omi which both bind to, and inactivate proteins of, the IAP-family. Permeability of the mitochondrial membrane is controlled by a tight balance between pro- and anti-apoptotic members of the bcl-2 family of proteins [1]. The pro-apoptotic members comprise proteins such as Bax, Bak Bad which contain three Bcl-2 homology domains (BH1-3) and proteins with only one domain (BH-3) such as Bid, Bim, Puma and Noxa. The anti-apoptotic members are Bcl-2, Bcl-X_L, Bcl-w and Mcl-1. Bcl-2 and Bcl-X_L form stable complexes with the pro-apoptotic BH-3 domain only proteins, thereby preventing the activation and translocation of Bax and Bak to the mitochondria. This balance of pro- and anti-apoptotic members of the bcl-2 family of proteins is influenced by p53 which gets activated upon cellular stress. P53 induces transcriptional activation of the pro-apoptotic Bax and Puma, thereby shifting the balanced network of bcl2-family proteins towards apoptosis [1,5]. Since most chemotherapeutic agents induce intracellular damage, they induce apoptosis via the intrinsic pathway. Disruption of the intrinsic pathway therefore often leads to chemoresistance. The causes can be manifold, such as mutations in pro-apoptotic proteins, e.g. p53, or Bax, or overexpression of anti-apoptotic protein, e.g. bcl-2 or survivin.

In the extrinsic apoptotic pathway, apoptosis is induced by the activation of cell surface receptors belonging to the death receptor family [1,6]. This family comprises TNF-R1, Fas (also called CD95 or APO-1), DR3, TRAIL-receptors 1 and 2 (also called DR4 and DR5) and DR6. Binding of their respective ligand leads to trimerization of the death receptors, resulting in a conformational change of the intracellular 'death domain', and allowing it to bind to an adaptor molecule which is FADD for Fas, TRAIL-R1 and R-2, and TRADD for TNF-R1. The bound adaptor molecules than recruit and activate procaspases-8 and -10. The complex of death receptor, adaptor protein and initiator caspase is referred to as death inducing signaling complex (Disc). Caspases-8 and -10 activate effector caspases and the pro-apoptotic bcl-2 family protein bid. In cells in which activation of death receptors generate large amounts of active caspase-8 and/or -10, sufficient activation of effector-caspases leading to apoptosis ensues (type I cells). In cells with smaller generation of caspase-8 and/or -10, activation of the intrinsic pathway via bid is necessary for the induction of apoptosis (type II cells). As in the intrinsic pathway, activation of p53 modulates the extrinsic pathway towards apoptosis. Activated p53 results in transactivation of death receptors Fas and TRAIL-R2. Resistance to the extrinsic apoptotic pathway can occur at various levels. For example, at the receptor level there are TRAIL-R3 and R-4 which do not contain a death domain and can sequester TRAIL from the apoptosis inducing receptors TRAIL-R1 and -R2. Overexpression of the protein FLIP has been shown to prevent binding of the adaptor FADD to procaspase-8 and -10. Mutations in Fas as well as absent expression of death receptors or caspases-8 and -10 are also known causes of resistance to the induction of apoptosis via the extrinsic pathway.

In the following, the apoptotic pathways in malignant bone tumors are described in detail. Insight into which pathways are intact, and how deficient pathways can be restored, could be of potential value for the design of new treatment concepts.

II. OSTEOSARCOMA

A. The Fas/Fas Ligand Pathway

Fas surface expression is found in the majority of OS cell lines [7]. Hamada *et al.* detected Fas surface expression in 10 out of 14 OS cell lines examined; in the remaining four cell lines, Fas was only detected in the cytoplasm. Only two out of 14 cell lines were susceptible to apoptosis by anti-Fas antibody. Co-incubation with the protein-synthesis inhibitor cycloheximide resulted in Fas-mediated apoptosis of 10 cell lines. Similar results were observed by Fellenberg *et al.* [8]. Whereas all three OS cell lines had surface expression of Fas, anti-Fas antibody alone was not able to induce apoptosis. Co-incubation with cyloheximide or incubation with TNF rendered OS cells sensitive to Fas-mediated apoptosis. Interestingly, OS cell lines produced a soluble form of Fas which was able to protect Jurkat cells from anti-Fas antibody mediated apoptosis. Inaba *et al.* analyzed the effect of interferon-gamma on Fas-mediated apoptosis in four OS cell lines [9]. Interferon-gamma increased Fas- and caspase-8 expression in all four cell lines. Whereas interferon-gamma or anti-Fas-antibody alone only caused minimal apoptosis, the combination of both substances resulted in marked apoptosis.

Loss of Fas expression has been linked to tumor progression in various cancers. Gordon *et al.* investigated the role of the Fas-signaling pathway on the development of metastases in osteosarcoma (OS). By selection of variants of the OS cell line SAOS, with different degrees of Fas expression as well as by transfection of Fas, they were able to show that the degree of Fas expression inversely correlated with the metastatic potential of the cell line variants in a mouse xenograft model. In addition, using a murine osteosarcoma model they could show that primary tumors expressed high levels of Fas, whereas no expression of Fas was present in actively growing lung metastases [10]. Gordon and colleagues hypothesize that Fas-expressing OS cells are eliminated from the lungs through the induction of apoptosis by Fas ligand expressing pulmonary epithelial cells. Similarly, when analyzing Fas expression in pulmonary metastases from patients with OS, they found that 60% of tumors did not express Fas and only 32% showed weak expression by immunohistochemistry. Whereas disruption of the Fas pathway by transfection of K7M2 murine OS cells with a dominant-negative FADD mutant resulted in a higher number of pulmonary metastases, inhalation of gemcitabine by mice upregulated Fas expression of pulmonary nodules, and reduced tumor growth [11]. Also, Fas expression in OS cells was shown to be upregulated by IL-12 [12]. Intranasal gene therapy with the IL-12 gene of SAOS-bearing mice xenografts and treatment with ifosfamide which upregulates the expression of Fas ligand in OS cells, inhibited the formation of lung metastases.

B. The TRAIL Pathway

In primary osteosarcomas and osteosarcoma cell lines sequence variations in the TRAIL-R1 gene but not TRAIL-R2 or FADD gene have been described [13]. Since these sequence variations are homozygous in 15% of tumor samples and cell lines but not in control cells, it is suggested that they influence ligand-receptor interactions and subsequent apoptosis induction. TRAIL signaling in osteosarcoma has been studied by various groups *in vitro*. In contrast to ES cells, only a minority of osteosarcoma cell lines are sensitive to TRAIL-mediated apoptosis [14]. Incubation of resistant cell lines with cytotoxic drugs doxorubicin, cisplatin and etoposid but not methotrexate or cyclophosphamide could sensitize them to TRAIL-mediated apoptosis. No effect of TRAIL alone or in combination with cytotoxic drugs could be observed in human osteoblasts [14,15]. The sensitizing effect of doxorubicin and cisplatin to TRAIL in osteosarcoma cells has been further analyzed in U2OS cells and was shown to rely on the downregulation of the inhibitory apoptotic protein X-IAP, an inhibitor of caspases-3 and -9 [16]. Whereas the execution of apoptosis in OS cells by TRAIL is caspase-dependent, apoptosis induction has been shown not to be dependent on FADD and caspase-8 in U2OS cells [17]. Inhibition of the two proteins with siRNA did not protect from TRAIL-mediated apoptosis. In contrast, inhibition of BID or cathepsin B, which has been shown to mediate TRAIL-induced apoptosis in oral cancer cells, prevented apoptosis by TRAIL. In cell line BTK-143, however, TRAIL-mediated apoptosis could be prevented by a transfection of a dominant-negative form of FADD [14]. This suggests a diversity in the TRAIL-signaling pathyway, even in one tumor entity. Resistance to TRAIL was acquired *in vitro* by BTK-143 cells through expression of TRAIL-R4. This receptor lacks a functional death domain and cannot mediate apoptosis. Sensitivity against TRAIL could be restored by blocking TRAIL-R4 with a specific antibody and by the incubation of cells with doxorubicin, etoposid and cisplatin [18]. Cenni *et al.* analyzed the TRAIL-sensitivity of OS cell line U2OS and an MDR-expressing subline. Both clones expressed TRAIL-receptors to a similar amount. While the parent clone was TRAIL-resistant, the MDR-expression clone was TRAIL-sensitive. Analysis of post-receptor events revealed that TRAIL-responsiveness inversely correlated with activation of Akt. Expression of a constitutively active Akt in MDR-U2OS decreased TRAIL-sensitivity [19].

C. Drug-induced Apoptosis

Fellenberg *et al.* demonstrated that chemotherapeutics doxorubicin, methotrexate and cisplatin induced apoptosis in three different OS cell lines (HOS/TE-85, MG63, Saos-2) [8]. Induction of apoptosis resulted in the reduction of the mitochondrial potential and cytochrome c release into the cytoplasm and was caspase-dependent. No increase in the expression of Fas or induction of FasL expression by chemotherapeutics was observed. However, all four cell lines were either *p53* null or expressed mutant *p53*, while Fas expression has been shown to be upregulated by wt *p53* in various cell systems. Also, no inhibition of drug-induced apoptosis was seen when an anti-FasL antibody was added.

1. PACLITAXEL
Paclitaxel induces cytotoxicity through inhibition of microtubuli formation. In the OS cell line U2OS paclitaxel induces G2/M arrest and apoptosis via the activation of

caspase-3. Also, caspase-3 mRNA expression is increased after incubation of cells with paclitaxel [20].

2. HISTONE-DEACETYLASE INHIBITORS
Histone acetylation is regulated by the balance of histone acetyltransferase (HAT) and histone deacetylase (HDAC) and plays an important role in regulating gene expression by modulating chormatine structure. HDAC inhibitors can cause a variety of biological effects such as cell cycle arrest, apoptosis and differentiation. In osteosarcoma cells the HDAC inhibitor FR901228 has been shown to downregulate FLIP by inhibiting generation of FLIP mRNA, thereby sensitizing Fas-resistant OS cell lines to Fas-mediated apoptosis [21]. In another study, valproic acid was found to decrease the secretion of soluble Fas by OS cell lines and to sensitize cell lines against Fas-mediated apoptosis [22].

3. PROTEASOME INHIBITORS
The ubiquitine-proteasome system plays a major role in cell proliferation and cell death. Its inhibition by proteasome inhibitors offers a new therapeutic strategy for cancer treatment. The proteasome inhibitor MG132 induced apoptosis in OS cell line SaOS-2 via an increase in levels of reactive oxygen species (ROS), mitochondrial membrane depolarization with release of cytochrome c and subsequent caspase activation. Introduction of the RB gene into SaOS-2 cells had a protective influence, possibly due to increased levels of Bcl-2, whereas introduction of p53 potentiated the apoptotic effect of MG132 [23].

4. FLAVOPIRIDOL
Flavopiridol is a pan-cyclin-dependent kinase (CDK) inhibitor that induces cell cycle arrest and apoptosis in many cancer cells. Flavopiridol induced apoptosis in ES cell line WE-68 and OS cell line MNNG [24]. Apoptosis was also observed in P-glycoprotein and multidrug resistance-associated protein 1 overexpressing subclones which were resistant to adriamycin. Flavopiridol caused release of mitochondrial cytochrome c and activation of caspases-9, -3 and -8. Apoptosis was inhibited by pan-caspase and caspase-3 inhibitor, but not caspase-8 inhibitor, suggesting activation of the intrinsic pathway.

5. ZOLEDRONIC ACID
Zoledronic acid (ZOL) is a biphosphonate which inhibits osteoclast-mediated bone resorption. In addition, ZOL inhibits proliferation and induces apoptosis in various tumor cell lines. In OS cells, ZOL has been shown to activate an intra-S DNA checkpoint with an increase in P-ATR, P-chk1, Wee 1, and P-cdc2 and a decrease in cdc25, independent of the p53 and Rb status [25]. Induction of apoptosis has been demonstrated to be caspase-independent and to be characterized by increased mitochondrial permeability with translocation of apoptosis-inducing factor (AIF) and

endonuclease G from a mitochondrial to a perinuclear location. In an orthotopic OS mouse xenograft model, ZOL resulted in the inhibition of primary tumor growth and the reduction of lung metastases of SaOS-2 tumor-bearing mice [26]. ZOL also inhibited the formation of lung metastases in a murine osteosarcoma model using the cell line POS-1 [27].

6. STATINS

Statins are cholesterol-lowering agents which have been found to trigger cell death in a variety of tumor cells. Statins inhibit the 3-hydroxy-3-methylglutaryl-coenzyme A (HMG-CoA) reductase that catalyses the conversion of HMG-CoA into mevalonate during cholesterin biosynthesis. Blocking this pathway by statins results in decreased prenylation of proteins, such as small G proteins, altering cell growth and survival. Fromigue *et al.* demonstrated that lipophilic statins induced apoptosis in OS cell lines SaOS-2 and OHS4 by inactivation of the small G-protein RhoA. Inactivation of RhoA resulted in decreased levels of p42/p44-MAPKs, Bcl-2 and Mcl-1 [28].

7. INHIBITION OF GLUTATHIONE S-TRANSFERASE P1 (GSTP)

GSTP is one of the cytosolic glutathione transferases and detoxifies a wide variety of electrophilic compounds including certain anticancer agents. Overexpression of GSTP1 has been linked to chemoresistance in various cancers [29]. When establishing a series of cisplatin-resistant osteosarcoma cell lines, Pasello *et al.* found that resistance to cisplatin was mainly associated with an increase of both the intracellular level and enzymatic activity of GSTP1 [30]. Overexpression of GSTP1 in osteosarcoma cells caused cells to be more resistant to doxorubicin and cisplatin, whereas GSTP1 suppression by siRNA resulted in growth inhibition and an increase in apoptosis to both drugs [31]. Treatment of cisplatin-resistant osteosarcoma cell lines with the GSTP1-inhibitor 6-(7-nitro-2,1,3-benozoxydiazol-4ylthio)hexanol (NBDHEX) sensitized cells to cisplatin cytotoxicity *in vitro* [30]. Analyzing 34 patients with high-grade osteosarcoma, increased expression of GSTP1 was associated with a significantly higher relapse rate and worse clinical outcome [30].

D. Apoptosis-relevant Genes as Prognostic Markers

Mutations in the tumor suppressor gene *p53* are found in 20–60% of patients with sporadic osteosarcoma [32–34]. Whereas *p53* mutations are associated with an aggressive tumor phenotype, chemoresistance and poor outcome in a variety of malignancies, a large prospective study did not find an influence of *p53* mutations on chemoresistance and clinical outcome in osteosarcoma [35]. In a smaller study, 35 primary osteosarcoma specimens were analyzed for the expression of p53, bax and bcl-2 by immunohistochemistry. None of the parameters studied correlated with prognosis. However, patients who were bax + /bcl-2/p53+ had a significantly lower 4-year disease-free survival than other patients [35]. Survivin is a member of the inhibitor of apoptosis protein (IAP) family. It inhibits apoptosis by binding directly to both caspases-3 and -7. When analyzing the initial biopsy specimen of 22 patients with OS, Osaka *et al.* could demonstrate that patients with metastases had significantly higher mRNA levels of survivin than patients without metastases, and that the 5-year survival of patients with high survivin levels was significantly lower than the one for patients with low survivin levels [36].

III. APOPTOSIS IN EWING'S SARCOMA

A. The Fas/Fas Ligand Pathway

Expression of FasL by immunohistochemistry has been reported in 62.5% and Fas in 79.4% of primary Ewing's sarcoma (ES) [37]. A higher expression of FasL (95%) has been found in metastatic tumors, suggesting an association with a metastastic phenotype. In ES cell lines, apoptosis through the Fas signaling pathway could only be induced in 30% of Fas-expressing cell lines [38]. When cells were treated with a combination of an anti-Fas antibody and the protein synthesis inhibitor cycloheximide, seven out of nine cell lines became Fas-sensitive. As in primary cells, simultaneous expression of Fas and FasL in cell lines was observed, even in Fas-sensitive cells. Expression of FasL was strictly confined to the cytoplasm in one report, whereas transmembrane expression and secretion of soluble FasL by metalloproteinase into the supernatant was also observed by another group [38,39]. Inhibition of FasL shedding by matrixmetalloproteinase-inhibitors resulted in Fas-mediated apoptosis in Fas-sensitive ES cell lines [40].

Zhou *et al.* demonstrated that transfection of ES cell line TC71 with an adenovirus carrying cDNA of the IL-12 gene upregulated Fas expression [41]. Whether transfected cells became sensitive to Fas-mediated apoptosis, however, has not been shown. Intratumoral injection of adenovirus murine IL-12 into mice bearing xenografts of ES cell line TC71 inhibited tumor growth of primary tumor as well as growth of an untreated tumor on the contralateral side [42]. Immunohistochemistry of treated tumors demonstrated increased expression of Fas, FasL as well as tumor cell apoptosis.

B. The TRAIL Pathway

Ewing's sarcoma cells do express receptors for TRAIL. Mitsiades *et al.* found that 94% of tumors from patients with ES expressed TRAIL-R1 and 75% TRAIL-R2 by immunohistochemistry [39]. Either one of the TRAIL receptors was expressed by 97%. In contrast to the Fas-signaling pathway, the TRAIL pathway seems to be intact in the majority of ES cells and its activation leads to apoptosis in about 80% of ES cell lines examined [39,43–45]. Resistance to TRAIL in ES cell lines has so far only been linked to deficient expression of caspase-8 [43,46]. Heterogeneous expression of caspase-8, however, has also been observed in tumors from patients with ES and therefore could be a major obstacle to the success of TRAIL-receptor targeted therapy. We have shown that 25% of tumors from patients with ES had less than 50% of tumor cells expressing caspase-8 [46]. As in neuroblastoma, the lack of expression of caspase-8 is due to methylation within the caspase-8 gene [47]. A means to re-express caspase-8 in ES tumor cells could be the application of interferon-gamma. We were able to show that interferon-gamma in concentrations of 10–20 U/ml leads to re-expression of caspase-8 in ES cell lines and sensitizes cell lines to TRAIL-mediated apoptosis [46]. Since in humans interferon-gamma concentrations of up to about 80U/ml can be achieved, the therapeutic application of interferon-gamma in patients with ES could upregulate caspase-8 expression in tumors and make them amenable to therapy with TRAIL-receptor agonists. TRAIL is also able to suppress the growth of Ewing's tumors in an orthotopic ES xenograft model in which tumor cells were injected into the gastrognemius muscle [48]. Interestingly, when the tumor-bearing extremities were amputated and mice were followed up for the development of metastases, those initially treated with TRAIL or vehicle died within 2 months of metastases. In contrast, treatment with interferon-gamma alone or in combination with TRAIL did significantly decrease the incidence of metastatic disease with 60% of the mice treated with TRAIL and interferon-gamma still being alive at the end of the 6-month observation period.

C. CD-99-induced Apoptosis

The CD99 antigen is consistently expressed in ES and therefore used as a marker to distinguish ES from other small blue round cell tumors [49]. It has been shown to be involved in the transendothelial migration of human neutrophils [50]. It is expressed in cells of all leukocyte lineages. The degree of expression is high in immature bone marrow precursors, diminishes with differentiation of cells and is low in peripheral blood cells [51]. Since CD99 is highly and consistently expressed in ES, it represents an attractive target for therapeutic intervention. Ligation of CD99 with a specific antibody leads to rapid aggregation of cells and caspase-independent apoptosis [52]. Apoptosis can be inhibited by silencing of the zyxin gene, which codes a protein involved in the regulation of the actin cytoskeleton and of which expression gets upregulated after CD99 engagement. Simultaneous administration of an anti-CD99 antibody with doxorubicin had a synergistic effect on the inhibition of cell growth *in vitro*. In athymic mice the combination of anti-CD99 and doxorubicin proved to be more active in inhibiting the growth of primary tumors as well as reducing the number of lung and bone metastases than each component alone [53].

D. Drug-induced Apoptosis

A role for the Fas/FasL pathway in doxorubicin-mediated cytotoxicity has been shown by Mitsiades [40]. Doxorubicin-mediated apoptosis was reduced in cells of the ES cell line SK-N-MC either by a soluble form of Fas, acting as a decoy inhibitor of membrane-bound Fas or by matrix metalloproteinase-7 through cleavage of membrane-bound FasL. However, no role for caspase-8 in doxorubicine or etoposide-induced apoptosis has been demonstrated in ES cell lines A4573 and JR [46]. Both cell lines do not express initiator caspases-8 and -10, required for death receptor-mediated apoptosis. Transfection of wt caspase-8 or induction of caspase-8 expression by interferon-gamma did not alter their sensitivity to drug-mediated apoptosis. In patients with ES, caspase-8 expression of primary tumors did not correlate with event-free or overall survival.

1. TREOSULFAN

Treosulfan is a bifunctional alkylating agent which is structurally related to busulfan. In contrast to busulfan, treosulfan causes less adverse effects in patients, even allowing high-dose chemotherapy in previously irradiated patients. Treosulfan has been shown in a mouse xenograft model to be more active against ES xenografts than busulfan. Apoptosis is induced via the intrinsic pathway and involves caspase-9 and the effector-caspase-3 [54].

2. FENRETINIDE

Fenretinide is a synthetic vitamin A analog. It induces apoptosis in ES cell lines at concentrations achievable *in vivo* and slows the growth of ES xenograft in nude mice [55, 56]. Myatt *et al.* investigated the induction of apoptosis by fenretinide in ES cells. Fenretinide led to the accumulation of reactive oxygen species (ROS) within 5 minutes. This was followed by the activation of p38^{MAPK}. An increase in the mitochondrial membrane permeability and release of cytochrome c was observed after 8 hours and dependent on ROS and the activation of p38 ^{MAPK} [56].

3. ZOLEDRONIC ACID

Zoledronic acid (ZOL) has been shown to induce apoptosis in ES cell line TC71. Apoptosis was increased in a synergistic way with paclitaxel [57]. In a mouse xenograft model, in which TC71 tumor cells were injected intratibially, ZOL alone inhibited the development of bone tumors. Whereas paclitaxel alone had no inhibiting effect on the development of primary tumors, the combination therapy of ZOL and paclitaxel led to tumors in only 22% of mice versus 89% in the control group.

4. PROTEASOME INHIBITORS

ES cell lines were found to be highly sensitive to the proteasome inhibitor bortezomib *in vitro*. Bortezomib was able to induce apoptosis via activation of caspase-3, cleavage of PARP and induction of p21 and p27. In addition, it exhibited synergistic activity with TRAIL in some ES cell lines [58].

E. Apoptosis-relevant Genes as Prognostic Markers

Aberrations in p53 have been found in about 10% of tumor samples from patients with ES either by aberrant expression detected by immunohistochemistry or by molecular methods [59–62]. In contrast, the majority of ESFT cell lines contain alterations of p53, indicating selective pressure in the process of establishing *in vitro* growth [63]. In several studies, p53 overexpression has been associated with a significantly poorer survival [31,59,60]. Ewing's tumors containing either p53 or p16/p14ARF alterations showed a poor histological response to chemotherapy [31]. When wild-type p53 was reintroduced by adenoviral transfection into cells of the ES cell line RH1, which contains mutp53, the transfected cells showed decreased viability and increased sensitivity to the chemotherapeutic agents cisplatin and doxorubicin [64].

IV. APOPTOSIS IN CHONDROSARCOMA

Chondrosarcomas do not usually respond to chemotherapy. Tumors are also relatively radiotherapy-resistant, requiring doses >60 Gy. Radiotherapy has been shown to upregulate the expression of the anti-apoptotic Bcl-2, Bcl-xL, and XIAP. When expression of these genes was inhibited using specific small interfering RNAs (siRNAs), radiosensitivity markedly increased [65]. The chondrosarcoma cell line HTB-94 has been shown to be resistant to apoptosis via TRAIL [66]. However, co-incubation with doxorubicin sensitizes cells to TRAIL-mediated apoptosis. The mechanism of this has not yet been elucidated.

References

1. C. Borner, The Bcl-2 protein family: sensors and check-points for life-or-death decisions, Mol Immunol 39 (2003) 615–647.
2. Y. Pommier, O. Sordet & S. Antony, et al., Apoptosis defects and chemotherapy resistance: molecular interaction maps and networks, Oncogene 23 (2004) 2934–2949.
3. I.N. Lavrik, A. Golks & P.H. Krammer, Caspases: pharmacological manipulation of cell death, J Clin Invest 115 (2005) 2665–2672.
4. G.S. Salvesen & C.S. Duckett, IAP proteins: blocking the road to death's door, Nat Rev Mol Cell Biol 3 (2002) 401–410.
5. K.M. Ryan, A.C. Phillips & K.H. Vousden, Regulation and function of the p53 tumor suppressor protein, Curr Opin Cell Biol 13 (2001) 332–337.
6. I. Lavrik, A. Golks & P.H. Krammer, Death receptor signaling, J Cell Sci 118 (2005) 265–267.
7. T. Hamada, S. Komiya & H. Yano, et al., Modulation of fas-mediated apoptosis in osteosarcoma cell lines, Int J Oncol 15 (1999) 1125–1131.
8. J. Fellenberg, H. Mau & S. Nedel, et al., Drug-induced apoptosis in osteosarcoma cell lines is mediated by caspase activation independent of CD95-receptor/ligand interaction, J Orthop Res 18 (2000) 10–17.
9. H. Inaba, M. Glibetic & S. Buck, et al., Interferon-gamma sensitizes osteosarcoma cells to Fas-induced apoptosis by up-regulating Fas receptors and caspase-8, Pediatr Blood Cancer 43 (2004) 729–736.
10. N. Gordon, C.A. Arndt & D.S. Hawkins, et al., Fas expression in lung metastasis from osteosarcoma patients, J Pediatr Hematol Oncol 27 (2005) 611–615.
11. N. Gordon, N.V. Koshkina & S.F. Jia, et al., Corruption of the Fas pathway delays the pulmonary clearance of murine osteosarcoma cells, enhances their metastatic potential, and reduces the effect of aerosol gemcitabine, Clin Cancer Res 13 (2007) 4503–4510.
12. E.A. Lafleur, S.F. Jia & L.L. Worth, et al., Interleukin (IL)-12 and IL-12 gene transfer up-regulate Fas expression in human osteosarcoma and breast cancer cells, Cancer Res 61 (2001) 4066–4071.
13. M.J. Dechant, J. Fellenberg & C.G. Scheuerpflug, et al., Mutation analysis of the apoptotic 'death-receptors' and the adaptors TRADD and FADD/MORT-1 in osteosarcoma tumor samples and osteosarcoma cell lines, Int J Cancer 109 (2004) 661–667.
14. A. Evdokiou, S. Bouralexis & G.J. Atkins, et al., Chemotherapeutic agents sensitize osteogenic sarcoma cells, but not normal human bone cells, to Apo2L/TRAIL-induced apoptosis, Int J Cancer 99 (2002) 491–504.
15. G.J. Atkins, S. Bouralexis & A. Evdokiou, et al., Human osteoblasts are resistant to Apo2L/TRAIL-mediated apoptosis, Bone 31 (2002) 448–456.
16. P. Mirandola, I. Sponzilli & G. Gobbi, et al., Anticancer agents sensitize osteosarcoma cells to TNF-related apoptosis-inducing ligand downmodulating IAP family proteins, Int J Oncol 28 (2006) 127–133.
17. T.O. Garnett, M. Filippova & P.J. Duerksen-Hughes, Bid is cleaved upstream of caspase-8 activation during TRAIL-mediated apoptosis in human osteosarcoma cells, Apoptosis 12 (2007) 1299–1315.
18. S. Bouralexis, D.M. Findlay & G.J. Atkins, et al., Progressive resistance of BTK-143 osteosarcoma cells to Apo2L/TRAIL-induced apoptosis is mediated by acquisition of DcR2/TRAIL-R4 expression: resensitisation with chemotherapy, Br J Cancer 89 (2003) 206–214.
19. V. Cenni, N.M. Maraldi & A. Ruggeri, et al., Sensitization of multidrug resistant human ostesarcoma cells to Apo2 Ligand/TRAIL-induced apoptosis by inhibition of the Akt/PKB kinase, Int J Oncol 25 (2004) 1599–1608.
20. K.H. Lu, K.H. Lue & M.C. Chou, et al., Paclitaxel induces apoptosis via caspase-3 activation in human osteogenic sarcoma cells (U-2 OS), J Orthop Res 23 (2005) 988–994.

21. K. Watanabe, K. Okamoto & S. Yonehara, Sensitization of osteosarcoma cells to death receptor-mediated apoptosis by HDAC inhibitors through downregulation of cellular FLIP, Cell Death Differ 12 (2005) 10–18.

22. K. Yamanegi, J. Yamane & M. Hata et al., Sodium valproate, a histone deacetylase inhibitor, decreases the secretion of soluble Fas by human osteosarcoma cells and increases their sensitivity to Fas-mediated cell death. J Cancer Res Clin Oncol Dec 9 (2008) [E-pub ahead of print].

23. M. Lauricella, A. D'Anneo & M. Giuliano, et al., Induction of apoptosis in human osteosarcoma Saos-2 cells by the proteasome inhibitor MG132 and the protective effect of pRb, Cell Death Differ 10 (2003) 930–932.

24. Y. Li, K. Tanaka & X. Li, et al., Cyclin-dependent kinase inhibitor, flavopiridol, induces apoptosis and inhibits tumor growth in drug-resistant osteosarcoma and Ewing's family tumor cells, Int J Cancer 121 (2007) 1212–1218.

25. B. Ory, F. Blanchard & S. Battaglia, et al., Zoledronic acid activates the DNA S-phase checkpoint and induces osteosarcoma cell death characterized by apoptosis-inducing factor and endonuclease-G translocation independently of p53 and retinoblastoma status, Mol Pharmacol 71 (2007) 333–343.

26. C.R. Dass & P.F. Choong, Zoledronic acid inhibits osteosarcoma growth in an orthotopic model, Mol Cancer Ther 6 (2007) 3263–3270.

27. B. Ory, M.F. Heymann & A. Kamijo, et al., Zoledronic acid suppresses lung metastases and prolongs overall survival of osteosarcoma-bearing mice, Cancer 104 (2005) 2522–2529.

28. O. Fromigue, E. Hay & D. Modrowski, et al., RhoA GTPase inactivation by statins induces osteosarcoma cell apoptosis by inhibiting p42/p44−MAPKs-Bcl-2 signaling independently of BMP-2 and cell differentiation, Cell Death Differ 13 (2006) 1845–1856.

29. D.M. Townsend & K.D. Tew, The role of glutathione-S-transferase in anti-cancer drug resistance, Oncogene 22 (2003) 7369–7375.

30. M. Pasello, F. Michelacci & I. Scionti, et al., Overcoming glutathione S-transferase P1-related cisplatin resistance in osteosarcoma, Cancer Res 68 (2008) 6661–6668.

31. H.Y. Huang, P.B. Illei & Z. Zhao, et al., Ewing sarcomas with p53 mutation or p16/p14ARF homozygous deletion: a highly lethal subset associated with poor chemoresponse, J Clin Oncol 23 (2005) 548–558.

32. N. Gokgoz, J.S. Wunder & S. Mousses, et al., Comparison of p53 mutations in patients with localized osteosarcoma and metastatic osteosarcoma, Cancer 92 (2001) 2181–2189.

33. T. Tsuchiya, K. Sekine & S. Hinohara, et al., Analysis of the p16INK4, p14ARF, p15, TP53, and MDM2 genes and their prognostic implications in osteosarcoma and Ewing sarcoma, Cancer Genet Cytogenet 120 (2000) 91–98.

34. J.S. Wunder, N. Gokgoz & R. Parkes, et al., TP53 mutations and outcome in osteosarcoma: a prospective, multicenter study, J Clin Oncol 23 (2005) 1483–1490.

35. M.K. Kaseta, L. Khaldi & I.P. Gomatos, et al., Prognostic value of bax, bcl-2, and p53 staining in primary osteosarcoma. J Surg Oncol 97(3) (2008) 259–266.

36. E. Osaka, T. Suzuki & S. Osaka, et al., Survivin expression levels as independent predictors of survival for osteosarcoma patients, J Orthop Res 25 (2007) 116–121.

37. N. Mitsiades, V. Poulaki & V. Kotoula, et al., Fas ligand is present in tumors of the Ewing's sarcoma family and is cleaved into a soluble form by a metalloproteinase, Am J Pathol 153 (1998) 1947–1956.

38. H.U. Kontny, T.M. Lehrnbecher & S.J. Chanock, et al., Simultaneous expression of Fas and nonfunctional Fas ligand in Ewing's sarcoma, Cancer Res 58 (1998) 5842–5849.

39. N. Mitsiades, V. Poulaki & C. Mitsiades, et al., Ewing's sarcoma family tumors are sensitive to tumor necrosis factor-related apoptosis-inducing ligand and express death receptor 4 and death receptor 5, Cancer Res 61 (2001) 2704–2712.

40. N. Mitsiades, W.H. Yu & V. Poulaki, et al., Matrix metalloproteinase-7-mediated cleavage of Fas ligand protects tumor cells from chemotherapeutic drug cytotoxicity, Cancer Res 61 (2001) 577–581.

41. Z. Zhou, E.A. Lafleur & N.V. Koshkina, et al., Interleukin-12 up-regulates Fas expression in human osteosarcoma and Ewing's sarcoma cells by enhancing its promoter activity, Mol Cancer Res 3 (2005) 685–691.

42. S.F. Jia, X. Duan & L.L. Worth, et al., Intratumor murine interleukin-12 gene therapy suppressed the growth of local and distant Ewing's sarcoma, Cancer Gene Ther 13 (2006) 948–957.

43. H.U. Kontny, K. Hammerle & R. Klein, et al., Sensitivity of Ewing's sarcoma to TRAIL-induced apoptosis, Cell Death Differ 8 (2001) 506–514.

44. A. Kumar, A. Jasmin & M.T. Eby, et al., Cytotoxicity of Tumor necrosis factor related apoptosis-inducing ligand towards Ewing's sarcoma cell lines, Oncogene 20 (2001) 1010–1014.

45. F. Van Valen, S. Fulda & B. Truckenbrod, et al., Apoptotic responsiveness of the Ewing's sarcoma family of tumours to tumour necrosis factor-related apoptosis-inducing ligand (TRAIL), Int J Cancer 88 (2000) 252–259.

46. A. Lissat, T. Vraetz & M. Tsokos, et al., Interferon-gamma sensitizes resistant Ewing's sarcoma cells to tumor necrosis factor apoptosis-inducing ligand-induced apoptosis by up-regulation of caspase-8 without altering chemosensitivity, Am J Pathol 170 (2007) 1917–1930.

47. S. Fulda, M.U. Kufer & E. Meyer, et al., Sensitization for death receptor- or drug-induced apoptosis by re-expression of caspase-8 through demethylation or gene transfer, Oncogene 20 (2001) 5865–5877.

48. M.S. Merchant, X. Yang & F. Melchionda, et al., Interferon gamma enhances the effectiveness of tumor necrosis factor-related apoptosis-inducing ligand receptor agonists in a xenograft model of Ewing's sarcoma, Cancer Res 64 (2004) 8349–8356.

49. H. Kovar, M. Dworzak & S. Strehl, et al., Overexpression of the pseudoautosomal gene MIC2 in Ewing's sarcoma and peripheral primitive neuroectodermal tumor, Oncogene 5 (1990) 1067–1070.

50. O. Lou, P. Alcaide & F.W. Luscinskas, et al., CD99 is a key mediator of the transendothelial migration of neutrophils, J Immunol 178 (2007) 1136–1143.

51. M.N. Dworzak, G. Fritsch & P. Buchinger, et al., Flow cytometric assessment of human MIC2 expression in bone marrow, thymus, and peripheral blood, Blood 83 (1994) 415–425.

52. V. Cerisano, Y. Aalto & S. Perdichizzi, et al., Molecular mechanisms of CD99-induced caspase-independent cell death and cell-cell adhesion in Ewing's sarcoma cells: actin and zyxin as key intracellular mediators, Oncogene 23 (2004) 5664–5674.

53. K. Scotlandi, S. Perdichizzi & G. Bernard, et al., Targeting CD99 in association with doxorubicin: an effective combined treatment for Ewing's sarcoma, Eur J Cancer 42 (2006) 91–96.

54. S. Werner, A. Mendoza & R.A. Hilger, et al., Preclinical studies of treosulfan demonstrate potent activity in Ewing's sarcoma, Cancer Chemother Pharmacol 62 (2007) 19–31.

55. S. Batra, C.P. Reynolds & B.J. Maurer, Fenretinide cytotoxicity for Ewing's sarcoma and primitive neuroectodermal tumor cell lines is decreased by hypoxia and synergistically enhanced by ceramide modulators, Cancer Res 64 (2004) 5415–5424.

56. S.S. Myatt, C.P. Redfern & S.A. Burchill, p38MAPK-Dependent sensitivity of Ewing's sarcoma family of tumors to fenretinide-induced cell death, Clin Cancer Res 11 (2005) 3136–3148.

57. Z. Zhou, H. Guan & X. Duan, et al., Zoledronic acid inhibits primary bone tumor growth in Ewing sarcoma, Cancer 104 (2005) 1713–1720.

58. G. Lu, V. Punj & P.M. Chaudhary, Proteasome inhibitor Bortezomib induces cell cycle arrest and apoptosis in cell lines derived from Ewing's sarcoma family of tumors and synergizes with TRAIL, Cancer Biol Ther 7 (2008) 603–608.

59. A. Abudu, D.C. Mangham & G.M. Reynolds, et al., Overexpression of p53 protein in primary Ewing's sarcoma of bone: relationship to tumour stage, response and prognosis, Br J Cancer 79 (1999) 1185–1189.

60. E. de Alava, C.R. Antonescu & A. Panizo, et al., Prognostic impact of P53 status in Ewing sarcoma, Cancer 89 (2000) 783–792.

61. R. Hamelin, J. Zucman & T. Melot, et al., P53 mutations in human tumors with chimeric EWS/FLI-1 genes, Int J Cancer 57 (1994) 336–340.

62. H. Komuro, Y. Hayashi & M. Kawamura, et al., Mutations of the p53 gene are involved in Ewing's sarcomas but not in neuroblastomas, Cancer Res 53 (1993) 5284–5288.

63. H. Kovar, A. Auinger & G. Jug, et al., Narrow spectrum of infrequent p53 mutations and absence of MDM2 amplification in Ewing tumours, Oncogene 8 (1993) 2683–2690.

64. H. Ganjavi, M. Gee & A. Narendran, et al., Adenovirus-mediated p53 gene therapy in pediatric soft-tissue sarcoma cell lines: sensitization to cisplatin and doxorubicin, Cancer Gene Ther 12 (2005) 397–406.

65. D.W. Kim, S.W. Seo & S.K. Cho, et al., Targeting of cell survival genes using small interfering RNAs (siRNAs) enhances radiosensitivity of Grade II chondrosarcoma cells, J Orthop Res 25 (2007) 820–828.

66. S. Tomek, W. Koestler & P. Horak, et al., Trail-induced apoptosis and interaction with cytotoxic agents in soft tissue sarcoma cell lines, Eur J Cancer 39 (2003) 1318–1329.

Index

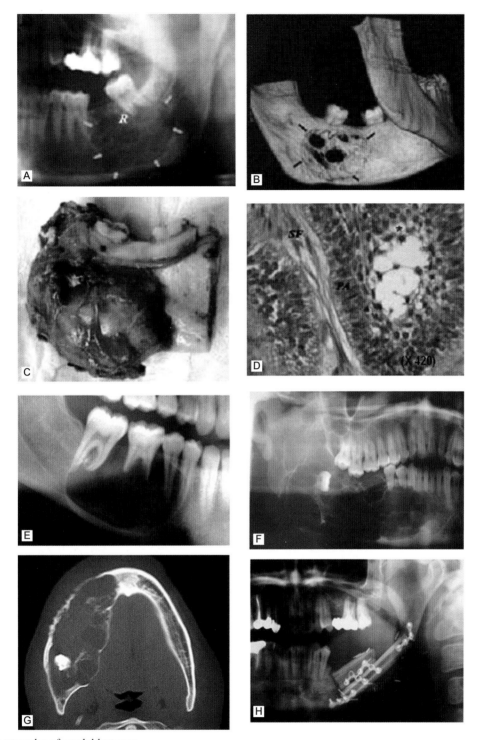

PLATE 1   Three examples of ameloblastoma:
- Left mandibular corpus ameloblastoma: panoramic view (A) and tridimentionnal cephalic scanography (B). Macroscopic sample showing a soft tissue invasion (C) and the follicular histologic aspect of the same lesion (D): PA (ameloblastic celluar type), SF (mesenchymal tissue).
- Right mandibular corpus unicystic ameloblastoma: panoramic view (E).
- Voluminous left parasymphyseal, mandibular corpus and ramus multicystic ameloblastoma: panoramic view (F) and axial scanographic slide (G).
- Radical resection of a mandibular ameloblastoma (in the left molar, angular and ramus mandibular regions): dental panoramic after a left mandibular reconstruction by a double barrel fibula-free flap (H).

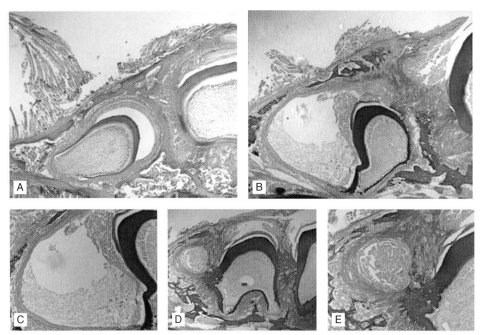

PLATE 2 Molar structures in wild-type and Msx2 −/− mice at 21 days. The second (M2) and third (M3) molars are evidenced in the mandible of Msx2 +/+ (A) and Msx2 −/− (B) mice. In Msx2 −/− mice, the enamel organ is not formed properly and gives rise to epithelial cystic structures (B–E). In the distal area of the third molar, epithelial cells delaminate (C). In the distal area of crown-root junction in the second molar, an epithelial cyst is visible (D and enlargement in E).

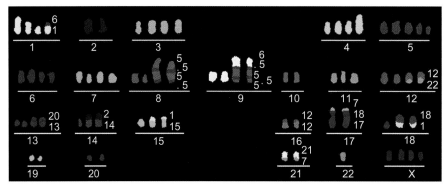

PLATE 3 Typical osteosarcoma karyotype as analyzed by spectral karyotyping (SKY) derived from short-term culture of patient tumor (reported in ref. 81). Of note is the high frequency of duplicated complex structural chromosome aberrations such as translocations t(8;18), t(7;17;18) present in this near tetraploid karyotype. These findings indicate that multiple chromosomal translocations in this tumor occurred at high frequency and took place in a diploid progenitor prior to tetraploidization. This process is likely ongoing as alterations such as t(1;6) and t(12;22) are present singly in the tetraploid cells.

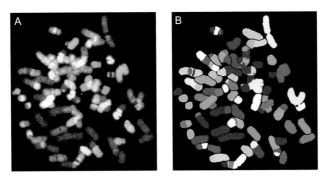

PLATE 4 An example of metaphase chromosomes from osteosarcoma after hybridization with 24 differentially labeled whole-chromosome painting probes. (A) Spectra-based display colors and (B) spectral classification from the same metaphase.

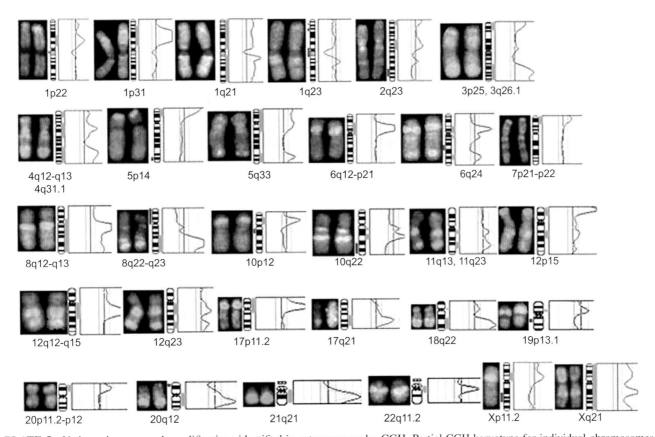

1p22 1p31 1q21 1q23 2q23 3p25, 3q26.1

4q12-q13
4q31.1 5p14 5q33 6q12-p21 6q24 7p21-p22

8q12-q13 8q22-q23 10p12 10q22 11q13, 11q23 12p15

12q12-q15 12q23 17p11.2 17q21 18q22 19p13.1

20p11.2-p12 20q12 21q21 22q11.2 Xp11.2 Xq21

PLATE 5 Various chromosomal amplifications identified in osteosarcoma by CGH. Partial CGH karyotype for individual chromosomes (left) and corresponding ratio profiles showing high-level amplifications. The vertical red and green bars on the right of the ideogram indicate the threshold values of 0.80 and 1.20 for loss and gain respectively.

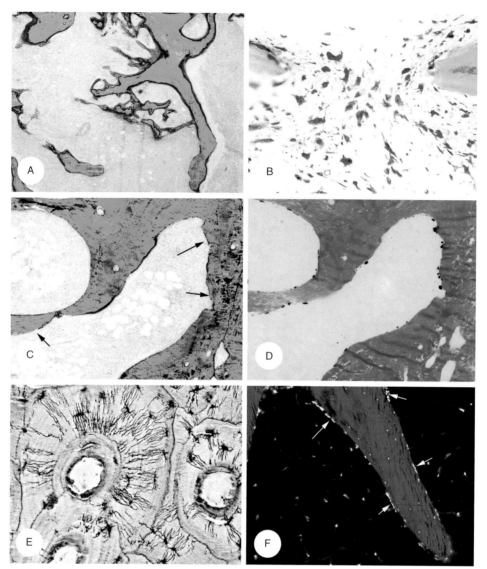

PLATE 6 (A) Bone biopsy in a patient with prostatic adenocarcinoma. The bone marrow is completely invaded by the tumor but cells are lightly stained. On the contrary, osteoid is well demonstrated in red and calcified bone matrix in green. Note the extended bone metaplasia. Modified Goldner's trichrome. Original magnification ×100. (B) TRAcP stained cells in the bone marrow of a patient with a metastatic breast cancer. Note the considerable osteoclastogenesis occurring in the tumor stroma with numerous osteoclasts. Original magnification ×200. (C) Bone biopsy from a patient with multiple myeloma with extended eroded surfaces (arrowed). Modified Goldner's trichrome. Original magnification ×100. (D) Paired section of the same case with histoenzymatic identification of osteoclasts by their TRAcP content. (E) Argentophilic proteins (osteopontin) in the resting lines, osteocytes lacunae and canaliculi and NORs of the nuclei. Modified AgNOR method. Original magnification ×100. (F) Nuclei of living cells stained with Hoechst 33342 (brilliant green) and bone matrix counter-stained in red. Lining cells are arrowed. Fluorescence microscopy. Original magnification ×100.

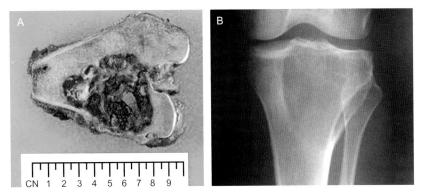

PLATE 7 A distal femoral resection showing the macroscopic appearance of a giant cell tumor of bone. There is extensive hemorrhage and necrosis. Note the subarticular site in a long bone in which the epiphysis is closed (A). The radiographic appearance of a typical giant cell tumor of the proximal tibia: this expansile lytic tumor is sited in the subarticular area in a skeletally mature individual. Also note the absence of a periosteal reaction (B). These tumors generally are without a sclerotic margin (a narrow zone of transition) and if present is seldom complete. Septa may be seen in the lesion in 33–57% of patients; these represent non-uniform growth of the tumor rather than true septa.

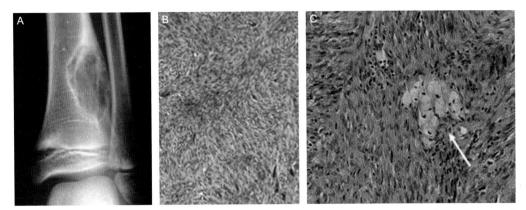

PLATE 8 A non-ossifying fibroma in a young patient with neurofibromatosis type 1. In contrast to a giant cell tumor, the non-ossifying fibroma is sited in the metadiaphysis of the bone, has a sclerotic rim surrounding the central lytic area and is most often present in a growing child (skeletally immature) (A). Microscopic appearance of a non-ossifying fibroma showing bland fibroblastic cells in a storiform arrangement (B) in which clusters of foamy histiocytes are seen (arrow) (C).

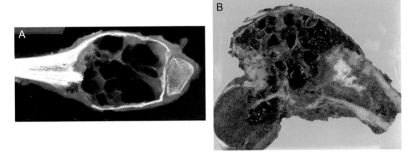

PLATE 9 This radiographic image of a fine cut slab shows the typical appearance of a primary aneurysmal bone cyst (A). The findings consist of a central expansive lytic lesion, appearing cystic as a result of fine septae. The macroscopic appearance of an aneurysmal bone cyst involving the greater trochanter (B).

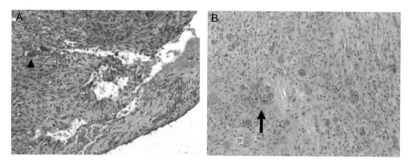

PLATE 10   Hematoxylin and eosin sections of pigmented villonodular synovitis/tenosynovial giant cell tumor. This osteoclast-rich tumor generally contains a more fibroblastic population compared to that seen in giant cell tumors and the osteoclasts (arrow heads) are more scattered throughout the fibroblastic cells (A). Hemosiderin is also a common finding (arrows) (B).

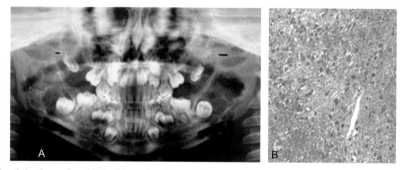

PLATE 11   A radiograph of the jaw of a child with a cherubism phenotype but who has a *PTPN11* mutation (Noonan syndrome). Note the bilateral symmetric radiolucent bubbly appearance of the mandible and maxilla (arrows) (A). The histology shows an osteoclast-rich lesion with features not dissimilar to that of a non-ossifying fibroma: there is a fibroblastic population of cells in which osteoclasts are scattered (B).

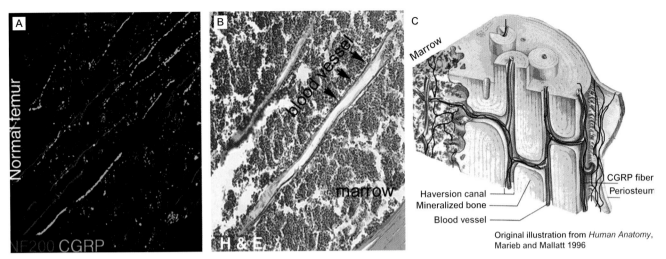

PLATE 12 Innervation of bone. Histophotomicrographs of (A) confocal and (B) histologic serial images of normal bone. Note the extensive myelinated (red, NF200) and unmyelinated (green, CGRP) nerve fibers within bone marrow which appear to course along blood vessels (arrowheads, B). (C) Schematic diagram demonstrating the innervation within periosteum, mineralized bone and bone marrow. All three tissues may be sensitized during the various stages of bone cancer pain.

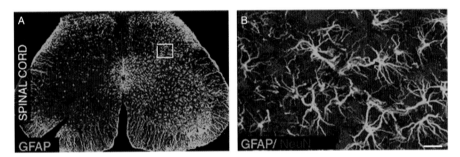

PLATE 13 Neurochemical changes in the spinal cord and dorsal root ganglia (DRG) in bone cancer pain. (A) Confocal imaging of glial fibrillary acidic protein (GFAP) expressed by astrocytes in a spinal cord of a tumor-bearing mouse. Note increased expression only on side ipsilateral to tumorous limb. (B) High power magnification of spinal cord showing hypertrophy of astrocytes (green) without changes in neuronal numbers (red, stained with neuronal marker, NeuN).

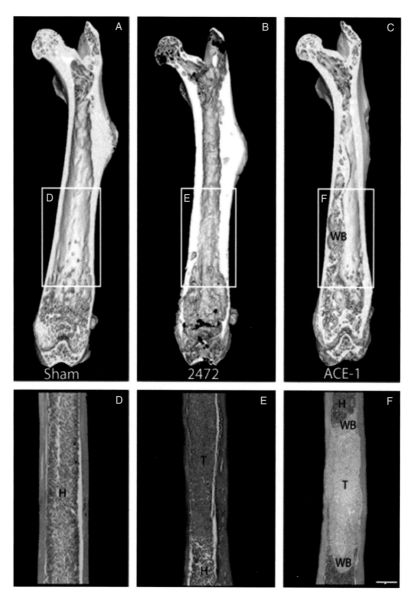

PLATE 14 Bone remodeling and tumor growth in the 2472 sarcoma and ACE-1 prostate carcinoma-injected femurs have different characteristics depending on the osteolytic or osteoblastic component of the tumor cells as assessed by μCT imaging and hematoxilin and eosin (H&E) staining. Sham-injected femurs present relative absence of bone formation or bone destruction (A, D). The 2472 sarcoma-injected femurs display a primarily osteolytic appearance visible as regions absent of trabecular bone at the proximal and distal heads (B) as well as replacement of normal hematopoietic cells by tumor cells (E). The ACE-1 prostate carcinoma-injected femurs mainly present an osteoblastic appearance which is characterized by pathologic bone formation in the intramedullary space (C) surrounding pockets of tumor cells which generate diaphyseal bridging structures (F). A–F: Scale bar, 0.5 mm. T, tumor; H, normal hematopoietic cells; WB, ACE-1-induced woven bone formation.

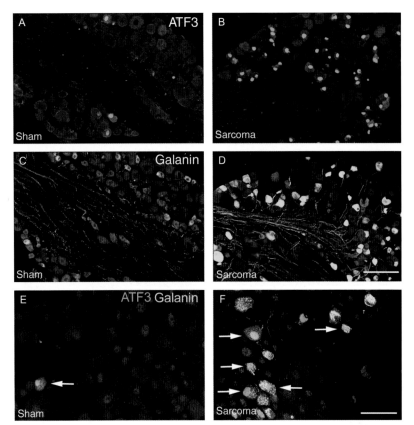

PLATE 15 Activated transcription factor-3 (ATF-3) and galanin are up-regulated in primary sensory neurons that innervate the tumor-bearing femur 14 days following injection of osteolytic sarcoma cells into intramedullary space of the femur. Neurons in the sham-vehicle L2 dorsal root ganglia express low levels of both activating transcription factor-3 (A) or the neuropeptide galanin (C), whereas 14 days following injection and confinement of sarcoma cells to the marrow space there is a marked up-regulation of both ATF-3 (B) and galanin (D) in sensory neurons in the L2 dorsal root ganglia ipsilateral to the tumor-bearing bone. Many sensory neurons which show an up-regulation of galanin in response to tumor-induced injury of sensory fibers in the bone also show an up-regulation of ATF-3 in their nucleus (compare E vs. F, arrows). These data suggest tumor cells invading the bone injure the sensory nerve fibers that normally innervate the tumor bearing bone. Scale bar = 200 μm (A–D), Scale bar = 100 μm (E, F).

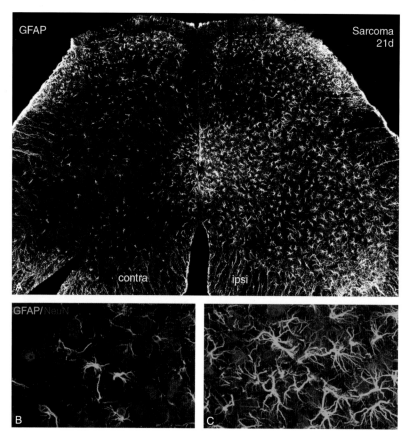

PLATE 16 Confocal images showing the increase in the astrocyte marker glial fibrillary acidic protein (GFAP) in a mouse with bone cancer pain in the right femur. Coronal sections of the L4 spinal cord 21 days following injection of osteolytic sarcoma cells into the intramedullary space of the femur. In (A) the GFAP is bright orange and in (B&C) GFAP is green and the NeuN staining (which labels neurons) is in red. A low power image (A) shows that the up-regulation of GFAP is almost exclusively ipsilateral to the femur with the intraosseous tumor. Higher magnification of GFAP contralateral (B) and ipsilateral (C) to the femur with cancer shows that on the ipsilateral side, there is marked hypertrophy of astrocytes characterized by an increase in both the size of the astrocyte cell bodies and the extent of the arborization of their distal processes. Additionally, this increase in GFAP (green) is observed without a detectable loss of neurons, as NeuN (red) labeling remains unchanged. These images, from 60 μm thick tissue, are projected from six optical sections acquired at 4 μm intervals with a 20× lens, scale bar = 200 μm (A), are projected from 12 optical sections acquired at 0.8 μm intervals with a 60× lens, scale bar = 30 μm (B&C).

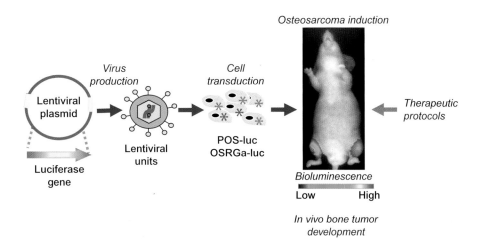

PLATE 17 *In vivo* bioluminescence imaging to follow and quantify the progression or regression of bone tumor in response to therapeutic protocols. By cloning the firefly luciferase gene into a lentiviral plasmid, it is possible to produce lentiviral units which are highly efficient to stably transfer the transgene luciferase into various tumor cell types, including murine POS and rat OSRGa osteosarcoma cells. These cells are then injected into mice/rats to develop the corresponding osteosarcoma model. The measurement of *in vivo* bioluminescence further allows us to quantify tumor progression, regression or recurrence, together with pulmonary metastases dissemination in response to the applied therapeutic protocol.

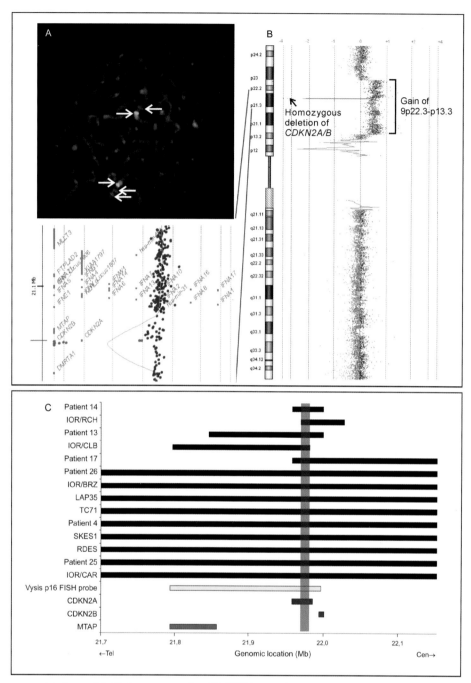

PLATE 18 Homozygous deletions of 9p21.3, encompassing CDKN2A gene locus, are common in Ewing's sarcoma family of tumors. Homozygous 9p21.3 deletions, harboring *CDKN2A* locus coding for p16 and p14 tumor suppressor proteins, are frequent in the Ewing's sarcoma patient and cell line samples. Inactivation of *CDKN2A* by deletions, point mutations or by promoter methylation is also a common and early event in other bone tumors like chondrosarcoma, osteosarcoma and chordoma. (A) Narrowest microdeletions (<190 kb) in 9p21.3 can create false negative results by using commercial FISH probes, as shown in FISH analysis on Ewing's sarcoma cell lines (IOR/RCH). FISH results show that one *CDKN2A* locus is gained as indicated by three red signals (arrows to left) in the sample. For experimental details see Ref. [107]. (B) Array CGH analysis with high-resolution oligo-microarray (244,000 probes) on the same IOR/RCH Ewing's sarcoma cell line shows that within the gain of 9p22.3-p13.3, there is a homozygous deletion of 9p21.3. The size of homozygous deletion is 58 kb and it harbors only genes *CDKN2A* and *CDKN2B*. (C) Genomic locations of 9p deletions in Ewing's sarcoma patients and cell line samples arranged by their size. Genes *CDKN2A* (yellow), *CDKN2B* (red) and *MTAP* (green), their sizes and locations are also indicated in the figure. The smallest overlapping region of deletion (12,2kb), which is indicated by purple bar, is much smaller than the size of the most commonly used commercial FISH probe (Vysis p16 FISH probe). This commercial FISH probe is ~190kb in size and it covers genes *CDKN2A*, *CDKN2B* and *MTAP*, explaining the false negative results seen in FISH analysis (see A). (A) and (B) reproduced from *Cytogenetic Genome Research* (2007), **119**, 21–26, by permission of S. Karger AG, Basel.